M.

INTERVENTIONAL ELECTROPHYSIOLOGY

SECOND EDITION

INTERVENTIONAL ELECTROPHYSIOLOGY

• • •

SECOND EDITION

EDITOR

IGOR SINGER, M.B.B.S., F.R.A.C.P., F.A.C.P., F.A.C.C., F.A.C.A.

Professor of Medicine
Chief, Arrhythmia Service
Director, Cardiac Electrophysiology and Pacing
University of Louisville School of Medicine
Louisville, Kentucky

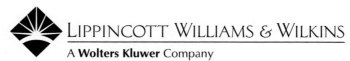

A **Wolters Kluwer** Company
Philadelphia • Baltimore • New York • London
Buenos Aires • Hong Kong • Sydney • Tokyo

Acquisitions Editor: Ruth W. Weinberg
Developmental Editor: Leah Hayes
Production Manager: Toni Ann Scaramuzzo
Production Editor: Michael Mallard
Manufacturing Manager: Benjamin Rivera
Cover Designer: Futuristic Graphics and Multimedia, Inc.
Compositor: Maryland Composition
Printer: Maple Press

© 2001 by LIPPINCOTT WILLIAMS & WILKINS
530 Walnut Street
Philadelphia, PA 19106 USA
LWW.com

All rights reserved. This book is protected by copyright. No part of this book may be reproduced in any form or by any means, including photocopying, or utilized by any information storage and retrieval system without written permission from the copyright owner, except for brief quotations embodied in critical articles and reviews. Materials appearing in this book prepared by individuals as part of their official duties as U.S. government employees are not covered by the above-mentioned copyright.
Printed in the USA

Library of Congress Cataloging-in-Publication Data

Interventional electrophysiology/editor, Igor Singer.—2nd ed.
   p.; cm.
   Includes bibliographical references and index.
   ISBN 0-7817-2333-7
   1. Arrhythmia—Treatment. 2. Arrhythmia—Surgery. 3. Implantable cardioverter-defibrillators. 4. Cardiac pacing. I. Singer, Igor.
   [DNLM: 1. Arrhythmia—Surgery. 2. Catheter Ablation—methods. 3. Defibrillators, Implantable. 4. Electrophysiology—methods. 5. Pacemaker, Artificial. WG 330 I635 2001]
   RC685.A65 I582 2001
   616.1′2806—dc21
                                                     00-067799

   Care has been taken to confirm the accuracy of the information presented and to describe generally accepted practices. However, the authors, editors, and publisher are not responsible for errors or omissions or for any consequences from application of the information in this book and make no warranty, expressed or implied, with respect to the currency, completeness, or accuracy of the contents of the publication. Application of this information in a particular situation remains the professional responsibility of the practitioner.
   The publisher does not use the registered trademark symbol (®) when referring to trademarked drugs or devices, however all rights are reserved.
   The authors, editors, and publisher have exerted every effort to ensure that drug selection and dosage set forth in this text are in accordance with current recommendations and practice at the time of publication. However, in view of ongoing research, changes in government regulations, and the constant flow of information relating to drug therapy and drug reactions, the reader is urged to check the package insert for each drug for any change in indications and dosage and for added warnings and precautions. This is particularly important when the recommended agent is a new or infrequently employed drug.
   Some drugs and medical devices presented in this publication have Food and Drug Administration (FDA) clearance for limited use in restricted research settings. It is the responsibility of the health care provider to ascertain the FDA status of each drug or device planned for use in their clinical practice.

THIS BOOK IS DEDICATED TO MY BELOVED WIFE SYLVIA ANN,

TO MY CHILDREN JUSTIN, JESSICA AND CHRISTINA,

AND TO MY PARENTS DR. D. SINGER AND IVAN SINGER.

CONTENTS

Contributors ix
Preface xv

SECTION I: INTERVENTIONAL TECHNIQUES FOR ABLATION OF TACHYCARDIAS

1. **Morphologic Features of Normal and Abnormal Conduction Systems** 3
   Bruce M. McManus, Salima Harji, Shelley M. Wood

2. **Organization of the Interventional Laboratory** 57
   David E. Adams

3. **Catheterization and Electrogram Recordings** 77
   Igor Singer

4. **Catheter Designs for Interventional Electrophysiology** 103
   John Gaiser

5. **Cardiac Mapping Systems and Their Use to Treat Tachyarrhythmias** 163
   Gregory P. Walcott, Raymond E. Ideker

6. **Ablation of Left-Sided Accessory Pathways: The Retrograde Aortic Versus the Transseptal Approach** 173
   Huagui Li, Robert A. Schweikert, Andrea Natale

7. **Ablation of Right Free Wall and Atriofascicular Accessory Pathways** 193
   Gery Tomassoni, Logan Kanagaratnam, Walid Saliba, Robert A. Schweikert, Andrea Natale

8. **Catheter Ablation of Posteroseptal Accessory Pathways** 221
   Fred Morady

9. **Catheter Ablation of Anteroseptal and Midseptal Accessory Pathways** 237
   Hugh Calkins, Ronald D. Berger

10. **Modification of the Atrioventricular Node for Management of Atrioventricular Nodal Reentrant Tachycardia** 255
    Dennis W. X. Zhu

11. **Ablation of Atrial Tachycardias** 289
    Jeffrey E. Olgin

12. **Atrial Fibrillation Ablation: Present and Future** 313
    Boaz Avitall, Vinay Malhotra, Arvydas Urbonas, Dalia Urboniene, and Scott C. Millard

13. **Ablation of Idiopathic Left Ventricular Tachycardia, Right Ventricular Outflow Tachycardia, and Bundle Branch Reentry Tachycardia** 343
    William M. Miles, Raul D. Mitrani

14. **Radiofrequency Catheter Ablation of Ventricular Tachycardia in Patients with Coronary Artery Disease** 373
    Ross D. Fletcher, Pamela Karasik

15. **Surgical Techniques for Ablation of Supraventricular Tachycardias** 409
    Gerard M. Guiraudon, George J. Klein, and Raymond Yee

16. **Surgical Approach to Atrial Flutter and Atrial Fibrillation** 433
    T. Bruce Ferguson, Jr., James J. McKinnie

17. **Role of Intraoperative Mapping in Ventricular Arrhythmia Surgery** 463
    John M. Miller, Gregory T. Altemose, Mark A. Coppess, and Yousuf Mahomed

18. **Ventricular Tachycardia Surgical Techniques** 481
Gerard M. Guiraudon, George J. Klein, Colette M. Guiraudon

SECTION II: ADVANCES IN IMPLANTABLE CARDIOVERTER DEFIBRILLATORS AND PACEMAKER THERAPY

19. **Implantation of Cardioverter-Defibrillators in the Electrophysiology Laboratory** 491
Adam Zivin, Gust H. Bardy

20. **Defibrillation Waveforms** 507
Jian Huang, Raymond E. Ideker

21. **Dual-Chamber Sensing and Detection for Implantable Cardioverter-Defibrillators** 523
Jeffrey M Gillberg, Walter H. Olson

22. **Atrial Defibrillation with Implantable Cardioverter-Defibrillators** 571
Steven D. Girouard, Milton M. Morris, Hendrik Lambert, Ulrich Michel, Michael E. Benser, Bruce H. KenKnight, Douglas J. Lang

23. **Tiered Therapy for Implantable Cardioverter-Defibrillators: Underlying Principles and Clinical Implications** 597
Milton M. Morris, Stephen J. Hahn, Stephen P. McQuillan, Bruce H. KenKnight, Lynn S. Elliott, James O. Gilkerson, Lorenzo A. DiCarlo

24. **Atrial Defibrillators** 619
Johan E.P. Waktare, A. John Camm

25. **Clinical Results with Investigational Implantable Cardioverter-Defibrillators** 631
Werner Jung, Berndt Lüderitz

26. **Clinical Results with Implantable Cardioverter-Defibrillators** 653
Seah Nisam

27. **Randomized Clinical Trials of Implantable Cardioverter-Defibrillators for Prophylaxis of Sudden Cardiac Death** 663
David S. Cannom

28. **What is the Role for Pharmacologic Therapy for Sustained Ventricular Tachyarrhythmias?** 685
L. Brent Mitchell

29. **Future Implantable Cardioverter-Defibrillator Technologies** 701
Edwin G. Duffin

30. **Implantation Techniques for Single- and Dual-Chamber Pacemakers** 713
Peter H. Belott

31. **Clinical Trials in Cardiac Pacing** 765
Kenneth A. Ellenbogen, Mark A. Wood

32. **New and Evolving Indications for Cardiac Pacing** 781
S. Serge Barold

33. **Is There a Role for Cardiac Pacing in Vasodepressor Syncope?** 809
David G. Benditt, Nemer Samniah, Gerard Fahy, Keith G. Lurie, Scott Sakaguchi

34. **Extraction of Transvenous Pacemaker and Defibrillator Leads** 819
Ayman S. Al-Khadra, Bruce L. Wilkoff

Index 843

CONTRIBUTORS

David E. Adams, B.S.E.E.
Director, Biomedical Engineering
Department of Medicine
Krannert Institute of Cardiology
Indiana University School of Medicine
Indianapolis, Indianapolis

Ayman S. Al-Khadra, M.D.
Cosultant Cardiac Electrophysiologist
Prince Sultan Cardiac Center
Riyadh, Saudi Arabia

Gregory T. Altemose, M.D.
Assistant Professor of Medicine
Krannert Institute of Cardiology
Indiana University School of Medicine
Indianapolis, Indiana

Boaz Avitall, M.D., Ph.D.
Professor of Medicine
Director, Clinical and Research Cardiac Electrophysiology
University of Illinois College of Medicine
Chicago, Illinois

Gust H. Bardy, M.D.
Professor of Medicine
University of Washington
University Hospital
Seattle, Washington

S. Serge Barold, M.B.B.S., F.R.A.C.P., F.A.C.C., F.E.S.C.
Clinical Professor of Medicine Emeritus
University of Rochester School of Medicine and Dentistry
Rochester, New York
Electrophysiology Institute
Broward General Hospital
Ft. Lauderdale, Florida

Peter H. Belott, M.D., F.A.C.C.
Clinical Instructor
University of California at San Diego School of Medicine
Director, Pacemaker Center
El Cajon, California

David G. Benditt, M.D.
Professor of Medicine
Cardiac Arrhythmia Center
University of Minnesota
Minneapolis, Minnesota

Michael E. Benser, Ph.D.
Sr. Scientist, Atrial Arrhythmia Research
Department of Therapy Research
Guidant Corporation
St. Paul, Minnesota

Ronald D. Berger, M.D., Ph.D.
Associate Professor of Medicine
Department of Medicine/Cardiology
Johns Hopkins University
Associate Director of Electrophysiology
Johns Hopkins Hospital
Baltimore, Maryland

Hugh Calkins, M.D.
Professor of Medicine
Department of Medicine/Cardiology
Johns Hopkins University
Director of Electrophysiology
Johns Hopkins Hospital
Baltimore, Maryland

A. John Camm, M.D., F.R.C.P., F.E.S.C., F.A.C.C.
Professor of Clinical Cardiology
Department of Cardiological Sciences
St. George's Hospital Medical School
London, United Kingdom

David S. Cannom, M.D.
Medical Director of Cardiology
Hospital of the Good Samaritan
Los Angeles, California

Mark A. Coppess, M.D.
Senior Fellow in Electrophysiology
Krannert Institute of Cardiology
Indiana University School of Medicine
Indianapolis, Indiana

CONTRIBUTORS

Lorenzo A. DiCarlo, M.D.
Director, Medical Sciences
Guidant Corporation
St. Paul, Minnesota

Edwin G. Duffin, Ph.D.
Bakken Fellow
Medtronic, Incorporated
Minneapolis, Minnesota

Kenneth A. Ellenbogen, M.D.
Professor of Medicine
Director, Clinical Electrophysiology and Pacing
Department of Cardiology
Medical College of Virginia
Richmond, Virginia

Lynn S. Elliott, B.S.E.E., M.S.S.W.E.
Vice President Product Development
Guidant Cardiac Rhythm Management
St. Paul, Minnesota

Gerard Fahy, M.D.
Assistant Professor of Medicine
Cardiac Arrhythmia Center
University of Minnesota
Minneapolis, Minnesota

T. Bruce Ferguson, Jr., M.D.
Clinical Associate Professor of Surgery
Tulane University School of Medicine
Professor of Surgery and Physiology
Louisiana State University Health Science Center
New Orleans, Louisiana

Ross D. Fletcher, M.D.
Professor of Medicine
Georgetown University
Chief of Staff
Veterans Administration Medical Center
Washington, D.C.

John Gaiser
Vice President, Research and Development
Medtronic Cardiorhythm
San Jose, California

James O. Gilkerson, D.V.M.
Clinical Advisor, Advanced Tachy Design
Guidant Corporation
Saint Paul, Minnesota

Jeffrey M. Gillberg, M.S.
Senior Staff Scientist
Medtronic, Incorporated
Fridley, Minnesota

Steven D. Girouard, Ph.D.
Department of Therapy Research
Guidant Corporation
St. Paul, Minnesota

Colette M. Guiraudon, M.D.
Professor of Pathology
University of Western Ontario
London, Ontario, Canada

Gerard M. Guiraudon, M.D., F.R.C.S., F.A.C.C.
Professor of Surgery
State University of New York at Buffalo
Buffalo, New York
Director, Clinical Trials
Cardiovascular Device Division
University of Ottawa Heart Institute
Ottawa, Ontario, Canada

Stephen J. Hahn, Ph.D.
Senior Principal Research Engineer
Tachycardia Therapy Research
Cardiac Rhythm Management Division
Guidant Corporation
St. Paul, Minnesota

Salima Harji, B.Sc, M.H.S.c.
Research and Education Coordinator
Cardiovascular Registry
University of British Columbia-St. Paul's Hospital
Providence Health Care
Vancouver, British Columbia, Canada

Jian Huang, M.D., Ph.D.
Department of Medicine
Division of Cardiology
Cardiac Rhythm Laboratory
University of Alabama at Birmingham
Birmingham, Alabama

Raymond E. Ideker, M.D., Ph.D.
Departments of Medicine, Physiology, and Biomedical Engineering
Division of Cardiology
Cardiac Rhythm Laboratory
University of Alabama at Birmingham
Birmingham, Alabama

Werner Jung, M.D., F.E.S.C.
Chief, Department of Cardiology
Klinik für Innere Medizin III
Klinikum der Stadt Villingen-Schwenningen
Villingen, Germany

Logan Kanagaratnam, M.D.
Division of Cardiology
The Cleveland Clinic Foundation
Cleveland, Ohio

Pamela Karasik, M.D.
Associate Professor of Medicine
Department of Cardiology
Georgetown University
Assistant Director of Clinical Electrophysiology
Veterans Administration Medical Center
Washington, D.C.

Bruce H. KenKnight, Ph.D.
Director, Heart Failure and Atrial Arrhythmia Management
Guidant Corporation
St. Paul, Minnesota

George J. Klein, M.D., F.R.C.P.C., F.A.C.C.
Professor of Medicine
University of Western Ontario
London Health Science Center
London, Ontario, Canada

Hendrik Lambert, Ph.D.
Field Clinical Engineer Manager
Guidant Europe N.V./S.A.
Diegem, Belgium

Douglas J. Lang, Ph.D.
Director, Brady and Tachy Therapy Research
Guidant Corporation
St. Paul, Minnesota

Huagui Li, M.D., Ph.D.
Associate Professor
Department of Medicine
Creighton University
St. Joseph Hospital
Omaha, Nebraska

Berndt Lüderitz, M.D., F.E.S.C., F.A.C.C.
Professor of Medicine
Head, Department of Medicine and Cardiology
Division of Cardiology
University of Bonn
Bonn, Germany

Keith G. Lurie, M.D.
Associate Professor of Medicine
Co-director, Cardiac Arrhythmia Center
University of Minnesota
Minneapolis, Minnesota

Yousuf Mahomed, M.D.
Professor of Surgery
Department of Cardiothoracic Surgery
Indiana University School of Medicine
Director of Adult Cardiac Services
Department of Surgery-Cardiothoracic Surgery
Indiana University Medical Center
Indianapolis, Indiana

Vinay Malhotra, M.D.
The University of Illinois at Chicago
Department of Medicine
Section of Cardiology
Chicago, Illinois

James J. McKinnie, M.D.
Associate Professor of Medicine
Director, Section of Electrophysiology
Tulane University School of Medicine
New Orleans, Louisiana

Bruce M. McManus, M.D., Ph.D.
Professor and Head
Department of Pathology and Laboratory Medicine
University of British Columbia-St. Paul's Hospital
Providence Health Care
Vancouver, British Columbia, Canada

Stephen P. McQuillan, M.S.
Manager/Clinical Programs
Guidant Corporation
St. Paul, Minnesota

Ulrich Michel, B.S.B.M.E.
Director Clinical Programs CRM Europe
Guidant Europe N.V./S.A.
Diegem, Belgium

William M. Miles, M.D.
Voluntary Professor of Medicine
University of Miami School of Medicine
Miami, Florida
Consulting Electrophysiologist
Southwest Florida Heart Group
Fort Myers, Florida

Scott C. Millard, B.S.E.E.
Department of Medicine
Section of Cardiology
The University of Illinois at Chicago
Chicago, Illinois

John M. Miller, M.D.
Professor
Department of Medicine
Cardiovascular Division
Indiana University School of Medicine
Director, Clinical Cardiac Electrophysiology
Krannert Institute of Cardiology
Indianapolis, Indiana

L. Brent Mitchell, M.D., F.R.C.P.C., F.A.C.C.
Professor and Head, Division of Cardiology
Department of Medicine
University of Calgary
Calgary, Alberta, Canada

Raul D. Mitrani, M.D.
Division of Cardiology
University of Miami
Miami, Florida

Fred Morady, M.D.
Professor of Internal Medicine
Director, Clinical Electrophysiology Laboratory
Division of Cardiology
The University of Michigan
Ann Arbor, Michigan

Milton M. Morris, Ph.D.
Manager, Atrial Arrhythmia Research
Department of Therapy Research
Guidant Corporation
St. Paul, Minnesota

Andrea Natale, M.D.
Professor of Medicine
Ohio State University
Director, Electrophysiology Laboratories
Section of Pacing and Electrophysiology
Department of Cardiology
Cleveland Clinic Foundation
Cleveland, Ohio

Seah Nisam, B.S.E.E.
Director, Medical Sciences
Guidant Corporation
Diegem, Belgium

Jeffrey E. Olgin, M.D.
Assistant Professor of Medicine
Indiana University School of Medicine
Krannert Institute of Cardiology
Indianapolis, Indiana

Walter H. Olson, M.D.
Senior Research Fellow
Bakken Foundation, Tachyarrhythmia Research
Medtronic, Incorporated
Fridley, Minnesota

Scott Sakaguchi, M.D.
Assistant Professor
Department of Internal Medicine
Fairview-University Medical Center
University of Minnesota
Minneapolis, Minnesota

Walid Saliba, M.D.
Staff Cardiologist
The Cleveland Clinic Foundation
Cleveland, Ohio

Nemer Samniah, M.D.
Post-Graduate Fellow
Clinical Cardiac Electrophysiology
Cardiac Arrhythmia Center
University of Minnesota Medical School
Minneapolis, Minnesota

Robert A. Schweikert, M.D.
Assistant Staff
Department of Cardiology
The Cleveland Clinic Foundation
Cleveland, Ohio

Igor Singer, M.B.B.S., F.R.A.C.P., F.A.C.P., F.A.C.C., F.A.C.A.
Professor of Medicine
Chief, Arrhythmia Service
Director, Cardiac Electrophysiology and Pacing
University of Louisville School of Medicine
Louisville, Kentucky

Gery Tomassoni, M.D.
Staff Cardiologist
Central Baptist Hospital
Lexington, Kentucky

Arvydas Urbonas, M.D.
Research Specialist
Department of Medicine
Section of Cardiology
The University of Illinois at Chicago College of Medicine
Chicago, Illinois

Dalia Urboniene, M.D.
Research Specialist
Department of Medicine
Section of Cardiology
The University of Illinois at Chicago College of Medicine
Chicago, Illinois

Johan E.P. Waktare, M.B., M.R.C.P.
Specialist Registrar
St. George's Hospital
London, United Kingdom

Gregory P. Walcott, M.D.
Assistant Professor
Department of Medicine
Division of Cardiology
University of Alabama-Birmingham
Birmingham, Alabama

Bruce L. Wilkoff, M.D.
Associate Professor
Department of Internal Medicine
The Ohio State University
Director, Cardiac Pacing and Tachyarrhythmia Devices
The Cleveland Clinic Foundation
Department of Cardiology
Cleveland, Ohio

Mark A. Wood, M.D.
Associate Professor of Medicine
Division of Cardiology
Medical College of Virginia
Richmond, Virginia

Shelley M. Wood, B.A., M.J.
Medical Journalist
Kelowna, British Columbia, Canada

Raymond Yee, M.D.
Professor of Medicine
The University of Western Ontario
Director, Arrhythmia Service
London Health Sciences Center
London, Ontario, Canada

Dennis W.X. Zhu, M.D., F.A.C.C.
Attending Cardiac Electrophysiologist
Minnesota Heart Clinic
Minneapolis, Minnesota
Formerly, Director, Clinical Cardiac Electrophysiology
Baylor College of Medicine
Houston, Texas

Adam Zivin, M.D.
Assistant Professor
Department of Medicine
Division of Cardiology/Arrhythmia Service
University of Washington School of Medicine
Seattle, Washington

PREFACE

Interventional electrophysiology is a subspecialty of cardiology dedicated to the therapy of complex arrhythmias using catheter-based interventions, implantable devices and cardiac surgical techniques. This subspecialty did not exist prior to the advent of intracardiac electrogram recordings, which became possible after 1968, when the first His bundle potential was recorded. Prior to this landmark event diagnostic decisions regarding arrhythmias were primarily based on surface electrocardiographic (ECG) recordings and deductive reasoning. A rapid evolution followed this remarkable discovery with the development of multi-catheter intracardiac recordings, the advent of programmed stimulation, development of sophisticated recording equipment, and evolution of computerized techniques for recording and analysis of arrhythmias.

Cardiac surgeons initially developed techniques designed to interrupt reentrant circuits. These techniques were subsequently adapted to catheter-based approaches designed to achieve the same end result with less morbidity and discomfort to the patient. Evolution in catheter designs, development of radiofrequency ablative therapy and evolution of cardiac pacemakers and implantable cardioverter-defibrillators have transformed interventional electrophysiology to a fast growing subspecialty of cardiology.

The first pacemakers became available in 1950's. Implantable cardioverter-defibrillators (ICDs) were introduced to the clinical arena in 1980. Since those early pioneering days, pacing and ICD therapies have evolved rapidly. Pacemaker and ICD technologies are increasingly more complex, and the device-based therapies overlapping. ICDs are now capable of treating bradyarrhythmias as well as ventricular and atrial tachyarrhythmias. With the development of microchips, microcircuits, smaller capacitors, and more efficient power sources biomedical engineers have succeeded in dramatically reducing the size and the volume of ICDs and pacemakers. Whereas pacemakers and ICDs were initially implanted by cardiothoracic surgeons, they are now implanted by interventional electrophysiologists. Smaller, more flexible leads and reduced volume and size of pacemakers, and ICDs have made the implantation procedure much simpler. With a limited surgical exposure and with conscious sedation, it is now more practical and economical to implant pacemakers and ICDs in an interventional electrophysiology laboratory setting. Innovations in catheter-based interventions and device therapies have imposed formidable new challenges to interventional electrophysiologists. They are required to master new procedural skills, and keep up with a torrid pace of technological advances.

The first edition of *Interventional Electrophysiology* was published in 1997. The stated goal of the textbook was to fill a perceived need for a unified text designed to teach the procedural aspects of interventional electrophysiology. Thus, the textbook was primarily written for cardiology and electrophysiology trainees, practicing electrophysiologists, cardiologists, and others involved in the care of patients with cardiac arrhythmias. Based on the feedback received to date, *Interventional Electrophysiology* was enthusiastically received and widely read by the targeted audience. Since its publication, the art and the science of interventional electrophysiology has continued to evolve at an ever increasing pace. Thus, new techniques have evolved for the analysis and the recording and display of multiple electrograms, such as non-contact mapping, electromechanical mapping, three dimensional displays, catheter-based electrode arrays and other sophisticated techniques. In parallel, ICDs have continued to evolve. Dual-chamber capabilities for monitoring and treating ventricular and atrial arrhythmias have been added to ICDs. These devices have shrunk in size considerably, and new indications for ICD therapy have been recognized. Controlled clinical trials have established superiority of ICDs for prophylaxis of primary sudden cardiac death compared to antiarrhythmic drug therapy.

These developments have stimulated the editor to update the textbook, in an effort to maintain it as a current and authoritative resource.

The second edition of *Interventional Electrophysiology* is structured in two parts:

Part I is focused on interventional catheter-based approaches to ablation of accessory pathways, atrioventricular nodal reentrant tachycardias, atrial flutter, atrial fibrillation, and ventricular tachycardia. Each chapter discusses newer techniques and approaches as well as the established techniques. Electrophysiologic mechanisms of tachycardias, ablation techniques, and outcomes of each approach are presented. Individual chapters are devoted to discussion of anatomic basis of arrhythmias, the organization of an interventional electrophysiology laboratory, cardiac catheterization techniques relevant to electrophysiologists, and catheter designs for interventional electrophysiology.

In recognition of a diminishing, but still an important supportive role of cardiac surgery for therapy of reentrant arrhythmias, discussion of surgical aspects of ablation is included. Important aspects of supraventricular and ventricular arrhythmia ablation and the maze procedure for atrial fibrillation are discussed and updated.

Part II devoted to an extensive discussion of device-based therapies. Since pacing and ICD therapies have merged significantly, it seems appropriate for these therapies to be discussed together. The intent here is not to provide an exhaustive encyclopedic coverage of all aspects of pacing and ICD therapy, but to focus on the procedural aspects, newer technologies and developments in these rapidly evolving technological fields.

Implantation techniques for ICDs and pacemakers are presented in detail. Technological advances for dual-chamber ICDs, such as dual-chamber detection, atrial defibrillation and tiered therapies are covered extensively. Clinical results with conventional and investigational devices, randomized clinical trials with ICDs and future technological advances in ICD technologies are discussed. Newer indications and clinical trials in pacing are covered in individual chapters. Finally, lead extraction techniques, an increasingly important subject with the explosion of device implants, is updated for the second edition of the textbook.

Much of the textbook has been revised and updated. Several new authors have contributed chapters for the second edition of the textbook, and many others have updated their contributions. As in the first edition, an effort was maintained throughout the text to emphasize and adhere to the practical, procedural aspects of interventional electrophysiology and to provide ample illustrations, guiding the operator through the procedures step by step.

It is my hope that this textbook will continue to be a valuable teaching resource for practicing electrophysiologists, interventional cardiologists, and cardiology fellows for years to come.

I wish to express my gratitude to all authors and contributors who have worked hard and made the second edition of *Interventional Electrophysiology* possible.

Igor Singer, *M.B.B.S., F.R.A.C.P., F.A.C.P., F.A.C.C., F.A.C.A.*
Professor of Medicine
Chief, Arrhythmia Service
Director, Cardiac Electrophysiology and Pacing
University of Louisville School of Medicine
Louisville, Kentucky

ACKNOWLEDGMENT

THE EDITOR ACKNOWLEDGES THE CONTRIBUTION OF FUTURISTIC GRAPHICS AND MULTIMEDIA, INC. FOR ARTWORK AND GRAPHICS DEVELOPMENT.

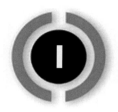

INTERVENTIONAL TECHNIQUES FOR ABLATION OF TACHYCARDIAS

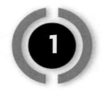

MORPHOLOGIC FEATURES OF NORMAL AND ABNORMAL CONDUCTION SYSTEMS
• • •

BRUCE M. MCMANUS, SALIMA HARJI, SHELLEY M. WOOD

⦿ HISTORICAL SYNOPSIS: DISCOVERY OF THE CARDIAC CONDUCTION SYSTEM

In 1845, Johannes Purkinje published a landmark paper in which he offered a microscopic description of ventricular fibers that were distinct from typical cardiac muscle fibers, providing the first documented histologic description of a component of the cardiac conduction system. Purkinje did not understand the physiologic significance of the fibers that would later bear his name. He inadvertently classified them as "cartilage," although stating that they were integral to the heart's "apparatus of motion." Understanding of the complex electrophysiologic properties and processes of the cardiovascular system grew immensely in the period after his important observation. Among the relevant observations by contemporaries, the essential role of action potential propagation as a requisite event before each contraction of cardiac muscle was established by Augustus Desire Waller (1). Within 50 years of Purkinje's discovery, Kent described aspects of the atrioventricular junctional area, His found the penetrating bundle, and Tawara applied his genius to detailed descriptions of the atrioventricular (AV) node. Today, almost a century later, the combined expertise of cardiologists, basic electrophysiologists, cell biologists, and pathologists has produced an elaborate picture of the cardiac conduction system, the heart's normal physiologic and electrical function, and the pathobiology underlying rhythm disturbances and aberrant conduction.

Wilhelm His, Jr., in his published work of 1843, *Embryonic Cardiac Activity and its Significance for Adult Heart Movement Theory,* described the physiologic consequence of separating the atrium from the ventricle: disruption of cardiac rhythm in the region of the septum. Based on these experimental findings, His concluded that the ventricle received atrial impulses primarily by way of a centrally located pathway. In contrast to His, a contemporary, Albert Kent, proposed that multiple muscular bridges located along the periphery of the atria carried the atrial impulse to the ventricle in the normal heart. These fibers (i.e., Mahaim fibers), now known to occur only in hearts with preexcitation, are sometimes designated as the bundle of Kent-Paladino, based on Kent's efforts and Giovanni Paladino's early suggestion of muscle fibers around the atrioventricular valves in 1876.

In 1906, Suano Tawara, under the tutelage of Ludwig Aschoff, described the anatomic and histologic relationships of the AV node in a monograph published in German. This landmark work was translated into English in 1998 (2) and is discussed in some depth by Anderson and Ho (3) in their appraisal of knowledge regarding the cardiac conduction system. Tawara provided elegant detail of the AV node, the segregation of the atrioventricular conduction system originating at the atrioventricular node into two main branches, the His conduction system, and the proximal Purkinje network. Only the later work by Inoue and Becker (4) postulated the critical importance of posterior extensions of the AV node to arrhythmogenesis. Koch described important anatomic landmarks relevant to the AV node (1909), landmarks that have emerged with greater relevance in an era of successful electrophysiologic intervention.

All that remained was identification of the anatomic structure responsible for initiating the cardiac impulse. Almost concurrent with identification of the AV node, Arthur Keith and his student Martin Flack described a "primitive" muscle mass at the right superior vena caval–right atrial junction, which they called the *sinoauricular node* in 1907. The observations of Keith and Flack were prompted by Wenckebach's exploration of heart innervation and his suggestion that the heart beat might originate in the region that eventually was shown to be the seat of the sinoatrial node. In 1909, Thorel put forward the still debated, highly controversial concept of specialized conduction pathways linking the sinoatrial node and the AV node. The best evidence available (3) definitively shows that the preferential conduction from the sinoatrial node to AV node is through orientation and alignment of working myocardial bundles, not by "specialized tissues" as suggested by Racker (1947). In 1916, Jean Bachmann described the possibility of bundles of interatrial conducting fibers, later referred to as *Bachmann's bundle,* as being responsible for conveying the cardiac impulse from the right atrium to the left atrium. This also turns out to be a physiologic paradigm and not one related to anatomically specialized tissues.

By the early part of the 20th century, all major components and pathways of the cardiac conduction system had been identified or postulated. The ideas brought forth during the dynamic exploratory period form the basis for our modern understanding of the function and morphology of the cardiac conduction system. Works by Lüderitz (5) and Anderson and Ho (3) offer a comprehensive historical and contextual discussion of the cardiac conduction system and arrhythmias.

◉ CLASSIFICATION OF CARDIAC ARRHYTHMIAS

Cardiac arrhythmias result from abnormal impulse initiation or conduction. The abnormal impulse can be automatic or triggered by early or delayed afterdepolarizations. A critically placed block or unidirectional block may permit ordered or disordered reentry and abnormal conduction. Generally speaking, abnormal rhythms are rapid (regular or irregular) or slow. Classification of arrhythmias outlined by Hoffman (6) provides a framework for understanding the various subtypes of arrhythmias and their mechanisms of action.

Supraventricular tachycardias include atrial tachycardias arising from the sinoatrial node, automatic atrial (working myocardium) tachycardias, intraatrial reentrant tachycardias (IART), and possibly triggered atrial tachycardias. Tracy (7) depicts the typical locations of ectopic foci associated with automatic atrial tachycardias; the atrial appendages, junction of the left atrium and pulmonary veins, free walls, and interatrial septum. IART encompass atrial flutter and fibrillation, atrioventricular reentrant tachycardia (AVRT), and AV nodal reentrant tachycardias (AVNRT). The latter two atrial tachycardias involve a reentrant circuit that includes an accessory pathway or an atrioventricular nodal pathway. AVRT involves propagation through an accessory atrioventricular pathway, and AVNRT requires dual input from atrioventricular internodal pathways. A later section of this chapter describes the anatomic substrates responsible for supraventricular tachycardias (7–9).

◉ DEVELOPMENT OF THE CARDIAC CONDUCTION SYSTEM

An understanding of the normal development of cardiac structures in the fetus and infant can help us to appreciate how conduction abnormalities arise, particularly in the context of well-documented congenital anomalies or syndromes (10–12). A more comprehensive discussion of embryologic changes pertaining to the conduction system is available elsewhere (13–15). Briefly, the primordium of the sinoatrial node can be seen in the position it will assume postnatally after cardiac looping has occurred. After cardiac chamber septation, the embryonic ring forms and is composed of outer sulcus tissue, inner cushion tissue, and interposed ring tissue. In the developing human fetus, the atrial and ventricular myocardium are not anatomically separated initially. Sulcus tissue must grow into the atrioventricular junction, isolating atria from ventricles before this development. However, the atrioventricular junction appears to produce a slight delay between atrial and ventricular depolarizations, thereby modulating cardiac rhythm during the development of the heart chambers. The penetrating bundle and bundle branches are separated from the ventricular myocardium by an extended sheath of sulcal tissue. With time, the conductive primordium overlying the septal surfaces of the ventricles extends, forming the distal bundles and Purkinje system. With the continuity of the atrioventricular axis established, a remnant of sulcal tissue normally adopts an insulating, protective role for the remainder of postnatal life.

Ectopic atrioventricular connections are found commonly in fetal hearts, however these are usually severed during development of the central fibrous body and valve annuli. Persistence of these ectopic fibers beyond infancy can serve as the basis for preexcitation in adult hearts.

Early during cardiac morphogenesis, the primary heart tube develops from the mesoderm and moves blood forward by way of unidirectional, slow-conducting, peristaltic contractions (16). Progression of contractile waves in the fashion described ensures that the downstream outflow tract segment, the future site of the ventricles, does not contract prematurely before contraction terminates in the area of the inflow tract, future site of the atria. The latter area, with the highest beat frequency and pacemaker activity contributes to the maintenance of unidirectional distribution of contractions toward the ventricular segment. Moreover, the slow-conducting sinoatrial and atrioventricular tissues originate from the inflow tract along with the atrioventricular canal. The fast-conducting ventricular conduction system, composed of the His bundle, left and right bundle branches, and Purkinje fibers, develops from the trabecular ventricular tissue. Separation of the slow- and fast-conducting pathways contributes to the atrial-ventricular dysharmony established early in development.

Origin of conductive tissues in the heart continues to be of great interest. Experimental findings fail to support unequivocally the notion that the cardiac conduction system originates from an extracardiac source such as neural crest cells. For instance, adult-like electrograms have been obtained for chicken hearts less than 4 days of age, but neural crest cells migrate into chicken hearts at 4 days of development (17,18). These migrant cells most likely do not facilitate developmentally the sequential activation of the atria and ventricles observable by such time (19,20). Similarly, the function of the sinoatrial and atrioventricular nodes, as represented on the electrogram, occurs before the time neural crest cells migrate into the heart (21,22). Moreover, genetic, molecular, functional, and morphologic evidence supports the concept that the trabecular ventricular component, instead of an extracardiac source, gives rise to the entire ventricular conduction system. For example, mice carrying a loss-of-function mutation in neuregulin, neuregulin receptors Erb2 or Erb4, or retinoic X receptor-α genes die prematurely from conduction disturbances (23). Because all such genes play a role in signal transduction pathways responsible for the development and formation of ventricular trabeculae, it seems reasonable to suggest that ventricular trabeculae give rise to the ventricular conduction system.

The myogenic versus neurogenic origin of Purkinje fibers is a discussion that has received much attention. Cell lineage data support the proposition that Purkinje fibers are descendants of a subset of developing cardiomyocytes (24). This subset of cardiomyocytes appears to undergo molecular switching such that they express myofibrillar proteins normally expressed by skeletal muscle, such as skeletal muscle-specific myosin binding protein-H (25). This molecular switching must in part determine how cells destined to become nodal cells or cells of the ventricular conduction system avoid becoming working myocardial cells. Molecular switching involves augmented expression of the calcium-release channel/type-I inositol triphosphate receptor, γ-enolase, $\alpha 2$ and $\alpha 3$ isoforms of the sodium pump (Na^+,K^+-ATPase), G protein α-subunit, and the angiotensin type 2 receptor subtype. These proteins are expressed at higher levels in specialized nodal and ventricular conduction cells than in myocardial cells (15). The "switch" responsible for differentiation of cardiomyocytes to nodal myocytes results in disorganized actin and myosin filaments, underdevelopment of the sarcoplasmic reticulum, and a smaller cell size (26).

Gourdie and colleagues (27) propose that coronary hemodynamics play a role in the cardiac myocyte differentiation pathway. In particular, they argue that endothelin (EDN), a shear stress–induced cytokine, released from the arterial system within the myocardium stimulates differentiation of primitive cardiac myocytes into conduction myocytes. These investigators base their proposition in part on the finding that differentiating myocytes virtually all express EDN receptors, and transgenic deletion of the *EDN1* gene results in abnormal heart development (28,29). They also showed *in vitro* that recombinant EDN1 induces differentiation of cardiac myocytes isolated from chick embryos into cells displaying a Purkinje fiber phenotype (30). They further demonstrated that cardiac myocytes adjacent to coronary arteries are recruited to become periarterial Purkinje fibers, supporting a role for coronary hemodynamics in the differentiation process.

Structural variability in the cardiac conduction system acquired during the developmental stage may not necessarily serve as substrates for arrhythmias or lead to sudden death in children or adults. Paz Suá-Mier and Gamallo (31) demonstrated that persistent fetal dispersion of the AV node and fragmentation of the His bundle, anatomic variants commonly thought to be substrates for arrhythmias and sudden death, were more common in 98 adult, control autopsy hearts than in 249 autopsy hearts from sudden cardiac death patients (137 ischemic heart disease, 48 nonischemic heart disease, 64 unexplained sudden cardiac deaths). Of the control hearts, 40.8% and 47.7% exhibited persistent fetal dispersion of the AV node and fragmentation of the His bundle, respectively.

Similarly, Paz Suá-Mier and Aguilera (32) demonstrated that structural "abnormalities" of the cardiac conduction system might not necessarily be responsible for sudden death in infants. In particular, these investigators assessed the histology of the conduction system in 87 sudden infant death syndrome (SIDS) babies between 15 days and 1 year of age. The heart tissues were divided into three groups: SIDS exhibiting typical histopathologic findings (group I), SIDS exhibiting mild lesions insufficient to explain sudden death (group II), and sudden unexplained deaths considered to be controls (group III). Fetal dispersion of the AV node or His bundle (or both) and the left-sided His bundle were present in all three study groups at a high frequency. The researchers concluded that these structural variations were normal. However, these same investigators identified fasciculoventricular tracts at a higher frequency in the SIDS group compared with the other groups (7 in group I, 1 in group II, and 0 in group III). They speculated that these accessory pathways might be responsible for sudden death in such infants.

Kelmanson and colleagues (33) provided evidence to suggest that the abnormal or delayed cardiac development seen in premature infants is associated with a greater risk of cardiac arrhythmias. They compared the birth weights of 31 children between 1 and 15 years of age who had accessory pathways of conduction in the heart and inducible reciprocating supraventricular tachycardia with the birth weights of a control group consisting of 62 matched, healthy children. They discovered that children with a low birth weight ($<2,500$ g) are at a higher risk of arrhythmias. Compared with other variables, including preterm birth, maternal age, birth order, maternal smoking during pregnancy, and gynecologic disease, low birth weight was the most reliable predictor of the risk of arrhythmia. The researchers speculated that retarded maturation of the cardiac conduction system is a consequence of an overall low birth weight and heart weight, setting the stage for cardiac arrhythmias. Much debate still surrounds the notion that structural abnormalities in the cardiac conduction system cause sudden death in infants, and more work is needed.

MAJOR COMPONENTS OF THE CARDIAC CONDUCTION SYSTEM: NORMAL ANATOMY

Sinus Node

The sinus node (i.e., sinoatrial node) in the adult heart is described as an upside-down teardrop measuring

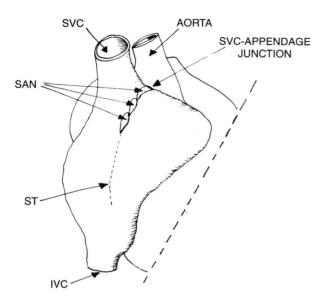

FIGURE 1-1. Location of the sinoatrial node (SAN) in the sulcus terminalis at the superior vena cava–right atrial appendage junction. The node is typically constant in its position in an anatomically normal heart, lapping over the roof peak of the right atrial appendage in certain hearts. ST, sulcus terminalis; IVC, inferior vena cava; SVC, superior vena cava.

up to 1.5 × 0.5 × 0.3 cm and located in the epicardial groove of the sulcus terminalis at the junction of the superior vena cava and the right atrium (34) (Figs. 1-1 and 1-2). The specificity of this description, however, can be misleading because the shape and position of the node appear to vary according to the shape of the sulcus terminalis and, to some degree, the variable positioning and extent of its arterial supply (Fig. 1-3). In infants, the node may apparently extend toward the inferior vena cava (35). Appreciation of the sinoatrial node as a "region" of pacemaker cells, originally hypothesized by Karl Wenckebach and confirmed by physiologists, may reduce the potential for accidental damage during surgery or manipulation. Proposed approaches to determining the exact location of the node include the cavoauricular incision described by Calmat Par and colleagues (36), identification of the curved sinoatrial "notch" reported by He (35), and localization of the antrum atria dextri.

Postganglionic parasympathetic nerve fibers in the epicardium surround and innervate the node. The sinoatrial node receives input from adrenergic and cholinergic nerves. Histologic examination of the node reveals small, pale, whorled, interwoven muscle cells and interspersed collagenous connective tissue elements (Fig. 1-4). Light microscopy permits differ-

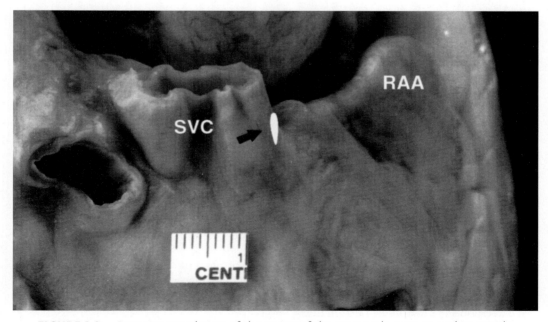

FIGURE 1-2. Posterior-septal view of the region of the sinus node, seen as a white upside-down teardrop *(arrow)*. RAA, right atrial appendage; SVC, superior vena cava.

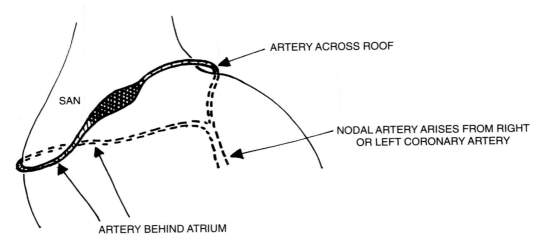

FIGURE 1-3. The typical anteroposterior and posteroanterior course of the sinus node artery running through the long axis of the sinoatrial node (SAN).

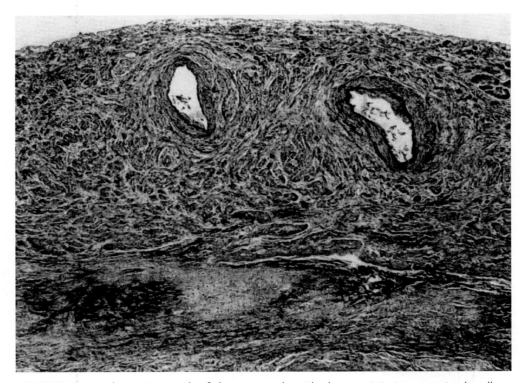

FIGURE 1-4. Photomicrograph of the sinus node with characteristic interweaving bundles of sinus node cardiocytes and connective tissue, both of which surround branches of the sinus node artery. The epicardial surface of the right atrium is located near the top of the photograph, illustrating the proximity of the node to the epicardium. Similar proximity exists for the endocardium in the antrum atria dextri.

entiation of apparent pacemaking cells, transitional cells, and atrial working muscle cells.

The sinoatrial node artery arises from the left or right (55%) circumflex coronary artery and resides along the sulcus terminalis. Its central location within the sinoatrial node and perhaps its proximity to the aorta permit modulation of sinoatrial node activity according to aortic pressure and pulsations. Some patients exhibiting thickening and obliteration of the sinoatrial node artery lumen may exhibit arrhythmic disturbances that lead to sudden death (14).

The origin of the sinus impulse is dynamic and relies on intranodal and extranodal factors. Schuessler and coworkers (37) proposed the presence of a dominant pacemaker within the node and a limited number of exit sites from the sinoatrial node. The intranodal component arises instantaneously from multiple origins and may sometimes shift, leading to a complex conduction pattern out of the node. Extranodal pacemaker cells may override the dominant intranodal pacemaker, thereby posing a challenge during surgical or ablative therapies. For instance, patients undergoing the first version of the Maze procedure for atrial arrhythmias experienced a depressed heart rate during exercise based on the interference of pacemaker cells from outside the sinoatrial node (38). Similarly, ablation of areas deemed responsible for sinus tachycardia may not be sufficient, because the impulse may reemerge from an otherwise unsuspected extranodal source.

Internodal Tracts

Anatomic distinction of internodal tracts is of great interest. Sherf and James (39) propose the presence of three internodal tracts: the anterior, middle, and posterior internodal pathways. The anterior pathway corresponds to Bachmann's bundle, and the posterior pathway corresponds to the crista terminalis and eustachian ridge as reviewed by James (14). One pathway connects the sinoatrial node to the left atrium. These tracts lack insulation from the surrounding myocardium. Until recently, no one had demonstrated the presence of discrete internodal tracts that were histologically distinguishable from the surrounding myocardium. However, Blom and colleagues (40) obtained positive staining for the HNK-1 epitope along a tract located in the region corresponding to the proposed posterior pathway. The remaining two tracts that stained positively for HNK-1 reside in regions that do not exactly match the other two pathways proposed by Sherf and James. These investigators obtained HNK-1–positive staining around the orifice of the common pulmonary vein and in parts of the sinus venosus myocardium. The myocardium surrounding the orifices of the pulmonary veins contain the foci commonly associated with ectopic atrial tachycardia (i.e., atrial fibrillation) (41). The researchers speculated that the HNK-1–positive staining region located around the pulmonary vein may correspond to these arrhythmic foci. Similarly, the investigators speculated that the positive staining located in parts of the sinus venosus may correspond to those foci associated with abnormal right atrial automaticity. Hirao and associates (42) provided evidence that multiple, rather than dual, AV node inputs exist.

Atrioventricular Nodal Axis

The AV node can be considered as three related regions: the compact node, the transitional zone, and the penetrating bundle (Fig. 1-5). The compact AV node has been described as shaped like a half oval and, fully formed, measuring approximately $1 \times 3 \times 5$ mm. Arterial supply normally originates as a branch of the right coronary artery at the crux of the heart, constituting the atrioventricular nodal artery; however, in certain hearts, the left circumflex artery may serve this function. Abuin (43) discovered that Kugel's artery and the right descending superior artery feed the AV node in a certain proportion of the population. The AV node is located epicardially, just underlying the right atrial epicardium posteriorly, anterior to the nodal artery and between the coronary sinus and the medial tricuspid valve leaflet, and posterosuperior to the membranous septum. Koch's triangle is a useful anatomic landmark for identifying the location of the compact node, delineated leftward by the intersection of the eustachian valve and the tricuspid valve annulus, with the ostium of the coronary sinus

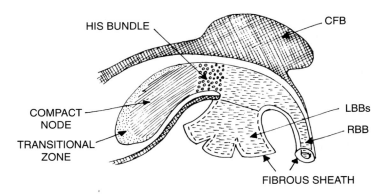

FIGURE 1-5. Atrioventricular node, His bundle, and proximal left and right bundle branches. The central fibrous body (CFB) is adjacent to the atrioventricular nodal complex, and in continuity with the rest of the fibrous skeleton, it provides a protective sheath to insulate the upper reaches of the transitional and compact node from the distal ventricular contact points of the left bundle branch (LBB) and right bundle branch (RBB).

forming the rightward base of the triangle (Fig. 1-6). The node is located at the apex of Koch's triangle and abutted by the annulus fibrosis and Todaro's tendon (Fig. 1-7). The latter reflects the condensation of connective tissue in the thebesbian and eustachian valves, which is in essence a lengthy, slender commissure. The AV node projects leftward into the His bundle at the apex of Koch's triangle and merges this conductive axis with ventricular tissue below the intersection of Todaro's tendon and the central fibrous body.

The notion of a "compact" AV node refers to the most easily histologically distinguishable tissue within a continuous axis of specialized tissue. It is made up of interconnecting fasciculi of small cells, morphologically comparable to the interlacing myofibers of the sinoatrial node. Unlike the sinoatrial node, the AV node lacks a consistently located central artery. Small archipelagos of these nodal cells frequently extend from the compact node into the central fibrous body. From the compact body of the node, two extensions made up of identical cells run posteriorly from the node and branch to approach the mitral and tricuspid annuli. Inoue and Becker (4) described the configuration of the generally forgotten AV nodal posterior extensions. The AV node traditionally has been depicted as blunt ended. However, of 21 autopsy hearts inspected, 13 had prominent rightward and leftward extensions, 7 had rightward extensions exclusively, and 1 had a leftward extension exclusively. These researchers further propose that the extensions may serve as the substrate for the "slow pathway" in the circuit associated with AVNRT. However, Sanchez-Quintana and colleagues (44) showed that two autopsied hearts from patients who underwent successful ablation for AVNRT showed only short posterior extensions of the compact AV node. In an investigation of the arrangement of superficial atrial muscle fibers in the triangle of Koch and their influence on AVNRT, they demonstrated that the arrangement of these fibers varied in 16 autopsy hearts from adults who died of noncardiac diseases. They also showed

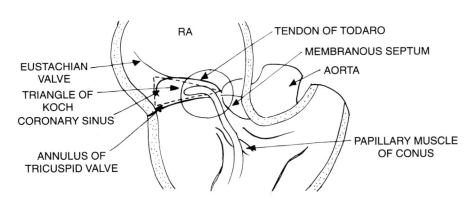

FIGURE 1-6. Cutaway view of right-sided cardiac chambers, displaying the essential anatomic landmarks of the atrioventricular node and His bundle system. Situated at the apex of the triangle of Koch is the atrioventricular node; the His bundle courses through the fibrous skeleton, giving rise to the proximal bundle branches and inferior to the membranous septum. RA, right atrium.

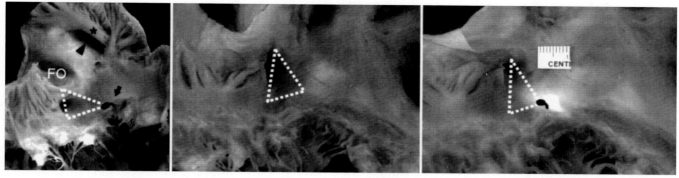

FIGURE 1-7. A: Opened right atrium and ventricle illustrate *(dotted lines)* the triangle of Koch, including the typical location of the atrioventricular node and proximal His bundle at its apex *(arrow)*. Other relevant landmarks include the tendon of Todaro as a confluence of the eustachian and thebesian valves, the coronary sinus at the posterior boundary of the triangle of Koch, the fossa ovale (FO) region, the entry site of the superior vena cava *(arrowhead)*, and the crista terminalis *(star)*. The posterior leaflet of the tricuspid valve defines the lowest margin of the triangle of Koch by its point of attachment. B and C: The triangle of Koch is foreshortened because of the angle of viewing. C: The membranous septum has been transilluminated, illustrating its intimate relationship to the atrioventricular node *(black)*.

that the site of successful ablation in two patients with AVNRT was distant from the compact atrioventricular node and, in one heart, included the inferior, slow pathway. Their work lends credence to the notion that the slow pathway may serve as an anatomic substrate for the reentrant circuit of AVNRT. They speculated that the arrangement of these fibers influences the route by which the circuit responsible for AVNRT approaches the atrioventricular node.

Transitional cells comprising a well-defined layer surround the compact node and inferior (posterior) extensions. The transitional zone is further differentiated by the three main approaches to the compact node that are designated as *superficial transitional cells*, which run anteriorly and inferiorly to the compact node; *posterior transitional cells*, which approach the node from the coronary sinus area; and *deep transitional cells*, which link the left atrium to the compact node. The transitional zone may be implicated in the dual atrioventricular nodal conduction seen in patients with atrioventricular junctional reentrant tachycardia.

The junction between the compact atrioventricular node and the penetrating atrioventricular bundle is designated as the point at which the axis of nodal cells penetrate the annulus fibrosis. Whereas the nodal cells of the compact AV node are in contact with the atrial myocardium (through the transitional cells), the cells of the atrioventricular bundle, although histologically similar to those of the compact node, are separated from the atrial myocardium by the annulus fibrosis. Tongues of tissue extending from the compact AV node into the central fibrous body and connecting the bundle axis to the ventricular septum or from the initial part of the bundle branches to the septal crest have been implicated as potential substrates for preexcitation and circus rhythm circuits. A comprehensive anatomic description of the atrioventricular conduction axis is available elsewhere (3).

His Bundle, Bundle Branches, and Purkinje Fibers

The penetrating bundle, or His bundle, is defined histologically as a continuation of the compact atrioventricular node, where it projects through the central fibrous body (Fig. 1-5) and descends along the posterior border of the membranous ventricular septum. The bundle itself is approximately 2 mm long and divided into three anatomic components. The proximal or nonpenetrating tract is located distal to the AV node. The middle or penetrating tract is embedded within the central fibrous body. The distal tract branches into the right and left bundle branches at the crest of the ventricular septum, with the right bundle branch continuing as an extension of the main bundle, sometimes running deep into the endomyocardium. On exiting the central fibrous body, the left bundle branch divides, forming additional multifasiculi. The Purkinje fibers, which act as extensions of the bundle branches, typically run in fine trabeculae within the immediate subendocardium of both ventricles. Purkinje fibers are only slightly larger than working myofibers in humans. They are readily observed in papillary muscles.

Cardiac Skeleton and Membranous Septum

The primary components of the cardiac conduction system and of the basic musculature of the heart are largely supported by the sturdy fibrocollagenous tissue that comprises the cardiac skeleton. The central fibrous body provides connective tissue continuity between the aortic, mitral, and tricuspid valves (Fig. 1-8). Extending posteroinferiorly and anteriorly from the central fibrous body is the left fibrous trigone, composed of firm bundles of connective tissue. The mitral and tricuspid valve annuli are essentially fibroelastic extensions of the left and right fibrous trigones, respectively. The membranous septum acts as an extension of the cardiac skeleton at the base of the ventricular septum. In forming a segment of the medial right atrial wall, the membranous septum acts as the primary supporting structure for the right aortic valve cusp. After the AV nodal tissue has penetrated the central fibrous body as the His bundle, the inferior margin of the membranous septum marks the course of the His bundle between the right and noncoronary aortic valve cusps.

Age-Related Changes Affecting the Cardiac Conduction System

Replacement of cell populations by fat and fibrous tissue occurs throughout the conduction system as part of the normal aging process. In the sinoatrial node, myocardial cells are replaced by fibrous tissue, with nodal cells persisting in the collagen and thicker

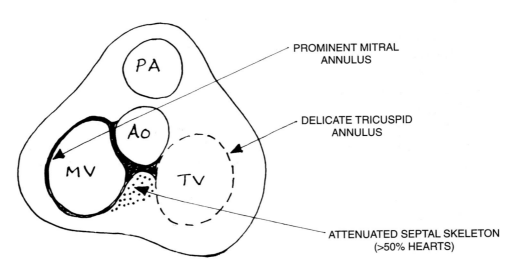

FIGURE 1-8. Transversely sectioned atrioventricular junctional region of a heart illustrates the relative completeness of the fibrous skeleton toward the left side of the heart and the relative delicacy of the corresponding right-sided skeleton. Typically, there is attenuation of the skeleton in the region of the posteroseptal space. The latter may be of practical relevance because several bypass tracts are detected by electrophysiologic mapping of this region. A greater number of bypass tracts, however, are located in the left lateral location, perhaps a surprising finding considering that the fibrous skeleton is more fully developed in this region than anywhere in the heart.

elastic cells developing around nodal myocytes. Aging in the AV node is characterized by fatty infiltration and an increase in nodal collagen and elastic tissue, with slight infiltration of mononuclear cells and degeneration of nodal myocytes. Atrial dilatation, myocyte atrophy, lipofuscin accumulation, and interstitial fibrosis in all four chambers of the heart may participate in arrhythmogenesis but are not unique to or even preferential to the conduction system.

However, Gottwald and coworkers (45) proposed that two factors related to the aging process influence the development of arrhythmias in otherwise normal hearts. Changes in cardiac hemodynamics and structural changes in cardiac tissue, such as deposition of collagen, impinge on normal conduction in the heart. They further concluded, based on their electrophysiologic and histologic examination of rabbit hearts, that aging causes the deposition of fat cells and connective tissue in ventricular tissue and in the atrioventricular node region and therefore causes a higher beat-to-beat variability. They also demonstrated that aging causes an increase in dispersion of the epicardial potential duration and atrioventricular conduction time, along with a decrease in local activation velocity. Spach (46) discusses aging in the context of gap junction distribution and arrhythmogenesis. With normal aging, gap junctions along the lateral edges of cardiac myocytes disappear and focally aggregate at the intercalated disks. The loss of lateral connections with aging appears in concert with microfibrosis and concomitant nonuniform anisotropy and possibly contributes to arrhythmogenesis. A more comprehensive discussion of the effects of aging on the conduction system is available elsewhere (47).

⦿ ABNORMAL ANATOMY OF THE CONDUCTION SYSTEM

Atresia

Atresia of the sinoatrial node is rare. It is usually seen when the predominant pacemaker is at the level of the atrioventricular or ventricular tissue. Interruption of conduction between the atria and ventricles is attributed to different origins of tissue in the crucial interface among conduction fibers of the His bundle, central fibrous body, and endocardial cushion tissue.

Displacement

Complex congenital cardiac malformations can affect the developmental positioning of the sinoatrial node. In particular, atrioventricular canal defects, transposition of the great arteries, and ventricular septal defects (VSDs) may lead to displacement of the sinoatrial node. Normally located along the sulcus terminalis anteriorly and over the rooftop junction of the right atrial appendage and the superior vena cava, the sinoatrial node may be congenitally displaced; it may project out of the sulcus terminalis and more toward the left side of the right atrial appendage.

Duplication

Duplication of the sinoatrial node can occur in situs ambiguous (i.e., atrial isomerism) of the heart. The anatomy of the heart with normal atria is usually classified as *situs solitus,* in which the morphologic right atrium is found on the right side of the body and the left on the left, or as *situs inversus,* in which the atria is arranged in an opposite fashion, effectively "mirroring" the arrangement in situs solitus. The abdominal viscera are also mirror-image compared with normal in situs inversus. *Situs ambiguous* describes a heart in which the atrial features fall neither into solitus nor inversus categories. Right isomerism describes a heart with duplication of right-sided structures; left isomerism describes a heart with duplication of left-sided structures. Duplication of the sinoatrial node can occur in right isomerism (48), creating alternative or competing pacemakers capable of producing a range of conduction disturbances. Similarly, duplication of the AV node has been documented. Attie and associates (49) reported four rare cases of congenitally corrected transposition associated with atrioventricular septal defect. They identified two AV nodes in one heart with a normal atrial arrangement. They detected abnormal conduction through the posterior node and normal conduction through the anterior node of this patient. A comprehensive review of the cardiac conduction system in situs ambiguous is available elsewhere (50).

Infection and Inflammation

Conduction disturbances can arise from a range of infections and other inflammatory conditions resulting from specific microbial or postinfectious processes or from an immune response. Lyme disease, Chagas' disease, and diphtheria are three of the most common infections exhibiting tropism for the heart, and cardiac sarcoidosis, and Wegener's granulomatosis commonly produce arrhythmic sequelae. Other bacterial causes of cardiac arrhythmias include syphilis and group A streptococci (51–53). Miyamoto and colleagues (54) reported a 59-year-old male who developed complete heart block in association with *Salmonella* prosthetic valve endocarditis, a reflection of the well-known arrhythmic consequences of valvular endocarditis (especially with regard to the aortic valve).

Enteroviruses are well known to cause cardiac arrhythmias based on their tropism for the heart. The role of other common human pathogenic viruses such as respiratory syncytial virus in the development of cardiac arrhythmias remains to be proven. Of the few documented occurrences of cardiac dysrhythmias associated with respiratory syncytial virus infection, the most common are supraventricular tachycardias and heart block (55,56). Thomas and coworkers (57) reported two infant patients with respiratory syncytial virus infection and severe dysrhythmias, including supraventricular tachycardias and malignant ventricular dysrhythmias such as ventricular tachycardia, torsade de pointes, and ventricular fibrillation. Similarly, Huang and associates (51) reported a single 7-week-old infant diagnosed with respiratory syncytial virus bronchiolitis and ventricular tachycardia. These observations suggest that respiratory syncytial virus may exhibit a more frequent affinity for the ventricular myocardium than previously believed.

Patients with cardiac sarcoidosis most often die because of an arrhythmia or conduction block and congestive heart failure (58,59). Veinot and Johnston (60) reported a patient with sudden death most likely attributable to cardiac sarcoidosis. They showed marked granulomatous inflammation in the region of the sinoatrial and atrioventricular nodes, as well as in the region of the ventricular septum, potential bases for the sudden arrhythmic death of this patient. Certain observations suggest that this disease selectively targets the conduction system (58,61,62).

Arrhythmogenic right ventricular dysplasia/cardiomyopathy (ARVD/C) is a heart muscle disease characterized by fibrofatty infiltration predominantly of the right ventricle and may be a common cause of sudden death in young people. Ventricular arrhythmias, particularly ventricular tachycardias, appear to be the most frequent cause of sudden death. Strands of surviving fibers most likely serve as the substrate for reentrant pathways and ensuing fatal arrhythmias in these patients (63,64). Several investigators propose that enteroviral infection plays an important role in the pathogenesis of ARVD/C, largely based on the high prevalence of inflammatory infiltrates reported in diseased myocardium (65–67). Grumbach and colleagues (68) provided further evidence to suggest that coxsackievirus infection of the myocardium may promote development of ARVD/C. They demonstrated the presence of enteroviral RNA in endomyocardial biopsies of three of eight patients with ARVD/C and the absence in a control group of five patients with noninflammatory heart disease using nested reverse-transcriptase polymerase chain reaction methods (RT-PCR). They also detected enteroviral RNA in 7 of 23 patients with myocarditis or dilated cardiomyopathy (DCM). These researchers speculate that enteroviral infection directly causes acquired ARVD/C in some instances and "precipitates the development of the disease in genetically predisposed patients" in other instances (68). Fornes and coworkers (69) examined the clinical characteristics and the pathologic features of hearts from 20 individuals who died suddenly of ARVD/C. They discovered that hearts from 60% of these patients had myocardial inflammatory infiltrates consisting of lymphocytes, and one heart had myocyte necrosis. They also provided evidence to suggest that physical and emotional stress precipitates fatal arrhythmic events in sudden ARVD/C related deaths.

Infarction

The nature and degree of conduction system disturbances in the setting of a myocardial infarction depends on the location of the infarct and the extent of scarring and related fibroelastosis (34). Archbald and associates (70) demonstrated a decline in the rate of severe conduction defects since the introduction of thrombolytic therapy based on their investigation of 1,225 consecutive patients with acute myocardial infarction treated between 1988 and 1994. They further speculate that the introduction of thrombolytic therapy most likely resulted in an overall decrease in the size of myocardial infarcts and the occurrence of conduction disturbances. Xing and Martins (71) discovered that the size of the ischemic zone in dogs, as determined from the electrograms obtained, did not substantially influence the occurrence or origin of arrhythmias. In particular, they recorded ventricular tachycardias using computer-assisted three-dimensional (3-D) mapping after occlusion of the left anterior descending artery and reperfusion in open chest dogs. Dogs with a small ischemic zone, compared with those with a large ischemic zone, did not differ with regard to the occurrence or homogeneity of ventricular tachycardia. Similar results were obtained after reperfusion. Ventricular fibrillation and ventricular tachycardia originated from Purkinje or endocardial sites, as determined by selective filtering and sampling of the electrograms obtained, regardless of the size of the ischemic zone.

Puljevic and colleagues (72) showed that QT dispersion increased significantly in relation to the severity of arrhythmia and postinfarction scar size in 303 patients assessed 3 months after myocardial infarction compared with 21 healthy subjects. Majumder and coworkers (73) detected an association between the anatomic location of the myocardial infarct and the type of ensuing conduction disturbance. These investigators assessed 45 anterior, 43 inferior, and 12 combined anterior and inferior myocardial infarction patients for the type of conduction disturbance present. Of these patients, 44 exhibited some type of conduction disturbance, and 56 experienced no disturbance. Inferior myocardial infarction patients displayed a higher incidence of conduction disturbance than anterior myocardial infarction patients. Inferior myocardial infarction patients experienced atrioventricular conduction disturbances, whereas anterior myocardial infarction patients experienced intraventricular conduction disturbances.

Mosseri and associates (74) showed that atherosclerosis in coronary arteries that feed the conduction system may lead to conduction disturbances. They compared the coronary anatomy and pathology in two groups of patients. The study group consisted of 43 patients who required implantation of a permanent pacemaker because of a conduction disturbance and had undergone coronary angiography. The control group consisted of patients with angiographically proven epicardial coronary artery disease who were matched with the study patients in regard to age, sex, extent of coronary occlusion, and other factors. Patients with permanent pacemakers had compromised blood flow to the septal branches and the right coronary artery. This pattern was significantly different from what was found in the control group, in whom blood flow to the right coronary artery was compromised with distal left anterior descending artery lesions.

Proposed pathologic conditions that further contribute to the development of arrhythmias after acute myocardial infarction include ischemia, inflammation, local autonomic denervation, local electrolyte imbalance, and elevated levels of free fatty acids and oxygen-derived free radicals (75,76). Comprehensive reviews of the types of arrhythmias that arise after myocardial infarction and their management strategies can be found elsewhere (75,77–79). Briefly, patients with previous myocardial infarction have the potential for developing multiple reentrant circuits in the area of scarring. These reentrant circuits include anatomic, leading circle, anisotropic, figure-eight, and spiral wave reentry, as discussed in a review by Skanes and Green (80). ST segment depression (denoting ischemia), premature contractions, ventricular tachycardia, fibrillation, and standstill are common arrhythmias resulting from acute, subacute, and chronic myocardial injury and the healing process.

Daleau and Deleze demonstrated that a steep transition from high to low input resistance along Purkinje fibers, as seen in localized regions of ischemia, leads to interruptions in conduction (81). These researchers induced focal and long-range internal resistance in Purkinje fibers by applying hepatanol. They subsequently showed that the internal resistance required to initiate conduction block was 50% less when hepatanol was applied over a short fiber segment compared with the application over a longer segment.

Lurie and colleagues (82) demonstrated that an increase in extracellular space, one consequence of ischemia and aging, dramatically alters electrical conduction. These investigators artificially induced an increase in extracellular space by infusing mannitol through canine blood-perfused AV nodal preparations. They subsequently detected an increase in the AV nodal or His-ventricular conduction time and the AV nodal effective refractory period. Other studies have demonstrated that the pathologic substrate for ventricular arrhythmias and concomitant nonuniform anisotropic dysynchronous conduction in the setting of myocardial infarction includes isolated, decoupled normal myocytes enmeshed in fibrous tissue (83,84). The decoupling of cell-to-cell connections between myocytes results in a zigzag pattern of conduction and leads to the initiation of reentrant arrhythmias (85). In an elaborate review of the influence of microfibrosis on the manifestation of arrhythmias, Spach and Boineau (86) propose that therapies designed to reestablish gap junctional cell-to-cell connections between myocytes may obviate conduction block and reentry.

Wu and colleagues (87) correlated activation patterns of reentry obtained during ventricular tachycardia using computer mapping techniques with increased fibrosis in five hearts from transplant recipients diagnosed with DCM. Such cardiomyopathy is characterized by significant interstitial replacement and perivascular fibrosis in ventricular myocardium (88–90). Tissue areas with lines of block, as determined by epicardial mapping, contained a significantly higher percentage of fibrous tissue than areas lacking lines of block. "The most common mode of initiation of reentry was epicardial breakthrough, followed by a line of conduction block parallel to the epicardial fiber orientation" (87). In this regard, the researchers speculate that fibrosis causes nonuniform anisotropy and preferential propagation in the longitudinal as opposed to the transverse direction. Consequent unidirectional block sets the stage for the development of reentrant circuitry. Similarly, de Bakker and coworkers (91) demonstrated that fibrosis accounted for abnormal conduction patterns and fractionated electrograms seen in explanted hearts from heart transplant recipients diagnosed with DCM. Pogwizd and colleagues (92) demonstrated that a focal mechanism possibly involving early afterdepolarizations or delayed afterdepolarizations instead of reentrant circuitry initiates subendocardial spontaneous ventricular tachycardias. Programmed stimulation may initiate reentry in patients with idiopathic cardiomyopathy undergoing heart transplantation as determined by 3-D intraoperative mapping. Histologic analysis of the explanted hearts revealed variable degrees of interstitial fibrosis at the sites of focal activation and ventricular tachycardia initiation. Fibrosis appeared to be restricted to areas of conduction delay or block.

Infiltration

Deposits of amyloid protein typically produce atrial fibrillation and heart block and, less commonly, ventricular arrhythmias. Amyloidosis is common in aged human hearts and can contribute to arrhythmogenesis at earlier ages in association with chronic inflammatory conditions and multiple myeloma or neoplasms. Reisinger and colleagues (93) demonstrated that the His-Purkinje system of AL amyloidosis patients is selectively impaired. In particular, they conducted an electrophysiologic study of 25 patients with biopsy-proven cardiac AL amyloid. They discovered that the sinoatrial and atrioventricular nodes functioned normally, but the infra-His (HV) conduction times were abnormal. HV prolongation was the sole independent predictor of sudden death in 23 of the patients who died during follow-up. Their results corroborate histologic findings that amyloid fibrils may preferentially or at least prominently infiltrate the His-Purkinje system (94,95). Rodriguez Reguero and associates (96) described a patient with cardiac amyloidosis who had neither rhythm nor conduction abnormalities. The heart and particularly the cardiac conduction system appears more readily affected in immunoglobulin-related (primary) amyloidosis compared with reactive (secondary) infiltration. However, Ahmed and coworkers (97) reported secondary amyloidosis involving the cardiac conduction system. A complete discussion of cardiac amyloidosis and its association with conduction disturbances can be found elsewhere (98).

Iron overload in the hearts of idiopathic hemochromatosis patients may lead to disruptions in normal cardiac conduction, perhaps most strikingly when iron deposits in proximity to components of the conduction system. Olson and colleagues (99) showed the presence of iron deposits within the AV node ($n = 6$) and absence in the sinoatrial node of 14 autopsied hearts from idiopathic hemochromatosis patients. Unfortunately, no mention was made of the presence or absence of conduction disturbances in these patients. Exogenous or endogenous hemochromatosis can lead to atrial flutter or fibrillation, sinus tachycardia, heart block, and syncope. Iron deposits and associated fibrosis are more common in the subepicardial region and in the AV node and less common in the subendocardial region and sinoatrial node. Fibrosis occurring from injury and necrosis accompanying iron deposits or as part of the normal aging process can act as a substrate for arrhythmogenesis.

Primary tumors, including rhabdomyomas (i.e., Purkinje cell tumors), and mesotheliomas (i.e., endotheliomas) are believed to produce heart block through tumor enlargement. Rhabdomyomas, also associated with paroxysmal arrhythmias, may be congenital in origin and are seen predominantly in children. Unger and associates (100) reported a 64-year-old woman who was diagnosed with primary cardiac lymphoma and presented with first-degree atrioventricular block and atrial fibrillation. Transesophageal echocardiography revealed a large extranodal tumor in the posteroinferior right atrium that extended to the inferior left atrial wall and compressed the coronary sinus and the inferior vena cava orifice. Van Hare and coworkers (101) provided evidence that tumors, particularly rhabdomyomas, contribute to the development of conduction disturbances by functioning as an accessory pathway. These researchers investigated the location of the cardiac tumor and accessory pathway in one infant and one adolescent patient, both of whom were diagnosed with multiple cardiac tumor lesions and conduction disturbances. There was close correspondence between the site of the intracardiac tumor and location of the accessory pathway; the tumor was subsequently treated with successful radiofrequency ablation. The researchers speculate that accessory pathways seen in patients with cardiac tumors, particularly rhabdomyomas, are not typical Kent bundles but may instead originate and extend from the cardiac tumor itself. Mesotheliomas normally affect the AV node, interrupting the conduction axis and resulting in block or atrial fibrillation.

⦿ MOLECULAR SUBSTRATES OF ARRHYTHMIAS

Antiarrhythmic Drugs

An appreciation of the mechanisms by which antiarrhythmic drugs exert their therapeutic effects provides clues with regard to the molecular basis of cardiac arrhythmogenesis. In a comprehensive review, Singh (102) describes the four classes of antiarrhythmic drugs developed. These drugs interfere with conduction by delaying fast sodium channel–mediated conduction (class I), blocking sympathetic stimulation (class II), prolonging repolarization (class III), or serving as calcium antagonists (class IV). These drugs exert their therapeutic action by impeding or enhancing ion channel conductance, whether sodium, potassium, or calcium channel conductance. A list of drugs used to treat specific types of arrhythmias can be found elsewhere (103).

The efficacy of class I drugs has been placed in disrepute in light of the shocking results from the Cardiac Arrhythmia Suppression Trial (CAST), a randomized placebo-controlled clinical trial. Data from this study demonstrated that encainide, flecainide, or moricizine (sodium channel blockers) increases rather than decreases mortality in post-myocardial infarction patients with ventricular ectopy (104,105). Class I drugs appear to sustain otherwise nonsustained reentrant circuits by slowing the rate of conduction, so much so that the circuit propagates through myocardium that has had sufficient time to recover electrically (80). Similar results were obtained in patients with cardiac arrest or atrial fibrillation (106–108). For this reason, class I drugs are rarely used to treat postmyocardial infarction ventricular arrhythmias.

In contrast, β-adrenoceptor blockade by class II agents appears to consistently reduce mortality in cardiac arrest survivors, patients with congenital long QT interval syndrome, myocardial infarction survivors, patients with implantable cardioverter-defibrillators for ventricular tachycardia or ventricular fibrillation, and postoperative cardiac patients (102). Class

II drugs remain the only drug of proven capability to reduce mortality in post-myocardial infarction patients. Recent results from the European Myocardial Infarct Amiodarone Trial (EMAIT) and Canadian Amiodarone Myocardial Infarction Arrhythmia Trial (CAMIAT) confirm this impression and show that amiodarone, a class III agent that simultaneously blocks adrenergic stimulation while lengthening repolarization, does not significantly reduce mortality in post-myocardial infarction patients compared with placebo (109,110). Moreover, the Survival with Oral d-Sotalol (SWORD) study showed that treatment with d-sotalol alone, a selective potassium channel blocker, increased mortality in patients with ventricular dysfunction (111). Roden (112) speculates that this increase in mortality rate may be attributed to the drug's ability to induce torsade de pointes, ventricular proarrhythmias believed to originate from the His-Purkinje network and possibly from a subset of myocardial cells located in the midventricular myocardium referred to as M cells (80,113). The final results of the Danish Investigation of Arrhythmia and Mortality on Dofetilide (DIAMOND) are still pending, but preliminary results suggest that dofetilide, another selective potassium channel blocker, did not alter mortality in patients with depressed left ventricular function compared with placebo. Sotalol and amiodarone, class III potassium channel blockers, control ventricular and supraventricular arrhythmias based on their ability to lengthen repolarization and refractoriness without slowing conduction in atria and ventricles, while blocking sympathetic innervation (114, 115). For this reason, use of d-sotalol is limited to patients without significant cardiac disease. The race is on to develop more selective and efficacious class III drugs for the treatment of arrhythmias.

Calcium Homeostasis and Arrhythmogenesis

Class IV drugs, or calcium antagonists, target one of the two types of plasma membrane channels of cardiac cells, as reviewed by Nattel (116) and Katz (117). Briefly, L-type plasma membrane calcium channels permit entry of calcium into the cytosol in response to membrane depolarization and, in so doing, stimulate the release of intracellular calcium through intracellular calcium-release channels: the ryanodine receptors and inositol triphosphate–activated calcium channels. In this way, L-type channels located in the sinoatrial node contribute to the maintenance of nodal pacemaker activity, and L-type channels in the AV node maintain atrioventricular conduction. T-type plasma membrane channels are located primarily in pacemaker cells and less so in cells of the atria and ventricles. They contribute to coupling of smooth muscle cell contraction and may regulate cell growth. The most widely used calcium channel antagonists in the treatment of supraventricular tachycardias include verapamil and diltiazem, both selective for L-type channels. T-type antagonists are not used in the clinical setting, but mibefradil, a novel T-type antagonist, appears effective in countering electrical remodeling and atrial fibrillation in dogs (118).

Abnormalities of calcium homeostasis in the heart, especially calcium overload, affect cardiac excitability and arrhythmogenesis by two major mechanisms: cell-to-cell uncoupling and triggered arrhythmias. The first mechanism plays a role in conduction block and in setting the stage for reentrant circuits, whereas the second involves the production of delayed afterdepolarizations by calcium activation of nonspecific cation channels and inward currents carried by the Na^+/Ca^{2+} exchanger (George Rozanski, personal communication, 1999).

Calcium plays a pivotal role in the propagation and perpetuation of arrhythmic processes, and therefore much effort has gone into the development of more efficacious calcium antagonists. Results from numerous studies suggest that prolonged tachycardia triggers changes in calcium loading and stimulates cellular dedifferentiation, hypertrophy, fibrosis, and cell death (119–122). For instance, Van Gelder and colleagues (123) demonstrated alterations in the level of mRNA encoding proteins and ion channels involved in calcium handling in patients suffering from persistent atrial fibrillation. They found that patients with atrial fibrillation lasting longer than 6 months had reduced levels of L-type calcium channel mRNA and inhibitory guanine nucleotide binding protein iα_2 mRNA. The investigators speculate that downregulation of channels involved in calcium regulation during atrial fibrillation causes changes in intracellular calcium levels and disruption of calcium-dependent pathways. These results further stress the importance of normalizing calcium levels in patients with arrhythmias.

In a review of antiarrhythmic drugs, Camm and Yap (103) discuss the characteristics of the ideal antiarrhythmic drug. Briefly, antiarrhythmic drugs should correct the problem responsible for the arrhythmia, not just compensate for the arrhythmia. The drug should directly target the cause of the arrhythmia, not downstream incidental pathways. The drug effects also should be site specific to exclude the possibility of toxic episodes.

Genetic Basis for Idiopathic Arrhythmias

Most arrhythmias occur in patients with structural heart disease, but certain patients with arrhythmias do not have structural heart disease. The genetic basis for idiopathic arrhythmias (i.e., primary and familial) continues to unfold, and new clues to the molecular substrates involved in arrhythmogenesis are forthcoming (124). Mutations within genes encoding various cardiac ion channels involved in normal conduction have been identified in patients with specific arrhythmic disorders. For instance, mutations within the genes encoding the cardiac sodium channel *(SCN5A)*, I_{Kr} potassium channel *(KCNH2)*, α-subunit of I_{Ks} potassium channel *(KCNQ1)*, or ancillary subunit for the I_{Ks} channel complex *(KCNE1)* are responsible for the autosomal dominant form of long-QT syndrome characterized by prolonged QT interval, torsade de pointes and sudden death (125). All such mutations lead to prolonged ventricular action potentials, which may cause early afterdepolarizations and torsade de pointes (126). The *LQT4* mutation has been mapped to chromosome 4, but the gene still remains to be identified. Mutation of the sodium channel gene *(SCN5A)*, which is defective in long-QT syndrome, also appears to cause at least one variant of the Brugada syndrome (127). The Brugada syndrome mutation causes a loss of function, and the long-QT syndrome mutation causes a gain of function.

A few other familial arrhythmic disorders have been mapped to specific chromosomes, but the genes have yet to be identified. For instance, familial bundle branch block has been mapped to a locus located on chromosome 19 (128,129). Some of the candidate genes include those for kallikrein, troponin T, and the histidine-rich Ca^{2+}-binding protein (125). Familial atrial fibrillation has been mapped to chromosome 10 (130).

Genetic factors also play a pivotal role in the development of familial arrhythmias associated with structural heart disease or heart failure. Grunig and colleagues (131) identified five phenotypes of familial DCM derived from observations of 48 index patients of a total of 445 with confirmed DCM. One familial phenotype was associated with early conduction defects. Families of six index patients (76 members in total) falling into the familial phenotypic group with early conduction defects exhibited a higher incidence of atrial fibrillation and atrioventricular block compared with members of other phenotypic groups. This condition has been mapped to chromosome 1 and 3 in two different families with atrioventricular block and AV node dysfunction, respectively, but the genes remain to be identified (124,132–134). Wang and associates (135) observed that mice carrying mutations within mitochondrial transcription factor A develop cardiac-specific, progressive respiratory chain deficiency, DCM, and atrioventricular heart conduction block. The same factor regulates transcription and replication of mitochondrial DNA in humans, mutation of which causes DCM, conduction defects, and features commonly associated with Kearns-Sayre syndrome.

ARVD/C is associated with life-threatening ventricular tachyarrhythmias originating from the right ventricle and is characterized by fibrofatty replacement that predominates in the right ventricular myocardium. The disease carries a sudden death rate of 2.5% per year (136). An autosomal dominant form has been mapped to four loci (14q23, 1q42, 14q12, and 2q32), and a recessive form (i.e., Naxos disease) has been mapped to 17q21 (124,137–141). Ahmad and coworkers (136) mapped another locus for ARVD/C to chromosome 3p23 in a family of more than 200 members, 10 of whom showed autosomal dominant signs of the condition. Candidate genes include those encoding a RAF serine-threonine protein kinase, a DNA-binding protein, and a protein-tyrosine phosphatase. Unfortunately, no genes have been identified.

Mutations in seven sarcomeric protein genes have been identified in families with familial hypertrophic cardiomyopathy-related arrhythmias. β-Myosin heavy chain, cardiac essential myosin light chain, cardiac regulatory myosin light chain, cardiac troponin T, α-tropomyosin, cardiac myosin-binding protein C, and cardiac troponin I have all been implicated (125). It is not surprising that sarcomere contractile performance is abnormal in affected patients. Priori and colleagues (125,142) further propose that arrhythmias in these patients may be a consequence of myocyte disarray, myocardial fibrosis, and myocyte hypertrophy. A subtype of familial hypertrophic cardiomyopathy that coexists with Wolff-Parkinson-White (WPW) syndrome has been mapped to chromosomes 7q3 and 19 (143,144). Multiple genes play a role in arrhythmogenesis.

The positive identification of genes responsible for primary familial arrhythmias in the presence and absence of structural heart disease opens up the possibility of molecular screening and diagnosis as well as the development of site-specific drugs. Other sources review the genetic mutations responsible for arrhythmias (124,125,142,145).

Role of Gap Junctions and Connexins in Arrhythmogenesis

Saffitz and colleagues (146) proposed that fibrosis in the context of myocardial ischemia contributes to the initiation of reentrant ventricular tachycardia through a change in the number and rearrangement of gap junctions. Myocytes and components of the conduction system probably alter their expression of connexins, gap junctional channel proteins that permit intercellular flow of ions, in response to stresses imposed by ischemic myocardial disease. As determined by knockout experiments, connexin 43 (Cx43), the principal gap junctional protein expressed in ventricular myocytes, and connexin 40 (Cx40), which is expressed in the cardiac conduction system, play a pivotal role in electrical coupling (147,148). The Cx40 null mice exhibit atrioventricular block and bundle branch block, whereas mice heterozygous for Cx43 null mutation have slowed ventricular conduction. Luke and Saffitz (149) further demonstrated a reduction in the number of cells connected by intercalated disks in tissue bordering infarcted tissue compared with normal tissue. Similarly, Peters and associates (150) demonstrated a 47% reduction in the gap junction surface area per unit cell volume and a decrease in Cx43 content in gap junctions in ischemic hearts. Kaprielian and colleagues (151) also demonstrated a reduction in Cx43 content in gap junctions in biopsies taken from "reversibly ischemic" segments based on digital image processing techniques and confocal immunofluorescence microscopy. In light of these findings, the researchers speculated that Cx43 plays a dominant role in conduction and that downregulation of Cx43 contributes to the creation of anatomic substrates of abnormal conduction and arrhythmogenesis.

The redistribution of gap junctions also strongly influences the development of conduction disturbances. For instance, Luke and Saffitz (149) demonstrated selective reduction in the number of side-to-side connections and preservation, for the most part, of the number of end-to-end connections in adjacency to infarcted tissue compared with normal tissue. Saffitz and coworkers (146) proposed that changes in the rate of connexin turnover by the lysosomal or cytoplasmic ubiquitin-proteosomal pathways may account for the redistribution observed. In this regard, the investigators argue that the redistribution of gap junctions and partial uncoupling of cardiac myocytes promotes a zigzag pattern of conduction and reduced conduction velocity. In this state of general anisotropy, wavefronts preferentially travel in the longitudinal direction, rather than the transverse direction, and may reenter postrefractory tissue, thereby setting the stage for the initiation of reentrant tachycardias.

Until recently, investigators had observed the redistribution of gap junctions after ischemic injury during the period late after infarction, when fibrotic scarring had taken place (149,152). It is well established that fibrotic scarring interrupts the integrity of gap-junctional connections between myocytes and, in so doing, sets the stage for anisotropic conduction and the initiation of arrhythmias. However, Peters and associates (153) showed redistribution of Cx43 as little as 4 days after infarction in the epicardial border zone. They correlated the location of reentrant ventricular tachycardia in the surviving subepicardial myocardial layer with the location of Cx43 by immunohistochemistry. The researchers concluded that the redistribution of gap junctions after ischemic injury causes nonuniform anisotropy early in the absence of fibrotic scarring. Spach (46) proposes that therapeutic agents designed to reestablish gap junction connections may cure and even prevent arrhythmias. Comprehensive discussions of the molecular basis of anisotropy in the context of myocardial ischemia (154–156) and of the distribution of connexins in the heart and conduction system can be found elsewhere (157–160).

● CONGENITAL CARDIAC MALFORMATIONS ASSOCIATED WITH ARRHYTHMOGENESIS PREOPERATIVELY AND POSTOPERATIVELY

Accessory pathways are frequently found in otherwise normal hearts and are also associated with a number of grossly evident cardiovascular malformations. Moreover, an underlying, sometimes asymptomatic congenital malformation of the heart can itself represent an important risk factor for arrythmogenesis and sudden death. Several well-defined congenital conditions involve a fundamental malalignment of the principal conduction components, which affects the electrical activation patterns of the heart. For the electrophysiologist, a knowledge of common congenital abnormalities is important because of the conduction patterns related to the malformations themselves and because of the conduction disturbances that can arise after the patient has undergone corrective surgery. For instance, ventricular surgery, including repair of VSD, tetralogy of Fallot (TOF), and atrioventricular canal, may result in conduction disturbances, atrioventricular block, and ventricular arrhythmias (161). Similarly, any type of atriotomy may cause postoperative atrial arrhythmias (162). Virtually all atriotomies involve the intercaval region between the crista terminalis and the right pulmonary veins. IART is prevalent among patients who undergo surgery for a congenital heart defect (163). Triedman and colleagues (164) characterized the mechanism of IART in eight patients who underwent congenital heart surgery using recordings from a multipolar basket recording catheter; it was an arrhythmia with a mechanism distinct from that found in common atrial flutter and involved native and surgically created zones of conduction block. One percent of patients who undergo surgery for congenital heart disease experience complete heart block, as reviewed by Bonatti and coworkers (165).

Several investigators have sought to determine the risk of late sudden cardiac death after operation for congenital heart defects and the factors associated with this increased risk of sudden death. Silka and colleagues (166) determined the incidence and cause of sudden death in 3,589 patients undergoing operation for a heart defect between 1958 and 1996. They identified 41 late sudden deaths in this study population, 37 of which occurred in patients with aortic stenosis, coarctation, transposition of the great arteries, or TOF. Arrhythmia was cited as the cause of sudden death in 30 of the 37 study patients, and they further demonstrated that the risk of late sudden death increased incrementally 20 years after operation for TOF, aortic stenosis, and coarctation. The investigators concluded that the risk of late sudden death after operation for a congenital heart defect is 25 to 100 times greater than that found in an age-matched control population. Patients with cyanotic or left heart obstructive lesions experience the greatest risk of sudden death. Reddy and colleagues (167) provide evidence to suggest that delaying surgical repair of congenital heart defects in low-birth-weight infants confers a higher mortality rate.

Congenital Complete Atrioventricular Block

Impairment of conduction through the atrioventricular junction tissues can be present at birth or result from a number of acquired diseases. James and associates (168) suggested that apoptosis may be responsible for the gradual development of complete heart block. Histologic examination of hearts from three subjects who died suddenly revealed similar abnormalities in the sinoatrial node, internodal and interatrial pathways, and AV node. The sinoatrial node was nearly destroyed in all the hearts and lacked any signs of fibrosis, infiltration, or inflammatory degeneration, but numerous Tdt-mediated UTP Nick End Labeled (TUNEL)-positive cells were observed in all hearts studied. True congenital block, resulting from a developmental anomaly that is intrinsic to the AV node or branches, must be distinguished from congenital conditions in which block results from well-defined structural malformations. The latter include congenitally corrected transposition, in which a malalignment of the atrial and ventricular septa can produce atrioventricular conduction disturbances, or atrioventricular septal defects and double-inlet left ventricle, in which a deficiency or absence of the right ventricle results in block. Kertesz and colleagues (169) have outlined the association between congenital complete atrioventricular block (CCAVB) and congenital heart disease. About one third of patients with CCAVB are diagnosed with some form of congenital heart disease, with L-transposition of the great arteries being the most frequent defect (170,171). Similarly, 53% of fetuses with CCAVB are diagnosed with an associated congenital heart disease, with left atrial isomerism being the most common defect (172).

When no major cardiac malformations are associated with conduction block, fibrosis and fatty replacement of the conduction tissue occur in three morphologic settings, as outlined by Chow and colleagues (173). In atrial-axis discontinuity, the atrial myocardium fails to contact the atrioventricular specialized conduction axis, and nodoventricular discontinuity is marked by a break in the axis responsible for conduction between the compact AV node and the ventricular conduction tissue. Intraventricular discontinuity occurs in instances of discontinuity between the branching bundle and the bundle branches.

Kaplan and coworkers (174) described a patient with complete atrioventricular block who underwent mediastinal irradiation 8.5 years before death. These researchers detected extensive fibrosis of the approaches to the sinoatrial and AV nodes, the atria, the atrial septum, the tricuspid, mitral and aortic valves, the atrioventricular junction, the ventricular septum, and in the ventricles surrounding the conduction system. They concluded that cardiac fibrosis in this patient was caused by previous mediastinal irradiation and not by atherosclerotic coronary artery disease, which is another consequence of mediastinal irradiation. Atrioventricular block from coronary artery disease is typically characterized by fibrodegenerative changes in the branching bundle, the left bundle branch, and the second portion of the right bundle branch. These investigators identified 26 of 39 patients who developed atrioventricular block or trifascicular block after radiation therapy in a review of published experience.

Accessory Pathways

The existence of accessory or anomalous pathways that "short circuit" the normal conduction pathway from the sinoatrial node through to the ventricular myocardium can produce preexcitation. In the human fetus, accessory atrioventricular connections are common, rarely producing disturbances that are clinically apparent, and they are normally severed during postnatal development. When accessory pathways crossing the atrioventricular ring tissue persist beyond the normal developmental period, the delay-producing activity of the compact AV node is bypassed, and additional or conflicting wavefronts of activation are produced. The result may be preexcitation, detected clinically as atrial fibrillation, ventricular fibrillation, or complete heart block. Accessory pathways, although associated with several gross congenital abnormalities, are also common in otherwise normal hearts.

Classification of Accessory Pathways

Researchers have studied aberrant electrical links between the atrial and ventricular myocardium for more than a century. In 1983, Davies and associates (13) summarized the observations gleaned from their own work and that of their predecessors and defined five types of anomalous connections capable of producing preexcitation (Fig. 1-9). The most common of these are accessory atrioventricular connections that exist outside the specialized atrioventricular junctional tissues, spanning from atria to ventricles. Two other categories link the atrioventricular node and His bundle to the ventricular septal musculature, and these are denoted as nodoventricular or fasiculoventricular connections. Differentiation of the latter pathways is made on the basis of their starting points, with the former originating in the compact node and the latter originating in the bundle or proximal bundle branches. The fourth possibility for an accessory tract is an atriofascicular pathway composed of atrial fibers

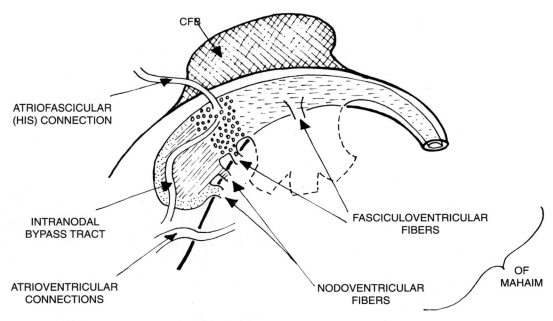

FIGURE 1-9. Atrioventricular nodal region shows the possible perinodal and remote atrioventricular bypass tracts. Fibers of Mahaim have been localized more remotely from the node-His axis than depicted in this diagram.

that connect with the His bundle or branches, penetrating the collagenous insulation provided by the central fibrous body. Intranodal bypass tracts, which also take their point of departure from within the atria, circumvent the main delay-producing region by joining the atrioventricular junctional tissues distal to the compact node but before the bundle penetrates the central fibrous body.

Reviews have focussed on the course and location of accessory pathways (175,176). Accessory pathways are often classified according to their anatomic connections—atrionodal, atrio-His, atrioventricular, or nodoventricular—as proposed by the European Study Group for Pre-excitation (177). Similarly, accessory pathways may be classified according to their point of insertion. For instance, they may insert in the right or left atrium or in the AV nodal junction. Discussions of the anatomy of the atrioventricular junction as it pertains to ventricular preexcitation can be found elsewhere (178).

The atrioventricular junction surrounds the orifices of the mitral and tricuspid valves. Anomalous conduction pathways exist within the atrioventricular junction and contribute to aberrant ventricular preexcitation. For example, the muscular accessory pathways responsible for the WPW syndrome reside in the left, septal, or right junctions in this region. Cain and colleagues (179,180) documented the regional distribution of accessory pathways, observing that 58% are found in the left free wall, 24% in the posteroseptal site, 13% in the right free wall, and 5% in the anterior septal site. "Specific muscular connections are found in the presence of Purkinje cell tumors, diverticula of the coronary sinus, or when taking origin from nodes of Kent at the acute margin of the ventricular mass" (178). The latter fibers usually constitute the Mahaim conduction unit. Okishige and colleagues (181) described the electrophysiologic properties of Mahaim pathways found in seven patients and their experience in ablating these pathways. All seven patients were diagnosed with a right-sided atriofascicular or atrioventricular pathway exhibiting decremental properties. The researchers successfully ablated the Mahaim pathway in all but one patient by identifying and subsequently targeting sites of Mahaim spiked potentials located along the tricuspid annulus. The investigators propose that the Mahaim pathway consists of two portions: "one shows decremental conduction, and the other shows a rate-independent conduction property like that of the usual Kent bundle"

(181). In a letter to the editor, Anderson (182) argued that Okishige and coworkers (181) inappropriately used "usual Kent bundle" to describe the distal segment of the Mahaim pathway, because Kent bundles may or may not bear resemblance to the node-like remnants originally described by Kent (183).

Unlike the previously mentioned accessory pathways, the slow and fast pathways residing in the atrioventricular region are composed of myocardial cells and lack any specialized component. Anderson and Ho (178) think the orientation of these myocardial fibers predisposes the fiber to a particular direction of electrical conduction. A sophisticated discussion of the anatomic factors that affect propagation and recovery in the conduction system is available elsewhere (184). Briefly, fiber orientation, transmural rotation of fiber direction, and transmural obliqueness of fiber direction affect excitation and recovery.

Tai and colleagues (185) described the orientation and electrophysiologic properties of fibers constituting left free wall accessory pathways using coronary sinus mapping and radiofrequency ablation by means of a retrograde ventricular approach. They investigated 96 consecutive patients with a single left free wall accessory pathway who underwent radiofrequency ablation. They showed that 72 of the 96 left free wall pathways had an oblique course of fiber orientation, 42 of which had proximal excursion (i.e., atrial insertion site distal to the ventricular insertion site of the accessory pathway) and 30 of which had distal excursion (i.e., atrial insertion site proximal to the ventricular insertion site of the accessory pathway). The remaining 24 patients had directly aligned atrial and ventricular insertion sites. They also demonstrated that retrograde conduction was poorest in patients with proximal excursion. Accessory pathways at the more posterior locations correlated with a higher incidence of proximal excursion, whereas anteriorly located pathways had a higher incidence of distal excursion. These researchers concluded that fiber orientation may have clinical implications in radiofrequency ablation. The importance of differentiating between the different sites and insertion points of bypass tracts has been underscored in numerous investigations and clinical observations.

Accessory pathways are further differentiated electrophysiologically based on the direction of impulse conduction (176). For instance, nondecremental bypass tracts (i.e., Kent bundles) conduct impulses in antegrade, retrograde, and both directions. Decremental pathways conduct impulses antegradely exclusively, as is the case with Mahaim fibers, or retrogradely exclusively, as is the case in permanent junctional reciprocating reentrant tachycardia

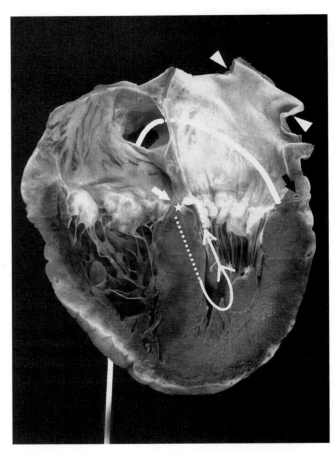

FIGURE 1-10. Four-chamber echocardiographic view of the posterointerior half of a human heart illustrates two routes for ablation catheters to reach atrioventricular bypass tracts in the left side of the heart. The passage of a catheter retrograde from the aorta and up underneath the medial posterior mitral leaflet may provide access to certain pathways adjacent to the posteroseptal space *(dashed arrow)*. More lateral pathways may be reached using a transseptal atrial approach, introducing the catheter by way of the inferior vena cava. The AV node *(white arrow)*, left circumflex coronary artery *(arrowhead)*, and coronary vein *(black arrow)* are shown. The relevance of the proximity of latter structures is related to the potential damage when radiofrequency energy is delivered to the site of a bypass tract. Ablation lesions usually are larger than originally anticipated, and neighboring structures must be considered.

(PJRT). The antegrade decremental tracts are further subdivided into long and short pathways. Most of these pathways have a proximal insertion point on the tricuspid annulus (i.e., atrioventricular pathways) or on the AV node (i.e., nodoventricular pathways).

Left free wall pathways are usually ablated at the point of ventricular insertion, which is believed to be the "weak link" in left-sided pathways (186). The ablation catheter may be advanced into the left ventricle across the aortic valve in a retrograde direction (Fig. 1-10). The catheter tip is then wedged beneath the mitral valve annulus, affording a stable position. When ablation of the region of ventricular insertion region fails to interrupt aberrant conduction, an atrial approach is used in which the ablation catheter is advanced across the mitral valve into the left atrium. A third approach, targeting the interface between the left atrium and the anomalous pathway, is to access the left atrium by a transseptal approach (Fig. 1-10). Ablation delivered from within the coronary sinus can be used in the rare occurrence of a subepicardial left free wall pathway (186). Ablation of right free wall pathways is approached from the atrial aspect of the tricuspid valve, targeting the "weak" atrial insertion point. The difficulty in achieving a stable catheter position is cited as the primary reason for failed ablation of right-sided pathways, frequently necessitating repeat sessions (186).

Experience with surgical and ablation procedures for septal pathways in general and posteroseptal pathways in particular emphasize the complexity of the surrounding architecture (187–189) (Fig. 1-11) and the specificity required for isolating an aberrant pathway (190–193). Posteroseptal pathways are typically located between the insertion of the atrial extension of the membranous septum into the right fibrous trigone anteriorly and the epicardium overlying the crux of the heart posteriorly. Laterally, posteroseptal pathways are bound by the walls of the left and right atria. This pyramidal space contains Todaro's tendon, the atrioventricular nodal artery, epicardial fat, and the proximal portion of the coronary sinus, and it is immediately adjacent to the triangle of Koch (179). Most posteroseptal pathways appear to course in a right atrial to left ventricle direction. Nearby, certain bypass pathways map to "diverticula" in the deep coronary sinus at the connecting site for the posterior coronary vein (Fig. 1-12). Anterior septal pathways

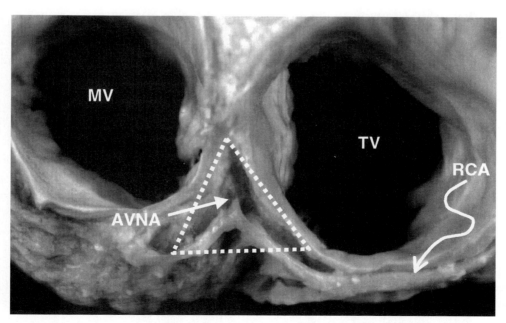

FIGURE 1-11. The posteroseptal space is viewed from a superior aspect. The site of penetration of the atrioventricular nodal artery (AVNA) into the posteroseptal space is shown (arrow). A substantial number of bypass tracts are located in this region. MV, mitral valve; RCA, right coronary artery; TV, tricuspid valve.

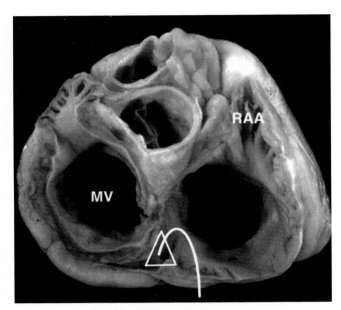

FIGURE 1-12. Superior view of heart with atria unroofed illustrates the approximate location of the posteroseptal space *(triangle)* and the approximate position of a catheter entering the ostium of the coronary sinus and projecting to a site of a potential coronary sinus diverticulum. Such diverticula are deemed to be the site of uncommon bypass tracts. MV, mitral valve; RAA, right atrial appendage.

are much less common than posteroseptal pathways. They are normally located just anterior to the atrioventricular node and anterosuperior to the bundle of His. They pass through the fat pad separating the atrioventricular insertion of the right coronary artery and the right and left fibrous trigone of the cardiac skeleton (179,186). Ablation is usually conducted via the right atrium using a jugular venous approach. During the past 10 years, several groups have reported an additional "intermediate septal pathway" that differs from an anterior septal pathway that inserts in the anteromedial right atrium and activates the ventricular septum anteriorly and from a posteroseptal pathway that inserts near the ostium of the coronary sinus and activates the right and left ventricles more posteriorly (193,194).

Tai and associates (195) review the anatomic features, the electrophysiologic characteristics, and radiofrequency ablation of septal accessory pathways. They focus attention on the anteroseptal, midseptal, para-Hisian, and posteroseptal pathways located in the complex atrioventricular septal region, all of which display electrocardiographic and electrophysiologic characteristics that differ from those of free wall accessory pathways. They further highlight numerous experiments demonstrating that "radiofrequency catheter ablation using the titration method and endocardial approach without entrance into the coronary sinus is effective in eliminating most of the septal accessory pathways without impairment of atrioventricular conduction" (195). Successful ablation of some posteroseptal pathways requires entrance into the coronary sinus, suggesting an epicardial route for the pathway (196). Aguinaga and colleagues (197) also demonstrated successful ablation of septal accessory pathways in 36 patients with the permanent form of junctional reciprocating tachycardia. They applied radiofrequency energy at "the site of earliest retrograde atrial activation during ventricular pacing or during reciprocating tachycardia" (197). Most accessory pathways in these patients were located in the posteroseptal zone (32 posteroseptal, 2 right midseptal, 1 right posterolateral, 1 left anterolateral).

Acquired cardiac malformations, including areas of scarring, aneurysm formation, or hypertrophy, can also act as anatomically discreet electrical pathways between the atria and ventricles or related conduction tissue, producing rhythm disturbances. They may also be amenable to ablation.

Wolff-Parkinson-White Syndrome and Variants

Accessory pathways are the underlying cause of the WPW syndrome. Described in the early 20th century (198) and in more detail by the investigators for whom the syndrome is named (199), WPW is an electrophysiologic condition characterized by a normal electrocardiogram and short PR intervals with functional bundle branch block. Paroxysmal tachycardia and paroxysmal atrial fibrillation or flutter are the common arrhythmic manifestations. The WPW syndrome is often observed in normal hearts, but it may also be associated with specific congenital malformations, including Ebstein's anomaly, mitral valve prolapse, and cardiomyopathy.

Investigators have defined several variants of the WPW syndrome that are also related to the presence of one or more accessory pathways. The most common of these is the so-called silent WPW syndrome or concealed bypass tract in which the pathway is only capable of retrograde conduction and cannot therefore be identified by a surface electrocardiogram nor be mapped to the ventricular insertion point by conventional methods. PJRT has also been identified as a subset of the WPW syndrome. In this condition, an accessory pathway, frequently located in the posteroseptal area, conducts in a retrograde direction and is conspicuous for its unusually slow conduction and atrial insertion at the coronary sinus ostium. The atrioventricular junctional region, including the compact node and His bundle, acts as the anterograde limb. A major clue to the presence of accessory pathway PJRT is incessant supraventricular tachycardia with a long R-P interval, narrow QRS complex, and inverted P waves in inferior leads (200). Caution must be exercised in ablating such a posteroseptal accessory pathway because of its proximity to the atrioventricular junctional region (200).

Plumb (201) highlighted some of the important anatomic landmarks and mapping procedures used for catheter ablation for the WPW syndrome. He emphasized the results obtained by electrophysiologic mapping and the different accessory pathways and insertion points with which these results are frequently associated. Percutaneous, vascular, multipolar electrode catheters are used to record the pacing of the atria and ventricles and to confirm the number and location of accessory pathways. The advent of large-tip deflectable electrode catheters has enabled the ablationist to map the aberrant pathway and deliver the radiofrequency current within the same session (202).

A variant form of the WPW syndrome is associated with hypertrophic cardiomyopathy and intraventricular conduction abnormalities and is inherited in an autosomal dominant fashion. Mehdirad and colleagues (203) described the electrophysiologic characteristics of accessory atrioventricular connections in four related individuals with ventricular preexcitation, abnormal intraventricular conduction or ventricular hypertrophy (or both), and a total of seven atrioventricular connections. The investigators demonstrated for the first time that preexcitation in this form of WPW syndrome resulted from accessory atrioventricular connections. The location and electrophysiologic characteristics of these connections were similar to those found in isolated WPW.

Lown-Ganong-Levine Syndrome

Accessory bypass tracts linking the bundle of His directly to the atrium or linking the atrial septum directly to the ventricular septum are speculated to produce the arrhythmias seen in the Lown-Ganong-Levine syndrome. Earlier investigations of this condition have not been comprehensively expanded in recent years (204,205).

Postoperative Issues in Radiofrequency Ablation

In the three decades that have passed since the first surgical ablation for an accessory pathway associated with WPW syndrome, nonsurgical, percutaneous catheter-based ablation techniques have revolutionized the treatment and cure of patients with a wide range of conduction disturbances. An overview of radiofrequency catheter ablation in the treatment of cardiac arrhythmias is available elsewhere (206,207). Briefly, an electrode-catheter is introduced into a peripheral blood vessel and is guided into a cardiac chamber in which it detects abnormal patterns of electric activity. After these sites have been identified, the catheter is positioned such that thermal energy is transferred from the catheter tip through the target tissue to a pad electrode applied to the surface of the body. The resistance of the tissue to the electric current causes tissue desiccation and coagulation. Direct current (DC) ablation has been largely supplanted by radiofrequency ablation, which is widely used to target accessory pathways, the AV nodal junction, and AV node. Radiofrequency ablation is, however, a relatively new technique, and the risk factors associated with the procedures and the late postoperative sequelae are only gradually emerging.

Much of the literature discussing successes and failures of radiofrequency ablation emphasizes the recurrence of conduction disturbances after radiofrequency ablation for WPW syndrome, Mahaim fibers (i.e., nodoventricular fibers), or other preexcitation syndromes (208–217). The incidence of recurring arrhythmias after ablation has been estimated to be as much as 12% (218), with the condition often returning in less than 24 hours. In most instances, recurrent conduction along a previously ablated pathway manifests within 2 months (210), and a second ablation session usually succeeds in permanently interrupting the recalcitrant bypass tract. One study reported that initial recurrence of aberrant conduction within 24 hours of ablation may cease spontaneously over ensuing weeks (219).

Investigators in major electrophysiology and pacing centers have attempted to pinpoint issues that may account for or contribute to failed interruption of an accessory pathway (186,201,208,210,218–222). In general, postablation arrhythmias appear to be more common in younger patients, in patients with multiple accessory pathways, or in patients whose initial ablation session is particularly long and complex (218). Right free wall and septal pathways fall into this category and carry a higher risk of postablation recurrence (210,218). Langberg and coworkers (218) reported that 14 patients of 200 receiving radiofrequency ablation for an accessory pathway experienced conduction recurrence along the accessory pathway. They also noticed a trend, substantiating a previous claim by Twidale and colleagues (210), of increased conduction recurrence along an accessory pathway in regions where the ablation electrode failed to record accessory pathway potentials during the initial catheter probing. Other investigators have corroborated this finding (208). A second predictor of recurrent accessory pathway conduction appears to be an absence of recorded antegrade conduction (208,210).

Langberg and associates (218) proposed that the disproportionately higher incidence of recurrence in right-sided and septal pathways may in part be caused by the specific positioning of the catheter as dictated by the ablation site. Because left-sided accessory pathways are often ablated by "wedging" the catheter tip between the mitral valve annulus and the left ventricle, the radiofrequency current can be delivered with a high degree of stability and accuracy. In contrast, catheters placed against the tricuspid annulus cannot achieve the same contact pressure and stability because of endocardial shifting caused by normal cardiac or respiratory motion (218).

Chugh and colleagues (223) provide evidence to suggest that the orientation of the catheter tip affects lesion size. These researchers compared the influence of electrode length on lesion size under conditions of parallel tip-tissue orientation or perpendicular orientation as determined by biplane fluoroscopy and intracardiac electrocardiography in 20 closed-chested dogs. They discovered that lesion size increased with increasing electrode length when the catheter tip was parallel to the endocardial surface.

Laohaprasitiporn and colleagues (224) investigated whether permanence of radiofrequency ablation correlates with successful ablation of the optimal target site identified on the electrogram. They retrospectively compared 42 transiently successful radiofrequency applications with 49 permanently successful radiofrequency applications in 58 patients. They correlated the time to success of interrupting accessory pathway conduction with permanence of successful radiofrequency ablation during temperature-controlled radiofrequency ablation. In particular, "time to interruption of accessory pathway conduction less than 2.3 seconds after the onset of radiofrequency application was predictive of the permanence of successful radiofrequency applications" (224). The investigators speculated that a shorter time to success of ablation indicates proximity of the catheter tip and the accessory pathway. In light of these findings, the researchers favor termination of radiofrequency application if accessory pathway conduction is not rapidly interrupted.

Several research papers have focussed on electrode temperature and tissue heating in relation to recurrent conduction (218,225,226). Several groups have proposed that lower electrode temperatures may result in insufficient or transient interruption of conduction along an aberrant pathway. The intensity of heat at the point of application diminishes after the temperature at the electrode reaches 100°C because of the formation of an adherent coagulum. The coagulum resists electrical conduction, preventing the formation of large, deep ablation lesions. Delacretaz and coworkers (227) investigated the impact of reducing the electrode tip temperature by irrigation with saline during current application on the ablation lesion size and depth. They demonstrated that saline irrigation generated moderately large lesions that penetrated deep into fibrotic myocardium in two patients who underwent catheter ablation before heart transplantation. The investigators speculated that saline irrigation may optimize catheter ablation of ventricular reentrant circuits in regions of infarction. Similarly, Jais and colleagues (228) demonstrated bidirectional isthmus block in 12 patients who previously underwent unsuccessful conventional radiofrequency ablation for common atrial flutter using an irrigated-tip catheter and temperature-controlled radiofrequency energy delivery. In particular, 13 of 170 patients showed signs of recurrent, resistant atrial flutter after conventional radiofrequency ablation. The researchers speculated that tip irrigation permits higher catheter tip temperatures and tissue temperatures.

Strickberger and associates (229) investigated the clinical utility of higher temperatures to ablate the slow pathway responsible for AVNRT. Temperatures between 48°C and 50°C are commonly used to ablate the slow pathway associated with AVNRT, and temperatures on the order of 60°C are used to ablate accessory pathways and atrioventricular conduction (230–232). They demonstrated a 76% primary success rate in patients randomized to undergo 48°C slow pathway ablation for AVNRT and a 100% primary success rate in patients randomized to undergo 60°C ablation. However, 24.6% of the 48°C patients experienced ventriculoatrial block, compared with 37.2% of the 60°C patients. The investigators argued that higher temperatures should be used to treat AVNRT provided there is close monitoring of ventriculoatrial conduction, because they failed to detect a significant increase in the incidence of atrioventricular block with higher temperatures. At 9.9 ± 4.2 months follow-up, only one 48°C patient experienced recurrence of AVNRT.

A study by Langberg and associates (218) found no difference in electrode temperatures at successful ablation sites compared with sites of recurrent conduction. They suggested, however, that imprecise positioning of the catheter for a particular pathway or an ablation target located in a middle myocardial or epicardial region can lead to inaccurate assumptions about the exact temperature reaching the intended lesion site. Tissue temperature drops significantly with increased distance from the exact point of electrode contact, and the correlation between a higher recurrence of conduction and specific accessory pathway locations may be linked to inadequate heating of the intended target. Greater accuracy in accessing or pinpointing anomalous conduction locales will stem from increasing understanding of conduction system anatomy and ongoing refinements to ablation technology.

Equally important to electrophysiologists is the issue of catheter-induced mechanical trauma and the impact of the catheter itself and the lesions it induces on future electrical and hemodynamic activity. Most investigators agree that arrhythmias after ablation usually result from an unsuccessful first ablation attempt and are not caused by the procedure. Lev and Bharati (233), however, postulated that inflammatory changes resulting from radiofrequency ablation might provide a "nidus" for future arrhythmic events. Others have suggested that small, homogenous, catheter-induced lesions in the adjacent myocardium may lead to late contractility and conduction disturbances (201). The possibility that other forms of catheter-induced damage could form the substrate for conduction disturbances has not been comprehensively explored. Chiang and colleagues (234), in a review of 666 patients, documented 17 with catheter-induced mechanical trauma. They suggested that the traumatized tissues might be temporarily or permanently damaged by the electrode tip or shaft; revival of traumatized tissues may account for the recurrence of conduction along an accessory pathway. King and colleagues (235) reviewed the incidence of AV nodal block (AVNB) caused by catheter positioning in 613 patients undergoing radiofrequency ablation for AVNRT or AVRT. They reported that AVNB due to mechanical trauma occurred in 10 patients (1.6%) during positioning of a stiff, large-tipped, steerable catheter in the junctional area, but in all cases, it resolved after repositioning of the catheter. Mechanical trauma, coronary artery blockage, myocardial perforation, pericardial bleeding, and thromboembolism have resulted from radiofrequency ablation catheters (201,202,234,236–238); however, these complications are uncommon.

Friedman and coworkers (239) addressed the effects of radiofrequency ablation on the autonomic nervous system. They proposed that transient atrioventricular block and sinus bradycardia during application of radiofrequency current and inappropriate sinus tachycardia after ablation for AV node modification or an accessory pathway may result from a loss of parasympathetic influence on the sinoatrial node. Previous reports (240,241) addressing this issue also support the claims put forward by Friedman's group. Denervation of the ventricular myocardium has not yet been reported; however, as the researchers suggested (239), newer, more powerful ablation techniques, including saline-irrigated ablation and cryoablation capable of producing transmural ventricular lesions may lead to denervation supersensitivity and arrhythmogenesis. Schmitt and colleagues (242) provided evidence to suggest that radiofrequency ablation does not hinder sympathetic innervation of the heart. They failed to detect abnormalities in the uptake of the catecholamine analog carbon-11-hydroxyephedrine by sympathetic nerve terminals as determined by positron emission tomography after radiofrequency ablation in nine patients with supraventricular tachycardia. In light of these results, they concluded that radiofrequency ablation does not compromise sympathetic function or cardiac innervation.

Conventional radiofrequency ablation fails when an epicardial site serves as the origin of a conduction disturbance, as is the case with some ventricular tachycardias. Fourteen percent of ventricular tachycardias in patients with chronic myocardial infarction are characterized by a reentrant circuit located in the subepicardial layer (243). Endocardial pulses of radiofrequency energy often fail to effectively destroy epicardial tissue because the temperature of the distant epicardial tissue rarely reaches effective temperatures. Sosa and colleagues (244) investigated the utility of a transthoracic technique to perform epicardial catheter ablation and mapping. These investigators were the first to demonstrate the effective and safe application of radiofrequency energy without the need for thoracotomy in six patients with ventricular tachycardia or Chagas' disease. Similarly, Watanabe and associates (245) created grossly well-demarcated radiofrequency lesions on the epicardial surface of five mongrel dog hearts using a new ablation probe for thoracoscopic surgery. They introduced a thoracoscope through the 7th intercostal space and effectively delivered radiofrequency energy on the nonvascular ventricular wall of canine beating hearts.

Calkins and coworkers (246) investigated the safety and efficacy of radiofrequency catheter ablation in 1,050 patients (adults and children) who underwent ablation of AVNRT, an accessory pathway, or the atrioventricular junction. Ablation was successful in 996 patients. The success rate was greatest in patients who underwent ablation of the atrioventricular junction, lowest in instances of ablation of an accessory pathway, and in-between in instances of ablation of the atrioventricular junction. Left free wall accessory pathway, atrioventricular junction, or AVNRT ablation and experience of a particular center predicted ablation success, whereas right free wall, posteroseptal, septal, and multiple accessory pathways predicted arrhythmia recurrence. These results can be explained on the basis of the "target-dependent differences in the effectiveness of tissue heating" (246). Structural heart disease and the presence of multiple targets predicted the development of complications, whereas lower ejection fraction and atrioventricular junction ablation predicted an increased risk of death. Complete atrioventricular block was the most common complication and is an important risk to consider when ablating areas along the septal aspect of the tricuspid valve. Moreover, the requirement for ablation of multiple targets results in longer procedure times and an increased risk of error.

Ebstein's Anomaly

In Ebstein's anomaly, the septal and posterior (inferior) tricuspid valve leaflets are displaced caudally, with the point of maximum displacement located in the commissure between the two leaflets found at the posterior border of the ventricular septum. The anterior leaflet is usually enlarged and attaches posteroinferiorly to the bridge between the trabecular and inlet portions of the right ventricle. The orifice of the valve is displaced apically into the right ventricle near the junction of the inlet and trabecular regions. In congenitally corrected transposition of the great arteries (CCTGA), Ebstein's anomaly can affect the left atrioventricular valve (essentially, the displaced tricuspid valve). Dilatation of the right atrium and enlargement of the right atrioventricular junction results in a prominent eustachian valve.

The downward displacement of the valve effectively divides the ventricle into an atrialized posterior ventricle that acts as an inlet and the trabecular and outlet portions that operate as the functional ventricle. Additional congenital abnormalities commonly associated with Ebstein's anomaly of the tricuspid valve include atrial septal defect (ASD), patent foramen ovale, right atrial enlargement, and myocardial abnormalities.

Preexcitation is common in patients with Ebstein's anomaly and is usually caused by the existence of one or more accessory pathways. One study claims that as many as 15% of patients with Ebstein's anomaly experience supraventricular tachycardia, which is most frequently associated with WPW syndrome (247,248). Enhanced AV nodal conduction and dual AV nodal physiology have also been reported (249).

Cappato and colleagues (250) explored the role of radiofrequency catheter ablation for accessory pathways associated with Ebstein's anomaly. They observed that the abnormal morphology, including the atrialized right ventricle and associated conduction irregularities, complicate electrophysiologic mapping and ablation. The higher incidence of failed accessory pathway ablation probably is caused by the structural complexity of the disease. Reich and associates (251) described the radiofrequency ablation success in 65 Ebstein's anomaly patients with 82 typical accessory pathways, 17 other supraventricular tachycardias, and 1 ventricular arrhythmia. Of the patients with an accessory pathway, 34 had a single accessory pathway, 9 had multiple accessory pathways, 6 had a single accessory pathway plus a nonaccessory pathway mechanism, and 6 had nonaccessory pathway mechanisms. Reich and coworkers (251) also demonstrated that body surface area less than 1.7 m^2 and a mild degree of tricuspid regurgitation independently predicted acute success of radiofrequency ablation in 65 pediatric patients with Ebstein's anomaly, whereas body surface area less than 1.7 m^2 predicted long-term success. They further explained that proper catheter placement is difficult during radiofrequency ablation in these patients because of the large right atrium, downward displacement of the tricuspid valve, and presence of multiple accessory pathways. The researchers speculated that a smaller right atrium inferred from a smaller body surface area positively influences the success rate. In light of these unusual anatomic and structural considerations, catheter approach by way of the superior or inferior vena cava and the hepatic vein appears to improve results (252). In contrast to other studies, they also demonstrated that the location of the pathway, the presence of associated congenital heart disease, the presence of multiple pathways, and the operator's experience did not influence the long-term or short-term success rate.

Septal Defects

Malformations involving the atrioventricular septal junction fall into the category of ASDs. These defects include isolated ASDs, which are in some way characterized by an opening between the left and right atria, and atrioventricular canal defects (or endocardial cushion defects), which result from incomplete embryologic partitioning of the atrioventricular canal. The most common arrhythmias associated with unoperated ASDs are atrial fibrillation and flutter, although supraventricular tachycardia has also been reported (253–256). Incomplete development of the endocardial primordia is suspected to be the cause of most electrophysiologically problematic ASDs; most involve incomplete or abnormal development of the lower portion of the atrial septum, the inflow portion of the ventricular septum, or the atrioventricular valves. The two principal ASDs of relevance to this discussion are ostium primum defects (i.e., partial atrioventricular canal) and complete ASDs (i.e., common orifice or common atrioventricular canal). The former refers to a septal malformation that extends to the atrioventricular valves and normally involves a cleft mitral valve with leaflets that are fused to a deficient ventricular septum, preventing communication at that level. The latter type arises from a lack of fusion between the anterior and posterior leaflets on the septal crest, resulting in failed differentiation of the primitive canal into two discrete atrioventricular apertures. The AV node can be hypoplastic or displaced as a result of a deficient atrial septum. Backward displacement of the compact node and associated tissues can result in early posterior activation. VSDs may be as common as ASDs but do not carry the same potential for arrhythmogenesis. Of 188 adults between the ages of 17 and 72 years with small, nonsurgically repaired VSDs, 8.5% exhibited age-related symptomatic arrhythmias, with atrial fibrillation being the most common arrhythmia observed (257).

Postoperative arrhythmias after ASD repair can occur immediately after surgery or late postoperatively and vary depending on the age of the patient. In children, junctional escape rhythms, atrioventricular dissociation, and ectopic atrial rhythm (i.e., sick sinus syndrome) are common in the early postoperative period, whereas adults typically present with atrial flutter. Late postoperatively, tachyarrhythmias are reasonably common in adults and children. Atrioventricular block has occasionally been observed in adults early and late postoperatively. The most common conduction system disturbance seen after repair of an atrioventricular septal defect is right bundle branch block. AV node and His-Purkinje conduction delays are also common soon after surgery. Up to one third of all patients undergoing repair of an ASD experience complete heart block. Surgery for VSDs in the region of the membranous septum frequently results in right bundle branch block, with past reports citing an incidence of up to 100% (258–261). Ventricular tachycardia, atrial flutter, atrial fibrillation, paroxysmal supraventricular tachycardia, and junctional tachycardia have also been reported (262–264).

Tetralogy of Fallot

An anterior malalignment of the infundibular septum is responsible for the four coexistent congenital malformations that comprise the TOF: VSD, infundibular pulmonary stenosis, overriding of the ventricular septum by the aortic valve, and right ventricular hypertrophy (265). The VSD in TOF can be an infundibular perimembranous defect or infundibular muscular type. The former is more common. Depending on the nature of the septal defect, the conduction system is normally unaffected, although right bundle branch block has been reported. Postoperatively, however, repaired TOF can be associated with a number of conduction disturbances, including right bundle branch block, sinoatrial node dysfunction, ventricular arrhythmias, and complete heart block (266–274).

Hemorrhage, necrosis, and inflammatory changes resulting from surgery are believed to be responsible for most conduction problems in patients undergoing surgical repair (259); however, the multifactoral nature of the malformation and the surgical steps required for its repair make it difficult to pinpoint the precise conditions responsible for arrhythmogenesis. As Ross (269) pointed out, no classification system exists for determining the severity of a given malformation or for cataloging the anatomic variability that exists between patients. Nevertheless, a growing number of clinical reports and experimental models have identified issues that appear to be important. For example, several studies have indicated that age at the time of surgery is an important factor in determining the risk of sudden death, although the cause of death is a subject of ongoing debate. Postoperative sudden death of children and adolescents may be caused by heart block (275,276) or ventricular arrhythmias and tachyarrhythmias (273,275–280). A study of adults (≥18 years) with previous corrective surgery suggested that conduction defects and rhythm disturbances were rare, potentially because of careful monitoring and correction of hemodynamic changes after surgery. Several investigators have proposed that ventricular arrhythmias are more prevalent in patients who undergo repair later as adolescents or young adults (268,274,277,281–283).

Sudden death occurring late after repair of TOF is most often attributed to a fatal ventricular arrhythmias (274). However, the prevalence of sustained ventricular tachycardia in patients with previous repair of TOF is low (284). Harrison and colleagues (284) sought to identify risk factors for ventricular arrhythmia in these patients by investigating the features associated with ventricular tachycardia in adult patients late after repair of TOF. They identified 18 patients with monomorphic ventricular tachycardia among 254 patients with long-standing repair of TOF. Most of the patients with monoform ventricular tachycardia exhibited outflow tract aneurysms or pulmonary regurgitation. The occurrence of ventricular ectopic beats in these patients compared with 192 arrhythmia-free patients after previous repair of TOF is higher. Based on this finding, the researchers proposed that pulmonary valve replacement, right ventricular aneurysmectomy, or both procedures in conjunction with ablation may lead to better arrhythmia management. Similarly, Gunal and associates (285) found a high prevalence of ventricular and supraventricular arrhythmias in 31 patients who underwent repair of TOF 1 month to 14 years before the investigation. In particular, 51% of the patients showed various degrees of ventricular arrhythmias, and 39% showed supraventricular arrhythmias. In light of these findings, the investigators recommended ambulatory monitoring of ventricular and supraventricular arrhythmias in patients who have undergone correction of TOF.

Different surgical approaches are thought to carry different degrees of arrhythmic risk. Dietl and co-workers (266) reported that the incidence of postoperative ventricular arrhythmias in adults was significantly higher when a right ventricular approach was used and lower with a right atrial procedure. In particular, their study and others (275,277,279,280) indicate that scarring in the right ventricle may serve as the site of origin for a reentrant mechanism resulting in ventricular tachycardia or may affect normal contractility and function of the right ventricle. Additional studies have qualitatively assessed aspects of different repair procedures and have highlighted issues that may increase the risk of postoperative arrhythmias or hemodynamics (271,286,287).

Univentricular Hearts

"Univentricular" hearts, lacking a ventricular septum between the right and left ventricular inlet structures, are categorized as left and right according to the morphologic orientation of the single, operative ventricle. Hearts with a single, morphologically right ventricle and rudimentary left ventricular chamber normally do not suffer from conduction disturbances, because the His bundle and node are able to develop normally. In single left ventricular hearts, however, the posterior AV node is typically hypoplastic and detached from the ventricular musculature. An anterior atrioventricular pathway forms in lieu of the His bundle, which would ordinarily connect with the posterior AV node. Prolonged PR interval, potentially culminating in complete heart block, is observed in left-sided univentricular hearts with a rudimentary right-sided chamber. The Fontan operation and modified versions thereof "permit direct communication between systemic venous return and the pulmonary arteries in the absence of a functional pulmonary arterial ventricle" (162). Postoperative atrial arrhythmias are commonly found in these patients as demonstrated by Driscoll and colleagues (288). They reported that 20% of patients ($n = 352$) who underwent this operation at the Mayo Clinic required antiarrhythmic drugs, pacemaker implantation, or both at 5 to 15 years of follow-up. Gelatt and associates (289) and Paul and coworkers (290) showed that the incidence of atrial arrhythmia is higher for those patients undergoing direct atriopulmonary connection than patients undergoing total cavopulmonary connections or connection of the right atrium to the right ventricle.

Transposition of the Great Arteries

Congenitally corrected transposition of the great arteries (CCTGA) embodies a physiologic "correction" of a malalignment of the atrial and ventricular septa. The morphologic left ventricle is situated on the right and *vice versa,* and the L-transposed aorta connects to the morphologic right ventricle on the left side, and the pulmonary trunk connects to the left ventricle on the right side. In CCTGA, the AV node is separated from the inlet septum, usually as a result of an expansive membranous septum or a VSD. Typically, a second atrioventricular bundle forms, descending anteriorly to reach the trabecular septum. This nonbranching bundle from the anomalous AV node can become fibrotic with aging, leading to atrioventricular block. Additional accessory pathways are often associated with CCTGA and can lead to preexcitation syndromes. Additional conduction disturbances have been reported, including premature atrial depolarization, junctional escape rhythms, sinoatrial block, and sinus bradycardia.

A procedure aimed at rechanneling the pulmonary and systemic venous drainage in hearts with complete transposition of the great arteries was developed by Mustard (291) in 1964. The Mustard operation involves a right atriotomy, an atrial septectomy, and placement of a pant-legs–shaped patch (162). The Senning operation involves a "right atriotomy, a left atriotomy just rightward of the right pulmonary veins, and mobilization of the atrial septum to create a systemic venous tube directing both caval returns to the mitral valve" (162). This operation differs from the Mustard operation in the use of native cardiac tissue. The Mustard operation is associated with a general deterioration of normal sinus rhythm and an increased incidence of sick sinoatrial node syndrome based on inferred damage to the sinoatrial node or its blood supply. Similar features have been observed in patients after the Senning operation.

After undergoing decades of modification, the preferred method for reconstructing a heart with complete TGA is an arterial switch operation (292). Although postsurgical arrhythmias are still reported, refinement of surgical techniques has greatly reduced the number of postoperative conduction disturbances (259). Physiologic alterations implicated in arrhythmogenesis after surgery include intraoperative damage to the sinoatrial node, sinoatrial node artery, or AV nodal tissue. Supraventricular arrhythmias, such as premature atrial complexes, atrial flutter, atrial fibrillation, ectopic atrial rhythms, slow junctional rhythms, junctional ectopic tachycardia, sick sinus syndrome, and less commonly, atrioventricular block, have been reported (259,293,294) after atrial switch operations.

Treatment of Arrhythmias Developing after Surgery for Congenital Heart Disease

After surgery for complex congenital heart disease, patients are at high risk for developing atrial arrhythmias if prominent regions of conduction block occur within the atria. For instance, many patients require placement of an atrial pacing system after the Mustard, Senning, or Fontan operations for reasons related to sinus bradycardia. Likewise, antitachycardia pacing and medical therapy are most often used to treat patients who develop atrial tachyarrhythmias after these operations. Medical therapy for atrial reentry tachycardia and atrial flutter has low efficacy, as demonstrated by Garson and colleagues (295), but it is still standard practice. These researchers demonstrated a 38% success rate for medical therapy, with amiodarone exhibiting the highest efficacy (78%). Alternatively, radiofrequency ablation is being used to treat atrial flutter and atrial reentry tachycardia after congenital heart surgery based on its success in animal models. For instance, Triedman and colleagues (296) showed that ablation of the region located in the isthmus between the inferior vena cava and tricuspid annulus or in the high medial right atrium near the superior vena cava orifice in patients after the Fontan operation eliminated the critical zones of slow or protected conduction. They demonstrated clinical improvement in 7 of 10 children undergoing radiofrequency ablation for reentrant circuits after the Fontan-type operation. Similarly, Van Hare and associates (297) reported successful ablation of reentrant circuits in 10 patients after the Mustard or Senning operations. Kanter and Garson (162) propose that surgical incisions made at the time of surgery for congenital defects may protect against ensuing arrhythmias.

Management of Patients with Congenital Heart Disease and Accessory Pathways

Of the pediatric patients reported to the Pediatric Radiofrequency Ablation Registry, 10% have associated congenital heart disease (298). When treating patients with congenital heart disease and coexisting accessory pathways, the electrophysiologist and pediatric cardiologist can choose from a variety of management options. Nonpharmacologic therapies appear to be the accepted form of therapy based on the risk of proarrhythmias and hemodynamic concerns such as poor cardiac output in patients with congenital heart disease. The question then becomes whether to ablate the pathway before surgery, during surgery, or not at all. In most instances, ablation is required based on the risk of activating an otherwise dormant supraventricular tachycardia after surgery. Van Hare (299) reviewed technical factors such as venous and arterial access, visceral situs, location of the atrioventricular conduction structures, and defect-specific factors to consider before ablating accessory pathways in patients with associated congenital heart disease.

● EMERGING ISSUES IN CONDUCTION SYSTEM MORPHOLOGY

Slow and Fast Pathways of the Atrioventricular Node: Implications for the Treatment of Atrioventricular Node Reentry Tachycardia

The observations by Scherf and Shookhoff in 1926 of "returning" atrial impulses in animal models has fueled more than seven decades of research into the reentrant tachycardias of the AV nodal region. The concept of "dual" nodal pathways within the atrioventricular junction, explored by Moe and colleagues throughout the 1950s and 1960s, has grown increasingly complex. During the ensuing years, investigators put forth the concept of a functional dissociation of the AV node into slow and fast pathways. These pathways form the basis for AVNRT, with one pathway acting as the retrograde reentry route for conduction impulses to reactivate the atria. In the most common form of AVNRT, anterograde conduction occurs over the "slow" AV nodal pathway, and the "fast" pathway provides the route for retrograde conduction. This form is generally referred to as slow/fast AVNRT. Less common is fast/slow AVNRT, in which antegrade conduction occurs over the fast pathway with the retrograde return by the slow pathway. A third, rare form of AVNRT involves two slow pathways, one of which provides the antegrade route and the other the retrograde route. Several groups (300,301) have proposed that AVNRT involves multiple intranodal and perinodal tissues that operate as functional slow and fast routes. Anselme and coworkers (302) showed the presence of a lower common pathway within the AV node during AVNRT. This pathway, they argue, resides between the reentrant circuit and the His bundle.

The application of intracardiac mapping and catheter ablation techniques in the diagnosis and treatment of AVNRT (the latter through AV node modification) has permitted electrophysiologists to gain a clearer understanding of reentry circuits and potential "routes" for slow and fast, anterograde and retrograde conduction. The anatomic delimitations of the reentrant circuits, however, continue to be a major point of contention in AVNRT research and patient care. The perinodal atrium, compact AV node, and proximal His bundle may be involved electrophysiologically.

For several years, investigators have debated whether functional dissociation of the AV nodal conduction into fast and slow pathways has any anatomic correlate (303–306). The possibility that reentry circuits involve tissues outside of the compact node has been explored by a number of groups and continues to be a major research focus. Kadish and Goldberger (303) argue that the approaches to the AV node, identified as being part of reentry circuits, are anatomically distinct with different conduction system components. Several investigators have suggested that the functional fast and slow pathways may be located anatomically within the differentiated tissues of the transitional zone surrounding the compact node, with the superficial transitional cells forming part of the fast pathway and the posterior zone constituting part of the slow pathway (305,307). Success of ablation sessions that have targeted the approach to the AV node seems to uphold these claims (308–311). An earlier study (312) reported that patients with dual AV nodal conduction demonstrated distinct atrial insertion points for slow and fast pathways during retrograde conduction. Using intracardiac mapping, Sung and colleagues (312) located the retrograde atrial exit of the fast AV node pathway at the low septal region of the right atrium near the His bundle recording site. The retrograde atrial exit of the slow AV node pathway was localized in or near the coronary sinus ostium, inferior and posterior to the exit of the fast AV node pathway (Fig. 1-13). A broad tissue region is postulated to be the upper point of connection between the fast and slow pathways (312). Tondo and associates (313) also explored the atrial component of the AV nodal reentrant circuit, focusing primarily on the coronary sinus as an ablation target. They reported that the atrial muscle within the coronary sinus or adjacent myocardium might form part of the reentry route in certain patients (313). Additional reports have corroborated these observations (314,315). Likewise, observations that reentrant tachycardias of the atrioventricular region can persist despite a 2:1 conduction block superior to the His bundle (316–318) support the hypothesis that the "lower turnaround point" where the two pathways converge may be located within or close to the His bundle. Patterson and Scherlag (319) demonstrated experimentally longitudinal dissociation of the posterior input of the AV node (i.e., slow pathway) at slow heart rates and their involvement in the initiation of AVNRT. Decreases in the atrial cycle of superfused rabbit atrioventricular junction caused circus movement within the transitional cells located in the region separating the two dissociated pathways.

Yamane and coworkers (320) investigated the optimal target site for slow atrioventricular nodal path-

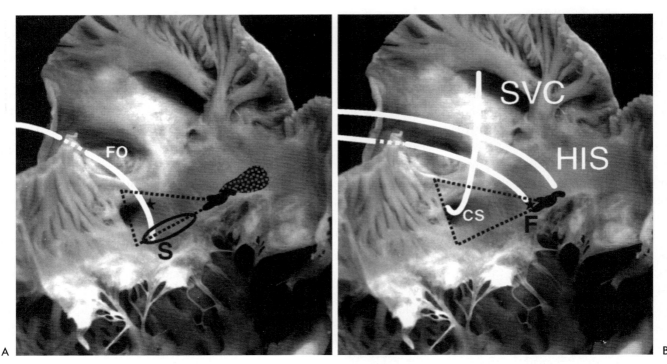

FIGURE 1-13. Views of the opened right atrium and right ventricle in which the slow **(A)** and fast **(B)** pathways for atrioventricular reentrant tachycardia are depicted as sites for possible ablation. **A:** The oblong region for the slow (S) pathway may be a site for ablation, as well as at the anterior margin of the coronary sinus *(star)*. Koch's triangle is outlined with the atrioventricular node adjacent to the septal leaflet of the tricuspid valve and inferoposterior to the membranous septum *(shaded region)*. The fossa ovale (FO) is also denoted. **B:** With the same photograph, representation is provided of an ablation catheter for the fast (F) pathway *(star)*, a His recording catheter, and a catheter in the ostium of the coronary sinus (CS). The coronary sinus catheter enters through the superior vena cava (SVC). The atrioventricular node is represented with a short posterior leftward extension and a longer rightward extension. (From McManus BM. In: Singer I, Barold SS, Camm AJ, eds. *Nonpharmacological therapy of arrhythmias for the 21st century: the state of the art.* Armonk, NY: Futura Publishing, 1998, with permission.)

way ablation in the treatment of AVNRT. Ablation of the slow pathway has been difficult because of variations in the size and shape of Koch's triangle, the major landmark used. Until recently, the site of radiofrequency ablation was determined by an extensive electrogram-guided mapping method that started at the bottom of Koch's triangle and progressed toward the middle part of the triangle until the AVNRT was eliminated. These investigators compared the success of radiofrequency ablation in a group of 60 patients undergoing this form of treatment with that in a group of 59 patients who underwent a predetermined focal mapping method. A restricted area around the upper margin of the coronary sinus ostium was mapped and ablated, and coronary sinus venography was subsequently performed to determine the location of the successful ablation site. They discovered that patients undergoing this new method required fewer radiofrequency applications and a lower level of energy for successful ablation. Success rates for the groups did not differ. The successful ablation site with this new method was localized in the area within 5 mm above and below the level of the upper margin of the coronary sinus ostium along the tricuspid annulus. The investigators further speculated that the rightward posterior extensions of the atrioventricular node documented by Inoue and Becker (4) may serve as the substrate for arrhythmias in the target site.

A reentrant circuit comprising of the slow and fast nodal pathway is responsible for AVNRT in 15% of children with supraventricular tachycardia (321,322). Radiofrequency ablation has not been widely used to treat children with supraventricular tachycardias because of the high risk of damaging the AV node while trying to ablate the slow pathway. By knowing the dimensions of Koch's triangle, the length of the tricuspid annulus segment along which current can be applied without damaging the AV node can be calculated. Until recently, the dimensions of Koch's triangle in young patients was unknown. Francalanci and colleagues (323) showed that the cathetus of Koch's triangle is about one half of the tricuspid valve diameter in young patients (average age, 3 months; range, 1 day to 14 years; $n = 69$). With this relationship in mind and knowing the diameter of the tricuspid valve, the investigators believe it is possible to calculate where the slow pathway and Koch's triangle reside along the tricuspid annulus. However, Goldberg and associates (324) demonstrated that the dimensions of Koch's triangle in children varies directly with the patient's weight, height, body surface area, age, and heart weight. They showed that the length of Koch's triangle may be shorter than the diameter of lesions (5 to 7 mm) produced by a standard 4-mm tip of an radiofrequency ablation catheter in children smaller than 0.6 m^2 or 15 kg. In light of their findings, these investigators strongly discourage catheter ablation in the area of Koch's triangle in these children. The dimensions of Koch's triangle do not correlate with body surface area in adults (325).

Radiofrequency Catheter Ablation for Atrial Fibrillation and Atrial Flutter

Surgical strategies for atrial fibrillation, including the corridor and MAZE procedures, revolve around the creation of nonconductive boundaries that prevent reentry of wavelet circulation by anatomically limiting the contiguous tissue area required by reentrant circuits. The MAZE procedure, having undergone several refinements, affords high success rates and long-term cure. For instance, the MAZE III procedure involves "creating atriotomies that block potential reentrant circuits" and may be the best surgical method for the treatment of medically refractory atrial fibrillation (326,327). Lee and coworkers (327) created the lesions of the MAZE III without the support of cardiopulmonary bypass using a tunnel technique in a canine model. The procedure restores the synchrony of the atria and ventricles and reestablishes sinoatrial node control of ventricular rate by serial partitioning of both atria. Antz and colleagues (328) confirmed the existence of electrical conduction between the right and left atria by the musculature of the coronary sinus and further speculated that this pathway plays an important role in the propagation of impulses during sustained atrial fibrillation. They stressed the importance of severing this connection in the surgical MAZE procedure. The major shortcomings of the MAZE procedure as an open heart surgery are its cost and associated risks. A review of common surgical strategies used to treat atrial fibrillation is available elsewhere (329).

Attempts to design catheter-based methods to achieve the same linear, nonconductive barriers to intraatrial reentry are being explored. However, catheter ablation is restricted to the right atrium because of the high risk of thromboembolism associated with extensive lesions in the left atrium (330). Zhou and associates (331) determined the incidence of thromboembolic complications in radiofrequency catheter ablation to be as high as 0.6%. The incidence rises when radiofrequency catheter ablation is performed in the left atrium (1.8%) and rises even further in the context of ventricular tachycardia (2.8%). However, Kottkamp and coworkers (332) demonstrated the successful ablation of left atrial "anchor" reentrant circuits in 12 patients with chronic atrial fibrillation. They created radiofrequency lesions between the "mitral annulus and the left lower pulmonary vein, further to the left upper pulmonary vein, from there to the right upper pulmonary vein, and finally to the right lower pulmonary vein" using a right atrial-transeptal approach (332). At 11 months follow-up, chronic atrial fibrillation was successfully ablated in 9 of the 11 patients; 1 patient died postoperatively.

Avitall and colleagues (333) reported successful interruption of atrial fibrillation in dogs using radiofrequency-induced lesions to "compartmentalize" the right atrium. Likewise, Haissaguerre and associates (220) reported successful ablation of atrial fibrillation through the creation of serial, vertical lesions along the posterior wall of the right atrium; a second series along the lateral wall of the right atrium; and a third series along the anterior wall of the right atrium. It is generally agreed that the atria as a whole participate in the perpetuation of atrial fibrillation, but Konings and coworkers (334) found that not all atrial regions participate equally. Kumagai and colleagues (335) showed in dogs that a reentrant circuit localized to the septum may represent the principal participant in the propagation of atrial fibrillation. Similarly, Gaita and associates (336) demonstrated that radiofrequency application predominantly in the septal region was more frequently successful in patients who exhibited an irregular activation pattern in the septal region as determined by right atrial mapping. Likewise, radiofrequency application in the septal region failed in those patients who exhibited similar irregular activation patterns in the lateral and septal region. Baker and coworkers (337) have reviewed nonpharmacologic approaches used in the management of atrial arrhythmias and newer avenues of therapy being explored.

Despite advances, atrial fibrillation is the only remaining supraventricular tachycardia not completely curable by catheter ablation, most likely because atrial fibrillation typically involves multiple, unstable reentrant wavelets rather than a single reentrant circuit as with atrial flutter. It is difficult to pinpoint the exact location of these fleeting wavelets, and their isolation by catheter ablation poses even more technical challenges. Curative procedures for atrial fibrillation and those for atrial flutter are predicated on the creation of long, linear lesions according to the widespread topography of the circuit involved. Two strategies are used to create these lesions, one of which involves dragging a standard-tip catheter during radiofrequency ablation. The other involves sequential application of radiofrequency energy through multiple, small, ring electrodes along a catheter. Both methods are time consuming, and efforts are underway to improve the efficacy of catheter ablation in the context of atrial fibrillation. Focal catheter ablation has been shown to cure atrial fibrillation in some patients. Jais and colleagues (338) reported nine patients with rare paroxysmal focal atrial fibrillation who were cured by discrete radiofrequency energy applications.

Haissaguerre and associates (339) provided evidence that discontinuous catheter lesions may be responsible for proarrhythmias seen in patients who undergo ablation for atrial fibrillation. Mitchell and coworkers (340) demonstrated that gaps less than 5 mm long may lead to conduction block during atrial pacing and atrial fibrillation, but gaps greater than 5 mm rarely produce conduction block. These researchers monitored conduction during atrial pacing and fibrillation in seven dogs that underwent discontinuous linear epicardial ablation in the right atrial free wall. Multielectrode catheters create long, linear, and continuous radiofrequency lesions in animals, but proarrhythmia after ablation using these catheters has yet to be determined (341). For instance, Roithinger and colleagues (342) demonstrated that a tip-deflectable multielectrode catheter guided by intracardiac echocardiography effectively creates long, linear, gap-free lesions in the canine left atrium. Similarly, Olgin and associates (343) demonstrated that a multielectrode catheter consisting of four coils created long, linear, continuous, and discrete lesions in six pigs as determined by histologic examination of right atrial tissue. Epicardial mapping revealed that these lesions resulted in complete conduction block across the lesions in all animals. Unfortunately, the use of multielectrode catheters requires a long procedure time. The efficacy of multielectrode catheters has been investigated in the context of atrial flutter. Anfinsen and coworkers (344) created longer radiofrequency lesions in the inferior vena cava–tricuspid valve isthmus and right atrial free wall of 16 pigs using a bipolar electrode compared with a unipolar electrode. The investigators propose increasing the distance between the two electrodes in the bipolar mode and lend credence to the efficacy of multielectrode catheters.

Mehdirad and colleagues (345) investigated the possibility of using a longer-tip electrode to create larger radiofrequency lesions in the canine tricuspid valve annulus by a dragging method to treat atrial flutter. Increasing the electrode tip length reduced the amount of dragging time and thereby the procedure time. Moreover, longer tips permitted greater tissue cooling because of the increased tip surface area and the removal of more heat by blood flowing past the application site. This resulted in a lower impedance rise, allowed higher power settings, and formed larger lesions. However, when the cooling effect is excessive, lesion size decreases dramatically. These researchers created substantially larger and deeper lesions using an 8-mm-long tip compared with a 4-mm-long tip, as determined by histologic examination of radiofrequency lesions from 10 canines. Likewise, Grumbrecht and associates (346) demonstrated that, with increasing flow velocity at the catheter tip, the tissue temperature, lesion depth, and amount of energy required to create lesions increases because of the blood cooling effect at the point of application. They further demonstrated that pulsed radiofrequency energy delivery created deeper lesions, because more total energy was delivered at comparable electrode temperatures in this mode compared with the continuous mode.

In addition to multielectrode catheters, other unconventional catheters used to create linear continuous lesions include expandable-loop catheters (347). Avitall and coworkers (347) showed that an adjustable-loop catheter could create continuous, linear, atrial lesions up to 16 cm long in 33 dogs using one of three power titration protocols and without creating perforations or causing valvular damage. They speculated that the design of the catheter permitted the creation of loops in the atria and allowed atrial tissue to be forced firmly around the catheter loop, ensuring optimal tissue contact. Treatment with this particular catheter never generated atrial fibrillation in any of the dogs, but atrial flutter was inducible in three dogs after lesion formation, suggesting reentry around an incomplete lesion.

Radiofrequency current can be used to modify atrioventricular conduction and reduce the maximum ventricular rate during atrial tachyarrhythmias while maintaining normal atrioventricular conduction (348, 349). Unfortunately, this procedure fails to generate consistent results among investigators. When the procedure results in reduced ventricular rate, investigators speculate that the procedure involves destruction of the slow pathway (350,351). However, Garrigue and colleagues (352) suggest otherwise in a study in which they surgically dissociated the AV node from its posterior approach to determine the role of slow pathway input during atrial fibrillation. They demonstrated that posteroseptal surgical cuts did not destroy slow pathway input or reduce ventricular rate in eight rabbit heart atrial–AV node preparations. However, the His bundle region remains an anatomic focus of radiofrequency ablation for atrial fibrillation associated with rapid ventricular rates.

If modification of atrioventricular conduction fails to reduce ventricular rate, patients typically undergo complete AV node destruction and permanent pacing. Catheter ablation of the atrioventricular conduction system and subsequent pacemaker implantation represent the most widely accepted form of treatment for atrial fibrillation that is refractory to medical therapy. Until recently, the outcome of this procedure had not been studied, and its effect on quality of life indices was unknown. The Ablate and Pace Trial sought to assess "the effects of catheter ablation of the atrioventricular conduction system and permanent pacemaker implantation on health-related quality of life, survival, exercise capacity, and ventricular function in 156 patients with symptomatic atrial fibrillation" (353). They demonstrated an overall improvement in quality of life in these patients, as well as improved left ventricular ejection fraction in patients with impaired left ventricular systolic function and persistent atrial fibrillation. Similarly, Marshall and associates (354) demonstrated the superiority of ablation of the AV node and pacing over medical therapy in patients with drug-refractory paroxysmal atrial fibrillation. They performed AV node ablation in 37 patients and subsequently randomized them to dual-chamber mode-switching (DDDR/MS) or single-chamber, rate responsive (VVIR) pacing. Compared with the 19 patients randomized to receive medical therapy alone, the ablate and pace group, particularly the DDDR/MS pacing group, experienced greater improvements in quality of life.

Mazgalez and coworkers (355) investigated the possibility of nonsurgically reducing the ventricular rate during atrial fibrillation through acetylcholine mediated postganglionic vagal stimulation of the AV node. They induced atrial fibrillation in 11 atrial–AV node rabbit heart preparations by random high right atrial pacing and obtained microelectrode recordings of cellular action potentials after direct injection of acetylcholine into the AV node. They demonstrated a progressive decrease in ventricular rate with progressive increases in postganglionic vagal stimulation.

These investigators demonstrated that slow and fast AV nodal pathways conduct through an acetylcholine-mediated depression of the AV node and, in so doing, maintain basal conduction to the bundle of His.

Atrial flutter differs from atrial fibrillation in involvement of a single macroreentrant circuit localized within the right atrium, as is reviewed elsewhere (356). Briefly, anatomic barriers, particularly the isthmus of atrial tissue bordered by the inferior vena cava and the tricuspid annulus, serve as the substrate for atrial flutter. In patients with atrial flutter, this region contains a zone of slow conduction and an area of unidirectional conduction block, two prerequisites for the formation of reentrant circuits. Arenal and colleagues (357) demonstrated the presence of rate-dependent transversal conduction block at the crista terminalis in patients with typical atrial flutter. Atrial flutter can be classified as counterclockwise typical atrial flutter, clockwise typical flutter, true atypical atrial flutter, or incisional reentrant atrial tachycardia (356). Lesh and associates (358) summarized many of the observations made by investigators over the past 80 years regarding the anatomic delineation of reentrant circuits implicated in atrial flutter (Fig. 1-14). They found that macroscopic anatomic regions play a key role in determining circuit boundaries. Olgin and coworkers (359) demonstrated that the entire crista terminalis and its continuation as the eustachian ridge form the posterior barrier in atrial flutter, whereas the tricuspid annulus acts as the anterior barrier (360). In a different series, Guiraudon and colleagues (361) have identified the narrow isthmus of tissue found between the inferior vena cava and the tricuspid annulus as the region of slow conduction. Shah and associates (362) demonstrated variations in the right atrial circuit of 17 patients with common atrial flutter using correlative 3-D mapping. They detected constant activation through the cavotricuspid isthmus. Likewise, Anselme and coworkers (363) further implicated the inferior vena cava–tricuspid annulus isthmus as the substrate for common atrial flutter in a study in which they followed 54 patients with atrial flutter and 29 patients with atrial flutter and fibrillation after complete bidirectional inferior vena cava–tricuspid annulus isthmus block. Of all the patients who underwent ablation, only one patient

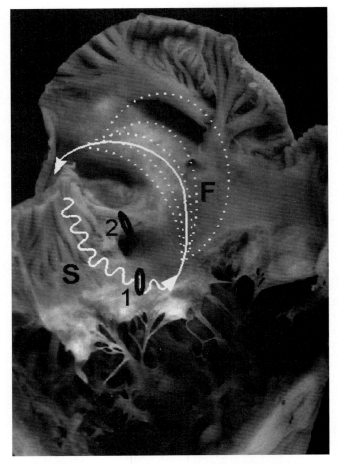

FIGURE 1-14. View of an opened right atrium and right ventricle illustrates potential routes of slow (S) and fast (F) pathways in atrial flutter. At 1 and 2, the preferred sites for successful ablation of an atrial flutter pathway are denoted. (From McManus BM. In: Singer I, Barold SS, Camm AJ, eds. *Nonpharmacological therapy of arrhythmias for the 21st century: the state of the art.* Armonk, NY: Futura Publishing, 1998, with permission.)

showed clinical signs of recurrent atrial flutter 6 months after ablation. However, a significant number of patients complained of persistent palpitations even after catheter ablation of common atrial flutter. The researchers provided evidence that these palpitations primarily resulted from atrial fibrillation, not recurrent atrial flutter, thereby underscoring the clinical benefit of catheter ablation in this region. Similarly, Shah and colleagues (364) demonstrated that recurrent atrial flutter in 18 of 21 patients who underwent previous ablation in the inferior vena cava–tricuspid annulus isthmus occurred primarily because of the presence of a single, discrete gap in the ablation line through which conduction may traverse. They further showed that these gaps can be identified on electrograms as a single or fractionated potential spanning the isoelectric interval of adjacent double potentials. These gaps can be ablated selectively without again ablating previously ablated tissue because ablated tissue exhibits a unique pattern of excitation on the electrogram that is distinct from that of the gap. Other investigators also cured atrial flutter by catheter ablation in the region of the right atrial isthmus, further implicating this region as the substrate of common atrial flutter (365,366).

Cabrera and associates (367) characterized the arrangement and orientation of the atrial myocardial fibers residing in the critical region of the right atrial isthmus. They demonstrated marked variation in the arrangement of subendocardial fibers in 28 normal hearts, as well as the presence of recesses and membranous areas in some hearts. They also discovered that the posterior sector contains predominantly fibrous tissue and the subendocardial fibers intersect at the confluence between the middle and anterior sectors in most specimens. In light of these findings, they argue that ablative lesions need not extend into the posterior region when treating patients with atrial flutter by catheter ablation. Constructing a continuous line of radiofrequency lesions between the tricuspid valve and the eustachian ridge may not be necessary.

Pathology of Ablation Lesions: Radiofrequency and Alternative Energy Sources

Our understanding of tissue destruction in radiofrequency ablation is based on a number of animal models and clinical observations (225,231,368) that indicate the injury process is thermally mediated. In one study, guinea pig papillary muscle subjected to temperatures of 45°C or higher demonstrated increased resting tension, and at temperatures of 50°C or above, they showed signs of irreversible myocardial contracture (369). One group (369) has postulated that hyperthermally mediated injury damages plasma membranes, permitting influx of extracellular sodium and calcium that results in depolarization and increased myocardial resting tension, respectively. Intracellular buffering systems are also affected by excessive heat; activity of adenosine triphosphatase in the sarcoplasmic reticulum is suppressed at temperatures in excess of 50°C (370). Nath and coworkers (371) have reviewed the biophysics of radiofrequency energy delivery, tissue effects of radiofrequency ablation, and pathology of radiofrequency lesions.

Studies of myocardial macrovasculature in animals indicate that cellular damage induced through tissue heating is linked to compromised vessel function and perfusion. Histologic examination reveals microvascular swelling and disruption, intravascular thrombosis, and neutrophil adherence to vessel walls. As recently proposed (369), early and late changes in tissue conductivity may result from recovery and reperfusion of an area after ablation, or loss of aberrant conduction in an initially resilient pathway may be a late effect of impaired vascular function. Vascular preservation appears to be greater after DC ablation than radiofrequency ablation, providing one reason for a higher incidence of conduction interruption when radiofrequency energy is employed (372).

In their comprehensive review, Nath and Haines (369) characterized the gross and pathologic features of lesions produced by radiofrequency ablation and compared the pathophysiologic effects and efficacy of alternative methods of ablation, with most work having been done in animal models. Briefly, the endocardium after radiofrequency ablation may be slightly deformed and pale, although hemorrhage is not uncommon. Charring can occur if ablation temperatures exceed 100°C or occur after a swift increase in electrical impedance (369). Early microscopic study reveals distinct, pale, necrotic lesions surrounded by hemorrhagic tissue (Fig. 1-15). After 5 days, this peripheral hemorrhaging is accompanied by inflammatory infiltrates encircling a well-differentiated nidus of coagulation necrosis. Within 2 months after ablation, lesions are considerably smaller and made up of granulation and fibrous tissue, fat cells, cartilaginous tissue, and a chronic inflammatory infiltrate (369).

Until recently, few studies described the pathology and size of radiofrequency lesions in humans. Leonelli and colleagues (373) described the pathologic changes associated with radiofrequency ablation of the tricuspid valve–inferior vena cava isthmus in a patient who

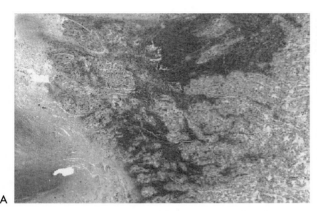 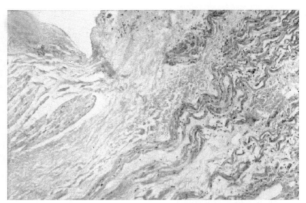

FIGURE 1-15. Photomicrographs of a region in which hemorrhage and necrosis were induced by radiofrequency ablation. **A:** There are areas of coagulative necrosis adjacent to large areas of hemorrhage *(darker staining)* (hematoxylin and eosin stain; original magnification ×25). **B:** Areas of necrosis can be highlighted using an antibody to muscle-specific actin (MSA), with which no immunoreactivity is present in injured tissue adjacent to deeply staining viable myocytes (muscle-specific actin staining; original magnification ×25). (From McManus BM. Morphological features of normal and abnormal conduction system: essentials for interventional electrophysiologists. In: Singer I, Barold SS, Camm AJ, eds. *Nonpharmacological therapy of arrhythmias for the 21st century: the state of the art.* Armonk, NY: Futura Publishing, 1998, with permission.)

underwent heart transplantation 4 months after atrial flutter ablation. They correlated conduction block across the right atrial isthmus with full-thickness fibrosis, loss of cardiomyocytes, and absence of surviving muscle in this region. They further speculated that these findings accounted for complete conduction block observed in the patient. Similarly, Vassilikos and associates (374) reported a patient with WPW syndrome who experienced recurrence of tachycardia 1 month after initially successful radiofrequency ablation. Histologic examination revealed incomplete disruption of the accessory pathway. They identified the pathway of the accessory pathway band and speculated that edematous changes at the time of radiofrequency ablation prevented conduction through the intact accessory pathway in both directions. Once healed, retrograde conduction resumed in absence of severe lesions at the atrial insertion site, whereas antegrade conduction halted because of the presence of extensive lesions at the ventricular insertion site.

Grubman and coworkers (375) described the pathologic appearance of radiofrequency lesions in three patients who died 1 day, 7 days, or 9 months after radiofrequency ablation for postinfarction ventricular tachycardia. They discovered areas of focal inflammation and fibrin deposition in recent radiofrequency lesions and multiple foci of fibrosis and granulation in older radiofrequency lesions. The oldest radiofrequency lesion contained a dense band of fibrosis measuring 17 × 17 × 5 mm. Based on these findings, the investigators concluded that radiofrequency ablation of ischemic ventricular tachycardia causes coagulation necrosis initially, inflammatory infiltration later on, and then fibrosis as seen in normal animal models. They speculate that the limited success rate associated with radiofrequency ablation of ischemic ventricular tachycardia may be attributable to the small radiofrequency lesion size compared with the size of the reentrant circuit involved. However, these researchers achieved larger radiofrequency lesion size compared with other investigators by creating a series of closely spaced lesions.

In electrophysiology centers, radiofrequency has replaced high- and low-energy DC technology and has become the modality of choice for catheter ablation. Power-regulated and temperature-controlled radiofrequency ablation permits the titration of power, ensuring that the tissue-electrode interface reaches effective temperatures. For instance, Strickberger and colleagues (376) compared the efficacy of fixed-power radiofrequency ablation with power titration by temperature monitoring in 120 patients undergoing ablation of the slow pathway for AVNRT. They achieved a 72% primary success rate in patients undergoing fixed-power radiofrequency ablation and a 95% success rate in the temperature-monitored group. Both techniques generated a temperature of approximately 50°C, with the temperature-monitored group experiencing slightly higher temperatures. The investigators speculated that a slight increase in temperature most likely accounts for the higher success rate in the temperature-monitored group.

However, patients undergoing radiofrequency ablation may experience complications from radiation exposure during fluoroscopy-based imaging of catheter movement and positioning (377). Radiofrequency ablation suffers from long procedure times and extended fluoroscopy times. Multiple intrasessional and sometimes intersessional radiofrequency applications are required in most instances to cure the arrhythmia. Radiofrequency ablation also fails in most instances to create the long, continuous, linear lesions required to redirect electrical impulses associated with atrial fibrillation and flutter. Radiofrequency ablation has yet to cure ventricular tachycardia and fibrillation, both of which originate in the thick walls of the ventricles. Radiofrequency ablation is restricted in its use and is successful in the treatment of selective types of arrhythmias, such as supraventricular arrhythmias. Moreover, radiofrequency ablation fails to create lesions large and deep enough based on the large dispersive nature of the surface electrode and dissipation of energy through neighboring tissue.

Despite ongoing research into other energy sources—including laser energy, microwave ablation, ultrasound, and cryoablation—no alternative forms of energy delivery have surpassed existing radiofrequency ablation techniques. However, transcatheter laser ablation represents a feasible and attractive alternative to radiofrequency-based ablation because of the larger lesion size attainable with the use of lasers and the shorter procedure times (378). Weber and associates (379) reported the first clinical results with laser catheter ablation in the treatment of the common type of AVNRT in 10 consecutive patients. These researchers successfully irradiated the posteroinferior AV nodal area between the tricuspid valve ring and coronary sinus ostium without disrupting atrioventricular conduction using catheter-directed, continuous-wave, neodymium-doped yttrium-aluminum-garnet (Nd:YAG) laser light. All tachycardias were noninducible after irradiation, and the patients did not experience any complications or recurrent arrhythmias in a follow-up at 12 to 35 months. Despite this reported success, laser-based ablation is limited by technical considerations, especially the possibility of tissue perforation or dissection and its cost.

Ultrasound energy offers the advantage of noninvasive, extracorporeal delivery of energy to target sites within the heart. Ultrasound energy is propagated as a mechanical wave by the motion of particles within the medium and is converted into heat by the compression and rarefaction of the particles. He and coworkers (380) created ultrasound lesions *in vitro* and *in vivo* in the canine system using a small ultrasound transducer mounted on the tip of an intracardiac catheter. Previously, it was thought that a small transducer would fail to produce sufficient energy for generation of effective lesions. These investigators demonstrated otherwise and showed a linear relationship between increasing power and lesion depth. Histologic examination of the lesions revealed well-circumscribed lesions and a clear border between necrotic areas and intact cell layers. Likewise, Strickberger and colleagues (381) demonstrated the successful noninvasive extracorporeal ablation of the atrioventricular junction within the beating heart of 10 open-chested dogs using high-intensity focused ultrasound. They used diagnostic 2-D ultrasound to identify target sites and created complete atrioventricular block by gating the cardiac cycle to the application of ultrasound energy. Histologic analysis revealed that they selectively targeted the atrioventricular junction, as seen by the presence of well demarcated lesions, without damaging adjacent cardiac tissue. The lesion depth and size were similar to those obtained by radiofrequency catheter ablation.

Microwave catheters appear to be more efficacious in the treatment of atrial flutter and fibrillation, because these catheters deliver higher-power energy deeper and over a greater distance than radiofrequency ablation catheters. Microwave catheters create lesions by producing heat exclusively through electromagnetic radiation, whereas radiofrequency catheters rely on electric current flow between two electrodes to produce destructive heat energy. Liem and associates (382) investigated the possibility of using microwave energy to create linear lesions across the inferior vena cava–tricuspid annulus isthmus in the treatment of atrial flutter. They created bidirectional isthmus block in seven canines after an average of 2.7 ablations and unidirectional block in one canine after five ablations without causing coronary vascular or other structural damage. Histologic evaluation revealed hemorrhage, necrosis, degeneration, and fragmentation of the atrial myocardium. Despite their advantages, microwave catheter systems suffer the possibility of radiation leaks and power reflecting back into the catheter and potentially causing harm to the patient.

Because the dimensions of microwave lesions vary considerably, effort has gone into devising detection systems for the assessment of microwave lesion formation. Current fluoroscopic imaging techniques pose health hazards to the patient and physician because of the high level of radiation exposure associated with the procedure (377). For this reason, Tardif and coworkers (383) investigated whether intracardiac echocardiography could be used to monitor lesion formation during microwave catheter ablation *in vitro* in bovine left ventricles. These researchers demonstrated that intracardiac echocardiography failed to predict lesion dimension but succeeded in discriminating small from large lesions, as confirmed by pathologic evaluation of the lesions. Intracardiac guidance during microwave ablation provided information with regard to tissue-electrode contact, lesion formation, and lesion location. Other sources have reviewed microwave technology in the context of catheter design and ablation (384,385).

Dubuc and colleagues (386) demonstrated the successful use of a transvenous, hand-held, steerable cryoablation catheter containing halocarbon 502 to ablate the right and left ventricles in six dogs. Histologic examination revealed the absence of lesions when the temperature was cooler than $-30°C$ and the presence of 26 well-demarcated lesions when the temperature was warmer than $-30°C$. Likewise, Rodriguez and associates (387) created permanent complete atrioventricular block in four of six mongrel dogs using two applications of 5 minutes each using a steerable cryoablation catheter containing N_2O. The remaining two dogs showed permanent right bundle branch block and transient complete A-V block, respectively. Histologic evaluation revealed that the cryolesions were discrete and contained homogeneous fibrotic transmural tissue lacking viable myocytes, whereas radiofrequency lesions in two dogs contained less homogeneous fibrotic tissue interspersed among viable myocytes. The investigators speculated that cryolesions may not serve as arrhythmogenic substrates because of their homogenous nature, whereas radiofrequency lesions may serve as arrhythmogenic substrates based on their inhomogeneity. However, cryolesions have yet to reach sizes comparable to those of radiofrequency lesions. New cryocatheters must transport energy more effectively and create lower temperatures in the tissue to compensate for the fact that the circulating warm blood attenuates the cooling effect. Studies have already demonstrated that the size of cryolesions depends on the cryoprobe temperature and diameter, as well as the exposure time and temperature of the myocardium. Hoekstra and coworkers (388) devised a method based on monitoring the isothermic period after transcatheter cryoablation to predict cryolesion size. They correlated the duration of the constant-temperature plateau or the $0°C$ isothermic period, measured by the catheter tip feedback thermocouple, with lesion volume determined histologically in seven anesthetized pigs. All these *in vivo* studies demonstrate the potential efficacy of alternative forms of energy to treat cardiac arrhythmias.

A comprehensive examination of alternative ablation methods is beyond the scope of this chapter, but it is important to emphasize that radiofrequency ablation, although highly successful and relatively inexpensive, does have its drawbacks. In particular, the small lesions that radiofrequency produces are implicated in the failure of ablation to effectively or lastingly block conduction. New developments in catheter design aimed at improving maneuverability and stability may help to optimize radiofrequency lesion size and placement. Microwave and ultrasound can produce larger, discrete lesions; however, these techniques are limited by existing methods of safe and effective energy delivery. It seems likely that, with time and technologic refinements, different energy sources may be used in different anatomic settings or conditions.

● CONCLUSIONS

Management of patients with automaticity and conduction abnormalities has improved dramatically over the last two decades. An understanding of the technology, anatomy, potential sequelae, and opportunities for innovation will continue to advance the field. Closer interaction among electrophysiologists, pathologists, and cell biologists can help to clarify the remaining structure-function conundrums that underlie arrhythmogenesis and its therapies.

● ACKNOWLEDGEMENTS

The authors wish to express their gratitude to Drs. John Yeung, John Kugler, Charles Kerr, Igor Singer, George Rozanski, and Jeff Saffitz for their suggestions, feedback and advice. We also thank Albert Lee, Stuart Greene, Janet Wilson, and Jennifer Hards for their artistic and photographic expertise.

REFERENCES

1. Waller AD. A demonstration on man of electromotive changes accompanying the heart's beat. *J Physiol (Lond)* 1887;8:229–234.
2. Suma K, Shimada M. *The conduction system of the mammalian heart* [Translated from German by Sunao Tawara]. London: Imperial College Press, 1998.
3. Anderson RH, Ho SY. The architecture of the sinus node, the atrioventricular conduction axis, and the internodal atrial myocardium [Review]. *J Cardiovasc Electrophysiol* 1998;9:1233–1248.
4. Inoue S, Becker AE. Posterior extensions of the human compact atrioventricular node: a neglected anatomic feature of potential clinical significance [published erratum appears in *Circulation* 1998;97:1216]. *Circulation* 1998;97:188–193.
5. Lüderitz B. History of the disorders of cardiac rhythm. Armonk, NY: Futura Publishing, 1995.
6. Hoffman BF. Cardiac arrhythmias: what do we need to know about basic mechanisms? [Review]. *J Cardiovasc Electrophysiol* 1999;10:414–416.
7. Tracy CM. Catheter ablation for patients with atrial tachycardia [Review]. *Cardiol Clin* 1997;15:607–621.
8. Obel OA, Camm AJ. Supraventricular tachycardia: ECG diagnosis and anatomy [Review]. *Eur Heart J* 1997;18:C2–C11.
9. Obel OA, Camm AJ. Accessory pathway reciprocating tachycardia [Review]. *Eur Heart J* 1998;19:E13–E24, E50–51.
10. Rajadurai VS, Menahem S. Fetal arrhythmias: a 3-year experience. *Aust N Z J Obstet Gynaecol* 1992;32:28–31.
11. Reed KL. Fetal arrhythmias: etiology, diagnosis, pathophysiology, and treatment [Review]. *Semin Perinatol* 1989;13:294–304.
12. Colvin EV. Cardiac embryology. In: Garson JA, Bricker JT, McNamara DG, eds. *The science and practice of pediatric cardiology*. Philadelphia: Lea & Febiger, 1990:71.
13. Davies MJ, Anderson RH, Becker AE. *The conduction system of the heart*. London: Butterworths, 1983.
14. James TN. Cardiac conduction system: fetal and postnatal development. *Am J Cardiol* 1970;25:213–226.
15. Moorman AF, de Jong F, Denyn MM, Lamers WH. Development of the cardiac conduction system [Review]. *Circ Res* 1998;82:629–644.
16. Moorman AF, de Jong F, Lamers WH. Development of the conduction system of the heart [Review]. *Pacing Clin Electrophysiol* 1997;20:2087–2092.
17. Lieberman M, Paes de Carvalho A. The electrophysiological organization of the embryonic chick heart. *J Gen Physiol* 1965;49:351–363.
18. Kirby ML, Weidman TA, McKenzie JW. An ultrastructural study of the cardia ganglia in the bulbar plexus of the developing chick heart. *Dev Neurosci* 1980;3:174–184.
19. Kirby ML, Kumiski DH, Myers T, et al. Backtransplantation of chick cardiac neural crest cells cultured in LIF rescues heart development. *Dev Dyn* 1993;198:296–311.
20. Kirby ML, Stewart DE. Neural crest origin of cardiac ganglion cells in the chick embryo: identification and extirpation. *Dev Biol* 1983;97:433–443.
21. Van Mierop LH. Location of pacemaker in chick embryo heart at the time of initiation of heartbeat. *Am J Physiol* 1967;212:407–415.
22. Satin J, Fujii S, DeHaan RL. Development of cardiac beat rate in early chick embryos is regulated by regional cues. *Dev Biol* 1988;129:103–113.
23. Dyson E, Sucov HM, Kubalak SW, et al. Atrial-like phenotype is associated with embryonic ventricular failure in retinoid X receptor alpha −/− mice. *Proc Natl Acad Sci U S A* 1995;92:7386–7390.
24. Gourdie RG, Mima T, Thompson RP, Mikawa T. Terminal diversification of the myocyte lineage generates Purkinje fibers of the cardiac conduction system. *Development* 1995;121:1423–1431.
25. Alyonycheva T, Cohen-Gould L, Siewert C, et al. Skeletal muscle-specific myosin binding protein-H is expressed in Purkinje fibers of the cardiac conduction system. *Circ Res* 1997;80:665–672.
26. Canale ED, Campbell GR, Smolich JJ, Campbell JH. *Cardiac muscle*. Berlin: Springer-Verlag, 1986.
27. Gourdie RG, Kubalak S, Mikawa T. Conducting the embryonic heart: orchestrating development of specialized cardiac tissues [Review]. *Trends Cardiovasc Med* 1999;9:18–26.
28. Clouthier DE, Hosoda K, Richardson JA, et al. Cranial and cardiac neural crest defects in endothelin-A receptor-deficient mice. *Development* 1998;125:813–824.
29. Kurihara Y, Kurihara H, Suzuki H, et al. Elevated blood pressure and craniofacial abnormalities in mice deficient in endothelin-1. *Nature* 1994;368:703–710.

30. Gourdie RG, Wei Y, Kim D, et al. Endothelin-induced conversion of embryonic heart muscle cells into impulse-conducting Purkinje fibers. *Proc Natl Acad Sci U S A* 1998;95:6815–6818.
31. Paz Suarez-Mier MP, Gamallo C. Atrioventricular node fetal dispersion and His bundle fragmentation of the cardiac conduction system in sudden cardiac death. *J Am Coll Cardiol* 1998;32:1885–1890.
32. Paz Suarez-Mier MP, Aguilera B. Histopathology of the conduction system in sudden infant death. *Forensic Sci Int* 1998;93:143–154.
33. Kelmanson IA, Adrianov AV, Zolotukhina TA. Low birth weight and risk of cardiac arrhythmias in children. *J Cardiovasc Risk* 1998;5:47–51.
34. McManus BM, Wood SM. Key morphological features of the normal and abnormal, modified and unmodified conduction system. In: Singer I, ed. *Interventional electrophysiology*. Baltimore: Williams & Wilkins, 1997:133.
35. He BM, Tan YX, Cheng M, Cui YQ. The surgical anatomy of the sinoatrial node. *Surg Radiol Anat* 1991;13:123–128.
36. Calmat A, Hammou JC, Chomette G, et al. Precise localization of the sino-atrial node [French]. *Arch Mal Coeur Vaiss* 1973;66:855–862.
37. Schuessler RB, Boineau JP, Bromberg BI. Origin of the sinus impulse [Review]. *J Cardiovasc Electrophysiol* 1996;7:263–274.
38. Cox JL, Boineau JP, Schuessler RB, et al. Electrophysiologic basis, surgical development, and clinical results of the maze procedure for atrial flutter and atrial fibrillation [Review]. *Adv Card Surg* 1995;6:1–67.
39. Sherf L, James TN. Fine structure of cells and their histologic organization within internodal pathways of the heart: clinical and electrocardiographic implications [Review]. *Am J Cardiol* 1979;44:345–369.
40. Blom NA, Gittenberger-de Groot AC, DeRuiter MC, et al. Development of the cardiac conduction tissue in human embryos using HNK-1 antigen expression: possible relevance for understanding of abnormal atrial automaticity. *Circulation* 1999;99:800–806.
41. Walsh EP, Saul JP, Hulse JE, et al. Transcatheter ablation of ectopic atrial tachycardia in young patients using radiofrequency current. *Circulation* 1992;86:1138–1146.
42. Hirao K, Scherlag BJ, Poty H, et al. Electrophysiology of the atrio-AV nodal inputs and exits in the normal dog heart: radiofrequency ablation using an epicardial approach. *J Cardiovasc Electrophysiol* 1997;8:904–915.
43. Abuin G, Nieponice A. New findings on the origin of the blood supply to the atrioventricular node: clinical and surgical significance. *Tex Heart Inst J* 1998;25:113–117.
44. Sanchez-Quintana D, Davies DW, Ho SY, et al. Architecture of the atrial musculature in and around the triangle of Koch: its potential relevance to atrioventricular nodal reentry. *J Cardiovasc Electrophysiol* 1997;8:1396–1407.
45. Gottwald M, Gottwald E, Dhein S. Age-related electrophysiological and histological changes in rabbit hearts: age-related changes in electrophysiology. *Int J Cardiol* 1997;62:97–106.
46. Spach MS. Anisotropy of cardiac tissue: a major determinant of conduction? *J Cardiovasc Electrophysiol* 1999;10:887–890.
47. Thompson CJ. Dysrhythmia formation in the older adult [Review]. *Crit Care Nurs Q* 1996;19:23–33.
48. Van Mierop LHS, Wiglesworth FW. Isomerism of the cardiac atria in asplenia syndrome. *Lab Invest* 1962;11:1303–1315.
49. Attie F, Iturralde P, Zabal C, et al. Congenitally corrected transposition with atrioventricular septal defect. *Cardiol Young* 1998;8:472–478.
50. Dickinson DF, Wilkinson JL, Anderson KR, et al. The cardiac conduction system in situs ambiguus. *Circulation* 1979;59:879–885.
51. Huang M, Bigos D, Levine M. Ventricular arrhythmia associated with respiratory syncytial viral infection. *Pediatr Cardiol* 1998;19:498–500.
52. Moral L, Majo J, Rubio EM, et al. Unsuspected rheumatic heart underlying group B streptococcal endocarditis at the age of 20 months. *Eur J Pediatr* 1992;151:745–747.
53. Becherer P, Gutsch D, Fischer J. Ventricular arrhythmia in secondary syphilis [Letter]. *Lancet* 1990;336:382–383.
54. Miyamoto MI, Hutter AM Jr, Blum JH, Torchiana DF. Cardiac conduction abnormalities preceding transoesophageal echocardiographic evidence of perivalvar extension of infection in a case of *Salmonella* prosthetic valve endocarditis. *Heart* 1997;78:416–418.
55. Donnerstein RL, Berg RA, Shehab Z, Ovadia M. Complex atrial tachycardias and respiratory syncytial virus infections in infants. *J Pediatr* 1994;125:23–28.
56. Bairan AC, Cherry JD, Fagan LF, Codd JE Jr. Complete heart block and respiratory syncytial virus infection. *Am J Dis Child* 1974;127:264–265.
57. Thomas JA, Raroque S, Scott WA, et al. Successful treatment of severe dysrhythmias in infants with respiratory syncytial virus infections: two cases and a literature review [Review]. *Crit Care Med* 1997;25:880–886.
58. Ogbuihi S, Fechner G, Brinkmann B. Sudden death due to cardiac sarcoidosis in a case of suspected homicide. *Int J Legal Med* 1993;106:99–102.
59. Bajaj AK, Kopelman HA, Echt DS. Cardiac sarcoidosis with sudden death: treatment with the automatic implantable cardioverter defibrillator. *Am Heart J* 1988;116:557–560.
60. Veinot JP, Johnston B. Cardiac sarcoidosis—an occult cause of sudden death: a case report and literature review [Review]. *J Forensic Sci* 1998;43:715–717.
61. Lie JT, Hunt D, Valentine PA. Sudden death from cardiac sarcoidosis with involvement of conduction system. *Am J Med Sci* 1974;267:123–128.
62. Abeler V. Sarcoidosis of the cardiac conducting system. *Am Heart J* 1979;97:701–707.
63. Jaoude SA, Leclercq JF, Coumel P. Progressive ECG changes in arrhythmogenic right ventricular disease: evidence for an evolving disease. *Eur Heart J* 1996;17:1717–1722.
64. Dec GW, Fuster V. Idiopathic dilated cardiomyopathy [Review]. *N Engl J Med* 1994;331:1564–1575.
65. Basso C, Thiene G, Corrado D, et al. Arrhythmogenic right ventricular cardiomyopathy: dysplasia, dystrophy, or myocarditis? *Circulation* 1996;94:983–991.
66. Fontaine G, Fontaliran F, Frank R, et al. Arrhythmogenic right ventricular dysplasia. A new clinical entity [French]. *Bull Acad Natl Med* 1993;177:501–512, discussion 512–514.
67. Hisaoka T, Kawai S, Ohi H, et al. Two cases of chronic myocarditis mimicking arrhythmogenic right ventricular dysplasia. *Heart Vessels Suppl* 1990;5:51–54.
68. Grumbach IM, Heim A, Vonhof S, et al. Coxsackievirus genome in myocardium of patients with arrhythmogenic right ventricular dysplasia/cardiomyopathy. *Cardiology* 1998;89:241–245.
69. Fornes P, Ratel S, Lecomte D. Pathology of arrhythmogenic right ventricular cardiomyopathy/dysplasia—an autopsy study of 20 forensic cases. *J Forensic Sci* 1998;43:777–783.
70. Archbold RA, Sayer JW, Ray S, et al. Frequency and prognostic implications of conduction defects in acute myocardial infarction since the introduction of thrombolytic therapy. *Eur Heart J* 1998;19:893–898.
71. Xing D, Martins JB. The relationship between myocardial is-

chemic size and ventricular arrhythmia during ischemia-reperfusion in the dogs [Abstract]. *J Invest Med* 1998;46:269A.
72. Puljevic D, Smalcelj A, Durakovic Z, Goldner V. Effects of postmyocardial infarction scar size, cardiac function, and severity of coronary artery disease on QT interval dispersion as a risk factor for complex ventricular arrhythmia. *Pacing Clin Electrophysiol* 1998;21:1508–1516.
73. Majumder AA, Malik A, Zafar A. Conduction disturbances in acute myocardial infarction: incidence, site-wise relationship and the influence on in-hospital prognosis. *Bangladesh Med Res Counc Bull* 1996;22:74–80.
74. Mosseri M, Izak T, Rosenheck S, et al. Coronary angiographic characteristics of patients with permanent artificial pacemakers. *Circulation* 1997;96:809–815.
75. Aufderheide TP. Arrhythmias associated with acute myocardial infarction and thrombolysis [Review]. *Emerg Med Clin North Am* 1998;16:583–600, viii.
76. Antman EM, Braunwald E. Acute myocardial infarction. In: Braunwald E, ed. *Heart disease: a textbook of cardiovascular medicine,* 5th ed. Philadelphia: WB Saunders, 1997:1245.
77. Podrid PJ. Arrhythmias after acute myocardial infarction. Evaluation and management of rhythm and conduction abnormalities [Review]. *Postgrad Med* 1997;102:125–128, 131–134, 137–139.
78. Ducceschi V, Di Micco G, Sarubbi B, et al. Ionic mechanisms of ischemia-related ventricular arrhythmias [Review]. *Clin Cardiol* 1996;19:325–3231.
79. Mehta D, Curwin J, Gomes JA, Fuster V. Sudden death in coronary artery disease: acute ischemia versus myocardial substrate [Review]. *Circulation* 1997;96:3215–3223.
80. Skanes AC, Green MS. What have clinical trials taught us about proarrhythmia? [Review]. *Can J Cardiol* 1996;12:20B–26B.
81. Daleau P, Deleze J. Conduction block in Purkinje fibers by homogeneous versus localized decrease of the gap junction conductance. *Can J Physiol Pharmacol* 1998;76:630–641.
82. Lurie KG, Sugiyama A, McKnite S, et al. Modulation of AV nodal and Hisian conduction by changes in extracellular space. *Am J Physiol* 1999;276:H953–H960.
83. Fenoglio JJ Jr, Pham TD, Harken AH, et al. Recurrent sustained ventricular tachycardia: structure and ultrastructure of subendocardial regions in which tachycardia originates. *Circulation* 1983;68:518–533.
84. de Bakker JM, van Capelle FJ, Janse MJ, et al. Reentry as a cause of ventricular tachycardia in patients with chronic ischemic heart disease: electrophysiologic and anatomic correlation. *Circulation* 1988;77:589–606.
85. Wit AL, Dillon SM, Coromilas J, et al. Anisotropic reentry in the epicardial border zone of myocardial infarcts [Review]. *Ann N Y Acad Sci* 1990;591:86–108.
86. Spach MS, Boineau JP. Microfibrosis produces electrical load variations due to loss of side-to-side cell connections: a major mechanism of structural heart disease arrhythmias [Review]. *Pacing Clin Electrophysiol* 1997;20:397–413.
87. Wu TJ, Ong JJ, Hwang C, et al. Characteristics of wave fronts during ventricular fibrillation in human hearts with dilated cardiomyopathy: role of increased fibrosis in the generation of reentry. *J Am Coll Cardiol* 1998;32:187–196.
88. Anderson KR, Sutton MG, Lie JT. Histopathological types of cardiac fibrosis in myocardial disease. *J Pathol* 1979;128:79–85.
89. Schwarz F, Mall G, Zebe H, et al. Quantitative morphologic findings of the myocardium in idiopathic dilated cardiomyopathy. *Am J Cardiol* 1983;51:501–506.
90. Unverferth DV, Baker PB, Swift SE, et al. Extent of myocardial fibrosis and cellular hypertrophy in dilated cardiomyopathy. *Am J Cardiol* 1986;57:816–820.
91. de Bakker JM, van Capelle FJ, Janse MJ, et al. Fractionated electrograms in dilated cardiomyopathy: origin and relation to abnormal conduction. *J Am Coll Cardiol* 1996;27:1071–1078.
92. Pogwizd SM, McKenzie JP, Cain ME. Mechanisms underlying spontaneous and induced ventricular arrhythmias in patients with idiopathic dilated cardiomyopathy [clinical trial]. *Circulation* 1998;98:2404–2414.
93. Reisinger J, Dubrey SW, Lavalley M, et al. Electrophysiologic abnormalities in AL (primary) amyloidosis with cardiac involvement. *J Am Coll Cardiol* 1997;30:1046–1051.
94. James TN. Pathology of the cardiac conduction system in amyloidosis. *Ann Intern Med* 1966;65:28–36.
95. Ridolfi RL, Bulkley BH, Hutchins GM. The conduction system in cardiac amyloidosis: clinical and pathologic features of 23 patients. *Am J Med* 1977;62:677–686.
96. Rodriguez Reguero J, Iglesias Cubero G, Rubin J. Primary amyloidosis and syncope. *Int J Cariol* 1997;58:185–187.
97. Ahmed Q, Chung-Park M, Mustafa K, Khan MA. Psoriatic spondyloarthropathy with secondary amyloidosis [Review]. *J Rheumatol* 1996;23:1107–1110.
98. Hesse A, Altland K, Linke RP, et al. Cardiac amyloidosis: a review and report of a new transthyretin (prealbumin) variant [Review]. *Br Heart J* 1993;70:111–115.
99. Olson LJ, Edwards WD, McCall JT, et al. Cardiac iron deposition in idiopathic hemochromatosis: histologic and analytic assessment of 14 hearts from autopsy. *J Am Coll Cardiol* 1987;10:1239–1243.
100. Unger P, Kentos A, Cogan E, et al. Primary cardiac lymphoma: diagnosis by transvenous biopsy under transesophageal echocardiographic guidance. *J Am Soc Echocardiogr* 1998;11:89–91.
101. Van Hare GF, Phoon CK, Munkenbeck F, et al. Electrophysiologic study and radiofrequency ablation in patients with intracardiac tumors and accessory pathways: is the tumor the pathway? *J Cardiovasc Electrophysiol* 1996;7:1204–1210.
102. Singh BN. Current antiarrhythmic drugs: an overview of mechanisms of action and potential clinical utility [Review]. *J Cardiovasc Electrophysiol* 1999;10:283–301.
103. Camm AJ, Yap YG. What should we expect from the next generation of antiarrhythmic drugs? [Review]. *J Cardiovasc Electrophysiol* 1999;10:307–317.
104. Anonymous. Effect of the antiarrhythmic agent moricizine on survival after myocardial infarction. The Cardiac Arrhythmia Suppression Trial II Investigators [Clinical trial]. *N Engl J Med* 1992;327:227–233.
105. Cardiac Arrhythmia Suppression Trial (CAST) Investigators. Preliminary report: effect of encainide and flecainide on mortality in a randomized trial of arrhythmia suppression after myocardial infarction [Clinical trial]. *N Engl J Med* 1989;321:406–412.
106. Hallstrom AP, Cobb LA, Yu BH, et al. An antiarrhythmic drug experience in 941 patients resuscitated from an initial cardiac arrest between 1970 and 1985. *Am J Cardiol* 1991;68:1025–1031.
107. Coplen SE, Antman EM, Berlin JA, et al. Efficacy and safety of quinidine therapy for maintenance of sinus rhythm after cardioversion: a meta-analysis of randomized control trials [clinical trial]. *Circulation* 1990;82:1106–1116.
108. Flaker GC, Blackshear JL, McBride R, et al. Antiarrhythmic drug therapy and cardiac mortality in atrial fibrillation. The Stroke Prevention in Atrial Fibrillation Investigators [Clinical trial]. *J Am Coll Cardiol* 1992;20:527–532.
109. Cairns JA, Connolly SJ, Roberts R, Gent M. Randomised trial of outcome after myocardial infarction in patients with frequent or repetitive ventricular premature depolarisations: CAMIAT. Canadian Amiodarone Myocardial Infarction Ar-

109. rhythmia Trial Investigators [Clinical trial] [published erratum appears in *Lancet* 1997;349:1776]. *Lancet* 1997;349:675–682.
110. Julian DG, Camm AJ, Frangin G, et al. Randomised trial of effect of amiodarone on mortality in patients with left-ventricular dysfunction after recent myocardial infarction: EMIAT. European Myocardial Infarct Amiodarone Trial Investigators [Clinical trial]. *Lancet* 1997;349:667–674.
111. Waldo AL, Camm AJ, deRuyter H, et al. Effect of D-sotalol on mortality in patients with left ventricular dysfunction after recent and remote myocardial infarction. The SWORD Investigators: Survival with Oral D-Sotalol [Clinical trial]. *Lancet* 1996;348:7–12.
112. Roden DM. Mechanisms and management of proarrhythmia [Review, clinical trial]. *Am J Cardiol* 1998;82:49I–57I.
113. Okazaki O, Wei D, Harumi K. A simulation study of Torsade de Pointes with M cells. *J Electrocardiol* 1998;31:145–1451.
114. Kodama I, Kamiya K, Toyama J. Cellular electropharmacology of amiodarone [Review]. *Cardiovasc Res* 1997;35:13–29.
115. Singh BN. Controlling cardiac arrhythmias with sotalol, a broad-spectrum anti-arrhythmic with beta-blocking effects and class III activity. *Am J Cardiol* 1990;765:1A–84A.
116. Nattel S. The molecular and ionic specificity of antiarrhythmic drug actions [Review]. *J Cardiovasc Electrophysiol* 1999;10:272–282.
117. Katz AM. Calcium channel diversity in the cardiovascular system [Review]. *J Am Coll Cardiol* 1996;28:522–529.
118. Fareh S, Thibault B, Nattel S. Treatment with a T-type calcium channel blocker prevents atrial fibrillation caused by tachycardia-induced atrial remodeling [Abstract]. *Circulation* 1998;98:I-210.
119. Ausma J, Wijffels M, Thone F, et al. Structural changes of atrial myocardium due to sustained atrial fibrillation in the goat. *Circulation* 1997;96:3157–3163.
120. Morillo CA, Klein GJ, Jones DL, Guiraudon CM. Chronic rapid atrial pacing: structural, functional, and electrophysiological characteristics of a new model of sustained atrial fibrillation. *Circulation* 1995;91:1588–1595.
121. Davies MJ, Pomerance A. Pathology of atrial fibrillation in man. *Br Heart J* 1972;34:520–525.
122. Mary-Rabine L, Albert A, Pham TD, et al. The relationship of human atrial cellular electrophysiology to clinical function and ultrastructure. *Circ Res* 1983;52:188–199.
123. Van Gelder IC, Brundel BJ, Henning RH, et al. Alterations in gene expression of proteins involved in the calcium handling in patients with atrial fibrillation. *J Cardiovasc Electrophysiol* 1999;10:552–560.
124. Brugada R, Roberts R. The molecular genetics of arrhythmias and sudden death [Review]. *Clin Cardiol* 1998;21:553–560.
125. Priori SG, Barhanin J, Hauer RN, et al. Genetic and molecular basis of cardiac arrhythmias: impact on clinical management part III [Review]. *Circulation* 1999;99:674–681.
126. Janse MJ, Wilde AA. Molecular mechanisms of arrhythmias [Review]. *Rev Port Cardiol* 1998;17:II41–II46.
127. Chen Q, Kirsch GE, Zhang D, et al. Genetic basis and molecular mechanism for idiopathic ventricular fibrillation. *Nature* 1998;392:293–296.
128. de Meeus A, Stephan E, Debrus S, et al. An isolated cardiac conduction disease maps to chromosome 19q. *Circ Res* 1995;77:735–740.
129. Brink PA, Ferreira A, Moolman JC, et al. Gene for progressive familial heart block type I maps to chromosome 19q13. *Circulation* 1995;91:1633–1640.
130. Brugada R, Tapscott T, Czernuszewicz GZ, et al. Identification of a genetic locus for familial atrial fibrillation. *N Engl J Med* 1997;336:905–911.
131. Grunig E, Tasman JA, Kucherer H, et al. Frequency and phenotypes of familial dilated cardiomyopathy. *J Am Coll Cardiol* 1998;31:186–194.
132. Kass S, MacRae C, Graber HL, et al. A gene defect that causes conduction system disease and dilated cardiomyopathy maps to chromosome 1p1-1q1. *Nat Genet* 1994;7:546–551.
133. Durand JB, Bachinski LL, Bieling LC, et al. Localization of a gene responsible for familial dilated cardiomyopathy to chromosome 1q32. *Circulation* 1995;92:3387–3389.
134. Olson TM, Keating MT. Mapping a cardiomyopathy locus to chromosome 3p22-p25. *J Clin Invest* 1996;97:528–532.
135. Wang J, Wilhelmsson H, Graff C, et al. Dilated cardiomyopathy and atrioventricular conduction blocks induced by heart-specific inactivation of mitochondrial DNA gene expression. *Nat Genet* 1999;21:133–137.
136. Ahmad F, Li D, Karibe A, et al. Localization of a gene responsible for arrhythmogenic right ventricular dysplasia to chromosome 3p23. *Circulation* 1998;98:2791–2795.
137. Coonar AS, Protonotarios N, Tsatsopoulou A, et al. Gene for arrhythmogenic right ventricular cardiomyopathy with diffuse nonepidermolytic palmoplantar keratoderma and woolly hair (Naxos disease) maps to 17q21. *Circulation* 1998;97:2049–2058.
138. Rampazzo A, Nava A, Danieli G. The gene for arrhythmogenic right ventricular cardiomyopathy maps to chromosome 14q23-q24. *Hum Mol Genet* 1994;3:959–962.
139. Rampazzo A, Nava A, Erne P, et al. A new locus for arrhythmogenic right ventricular cardiomyopathy (ARVD2) maps to chromosome 1q42-q43. *Hum Mol Genet* 1995;4:2151–2154.
140. Severini GM, Krajinovic M, Pinamonti B, et al. A new locus for arrhythmogenic right ventricular dysplasia on the long arm of chromosome 14. *Genomics* 1996;31:193–200.
141. Rampazzo A, Nava A, Miorin M, et al. ARVD4, a new locus for arrhythmogenic right ventricular cardiomyopathy, maps to chromosome 2 long arm. *Genomics* 1997;45:259–263.
142. Priori SG, Barhanin J, Hauer RN, et al. Genetic and molecular basis of cardiac arrhythmias; impact on clinical management. Study group on molecular basis of arrhythmias of the working group on arrhythmias of the European society of cardiology [Review]. *Eur Heart J* 1999;20:174–195.
143. MacRae CA, Ghaisas N, Kass S, et al. Familial hypertrophic cardiomyopathy with Wolff-Parkinson-White syndrome maps to a locus on chromosome 7q3. *J Clin Invest* 1995;96:1216–1220.
144. Kimura A, Harada H, Park JE, et al. Mutations in the cardiac troponin I gene associated with hypertrophic cardiomyopathy. *Nat Genet* 1997;16:379–382.
145. Priori SG, Barhanin J, Hauer RN, et al. Genetic and molecular basis of cardiac arrhythmias: impact on clinical management parts I and II [Review]. *Circulation* 1999;99:518–528.
146. Saffitz JE, Schuessler RB, Yamada KA. Mechanisms of remodeling of gap junction distributions and the development of anatomic substrates of arrhythmias [Review]. *Cardiovasc Res* 1999;42:309–317.
147. Guerrero PA, Schuessler RB, Davis LM, et al. Slow ventricular conduction in mice heterozygous for a connexin43 null mutation. *J Clin Invest* 1997;99:1991–1998.
148. Simon AM, Goodenough DA, Paul DL. Mice lacking connexin40 have cardiac conduction abnormalities characteristic of atrioventricular block and bundle branch block. *Curr Biol* 1998;8:295–298.
149. Luke RA, Saffitz JE. Remodeling of ventricular conduction pathways in healed canine infarct border zones. *J Clin Invest* 1991;87:1594–1602.
150. Peters NS, Green CR, Poole-Wilson PA, Severs NJ. Reduced

content of connexin43 gap junctions in ventricular myocardium from hypertrophied and ischemic human hearts. *Circulation* 1993;88:864–875.
151. Kaprielian RR, Gunning M, Dupont E, et al. Downregulation of immunodetectable connexin43 and decreased gap junction size in the pathogenesis of chronic hibernation in the human left ventricle. *Circulation* 1998;97:651–6560.
152. Smith JH, Green CR, Peters NS, et al. Altered patterns of gap junction distribution in ischemic heart disease: an immunohistochemical study of human myocardium using laser scanning confocal microscopy. *Am J Pathol* 1991;139:801–821.
153. Peters NS, Coromilas J, Severs NJ, Wit AL. Disturbed connexin43 gap junction distribution correlates with the location of reentrant circuits in the epicardial border zone of healing canine infarcts that cause ventricular tachycardia. *Circulation* 1997;95:988–996.
154. Saffitz JE, Davis LM, Darrow BJ, et al. The molecular basis of anisotropy: role of gap junctions [Review]. *J Cardiovasc Electrophysiol* 1995;6:498–510.
155. Peters NS. New insights into myocardial arrhythmogenesis: distribution of gap-junctional coupling in normal, ischaemic and hypertrophied human hearts [Review]. *Clin Sci (Colch)* 1996;90:447–452.
156. Saffitz JE, Yamada KA. Do alterations in intercellular coupling play a role in cardiac contractile dysfunction? [Editorial]. *Circulation* 1998;97:630–632.
157. Davis LM, Rodefeld ME, Green K, et al. Gap junction protein phenotypes of the human heart and conduction system [published erratum appears in *J Cardiovasc Electrophysiol* 1996;7:383–385]. *J Cardiovasc Electrophysiol* 1995;6:813–822.
158. Kwong KF, Schuessler RB, Green KG, Laing JG, et al. Differential expression of gap junction proteins in the canine sinus node. *Circ Res* 1998;82:604–612.
159. Coppen SR, Dupont E, Rothery S, Severs NJ. Connexin45 expression is preferentially associated with the ventricular conduction system in mouse and rat heart. *Circ Res* 1998;82:232–243.
160. Gros DB, Jongsma HJ. Connexins in mammalian heart function [Review]. *Bioessays* 1996;18:719–730.
161. Friedli B, Faidutti B, Oberhansli I, Rouge JC. Late results of surgery for congenital heart defects. *Helv Chir Acta* 1991;57:533–543.
162. Kanter RJ, Garson A Jr. Atrial arrhythmias during chronic follow-up of surgery for complex congenital heart disease [Review]. *Pacing Clin Electrophysiol* 1997;20:502–511.
163. Rhodes LA, Walsh EP, Gamble WJ, et al. Benefits and potential risks of atrial antitachycardia pacing after repair of congenital heart disease. *Pacing Clin Electrophysiol* 1995;18:1005–1016.
164. Triedman JK, Jenkins KJ, Colan SD, et al. Intra-atrial reentrant tachycardia after palliation of congenital heart disease: characterization of multiple macroreentrant circuits using fluoroscopically based three-dimensional endocardial mapping. *J Cardiovasc Electrophysiol* 1997;8:259–270.
165. Bonatti V, Agnetti A, Squarcia U. Early and late postoperative complete heart block in pediatric patients submitted to open-heart surgery for congenital heart disease [Review]. *Pediatr Med Chir* 1998;20:181–186.
166. Silka MJ, Hardy BG, Menashe VD, Morris CD. A population-based prospective evaluation of risk of sudden cardiac death after operation for common congenital heart defects. *J Am Coll Cardiol* 1998;32:245–251.
167. Reddy VM, McElhinney DB, Sagrado T, et al. Results of 102 cases of complete repair of congenital heart defects in patients weighing 700 to 2500 grams. *J Thorac Cardiovasc Surg* 1999;117:324–331.
168. James TN, St Martin E, Willis PW 3rd, Lohr TO. Apoptosis as a possible cause of gradual development of complete heart block and fatal arrhythmias associated with absence of the AV node, sinus node, and internodal pathways. *Circulation* 1996;93:1424–1438.
169. Kertesz NJ, Fenrich AL, Friedman RA. Congenital complete atrioventricular block [Review]. *Tex Heart Inst J* 1997;24:301–307.
170. Michaelsson M, Engle MA. Congenital complete heart block: an international study of the natural history [Review]. *Cardiovasc Clin* 1972;4:85–101.
171. Pinsky WW, Gillette PC, Garson A Jr, McNamara DG. Diagnosis, management, and long-term results of patients with congenital complete atrioventricular block. *Pediatrics* 1982;69:728–733.
172. Schmidt KG, Ulmer HE, Silverman NH, Kleinman CS, Copel JA. Perinatal outcome of fetal complete atrioventricular block: a multicenter experience. *J Am Coll Cardiol* 1991;17:1360–1366.
173. Chow LT, Cook AC, Ho SY, et al. Isolated congenitally complete heart block attributable to combined nodoventricular and intraventricular discontinuity. *Hum Pathol* 1998;29:729–736.
174. Kaplan BM, Miller AJ, Bharati S, et al. Complete AV block following mediastinal radiation therapy: electrocardiographic and pathologic correlation and review of the world literature [Review]. *J Interv Card Electrophysiol* 1997;1:175–188.
175. Tai YT, Lau CP. Patterns of radiofrequency catheter ablation of left free-wall accessory pathways: implications for accessory pathway anatomy. *Clin Cardiol* 1993;16:644–652.
176. Pitzalis MV, Luzzi G, Anaclerio M, Rizzon P. Radiofrequency catheter ablation of atrio-ventricular accessory pathways [Review]. *Rev Port Cardiol* 1998;17:III15–III22.
177. Anderson RH, Becker AE, Brechenmacher C, et al. Ventricular preexcitation: a proposed nomenclature for its substrates. *Eur J Cardiol* 1975;3:27–36.
178. Anderson RH, Ho SY. Anatomy of the atrioventricular junctions with regard to ventricular preexcitation [Review]. *Pacing Clin Electrophysiol* 1997;20:2072–2076.
179. Cain ME, Luke RA, Lindsay BD. Diagnosis and localization of accessory pathways [Review]. *Pacing Clin Electrophysiol* 1992;15:801–824.
180. Cain ME, Cox JL. Surgical treatment of supraventricular arrhythmias. In: Platia E, ed. *Management of cardiac arrhythmias: the nonpharmacologic approach*. Philadelphia: JB Lippincott, 1987:304.
181. Okishige K, Goseki Y, Itoh A, et al. New electrophysiologic features and catheter ablation of atrioventricular and atriofascicular accessory pathways: evidence of decremental conduction and the anatomic structure of the Mahaim pathway [Clinical trial]. *J Cardiovasc Electrophysiol* 1998;9:22–33.
182. Anderson RH. Mahaim pathway [Letter]. *J Cardiovasc Electrophysiol* 1998;9:448–489.
183. Kent AFS. The structure of the cardiac tissues at the auriculoventricular junction. *J Physiol* 1913;47:17–18.
184. Taccardi B, Lux RL, Ershler PR, et al. Anatomical architecture and electrical activity of the heart [Review]. *Acta Cardiol* 1997;52:91–105.
185. Tai CT, Chen SA, Chiang CE, et al. Identification of fiber orientation in left free-wall accessory pathways: implication for radiofrequency ablation. *J Interv Card Electrophysiol* 1997;1:235–241.
186. Schluter M, Kuck KH. Radiofrequency current therapy of supraventricular tachycardia: accessory atrioventricular pathways [Review]. *Pacing Clin Electrophysiol* 1993;16:643–648.
187. Edwards FH, Weston L. Surgical management of posteroseptal

accessory atrioventricular pathways. *Ann Thorac Surg* 1992;53: 321–325.
188. Davis LM, Byth K, Ellis P, et al. Dimensions of the human posterior septal space and coronary sinus. *Am J Cardiol* 1991; 68:621–625.
189. Cox JL. Anatomy of the "posterior septal space" [Editorial]. *Am J Cardiol* 1991;68:675–677.
190. Wen MS, Yeh SJ, Wang CC, et al. Radiofrequency ablation therapy of the posteroseptal accessory pathway. *Am Heart J* 1996;132:612–620.
191. Dhala AA, Deshpande SS, Bremner S, et al. Transcatheter ablation of posteroseptal accessory pathways using a venous approach and radiofrequency energy. *Circulation* 1994;90: 1799–1810.
192. Sealy WC, Mikat EM. Anatomical problems with identification and interruption of posterior septal Kent bundles. *Ann Thorac Surg* 1983;36:584–595.
193. Sealy WC, Gallagher JJ. The surgical approach to the septal area of the heart based on experiences with 45 patients with Kent bundles. *J Thorac Cardiovasc Surg* 1980;79:542–551.
194. Epstein AE, Kirklin JK, Holman WL, et al. Intermediate septal accessory pathways: electrocardiographic characteristics, electrophysiologic observations and their surgical implications. *J Am Coll Cardiol* 1991;17:1570–1578.
195. Tai CT, Chen SA, Chiang CE, Chang MS. Characteristics and radiofrequency catheter ablation of septal accessory atrioventricular pathways [Review]. *Pacing Clin Electrophysiol* 1999; 22:500–511.
196. Beukema WP, Van Dessel PF, Van Hemel NM, Kingma JH. Radiofrequency catheter ablation of accessory pathways associated with a coronary sinus diverticulum. *Eur Heart J* 1994;15: 1415–1218.
197. Aguinaga L, Primo J, Anguera I, et al. Long-term follow-up in patients with the permanent form of junctional reciprocating tachycardia treated with radiofrequency ablation. *Pacing Clin Electrophysiol* 1998;21:2073–2078.
198. Cohn AE, Fraser FR. Paroxysmal stimulation of the vagus nerves by pressure. *Heart* 1913–1914;4:93.
199. Wolff L, Parkinson J, White PD. Bundle-branch block with short P-R interval in healthy young people prone to paroxysmal tachycardia. *Am Heart J* 1930;5:685–704.
200. Shih HT, Miles WM, Klein LS, et al. Multiple accessory pathways in the permanent form of junctional reciprocating tachycardia. *Am J Cardiol* 1994;73:361–367.
201. Plumb VJ. Catheter ablation of the accessory pathways of the Wolff-Parkinson-White syndrome and its variants [Review]. *Prog Cardiovasc Dis* 1995;37:295–306.
202. Kay GN, Epstein AE, Dailey SM, Plumb VJ. Role of radiofrequency ablation in the management of supraventricular arrhythmias: experience in 760 consecutive patients [Review]. *J Cardiovasc Electrophysiol* 1993;4:371–389.
203. Mehdirad AA, Fatkin D, DiMarco JP, et al. Electrophysiologic characteristics of accessory atrioventricular connections in an inherited form of Wolff-Parkinson-White syndrome. *J Cardiovasc Electrophysiol* 1999;10:629–635.
204. James TN. Morphology of the human atrioventricular node, with remarks pertinent to its electrophysiology. *Am Heart J* 1961;62:756–771.
205. Douglas JE, Mandel WJ, Danzig R, Hayakawa H. Lown-Ganong-Levine syndrome. *Circulation* 1972;45:1143–1144.
206. Knight BP, Morady F. Catheter ablation of accessory pathways [Review]. *Cardiol Clin* 1997;15:647–660.
207. Morady F. Radio-frequency ablation as treatment for cardiac arrhythmias [Review]. *N Engl J Med* 1999;340:534–544.
208. Chen SA, Chiang CE, Tsang WP, et al. Recurrent conduction in accessory pathway and possible new arrhythmias after radiofrequency catheter ablation. *Am Heart J* 1993;125:381–387.
209. Gursoy S, Schluter M, Kuck KH. Radiofrequency current catheter ablation for control of supraventricular arrhythmias [Review]. *J Cardiovasc Electrophysiol* 1993;4:194–205.
210. Twidale N, Wang XZ, Beckman KJ, et al. Factors associated with recurrence of accessory pathway conduction after radiofrequency catheter ablation. *Pacing Clin Electrophysiol* 1991;14: 2042–2048.
211. Klein GJ, Bashore TM, Sellers TD, et al. Ventricular fibrillation in the Wolff-Parkinson-White syndrome. *N Engl J Med* 1979; 301:1080–1085.
212. Bockeria LA, Chigogidze NA, Golukhova EZ, Artjukhina TV. Diagnosis and surgical treatment of tachycardias in patients with nodoventricular fibers. *Pacing Clin Electrophysiol* 1991;14: 2004–2009.
213. Ellenbogen KA, Ramirez NM, Packer DL, et al. Accessory nodoventricular (Mahaim) fibers: a clinical review. *Pacing Clin Electrophysiol* 1986;9:868–884.
214. Moss AJ. Clinical significance of ventricular arrhythmias in patients with and without coronary artery disease [Review]. *Prog Cardiovasc Dis* 1980;23:33–52.
215. Gallagher JJ, Pritchett EL, Sealy WC, et al. The preexcitation syndromes [Review]. *Prog Cardiovasc Dis* 1978;20:285–327.
216. Short DS. The syndrome of alternating bradycardia and tachycardia. *Br Heart J* 1954;16:208.
217. MacWilliam JA. Some applications of physiology to medicine. II. Ventricular fibrillation and sudden death. *Br Heart J* 1923; 2:215.
218. Langberg JJ, Calkins H, Kim YN, et al. Recurrence of conduction in accessory atrioventricular connections after initially successful radiofrequency catheter ablation. *J Am Coll Cardiol* 1992;19:1588–1592.
219. Wagshal AB, Pires LA, Mittleman RS, et al. Early recurrence of accessory pathways after radiofrequency catheter ablation does not preclude long-term cure. *Am J Cardiol* 1993;72: 843–846.
220. Haissaguerre M, Fischer B, Labbe T, et al. Frequency of recurrent atrial fibrillation after catheter ablation of overt accessory pathways. *Am J Cardiol* 1992;69:493–497.
221. Morady F, Strickberger A, Man KC, et al. Reasons for prolonged or failed attempts at radiofrequency catheter ablation of accessory pathways. *J Am Coll Cardiol* 1996;27:683–689.
222. Huang JL, Chen SA, Tai CT, et al. Long-term results of radiofrequency catheter ablation in patients with multiple accessory pathways. *Am J Cardiol* 1996;78:1375–1379.
223. Chugh SS, Chan RC, Johnson SB, Packer DL. Catheter tip orientation affects radiofrequency ablation lesion size in the canine left ventricle. *Pacing Clin Electrophysiol* 1999;22: 413–420.
224. Laohaprasitiporn D, Walsh EP, Saul JP, Triedman JK. Predictors of permanence of successful radiofrequency lesions created with controlled catheter tip temperature. *Pacing Clin Electrophysiol* 1997;20:1283–1291.
225. Nath S, Lynch CD, Whayne JG, Haines DE. Cellular electrophysiological effects of hyperthermia on isolated guinea pig papillary muscle: implications for catheter ablation. *Circulation* 1993;88:1826–1831.
226. Hirao K, Sato T, Otomo K, et al. The response of atrioventricular junctional tissue to temperature. *Jpn Circ J* 1994;58: 351–361.
227. Delacretaz E, Stevenson WG, Winters GL, et al. Ablation of ventricular tachycardia with a saline-cooled radiofrequency catheter: anatomic and histologic characteristics of the lesions in humans. *J Cardiovasc Electrophysiol* 1999;10:860–865.

228. Jais P, Haissaguerre M, Shah DC, et al. Successful irrigated-tip catheter ablation of atrial flutter resistant to conventional radiofrequency ablation [Clinical trial]. *Circulation* 1998;98: 835–838.
229. Strickberger SA, Tokano T, Tse HF, et al. Target temperatures of 48°C versus 60°C during slow pathway ablation: a randomized comparison. *J Cardiovasc Electrophysiol* 1999;10:799–803.
230. Strickberger SA, Zivin A, Daoud EG, et al. Temperature and impedance monitoring during slow pathway ablation in patients with AV nodal reentrant tachycardia [Clinical trial]. *J Cardiovasc Electrophysiol* 1996;7:295–300.
231. Langberg JJ, Calkins H, el-Atassi R, et al. Temperature monitoring during radiofrequency catheter ablation of accessory pathways. *Circulation* 1992;86:1469–1474.
232. Nath S, DiMarco JP, Mounsey JP, et al. Correlation of temperature and pathophysiological effect during radiofrequency catheter ablation of the AV junction [Clinical trial]. *Circulation* 1995;92:1188–1192.
233. Bharati S, Lev M. *The cardiac conduction system in unexplained sudden death.* Mount Kisco, NY: Futura Publishing, 1990.
234. Chiang CE, Chen SA, Wu TJ, et al. Incidence, significance, and pharmacological responses of catheter-induced mechanical trauma in patients receiving radiofrequency ablation for supraventricular tachycardia. *Circulation* 1994;90:1847–1854.
235. King A, Wen MS, Yeh SJ, et al. Catheter-induced atrioventricular nodal block during radiofrequency ablation. *Am Heart J* 1996;132:979–985.
236. Willems S, Shenasa M, Borggrefe M, et al. Unexpected emergence of manifest preexcitation following transcatheter ablation of concealed accessory pathways. *J Cardiovasc Electrophysiol* 1993;4:467–472.
237. Jackman WM, Wang XZ, Friday KJ, et al. Catheter ablation of accessory atrioventricular pathways (Wolff-Parkinson-White syndrome) by radiofrequency current [Clinical trial]. *N Engl J Med* 1991;324:1605–1611.
238. Epstein MR, Knapp LD, Martindill M, et al. Embolic complications associated with radiofrequency catheter ablation. Atakr Investigator Group [Clinical trial]. *Am J Cardiol* 1996;77: 655–658.
239. Friedman PL, Stevenson WG, Kocovic DZ. Autonomic dysfunction after catheter ablation [Review]. *J Cardiovasc Electrophysiol* 1996;7:450–459.
240. Ehlert FA, Goldberger JJ, Brooks R, et al. Persistent inappropriate sinus tachycardia after radiofrequency current catheter modification of the atrioventricular node. *Am J Cardiol* 1992; 69:1092–1095.
241. Kokovic DZ, Harada T, Shea JB, et al. Alterations of heart rate and of heart rate variability after radiofrequency catheter ablation of supraventricular tachycardia: delineation of parasympathetic pathways in the human heart. *Circulation* 1993;88: 1671–1681.
242. Schmitt C, Meyer C, Kosa I, et al. Does radiofrequency catheter ablation induce a deterioration in sympathetic innervation? A positron emission tomography study. *Pacing Clin Electrophysiol* 1998;21:327–330.
243. Kaltenbrunner W, Cardinal R, Dubuc M, et al. Epicardial and endocardial mapping of ventricular tachycardia in patients with myocardial infarction: is the origin of the tachycardia always subendocardially localized? *Circulation* 1991;84:1058–1071.
244. Sosa E, Scanavacca M, D'Avila A, et al. Endocardial and epicardial ablation guided by nonsurgical transthoracic epicardial mapping to treat recurrent ventricular tachycardia [Clinical trial]. *J Cardiovasc Electrophysiol* 1998;9:229–239.
245. Watanabe G, Misaki T, Nakajima K, et al. Thoracoscopic radiofrequency ablation of the myocardium. *Pacing Clin Electrophysiol* 1998;21:553–558.
246. Calkins H, Yong P, Miller JM, et al. Catheter ablation of accessory pathways, atrioventricular nodal reentrant tachycardia, and the atrioventricular junction: final results of a prospective, multicenter clinical trial. The Atakr Multicenter Investigators Group [Clinical trial]. *Circulation* 1999;99:262–270.
247. Kocheril AG, Rosenfeld LE. Radiofrequency ablation of an accessory pathway in a patient with corrected Ebstein's anomaly. *Pacing Clin Electrophysiol* 1994;17:986–990.
248. Mair DD. Ebstein's anomaly: natural history and management [Editorial]. *J Am Coll Cardiol* 1992;19:1047–1048.
249. Porter CJ. Ebstein's anomaly of the tricuspid valve. In: Garson JA, Bricker JT, McNamara DG, eds. *The science and practice of pediatric cardiology.* Philadelphia: Lea & Febiger, 1990:1134.
250. Cappato R, Schluter M, Weiss C, et al. Radiofrequency current catheter ablation of accessory atrioventricular pathways in Ebstein's anomaly. *Circulation* 1996;94:376–383.
251. Reich JD, Auld D, Hulse E, et al. The Pediatric Radiofrequency Ablation Registry's experience with Ebstein's anomaly. Pediatric Electrophysiology Society. *J Cardiovasc Electrophysiol* 1998;9:1370–1377.
252. Fischbach P, Campbell RM, Hulse E, et al. Transhepatic access to the atrioventricular ring for delivery of radiofrequency energy. *J Cardiovasc Electrophysiol* 1997;8:512–516.
253. Dave KS, Pakrashi BC, Wooler GH, Ionescu MI. Atrial septal defect in adults. Clinical and hemodynamic results of surgery. *Am J Cardiol* 1973;31:7–13.
254. Gault JH, Morrow AG, Gay WA, et al. Atrial septal defect in patients over the age of 40. *Circulation* 1968;37:261–272.
255. Kuzman WJ, Yuskis AS. Atrial septal defects in the older patient simulating acquired valvular heart disease. *Am J Cardiol* 1965;15:303.
256. Saksena FB, Aldridge HE. Atrial septal defect in the older patient: a clinical and hemodynamic study in patients operated on after age 35. *Circulation* 1970;42:1009–1020.
257. Neumayer U, Stone S, Somerville J. Small ventricular septal defects in adults. *Eur Heart J* 1998;19:1573–1582.
258. Kulbertus HE, Coyne JJ, Hallidie-Smith KA. Conduction disturbances before and after surgical closure of ventricular septal defect. *Am Heart J* 1969;77:123–131.
259. Vetter VL, Horowitz LN. Electrophysiologic residua and sequelae of surgery for congenital heart defects [Review]. *Am J Cardiol* 1982;50:588–604.
260. Dickens I, Maranhao V, Goldbert H. Right bundle branch block: a vectorcardiographic and electrocardiographic study of ventricular septal defect following open heart surgery. *Circulation* 1959;20:201.
261. Okoroma EO, Guller B, Maloney JD, Weidman WH. Etiology of right bundle-branch block pattern after surgical closure of ventricular-septal defects. *Am Heart J* 1975;90:14–18.
262. Perloff JK. *The clinical recognition of congenital heart disease.* Philadelphia: WB Saunders, 1987.
263. Clark DS, Hirsch HD, Tamer DM, Gelband H. Electrocardiographic changes following surgical treatment of congenital cardiac malformations. *Prog Cardiovasc Dis* 1975;17:451–465.
264. Sasaki R, Theilen EO, January LE. Cardiac arrhythmias associated with the repair of atrial and ventricular septal defects. *Circulation* 1958;18:909–915.
265. Anderson RH, Becker AE. *Pathology of congenital heart disease.* London: Butterworths, 1981.
266. Dietl CA, Cazzaniga ME, Dubner SJ, et al. Life-threatening arrhythmias and RV dysfunction after surgical repair of tetralogy of Fallot: comparison between transventricular and

transatrial approaches [Clinical trial]. *Circulation* 1994;90: II7–II12.
267. Cullen S, Celermajer DS, Franklin RC, et al. Prognostic significance of ventricular arrhythmia after repair of tetralogy of Fallot: a 12-year prospective study. *J Am Coll Cardiol* 1994;23: 1151–1155.
268. Joffe H, Georgakopoulos D, Celermajer DS, et al. Late ventricular arrhythmia is rare after early repair of tetralogy of Fallot. *J Am Coll Cardiol* 1994;23:1146–1150.
269. Ross BA. From the bedside to the basic science laboratory: arrhythmias in Fallot's tetralogy. *J Am Coll Cardiol* 1993;21: 1738–1740.
270. Dreyer WJ, Paridon SM, Fisher DJ, Garson A Jr. Rapid ventricular pacing in dogs with right ventricular outflow tract obstruction: insights into a mechanism of sudden death in postoperative tetralogy of Fallot. *J Am Coll Cardiol* 1993;21: 1731–1737.
271. Murphy JG, Gersh BJ, Mair DD, et al. Long-term outcome in patients undergoing surgical repair of tetralogy of Fallot. *N Engl J Med* 1993;329:593–599.
272. Rosenthal A. Adults with tetralogy of Fallot—repaired, yes; cured, no [Editorial]. *N Engl J Med* 1993;329:655–656.
273. Waien SA, Liu PP, Ross BL, et al. Serial follow-up of adults with repaired tetralogy of Fallot. *J Am Coll Cardiol* 1992;20: 295–300.
274. Chandar JS, Wolff GS, Garson A Jr, et al. Ventricular arrhythmias in postoperative tetralogy of Fallot [Clinical trial]. *Am J Cardiol* 1990;65:655–661.
275. Deanfield JE, Ho SY, Anderson RH, et al. Late sudden death after repair of tetralogy of Fallot: a clinicopathologic study. *Circulation* 1983;67:626–631.
276. James FW, Kaplan S, Chou TC. Unexpected cardiac arrest in patients after surgical correction of tetralogy of Fallot. *Circulation* 1975;52:691–695.
277. Kobayashi J, Hirose H, Nakano S, et al. Ambulatory electrocardiographic study of the frequency and cause of ventricular arrhythmia after correction of tetralogy of Fallot. *Am J Cardiol* 1984;54:1310–1313.
278. Gillette PC, Yeoman MA, Mullins CE, McNamara DG. Sudden death after repair of tetralogy of Fallot: electrocardiographic and electrophysiologic abnormalities. *Circulation* 1977; 56:566–571.
279. Kavey RE, Blackman MS, Sondheimer HM. Incidence and severity of chronic ventricular dysrhythmias after repair of tetralogy of Fallot. *Am Heart J* 1982;103:342–350.
280. Horowitz LN, Vetter VL, Harken AH, Josephson ME. Electrophysiologic characteristics of sustained ventricular tachycardia occurring after repair of tetralogy of Fallot. *Am J Cardiol* 1980;46:446–452.
281. Garson A Jr, Gillette PC, Gutgesell HP, McNamara DG. Stress-induced ventricular arrhythmia after repair of tetralogy of Fallot. *Am J Cardiol* 1980;46:1006–1012.
282. Deanfield JE, McKenna WJ, Presbitero P, et al. Ventricular arrhythmia in unrepaired and repaired tetralogy of Fallot: relation to age, timing of repair, and haemodynamic status. *Br Heart J* 1984;52:77–81.
283. Marie PY, Marcon F, Brunotte F, et al. Right ventricular overload and induced sustained ventricular tachycardia in operatively "repaired" tetralogy of Fallot. *Am J Cardiol* 1992;69: 785–789.
284. Harrison DA, Harris L, Siu SC, et al. Sustained ventricular tachycardia in adult patients late after repair of tetralogy of Fallot. *J Am Coll Cardiol* 1997;30:1368–1373.
285. Gunal N, Tokel K, Kahramanyol O, et al. Incidence and severity of arrhythmias and conduction disturbance after repair of tetralogy of Fallot. *Turk J Pediatr* 1997;39:491–498.
286. Katz NM, Blackstone EH, Kirklin JW, et al. Late survival and symptoms after repair of tetralogy of Fallot. *Circulation* 1982; 65:403–410.
287. Fuster V, McGoon DC, Kennedy MA, et al. Long-term evaluation (12 to 22 years) of open heart surgery for tetralogy of Fallot. *Am J Cardiol* 1980;46:635–642.
288. Driscoll DJ, Offord KP, Feldt RH, et al. Five- to fifteen-year follow-up after Fontan operation. *Circulation* 1992;85: 469–496.
289. Gelatt M, Hamilton RM, McCrindle BW, et al. Risk factors for atrial tachyarrhythmias after the Fontan operation. *J Am Coll Cardiol* 1994;24:1735–1741.
290. Paul T, Ziemer G, Luhmer L, et al. Early and late atrial dysrhythmias after modified Fontan operation. *Pediatr Med Chir* 1998;20:9–11.
291. Mustard WT. Successful two-stage correction of transposition of the great vessels. *Surgery* 1964;55:469–472.
292. Webb GD, McLaughlin PR, Gow RM, Liu PP, Williams WG. Transposition complexes [Review]. *Cardiol Clin* 1993; 11:651–664.
293. Braunstein PW Jr, Sade RM, Gillette PC. Life-threatening postoperative junctional ectopic tachycardia [Review]. *Ann Thorac Surg* 1992;53:726–728.
294. Mair DD, Danielson GK, Wallace RB, McGoon DC. Long-term follow-up of Mustard operation survivors. *Circulation* 1974;50:II46–II53.
295. Garson A Jr, Bink-Boelkens M, Hesslein PS, et al. Atrial flutter in the young: a collaborative study of 380 cases. *J Am Coll Cardiol* 1985;6:871–878.
296. Triedman JK, Saul JP, Weindling SN, Walsh EP. Radiofrequency ablation of intra-atrial reentrant tachycardia after surgical palliation of congenital heart disease. *Circulation* 1995;91: 707–714.
297. Van Hare GF, Lesh MD, Ross BA, et al. Mapping and radiofrequency ablation of intraatrial reentrant tachycardia after the Senning or Mustard procedure for transposition of the great arteries. *Am J Cardiol* 1996;77:985–991.
298. Kugler JD, Danford DA, Deal BJ, et al. Radiofrequency catheter ablation for tachyarrhythmias in children and adolescents. The Pediatric Electrophysiology Society. *N Engl J Med* 1994; 330:1481–1487.
299. Van Hare GF. Radiofrequency ablation of accessory pathways associated with congenital heart disease [Review]. *Pacing Clin Electrophysiol* 1997;20:2077–2081.
300. Shakespeare CF, Anderson M, Camm AJ. Pathophysiology of supraventricular tachycardia. *Eur Heart J* 1993;14:2–8.
301. Swiryn S, Bauernfeind RA, Palileo EA, et al. Electrophysiologic study demonstrating triple antegrade AV nodal pathways in patients with spontaneous and/or induced supraventricular tachycardia. *Am Heart J* 1982;103:168–176.
302. Anselme F, Poty H, Cribier A, et al. Entrainment of typical AV nodal reentrant tachycardia using para-Hisian pacing: evidence for a lower common pathway within the AV node. *J Cardiovasc Electrophysiol* 1999;10:655–661.
303. Kadish A, Goldberg J. Ablative therapy for atrioventricular nodal reentry arrhythmias [Review]. *Prog Cardiovasc Dis* 1996; 37:273.
304. Shah DC, Jais P, Gencel L, et al. Radiofrequency catheter ablation for AV nodal reentrant tachycardias (AVNRT) [Review]. *Indian Heart J* 1996;48:231–239.
305. Sung RJ, Lauer MR, Chun H. Atrioventricular node reentry: current concepts and new perspectives [Review]. *Pacing Clin Electrophysiol* 1994;17:1413–1430.

306. McGuire MA, Janse MJ. New insights on anatomical location of components of the reentrant circuit and ablation therapy for atrioventricular junctional reentrant tachycardia [Review]. *Curr Opin Cardiol* 1995;10:3–8.
307. Racker DK. Atrioventricular node and input pathways: a correlated gross anatomical and histological study of the canine atrioventricular junctional region. *Anat Rec* 1989;224:336–354.
308. Wu D, Yeh SJ, Wang CC, et al. Double loop figure-of-8 reentry as the mechanism of multiple atrioventricular node reentry tachycardias. *Am Heart J* 1994;127:83–95.
309. Spach MS, Josephson ME. Initiating reentry: the role of nonuniform anisotropy in small circuits [Review]. *J Cardiovasc Electrophysiol* 1994;5:182–209.
310. Akhtar M, Jazayeri MR, Sra J, et al. Atrioventricular nodal reentry: clinical, electrophysiological, and therapeutic considerations [Review]. *Circulation* 1993;88:282–295.
311. Fromer M, Shenasa M. Ultrarapid subthreshold stimulation for termination of atrioventricular node reentrant tachycardia. *J Am Coll Cardiol* 1992;20:879–883.
312. Sung RJ, Waxman HL, Saksena S, Juma Z. Sequence of retrograde atrial activation in patients with dual atrioventricular nodal pathways. *Circulation* 1981;64:1059–1067.
313. Tondo C, Beckman KJ, McClelland JH, et al. Response to radiofrequency catheter ablation suggests that the coronary sinus forms part of the reentrant circuit in some patients with atrioventricular nodal reentrant tachycardia [Abstract]. *Circulation* 1996;94[Suppl 1]:2220A.
314. Keim S, Werner P, Jazayeri M, et al. Localization of the fast and slow pathways in atrioventricular nodal reentrant tachycardia by intraoperative ice mapping. *Circulation* 1992;86:919–925.
315. Ross DL, Johnson DC, Denniss AR, et al. Curative surgery for atrioventricular junctional ("AV nodal") reentrant tachycardia [Editorial]. *J Am Coll Cardiol* 1985;6:1383–1392.
316. Chaoui R, Bollmann R, Hoffmann H, Goldner B. Fetal echocardiography: Part III. Fetal arrhythmia [Review]. *Zentralbl Gynakol* 1991;113:1335–1350.
317. Meinertz T, Hofmann T, Zehender M. Can we predict sudden cardiac death? [Review]. *Drugs* 1991;41:9–15.
318. Larsen L, Markham J, Haffajee CI. Sudden death in idiopathic dilated cardiomyopathy: role of ventricular arrhythmias [Review]. *Pacing Clin Electrophysiol* 1993;16:1051–1059.
319. Patterson E, Scherlag BJ. Longitudinal dissociation within the posterior AV nodal input of the rabbit: a substrate for AV nodal reentry. *Circulation* 1999;99:143–155.
320. Yamane T, Iesaka Y, Goya M, et al. Optimal target site for slow AV nodal pathway ablation: possibility of predetermined focal mapping approach using anatomic reference in the Koch's triangle. *J Cardiovasc Electrophysiol* 1999;10:529–537.
321. Denes P, Wu D, Dhingra RC, et al. Demonstration of dual A-V nodal pathways in patients with paroxysmal supraventricular tachycardia. *Circulation* 1973;48:549–555.
322. Ko JK, Deal BJ, Strasburger JF, Benson DW Jr. Supraventricular tachycardia mechanisms and their age distribution in pediatric patients. *Am J Cardiol* 1992;69:1028–1032.
323. Francalanci P, Drago F, Agostino DA, et al. Koch's triangle in pediatric age: correlation with extra- and intracardiac parameters. *Pacing Clin Electrophysiol* 1998;21:1576–1579.
324. Goldberg CS, Caplan MJ, Heidelberger KP, Dick M 2nd. The dimensions of the triangle of Koch in children. *Am J Cardiol* 1999;83:117–120, A9.
325. McGuire MA, Johnson DC, Robotin M, et al. Dimensions of the triangle of Koch in humans. *Am J Cardiol* 1992;70:829–830.
326. Cox JL, Boineau JP, Schuessler RB, et al. Modification of the maze procedure for atrial flutter and atrial fibrillation. I. Rationale and surgical results. *J Thorac Cardiovasc Surg* 1995;110:473–484.
327. Lee R, Nitta T, Schuessler RB, et al. The closed heart MAZE: a nonbypass surgical technique. *Ann Thorac Surg* 1999;67:1696–1702.
328. Antz M, Otomo K, Arruda M, et al. Electrical conduction between the right atrium and the left atrium via the musculature of the coronary sinus. *Circulation* 1998;98:1790–1795.
329. Guiraudon GM, Klein GJ, Yee R, Guiraudon CM. Surgery for supraventricular tachycardia. *Arch Mal Coeur Vaiss* 1996;89:123–127.
330. Hindricks G. The Multicentre European Radiofrequency Survey (MERFS): complications of radiofrequency catheter ablation of arrhythmias. The Multicentre European Radiofrequency Survey (MERFS) investigators of the Working Group on Arrhythmias of the European Society of Cardiology. *Eur Heart J* 1993;14:1644–1653.
331. Zhou L, Keane D, Reed G, Ruskin J. Thromboembolic complications of cardiac radiofrequency catheter ablation: a review of the reported incidence, pathogenesis and current research directions [Review]. *J Cardiovasc Electrophysiol* 1999;10:611–620.
332. Kottkamp H, Hindricks G, Hammel D, et al. Intraoperative radiofrequency ablation of chronic atrial fibrillation: a left atrial curative approach by elimination of anatomic "anchor" reentrant circuits. *J Cardiovasc Electrophysiol* 1999;10:772–780.
333. Avitall B, Hare J, Mughal K, et al. Ablation of atrial fibrillation in a dog model [Abstract]. *J Am Coll Cardiol* 1994;484:276A.
334. Konings KT, Smeets JL, Penn OC, et al. Configuration of unipolar atrial electrograms during electrically induced atrial fibrillation in humans. *Circulation* 1997;95:1231–1241.
335. Kumagai K, Khrestian C, Waldo AL. Simultaneous multisite mapping studies during induced atrial fibrillation in the sterile pericarditis model: insights into the mechanism of its maintenance. *Circulation* 1997;95:511–521.
336. Gaita F, Riccardi R, Calo L, et al. Atrial mapping and radiofrequency catheter ablation in patients with idiopathic atrial fibrillation: electrophysiological findings and ablation results. *Circulation* 1998;97:2136–2145.
337. Baker BM, Smith JM, Cain ME. Nonpharmacologic approaches to the treatment of atrial fibrillation and atrial flutter [Review]. *J Cardiovasc Electrophysiol* 1995;6:972–978.
338. Jais P, Haissaguerre M, Shah DC, et al. A focal source of atrial fibrillation treated by discrete radiofrequency ablation. *Circulation* 1997;95:572–576.
339. Haissaguerre M, Jais P, Shah DC, et al. Right and left atrial radiofrequency catheter therapy of paroxysmal atrial fibrillation. *J Cardiovasc Electrophysiol* 1996;7:1132–1144.
340. Mitchell MA, McRury ID, Everett TH, et al. Morphological and physiological characteristics of discontinuous linear atrial ablations during atrial pacing and atrial fibrillation. *J Cardiovasc Electrophysiol* 1999;10:378–386.
341. Packer D, Johnson S. Comparison of multielectrode catheter versus drag techniques for the creation of linear lesions in canine atrial fibrillation [Abstract]. *Circulation* 1997;96[Suppl I]:575.
342. Roithinger FX, Steiner PR, Goseki Y, et al. Low-power radiofrequency application and intracardiac echocardiography for creation of continuous left atrial linear lesions. *J Cardiovasc Electrophysiol* 1999;10:680–691.
343. Olgin JE, Kalman JM, Chin M, et al. Electrophysiological effects of long, linear atrial lesions placed under intracardiac ultrasound guidance. *Circulation* 1997;96:2715–2721.

344. Anfinsen OG, Kongsgaard E, Foerster A, et al. Bipolar radiofrequency catheter ablation creates confluent lesions at larger interelectrode spacing than does unipolar ablation from two electrodes in the porcine heart. *Eur Heart J* 1998;19: 1075–1084.
345. Mehdirad A, Gaiser J, Baker P, et al. Effect of catheter tip length and position on lesion volume in temperature controlled RF ablation in canine tricuspid valve annulus. *J Interv Card Electrophysiol* 1998;2:279–284.
346. Grumbrecht S, Neuzner J, Pitschner HF. Interrelation of tissue temperature versus flow velocity in two different kinds of temperature controlled catheter radiofrequency energy applications. *J Interv Card Electrophysiol* 1998;2:211–219.
347. Avitall B, Helms RW, Koblish JB, et al. The creation of linear contiguous lesions in the atria with an expandable loop catheter. *J Am Coll Cardiol* 1999;33:972–984.
348. Williamson BD, Man KC, Daoud E, et al. Radiofrequency catheter modification of atrioventricular conduction to control the ventricular rate during atrial fibrillation [published erratum appears in N Engl J Med 1995;332:479]. *N Engl J Med* 1994; 331:910–917.
349. Kunze KP, Schluter M, Geiger M, Kuck KH. Modulation of atrioventricular nodal conduction using radiofrequency current. *Am J Cardiol* 1988;61:657–658.
350. Chen SA, Lee SH, Chiang CE, et al. Electrophysiological mechanisms in successful radiofrequency catheter modification of atrioventricular junction for patients with medically refractory paroxysmal atrial fibrillation [Clinical trial]. *Circulation* 1996;93:1690–701.
351. Kreiner G, Heinz G, Siostrzonek P, Gossinger HD. Effect of slow pathway ablation on ventricular rate during atrial fibrillation. Dependence on electrophysiological properties of the fast pathway. *Circulation* 1996;93:277–283.
352. Garrigue S, Mowrey KA, Fahy G, et al. Atrioventricular nodal conduction during atrial fibrillation: role of atrial input modification. *Circulation* 1999;99:2323–2333.
353. Kay GN, Ellenbogen KA, Giudici M, et al. The Ablate and Pace Trial: a prospective study of catheter ablation of the AV conduction system and permanent pacemaker implantation for treatment of atrial fibrillation. APT Investigators. *J Interv Card Electrophysiol* 1998;2:121–135.
354. Marshall HJ, Harris ZI, Griffith MJ, et al. Prospective randomized study of ablation and pacing versus medical therapy for paroxysmal atrial fibrillation: effects of pacing mode and mode-switch algorithm [Clinical trial]. *Circulation* 1999;99: 1587–1592.
355. Mazgalev TN, Garrigue S, Mowrey KA, et al. Autonomic modification of the atrioventricular node during atrial fibrillation: role in the slowing of ventricular rate. *Circulation* 1999; 99:2806–2814.
356. Daoud EG, Morady F. Pathophysiology of atrial flutter [Review]. *Annu Rev Med* 1998;49:77–83.
357. Arenal A, Almendral J, Alday JM, et al. Rate-dependent conduction block of the crista terminalis in patients with typical atrial flutter: influence on evaluation of cavotricuspid isthmus conduction block [Clinical trial]. *Circulation* 1999;99: 2771–2778.
358. Lesh MD, Van Hare G, Kao AK, Scheinman MM. Radiofrequency catheter ablation for Wolff-Parkinson-White syndrome associated with a coronary sinus diverticulum. *Pacing Clin Electrophysiol* 1991;14:1479–1484.
359. Olgin JE, Kalman JM, Fitzpatrick AP, Lesh MD. Role of right atrial endocardial structures as barriers to conduction during human type I atrial flutter: activation and entrainment mapping guided by intracardiac echocardiography. *Circulation* 1995;92: 1839–1848.
360. Kalman JM, Olgin JE, Saxon LA, et al. The anterior barrier in human atrial flutter: role of the tricuspid annulus [Abstract]. *Circulation* 1995;92:406.
361. Guiraudon GM, Klein GJ, van Hemel N, et al. Atrial flutter: lessons from surgical interventions (musing on atrial flutter mechanism). *Pacing Clin Electrophysiol* 1996;19:1933–1938.
362. Shah DC, Jais P, Haissaguerre M, Chouairi S, et al. Three-dimensional mapping of the common atrial flutter circuit in the right atrium. *Circulation* 1997;96:3904–3912.
363. Anselme F, Saoudi N, Poty H, Douillet R, Cribier A. Radiofrequency catheter ablation of common atrial flutter: significance of palpitations and quality-of-life evaluation in patients with proven isthmus block. *Circulation* 1999;99:534–540.
364. Shah DC, Haissaguerre M, Jais P, et al. Simplified electrophysiologically directed catheter ablation of recurrent common atrial flutter [Clinical trial]. *Circulation* 1997;96:2505–2508.
365. Kirkorian G, Moncada E, Chevalier P, et al. Radiofrequency ablation of atrial flutter: efficacy of an anatomically guided approach. *Circulation* 1994;90:2804–2814.
366. Nakagawa H, Lazzara R, Khastgir T, et al. Role of the tricuspid annulus and the eustachian valve/ridge on atrial flutter. Relevance to catheter ablation of the septal isthmus and a new technique for rapid identification of ablation success. *Circulation* 1996;94:407–424.
367. Cabrera JA, Sanchez-Quintana D, Ho SY, et al. The architecture of the atrial musculature between the orifice of the inferior caval vein and the tricuspid valve: the anatomy of the isthmus. *J Cardiovasc Electrophysiol* 1998;9:1186–1195.
368. Whayne JG, Nath S, Haines DE. Microwave catheter ablation of myocardium in vitro: assessment of the characteristics of tissue heating and injury. *Circulation* 1994;89:2390–2395.
369. Nath S, Haines DE. Biophysics and pathology of catheter energy delivery systems [Review]. *Prog Cardiovasc Dis* 1995;37: 185–204.
370. Inesi G, Millman M, Eletr S. Temperature-induced transitions of function and structure in sarcoplasmic reticulum membranes. *J Mol Biol* 1973;81:483–504.
371. Nath S, DiMarco JP, Haines DE. Basic aspects of radiofrequency catheter ablation [Review]. *J Cardiovasc Electrophysiol* 1994;5:863–876.
372. Idikio HA, Humen DP. Fine structural alterations in radiofrequency energy-induced lesions in dog hearts: possible basis for reduced arrhythmic complications. *Can J Cardiol* 1991;7: 270–274.
373. Leonelli FM, Natale A, W OC. Human histopathologic findings following radiofrequency ablation of the tricuspid–inferior vena cava isthmus. *J Cardiovasc Electrophysiol* 1999;10:599–602.
374. Vassilikos VP, Ho SY, Wong CY, Nathan AW. Recurrence of accessory pathway conduction after successful radiofrequency ablation: histological findings. *J Interv Card Electrophysiol* 1997; 1:311–315.
375. Grubman E, Pavri BB, Lyle S, et al. Histopathologic effects of radiofrequency catheter ablation in previously infarcted human myocardium. *J Cardiovasc Electrophysiol* 1999;10:336–342.
376. Strickberger SA, Daoud EG, Weiss R, et al. A randomized comparison of fixed power and temperature monitoring during slow pathway ablation in patients with atrioventricular nodal reentrant tachycardia [Clinical trial]. *J Interv Card Electrophysiol* 1997;1:299–303.
377. Calkins H, Niklason L, Sousa J, et al. Radiation exposure during radiofrequency catheter ablation of accessory atrioventricular connections. *Circulation* 1991;84:2376–2382.
378. Borbola J. Transcatheter laser ablation of atrioventricular nodal

reentrant tachycardia—do we really need a newer energy source? [Editorial]. *Eur Heart J* 1997;18:357–358.
379. Weber HP, Kaltenbrunner W, Heinze A, Steinbach K. Laser catheter coagulation of atrial myocardium for ablation of atrioventricular nodal reentrant tachycardia: first clinical experience. *Eur Heart J* 1997;18:487–495.
380. He DS, Zimmer JE, Hynynen K, et al. Application of ultrasound energy for intracardiac ablation of arrhythmias. *Eur Heart J* 1995;16:961–966.
381. Strickberger SA, Tokano T, Kluiwstra JU, et al. Extracardiac ablation of the canine atrioventricular junction by use of high-intensity focused ultrasound [Clinical trial]. *Circulation* 1999;100:203–208.
382. Liem LB, Mead RH. Microwave linear ablation of the isthmus between the inferior vena cava and tricuspid annulus. *Pacing Clin Electrophysiol* 1998;21:2079–2086.
383. Tardif JC, Groeneveld PW, Wang PJ, et al. Intracardiac echocardiographic guidance during microwave catheter ablation. *J Am Soc Echocardiogr* 1999;12:41–47.
384. Lin JC. Catheter microwave ablation therapy for cardiac arrhythmias. *Bioelectromagnetics* 1999;[Suppl 4]:120–132.
385. Nevels RD, Arndt GD, Raffoul GW, et al. Microwave catheter design. *IEEE Trans Biomed Eng* 1998;45:885–890.
386. Dubuc M, Talajic M, Roy D, et al. Feasibility of cardiac cryoablation using a transvenous steerable electrode catheter. *J Interv Card Electrophysiol* 1998;2:285–292.
387. Rodriguez LM, Leunissen J, Hoekstra A, et al. Transvenous cold mapping and cryoablation of the AV node in dogs: observations of chronic lesions and comparison to those obtained using radiofrequency ablation. *J Cardiovasc Electrophysiol* 1998;9:1055–1061.
388. Hoekstra A, de Langen CD, Nikkels PG, et al. Prediction of lesion size through monitoring the 0°C isothermic period following transcatheter cryoablation. *J Interv Card Electrophysiol* 1998;2:383–389.

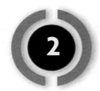

ORGANIZATION OF THE INTERVENTIONAL LABORATORY

• • •

DAVID E. ADAMS

◉ GENERAL LABORATORY AND STAFFING REQUIREMENTS

Personnel, equipment needs, types of studies, and facility construction must all be considered in organizing the interventional laboratory for clinical electrophysiologic studies. Addressing these concerns affects the safety, quality, and efficiency of any study or procedure performed. The interventional laboratory must be set up to accommodate a variety of needs, including conventional arrhythmia studies, ablation therapy, and device implantation. Certain aspects must be addressed regardless of the type of procedure being performed. Table 2-1 summarizes many of these common factors. Table 2-2 summarizes the North American Society of Pacing and Electrophysiology (NASPE) recommendations on cardiac ablation, especially those concerning personnel, facilities, and x-ray equipment (1). This set of guidelines is key to ensuring that cardiac ablations can be safely performed. Practitioners also must understand some of the theory behind the technologies used in the interventional laboratory. This chapter addresses these points and explains the basic theories of the technologies involved.

The most important aspect for performing safe, high-quality, and efficient studies is the presence of dedicated and adequately trained personnel. The numbers of personnel present and the roles they perform directly affect the facility size and equipment that are needed. In most situations, two physicians are required. The first is the primary electrophysiologist, who oversees the procedure; the second is a physician

TABLE 2-1 • GENERAL REQUIREMENTS

Patient
1. Subject to long, anxiety-producing, uncomfortable procedures
2. Exposed to hazards of radiography, invasive procedures, and drugs that alter conscious state, sensation, sympathetic activity, vascular tone, cardiac contractility, and myocardial electrical activity

Physician
1. Acquire and analyze electrophysiology data
2. Monitor interventions and effect on patient
3. Deal with any consequences of procedure
4. Provide appropriate management of patient

Nursing
1. Keep patient comfortable and reduce anxiety
2. Monitor vital signs
3. Administer drugs
4. Defibrillate or otherwise provide rescue support
5. Collect data from study

General
1. Minimize time of procedures
2. Maintain sterile environment
3. Minimize cost of procedure
4. Maximize safety of procedure

TABLE 2-2 • SUMMARY OF NASPE POLICY ON ABLATION LABORATORY REQUIREMENTS

Personnel Needs
  Physician
    (1) Certified electrophysiologist trained in catheter ablation
    (1) Physician or fellow adept at catheter manipulation
  Laboratory
    (1) Nurse or physician assistant to administer sedation and monitor patient
    (1) Nurse or technician to perform tasks related to ablation
Facilities
  Room
    a. Set up for invasive electrophysiologic studies
    b. Equipped to handle acute coronary complications (e.g., thrombus, spasm, cardiac tamponade)
  Support
    a. Cardiac surgical team
    b. Facilities for percutaneous transluminal coronary angioplasty
    c. Temporary and permanent pacemaker implantation
X-ray Requirements
  a. Minimum of rotatable C arm; biplane desirable but not necessary
  b. Video recording system of fluoroscopic images recommended
  c. State-of-the-art equipment to minimize radiation exposure
General Recommendations
  Devices used for ablation procedures should be used in a manner that conforms to hospital, local, and national regulations governing their application.

TABLE 2-3 • LIST OF EQUIPMENT

Emergency
  Defibrillators (2) with monitor (hands-free type)
  Temporary pacemaker
Vital Signs
  Surface electrocardiogram (physiologic recorder)
  Intraarterial pressure (physiologic recorder)
  Automatic blood pressure (noninvasive)
  Pulse oximeter
  Activated clotting time monitor (when heparin is given)
Miscellaneous
  Intravenous pumps
  Custom connecting cables
  Transport monitor
Data Recording
  Physiologic recording system
  Stimulator and isolators
  Radiograph with video storage
  Computer
Ablation
  Ablation generator
  Computer to run monitoring software

From Adams DE. Setting up the laboratory for ablation. In: Zipes, DP, ed. *Catheter ablation of arrhythmias.* Armonk, NY: Futura, 1994:83, with permission.

or fellow, who manipulates catheters. Adequate monitoring allows clinicians to follow catheter movement and the display of important data. Sedation of the patient is recommended, and a nurse or physician assistant administers the appropriate medications and monitors vital signs. A fourth person, a nurse or nurse-technician, performs other related tasks that are necessary during the procedure, including gathering data and providing appropriate supplies for the procedure. Room size must accommodate the movement of these four people as well as house the x-ray system and other needed equipment.

◉ LABORATORY EQUIPMENT

The equipment needed to conduct an electrophysiology study falls into several categories. Table 2-3 lists the minimum equipment required to perform the variety of studies encountered in the laboratory. Each device is grouped according to the type of function it performs.

Emergency rescue or life support equipment is the first category that is addressed. A functioning direct current (DC) defibrillator with monitor is required during all studies. A wide variety of commercially available units can provide adequate rescue capabilities. Regardless of the manufacturer, a hands-free, electrode patch system is preferred (2). One gelled patch is placed under the right scapula and the other on the left side at the level of the ventricular apex. A long patient cable connects the patches directly to the defibrillator. QRS synchronization can be provided by signals recorded from the patch or from a signal output from the physiologic recorder. This type of system provides excellent contact at the discharge surface, limits human intervention to the discharging of the defibrillator, and helps to maintain a sterile field. Because this is a frequently used rescue device, an identical defibrillator or one that can use the same patch system is recommended. A temporary pacemaker is also necessary for bradycardic situations. It serves as a backup to the laboratory stimulator and can be used during patient transportation.

Patient sedation is required because of the length of many procedures and the discomfort the patient encounters. Equipment is needed to monitor vital signs such as cardiac rhythm, blood pressure, and oxygen (O_2) saturation. The cardiac rhythm is usually displayed in several locations, including the physiologic recorder and the defibrillator system. The physiologic recorder usually provides conditioning for intraarterial pressures. The pressure channels must provide for single-step, electronic balancing and calibration of the pressure transducer. This is critical if adjustments in the transducer level must be made during the procedure. The pressure waveforms are displayed on the recorder's monitor along with digital displays of the systolic, diastolic, and mean pressure values. Some type of automatic, noninvasive blood pressure system is useful as a supplement to the intracardiac transducer. This provides a noninvasive means of pressure measurement when an intracardiac pressure is not needed. A pulse oximeter is used to monitor the patient's O_2 level (3). It is portable and can be easily located on a cart with other equipment. An activated clotting time (ACT) monitor determines clotting times when heparin is being given.

In the category of miscellaneous equipment, three items are listed in Table 2-3. For transporting the patient, the portable transport monitor allows observation of a minimal number of vital signs while the patient is being moved to his or her room and is still under the effects of sedation from the procedure. Rate-controlled drugs that are needed during the procedure are administered by the intravenous pumps. Custom connecting cables are essential items that are often overlooked. Many of the ablation catheters require extensions that are not available commercially to connect to recording systems. Cables are also needed to connect equipment together so that their outputs can be recorded.

The final two categories in Table 2-3 involve equipment to record data and provide the ablation energy. These devices are discussed in the following sections.

Recording Equipment

The physiologic recorder is the central device in the electrophysiology laboratory. It collects, stores, and displays all appropriate data; allows analysis of these data; and provides the requisite monitoring of the patient's vital signs. It can improve study efficiency and reduce procedure times if it performs all required tasks dependably. Special features and the minimum requirements to function as a useful tool during electrophysiology procedures are listed in Table 2-4.

The recorder must provide for display of a large number of input channels. Twelve surface leads allow the physician to monitor all characteristics of the surface electrocardiogram (ECG) (4). To eliminate the need for an external ECG machine, the signals of surface leads can be outputed to a printer. Twenty-four intracardiac channels allow viewing and analysis of the large number of electrograms that are required during many electrophysiologic procedures (5). This is especially true for some catheters that are used during ablation. Two pressure channels allow simultaneous monitoring of intracardiac pressures from different sites and provide for backup in case of a breakdown. Ground-referenced, single-ended, high-level signals are inputted and recorded by the DC channels. The output signals of external equipment fall into this category. DC channels are often overlooked by users and manufacturers. Ablation parameters such as power, temperature, and impedance can be recorded through these inputs. It can be difficult to determine radiofrequency energy initiation and performance without these channels displayed on the recorder. This arrangement also allows changes in electrograms to be viewed on the same screen on which the ablation signals are seen. Signal output from device programmers (e.g., intracardiac electrograms, marker channels) can be recorded through the DC inputs. This is critical if the laboratory is used to implant and test devices.

Table 2-4 lists essential input characteristics. All inputs must contain filtering to eliminate the noise generated by the radiofrequency energy used in ablations. This includes wavelengths around 500 kilohertz (kHz), the most commonly used frequency. Without this radiofrequency filtering, the surface and intracar-

TABLE 2-4 • PHYSIOLOGIC RECORDER: MINIMUM REQUIREMENTS

Input Types
  12 surface electrocardiographic leads
  24 intracardiac leads
  2 pressure channels
  4 direct current (DC) channels (high-level, single-ended, ground-referenced)
Output Types
  16 high-level outputs
Input Characteristics
  Radiofrequency filtered
  All but DC channels should be isolated and defibrillation-protected
  Adjustable low- and high-frequency filter settings
  Adjustable gain or input range settings
Display
  Large-screen, high-resolution, color display—multiple monitors desirable
  Main screen should display traces with labels, heart rate, pressure, stimulator connections
  Should be able to adjust channel gain and position from display screen and a setup screen
  Slave monitor for physician placing catheters
Features
  Separate amplifier module to allow remote location from rest of recorder
  User-friendly, computer-based switching of catheter poles for recording and stimulation
  Screen-based setup for channels acquired, displayed, gains, filter settings, limits, labeling, and coloring
  Optical storage of study data and some database to track patient studies stored on optical disks
  Efficient retrieval and display of acquired study traces
  Electronic calipers for making time measurements and comparisons
  Laser printer to print desired intervals of waveforms
  Minimum of 1-kHz sampling rate per channel and 10-bit resolution
  Capable of displaying all signal information (not just every *n*th data point)

From Adams DE. Setting up the laboratory for ablation. In Zipes DP, ed. *Catheter ablation of arrhythmias.* Armonk, NY: Futura, 1994:86, with permission.

diac signals are buried in bands of noise and are rendered unreadable. As with any cardiac monitor, all inputs are defibrillator protected and isolated from the power line ground. The DC inputs' grounding and other circuitry must be isolated from the other amplifier inputs that connect to the patient. If not, the power ground of the external signals can nullify the patient's isolation and provide a path for unsafe leakage or fault currents. Isolated patient inputs are never to be used to amplify and display external, ground-referenced signals (6–8).

Computer-based recorders provide a host of features that produce a user-friendly, orderly display of all the essential signals required to perform an electrophysiologic study (Fig. 2-1). Features can be modified as changes dictate, because programs determine most functions. Modular systems contribute even more versatility to the recording system. Modules are easily substituted when problems arise.

The patient junction boxes provide the interface to connect the wide variety of catheters to the amplifier. Excessive patient cable lengths contribute to floor clutter and interfere with recorded signals. These cable lengths should be minimized and routed close to the patient to ensure noise-free recordings and safety in moving around the patient. Remote amplifiers placed close to the patient table are an ideal solution. Manual switches on the patient junction box are employed by some systems to select which catheter poles are recorded and which are used to stimulate. A better solution is provided by computerized recorders. This setup allows electronic switching controlled by the operator at the main console. The main physician can easily check the setup for correctness and be assured that he or she is monitoring the desired signals.

The remote amplifier contains all the necessary electronics to process signals arriving at its inputs. All signals are provided with defibrillator protection and radiofrequency filtering before they are routed to the computer-controlled switching circuitry. The signals are then amplified, filtered for information content, and digitized for transmission to the main computer. The digitizing of patient data has produced extensive improvements in the acquisition, storage, presentation, and analysis of electrophysiology information.

Understanding the digitization process is essential for any physician relying on this type of system. By its nature, only samples at given intervals are stored. Figure 2-2 illustrates an ECG with samples taken at the encircled times. Each sample is taken at a fixed time interval. For the rate shown, there are plenty of samples for the baseline and the slower-moving P and T waves. The QRS does not have enough samples to adequately represent or reproduce its portion of

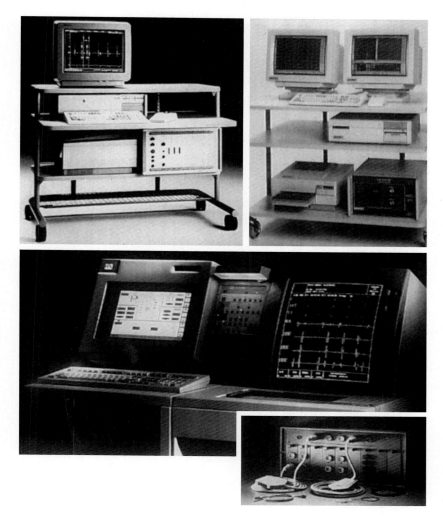

FIGURE 2-1. Three examples of computer-based physiologic recorders. The top two systems are modular systems. All systems use large monitors to display the electrophysiology traces.

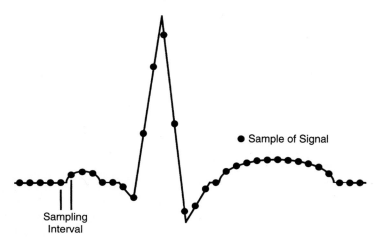

FIGURE 2-2. A digitally sampled waveform. Each sample is taken at the set sample interval. The sample interval must be small enough to ensure adequate reproduction of the signal. In this example, information in the QRS would be lost because of inadequate sampling rate.

the signal. To truly represent the signal, more samples must be taken using shorter sampling intervals. The sampling rate is crucial to ensure that important information is not lost. It is related to sampling interval by the following formula:

$$\text{Sampling rate} = 1/\text{Sampling interval}$$

The Nyquist sampling theory describes the signal-digitizing conditions that ensure adequate reproduction of a waveform with minimal signal loss. The signal must be digitized at a sampling rate twice the signal's highest frequency content. For electrophysiology, a signal must be sampled at a 1-kHz sampling rate for the required high-end frequency response of 500 Hz, minimizing the signal loss of most intracardiac signals (9,10). Physiologic recorders must sample many channels to acquire and display all the required data. Physical restrictions on digitizing hardware make it difficult or expensive to sample all channels simultaneously. Each channel must be sampled after some delay. Figure 2-3 demonstrates two methods typically used to satisfy these requirements. Method A shows each of channels 1 through 4 being sampled at a set frequency (i.e., sample interval), followed by a longer delay until the process repeats itself. The sum of these sample intervals and the delay makes up the channel interval. The sample interval is usually the maximum speed at which the converter can operate, minimizing skew (i.e., time delay error) between channels. The delay makes up the timing difference to bring each channel's sample rate to the desired timing period. This is represented by the following formula:

$$\text{Channel interval} = [(\text{Number of channels} - 1) \times \text{Sample interval}] + \text{Delay interval}$$

This requires special hardware to generate the required timing intervals. Method B illustrates an easier method to implement in the hardware. Only one sampling interval is used, and it is calculated by using the following formula:

$$\text{Sample interval} = \text{Channel interval}/\text{Number of channels}$$

Of the two approaches, method A illustrates the preferred sampling scheme. Timing measurement errors between channels are kept to a minimum while the channel interval is maintained. Researchers and practitioners must understand how the digitized data are represented. Table 2-5 describes how samples are stored in the computer. Each sample is converted to a number in binary format that includes a given number of bits (1 or 0). This number of bits determines how many different voltage levels (i.e., dynamic range) can be represented and the minimum resolution that can be measured. The table assumes a measurement range of -10 millivolts (mV) to $+10$ mV. With a 10-bit converter, 1,024 different voltage levels can be discerned with the minimum measured voltage level, or resolution, of 19.5 μV. By increasing the number of bits to 12, 4,096 levels can be realized with a resolution of 4.88 μV. The more bits are added, the more precisely measurements can be made. However, increased cost and slower converter times are associated with more bits. A minimum 10-bit analog-to-digital converter is recommended (11).

Once digitized, the signals are further processed to select gains and filter settings before being transmitted to the computer. The computer buffers the data, streaming them to the optical disk drive while simultaneously formatting for display and retrieving the data when review is desired. This is simpler and more

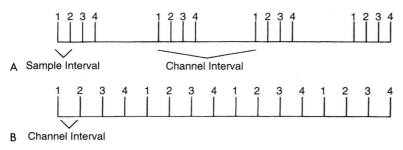

FIGURE 2-3. Two types of multiple channel-sampling methods. Method A minimizes the skew between channels (i.e., time delay error). A constant channel interval is maintained by adding a calculated delay after all channels are sampled. Method B is easier to implement but adds a set time delay error between each channel.

TABLE 2-5 • ANALOG TO DIGITAL CONVERSION

	Analog To Digital Conversion Values			
	10 Bit		12 Bit	
Input Voltage	Decimal	Binary	Decimal	Binary
−10.0 mV	−512	10 0000 0000	−2048	1000 0000 0000
−5.0 mV	−256	11 0000 0000	−1024	1100 0000 0000
−1.0 mV	−51	11 1100 1100	−204	1111 0011 0100
−19.5 μV (approx.)	−1	11 1111 1111	−4	1111 1111 1100
−4.88 μV (approx.)			−1	1111 1111 1111
0.0	0	11 0000 0000	0	0000 0000 0000
4.88 μV (approx.)			1	0000 0000 0001
19.5 μV (approx.)	1	00 0000 0001	4	0000 0000 0100
1.0 mV	51	00 0011 0011	204	0000 1100 1100
5.0 mV	256	01 0000 0000	1024	0100 0000 0000
10.0 mV	511	01 1111 1111	2047	0111 1111 1111

efficient than searching through rolls of tracings from a paper writer. Control of the display, analog output setup parameters, and responding to user inputs encompass the remainder of the computer's function.

Signal traces and other information are displayed on large, high-resolution, color monitors. Some systems use multiple monitors to ensure a full screen of real-time patient monitoring, and another screen is used for analysis or setup. The main screen displays the traces in different colors with labels, shows digital heart rate and blood pressure, and contains the menus to run the entire system. A trace's placement and size can be controlled from the main screen while current data are being monitored. Selection of catheter connections to the stimulator is changed and displayed. Different modes of operation are selected along with their appropriate display screens. This allows viewing of current data, review of stored data for analysis or comparison, and changing of system setup parameters. If the system uses one monitor, the screen is split between current data and the analysis or setup screen. In the analysis mode, electronic calipers measure time intervals between periods of interest. These measured points can be stored and reviewed as needed. Fixed time intervals can be stored on the calipers as parallel lines and compared with future intervals. Setup of recording channels and stimulator outputs is accomplished with on-screen programming instead of clumsy mechanical switchboxes. This allows convenient monitoring of the setup by the primary physician and increases efficiency. Catheter pole connections are easily routed to appropriate recording channels and stimulus isolator outputs. Parameters such as channels acquired, traces displayed, gains, filters, limits, labeling, and coloring are set and displayed on screen.

It is desirable to control the parameters for each channel individually. On many systems, they are controlled as blocks of channels. Unfortunately, this forces the user to set one block of channels for each type of signal recorded (i.e., bipolar and unipolar). This requires two blocks of intracardiac channels to record only two different signal types. The operator must access his or her recording needs to ensure that enough channels are provided for all situations. Enough intracardiac channels must exist to exploit some of the multipole ablation catheters that are in use today. Most systems provide a means to output the conditioned patient waveforms as high-level signals. The operator selects up to 16 recorder channels to link to the analog outputs. Intracardiac or surface leads can be routed to a stimulator's sense input or a defibrillator's ECG input, providing different sensing capabilities as needed.

Of special concern is the monitor's ability to display all pertinent deflection information. Even large, high-resolution displays have a limited number of horizontal data points that can display information. After the areas that are used for display configuration are removed, as few as 1,000 points may be left to display data. At a sample rate of 1 kHz, only 1 second of data could be displayed by plotting every point. To display more time, such as 2 seconds of data, only one half of the data points could be plotted. Instead of just displaying every other data point, an algorithm must exist to analyze all deflection information and ensure that it is reflected accurately in the traces on the screen.

A laser printer provides printouts of appropriate data when needed for charts or reports. All of these capabilities eliminate the need to record traces to a paper writer. This eliminates the cost of expensive photosensitive paper and the need for large storage areas to warehouse the recorded traces. The clumsiness of paper as a measurement tool is supplanted by the convenience of on-screen cursors.

Physiologic Stimulator

A programmable stimulator plays a key role in all electrophysiology studies. Precise timing pulses are generated in complex intervals and isolated as constant current pulses to stimulate the heart. The stimulator is used to induce arrhythmias and measure electrical characteristics of the conduction system. Table 2-6 lists the basic requirements of a stimulator as used in the interventional laboratory (12).

Multiple stimuli should be available. The S1 pulse provides basic pacing alone or as a group of train pulses. The end of the train triggers the remaining stimuli, S2 through S5. Four extra stimuli have proven adequate for clinical induction of arrhythmias. Pulse timing and width parameters are shown in the Table 2-6. Single-output stimulators can be used, but multiple-output devices allow multiple sites to be paced without changing the threshold levels. This results in more efficient pacing and removes any confusion about the appropriate threshold level at the different pacing sites.

A variety of pacing modes allows complete testing in the laboratory. Incremental pacing for atrioventricular and ventriculoatrial conduction determination is achieved by using the synchronous pacing mode. Arrhythmia induction is accomplished with synchronous pacing with prematures or sensing with prematures. These various modes are also used for verifying the location of accessory pathways (13). The delay from trigger pacing modes allows synchronization of the first beat of the train with a selected portion of the cardiac cycle. Burst mode is useful in interrupting some tachycardias and for inducing fibrillation. Figure 2-4 illustrates the timing sequence for the modes mentioned in Table 2-6.

Imaging System

The NASPE policy committee was particularly concerned with radiation exposure because of the length of the procedures and the time the patient and laboratory personnel are exposed to x-rays. Radiation exposure is especially a concern when older systems are in operation. Beam scatter and control can be a problem, and higher tube currents are used to enhance poor image quality. These factors lead to inappropriate levels of radiation exposure. If older systems are used, they must be properly maintained, calibrated, and fre-

TABLE 2-6 • STIMULATOR SPECIFICATIONS

Stimuli
 S1 (200–2000 msec cycle lengths)
 S2–S5 (10–1000 msec delay)
 0.1–9.9 msec duration (2 msec is the most common setting)
 0.1–10.0 mA amplitude (constant current)
 2–4 output channels
Modes
 Pace asynchronous
 Pace asynchronous with train/prematures
 Pace synchronous
 Delay from trigger pace synchronous with train/prematures
 Atrioventricular sequential
 Burst
 Sense with train/prematures
Other Features
 Digital sense rate display
 Digital burst rate display
 Stimuli/output switch matrix
 Train length selection
 Digital display of train count
 Pause length selection

Adapted from Adams DE. Setting up the laboratory for ablation. In Zipes DP, ed. *Catheter ablation of arrhythmias.* Armonk, NY: Futura, 1994:89, with permission.

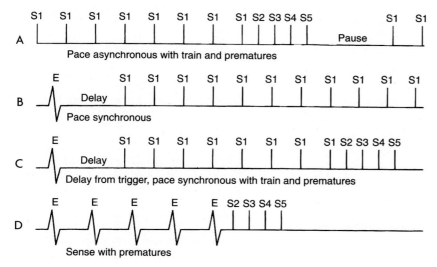

FIGURE 2-4. Examples of stimulation patterns. **A:** Asynchronous pacing with a train and prematures. The train of eight beats begins when the operator presses a start button. The final S1 pulse triggers the S2 delay period and then each of the other prematures, with a pause occurring after the last premature (in this case, S5). **B:** Synchronous pacing and pacing that begins at a set interval into the cardiac cycle. **C:** Start of a pacing train with prematures after a trigger and set delay. This allows the first paced beats to occur at a set time in the cardiac cycle. **D:** Prematures shown are triggered from a train of sensed beats.

quently checked for safety compliance. It is recommended that a state-of-the-art unit be used to eliminate these problems. Newer fluoroscopy systems have superior imaging capabilities. To allow mapping, a C arm is the minimally acceptable system, and a biplane configuration is desirable. The biplane arrangement decreases mapping times by minimizing the need to move the C arm, permitting simultaneous viewing of two planes. A video chain with digital capture or some type of printer allows documentation of catheter placements. Previous views can be compared with the views of later placements. A main monitor and slave monitor allow physicians to easily observe the movement of catheters.

Computer Requirements

A final piece of data acquisition equipment is a desktop computer in the laboratory. The computer can be based on any of the popular graphically based operating systems such as the Mac OS, Windows, or OS/2 Warp. All of these systems are fairly easy to learn and use. A wide variety of laboratory documentation needs can be satisfied with only a word processor and spreadsheet application. Laboratory data can be entered, reviewed, and printed. Forms are stored and printed as needed for informed patient consent. Figure 2-5 illustrates two spreadsheets designed to record data. The spreadsheet in Figure 2-5A is a pharmacologic log sheet that tracks all drugs administered to the patient. The spreadsheet in Figure 2-5B is an radiofrequency ablation log to track the number of radiofrequency burns, any measured parameters, and comments. Both screens display their information in easy-to-read format and can be printed after completion of the case for documentation.

Figures 2-6 and 2-7 illustrate a custom database that is used to track a wide variety of data sets for all types of procedures in the laboratory. Each panel represents a separate screen. Each screen can easily be called from any other screen. The screen in Figure 2-6A gives general information about the patient and lists any studies that have been performed. The screens in Figures 2-6B–D record different measurements that are made during the case. The screens in Figures 2-7A and 2-7B allow the tracking of all drugs administered during the study. For an ablation, the screens in Figures 2-7C and 2-7D record radiofrequency parameters and any comments. Fluoroscopy times are monitored and can be updated from any screen. The screen in Figure 2-6B shows a variety of reports that can be generated and printed.

Other convenient tools are a local area network (LAN) and a file server to store reports and other patient-related documents. The LAN provides a communication channel between the server and the laboratory or other related computers. The server is

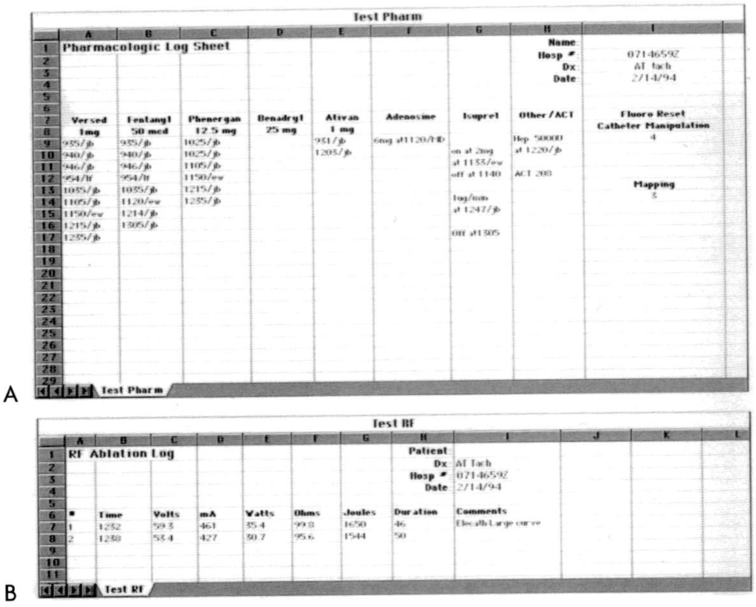

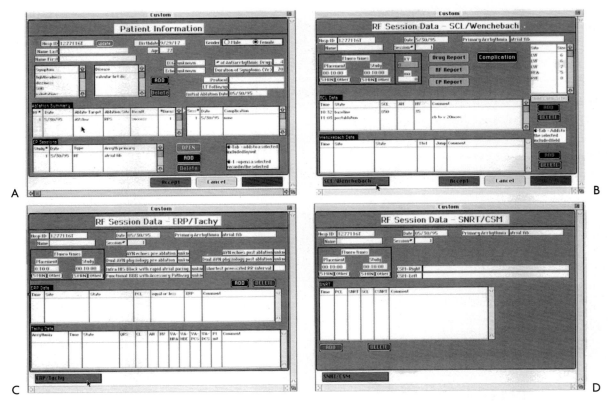

FIGURE 2-5. Two spreadsheets used to record information during an ablation. **A:** The spreadsheet logs all drugs administered during the study. **B:** The spreadsheet logs ablation interactions. Both screens can be saved as computer files and printed for placement in charts.

FIGURE 2-6. The first four screens of an electrophysiology study database. **A:** Screen A displays general patient information, any studies that have been performed, and a summary of any ablation sessions. **B and C:** These screens allow the entry and display of conduction system measurements. **D:** Catheter sites and fluoroscopy times are also recorded. A variety of reports can be generated by selecting the correct "button" on screen B.

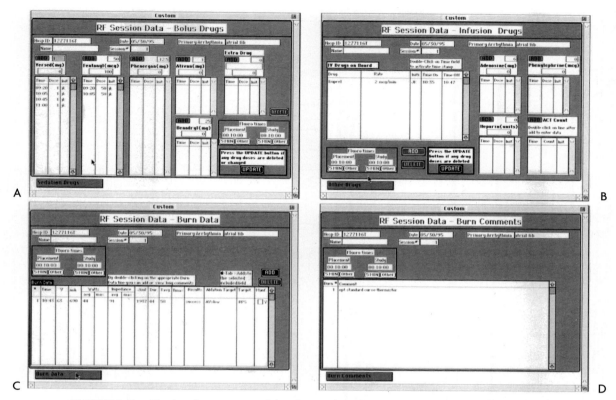

FIGURE 2-7. The last four screens of the electrophysiology study database. **A and B:** Screens A and B allow the tracking of pharmacologic agents administered to the patient. Separate doses are displayed along with totals for each drug and the nurse's initials. Activated clotting time (ACT) counts are recorded if heparin is being given. **C and D:** Screens C and D allow the entry and display of all ablation parameters and associated comments.

a computer with one or more disk drives to allow common storage areas that are accessible to any user who has a valid account. This allows remote retrieval of information at distant locations any time it is needed. This information can include past electrophysiology reports, discharge notes, or other documents that can aid in a study being performed.

Equipment Needs for Ablation

Catheter ablation has emerged as an important therapeutic tool for the management of patients with sustained supraventricular arrhythmias. Although DC energy can be used, radiofrequency energy sources are the primary mode of therapy (14–16). In general, these systems consist of an energy source, controls for this source, and a switching mechanism that allows the catheter tip to record electrograms or deliver energy. The following descriptions are examples of the functions that are implemented in a given device.

Direct Current Ablation

DC ablation is rarely used in modern laboratories, usually for ventricular ablation. No commercial devices are available for DC ablation, but modifying and manufacturing the needed equipment to perform these procedures are straightforward operations. All modifications and custom devices must be made by in-house engineering staff, be approved by the hospital and any other local authority (e.g., the institutional review board committee), and meet national regulations such as those covering leakage currents and patient isolation. A DC defibrillator serves as the energy source.

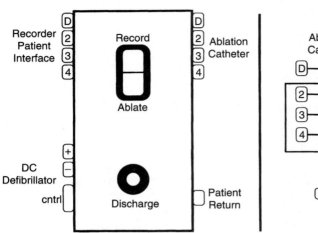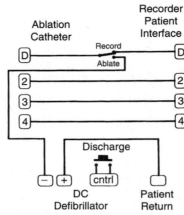

FIGURE 2-8. A simple switchbox allows the delivery of defibrillator energy as a source of ablation. (From Adams DE. Setting up the laboratory for ablation. In: Zipes DP, ed. *Catheter ablation of arrhythmias.* Armonk, NY: Futura, 1994, with permission.)

An extra paddle set is obtained, and the paddles are removed. The cathodal and anodal wires of the defibrillator output circuit and a pair of wires that engage the discharge circuit are exposed and can be wired to the DC ablation switchbox. Figure 2-8 illustrates a simple switchbox and the associated circuitry. The record/ablate switch's amperage rating is selected to handle currents delivered by the defibrillator. The cathode wire is soldered to the ablate position terminal on the ablate switch. The anode wire is soldered to the patient return connector. The distal catheter connection is soldered to the common terminal on the ablate switch; the other poles' connectors are wired to the appropriate recorder connectors. The record switch position terminal is soldered to the distal recorder connection. The ablate switch is set to ablate, and all personnel must be clear of the patient before the defibrillator is discharged.

Radiofrequency Ablation

Radiofrequency catheter ablation is the preferred method of therapy. Several systems are commercially available in the United States, including the EPT Cardiac Ablation Controller (EP Technologies, Inc., Sunnyvale, CA), the Medtronic Cardiorhythm Atakr Ablation System (Medtronic, Inc., Minneapolis, MN), and the Radionics Lesion Generator (Radionics, Inc. Burlington, MA). All three systems are shown in Figure 2-9. Table 2-7 describes several characteristics that all ablation systems should have.

Radiofrequency generators use an unmodified sinusoid in, with a frequency in the 500-kHz range (17). Heat generation during the ablation results from resistive heating of the myocardium and depends on

TABLE 2-7 • RADIOFREQUENCY GENERATOR: MINIMUM SPECIFICATIONS

General
  Radiofrequency (RF) output frequency (500-kHz sine wave)
  RF power delivery (50 W maximum)
  RF time setpoints (1–120 sec)
  Impedance limits for shutdown (40–50 Ω minimum and 250–300 Ω maximum)
  Appropriate safety features to limit maximum power and temperature as needed
  Digital display of time, measured power, measured impedance, and temperature
  Digital display of number of burns
  Patient interface with automatic switching of distal pole
  Analog outputs of power, impedance, and temperature signals
  Serial ASCII data output of power, impedance, and temperature values

Power Control
  RF power set points (1–50 W in 1-W increments)
  Digital display of power and time set points

Temperature Control
  Temperature set point (40–95°C in 1-degree increments)
  Digital display of temperature and time set points

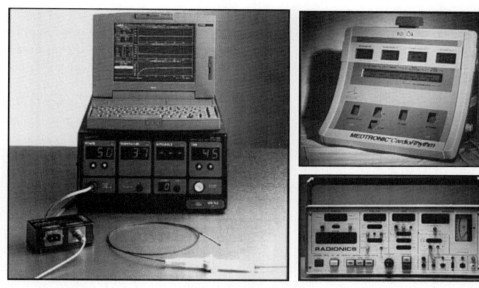

FIGURE 2-9. Three commercially available radiofrequency generator systems.

the current flow of the radiofrequency signal through the tissue (18,19). A tissue temperature of approximately 50°C must be achieved for irreversible injury to occur (19,20). Catheter-tip temperatures of 100°C or higher can cause formation of coagulum on the electrode tip, leading to an abrupt impedance rise, an abrupt fall in delivered current, and a severe decrease in tissue heating (19,21). This event necessitates removal of the catheter, cleaning of the tip, reintroduction of the catheter, and repositioning at the ablation target. To prevent the problem, several parameters must be monitored to ensure that a safe and efficacious ablation occurs. Traditionally, these measures included impedance, power, and time (22). Because of the importance of tissue temperature during radiofrequency ablation, temperature monitoring has been proposed as a measured parameter that can facilitate catheter ablation by ensuring adequate lesion formation, optimizing lesion size, and preventing coagulum formation on the catheter tip (19,21,23). Of these measured values, temperature has emerged as the primary parameter of importance. Tissue temperature is directly related to the success or failure of the ablation attempt because thermal injury is the primary mechanism of myocardial injury (19,20,24).

Figure 2-10 describes in simplified block diagrams the circuitry needed to monitor the appropriate radiofrequency parameters. Voltage, current, and temperature are measured, and all other parameters are generated. In Figure 2-10A, amplifier A1 uses a high-impedance voltage divider to measure a fraction of the radiofrequency voltage across the outputs. This is isolated, converted to a root-mean-square (RMS) value, and scaled to an appropriate level. The RMS signal has a very-low-frequency waveform and can be easily displayed or digitized at low sampling intervals. Amplifier A2 samples the radiofrequency current by using the current sensing resistor or sometimes a coil placed around the return. This signal is also isolated, converted to an RMS value, and scaled. A thermistor is used to measure temperature at the catheter tip. Amplifier A3 isolates the signal, converts the change in resistance to a linearized voltage, and scales the output. The thermistor placement is critical to correct temperature monitoring. This sensor is usually placed as close to the tip as possible and thermally isolated from the rest of the electrode. Even with these precautions, the temperature that is monitored by the system is only an approximation of the tissue temperature at the lesion site. The electrode temperature that is recorded represents a complex interaction of heat generated in the tissue interface, the radiofrequency field, and convective heat loss to surrounding blood and tissue (18,19,24,25). Although not ideal, it is the best system available.

The signals for power and impedance are derived

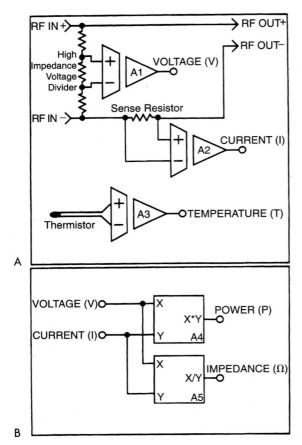

FIGURE 2-10. Diagrams of the analog block functions to be implemented in a radiofrequency (RF) control box. **A:** The high-impedance voltage divider provides a reduced signal to monitor and minimizes loading of the RF voltage waveform. A1 represents a group of discrete amplifiers that buffer the signal, convert it to its root-mean-square (RMS) value, and electrically isolate and scale the voltage to an appropriate value. A2 performs the same function for the RF current. A low-value, typically 0.1 to 1.0 Ω, resistor is used to translate the current to a voltage that represents the current. The relationship is described by V = IR, in which V is voltage, I is current, and R is resistance. A3 converts the variable resistance of the thermistor that senses temperature into a linear voltage and provides isolation. **B:** The voltage and current waveforms use analog function blocks to calculate the power and impedance signals and scale them to appropriate values. Power (W) is derived from the formula W = VI. Impedance (Ω) is calculated as Ω = V/I. (Adapted from Adams DE. Setting up the laboratory for ablation. In: Zipes DP, ed. *Catheter ablation of arrhythmias.* Armonk, NY: Futura, 1994, with permission.)

from the measured values of voltage and current. Given a sinusoidal signal and assuming resistive loads as the major component affecting our output, the following relationships can be used (26):

$$\text{Impedance} = \text{Voltage}/\text{Current}$$
$$\text{Power} = \text{Voltage} \times \text{Current}$$

These associations can be generated by using analog computational blocks as shown in Figure 2-10B or by mathematically processing digitized signals.

When a generator's output is started or terminated depends on an interaction of the operator and automatic relationships set by the operator or manufacturer. Figure 2-11 is a simplified block diagram of a digital control of the generator output. Block A represents a set-reset flip-flop. The output goes true when the start input is set and false when the stop input is set. This output turns on the generator and starts the time counter. Block C is the Boolean OR function and is set true if any of its inputs are true. It serves to sum all of the limit conditions that can stop the generator's output. The B blocks represent comparators, for which the output goes true whenever the X input is greater than the Y input. Otherwise, the output stays false. In this manner, the generator output is terminated whenever the time exceeds the set time, the impedance is outside the set minimum and maximum, the temperature is outside the preset minimum and maximum, or the operator pushes stop.

Radiofrequency Modes

Most radiofrequency generators can operate in a power mode. In this mode of operation, time duration is selected, limits on impedance or temperature are set or predetermined by the manufacture, and the desired power level is chosen. The generator outputs the set level of power while allowing the operator to see how the impedance and temperature levels are changing. If an adequate tip temperature is not reached quickly, the operator can terminate the delivered energy or adjust it. If the safety limits of the temperature or impedance settings are exceeded, automatic shutdown occurs.

Because temperature is critical to the success of

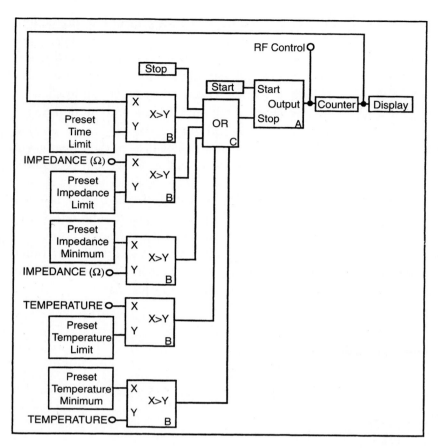

FIGURE 2-11. Block diagram of the minimal digital control necessary to control the radiofrequency (RF) energy source. The RF control signal is initiated by pressing the start button. This also initiates the digital counter that displays ablation duration time. Four situations should terminate delivery of energy: manually pressing the stop button, reaching the preset time limit, exceeding the preset impedance levels, or exceeding the preset temperature limits. The time limit is set by a comparator when the counter value exceeds the preset time. The impedance limit is set by one comparator if the calculated impedance exceeds the preset impedance maximum and by another if it falls below a preset minimum. The temperature limit is set by one comparator if the measured temperature exceeds the preset temperature maximum and by another if it falls below the preset temperature minimum. These six signals are logically "ORed" to reset the RF control when appropriate.

catheter ablation, a temperature mode of operation has been developed. This also has been called the closed-loop mode of operation. The impetus for using this method was to eliminate coagulum formation and to ensure target-tissue temperatures. Instead of the operator choosing a set power level, a temperature set point is selected. The generator then adjusts the power level and monitors the temperature output. Initially, the power is limited as heating begins. The generator then delivers a much larger output level, usually the maximum, as long as the difference between the set point and the monitored value is larger (10° to 12°C) than a manufacturer's determined level. After that difference is at or below the manufacturer's setting, power drops off. When the temperature difference becomes sufficiently small (2° to 3°C), a minimal amount of power is delivered to maintain temperature and to allow monitoring of other parameters. The generator ceases to deliver power if any of the safety limits are exceeded.

Limited clinical studies have shown that the temperature control mode has been somewhat successful (27). Coagulation formation was reduced significantly but not eliminated. Target temperatures were reached in only one third of the attempts, even though maximum output was delivered. Inadequate tissue-interface temperature monitoring was the primary factor in limiting this method (27). Tip contact, tip location, blood flow, and thermistor location all affect the accuracy of the temperature reading. They can compromise the system's ability to predict the temperature at the tissue interface. Further improvements in catheter design, temperature sensing technology, and ablation technique are needed to eliminate these concerns.

The temperature mode allows for full power delivery only until a preset temperature point is reached. Situations occur in which this is undesirable and the ability to limit power output is essential, including ablations in which damage may occur in collateral structures near the target, in areas where blood flow is limited (i.e., low blood flow can cause excessively quick temperature rises), and in patients with unusually thin cardiac walls. The ability to set a low power level in the power mode can provide safer and more effective treatment.

● INTERVENTIONAL LABORATORY LAYOUT

The layout of the laboratory can vary greatly and still meet all criteria for space, equipment placement, and personnel movement. The room size and shape are usually the limiting factors in any setup. Two laboratory configurations are the single room and a room with an attached control room. Figure 2-12 uses these layouts to illustrate various aspects of locating equipment in a laboratory.

The first equipment that is accommodated is the patient table and the x-ray equipment. These are purchased as a single system. The x-ray control panels are positioned along unused walls and out of the way of personnel flow. In some cases, they can be located in a small separate room. The head of the patient table is placed as close to a wall as the C arm or biplane configuration allows. Suction, O_2, other gases, and sufficient electrical outlets are located at appropriate levels on this wall. They are placed adjacent to the table head. The patient table's sides are positioned far enough from any given wall, cabinet, or other equipment to allow easy passage. A good minimum distance is 4 feet, which ensures that personnel can

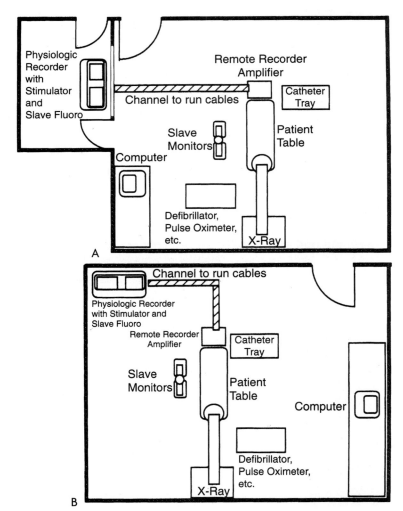

FIGURE 2-12. Two possible layouts for an interventional laboratory. (Adapted from Adams DE. Setting up the laboratory for ablation. In: Zipes DP, ed. *Catheter ablation of arrhythmias.* Armonk, NY: Futura, 1994, with permission.)

quickly move to an appropriate position, especially in an emergency.

The radiographic video system should consist of two monitors and a way to capture and print the fluoroscopic images. One monitor, along with the physiologic recorder's slave monitor, hangs from a movable, ceiling-mounted bracket. This allows the physician who is positioning the catheters to locate the monitors for the best viewing angles, regardless of the side of the table on which the physician stands or which catheter site he or she is attending. Viewing both monitors is critical. Small changes in catheter placement and all of the recorder's traces can be adequately monitored.

The remote amplifier for the physiologic recorder should be mounted as close as possible to the patient table. An ideal place is at the end of table, close to the patient's feet. If there is adequate room, the amplifier could be mounted under the table. The lengths of the cables for the surface ECG, pressure transducers, and intracardiac connections are thereby minimized, and the cables can be routed along the patient table as close to the patient as possible. Cable loops should be eliminated to minimize signal noise and remove floor clutter caused by excess cable trailing across the floor.

Connection of the remote amplifier to the main recorder console is accomplished with a floor channel or conduit. Isolating fiber-optic cable from the physiologic recorder and stimulator output cables are commonly routed in this way. In some cases, radiofrequency equipment cables can also use this channel. This eliminates floor clutter and protects all enclosed cables. Any electrical power cables should be run in separate conduits.

The main physician's equipment console consists of a variety of instruments, including the physiologic recorder, the slave monitor for the fluoroscopic imaging system, the physiologic stimulator, radiofrequency ablation devices, and other miscellaneous items. Devices are grouped together on a large cart or on permanent cabinets. Flow of traffic around the patient should not be impeded by the console's location. This grouping allows easy access and operation by the primary physician while maintaining the ability to monitor all recorded signals and vital signs. If the console is located in a separate room, adequate communications equipment is required to allow conversations between personnel in the two rooms. Adequate power receptacles and electrical circuits must exist to power all of the necessary electronic devices.

The rescue and vital signs monitoring equipment is located on a large, mobile cart near the patient's head. The location should allow ease of patient connections but still allow movement of the x-ray C arm, or biplanes. This equipment includes the primary and backup defibrillators, pulse oximeter, automatic blood pressure cuff, ACT monitor, and any other emergency supplies. Another large cart is needed for the sterile catheter tray. A small cart or mounting bar is needed if the ablation source must be located close to the patient.

Space must be allotted for the required drug carts, intravenous stands, and an adequate number of cabinets and countertops. The computer that is used for data logging is set on part of the cabinet tabletops. Location of the computer in the main room allows the attending nurse easy access. The nurse can then enter or retrieve appropriate information without leaving the patient unattended.

The many electronic devices in the interventional laboratory require special planning with regard to power- and air-handling requirements. The room design should include an adequate number of circuits and properly placed receptacles. Each device in the different groups should be plugged into its own receptacle. This ensures better grounding and minimizes the chance of overloading. The air-handling system must account for the total quantity of heat generated by all of the electronic devices used, thereby ensuring the comfort of patient and personnel and prolonging equipment life by maintaining a favorable operating temperature.

The planning phases of construction or remodeling must account for future uses of the electrophysiology laboratory. A clean room environment, similar to that of a surgical suite, is necessary for the implantation of pacemakers and other devices. Sterility is maintained by air-handling systems that implement positive-pressure ventilation and by filtering systems that eliminate airborne particulates. The National Fire Protection

Association codes specify minimum standards for hospital air-handling systems.

EQUIPMENT INTERCONNECTION

Considerations for the interconnection of equipment in the laboratory include the physiologic recorder, stimulator, ablation sources, transducers, and possibly the defibrillator. Figure 2-13 illustrates the device interconnections and the usual direction of signal flow.

There are three types of connections to the patient: the 12 leads of the surface ECG cable, the pressure transducer, and the intracardiac catheters. The ECG and the pressure transducer cable connect directly to an active amplifier interface. All but the ablating catheter plug directly into interface boxes that connect to the amplifier. The ablating catheter connects to an ablation-switching device that then connects to the amplifier interface boxes. This allows recording potentials from or energy delivery to this catheter.

All of the traces generated by the patient connections are usually available as high-level output signals. These can be connected to the sense input on a stimulator to use as a timing reference or serve as an input to the defibrillator to allow synchronization of the

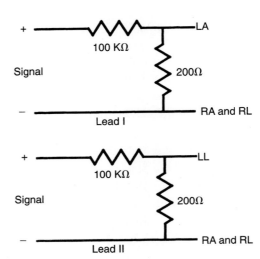

FIGURE 2-14. The circuit attenuates the outputs on the physiologic recorder. The signals can be connected to the defibrillator and monitor's electrocardiographic input. By selecting the appropriate lead, the unit can be synchronized by the recorder's output.

defibrillator output. Figure 2-14 shows a simple circuit that can be used to attenuate a high-level signal and allow connection to the defibrillator ECG input. High-level signals can also be connected to the recorder through special inputs. This arrangement allows traces from ablation sources (e.g., power, temperature, impedance) or device programmers (e.g.,

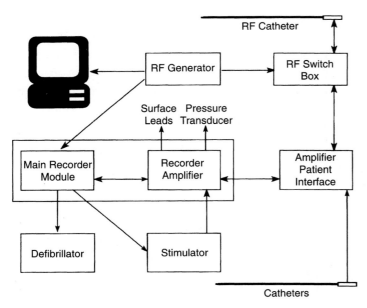

FIGURE 2-13. Interconnection diagram of ablation equipment, including a physiologic recorder, stimulator, radiofrequency (RF) energy source, defibrillator, and study catheters. Arrows indicate the flow of signals to and from each module. The isolated current outputs of the stimulator connect to the amplifier module to allow stimulus switching by the computer interface. The modules of the recorder system connect together as shown. The ablation delivery system can have separate units or have the generator and patient interface encased together. The ablation catheter is routed through the RF switchbox. The computer graphs the RF parameters as provided by the serial interface on the generator.

internal electrograms, marker channels) to be displayed on the recorder monitor.

The stimulator's isolated current outputs connect to the amplifier module or the patient interface box. The same matrix controls the catheter pole connections, allowing computer control of which poles are used for stimulation.

The ablation energy source can have high-level analog outputs that can be displayed on the recorder monitor. Most generators also have computer serial output ports that send digital information about the ablation system (e.g., impedance, power, temperature). An external computer can then provide real-time graphing of the signals, which facilitates monitoring of ablation parameters while energy is being delivered.

REFERENCES

1. NASPE Ad Hoc Committee on Catheter Ablation. Catheter ablation for cardiac arrhythmias, personnel, and facilities. *Pacing Clin Electrophysiol* 1992;15:715–721.
2. Josephson ME. *Clinical cardiac electrophysiology, techniques and interpretations*. Philadelphia: Lea & Febiger, 1993:10–11.
3. Geddes LA, Baker LE. *Principles of applied biomedical instrumentation*. New York: Wiley-Interscience, 1975:110–113.
4. Cooper MJ, Anderson KP, Mason JW. Invasive electrophysiologic studies. In: Zipes DP, Jalife J, eds. *Cardiac electrophysiology: from cell to bedside*. Philadelphia: WB Saunders, 1990:837.
5. Jackman WM, Kuck KH, Friday KJ, Lazzara R. Catheter recordings of accessory atrioventricular pathway activation. In: Zipes DP, Jalife J, eds. *Cardiac electrophysiology: from cell to bedside*. Philadelphia: WB Saunders, 1990:491–501.
6. Oakes JB. Electrical safety. In: Feinberg BN, Fleming DG, eds. *Handbook of clinical engineering*. Vol. 1. Boca Raton, FL: CRC Press, 1980:23—26.
7. Neuman MR. Biopotential amplifiers. In: Webster JG, ed. *Medical instrumentation: applications and design*. Boston: Houghton Mifflin, 1978:297–299.
8. Olson WH. Electrical safety. In: Webster JG, ed. *Medical instrumentation: applications and design*. Boston: Houghton Mifflin, 1978:667–697.
9. McGillem CD, Cooper GR. *Continuous and discrete signal and system analysis*. New York: Holt, Rinehart & Winston, 1974:167–170.
10. Josephson ME. *Clinical cardiac electrophysiology, techniques and interpretations*. Philadelphia: Lea & Febiger, 1993:9.
11. Smith WM, Wharton JM, Blanchard SM, et al. Direct catheter mapping. In: Zipes DP, Jalife J, eds. *Cardiac electrophysiology: from cell to bedside*. Philadelphia: WB Saunders, 1990:852–853.
12. Josephson ME. *Clinical cardiac electrophysiology, techniques and interpretation*. Philadelphia: Lea & Febiger, 1993:10.
13. Jackman WM, Kuck KH, Friday KJ, Lazzara R. Catheter recordings of accessory atrioventricular pathway activation. In: Zipes DP, Jalife J, eds. *Cardiac electrophysiology: from cell to bedside*. Philadelphia: WB Saunders, 1990:495–501.
14. Jackman WM, Wang X, Friday KJ, et al. Catheter ablation of accessory atrioventricular pathways (Wolff-Parkinson-White syndrome) by radiofrequency current. *N Engl J Med* 1991;324:1605–1611.
15. Jazayeri MR, Hempe SL, Sra JS, et al. Selective transcatheter ablation of the fast and slow pathways using radiofrequency energy in patients with atrioventricular nodal reentrant tachycardia. *Circulation* 1992;85:1318–1328.
16. Calkins H, Landberg J, Sousa J, et al. Radiofrequency catheter ablation of accessory atrioventricular connections in 250 patients. *Circulation* 1992;85:1337–1346.
17. Miles WH, Klein LS, Hackett FK. Catheter ablation for cardiac arrhythmias. *Curr Opinion Cardiol* 1993;8:75.
18. Shitzer A, Erez A. Controlled destruction and temperature distributions in biological tissues subjected to monoactive electrocoagulation. *J Biomech Eng* 1980;102:42–49.
19. Haines DE, Watson DD. Tissue heating during radiofrequency catheter ablation: a thermodynamic model and observations in isolated perfused and superfused canine right ventricular free wall. *Pacing Clin Electrophysiol* 1989;12:962–976.
20. Nath S, Lynch C, Whayne JG, Haines DE. Cellular electrophysiologic effects of hyperthermia on isolated guinea pig papillary muscle: implications for catheter ablation. *Circulation* 1993;88:1826–1831.
21. Hanes DE, Verow AF. Observations on electrode-tissue interface temperature and effect on electrical impedance during radiofrequency ablation of ventricular myocardium. *Circulation* 1990;82:1034–1038.
22. Borggrefe M, Hindricks G, Haverkamp W, et al. Radiofrequency ablation. In: Zipes DP, Jalife J, eds. *Cardiac electrophysiology: from cell to bedside*. Philadelphia: WB Saunders, 1990:998–999.
23. Hindricks G, Haverkamp W, Gulker H, et al. Radiofrequency coagulation of ventricular myocardium: improved prediction of lesion size by monitoring catheter tip temperature. *Eur Heart J* 1989;10:972–984.
24. Organ LW. Electrophysiologic principles of radiofrequency lesion making. *Appl Neurophysiol* 1976–1977;39:69–76.
25. Blouin LT, Marcus FI, Lampe L. Assessment of effects of radiofrequency energy field and thermistor location in an electrode catheter on the accuracy of temperature measurement. *Pacing Clin Electrophysiol* 1991;14:807–813.
26. Hayt WH, Kemmerly, JE. *Engineering circuit analysis*. New York: McGraw-Hill, 1971:306–307.
27. Calkins H, Prystowsky E, Carlson M, et al, for the Atakr Multicenter Investigators Group. Temperature monitoring during radiofrequency catheter ablation procedures using closed loop control. *Circulation* 1994;90:1279–1286.

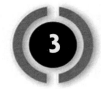

CATHETERIZATION AND ELECTROGRAM RECORDINGS
• • •
IGOR SINGER

◉ HISTORICAL PERSPECTIVE

The development of invasive vascular recording techniques is of relatively recent origin. Cardiac catheterization was first performed by Claude Barnard in a horse in 1844 (1). The first retrograde cardiac catheterization in humans is credited to Forssman, who in 1929 passed a catheter in himself from the left antecubital fossa to the right atrium with fluoroscopic guidance and documented the position of the catheter by a chest radiograph (2). As with many other scientific discoveries, Forssman's original intent was different from the ultimate application of this technique. His aim was to develop a therapeutic technique to deliver cardiac drugs directly into the cardiac chambers for treatment of cardiac emergencies. Criticism directed at him by his colleagues and peers, based on the unsubstantiated belief that this technique posed a danger to humans, led to his eventual abandonment of this technique.

Others, realizing the potential of Forssman's technique as a diagnostic tool, pursued the idea further. In 1930, Klein reported right-sided catheterization and measurement of cardiac output by Fick's principle (3). It was not until 1947 that Dexter reported measurement of oxygen saturation from the pulmonary capillary blood (4). Subsequent studies reported that the measurements of pressure from the capillary "wedge" position were a good estimate of pulmonary venous and left atrial pressure (5,6).

Retrograde left heart catheterization followed. In 1950, Zimmerman (7) and Limon-Lason (8) reported on the technique for retrograde left heart catheterization. The percutaneous technique was developed by Seldinger in 1953 (9). This technique was subsequently applied to left and right heart catheterization. Rapid development followed, including the transseptal catheterization technique by Ross (10) and Cope (11) and selective coronary arteriography by Sones and colleagues (12).

Selective coronary arteriography was modified for a percutaneous approach by Ricketts and Abrams in 1962 (13) and Judkins in 1967 (14). Evolution of cardiac catheterization from a diagnostic to an interventional technique occurred in 1977 with the first description of transluminal coronary angioplasty by Gruntzig and coworkers (15). In the past two decades, interventional techniques have evolved with breathtaking speed. In some cases, interventional intravascular techniques have replaced or supplanted cardiac surgical revascularization techniques as a primary therapeutic modality for management of myocardial ischemia and infarction. Development of more refined catheter techniques, thrombolytic drugs, intravascular stents, atherectomy catheters, and other invasive diagnostic techniques, such as angioscopy and intravascular ultrasound techniques, has revolutionized the diagnosis and treatment of coronary artery disease.

Development of invasive electrophysiologic techniques followed and paralleled the development of invasive intravascular catheterization techniques. Scherlag and associates (16) described the technique for recording His bundle activity in dogs and subsequently in humans in 1968. Independently, Durrer and colleagues and Coumel and coworkers described the technique of programmed electrical stimulation of the heart in 1967 (17,18). The technique of programmed electrical stimulation was combined with the His bundle recording technique by Wellens in 1971 (19). This led to elucidation of mechanisms of clinical tachycardias in humans and application of this knowledge to therapy for arrhythmias.

These early beginnings were followed by the use of multiple recordings and stimulation catheters in the heart chambers and elucidation of the normal and abnormal conduction and activation sequence during physiologic and pathologic tachycardias. Endocardial catheter-mapping techniques for localization of ventricular tachycardia (20), bypass tracts (21), atrioventricular (AV) node reentry tachycardia (22–24), and atrial flutter (25) have helped to elucidate these pathologic arrhythmias.

The impetus for the development of interventional electrophysiologic catheter techniques was provided by the realization that successful surgical ablation of accessory pathways (26), surgical resection of ventricular tachycardia (27), and curative surgery for AV node reentry tachycardia (28) were possible by focal destruction of tissues involved in reentry tachycardias. Further technologic developments, including flexible, maneuverable endocardial catheters, and suitable energy sources, provided the means to attempt ablative therapy with invasive intravascular electrode catheters. In this way, the modern era of interventional electrophysiology was ushered in.

Interventional catheter techniques have rapidly evolved over the past decade. Techniques for accessory pathway ablation (29), AV node modification (30,31), atrial flutter interruption (32), and ventricular tachycardia ablation (33,34) are all possible. Development of more refined mapping systems for electrophysiologic laboratory applications and further refinements and development of new energy sources are likely to result in further improvements in catheter ablation techniques.

Central to interventional electrophysiologic techniques is the ability to place intravascular catheters percutaneously to various right and left heart sites. Mapping and ablation require precision, with integration of knowledge of electrophysiologic principles, intimate knowledge of cardiac anatomy, and ability to deliver selective destructive lesions to pathologic reentry pathways without incurring damage to normal tissues.

In this chapter, cardiac catheterization techniques for interventional electrophysiologic procedures and principles for recording and processing electrograms, are discussed.

CARDIAC CATHETERIZATION TECHNIQUES

Femoral Artery and Vein Puncture

Femoral veins and arteries are the most common sites of entry used for cardiac catheterization of the right and left heart chambers for electrophysiologic recording, stimulation, and interventional procedures. Less commonly used sites are the subclavian and jugular veins.

The anatomic relationships of femoral arteries and veins are shown in Figure 3-1. The femoral artery typically lies at the midpoint of the inguinal ligament and is usually easily identified at the inguinal skin crease. Typically, the femoral vein is located alongside the artery, approximately one fingerbreath medial to the artery.

Adequate local anesthesia is administered before the vessel puncture. This point cannot be overemphasized. Poor anesthesia results in patient discomfort. Restlessness and lack of cooperation may exacerbate the risk of vascular complications. Appropriate anesthesia enhances the patient-doctor relationship and makes the procedure more comfortable and tolerable for the patient and the operator.

With three middle fingers of the left hand positioned alongside the femoral artery, with the topmost

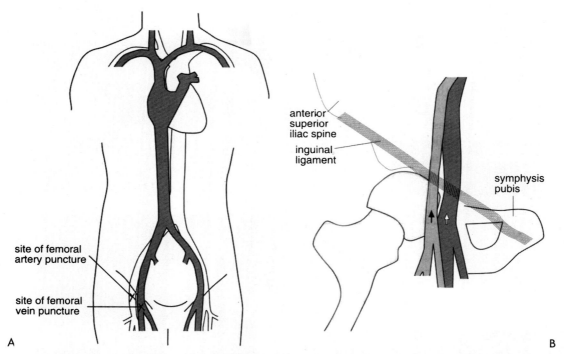

FIGURE 3-1. A: Relationship of arteries and veins, indicating the preferred sites for puncture of the right femoral artery and vein. **B:** Anatomic relationship of the right femoral artery and vein. The usual site for puncture of the femoral artery *(black arrow)* is below the inguinal ligament and approximately midway between the symphysis pubis and the anterior superior iliac spine. The femoral artery is lateral to the femoral vein, for which the puncture site *(white arrow)* is shown.

finger just below the inguinal ligament, the arterial course is identified. A linear intradermal wheal of 1% or 2% Nesacaine (chloroprocaine) or lidocaine is raised slowly with a 25- or 27-gauge needle at the chosen entry site.

With the left-hand fingers in place, a skin puncture is made over the femoral artery and vein with a no. 11 scalpel blade. With a 22-gauge needle, deeper tissues are anesthetized along the course of the entry. Gentle aspiration is applied to the syringe to identify entry into the lumen of the vessel. This is followed by additional injection of the anesthetic along the needle course. The needle must not be intravascular (i.e., identified by aspiration of blood into the syringe) before the injection of the anesthetic. If the needle is intravascular, it should be advanced more deeply until it passes through the posterior vessel wall. Additional anesthetic is infiltrated at that point to anesthetize the periosteum. Approximately 10 to 20 mL of anesthetic are usually required.

After the anesthesia is ensured, a small skin incision is enlarged by the use of a curved hemostat. This step minimizes the chance of crimping the intravascular sheath, which may cause vessel laceration.

Femoral Vein Puncture

Femoral vein puncture is accomplished while the middle three fingers of the left hand palpate and outline the course of the femoral artery below the inguinal ligament. A modified Seldinger or a Cook needle is introduced through the skin incision that was previously created. The needle is advanced along the anesthetized track at a 30- to 45-degree angle to the skin surface. Gentle suction is applied to the syringe as the needle is advanced until an abundant flashback of blood is encountered. The syringe and the needle are then depressed so that they are more parallel to the skin surface, which ensures that the needle tip lies

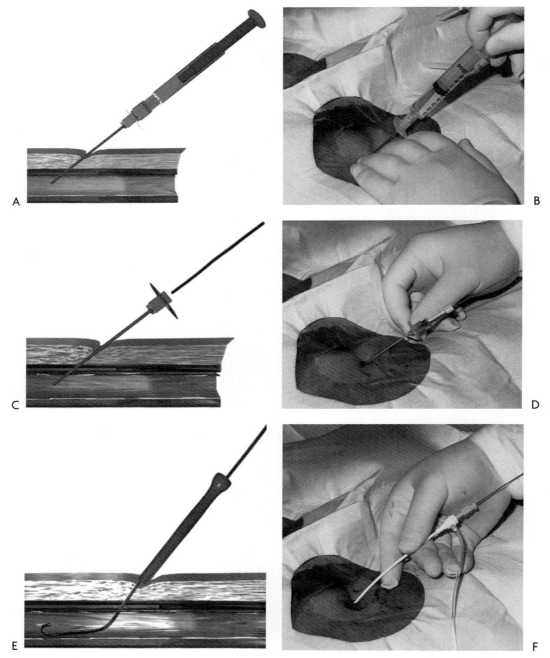

FIGURE 3-2. **A:** Technique for femoral vein puncture. The syringe is angled at approximately 30 to 45 degrees to the skin surface, parallel to the course of the artery, and approximately 1 cm medial to it. Aspiration of dark blood indicates that the needle is within the venous lumen. **B:** Example of a femoral vein puncture. **C:** The guide wire is advanced. No resistance should be encountered during the passage of the guide wire. **D:** Example of guide wire advancement. **E:** The sheath is advanced over the guide wire. The guide wire is removed, leaving the sheath in the vein lumen. **F:** Example of sheath advancement over the guide wire. (**B, D, E** from Singer I, Kupersmith J, eds. *Clinical manual of electrophysiology.* Baltimore: Williams & Wilkins, 1993:58, with permission.)

intravascularly. The syringe is then detached while the left hand stabilizes the hub of the needle. A 0.035- or 0.038-inch-diameter, J-tipped guide wire, which is provided with the introducer sheath, is advanced into the hub of the needle. The wire should slide forward through the vessel without perceptible resistance (Fig. 3-2). Fluoroscopy is usually not required unless resistance is encountered. The wire should not be advanced if resistance is encountered, because it may be extravascular or point downward at a sharp 180-degree angle. In that case, under fluoroscopic guidance, the guide wire is pulled back into the needle and redirected superiorly. The correct course of the guide wire may be confirmed by fluoroscopy.

Another common reason for failure to advance the guide wire is that the needle is positioned at a too-acute angle to the venous lumen, obstructing guide wire entry. This problem may be corrected by a downward depression of the needle so that the tip of the needle is placed intravascularly. If this maneuver fails, the guide wire should be removed, a clean syringe reattached to the needle, and the needle-syringe assembly slightly withdrawn or advanced until a free flow of blood is encountered. The guide wire should not be reintroduced unless a free flow of blood is ensured. If no free flow is encountered, the entire needle-syringe assembly is removed, and compression is applied at the puncture site for 3 to 5 minutes to ensure hemostasis. The landmarks should be rechecked before further attempts at venous puncture.

When the vein has been successfully entered, the guide wire is advanced and the needle is removed, leaving the guide wire in the intravascular position. The protruding wire is wiped clean of blood by a moistened gauze pad, and the free end is introduced into the distal end of a 6- or 7-Fr sheath. The guide wire is fed through the sheath until approximately 2 cm of the wire is protruding from the proximal part of the sheath. The assembly is then advanced with firm forward pressure and slight rotation. No force should be applied. If the sheath cannot be advanced, a dermotomy site may need to be enlarged with the curved hemostat. Occasionally, passage of the dilator without the sheath may be used to enlarge the tract before the passage of the entire sheath. Force must never be used.

When the sheath is intravascular and completely

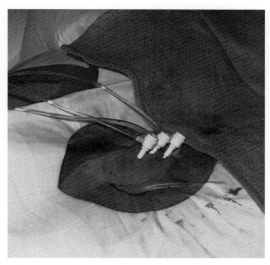

FIGURE 3-3. Three sheaths positioned within the femoral vein. (From Singer I, Kupersmith J, eds. *Clinical manual of electrophysiology.* Baltimore: Williams & Wilkins, 1993:59, with permission.)

advanced, the guide wire and the introducer are removed. The sheath is flushed with heparinized saline and connected by sterile tubing to normal saline solution. The sheath is continuously flushed with slow saline infusion. This helps to minimize the propensity to develop venous thrombosis. Ready access to the central circulation is also useful for administration of parenteral sedation and emergency drug administration.

Additional sheaths are introduced in an analogous manner with the entry sites positioned approximately 0.5 to 1 cm below each other in an imaginary line outlining the course of the deep femoral vein (Fig. 3-3). In this manner, up to three venous sheaths may be accommodated in a single vein. If more than three catheters are required or the right femoral vein is inaccessible, the left femoral vein may be used. A disadvantage of using the left femoral vein is that the course of the catheters is not as straight, requiring additional manipulation to place catheters in the right heart chambers. However, with maneuverable catheters, this may not be as much of a problem.

Femoral Artery Puncture

Femoral artery puncture is accomplished lateral to the venous puncture site immediately below the femoral crease. As described previously, three middle fingers of the left hand are used to outline the arterial course. The tip of the needle is introduced at the site where the maximal pulsation is felt. The open-lumen needle allows a pulsatile jet of blood to spurt from the hub when the needle has entered the arterial lumen. The needle may be advanced with the thumb and forefinger of both hands steadying the needle hub for better control (Fig. 3-4). While the thumb and the forefinger of the left hand steady the hub of the needle, the right hand is used to advance a 0.035- or 0.038-inch-diameter, J-tipped guide wire through the needle into

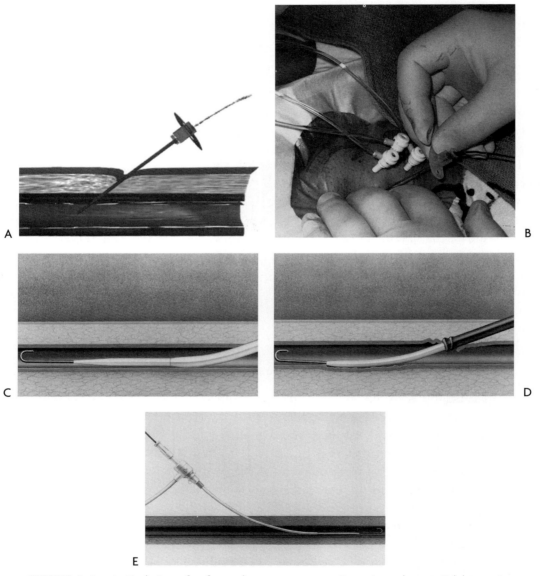

FIGURE 3-4. **A:** Technique for femoral artery puncture. Entry into the arterial lumen is signaled by the pulsatile flow of blood from the hub of the needle. **B:** Example of a femoral artery puncture. Three venous sheaths are positioned medial to the arterial sheath. (From Singer I, Kupersmith J, eds. *Clinical manual of electrophysiology.* Baltimore: Williams & Wilkins, 1993:59, with permission.) **C:** Adequate dermotomy is important because it permits a smooth advancement of the arterial sheath. **D:** Crimping of the sheath may produce intimal damage. **E:** Proper positioning of the arterial sheath (Fast Cath sheath, Daig). (Courtesy of Daig, Minetonka, MN.)

the arterial lumen. No resistance should be encountered. The guide wire should be advanced under fluoroscopic guidance. When correctly placed, it should be seen to the left of the spinal column.

If the passage of the guide wire meets slight resistance or if the patient complains of any discomfort, the subintimal position of the wire should be suspected. Alternatively, a kink in the iliac vessels or obstruction may be the cause. If subintimal dissection is suspected, the needle should be withdrawn, the wire wiped with a wet gauze, and a small-gauge cannula (5 Fr or less) passed over the guide wire. The guide wire is then removed. Injection of a small bolus of contrast by a control syringe positioned at the needle hub usually establishes the reason for obstruction. If a dissection is the cause, the cannula should be removed and hemostasis ensured by digital compression of the artery for 5 to 10 minutes. If dissection has occurred, a retrograde left heart catheterization should be attempted from another site (i.e., left femoral or brachial). If no dissection has occurred and the obstruction to the guide wire passage is caused by a kink in the artery or stenosis, other guide wires may be tried (i.e., floppy or movable core J-tipped or maneuverable guide wire). It is uncommon that a guide wire cannot be passed, unless there is a complete occlusion of the iliac vessel ipsilateral to the site of puncture. In that case, the contralateral femoral artery should be tried.

If difficulty in advancing the guide wire is encountered immediately beyond the needle tip, a slight downward depression of the needle hub should move the needle tip to a more intravascular position so that the guide wire does not strike the posterior arterial wall. At all times, the backflow of the blood must be pulsatile; otherwise, it is likely that the needle tip is not completely intravascular. Attention to these details can help to prevent vascular complications. Failure to enter the artery and advance the guide wire despite these maneuvers should prompt the operator to withdraw the needle and secure hemostasis by digital compression for 5 to 10 minutes before attempting another arterial puncture. Before the subsequent attempts, anatomic landmarks should be carefully rechecked, and the artery should be located by digital pressure.

When the guide wire has been advanced to the junction of the descending aorta and arch, the needle should be removed and the wire cleaned with a wet gauze. While an assistant holds the guide wire straight with minimal tension, a 5-Fr sheath or a Longdwell cannula is advanced. The guide wire is then removed, and the side arm of the sheath is flushed with heparinized saline. The arterial sheath should be attached to the pressure gauge by a continuous flush setup, and the arterial pressure is constantly monitored throughout the procedure. Continuous flushing with heparinized saline ensures the patency of the arterial sheath and prevents arterial thrombosis. My colleagues and I prefer to display the arterial waveform continuously throughout the procedure to help monitor the patency of the sheath and the arterial pressure. If retrograde left heart catheterization is required, the 5-Fr sheath or Longdwell cannula may be replaced by a larger sheath to accommodate mapping and ablation catheters.

Subclavian Vein Puncture

Subclavian vein puncture may be necessary when coronary sinus catheterization is desired. Left subclavian vein is most commonly used, because the convex curve of the catheter tends to be directed posteriorly, aiming at the coronary sinus ostium from this entry site. The Trendelenburg position facilitates subclavian vein entry by increasing venous return. A towel or rolled sheet can be placed longitudinally between the shoulder blades to raise the clavicles and facilitate subclavian vein cannulation.

The site of entry is just lateral to the ligament that connects the clavicle to the first rib. This lies approximately at the junction of the proximal two thirds and the distal one third of the clavicle. Adequate anesthesia is ensured by careful infiltration of 1% Nesacaine or lidocaine along the course of the intended subclavian vein puncture. A small incision in the skin is made with a no. 11 blade, and the site of entry is further enlarged with a curved hemostat. A Cook needle attached to a 10-mL syringe filled with 2 to 3 mL of saline is directed toward the sternal notch, parallel to the clavicle, and enters the space between

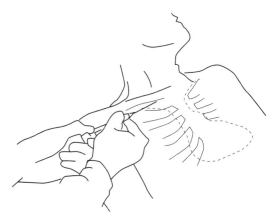

FIGURE 3-5. Technique for right subclavian vein puncture. A Cook needle attached to a saline-filled syringe is directed toward the sternal notch, parallel to the clavicle, and enters the space between the clavicle and the first rib.

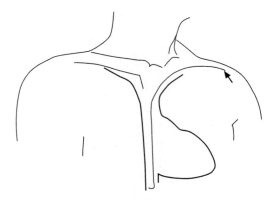

FIGURE 3-6. Fluoroscopic appearance of the guide wire (arrow), which is advanced from the left subclavian puncture site to the inferior vena cava.

the clavicle and the first rib (Fig. 3-5). The needle-syringe assembly should be advanced slowly and carefully with gentle aspiration. Entry into the subclavian vein is heralded by a gush of dark venous blood without pulsatile flow. At that point, the syringe is carefully detached while the needle is steadied with the left hand. A short 50-cm, J-tipped guide wire is then advanced. As with the femoral puncture, no resistance should be encountered. If resistance is encountered, the guide wire is extravascular and should be withdrawn, or the guide wire might have passed into the jugular vein. Using fluoroscopy, the guide wire should be pulled back and redirected to the superior vena cava. If the guide wire fails to pass at all, it should be withdrawn, the needle advanced or slightly pulled back until free flow of venous blood is seen in the syringe, and the wire re-advanced.

It is recommended that the guide wire be advanced into the inferior vena cava, which fluoroscopically lies to the right of the spinal column, to ensure that the guide wire has not been accidentally introduced into the subclavian artery (Fig. 3-6). At this point, the needle is removed, and a 6- or 7-Fr sheath is advanced over the guide wire. The wire is removed, and the side port is flushed with heparinized saline.

If bright red, pulsatile blood is aspirated, the needle has entered the subclavian artery. The needle should be removed, and digital pressure should be applied for 5 to 10 minutes to ensure hemostasis. A more medial site should then be selected. If air is aspirated, the pleural space has been entered, and the penetration has been too deep or too lateral. In a healthy person, a single puncture of the pleural space does not usually lead to a large pneumothorax, although in patients with obstructive airway disease, pneumothorax may ensue, requiring abandonment of this approach and, rarely, necessitating placement of a chest tube. Because this complication may require the operator to abandon the procedure entirely, it cannot be overemphasized that the selection of the subclavian puncture route should be reserved for cases in which it is absolutely necessary.

Internal Jugular Vein Puncture

The internal jugular vein is not a preferred site for most electrophysiologic procedures. For most patients, invasion of the neck area is unpleasant and may be perceived as more threatening. For prolonged procedures, it is often difficult to keep the neck area sterile and immobile for a sufficient period. Nevertheless, in certain circumstances, the internal jugular venous approach may offer some advantages, because it is generally free from most serious complications. A potential complication is inadvertent puncture of the carotid artery, resulting in neck hematoma and air embolism. However, there is far less risk of entering the pleural space and causing pneumothorax.

Positioning of a coronary sinus catheter and mapping catheter for right-sided accessory pathway ablations may be easier with this approach. Temporary pacemaker electrodes may be most easily positioned from this site so that the subclavian veins are preserved for the permanent pacemaker or defibrillator implant if that subsequently proves to be necessary.

The internal jugular vein is located anterior and lateral to the carotid artery and lies behind the clavicular head of the sternocleidomastoid muscle. The site of the puncture should be approximately 5 cm above the clavicle and medial to the lateral border of the sternocleidomastoid muscle. The Trendelenburg maneuver is helpful in distending the vein, making the stick more likely to encounter the vein and rendering the passage of the guide wire easier. The syringe and needle are held at an angle of 20 to 30 degrees, and the needle is directed lateral to the carotid artery through the muscle (Fig. 3-7). When the free flow of venous blood is encountered, the syringe is detached, the needle is stabilized, and a 50-cm-long, J-tipped guide wire is advanced. No resistance should be encountered during advancement of the guide wire. The needle is then removed, and the incision site may be slightly enlarged by the scalpel blade and curved hemostat before the sheath being advanced, as described previously.

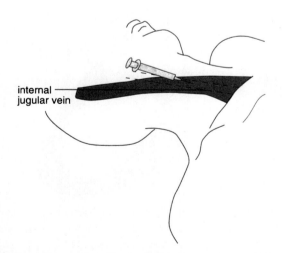

FIGURE 3-7. Technique for internal jugular vein puncture. The site of puncture is approximately 5 cm above the clavicle, lateral to and parallel to the course of the carotid artery.

If the carotid artery is inadvertently punctured, the needle should be withdrawn and digital pressure applied for 5 to 10 minutes before another attempt. Air embolism may be prevented by keeping the patient in the Trendelenburg position until the sheath is advanced.

Transseptal Left Atrial Catheterization

Transseptal catheterization has come back into vogue with the advent of radiofrequency ablation of the left accessory pathways. Its appeal derives from the fact that catheter manipulation may be easier from above the mitral annulus than with the retrograde transaortic approach. Some operators feel that seating of catheter from above the annulus for mapping and ablation may be easier when this approach is used.

Transseptal catheterization is accomplished from the right femoral venous approach. A transseptal dilator sheath assembly, a Brockenbrough needle, and a 150-cm wire are required for this technique (Fig. 3-8). The guide wire diameter should be between 0.028 and 0.032 inch. The transseptal sheath is composed of two parts: an inner dilator and the sheath. The outer sheath has an 8-Fr diameter and a hemostasis valve to prevent backflow of blood and air embolization.

After femoral vein puncture, a 0.032-inch-diameter, 150-cm-long, J-tipped guide wire is passed to the superior vena cava. The transseptal sheath is then passed over the guide wire to the superior vena cava, and the guide wire is withdrawn. The dilator sheath is flushed with heparinized saline, and the Brockenbrough transseptal needle is advanced to rest approximately 1 cm within the tip of the dilator. The assembly containing the sheath, dilator, and needle is oriented to point left and posteriorly and is slowly withdrawn as a unit to the right atrium. Proper positioning is ensured by orienting the hub arrow to a 4 o'clock position. The transseptal sheath tip is oriented toward the fossa ovalis in a shallow left anterior oblique view. Abrupt leftward movement of the dilator tip as the assembly is withdrawn identifies proper positioning for transseptal puncture. Proper positioning in the 30-degree right anterior oblique (RAO) view is ensured if the dilator tip rests anterior to the

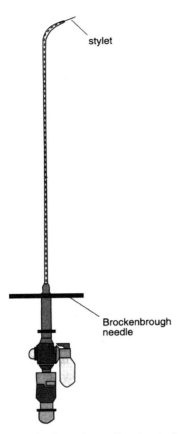

FIGURE 3-8. Brockenbrough needle. The shaft of the needle is not shown to scale.

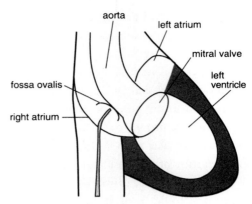

FIGURE 3-9. The diagram shows the positioning of the Brockenbrough needle for a transseptal puncture. In the right anterior oblique view, the aortic shadow is superimposed over the atria.

coronary sinus catheter in the fossa ovalis (Fig. 3-9). An arterial pigtail catheter positioned in the noncoronary cusp may be used to delineate the anterior extent of safe transseptal catheterization.

Gentle probing of the limbus is attempted before advancing of the Brockenbrough needle, in case a patent foramen ovale exists. If this is unsuccessful, the Brockenbrough needle is firmly but gently advanced within the sheath assembly. Transseptal puncture is accomplished under fluoroscopic guidance in a shallow left anterior oblique (LAO) view, because in the RAO view, an overlap is seen between the aortic root and the atria. Successful passage into the left atrium is sensed by a characteristic "give" to the catheter (Fig. 3-10). Confirmation of the left atrial entry may be made by recording of the pressure waveform. The dilator and the sheath are then gently advanced into the left atrium over the Brockenbrough needle. The sheath is further advanced over the dilator to the lateral left atrial wall. With the sheath stabilized at the femoral entry site, the dilator and the Brockenbrough needle are withdrawn. The sheath is then aspirated to prevent air embolization and flushed with heparinized saline. A deflectable 7-Fr catheter is passed through the sheath and used for mapping and ablation. After the catheter is properly positioned, a 5,000-IU bolus of heparin is administered, and heparinization is maintained with additional 1,000 to 2,000 IU of heparin boluses hourly for the duration of the procedure.

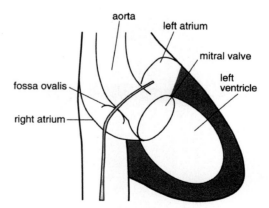

FIGURE 3-10. Transseptal puncture with advancement of the sheath into the left atrium. In the right anterior oblique view, the transseptal needle appears superimposed on the aortic shadow. The puncture should be accomplished in the shallow left anterior oblique view.

RADIOGRAPHIC EQUIPMENT

Radiographic and fluoroscopic equipment for electrophysiologic interventional laboratory should ideally provide biplane fluoroscopy and cine capabilities. The main and a slave monitor should be available to the operator to monitor catheter placements with simultaneous electrogram recordings. Digital video image capture should also be available. Radiation exposure should be carefully monitored and minimized.

FLUOROSCOPIC VIEWS

Optimal positioning of catheters for electrophysiologic studies and interventional procedures requires integration of knowledge of cardiac anatomy and radiographic correlates of these anatomic landmarks with intracardiac electrogram. An experienced operator visualizes intracardiac structures in three dimensions by integrating the visual input from these fluoroscopic projections. Three principal views are used for catheter positioning: AP (Fig. 3-11), right anterior

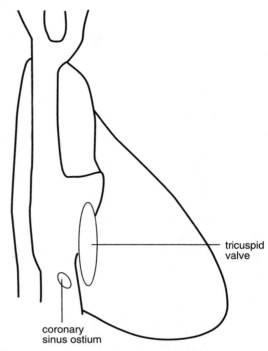

FIGURE 3-12. In the right anterior oblique fluoroscopic view, the tricuspid valve is seen almost side on. The superior margin of the tricuspid valve indicates the approximate position of the His bundle. The coronary sinus ostium lies posterior to the inferior margin of the tricuspid valve in this view.

oblique (RAO) (Fig. 3-12), and left anterior oblique (LAO) (Fig. 3-13).

Frontal View

The frontal view (i.e., anteroposterior) is used primarily during advancement and positioning of electrode catheters. Venous and arterial structures are best seen in this view because they generally run in the cephalocaudal direction. The tricuspid and mitral valves are seen obliquely in this view (Fig. 3-11). The right ventricular outflow tract is also best visualized in the anteroposterior view (Fig. 3-14).

Right Anterior Oblique View

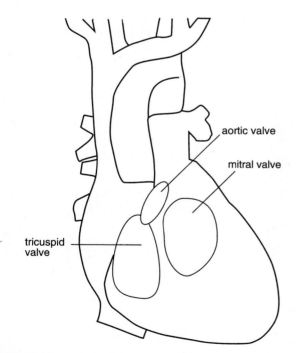

FIGURE 3-11. Anteroposterior fluoroscopic view of the heart shows the tricuspid, mitral, and aortic valves.

The RAO view is useful because tricuspid, mitral, and aortic valves are seen side on. In this view, the

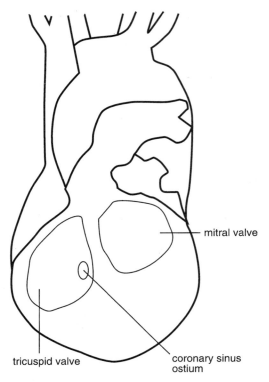

FIGURE 3-13. Left anterior oblique fluoroscopic view. In this view, the tricuspid and mitral valves may be mapped. The position of the coronary sinus ostium is also indicated. Passage of the catheter into the coronary sinus can be accomplished in this view with relative ease. The posterior aspect of the heart lies closest to the operator (anterior), the right margin of the heart is to the operator's left, and the left margin is to the right.

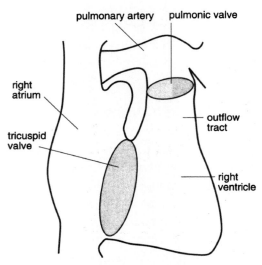

FIGURE 3-14. Fluoroscopic position of the right ventricular outflow tract and right ventricle in the anteroposterior view.

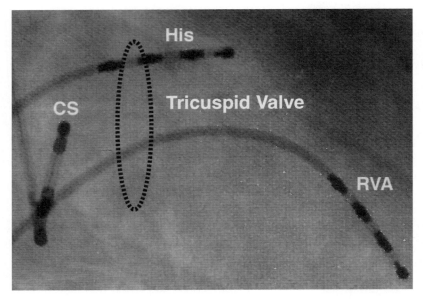

FIGURE 3-15. The right anterior oblique view shows the His bundle catheter in relation to the tricuspid annulus. The catheter lies at the superior margin of the annulus. The right ventricular and coronary sinus catheters are also shown.

His bundle is located at the most superior boundary of the tricuspid valve, snug to the intraventricular septum, so the catheter that is used for recording the His bundle is seen in profile (Fig. 3-15).

Positioning of the catheter in the aortic cusp, so that it is seen in profile before it is prolapsed into the left ventricular cavity, is best accomplished with this view. The left ventricle is displayed such that the base is formed by the mitral valve orifice and the apex by the outermost left lateral and inferior borders of the heart. Anterior-inferior walls and the apex of the left ventricle are best mapped in this view.

Left Anterior Oblique View

The LAO view positions the intraventricular septum in the middle of the cardiac shadow. The tricuspid and mitral valves are roughly circular structures in this view, with their posterior annuli located closest to the operator (anterior) and anterior borders farthest away (posterior). The lateral annulus of the tricuspid valve forms the right boundary of the heart shadow. Similarly, the lateral annulus of the mitral valve is located at the left heart border (Fig. 3-13). The septal aspects of both valves are located in the middle of the cardiac shadow. In this view, mapping of either valve may be optimally accomplished.

Another important landmark is the coronary sinus, which lies posteriorly and along the left lateral border of the heart. In this view, the coronary sinus catheter may be positioned and used for mapping of left accessory pathways (Fig. 3-16). Mapping of the septal, lateral, and basal portions of the left ventricle may best be accomplished in this view.

● CATHETER MANIPULATION TECHNIQUES

Techniques that are used for manipulation of electrode catheters are similar to those used for angiographic catheters. Gentleness and avoidance of force cannot be overemphasized, particularly for the electrode catheters, because they are generally stiffer and more likely to perforate thin venous structures or injure arterial intima. Flexible-tip catheters are easier to position, and they may in time replace the fixed-curve catheters entirely (Fig. 3-17).

Optimal electrode number and spacing depend on the purpose for which the catheters are used. Quadripolar catheters with 5- or 10-mm spacing are most commonly used. Pacing is accomplished from the distal pair and recording from the proximal electrode pair. Closer spacing (2 mm) is used for mapping with multipolar electrode catheters (i.e., octapolar or decapolar) in the coronary sinus or for recording of the proximal and distal His bundle during mapping pro-

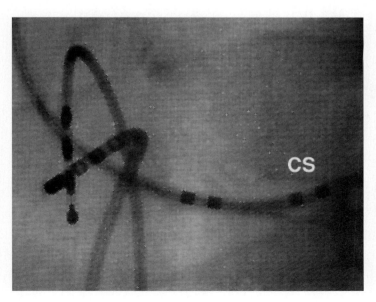

FIGURE 3-16. The coronary sinus catheter is shown in the left anterior oblique view.

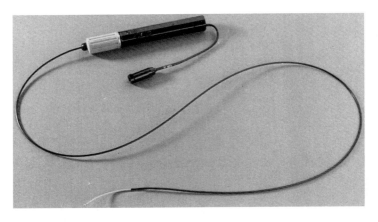

FIGURE 3-17. A steerable Livewire catheter. This type of catheter has the advantage of maneuverability and can be positioned more easily at various sites in the heart. (Courtesy of Daig, Minnetonka, MN.)

cedures (Fig. 3-18). For catheter ablation procedures, different curves are available to reach various sites within the cardiac chambers (Fig. 3-19).

Ablation catheters generally have a larger tip (4 mm) so that the energy is more efficiently distributed. They have flexible tips; are capable of independent tip rotation, flexion, and extension; and have different curvatures that are suitable for applications with small or large hearts.

Preformed vascular sheaths may be used in special circumstances for optimal positioning and mapping of the tricuspid and mitral annuli and to stabilize the catheters (Fig. 3-20). They may also be helpful for individuals with tortuous veins (particularly elderly patients), in whom catheter manipulation is often a technical challenge.

Manipulation of the catheters through the femoral and iliac veins and the inferior vena cava and into the right atrium may be achieved with relative ease by the use of deflectable-tip catheters. Even with the rigid catheters, this task is relatively straightforward in most patients. The catheter tip should be directed

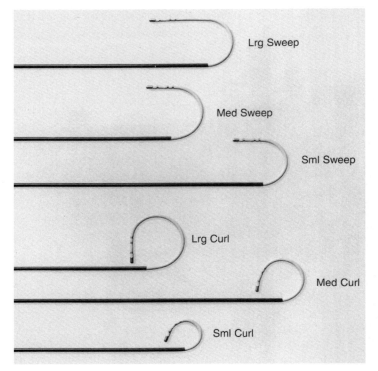

FIGURE 3-18. Steerable Livewire catheters, showing various sweeps and curls of the distal tip to reach diverse sites in the heart. (Courtesy of Daig, Minnetonka, MN.)

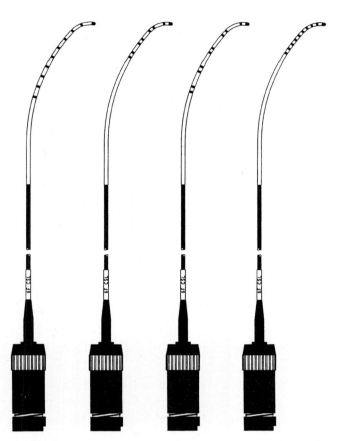

FIGURE 3-19. Coronary sinus catheters with different electrode spacings. Spacing of Response electrode arrays from left to right: 5, 2-5-2, 2-8-2, and 2 mm. (Courtesy of Daig, Minnetonka, MN.)

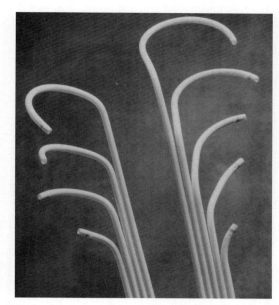

FIGURE 3-20. Intravascular sheaths used for positioning and stabilization of catheters during accessory pathway ablation. A complete set of Swartz Fast-Cath introducers is shown. (Courtesy of Daig, Minnetonka, MN.)

medially toward the spinal column, and when the venous branches are encountered, the catheter should be withdrawn slightly and redirected by gentle torquing and forward motion in the opposite direction. Electrophysiologic catheters usually are stiffer than most angiographic catheters, and the torque translation is therefore generally better. Smaller twists and turns of the catheter are generally more effective than more vigorous torquing.

The atrial catheter may be positioned at the junction of the superior vena cava and right atrium or in the right atrial appendage, where it is generally stable. The His catheter is positioned by prolapsing the catheter across the tricuspid valve into the right ventricle in the anteroposterior fluoroscopic position (Fig. 3-15), where the tricuspid valve is seen in a profile and the His bundle is located at its summit. The catheter is held in a profile in such a way that the convexity of the curve of the catheter is directed to the right atrium and the tip toward the left shoulder. The catheter is then withdrawn gently until it just crosses the spinal column, and a sharp triphasic signal is recorded from the proximal and distal electrodes between the atrial and ventricular electrograms, which should generally be equiphasic (Fig. 3-21). A clock torque of the catheter usually secures the catheter to the septum, where a larger His signal may be recorded.

The right ventricular catheter may be positioned in the apex or the outflow tract. We prefer the use of the deflectable tip catheter for the right ventricular recording and pacing because it is easier to maneuver it to the desired position. To position the catheter in the right ventricular outflow tract, a similar technique is used as for the positioning of the His catheter. Generally, further advancement of the catheter from the His portion with a slight clockwise and forward motion advances the catheter to the right ventricular outflow tract position. The tip of the catheter should be in close contact with the endocardium for effective stimulation. However, no undue pressure should be exerted on the catheter tip, because it may cause dis-

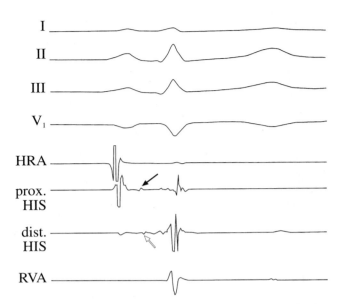

FIGURE 3-21. Electrogram recordings during sinus rhythm. From top to bottom: surface leads I, II, and III, V₁, high right atrium (HRA), proximal His (prox. His), distal His (dist. His), and right ventricular apex (RVA).

comfort to the patient and lead to perforation. Undue pressure may be recognized by excessive flexing of the catheter tip in either direction during the cardiac cycle when the tip is in contact with the endocardium. In that case, a 1- to 2-mm withdrawal of the catheter usually achieves optimal catheter-tissue contact.

Advancement of the catheter in the right ventricular apex is achieved by deflecting the tip downward when the catheter is prolapsed across the tricuspid valve (in the anteroposterior fluoroscopic view). An approximately 45- to 60-degree curvature is generally optimal. The catheter should be seen in a profile and then advanced. Generally, its tip then "seeks" the right ventricular apex. Sometimes, slight straightening of the curve after the catheter is in the ventricle may facilitate its advancement to the right ventricular apex position.

Positioning of the coronary sinus catheter may be accomplished from the right femoral position or from the left subclavian or jugular approach. With rigid catheters, the subclavian and jugular venous approaches are preferred. However, with the deflectable-tip catheters, the right femoral approach may be equally straightforward and has the advantage of avoiding the more risky and tedious approaches.

The coronary sinus is located in the medial posterior septum of the right atrium, and in the RAO view, it lies posterior to the inferior margin of the tricuspid valve (Fig. 3-12). In the LAO view (Fig. 3-13), it is located close to the posteromedial margin of the tricuspid valve, so the catheter tip is directed in the fluoroscopic anterior direction (posterior heart position) and to the left, paralleling the left heart margin (Fig. 3-16). Positioning of the coronary sinus catheter usually is easier from above, because the natural curve of the catheter tends to track in medial and slightly posterior directions toward the right atrial septum. Correct positioning and entry of the catheter are heralded by an easy give sensation and a typical silhouetting of the catheter along the left heart margin in the LAO view, accompanied by typical electrogram recordings, with sharp atrial and ventricular deflection of roughly equal amplitudes (Fig. 3-22). There should be no ventricular ectopy when the catheter is advanced into the coronary sinus, but if there is, passage of the catheter into the right ventricular outflow tract should be suspected.

Placement of the catheter in the left ventricle may be accomplished by the retrograde transaortic or transseptal approach. The transseptal approach was described earlier. For the transaortic approach, only deflectable-tip catheters should be used. The catheter should be advanced in the anteroposterior fluoroscopic view with the tip slightly flexed. When the junction of the arch and the descending aorta is en-

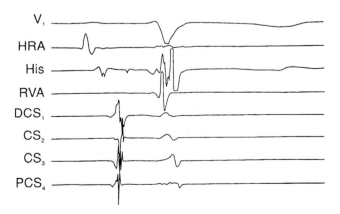

FIGURE 3-22. Coronary sinus (CS) recordings.

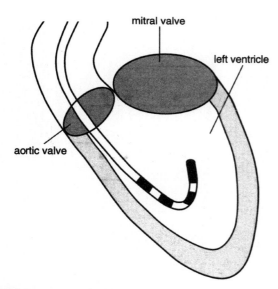

FIGURE 3-23. Technique for positioning of the catheter in the left ventricle. The catheter is prolapsed through the aortic valve while the tip curvature is maintained to minimize the risk of engaging the coronary artery and to facilitate prolapsing the catheter into the left ventricle.

countered, a sharp bend of the tip should be effected to create a loop. In the RAO view, the catheter should be directed with the loop pointing to the left in profile, and the catheter should be prolapsed across the aortic valve, analogous to the pigtail catheter used for left ventricular angiography. Asking the patient to take a breath in while the catheter is advanced usually is helpful for prolapsing the catheter across the aortic valve (Fig. 3-23). The loop helps to prevent inadvertent passage of the catheter tip into the left coronary artery, which could have disastrous consequences and cause coronary artery dissection. Before the arterial catheter entry, full heparinization should be effected. Further positioning in the left ventricular cavity depends on whether the catheter is used for accessory pathway ablation, ventricular mapping, or other purposes.

⊙ ELECTROPHYSIOLOGIC RECORDINGS

Organization of the interventional laboratory is described in Chapter 2. Recording of electrograms is accomplished with electrode catheters positioned at various locations in the heart. Typically, catheters are positioned in the right atrium, His bundle position, and right ventricular cavity for routine electrophysiologic studies. For evaluation of atrioventricular, AV nodal, and atrial tachycardias, a coronary sinus catheter also is required for assessment of left atrial activation timing and for pacing. Additional catheters may be required for interventional procedures, including the ablation catheter. For ventricular mapping and ablation, a left ventricular catheter also is required.

Physiologic Recorders

Physiologic recorders are used to display, store, and analyze electrograms and to monitor a patient's vital signs. At least five but preferably all 12 electrocardiographic channels can be recorded by using available physiologic recorders. At least 16 intracardiac channels may be displayed and recorded simultaneously; the number of channels is limited only by the number of available amplifiers and the screen size. Two pressure channels are capable of monitoring intracardiac and arterial pressures simultaneously. Direct current channels permit recording of ground-referenced signals, which are used by most external equipment. For example, external implantable cardioverter-defibrillator programmers or ablation equipment may be recorded by using these channels.

Filtering characteristics of the equipment are important to permit frequencies from below 1 MHz to 200 kHz. All inputs must be filtered for the range of frequencies used in radiofrequency ablations. All inputs must be protected from defibrillator discharges and must be properly grounded.

Computer-based recorders are preferable for interventional procedures. They allow for maximal flexibility and easy change of display (Fig. 3-24).

Catheters are connected to the physiologic recorders by the junction cables that provide the interface for connecting catheters to the amplifiers. The length of the cables should be minimized to decrease signal interference. Electronic switching by the computer is ideal, although manual switches are accept-

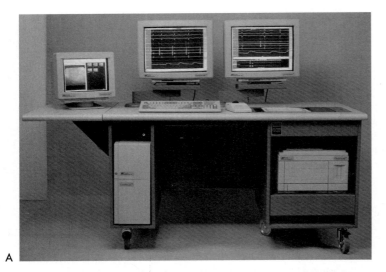

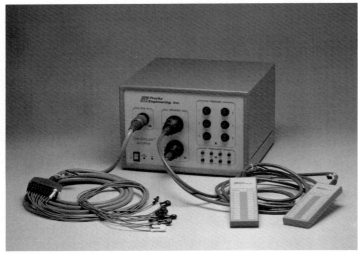

FIGURE 3-24. A: Computerized recording equipment. Two monitors are used for simultaneous recording of signals and for online analysis. Computer and printer are integrated in one system. B: Interface box for surface leads, intracardiac signals, and pressure channels for the CardioLab system. (Courtesy of Prucka Engineering, Inc., Houston, TX.)

able. Input protection for defibrillation and radiofrequency are provided before the signal processing by the amplifiers.

Signals are amplified, filtered, and digitized. They are then stored on an optical drive, from which they may be easily retrieved for display or analysis. Information is displayed on high-resolution color monitors that can display various channels in different colors. Two monitors or a split screen of a single monitor may be used for simultaneous data display and analysis.

Laser printers are used to output relevant data, limiting the use of reams of paper for data display and measurements. Recording of signals may be accomplished in unipolar or bipolar mode, and multielectrode catheters are commonly used to acquire simultaneous signals from the same electrode catheter.

Unipolar Electrograms

Unipolar recordings are based on recording of potential differences between a single electrode in contact with the extracellular space and an electrode placed at a distance from the heart (35). The approach of a depolarization wavefront toward an exploring electrode produces a positive deflection, and the passage away from the electrode produces a rapid deflection in the negative direction. The amplitude of the signal is proportional to the area of the dipole and the reciprocal value of the square of the distance between the dipole and the recording site (36,37).

Bipolar Electrograms

Bipolar recordings are acquired by measuring the potential difference between two closely spaced electrodes in direct contact with the endocardium. It represents a difference between two unipolar electrograms at each of the recording electrodes (38). The amplitude of the signal is inversely proportional to the third power of the distance between the recording electrodes and the moving dipole (39–41). If the activation wavefront is perpendicular to the recording electrodes, the amplitude is maximal. If the activation wavefront is parallel to the recording electrodes, it records a zero potential, because the electrodes record the same signal simultaneously (42).

Signal Recording

Computerized mapping systems are gradually replacing analog recorders. These were originally developed for intraoperative recordings and mapping to save operative time and produce more accurate activation maps during tachycardias. The advantages of such systems for signal acquisition and processing were easily appreciated by the clinical electrophysiologists, and similar systems have been developed for the use in the interventional electrophysiology laboratories. To be practical and useful, automatic activation detection algorithms have been devised for computerized applications.

For unipolar electrograms, most algorithms use the maximum downslope or largest negative downslope criteria. For bipolar electrograms, the maximum amplitude (V_{max}) of the bipolar electrogram and the maximum absolute amplitude are used (43,44) or the maximum absolute slope [$(dV/dt)_{max}$], the first elevation of more than 45 degrees from the baseline of the bipolar electrogram (45,46), the baseline crossing of the steepest slope (47–49) or morphologic algorithms are used (50).

Fractionated electrograms may be recorded after myocardial infarction and in patients with arrhythmogenic right ventricular dysplasia. They are called *fractionated* when they demonstrate several low-amplitude deflections, which are typically less than 1 mV (51). Late or fractionated electrograms may be recorded during sinus rhythm or during ventricular tachycardia. They are called *continuous electrical activity* when they persist during the entire cardiac cycle and are thought to represent electrical activity within the reentry circuit (52).

Cardiac Mapping

Cardiac mapping implies recording of electrical events from multiple electrodes positioned within the heart. Two essential steps are required for mapping: analysis of activation timing of each electrode site and creation of an isochronal map that represents a spatial model of the activation sequence. Activation mapping precision is therefore a function of the number of recorded electrode sites and the precision and speed of data acquisition and processing. Simple activation maps can be created by examining the activation wavefronts from several intracardiac sites simultaneously by using relatively few recording electrode sites or by looking at sequential electrograms recorded from a single bipolar pair of electrodes systematically moved from site to site and comparing the individual data points to a reference signal, such as the surface QRS or delta wave. With application of the computerized recording and processing techniques, it is expected that isochronal spatial mapping techniques may become a reality in electrophysiologic laboratories in the not too distant future.

Stimulator

Stimulators are multiple output devices that are capable of pacing the heart from at least two but preferably four independent locations (Fig. 3-25). They must be capable of asynchronous or synchronous pacing with variable output of 0.1 to 10 mA and 0.1- to 9.9-msec pulse duration. At least three independently programmable stimuli should be available on each channel,

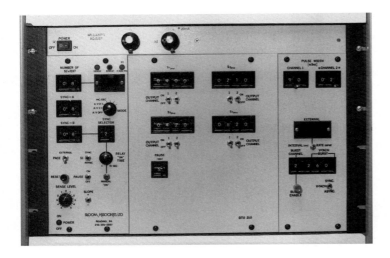

FIGURE 3-25. Bloom stimulator DTU 210 with two independent pacing channels and independently programmable burst pacing channel. (Courtesy of Bloom, Reading, PA.)

preferably up to five in at least 10-msec increments. Independently programmable burst overdrive pacing and a programmable antitachycardia pacing module should also be available.

The technique of programmed stimulation is beyond the scope of this chapter. A detailed discussion may be found elsewhere (53).

⦿ COMPLICATIONS OF INTERVENTIONAL ELECTROPHYSIOLOGIC STUDIES

Electrophysiologic studies and interventional techniques are remarkably safe, despite the fact that a significant number of patients have impaired left ventricular function and may have associated peripheral vascular disease. Fatal complications are rare. Death has been estimated to occur in fewer than 0.6% of electrophysiologic studies (54). This is comparable to the mortality associated with coronary angiography, which has been reported to occur in 0.1% to 0.3% of patients, depending on the patient mix (55,56). Complications that are associated with invasive electrophysiologic procedures may be classified as catheterization-related or caused by radiofrequency ablation.

Complications Related to Cardiac Catheterization

Complications related to cardiac catheterization can be largely avoided by good technique and careful patient selection. Electrophysiologic interventional techniques are absolutely contraindicated for patients with left main artery stenosis, unstable angina, and critical aortic stenosis. Careful consideration should also be given before using such procedures for patients with severe peripheral vascular disease. Consideration of risks and benefits should be weighed carefully for each invasive procedure, as well as the availability of less invasive options for diagnosis and therapy. The indications for the procedure should be clear, and risks should be minor compared with the potential benefits in each case. Potential difficulties should be anticipated rather than reacted to after they occur. In this way, most potential complications can be avoided. Despite these precautions, not all complications are avoidable even in the hands of the most experienced operators.

Prevention of fatal outcome for patients with risk factors such as severe left ventricular dysfunction (i.e., left ventricular ejection fraction $\leq 20\%$), advanced cerebrovascular and peripheral vascular disease, pulmonary insufficiency, and New York Heart Association (NYHA) functional class IV requires that the interventional techniques be coordinated with the backup surgical cardiothoracic team so that, if a serious complication occurs, the patient can easily be moved to a surgical suite for possible surgical intervention if necessary. The availability of angioplasty-capable personnel is also helpful in the event of, for example, coronary artery occlusion or spasm occurring during radiofrequency current delivery in the coronary sinus.

Local Vascular Complications

Vascular complications, including hemorrhage, arterial injury, and thrombophlebitis, have been reported in 0.7% of electrophysiologic studies (54). This is comparable to the vascular complication rates reported in the Registry report (56). It is quite remarkable that this is so, particularly because a typical electrophysiologic study requires multiple venous catheters and frequently requires arterial catheters, with longer vascular times (average of 2 to 3 hours per study and sometimes much longer for ablation procedures). Femoral venous thrombosis is a potential, although relatively rare, complication of electrophysiologic studies. It is most commonly seen in children and in patients who have undergone repeated procedures within a short time period. This is not particularly surprising, because up to three catheters may be positioned in a femoral vein for a relatively extended period. The potential for this complication can be minimized by a careful technique for vessel puncture, continuous saline infusion through the sheath throughout the study, and systemic heparinization. Treatment of this complication is similar to the therapy for idiopathic thrombophlebitis and includes bed rest and systemic heparinization for 7 to 10 days, followed by oral anticoagulation for up to 6 weeks.

Potential complications of the femoral arterial puncture and left heart catheterization include arterial thrombosis, distal embolization, false aneurysm, hematoma with vascular and neural compression, and delayed hemorrhage (55–60). Fortunately, these complications are rare, and the risk of their occurring can be minimized by careful technique.

Femoral arterial thrombosis requires urgent surgical intervention, because propagation of the thrombus distally may render late surgical intervention unsuccessful, leading to distal ischemia and the need for amputation. Distal embolization is rare with routine anticoagulation.

A false aneurysm may develop if compression is inadequate after the removal of the arterial sheath. These aneurysms are painful and pulsatile. Rupture may occur several days after the catheterization. Treatment of false aneurysms may require surgical intervention to correct the problem, although a technique for occlusion of the false aneurysm with ultrasound guidance has had a high rate of success.

Delayed hemorrhage most commonly results from poor clotting or from premature ambulation. Increased pressure from third-party payers to do same-day outpatient procedures with early ambulation may increase the frequency of this complication. Patients who are receiving aspirin or systemic anticoagulants are at a higher risk. We encourage at least 6 hours of bed rest after the procedure or longer when larger catheters and sheaths (7 or 8 Fr) are used. For outpatient procedures, we recommend 5- or 6-Fr catheters.

Arterial dissection may be caused by improper arterial puncture technique, particularly when the guide wire is advanced against resistance. Gentleness and lack of force during the guide wire and catheter advancement should help to minimize or prevent this complication. Dissection may be confirmed by contrast injection ipsilateral to the site of arterial puncture but occasionally may have to be diagnosed by retrograde arteriography from the contralateral femoral artery. Most frequently, dissections are benign when localized and may be managed conservatively. However, dissection may extend, compromise distal perfusion, and lead to vascular insufficiency. When this occurs, vascular percutaneous intervention may be required with angioplasty or, rarely, insertion of a vascular stent. Occasionally, surgical intervention may be required.

New-onset claudication after arterial puncture requires careful evaluation and arteriography to determine and correct the cause.

Perforation of the Heart or Vessels

Cardiac perforation has been reported in 0.15% of electrophysiologic studies (54). This rate is less than the perforation rates reported by the Cooperative Study on Cardiac Catheterization (55), which reported an incidence of 0.8%. This difference may reflect differences in patient populations or improvement in catheter design. Modern catheter designs allow for greater flexibility and torque control. The most common sites of perforation were the right atrium and the right ventricle. The greatest risk of perforation in our experience is in elderly women.

Perforation of the heart is the main hazard of the transseptal cardiac catheterization technique. The risk of this complication can be minimized by careful attention to details. Considerable experience is necessary with this technique. The technique should be avoided for patients with structural cardiac anomalies or kyphoscoliosis and restless or uncooperative patients.

Cardiac perforation may be accompanied by minimal symptoms and signs, or it may be a dramatic, life-threatening event. Unless heavily sedated, the patient with cardiac perforation usually complains of retrosternal or shoulder tip pain, dyspnea, and pain with breathing. This may be followed by hypotension and signs of pericardial tamponade. This requires immediate intervention, which consists of the reversal of anticoagulation, if pertinent, and pericardial aspiration with or without echocardiographic guidance. Occasionally, pericardiotomy is required, and perforation may require repair. More frequently, especially in younger patients, withdrawal of the catheter and careful observation may be all that is required, particularly when the right ventricular perforation is the cause. Clinical signs of tamponade, however, require immediate intervention.

Perforations of iliac veins, the inferior vena cava, iliac arteries, the abdominal aorta, and the subclavian artery have been reported and are usually caused by excessive force used in catheter manipulation. The dictum in catheter handling should be gentleness, avoidance of force, and attention to the patient's symptoms, particularly any complaints of pain during catheter manipulation. These warning symptoms should never be ignored.

Vasovagal Reactions

Vasovagal reactions are usually caused by inadequate local anesthesia in an anxious patient. The reaction is manifested by hypotension and bradycardia and is usually accompanied by nausea. The mechanism of the vasovagal response is thought to be sudden peripheral vasodilatation accompanied by vagal slowing of heart rate. Assumption of the Trendelenburg position with infusion of saline, with or without administration of atropine (0.5 to 1.0 mg), usually dramatically reverses the manifestations of this reaction. Vasovagal reaction should be reversed promptly; otherwise, it may progress to arrhythmias and cardiogenic shock, particularly in patients with severe ventricular dysfunction or severe coronary artery disease.

This reaction may also be seen in patients after the procedure, when the catheters and sheaths have been removed and the pressure is applied to the puncture sites, eliciting excessive discomfort. After the procedure, it is necessary to monitor the patient for the first 10 to 15 minutes before leaving the laboratory to ensure that the patient is stable.

Complications of the Subclavian Stick Technique

Pneumothorax

Pneumothorax is a potential complication of subclavian vein puncture. The incidence, as is true of the other potential complications, is a function of the operator's experience and training. It occurs rarely when a proper technique is used. It may be unrecognized at the time of its occurrence, especially if it is small. It is advisable to obtain a chest radiograph after the procedure, regardless of the presence or absence of symptoms that suggest pneumothorax.

When symptomatic, pneumothorax may be a dramatic event, heralded by cough, pleuritic chest pain, and occasionally hemoptysis and may be followed by hypotension and dyspnea, especially when it is associated with tension. In that case, immediate chest tube insertion is indicated to relieve tension. In an emergency and before chest tube insertion, a large-bore needle may be inserted into the pleural space to relieve tension while arrangements are made for the chest tube insertion. Most cases do not require chest tube insertion and resolve spontaneously unless the pneumothorax is large or associated with tension.

Hemothorax

Hemothorax may occur if a blood vessel is injured and a pneumothorax is also present. In the absence of a pleural puncture, the vessel is tamponaded, and the bleeding is usually limited. If there is no possibility of tamponade by the expanded lung, bleeding will continue, and hemothorax may result. This serious complication usually requires an immediate thoracotomy to stop the bleeding.

Subclavian Artery Puncture

Puncture of the subclavian artery is usually not a serious complication as long as it is recognized. When a subclavian stick is made, it is important to advance the guide wire to the inferior vena cava, which lies to the right of the spinal column, before the sheath is advanced. This approach ensures that the artery has not been inadvertently entered. At that point, withdrawal of the guide wire and digital compression can tamponade the bleeding. If arterial puncture has not been recognized and the sheath is advanced over the guide wire, serious bleeding or vessel injury may result.

Subclavian Arteriovenous Fistula

A subclavian arteriovenous fistula can occur if the anterior and posterior walls of the subclavian vein are punctured before the entry into the subclavian artery. It is important to puncture the anterior vein wall rather than advancing the needle through the vessel and then withdrawing it. A fistula may manifest late as a pulsatile, expanding mass, or it may be associated with an asymptomatic continuous murmur and thrill at the site of the original needle puncture.

Brachial Nerve Injury

Brachial nerve injury is a rare complication of the subclavian stick technique. More frequently, transient numbness of a finger or fingers on the ipsilateral side may follow the procedure because of the effect of the local anesthetic or because of transient neurapraxia caused by the needle puncture. Prognosis is usually excellent, and patient reassurance is usually all that is required.

Cerebrovascular Complications

Cerebrovascular complications are rarely associated with diagnostic electrophysiologic studies, because the catheters are most often positioned on the right side of the heart. However, with left-sided bypass tract ablations or left ventricular mapping and ablation, the potential for cerebral embolization is more significant. The transseptal technique may be associated with increased risk of embolization, and for transseptal and left heart catheterization, systemic anticoagulation is mandatory.

Cerebrovascular complications occurred in 0.2% of patients reported in the Cooperative Study of Cardiac Catheterization (55) and in 0.07% in the Registry report (56). The incidence of the cerebrovascular complications during interventional electrophysiologic procedures on the left side of the heart is likely to be comparable to the cardiac catheterization experience. Gentle catheter manipulation, adequate systemic anticoagulation, and avoidance of left ventricular catheter manipulation when a thrombus is known to be present in the left ventricle should help to minimize this risk.

Hypotension

Hypotension during the electrophysiologic study or interventional procedure may be caused by vasovagal reaction, hypovolemia, blood loss from vessel injury or pneumothorax, or delayed tamponade from cardiac perforation. Hypotension also may result from the administration of antiarrhythmic drugs, particularly the class IA agents, sedatives (e.g., midazolam), or narcotic analgesics.

In all cases, a careful search for the cause should be undertaken, and the problem should be corrected. Administration of normal saline with assumption of the Trendelenburg position is usually sufficient to correct hypotension, but pressors may occasionally be required to reverse the hypotension. Correction of the underlying cause, if it is related to vascular injury or pericardial tamponade, may require surgical intervention.

Myocardial Infarction

Myocardial infarction is rarely associated with interventional electrophysiologic techniques but may occur in patients with critical coronary artery disease. It may be precipitated by hypotension or by a prolonged episode of tachycardia.

Inadvertent advancement of the ablation catheter into the coronary artery and radiofrequency application at that site have been reported as a cause of coronary artery spasm or infarction. Treatment of acute myocardial infarction does not differ significantly from that of any cause. Exclusion of coronary artery spasm is important. Immediate coronary angiography and administration of intracoronary nitroglycerin are recommended. If this is unsuccessful, acute coronary angioplasty may be attempted. Rarely, acute coronary bypass surgery may be necessary to prevent infarction when the coronary occlusion results from the catheter-related coronary artery injury.

Complications Related to Radiofrequency Catheter Ablation

Radiofrequency catheter ablation shares all the vascular risks and potential complications of electrophysiologic studies. However, some unique complications may be associated with this technique. These include postablation chest pain, pericarditis, AV block, and radiation burns after prolonged procedures with long fluoroscopy exposures. These technique-related complications occur with different frequencies, depending on the site of ablation and the specific technique that is used.

CONCLUSIONS

Interventional electrophysiologic techniques are safe and effective when performed by an experienced operator. Although potential risks of the interventional procedures can and should be minimized by a careful technique and attention to detail, they cannot be entirely eliminated. The risk of an interventional procedure should always be balanced against the potential perceived benefit to the patient and risks and benefits of less-invasive alternatives. A well-equipped laboratory, trained personnel, and meticulous attention to detail are necessary to ensure optimal results.

REFERENCES

1. Cournard A. Cardiac catheterization: development of the technique, its contributions to experimental medicine, and its initial application in man. *Acta Med Scand Suppl* 1975;579:1–32.
2. Forssman W. Die Sondierung des rechten Herzens. *Klin Wochenschr* 1930;8:2085–2087.
3. Klein O. Bestimmung des zerkulatorischen minutens Volumen nach dem Fickschen Prinzip. *Munch Med Wochenschr* 1930;77:1311–1312.
4. Dexter L, Haynes FW, Burwell CS, et al. Studies of congenital disease. II. The pressure and oxygen content of blood in the right auricle, right ventricle, and pulmonary artery in control patients, with observations on the oxygen saturation and source of pulmonary "capillary" blood. *J Clin Invest* 1947;26:554–560.
5. Hellems HK, Haynes FW, Dexter L. Pulmonary capillary pressure in man. *J Appl Physiol* 1949;2:24–29.
6. Lagerlof H, Werko L. Studies on circulation of blood in man. *Scand J Clin Lab Invest* 1949;7:147–161.
7. Zimmerman HA, Scott RW, Becker ND. Catheterization of the left side of the heart in man. *Circulation* 1950;1:357–359.
8. Limon-Lason R, Bouchard A. El cateterismo intracardico; cathterzacion de las cavidades izquieredas en el hombre. Registro simultaneo de presion y electrocardiograma intercavetarios. *Arch Inst Cardiol Mex* 1950;21:271.
9. Seldinger SI. Catheter replacement of the needle in the percutaneous arteriography: a new technique. *Acta Radiol* 1953;39:368–376.
10. Ross J Jr. Transseptal left heart catheterization: a new method of left atrial puncture. *Ann Surg* 1959;149:395–401.
11. Cope C. Technique for transseptal catheterization of the left atrium: preliminary report. *J Thorac Surg* 1959;37:482–486.
12. Sones FM Jr, Shirey EK, Prondfit WL, Westcott RN. Cinecoronary angiography [Abstract]. *Circulation* 1959;20:773.
13. Ricketts HL, Abrams HL. Percutaneous selective coronary cine arteriography. *JAMA* 1962;181:620–624.
14. Judkins MP. Selective coronary arteriography: a percutaneous transluminal technique. *Radiology* 1967;89:815–824.
15. Gruntzig A, et al. Coronary transluminal angioplasty [Abstract]. *Circulation* 1977;56:II-319.
16. Scherlag BJ, Helfant RH, Damato AN, et al. A catheterization technique for recording His bundle stimulation and recording in the intact dog. *J Appl Physiol* 1968;25:425–428.
17. Durrer D, Schoo L, Schuilenburg RM, Wellens HJJ. The role of premature beats in the initiation and termination of supraventricular tachycardia in the WPW syndrome. *Circulation* 1967;36:644–662.
18. Coumel P, Cabrol C, Fabiato A, et al. Tachycardiamente par rythme réciproce. *Arch Mal Coeur Vaiss* 1967;60:1830–1840.
19. Wellens HJJ. *Electrical stimulation of the heart in the study and treatment of tachycardias.* Leiden: Stenfert Krosse, 1971.
20. Josephson ME, Horowitz LN, Farshidi A, et al. Recurrent sustained ventricular tachycardia. 2. Endocardial mapping. *Circulation* 1978;57:440–447.
21. Durrer D, Schuilenburg RM, Wellens HJJ. Preexcitation revisited. *Am J Cardiol* 1970;25:690–697.
22. Denes P, Dhingra RC, Chuquimia R, Rosen KM. Demonstration of dual A-V nodal pathways in patients with paroxysmal supraventricular tachycardia. *Circulation* 1973;43:549–555.
23. Rosen KM, Mehtra A, Miller RA. Demonstration of dual atrioventricular nodal pathways in man. *Am J Cardiol* 1974;33:291–294.
24. Wu D, Denes P, Wyndham C, et al. Demonstration of dual atrioventricular nodal pathways utilizing a ventricular extrastimulus in patients with atrioventricular nodal reentrant paroxysmal supraventricular tachycardia. *Circulation* 1975;52:789–798.
25. Waldo AL, MacLean WAH, Karp RB, et al. Entrainment and interruption of atrial flutter with atrial pacing: studies in man following open heart surgery. *Circulation* 1977;56:737–745.
26. Sealy WC, Hattler BC, Blumenschein SD, Cobb F. Surgical

treatment of Wolff-Parkinson-White syndrome. *Ann Thorac Surg* 1969;8:1–11.
27. Harken AH, Horowitz LN, Josephson ME. Surgical correction of recurrent sustained ventricular tachycardia following complete repair of tetralogy of Fallot. *J Thorac Cardiovasc Surg* 1980; 80:779–781.
28. Ross DL, Johnson DC, Dennis AR, et al. Curative surgery for atrioventricular junctional ("AV nodal") reentrant tachycardia. *J Am Coll Cardiol* 1985;6:1383–1392.
29. Jackman WM, Kuck KH, Naccarelli GV, et al. Radiofrequency current directed across the mitral annulus with bipolar epicardial-endocardial catheter electrode configuration in dogs. *Circulation* 1988;78:1288–1298.
30. Huang SKS, Lee MA, Bazgan ID, et al. Radiofrequency catheter ablation of atrioventricular junction for refractory supraventricular arrhythmias [Abstract]. *Circulation* 1988;78[Suppl 2]:II-156.
31. Langberg JJ, Chin MC, Rosenquist M, et al. Catheter ablation of the atrioventricular junction with radiofrequency energy. *Circulation* 1989;80:1527–1535.
32. Cosio FG, Lopez-Gil M, Goicolea A, et al. Radiofrequency ablation of the inferior vena cava–tricuspid valve isthmus in common atrial flutter. *Am J Cardiol* 1993;71:705–709.
33. Klein LS, Shih HT, Hackett FK, et al. Radiofrequency catheter ablation of ventricular tachycardia in patients without structural heart disease. *Circulation* 1992;85:1666–1674.
34. Stevenson WG, Khan H, Sager P, et al. Identification of reentry circuit sites during catheter mapping and radiofrequency ablation of ventricular tachycardia late after myocardial infarction. *Circulation* 1993;88:1647–1670.
35. Wilson FN, Johnston FD, Macleod AG, Barker PS. Electrocardiograms that represent the potential variations of a single electrode. *Am Heart J* 1934;9:447–458.
36. Shaefer H, Haas HG. Electrocardiography. In: Hamilton WF, Dow P, eds. *Handbook of physiology: circulation*. Vol I. Washington, DC: American Physiological Society, 1962:323–415.
37. Scher AM. The sequence of ventricular excitation. *Am J Cardiol* 1964;14:287–293.
38. Gallagher JJ, Kasell JH, Cox JL, et al. Techniques of intraoperative electrophysiologic mapping. *Am J Cardiol* 1982;49: 221–240.
39. Schaefer H, Trautwein W. Weitere versauche über die natur der erregungswelle im myokard des hundes. *Pflugers Arch* 1951; 253:152–164.
40. Durrer D, van der Tweel LH. The spread of the activation in the left ventricular wall of the dog, I. *Am Heart J* 1953;46: 683–691.
41. Frank R, Fontaine G, Piefitte M, Grosgogeat Y. Stimulation studies for the interpretation of delayed potentials. In: Schlepper M, Olsson B, eds. *Cardiac arrhythmias: diagnosis, prognosis, therapy. Proceedings of the First International Rhytmonorm-Congress*. Berlin: Springer-Verlag, 1983:53–61.
42. Clement E. Über eine neue methode zur untersuchung der fortleitung des erregungsvorganges in herzen. *Z Biol* 1912;58: 110–161.
43. Blanchard SM, Buhrman WC, Tedder M, et al. Concurrent activation detection from unipolar and bipolar electrodes [Abstract]. *Pacing Clin Electrophysiol* 1988;11:525.
44. Paul T, Moak JP, Morris C, Garson A Jr. Epicardial mapping: how to measure local activation? *Pacing Clin Electrophysiol* 1990; 13:285–292.
45. Kaplan DT, Smith JM, Rosenbaum D, Cohen RJ. On the precision of automated activation time estimation. *Comput Cardiol* 1988:101–104.
46. Scherlag BJ, Samet P, Helfant RH. His bundle electrogram: a critical appraisal of its uses and limitations. *Circulation* 1972;46: 601–613.
47. Josephson ME, Horowitz LN, Spielman SR, et al. Role of catheter mapping in the preoperative evaluation of ventricular tachycardia. *Am J Cardiol* 1982;49:207–220.
48. Cassidy DM, Vassalo JA, Marchlinski FE, et al. Endocardial mapping in humans in sinus rhythm with normal left ventricles: activation patterns and characteristics of electrograms. *Circulation* 1984;70:37–42.
49. Vassalo JA, Cassidy DM, Marchlinski FE, et al. Abnormalities of endocardial activation pattern in patients with previous myocardial infarction and ventricular tachycardia. *Am J Cardiol* 1986; 58:479–484.
50. Simpson EV, Ideker R, Smith WM. An automatic activation detector for bipolar cardiac electrograms. *Proceedings of the IEEE Engineering in Medicine and Biology 10th Annual International Conference*. 1988:113–114.
51. Ideker RE, Mirvis DM, Smith WM. Late, fractionated potentials [Editorial]. *Am J Cardiol* 1985;55:1614–1621.
52. Josephson ME, Horowitz LN, Farshidi A. Continuous local electrical activity: fact or artifact? [Editorial]. *Circulation* 1984; 70:529–532.
53. Singer I. Electrophysiologic study. In: Singer I, Kupersmith J, eds. *Clinical manual of electrophysiology*. Baltimore: Williams & Wilkins, 1993:52–67.
54. Horowitz LN, Kay HR, Kutalek SP, et al. Risks and complications of clinical cardiac electrophysiologic studies: a prospective analysis of 1000 consecutive patients. *J Am Coll Cardiol* 1987; 9:1261–1268.
55. Braunwald E, Swan HJC, eds. Cooperative studies on cardiac catheterization. *Circulation* 1968;Suppl:III-1.
56. Kennedy JW, et al. Complications associated with cardiac catheterization and angiography. *Cathet Cardiovasc Diagn* 1982;8: 5–11.
57. Judkins MP, Gander MP. Prevention of complications of coronary arteriography. *Circulation* 1974;49:599–602.
58. Eyer KM. Complications of transfemoral arteriography and their prevention using heparin. *Am Heart J* 1973;86:428.
59. Walker WJ, Mundall SL, Broderick HG, et al. Systemic heparinization for femoral percutaneous coronary arteriography. *N Engl J Med* 1973;288:826–828.
60. Brener BJ, Couch NP. Peripheral arterial complications of left heart catheterization and their management. *Am J Surg* 1973; 125:521–526.

CATHETER DESIGNS FOR INTERVENTIONAL ELECTROPHYSIOLOGY
• • •
JOHN GAISER

Radiofrequency catheter ablation has become the accepted first-line therapy for treatment of a variety of tachyarrhythmias. Under the heading of supraventricular tachycardia (SVT), radiofrequency catheter ablation is commonly used as a first-line therapy for atrioventricular (AV) junction ablation, AV node modification to treat AV nodal reentry tachycardia (AVNRT), and accessory pathway interruption, including Wolff-Parkinson-White syndrome. Although radiofrequency ablation for these indications has been common clinical practice worldwide for a number of years, the procedure and equipment for performing it have only recently been approved by the U.S. Food and Drug Administration. Radiofrequency catheter ablation was later used to treat atrial tachyarrhythmias directly, including ablation of ectopic atrial tachycardia (EAT) and atrial flutter. Early attempts at direct ablation of atrial fibrillation have been successfully undertaken as well. Radiofrequency catheter ablation has also been successfully used in the treatment of ventricular tachycardias (VTs).

As the clinical indications for catheter ablation have expanded beyond SVT, a wide variety of new catheter designs has been conceived, developed, and tested with the goal of addressing these new indications. Some of these designs have been successful, some have not been so successful, and others have yet to be fully evaluated. In the field of SVT ablation, many design improvements to current tools have been introduced to clinical practice, and additional innovations are planned. The driving forces for innovation have come from the medical community and from industry. Close cooperative effort between the two groups has produced the tools that most appropriately address clinical requirements. Close interaction among clinicians, engineers, and clinically trained industry personnel must be supported and enhanced if further device development is to proceed in a timely and efficient manner.

This chapter surveys catheter improvements and innovations that have recently been introduced to clinical practice, are currently in the animal or clinical investigational stage, or are in the concept or prototype stage. The discussion is organized according to the primary clinical indications for which radiofrequency catheter ablation is practiced or considered: SVT (i.e., accessory pathways, AV junction ablation, and AVNRT); atrial tachycardias (i.e., ectopic atrial tachycardias [EAT], atrial flutter, and atrial fibrillation); and ventricular tachycardias (i.e., idiopathic and ischemic or structural heart disease). New catheters for each clinical indication are further divided into tools for mapping and tools for ablation. A separate section covers intracardiac imaging catheters, which could find application in one or more of the clinical indications mentioned.

SUPRAVENTRICULAR TACHYCARDIA

Mapping

Mapping of SVTs has been conducted for the most part by using multiple reference catheters that are placed in select locations to detect key electrophysiologic signals plus a roving mapping/ablation catheter. The reference catheters are usually nonsteerable, meaning that they have a fixed distal curve. They typically are placed in locations such as the high right atrium, right ventricular apex, His bundle, and coronary sinus. High right atrium and right ventricular apex catheters generally have two or four electrodes. Some clinicians prefer hexapolar catheters for the His location, and 8-, 10-, or 12-electrode catheters are commonly used in the coronary sinus. The additional electrodes reduce the need for catheter repositioning to get the best possible signal. A variety of band spacing options is available to meet user preference, including 2-2-2, 2-5-2, and 5-5-5 mm.

Six French (Fr) is the most popular size for most nonsteerable reference catheters; 1 Fr equals approximately 0.013 inch or 0.33 mm. Specific preformed curve shapes are available to make anatomic positioning as straightforward as possible and to enhance catheter stability once positioned (Fig. 4-1). The typical steerable roving catheter is 7 or 8 Fr, with a deflectable tip for maneuverability and four electrodes. Most manufacturers provide a variety of curve sizes for access to various cardiac locations. Variations in tip stiffness are also available in some cases.

New catheter directions for SVT mapping include options in each of the following: electrode configuration, catheter size and shape, enhanced maneuverability, including deflectable designs, designs for specific clinical indications, options for thermal mapping, and enhanced mapping graphics.

Electrodes

Unipolar and bipolar electrograms are used in SVT mapping. In many cases of accessory pathway mapping, unipolar electrograms can provide important clues to identify successful ablation sites. Groups led by Haissaguerre, Grimm, Simmers, and Riccardi, among others, have described advantages of unipolar electrograms for accessory pathways ablation (1–4). This also applies for pace mapping of ventricular tachycardias, as reported by Kadish and associates (5). Bipolar electrograms provide the advantage of improved detection of low-amplitude signals from local sources while attenuating larger-amplitude signals from more distant sources (6). However, bipolar electrograms have lower spatial resolution, which can be crucial in ablating near the AV node. Unipolar recordings have better spatial resolution and can allow more accurate determination of activation time, but low-amplitude signals can be obscured by larger-amplitude signals from distant sources. The standard reference anode for unipolar electrograms is the Wilson central terminal on the electrogram recording equipment.

Kadish and associates and Jackman and associates reported that the signal-to-noise ratio for unipolar electrograms can be enhanced by placing the reference anode in the body, such as in the inferior vena cava (5,7). To provide the best possible unipolar mapping capability on a single catheter, some manufacturers provide a band electrode at a more proximal location on the mapping/ablation catheter shaft (e.g., 20 to 30 cm from the tip). This positions the proximal electrode in the vena cava or aortic arch when mapping on the right or left side of the heart, respectively. It is therefore possible to obtain improved unipolar

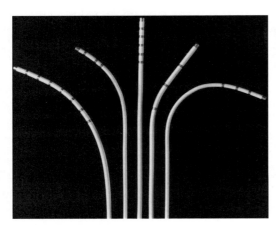

FIGURE 4-1. Commonly used curve shapes for fixed-curve reference diagnostic catheters. (Courtesy of Mansfield EP, Inc., Watertown, MA.)

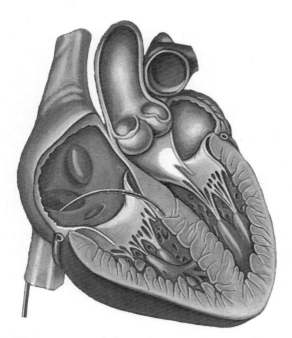

FIGURE 4-2. Special electrode spacing permits right ventricular pacing plus right ventricular and atrial recording from a single steerable catheter. (Courtesy of Cordis Webster, Inc., Baldwin Park, CA.)

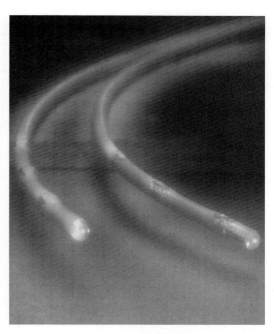

FIGURE 4-4. Fixed-curve and steerable versions of 12-pole orthogonal array catheters. (Courtesy of Cordis Webster, Inc., Baldwin Park, CA.)

electrogram signals by using these catheters without having to add another reference catheter.

Novel electrode positioning has also been used to create a "double-duty" catheter that permits recording and pacing at two anatomic locations using a single catheter (Fig. 4-2).

In an attempt to provide more precise spatial resolution and detect depolarization wavefronts in any possible direction for accessory pathway mapping, split-tip electrode and orthogonal array catheters have been developed (8,9) (Figs. 4-3 and 4-4). Catheters with orthogonal electrode arrays have found the most use in mapping left-sided accessory pathways when they are placed in the coronary sinus, as reported by Jackman and coworkers and Fogel and associates (7, 10,11). Linear electrode arrangements on mapping catheters amplify the component of the atrial or ventricular signal propagating parallel to the axis of the catheter. When a standard catheter is placed in the coronary sinus for mapping left-sided accessory pathways, the accessory pathway impulse, which travels at an angle to the recording dipole, is minimized and lost within the larger atrial or ventricular potential.

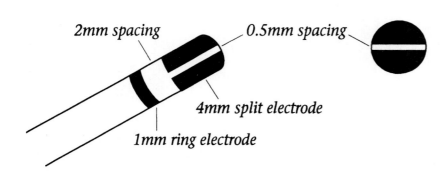

FIGURE 4-3. Split-tip electrode for improved recording of accessory pathway potentials in the orthogonal direction. (From Huang SK, ed. *Radiofrequency catheter ablation of cardiac arrhythmias.* Armonk, NY: Futura, 1995:574, with permission.)

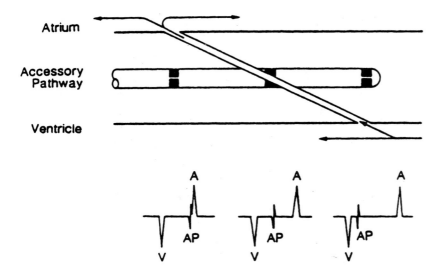

FIGURE 4-5. Schematic representation of an orthogonal electrode catheter positioned in the coronary sinus, with an accessory pathway connecting the ventricle and the atrium in an oblique fashion. The electrograms at the bottom of the figure represent those recorded from the proximal *(left)*, middle, and distal *(right)* orthogonal electrodes. During orthodromic reentrant tachycardia, a retrograde accessory pathway (AP) potential is recorded proximally close to the atrial insertion of the AP and distally close to the ventricular insertion site. (From Jackman WM, Friday KJ, Yeung-Lai-Wah JA, et al. New catheter technique for recording left free-wall accessory atrioventricular pathway fiber orientation. *Circulation* 1988;78:598–611, with permission.)

The orthogonal electrode arrangement (i.e., circumferential spacing, 90 or 180 degrees apart, in the same axial location) allows detection of accessory pathway potentials perpendicular to the catheter axis. This permits a detailed map to be constructed for atrial and ventricular insertions of the accessory pathway, which can theoretically be used to ablate the pathway with fewer radiofrequency applications (Fig. 4-5).

Catheter Size, Shape, and Construction

New tip shapes for nonsteerable mapping catheters are being developed to increase accessibility and improve stability. In addition to the standard coronary sinus-, Josephson-, Damato-, and Cournand-type curves, some manufacturers have released improved coronary sinus catheters with a double curve to permit easier access to the coronary sinus from a superior approach (Fig. 4-6).

Although 6-Fr catheters have been the standard for many years, several manufacturers have introduced 5-Fr, nonsteerable catheters (Fig. 4-7). Intended for pediatric and adult use, these catheters permit smaller introducer sheaths to be used. The 5-Fr catheters also generate less trauma to vessels, and they can sometimes be manipulated to locations where larger catheters cannot pass (e.g., middle cardiac vein). Some manufacturers have developed even smaller sizes (3 or 4 Fr). Concepts for introducing these very small catheters through a common introducer manifold have been implemented (Fig. 4-8).

Responding to clinicians' requests for catheters in a variety of convenient lengths, manufacturers have introduced catheters having lengths of 110 cm for left-sided access, 80 to 90 cm for right-sided or femoral vein access, and 65 cm or shorter for pediatric or superior venous access. Using the correct catheter length for a given situation reduces excessive shaft length outside the patient; this can maximize the catheter responsiveness.

Nonsteerable catheter construction has changed dramatically over the past few years. Traditionally, the most popular nonsteerable reference catheter has

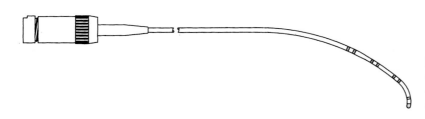

FIGURE 4-6. Octapolar 6-Fr catheter with a special double-radius curve shape to enhance access to the coronary sinus from a superior approach. (Courtesy of Daig Corporation, Minnetonka, MN.)

been the 6-Fr woven Dacron design. Forgiving, if unresponsive, maneuvering characteristics, conformability at body temperature, and familiarity through use in early training are all reasons that users cite to explain the popularity of this design. Initial attempts at providing alternative nonsteerable catheter designs (e.g., composites) met with limited acceptance because of poor stability or radically different behavior. Later composite catheter introductions were more successful because the designs provided improved torque response without sacrificing predictable performance. Composite catheter designs can be produced less expensively than woven Dacron, making it possible for manufacturers to sell them at a more competitive price.

Steerability

Special curves, smaller sizes, and composite shaft construction have made the placement of nonsteerable catheters easier. In some situations, however, none of these improvements provide enough maneuverability

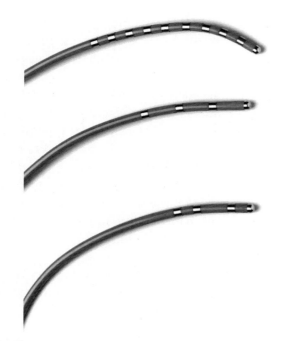

FIGURE 4-7. Assortment of 5-Fr fixed-curve reference diagnostic catheters, including quadripolar and decapolar models. (Courtesy of Medtronic CardioRhythm, Inc., San Jose, CA.)

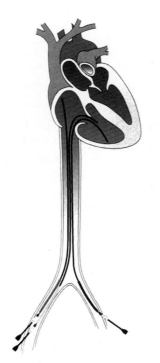

Competitive Diagnostic Catheters

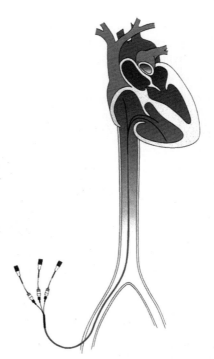

Cardiac Pathways Corporation Trio™ Multi-lumen Introducer and Ensemble™ Diagnostic Catheters

FIGURE 4-8. Three 2-Fr, fixed-curve reference diagnostic catheters are introduced through a single, long sheath inserted into the inferior vena cava. (Courtesy of Cardiac Pathways, Inc., Sunnyvale, CA.)

to reach desired locations. For these situations, steerable reference catheters are often used. For example, accessing the coronary sinus os from the femoral vein can be quite challenging with a nonsteerable catheter. Several manufacturers have introduced steerable octapolar and decapolar catheters for customers who prefer femoral access to the coronary sinus or for situations in which the superior access is not feasible. At some institutions, clinicians have chosen to use exclusively steerable reference catheters, reducing the number of catheters for the typical SVT case from three to four nonsteerables to one to three steerables. For some users, switching to steerables can provide overall device cost savings and reduced catheter manipulation or fluoroscopy time. The use of steerable catheters for mapping also facilitates certain specific procedures, including locating and pacing accessory pathways and mapping of certain atrial tachycardias.

Intracoronary Catheters

For special clinical indications such as Ebstein's anomaly, Cappato and colleagues have reported placing mapping catheters in the right coronary artery to provide a visual anatomic reference and electrogram information to improve chances for success in ablating accessory pathways (12). These coronary mapping catheters are typically very small and flexible and can contain a variety of electrode configurations. Intracoronary electrode catheters are discussed at greater length in the SVT ablation and ventricular tachycardia mapping sections of this chapter.

Thermal Mapping

Mapping of the AV junction using test burns to cause reversible tissue injury and then applying higher-power or longer-duration burns to permanently destroy tissue at the identified target has been described by Nath and associates and Cote and coworkers (13, 14). Applications of this technique to ventricular tachycardia mapping are discussed later in this chapter.

Enhanced Mapping Graphics

Activation mapping for SVT can take 1 to 3 hours on average, depending on the specific type of arrhythmia and patient. Electrophysiologic mapping systems have improved over the past several years, incorporating better filtering (especially for radiofrequency ablation interference), higher-resolution electrograms, and user-friendly tools for quicker determination of activation timing. Future enhancements to electrophysiologic mapping will include real-time graphic representation of activation maps for accurate and rapid localization of earliest activation times. These activation maps may be combined with a graphical display of anatomic information and catheter position. Although activation maps of this sort have been demonstrated to work for pacing stimuli in healthy hearts, the technology remains to be proven in patients with heart disease. More information regarding new mapping technologies is presented in the section on ventricular tachycardia mapping that follows.

Ablation

During the 8-year period that radiofrequency catheter ablation for SVT has been generally practiced, the first half saw relatively little innovative catheter development. In the early 1990s, however, a number of new electrophysiology catheter companies were formed with the express purpose of developing catheter ablation systems that could provide enhanced performance and safety. At the same time, clinicians were gaining considerable experience in catheter ablation and identifying specific unmet needs for new devices. As a result, the breadth of radiofrequency ablation catheters that are available to electrophysiologists has dramatically expanded in the past few years. Catheter manufacturers offer various steerable catheters aimed at specific anatomic locations, and numerous new designs aimed at improving efficacy have been introduced or proposed.

New catheter designs for SVT ablation include various options for curve size and shape and performance characteristics that are suited to particular locations, ideas for speeding up and simplifying the procedure, smaller catheters for pediatric and adult procedures, positioning sheaths for stability, alternative ablation electrodes, and incorporation of temperature or other feedback and control functions into radiofrequency generator and catheter systems.

Size, Shape, and Performance Options

Several catheter manufacturers have expanded their initial steerable ablation catheter offerings into families of products having different characteristics to meet specific needs. Most catheter manufacturers offer different curve sizes aimed at different locations in the heart. For example, manufacturers offer small curves that deflect to tighter radii for ablation of left-sided pathways on the mitral valve annulus from a retrograde approach. In this situation, the catheter tip must cross the aortic valve without causing damage and deflect to approximately 180 degrees to tuck up under the mitral valve in tight quarters. Manufacturers also offer larger curves for ablation of right freewall accessory pathways or for AVNRT ablation, where a long reach is needed.

In addition to curve size, different performance characteristics are also required for these two example sites. For the left side under the mitral valve, smooth torque transmission is a necessity because the catheter has gone through one 180-degree bend in the shaft around the aortic arch plus a second 180-degree bend at the tip. A more flexible shaft allowing precise maneuvering of the tip is required. For the right-sided freewall location, a high degree of tip stability and support is required. This requirement could translate into a stiffer shaft and tip with more body than the left-sided catheter.

Most catheter manufacturers provide wall charts or other reference materials that recommend catheters in their line having a particular curve size and shape for certain anatomic positions. Over the next few years, manufacturers will continue to broaden product lines with different tip or shaft flexibility options and curve sizes to match different applications. As a result, clinicians should have a formidable array of products from which to choose, with one to match nearly every clinical requirement.

In Vivo *Adjustment*

A more advanced concept for matching catheter characteristics to anatomic need is the *in vivo* adjustable catheter. Understanding that catheter users cannot always select the most appropriate catheter curve size in advance, some manufacturers have developed catheters that have an adjustable curve size (Fig. 4-9). Most of the adjustable catheter designs use an internal

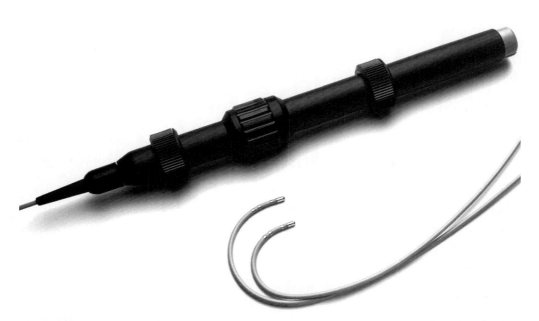

FIGURE 4-9. Multiple-curve catheter provides *in vivo* adjustments. The distal control deflects the tip, the middle control rotates the tip laterally, and the proximal control changes the radius of the tip curve. Sliding controls are lockable to maintain a preset tip position. (Courtesy of Medtronic CardioRhythm, Inc., San Jose, CA.)

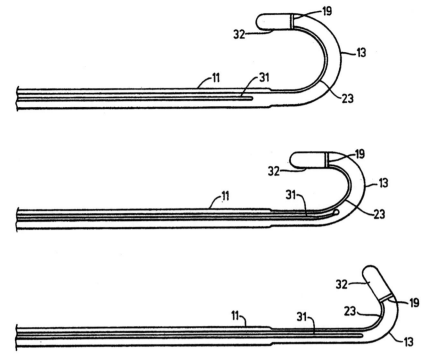

FIGURE 4-10. Sliding the stiffening mandrel within the catheter tip causes the curve size to change. (From Cimino W. Catheter for electrophysiological procedures. US Patent No 5,364,352, 1994, with permission.)

member that is moved back and forth to alter tip stiffness at a given position, which changes the curve size (Fig. 4-10). The change in tip stiffness afforded by this sliding member can also provide an important performance variable to allow the physician to adjust the catheter to meet situational requirements.

Anatomy-Specific Designs

In addition to adjustable designs, researchers and companies have developed catheters that are specialized for a particular location or procedure. One such commercially available catheter employs an adjustable-size loop, designed to place a ring of mapping electrodes in proximity to the tricuspid valve annulus tricuspid valve annulus (15) (Fig. 4-11). The size of the loop can be somewhat adjusted to fit a particular tricuspid valve annulus size. Another design proposed by Avitall and colleagues is a double-spline catheter, which has two arms joined at their proximal and distal extremities and the capability to expand or contract the opening between the splines (16) (Fig. 4-12).

An alternative to catheters designed for mapping the tricuspid annulus by the endocardium is a catheter designed for epicardial mapping from within the right coronary artery, which closely follows the tricuspid annulus in normal patients. Cappato and coworkers and Kuck and colleagues described the effective use of these catheters for Ebstein's anomaly and other applications (17–19). Over-the-guide-wire and rapid-exchange catheters intended for coronary artery map-

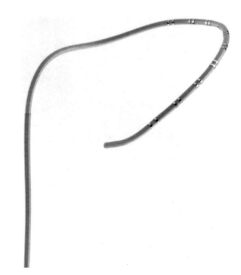

FIGURE 4-11. A 20-pole diagnostic catheter with a special shape for mapping the tricuspid valve annulus region. (Courtesy of Cordis Webster, Inc., Baldwin Park, CA.)

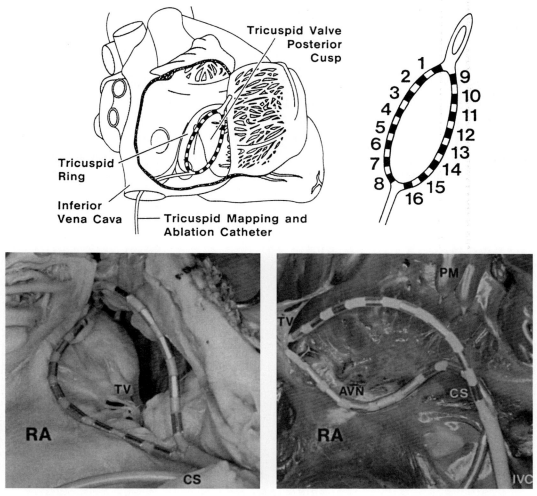

FIGURE 4-12. Expanding double-spline catheter with 16 × 4 mm wide bands for mapping and ablation. The shape can be adjusted *in vivo* to conform to tricuspid annulus region. (From Avitall B, Hare J, Krum D, Dhala A. The anatomical determinants for the design of intracardiac mapping and ablation catheters. *Pacing Clin Electrophysiol* 1994;17:141, with permission.)

ping have been developed by several manufacturers. These catheters tend to be very small, 2 or 3 Fr in diameter, with 2 to 12 mapping electrodes (Fig. 4-13). There are several disadvantages to right coronary artery mapping catheters. Electrophysiologists who are not trained for interventions in the coronary arteries are reluctant to use them unless absolutely necessary. Inserting devices into coronary arteries can cause acute effects such as spasm or perforation, and the trauma to the vessel intima may stimulate a healing

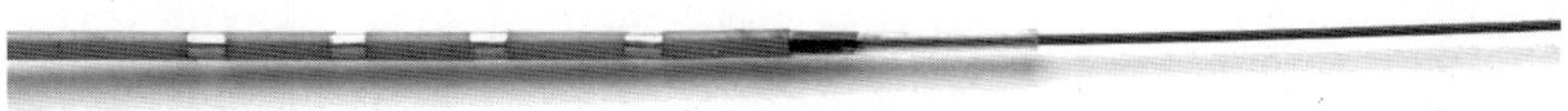

FIGURE 4-13. Diagnostic mapping electrode catheter for use in coronary arteries and veins: 2.5-Fr, over-the-guide wire, quadripolar version. (Courtesy of Medtronic CardioRhythm, Inc., San Jose, CA.)

response that could result in an artery-occluding lesion some years later.

For catheter-tip stability on the atrial side of the mitral valve annulus, several innovative catheter designs have been proposed. One such design from Avitall and associates involves a catheter with a pigtail distal end, having multiple band electrodes for mapping and ablation (20) (Fig. 4-14). This catheter was designed to be positioned in retrograde fashion across the mitral valve so that the secondary pigtail curve fits in the depression in the left atrium just above the mitral annulus. The multiple band electrodes are then used for mapping in the vicinity of the mitral valve and ablation from the appropriate electrode. Another anatomy-specific catheter, proposed and being developed by Kuck and colleagues, has the double-reverse curve of an Amplatz coronary guide catheter (Fig. 4-15). This special shape is intended to seat securely on the tricuspid or mitral valve annulus, creating a very stable tip electrode position for ablation of accessory pathways (Fig. 4-16). The proximal and distal curves can be made independently adjustable to match anatomy, and multiple ablation electrodes provide flexibility in the selection of lesion location.

Regarding Mahaim fiber ablation, surgical evidence from Guiraudon and coworkers (21) and elec-

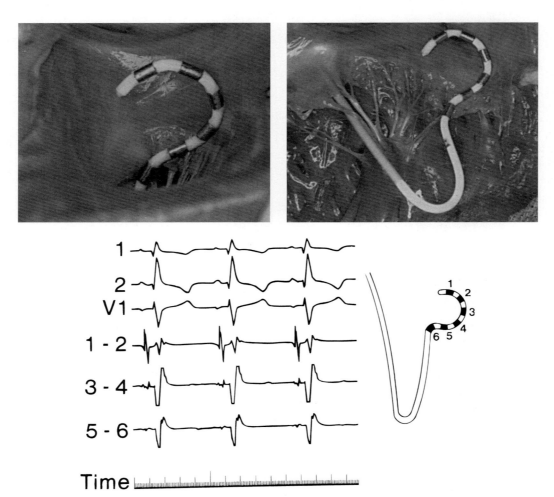

FIGURE 4-14. The pigtail catheter with 6 × 4 mm wide bands for mapping and ablation is designed to fit the left atrium just above the mitral valve annulus and to maintain a stable position. Electrograms from bands 1 through 6 show the transition from atrial to ventricular stimulus across the mitral ring. (From Avitall B, Hare J, Krum D, Dhala A. The anatomical determinants for the design of intracardiac mapping and ablation catheters. *Pacing Clin Electrophysiol* 1994;17:908–918, with permission.)

trophysiologic mapping data from Kuck and colleagues (22) confirm that many Mahaim fibers consist of a secondary AV node–like structure at or near the tricuspid annulus connecting to a His bundle–like structure having a ventricular or fascicular distal insertion. Other clinical ablation evidence from Grogin and associates points to an origin in the AV node or the slow AV nodal pathway for patients who have AVNRT and Mahaim tracts (23). The mapping bands on the primary curve of the Amplatz-type catheter can facilitate the mapping of these Mahaim fibers in the right ventricle. Another device aimed at improving Mahaim fiber mapping in the septal region is an octapolar catheter that has electrodes specially placed for electrogram recording and pacing of the His and right bundle branch (Fig. 4-17).

Brugada and Martinez-Alday and coworkers have observed that recording of discrete Mahaim potentials near the tricuspid annulus indicates an optimal site for ablation of Mahaim fibers (24,25). Most electrophysiologists report a preference for ablating the atrial insertion of Mahaim fibers (26). Miller and colleagues

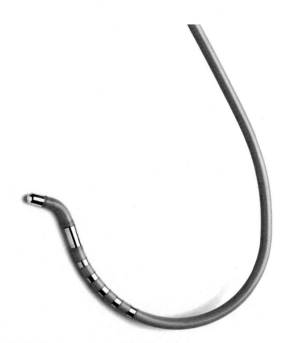

FIGURE 4-15. The Amplatz catheter has two ablation electrodes plus a series of bands for mapping ventricular insertion of Mahaim fibers. Curves are independently deflectable and designed to maintain a stable position on the tricuspid valve annulus. Other applications for similar designs include mapping and ablation on the mitral valve annulus. (Courtesy of Medtronic CardioRhythm, Inc., San Jose, CA.)

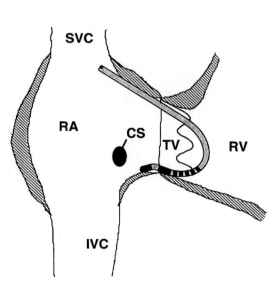

FIGURE 4-16. Amplatz catheter is shown in position, with ablation electrodes straddling the tricuspid valve annulus. (Courtesy of Medtronic CardioRhythm, Inc., San Jose, CA.)

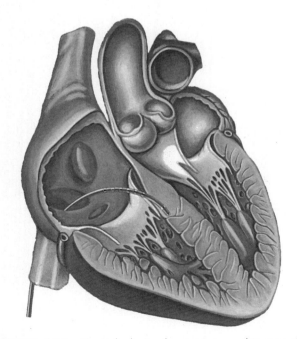

FIGURE 4-17. Special electrode spacing on this steerable catheter permits recording the His bundle electrogram (HBE) and pacing near this region. A second application is the recording of HBE and bundle branch electrograms from a single catheter. (Courtesy of Cordis Webster, Inc., Baldwin Park, CA.)

and Haissaguerre and associates reported success in ablating the ventricular insertion of Mahaim fibers (27,28). The ideal catheter for ablating Mahaim fibers may need atrial and ventricular ablation capability.

A final example of a catheter design with advantages for a particular anatomic situation is the open-lumen catheter, used by some to generate a clear fluoroscopic image of the coronary sinus and its branches (Fig. 4-18). Giorgberidze and coworkers and Chieng and colleagues showed that retrograde injection of radiopaque contrast agents into the coronary sinus can be especially helpful in attempting to navigate congenital abnormalities (29,30). Tebbenjohanns and coworkers have shown that the incidence of coronary sinus abnormalities approaches 50% for patients with posteroseptal pathways (31). As a modification to the open-lumen coronary sinus catheter, an occlusion balloon can provide even better visualization of complex coronary sinus anatomy. Arruda and associates observed that the addition of a balloon to better occlude the coronary sinus during angiography can reduce the amount of dye required and obviate subselective injection of contrast into venous branches (32).

Small-Size Catheters

Designed primarily for performing pediatric ablation, 5-Fr steerable ablation catheters are commercially available from several manufacturers (Fig. 4-19). Like their diagnostic counterparts, these catheters permit a smaller, less traumatic puncture site. For left-sided ablations, a smaller puncture site permits more aggressive anticoagulation. Shorter hospitalization after ablation is another potential advantage, with outpatient ablation a reasonable possibility. For pediatric applications, smaller catheters mean less risk of vessel and

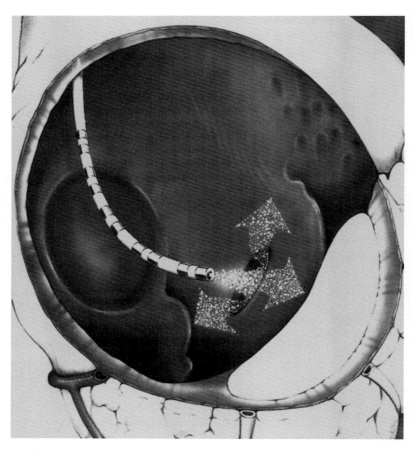

FIGURE 4-18. Open-lumen catheter permits contrast injection into the coronary sinus for detailed anatomy visualization. (Courtesy of Electro-Catheter Corporation, Rahway, NJ.)

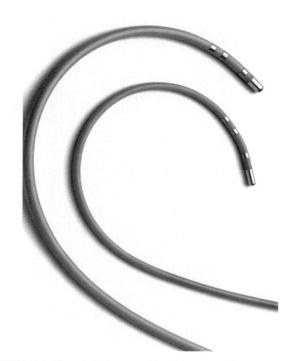

FIGURE 4-19. A 5-Fr, steerable ablation catheter next to a 7-Fr model. Temperature feedback is especially important with the 5-Fr size because of the increased possibility of impedance rise resulting from higher current density at the tip electrode relative to that of the 7-Fr size. (Courtesy of Medtronic CardioRhythm, Inc., San Jose, CA.)

valve damage. The smaller-tip electrode can create a more precise lesion, an advantage in young children for whom growth of lesions over time may be a concern (33).

For adults, more precise lesion control afforded by 5-Fr ablation catheters may reduce the likelihood of inadvertent complete heart block when ablating in the vicinity of the AV node. Until the advent of radiofrequency generators incorporating temperature monitoring and control, ablating with smaller-tip electrodes was hampered by poor tip electrode cooling, resulting in frequent impedance rise and coagulum formation. Real-time control of tip electrode temperature has made ablation with 5-Fr tip electrodes much more practical. Patient series by Kottkamp and colleagues (34,35) indicate that 5-Fr catheters may be used to ablate AVNRT and accessory pathways in adults with similar efficacy and reduced complications compared with 7-Fr catheters.

Another important potential application for 5-Fr ablation catheters is in the coronary sinus. Especially for posteroseptal pathways, the coronary sinus can provide a convenient (sometimes the only) avenue for ablation of epicardial pathway insertions, as reported by Langberg and coworkers and Giorgberidze and associates (36,37). The 7-Fr ablation catheters can be bulky and relatively stiff, limiting access to distal regions and branches of the coronary sinus. Their stiffness also can increase the risk of coronary sinus perforation. The 5-Fr ablation catheters can bring needed flexibility and maneuverability to bear on a difficult problem. The smaller lesion size afforded by the 5-Fr tip electrode can be beneficial in reducing overall trauma to the coronary sinus and nearby coronary arteries but may reduce efficacy in the ablation of more distant pathways.

Sheaths

For many years, the Brockenbrough needle and Mullins sheath have been necessary tools in performing transseptal punctures for mapping and ablation in the left atrium. Studies by Manolis and colleagues and Mittleman and coworkers indicated that, although the transaortic and transseptal approaches to left-sided ablation can be considered complementary, the transseptal approach may offer advantages in terms of success rate, radiation exposure, and complication rate (38,39). However, another study by Ma and associates showed little difference (40).

Some catheter manufacturers have developed and introduced long sheaths for the facilitation of catheter ablation in a variety of areas in the heart (Fig. 4-20). Ideally, the sheaths provide a stable platform from which the ablation catheter can be advanced, withdrawn, and torqued with precision. When using long sheaths, especially for ablation on the right side, some users claim that they can achieve improved tip-to-tissue contact, resulting in greater ablation efficiency and success. A variety of sheath curve designs are available, each intended to position a catheter at a specific location in the heart. All have the disadvantage of increasing the puncture site size by 1 or 2 Fr beyond the catheter shaft size. Sheaths are employed as a first-line adjunctive tool for some procedures or as a last resort, depending on physician preference. Additional sheath designs have been developed to fa-

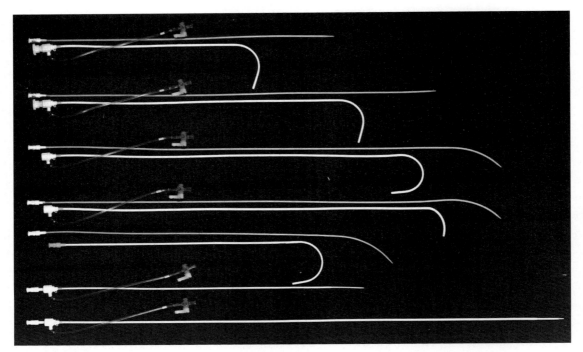

FIGURE 4-20. Assortment of long sheaths with various curve shapes for left and right heart applications. (Courtesy of Daig Corporation, Minnetonka, MN.)

cilitate ablation therapy for non-SVT clinical indications, such as atrial fibrillation (discussed below).

Ablation Electrodes

Haines and colleagues found that radiofrequency lesions increase in area and depth with increasing tip electrode radius (41). Likewise, lesion size has been shown to increase with increasing tip temperature and with tip length (42). Beginning in the late 1980s, tip electrodes for SVT ablation progressed from the original 2-mm-long, 7-Fr mapping tips to the 4-mm tips that are commonly in use today. Tips have grown to 6, 8, and 12 mm for certain specific applications, all with the intention of creating larger lesions (Fig. 4-21). A result of the move to larger ablation electrodes is a reduced likelihood of impedance rise and coagulum formation. Because the larger electrode has more surface area in tissue contact, the local current density is reduced. The lower current density produces a

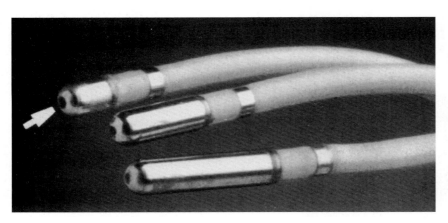

FIGURE 4-21. Electrodes with 4-, 8-, and 12-mm tips. The exposed thermistor temperature sensor (arrow) is mounted at the distal end of the tip. (From Langberg JJ, Gallagher M, Strickberger SA, Amirana O. Temperature-guided radiofrequency catheter ablation with very large distal electrodes. Circulation 1993; 88:245–249, with permission.)

lower temperature at the electrode-to-tissue interface and less heat conducted to the electrode. The larger electrode surface area that is in contact with blood provides greater cooling capacity. Both of these factors may reduce the occurrence of impedance rise. The same two factors can create larger lesions. First, the greater electrode surface area that is in contact with the tissue produces a larger volume of tissue that is resistively heated. Second, the increased cooling effect permits more radiofrequency energy to be delivered to the tissue for longer periods of time before an impedance rise occurs.

An animal study conducted by Langberg and coworkers demonstrated that increasing the length of a 7-Fr ablation electrode from 4 to 8 mm can quadruple lesion volume and double lesion depth (43) (Fig. 4-22). However, this study and another by Chan and associates showed that further increase in electrode length beyond 8 to 10 mm resulted in a decline in lesion size (43,44). Not surprisingly, larger electrodes required more power to achieve a desired tip temperature, and impedance monitored during radiofrequency ablation was inversely related to electrode size. A potential downside for larger tip electrodes is reduced spatial resolution for mapping. The two factors that can reduce impedance rises for large electrodes—lower current density and greater cooling effect—may also prevent adequate tissue heating in regions of high blood flow.

The 5-Fr tip electrodes, having reduced surface area and resulting higher current densities, are more efficient than 7-Fr tips, because they require less power to create a similar tip temperature. The 7-Fr electrodes are capable of carrying more power and therefore creating larger lesions. However, 5-Fr ablation electrodes may prove useful in situations in which high blood flow creates so much cooling that adequate tip temperatures cannot be achieved by using larger tips, assuming that a limited amount of radiofrequency power is available (e.g., 50 W).

Ablation catheter-tip electrodes have traditionally been constructed of platinum iridium for reasons of radiopacity, conductivity, and biocompatibility. Alternative materials have been prototyped and evaluated, including gold alloys. A study by Simmons and colleagues demonstrated that gold electrodes, because of their greater thermal conductivity, may be capable of delivering more power and creating larger lesions without impedance rise than platinum electrodes (45).

Other tip electrode innovations include peanut-shaped electrodes, designed to maintain a stable position on the tricuspid or mitral valve annulus (Fig. 4-23). The "saddle" portion of the electrode is designed

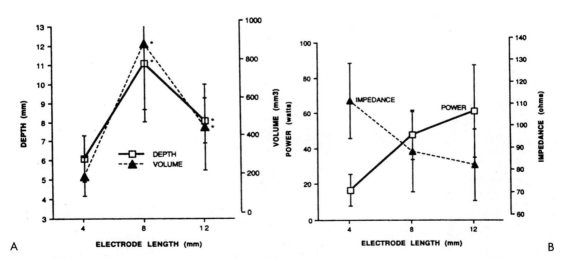

FIGURE 4-22. A: Mean maximal lesion depth and volume as a function of electrode length. B: Impedance and steady-state power as a function of electrode length. (From Langberg JJ, Gallagher M, Strickberger SA, Amirana O. Temperature-guided radiofrequency catheter ablation with very large distal electrodes. *Circulation* 1993;88:245–249, with permission.)

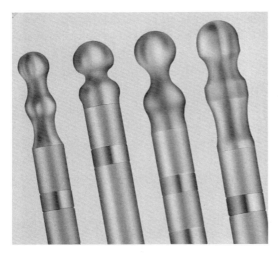

FIGURE 4-23. Examples of various peanut-shaped electrode configurations that are intended to improve stability of the tip electrode on a valve annulus. (Courtesy of EP Technologies, Inc., Sunnyvale, CA.)

to seat on the valve annulus to reduce slippage. Another potential advantage is increased current density because of the curvature.

Temperature Feedback

The first-generation radiofrequency ablation "system" that was in common use by the late 1980s combined 4-mm-tip, steerable, "diagnostic" catheters with radiofrequency generators that were originally developed for neurosurgical applications (Fig. 4-24). Although these radiofrequency generators can accept temperature sensor inputs, the catheters do not contain temperature sensors. This combination, still in use in some electrophysiology laboratories, requires the operator to manually control power delivered to the ablation electrode, based on observing impedance measured between the ablation electrode and an indifferent electrode. The potential for a sudden impedance rise during radiofrequency ablation when the tip electrode-to-tissue interface temperature reaches 100°C is well known (46) (Fig. 4-25). On observing the beginnings of an impedance rise, the operator must quickly reduce or shut off power to prevent coagulum formation. Because the impedance rise happens quickly, it is difficult to stop before significant coagulum is already present. In addition to watching for impedance rise, a small decline in impedance has been proposed as an earlier warning signal.

To provide the operator with additional information that is useful for predicting impedance rise, a second generation of radiofrequency ablation system was developed (Fig. 4-26). These systems use a temperature sensor in the catheter tip electrode, which provides tip temperature information during ablation. Some radiofrequency generators have an adjustable temperature limit, which can be set below 100°C to prevent impedance rise. The clinician manually adjusts power while observing the temperature. If the tip temperature reaches the preset limit, power is cut off.

Third-generation ablation systems have since emerged, in which closed-loop feedback is used to

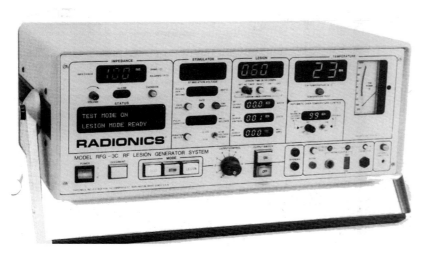

FIGURE 4-24. A radiofrequency generator is commonly used for cardiac ablation with catheters that do not monitor tip electrode temperature. Although the device has temperature inputs, no temperature sensor catheter has been approved by the U.S. Food and Drug Administration for this generator. (Courtesy of Radionics, Burlington, MA.)

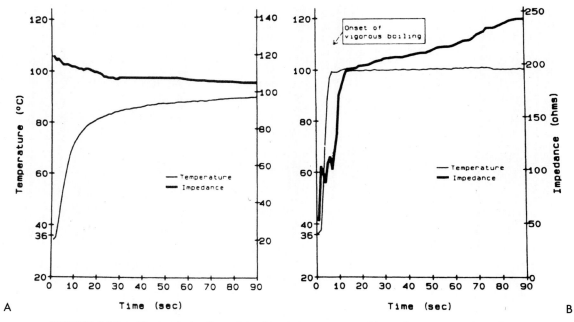

FIGURE 4-25. Electrode-to-tissue interface temperature and impedance versus time during radiofrequency ablation. **A:** A controlled, low-power delivery in which the temperature increases steadily to the 95°C maximum and the impedance drops by about 10 Ω. **B:** A higher-power delivery in which the temperature rapidly rises to 100°C, producing boiling at the electrode surface and a dramatic increase in electrical impedance. (From Nath S, Haines DE. Biophysics and pathology of catheter energy delivery systems. *Prog Cardiovasc Dis* 1995; 37:185–204, with permission.)

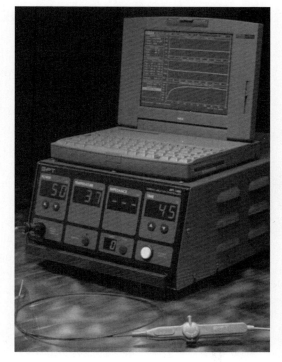

FIGURE 4-26. The radiofrequency (RF) ablation system consists of thermistor-tipped catheters and an RF generator that can monitor the catheter tip temperature during RF ablation. The system requires manual control of RF power to maintain the tip temperature at a desired level, but an upgrade for true temperature control capability is planned. Graphic display of ablation parameters (e.g., power, temperature, impedance) is available. (Courtesy of EP Technologies, Inc., Sunnyvale, CA.)

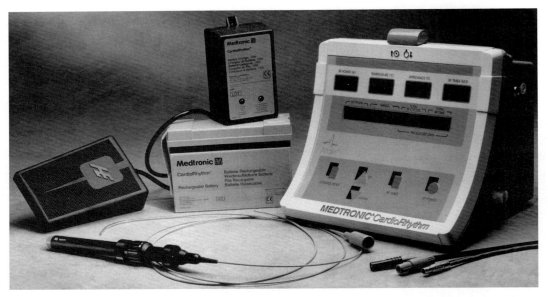

FIGURE 4-27. The radiofrequency (RF) ablation system comprises thermocouple-tipped catheters and an RF generator that can maintain catheter tip temperature at a preselected set point. RF power is automatically adjusted to compensate for variations in tip-to-tissue contact, blood flow, and other factors to maintain a constant tip temperature. Graphic display of ablation parameters is available. (Courtesy of Medtronic CardioRhythm, Inc., San Jose, CA.)

control tip temperature using a temperature sensor in the tip (Figs. 4-27 and 4-28). The operator determines the desired tip temperature, and power is automatically regulated to maintain that temperature. Because tip contact can vary rapidly over time in a beating heart, it is difficult to manually regulate power to keep temperature within a desired range. Local blood flow is different for various locations. Using an automatic power controller to maintain a desired tip temperature takes much of the workload off the operator. As a result, a significant reduction in impedance rise incidents and high temperature shutoff levels occur.

In vitro research by Nath and coworkers demonstrated that tissue temperature is a more accurate predictor of lesion size than is power delivered (46) (Fig. 4-29). Pires and associates demonstrated in dogs that controlling radiofrequency power to achieve a preset tip temperature had the potential for greater lesion size control and lower incidence of impedance rise than monitoring temperature with a preset power level (47). *In vitro* studies in a pulsatile flow tank by Chang and colleagues have demonstrated that variations in power that are required to achieve a constant tip electrode temperature can predict tip-to-tissue contact, depending on flow conditions (48). These data suggest that observing delivered power and temperature achieved may help predict ablation efficacy

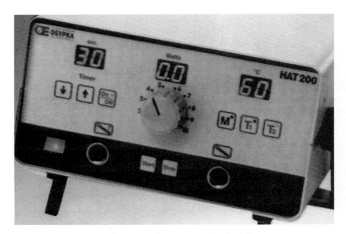

FIGURE 4-28. The radiofrequency (RF) ablation system includes thermistor-tipped catheters and an RF generator capable of automatically controlling tip temperature. Graphic display of ablation parameters is available. (Courtesy of Oscor Medical Corporation [Osypka, GmbH], Palm Harbor, FL.)

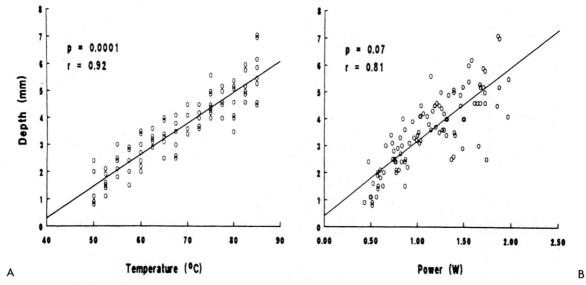

FIGURE 4-29. The linear relationship between the radiofrequency (RF) lesion depth and electrode-to-tissue interface temperature **(A)** and mean delivered power **(B)**. Temperature is a more accurate predictor of lesion size. (From Nath S, Haines DE. Biophysics and pathology of catheter energy delivery systems. *Prog Cardiovasc Dis* 1995;37:185–204, with permission.)

and control lesion size when performing clinical ablations using temperature control.

In clinical practice using closed-loop temperature control, data supporting a variety of potential benefits have been generated. These include lower incidence of impedance rise and coagulum, shorter procedure time, and less fluoroscopy time. Some of these data, collected in a clinical trial evaluating closed-loop temperature control, are summarized in Table 4-1 (49–52).

Temperature control ablation data collected by Calkins and coworkers have demonstrated that clinical success can be achieved at a variety of different temperatures and that the ability to achieve the temperature set point depends on the location (53). In another clinical series reported by Calkins and associates, higher tip electrode temperature predicted ablation success primarily at septal locations (54). Clinical data collected by Choi and colleagues have shown that real-time temperature control reliably allows the operator to tell the difference between ablation ineffectiveness due to inability to reach temperature and ineffectiveness due to incorrect positioning of the catheter tip (55).

TABLE 4-1 • TEMPERATURE CONTROL CLINICAL DATA

Study	Number Of Patients	Parameter Measured	Temp Control Mode	Power Control Mode Or System
Calkins et al. (49)	270	Coagulum	4%	22%
O'Connor et al. (50)	66 pediatric	Fluoro time	21 min	53 min
		Procedure	64 min	128 min
		Impedance rise	2.1%	55.6%
Gillette et al. (51)	174 vs. 277	Impedance rise	0.2 per patient	0.8 per patient
Farré et al. (52)	128	Radiofrequency burns	4.1 burns	8.6 burns

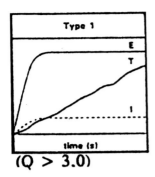 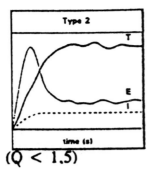 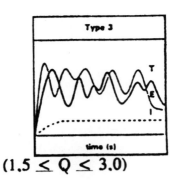

FIGURE 4-30. Plots showing type 1, 2, and 3 curves for temperature and power recorded during closed-loop temperature-controlled radiofrequency ablation. Type 1 was successful in 7.2% of applications. Type 2 was successful in 38.5% of applications. Type 3 was successful in 4.5% of applications. Type 2 was observed more often in left-sided accessory pathway (AP) ablation than in right-sided cases, which may explain why the number of applications was higher for right-sided APs in this series. (From Stellbrink C, Haltern G, Ziegert K, et al. Different temperature curves observed during temperature-guided radiofrequency ablation of accessory pathways correlate with application success [Abstract]. *Pacing Clin Electrophysiol* 1994;17:788, with permission.)

Tip temperature data recorded during clinical ablation of accessory pathways by Stellbrink and coworkers using a closed-loop temperature-controlled system showed good correlation of particular types of temperature curves with ablation success (56) (Fig. 4-30). When tip temperature rapidly plateaued near the set point and power quickly dropped off (type 2), tip contact proved to be good, and the resultant success rate was high. When high power was applied throughout the ablation or when power and temperature were oscillating (types 1 and 3), success was significantly lower. Carpinteiro and associates reported an unsuccessful attempt to use local electrogram characteristics to assess tip electrode contact at the tricuspid valve annulus. They concluded that a system that automatically regulates radiofrequency power to achieve the necessary temperature is needed in this location (57).

For all commercially available systems that monitor tip electrode temperature during radiofrequency ablation, the observed temperature generally represents the tip electrode temperature or sometimes the tip-to-tissue interface temperature, not the maximum tissue temperature, which can be several millimeters below the endocardial surface (58). This is especially true with high blood flow, as observed by Kongsgaard and colleagues (59). Although the tip electrode temperature may stabilize within seconds after radiofrequency energy is applied, the maximum tissue temperature continues to rise over 60 seconds or more (for any depth greater than 1 mm), as reported by Wittkampf and coworkers (60). Lesion growth can continue regardless of a stable tip electrode temperature.

An alternative to electronic temperature control is the use of Curie temperature materials in ablation electrodes. In these devices, heating can be accomplished by applying a time-varying magnetic field (61). Although this is an interesting possibility, significant issues remain to be resolved before this approach can be commercialized.

Commercially available radiofrequency generator systems with closed-loop temperature control may use fully digital or hybrid digital-analog control systems. One advantage of an analog control loop is continuous real-time monitoring of tip temperature information, rather than periodic sampling. Continuous monitoring can result in more rapid controller response to rapidly changing tip temperature, reducing the likelihood of temperature overshoot, impedance rise, and "popping" resulting from subendocardial microbubble formation.

Temperature Sensors and Placement

Two types of temperature sensors are used in commercially available ablation systems with temperature

TABLE 4-2 • TEMPERATURE SENSOR COMPARISON

Thermistor	Thermocouple
Temperature-sensitive resistor	Junction between two dissimilar metals
Can be small	Very small (two wires)
Requires external power	Self-powered
Larger signal	Smaller signal
Can be fragile (ceramic)	Very rugged (solder joint)
Moderate cost	Inexpensive
Possible self-heating errors	No self-heating

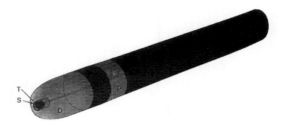

FIGURE 4-32. Schematic drawing of a commercially available catheter with temperature feedback. In this design, a thermistor insulated by a plastic sleeve is exposed at the distal tip of the electrode. (From Langberg JJ, Gallagher M, Strickberger SA, Amirana O. Temperature monitoring during radiofrequency catheter ablation of accessory pathways. *Circulation* 1992;86:1469–1474, with permission.)

feedback: the thermistor and the thermocouple. A thermistor is a resistor whose resistance changes with temperature. A thermocouple is a junction between two dissimilar metals that generates an electrical potential when the junction temperature is different from that of a reference junction (i.e., Seebeck effect). A comparison of features of the two types is shown in Table 4-2.

In addition to the type of sensor, there are differences in sensor placement between commercially available systems. Some manufacturers embed the temperature sensor inside the tip electrode (Fig. 4-31). This provides a measure of the average temperature of the tip electrode but does not necessarily indicate the maximum temperature at the tip electrode-to-tissue interface. Other manufacturers expose the temperature sensor at the distal end of the tip electrode, as well as thermally insulating the temperature sensor from the tip electrode itself (Fig. 4-32). Studies by Blouin and associates, Langberg and colleagues, and Wang and coworkers demonstrate that an exposed temperature sensor can measure the actual tissue interface temperature when the electrode is in end-on contact (62–64). Conversely, the temperature sensor measures the blood temperature when the tip is not in end-on contact with the tissue. The result is that the temperature sensor can underestimate the peak tip-to-tissue interface temperature by as much as 12°C for nonperpendicular orientation to the tissue, as reported by McRury and associates (65). The embedded sensor design, while providing an average tip temperature measurement, is independent of the tip-to-tissue contact angle.

Alternatives to Temperature Feedback

As an alternative to temperature monitoring for the control of impedance rise and coagulum formation, impedance monitoring continues to have its supporters. Remp and colleagues and Strickberger and coworkers have presented clinical evidence that a small (e.g., 5 to 15 Ω) decrease in impedance immediately precedes impedance rise and that this information can be used to effectively prevent coagulum formation (66,67). The study by Remp and associates showed that, although the sensitivity was 82% and the speci-

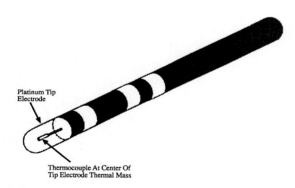

FIGURE 4-31. Schematic drawing of a commercially available catheter with temperature feedback. This design has a thermocouple positioned at the approximate center of thermal mass for the electrode. (From Calkins H, Prystowsky E, Carlson M, et al. Temperature monitoring during RF catheter ablation procedures using closed loop control. Atakr Multicenter Investigators Group. *Circulation* 1994;90:1279–1285, with permission.)

ficity was 80% for a 15-Ω impedance rise to predict impedance rise, the positive predictive value was only 18% (66). Hartung and colleagues proposed that the slope of the impedance curve during ablation could be used to estimate tip temperature and that a rapid change in impedance at the onset of radiofrequency could predict excessive heating. However, their data showed a positive predictive value for impedance rise of only 47% (68).

Hoffmann and associates and Strickberger and coworkers, among others, proposed that impedance monitoring is effective as a means of assessing the quality of tip electrode-to-tissue contact (69,70). Their evidence suggests that high impedance indicates good wall contact and that this information can be used to reduce the number of burns required for success by ensuring good contact before ablation and to reduce the incidence of impedance rises. Hoffmann and associates and Saul and colleagues proposed that preablation impedance monitoring at frequencies lower than the 500 kHz typically used for radiofrequency ablation (e.g., 40 to 50 Hz) may provide a more sensitive means for discriminating between good contact and noncontact (71,72). This approach could gain wider acceptance as systems employing more sophisticated impedance monitoring are commercialized. A closed-loop control system based on sensitive impedance monitoring could also become a reality.

ATRIAL FLUTTER

Mapping

There are two general schools of thought regarding mapping of "typical" atrial flutter. One group believes that global electrophysiologic mapping of the right atrium is the most effective method for identifying ablation targets, and the other group believes that a primarily anatomic approach is most efficient. Proponents of either approach may use both techniques, depending on the situation. For "atypical" atrial flutter (other than the antidromic version of typical atrial flutter), detailed mapping seems to be a necessity. Cosio and coworkers, Feld and associates, and others have suggested that typical atrial flutter comprises a large counterclockwise reentry circuit involving a sig-

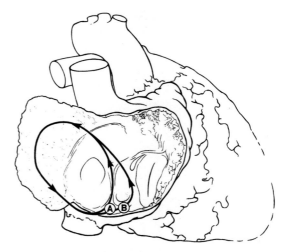

FIGURE 4-33. Schematic cutaway view of the right atrium from a right anterior oblique projection. The typical direction of activation during atrial flutter is shown. Commonly successful ablation sites include A and B. (From Feld GK, Fleck P, Chen PS, et al. Radiofrequency catheter ablation for the treatment of human type 1 atrial flutter. *Circulation* 1992;86:1233–1240.)

nificant portion of the right atrium and passing through an isthmus of slower conduction (73,74) (Fig. 4-33). The isthmus of tissue that represents the vulnerable portion of the typical flutter macro-reentrant circuit is located in the region between the tricuspid valve, inferior vena cava, and coronary sinus ostium. Opinions on the best target to ablate within this region vary. Arenal and colleagues suggested that atrial flutter might instead consist of macro-reentry around the tricuspid annulus (75).

In most procedures for ablating typical atrial flutter, a steerable, roving catheter is used to identify such markers as early potentials, fractionated electrograms, and double potentials in the region described previously. Another tool that is sometimes used to record the activation pattern of the right atrium more globally is a nonsteerable reference electrode catheter with many poles. This mapping catheter is typically looped across the roof of the right atrium and down the anterolateral wall (Figs. 4-34 and 4-35). After ablation, the catheter can be used to assess functional block across lesions by pacing from one side and looking for propagation. A third tool that is sometimes used for atrial flutter mapping is the 20-electrode loop catheter, which can be curved into a ring shape to approximate the tricuspid annulus (15) (Fig. 4-11). All three of

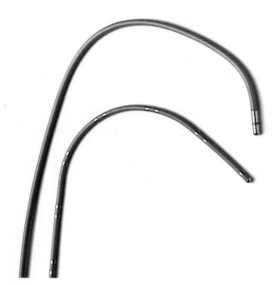

FIGURE 4-34. Two catheters developed for mapping and ablating atrial tachycardias, particularly atrial flutter. Above is a double-ablation electrode catheter with a curve designed to enhance tip stability at the inferior vena cava–tricuspid valve annulus isthmus. Below is a 6-Fr, 16-pole, fixed-curve catheter with a curve designed to fit across the roof of the right atrium for assessment of atrial activation. (Courtesy of Medtronic CardioRhythm, Inc., San Jose, CA.)

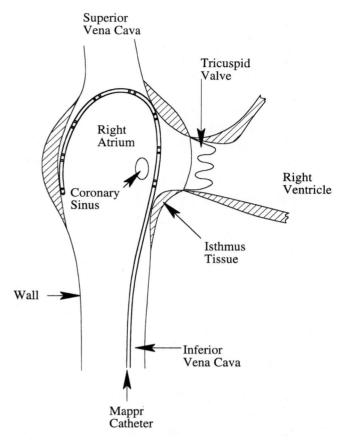

FIGURE 4-35. Schematic drawing shows the typical position of a 16-pole catheter for global activation assessment in the right atrium. (Courtesy of Medtronic CardioRhythm, Inc., San Jose, CA.)

these tools may also be useful for mapping atypical atrial flutter, for which no obvious anatomic approach is consistently effective. For atypical flutter involving the left atrium, improved catheters for mapping on the left side may also be required. Future tools for more extensive and quicker mapping of atypical atrial flutter may include regional multielectrode arrays for efficiently mapping a region of interest or atrium-filling basket arrays for global activation mapping.

Ablation

The usual anatomic ablation target for typical atrial flutter is a slow-conducting isthmus within or near a triangle formed by the tricuspid valve annulus inferior vena cava, and coronary sinus. Calkins and coworkers, after an abbreviated mapping protocol in this region, reported an acute ablation success rate of 81% for 16 patients (76). Fischer and associates, summarizing an 80-patient series, reported 70% acute success ablating along a line between the tricuspid valve annulus and inferior vena cava, 40% ablating between the tricuspid valve annulus and coronary sinus, and 10% ablating between the coronary sinus and inferior vena cava (77). Typical flutter ablation acute efficacies of 78% and 100%, respectively, were reported by Cosio and colleagues, using a primarily anatomic approach, and Feld and coworkers, using a more global mapping approach (73,74). Haissaguerre and associates reported an 89% initial success rate in 55 patients using the conservative anatomic approach of ablating all three legs of the triangle previously described (78). Results from a series of 18 patients reported by Rigden and colleagues, in which an anatomic approach was compared with mapping, indicate that the anatomic approach may have significant advantages in terms of success rate, number of burns, and fluoroscopic exposure (79).

Atrial flutter ablation, when performed with standard tools and the point ablation method, is time consuming and typically requires a larger number of burns than most SVT ablation techniques. It is generally accepted that longer lesions are required to create a complete conduction block across the critical isthmus. Most atrial flutter ablations today are accomplished by sequential ablations using a 4-mm electrode in multiple locations to create a linear burn or by using longer-tip electrodes for the same purpose. Several manufacturers provide standard ablation catheters with long-tip electrodes (i.e., 6, 8, or 10 mm) (Fig. 4-21). A clinical study conducted by Feld and coworkers demonstrated an increased success rate and lower recurrence rate for flutter ablation using 8-mm tips than using 4-mm tips (80). Lesh and associates reported an atrial ablation series in which success was achieved in four atrial flutter patients with a 10-mm tip in whom a 4-mm tip had previously failed (81).

For the 50-W radiofrequency generators that are available commercially, an 8- or 10-mm tip electrode length seems to be about the maximum for 7-Fr catheters, depending on local blood flow. Animal studies by Chan and colleagues using increasing electrode size for ablation in atrial tissue demonstrated that significantly larger lesions are possible as electrode length is increased from 4 to 10 mm, especially if the tip is maintained parallel to the endocardial tissue (44). However, the study also showed that lesion size diminishes for longer electrodes (Table 4-3).

On the basis of clinical atrial flutter ablation experience, some clinicians report that the high blood flows that are found in the right atrium may prevent even 8-mm tips from generating their maximum potential lesion size. To take full advantage of long-tip electrodes, some manufacturers are developing next-generation power supplies that are capable of delivering more than 50 W. Another approach to creating larger lesions is to use multiple electrodes. When radiofrequency is delivered simultaneously to several electrodes, they can function as a single larger electrode, generating larger, deeper lesions, as reported by Baal and coworkers (82). If simultaneous activation is not successful, the electrodes can be individually powered for greater current density per electrode.

In addition to the need for larger lesions for improved success in atrial flutter ablation, stability of the catheter tip is often a problem. Catheter instability can result from several factors, including the fluttering behavior of the atrium, AV ring movement with ventricular contraction, and patient breathing. Some manufacturers are developing special catheter shapes specifically to address this issue. One such example is a double-curve design proposed by Cosio and associates, which braces against the inferior vena cava wall and conforms to the tricuspid valve annulus-inferior vena cava isthmus, allowing the tip electrode to lie flat against the tissue. This catheter also employs double ablation electrodes for flexibility in lesion size generation (Figs. 4-34 and 4-36). A clinical series reported by Cosio and colleagues (83) indicates that use of this catheter may improve ablation success and efficiency for common atrial flutter. Other designs that are under study include shapes that are intended to facilitate ablation in the vicinity of the coronary sinus ostium.

Atrial flutter has a relatively high recurrence rate; "long-term" success has been reported variously as 80%, 56%, 58%, and 44% over different mean follow-

TABLE 4-3 • LARGE-TIP ELECTRODES FOR ATRIAL LESIONS

Orientation	Tip Length (mm)	Lesion Area (mm^2)	Lesion Depth (mm)	Lesion Volume (mm^3)
Perpendicular	4	31 ± 12	2.2 ± 0.3	63 ± 20
	6	45 ± 7	2.0 ± 0.2	90 ± 16
	10	42 ± 19	1.9 ± 0.7	78 ± 47
	12	55 ± 78	2.0 ± 0.9	31 ± 8
Parallel	4	59 ± 38	1.9 ± 0.3	114 ± 83
	6	70 ± 18	2.0 ± 1.0	155 ± 75
	10	99 ± 48	2.1 ± 0.5	214 ± 113
	12	70 ± 40	2.3 ± 0.6	159 ± 107

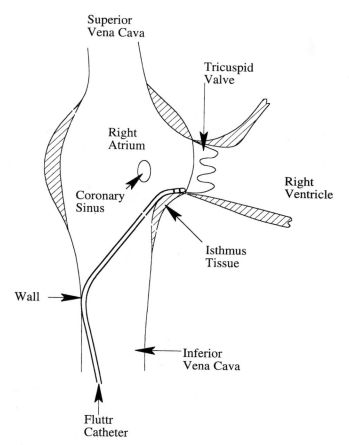

FIGURE 4-36. Schematic drawing shows the typical position of a flutter ablation catheter, with the proximal curve braced against the inferior vena cava wall and the distal curve conforming to the inferior vena cava–tricuspid valve annulus isthmus. Tip electrodes can be used for bipolar or unipolar mapping or for bipolar, single unipolar, or "dual-unipolar" ablation. (Courtesy of Medtronic CardioRhythm, Inc., San Jose, CA.)

up durations by several groups (73,74,76,77). Recurrence may stem from suboptimal lesions created during ablation; new catheter designs that succeed in creating larger or deeper lesions will likely reduce recurrence as well. More aggressive functional assessment of assumed lines of block after ablation can reduce the likelihood of recurrence. Some evidence for prediction of immediate and long-term success using electrophysiologic assessment criteria has been reported by Poty and coworkers, Nakagawa and associates, and Sarter and colleagues (84–86). Long-tip or multielectrode catheters, possibly coupled with high-power radiofrequency generators and augmented by convenient diagnostic tools, should significantly im-

prove the long-term success of atrial flutter ablation. Also of concern is the significant incidence of atrial fibrillation after successful atrial flutter ablation reported by Philippon and coworkers and Fischer and associates (87,88). Occurrence of atrial fibrillation after flutter ablation may be related to structural heart disease or a previous history of atrial fibrillation. Improved tools for flutter mapping ablation and postablation assessment may help to reduce the occurrence of atrial fibrillation after ablation of atrial flutter.

Ablation of reentrant atrial tachycardia resulting from surgical scars to correct congenital heart disease can be handled in much the same way as atrial flutter (i.e., an anatomic approach supplemented by mapping). If the anatomic boundaries that constrain electrical propagation through an isthmus of slow conduction are identified, a radiofrequency lesion that cuts across that isthmus can often terminate the tachycardia (81). The catheters that can work for these tachycardias depend on the size and location of the isthmus to be ablated. Imaging tools for accurate, real-time location of anatomic structures may prove to be indispensable for these anatomically based procedures.

Ectopic Atrial Tachycardia

Reports from the literature suggest that ectopic atrial tachycardias are caused by focal sites of abnormal automaticity, rather than large or multiple reentrant circuits (89). Available ablation catheters seem to be adequate for successful termination of many ectopic atrial tachycardias, if they can be mapped. Successful ectopic atrial tachycardia ablation series have been reported by the Walsh, Lesh,, Kall, and Shenasa groups and others (89–92). Shenasa and colleagues report that ectopic atrial tachycardias tend to cluster along the crista terminalis (92) (Fig. 4-37). Walsh and coworkers have seen right atrial ectopic atrial tachycardias mainly at the mouth of the right atrial appendage and left atrial foci near the pulmonary veins (89) (Fig. 4-38). Poty and associates observed that the success rate of radiofrequency ablation is lower in patients with multiple ectopic atrial tachycardia sites (93).

Catheters that facilitate tip positioning and good contact in the areas mentioned previously may provide the best results. One catheter feature that has

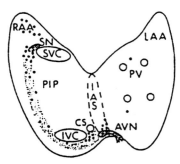

FIGURE 4-37. In a series of 35 patients with 38 discrete ectopic atrial tachycardia foci, 68% were in the right atrium. Of these, 76% originated along the crista terminalis from the sinus node to the atrioventricular node. (From Shenasa H, Merrill JJ, Hamer ME, Wharton JM. Distribution of ectopic atrial tachycardias along the crista terminalis: an atrial tachycardias [Abstract]. *Circulation* 1993:141, with permission.)

obvious value in delicate, thin-walled atrial structures is a flexible, atraumatic tip. An approach that has been reported by Weiss and colleagues and Brown and coworkers to successfully map and ablate ectopic atrial tachycardia is the encircling mapping technique, which involves the use of two steerable mapping catheters to progressively determine the point of earliest activation (94,95). Walsh and associates have suggested that mapping of ectopic atrial tachycardias may be facilitated by the use of multielectrode arrays, which are under investigation (89).

ATRIAL FIBRILLATION

Mapping

On the basis of the surgical success of Cox (96,97), an anatomically based endocardial catheter ablation procedure for chronic atrial fibrillation has been successfully pioneered by Swartz and colleagues (98). Haissaguerre and coworkers demonstrated a less aggressive, exclusively right atrial catheter ablation procedure for paroxysmal atrial fibrillation (99). Both of these promising early reports seem to point to an anatomically based atrial fibrillation ablation procedure. However, many researchers and clinicians believe that the procedure requires substantial simplification for catheter ablation of atrial fibrillation to become an established therapy. Considerable concern has been expressed regarding the sheer volume of atrial myocardium ablated in maze-type radiofrequency procedures. Fueling the controversy are questions regarding potential thromboembolic complications and the amount of atrial pumping contribution that can be obtained after such extensive radiofrequency ablation. To improve this anatomically based procedure, many think that optimization of the procedure through a better understanding of atrial fibrillation electrophysiology is required. To obtain these insights into atrial fibrillation, much more mapping research is required. This mapping research may also produce an alternative to the catheter maze procedure, such as identification of key sites necessary for the sustenance or even initiation of atrial fibrillation. Tackling these sites with radiofrequency ablation may be a more straightforward task than attempting to perform a catheter maze procedure or some variation.

One concept for rapid mapping of atrial tachycardias that has been proposed by more than one investigator is the multielectrode basket array. Although ablation of ectopic atrial tachycardias has been reasonably successful with current tools, a rapid method for obtaining simultaneous electrograms from

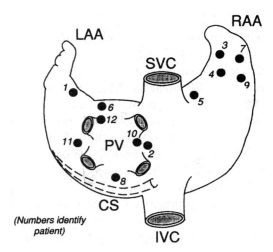

FIGURE 4-38. Successful ectopic atrial tachycardia ablation sites for 12 patients who were 19 years old or younger. Eleven patients in this series had a focal source for their arrhythmia that could often be eliminated by a single radiofrequency lesion. (From Walsh EP, Saul JP, Hulse JE, et al. Transcatheter ablation of ectopic atrial tachycardia in young patients using radiofrequency current. *Circulation* 1992;86:1138–1146, with permission.)

a large portion of the atrium may speed up some procedures, as suggested by Walsh and associates (89). Mapping and ablation of many atypical atrial flutters (from natural causes and resulting from surgical scars) and most atrial fibrillation have not been particularly successful. The kind of global activation pattern information that a basket may provide can be instrumental in the successful identification of ablation targets for these clinical indications. A particular embodiment of the basket concept that has been extensively evaluated in the atria of animals is a five-armed basket with 25 bipole pair electrodes that is deployed through a 10-Fr sheath (100). Figure 4-39 shows a four-armed version of this concept. The investigators of this device felt that, to be an effective mapping tool, a basket array catheter should have certain features:

- Comprise a large number of electrodes capable of sensing a substantial portion of the atrial surface
- Maintain stable electrode contact with the endocardium throughout the cardiac and respiratory cycles
- Not interfere with contraction of the heart or impede flow through it
- Not affect the electrical activity of the heart
- Collapse to a reasonable size for introduction into and removal from the heart

The catheter described previously was used in a series of 31 animals reported by Jenkins and colleagues (100), undergoing significant design iteration along the way. Early basket designs caused cardiac damage, but subsequent designs were improved.

Custom software was developed that displays the five intracardiac electrograms from each "spoke." An activation map using information from all five spokes was then superimposed on a fluoroscopic image of the basket. The investigators felt that the device design fulfilled the requirements described earlier and that the basket was ready for clinical evaluation. Triedman and coworkers reported that this basket catheter was safely deployed in the right atria of five humans, and electrograms were recorded (101). Although electrograms were recorded on only 66% of the available channels on average, it was felt that sufficient information could be collected for construction of useful activation maps.

Basket-style multielectrode array catheters continue to be investigated for use in atrial and ventricular mapping. Variations on the concept are being investigated at several sites. Some of the alternative designs are discussed in the section on ventricular tachycardia mapping. Although basket arrays show promise as mapping tools, safety concerns (e.g., perforation,

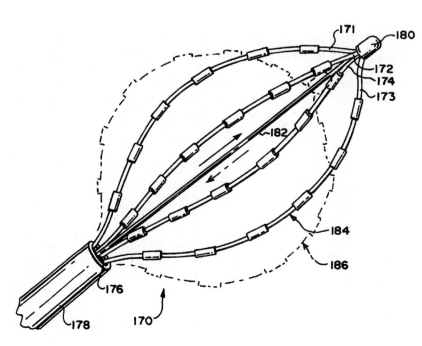

FIGURE 4-39. Drawing of a four-arm basket for atrial or ventricular mapping. Each strut contains six mapping electrodes. The basket is capable of expanding to a near-spherical shape or can collapse for withdrawal through a sheath. Other embodiments are possible, including five arms. (From Chilson DA. Intraventricular multielectrode cardiac mapping probe and method for using same. US Patent No 4,699,147, 1987, with permission.)

Ablation

Ablation therapy for atrial fibrillation can be categorized as the short-term, straightforward approach of controlling the ventricular response to atrial fibrillation (i.e., AV node ablation with pacemaker implantation or AV modification) or the longer-term challenge of direct ablation of atrial fibrillation. New devices for each of these therapies may be substantially different.

Reduction of Ventricular Response

AV node ablation and pacemaker implantation for controlling ventricular response rate to atrial fibrillation are successfully performed with current catheters (e.g., 4-mm tip) and radiofrequency power supplies (102). Many physicians consider the procedure to be a valuable palliative treatment for patients with drug-refractory, symptomatic atrial fibrillation. "Ablate and pace" is perhaps most applicable for elderly patients and those with left ventricular dysfunction resulting from the atrial fibrillation. Studies on direct current (DC) and radiofrequency ablation of the AV node followed by pacemaker implantation have shown significant improvement in systolic function, as measured by ejection fraction and other parameters (103–106). The procedural morbidity and mortality rates are acceptable, and quality of life is significantly improved for many of the patients who receive this treatment (107–109), but long-term reliance on an implantable device is an obvious disadvantage. As other options become available, this treatment will most certainly become less widely applied.

One alternative that does not require a permanent device implant is modification of the AV node to control ventricular rate response to atrial fibrillation. Some clinicians have reported the use of AV node modification to successfully control ventricular rate response using current commercially available tools (110–113). Results from a 10-patient series reported by Feld and associates in which modification of the AV node was 70% successful are summarized in Table 4-4 (114).

Most clinicians target the low midseptal or posteroseptal region of the right atrium, generally associated with the slow pathway location in patients with dual AV nodal physiology. This procedure is somewhat controversial, however, because of a significant risk of acute and delayed heart block (115) and difficulties for some groups in achieving earlier reported success rates (116). Evidence reported by Shenasa and col-

TABLE 4-4 • CLINICAL CHARACTERISTICS AND RESPONSES OF PATIENTS UNDERGOING RF CATHETER MODIFICATION OF THE ATRIOVENTRICULAR NODE FOR REFRACTORY ATRIAL FIBRILLATION AND RAPID VENTRICULAR RESPONSE

Patient No.	Male Or Female	Age	LVEF %	Max. HR Pre-RF	Max. HF Post-RF	Mean HR Pre-RF	Mean HR Post-RF	Min HR Post-RF
1	F	59	NL	190	112	120	75	50
2	M	59	NL	160	120	130	80	60
3	F	62	NL	150	120	130	80	50
4 (P)	M	69	NL	220	NA	120	NA	NA
5 (P)	F	64	NL	300	NA	130	NA	NA
6	M	68	NL	160	100	140	70	50
7	M	71	20	160	150	140	100	75
8 (A)	M	38	30	210	NA	120	NA	NA
9	M	75	30	160	133	110	90	40
10	M	54	NL	170	140	114	78	67
Mean ± SD		62 ± 10		164 ± 12	123 ± 16	128 ± 11	83 ± 10	54 ± 11

A, atrioventricular (AV) node modification unsuccessful, cardioversion performed after amiodarone loading; P, AV node modification unsuccessful, permanent pacemaker implanted after AV node ablation; LVEF, left ventricular ejection fraction; HR, heart rate; NL, normal limits; NA, not available.

facilitation of precise ablation in the vicinity of the AV node include high-density multielectrode arrays. One example is a coil-shaped catheter containing eight bipole pairs, covering an area of several square centimeters of endocardium near the node (Fig. 4-40). This slender array catheter is deployed through a steerable sheath. One design has a distal "anchor" for placement in the coronary sinus. The catheter can provide a detailed map of nodal anatomy so that the slow pathway can be clearly identified and the compact AV node can be avoided.

Direct Ablation to Terminate Atrial Fibrillation

Pioneering work by Swartz and Haissaguerre opened the door to percutaneous catheter ablation of atrial fibrillation. The early radiofrequency catheter ablation procedure reported by Swartz and coworkers is based on an anatomically guided surgical "maze" developed by Cox and associates (118) (Figs. 4-41 and

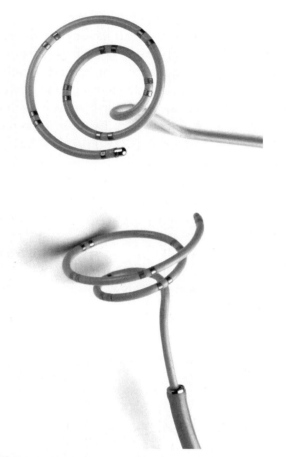

FIGURE 4-40. Coil-shaped regional array mapping catheter with 16 poles. When pressed against the endocardium, the shape-memory metal coil collapses flat for even electrode contact. The 3.5-Fr mapping catheter is delivered from an 8-Fr deflectable-tip sheath with tip electrode. (Courtesy of Medtronic CardioRhythm, Inc., San Jose, CA.)

leagues suggests that this approach may be most useful for patients with dual AV nodal physiology (117).

It may be that tools for very precise ablation are most applicable for AV node modification. Such tools may include very small tip electrodes (e.g., 2 mm/7 Fr, 4 mm/5 Fr) for the creation of small-area lesions, catheters with "micrometer" tip manipulation control, and radiofrequency generators with very precise control of energy delivery. An example of this lesion control technology that some manufacturers have adopted is the capability for limiting the maximum power delivered to the catheter, even when operating in temperature control mode. Other mapping catheters being developed that may prove useful for the

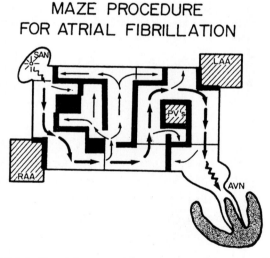

FIGURE 4-41. Schematic representation of the surgical maze procedure. Both atrial appendages are excised, and the pulmonary veins are isolated. Atrial incisions interrupt the conduction routes of the most common reentrant circuits and direct the sinus impulse from the sinus node to the atrioventricular node along a specified route. Except for the right atrial appendage, left atrial appendage, and pulmonary vein, the entire atrium is electrically activated by providing multiple blind alleys off the main conduction route from the sinoatrial node to the atrioventricular node. This preserves atrial transport function. (From Cox JL, Boineau JP, Schuessler RB, et al. A review of surgery for atrial fibrillation. *J Cardiovasc Electrophysiol* 1991;2:541–561, with permission.)

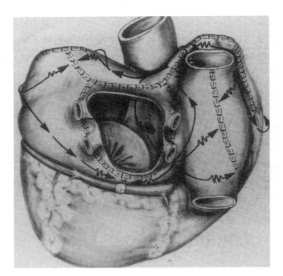

FIGURE 4-42. Anatomic representation of the maze procedure, showing propagation of a normal sinus rhythm beat. The impulse escapes from the sinus node region by traveling inferiorly and anteriorly around the base of the right atrium. Propagation continues around the anterior right atrium onto the top of the interatrial septum, where it splits into two wavefronts. One passes through the septum from anterior to posterior to activate the posteromedial left and right atria. The other wavefront continues around the base of the excised left atrial appendage to activate the posterolateral wall. All atrial myocardium is activated except the pulmonary vein orifices. (From Cox JL, Boineau JP, Schuessler RB, et al. A review of surgery for atrial fibrillation. *J Cardiovasc Electrophysiol* 1991;2:541–561, with permission.)

coworkers and Elvan and associates showed some promising results in this area, including reduced inducibility of atrial fibrillation by vagal stimulation and rapid pacing after application of epicardial radiofrequency lesions (125,126). Demonstration of conduction suppression across epicardially created radiofrequency linear lesions in dogs has been reported by Kempler and colleagues (127). Epicardial linear lesions have also been used by Elvan and coworkers to terminate atrial fibrillation in a rapid pacing model for chronic atrial fibrillation (128). In this study of three dogs, linear lesions were applied in an extensive series of maze-like locations involving the right and left atria (Fig. 4-43). These data may also have implications for the potential efficacy of an endocardial catheter-based atrial fibrillation maze ablation proce-

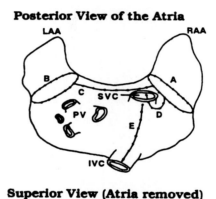

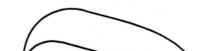

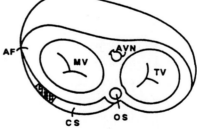

FIGURE 4-43. Diagram of epicardial RF lesions (A–E) performed in dogs. Lesions A and B are lesions around both atrial appendages. Lesion C connects A and B in the region of the transverse sinus. Lesion D extends from the medial superior vena cava (SVC) to A. Lesion E extends from the lateral SVC to the lateral inferior vena cava (IVC). A final ablation site was within the coronary sinus *(hatched area)*. (From Elvan A, Ridgen LB, Kisahuki A, et al. Radiofrequency catheter ablation of the atria reduces inducibility and duration of atrial fibrillation in dogs. *Circulation* 1995;91:2236, with permission.)

4-42) and further variations by Cox and others (119–122). Other surgical strategies for terminating atrial fibrillation include the "corridor" procedures of Guiraudon and others (123,124). The early radiofrequency ablation approach reported by Haissaguerre and colleagues is less involved than a full maze procedure and perhaps more limited in its applicability. To perform either of these radiofrequency catheter ablation procedures, it is assumed to be necessary to create linear lesions that are contiguous and transmural, but these assumptions have not been definitively proven.

Direct radiofrequency ablation of atrial fibrillation can be categorized in two ways. The first is epicardial ablation during surgery. Rather than the open heart surgery described by Cox, it may be as effective and safer to perform an epicardial maze procedure using radiofrequency catheters, without subjecting the patient to bypass. Animal experiments by Seifert and

dure. While interest and research in catheter-based treatments for atrial fibrillation gain momentum, Cox and others continue to modify the surgical maze procedure to make it less invasive. He has suggested that a combination of laparoscopic surgical techniques and transvenous catheter ablation might be the future of atrial fibrillation treatment (129).

An even less invasive and possibly more challenging approach to direct ablation of atrial fibrillation is an entirely percutaneous catheter procedure in which lesions are delivered only to the endocardial surface of the heart. Pioneering work in this area has generated tremendous excitement in the electrophysiology community. This area of research has attracted the attention of most device manufacturers, resulting in intensive device and procedure development. In an example of early atrial fibrillation ablation animal research, Avitall successfully rendered vagally mediated atrial fibrillation nonsustainable in a series of three dogs by creating endocardial radiofrequency linear lesions in the right atrium from the superior vena cava to the inferior vena cava and from the superior vena cava to the tricuspid valve (130).

Early Clinical Procedures

The clinical catheter maze procedure first introduced by Swartz and associates (98) comprised seven linear radiofrequency lesions. Three linear lesions were created on the right side: posterior inferior vena cava to the superior vena cava, along the crista terminalis, and tricuspid valve to the inferior vena cava. Four lesions were created on the left side after transseptal puncture: mitral valve to intraaortic septum; mitral valve to the caudal left atrium, separating the right and left pulmonary veins; parallel to mitral valve annulus, separating the anterior and posterior pulmonary veins; and one lesion on the interatrial septum. To create linear lesions, Swartz reported using long, specially shaped sheaths to position the tip of a standard 4-mm-tip ablation catheter at a particular location and then dragging the tip back toward the sheath, performing sequential ablations at several-millimeter increments, with a 15- to 20-second duration for each burn.

The procedure time for this endocardial maze procedure was initially reported to be as long as 15 hours with extremely high fluoroscopy exposure, but both are diminishing as experience is gained and tools are improved. Swartz observed that the atrial rhythm becomes progressively more organized as he proceeds through the lesions. In this early patient series, it was not possible to terminate chronic atrial fibrillation with right atrial lesions only. Tip electrode-to-tissue contact is of course critical in the Swartz procedure and critical to achieving good contact are the long sheaths. Several different sheath designs are used, some with curves in two planes. A later addition is the use of telescoping sheaths, which allow more configurations to be achieved with fewer unique sheaths. Clinical ablation data from Swartz suggest that chronic atrial fibrillation can be ablated with left atrial lesions alone.

The initial clinical catheter ablation case described by Haissaguerre and colleagues was a treatment for paroxysmal, rather than chronic, atrial fibrillation (99). The procedure described requires creating three intersecting linear lesions in the right atrium: two longitudinal and one transverse. Thirty sequential radiofrequency applications were delivered in the case (Fig. 4-44) by a 7-Fr, nonsteerable catheter with 14 ablation bands, each 4 mm wide and spaced apart by 3-mm gaps. The Haissaguerre procedure was obviously not an attempt to replicate the surgical maze procedure, but rather was a partitioning of the right atrium. Haissaguerre speculates that a variety of linear lesion locations may be successful in atrial fibrillation ablation, although he does think that it may be important that each lesion abut on another lesion or an anatomic obstacle that prolongs the line of block.

Haissaguerre states that the partitioning approach to atrial fibrillation termination relies on work by Moe and Allessie that demonstrated that atrial fibrillation is caused by multiple reentrant wavelets (131). According to this work, the greater the number of wavelets, the less feasible it is to terminate them simultaneously. Partitioning the available atrium should reduce the area available for completion of the circuits and thereby reduce the number of wavelets.

Later multipatient series on mapping and ablation of paroxysmal atrial fibrillation and chronic atrial fibrillation have been reported by Jaïs and coworkers (132) from the Haissaguerre group. Mapping data from these studies suggest that different atrial regions may be more or less important players in the sustenance of atrial fibrillation, which could have implica-

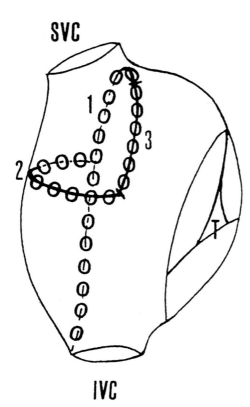

FIGURE 4-44. Diagram of the three linear lesions performed in the posterior *(dotted line)* and anterior *(solid line)* right atrium in humans. Each circle represents one electrode used for ablation. There is no assurance that the individual lesions produced at each site joined with others to produce a continuous line. (From Haissaguerre M, Gencel L, Fischer B, et al. Successful catheter ablation of atrial fibrillation. *J Cardiovasc Electrophysiol* 1994;5:1045–1052, with permission.)

Catheter Development and Animal Research

The multielectrode catheter approach used by Haissaguerre has a potential advantage over the drag technique used by Swartz in that significantly less catheter manipulation is required. Switching electrically between adjacent electrodes on a single catheter to create a long lesion seems simpler and quicker than physically moving a relatively small catheter tip along that same line. Two multielectrode, steerable ablation catheter designs that are being investigated for creating linear atrial lesions are shown in Figure 4-45. A possible disadvantage of the multielectrode catheter approach is obtaining assurance that all electrodes are in contact and can create adequate lesions, although good contact is by no means a certainty with the drag technique. Assessment of electrode-to-tissue contact can be performed by a number of techniques, including electrogram amplitude and quality, pacing from the ablation electrodes, preablation impedance measurements, temperature or impedance measurements during ablation, and visualization of contact using intracardiac ultrasound or other means.

Other investigators have reported numerous animal studies in which radiofrequency catheters were used to create linear lesions and ablate or modify atrial fibrillation (134). Haines and colleagues evaluated a deflectable catheter with three band ablation elec-

tions for optimal ablation catheter design. In these studies, paroxysmal atrial fibrillation patients showed more disorganization in smooth than in trabeculated right atrium, and chronic atrial fibrillation patients showed more disorganization in the left atrium than in the right atrium. Another study from the group (132) points out that linear lesions can unmask focal atrial fibrillation activity, which must then be ablated to achieve sinus rhythm. This raises the possibility that better mapping tools might help to identify focal sites before creation of linear lesions and that extensive maze procedures might be avoided in at least some cases. Another series on right atrial human atrial fibrillation ablation reported by Natale and associates (133) provides further evidence that drag lesions made by using standard catheters in sheaths can be effective for paroxysmal atrial fibrillation, although efficiency with these tools is still questionable.

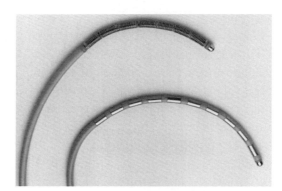

FIGURE 4-45. Two investigational ablation catheters capable of creating linear lesions. Both are 7-Fr catheters with deflectable tips. The lower catheter has 10 × 4 mm wide band electrodes separated by 3 mm for a total ablation segment length of 70 mm. The upper catheter has more closely spaced coil electrodes that have substantially greater flexibility. Both devices can incorporate individual thermocouples for each ablation electrode. (Courtesy of Medtronic CardioRhythm, Inc., San Jose, CA.)

trodes as a tool for creating linear lesions from the tricuspid valve annulus to the inferior vena cava that might be useful for treating atrial flutter and atrial fibrillation (135). The study demonstrated that ablation from multiple electrodes simultaneously was most effective when conducted in unipolar mode rather than bipolar mode. Haines and coworkers have evaluated a catheter that employs two splines that can be expanded outward to stabilize the catheter in the atrium, with a goal of creating good electrode-to-tissue contact (136). They reported performance for two alternative electrode configurations: multiple 3.5-mm-long bands and another with 12.5-mm-long coil electrodes. Both designs used temperature sensors in each ablation electrode for feedback on likely ablation success. Partially contiguous lesions were observed for both designs, with improved transmural contiguity produced by the coil design.

Avitall and associates reported success in creating linear lesions in canine ventricles using a catheter design with a segmented electrode composed of four 2-mm band electrodes, spaced 2 mm apart (137). The electrodes were powered sequentially with up to 30 W, resulting in contiguous lesions with an average length of 13 mm. Avitall and colleagues also reported using a 7-Fr, monorail sliding catheter system with 20 closely spaced 4-mm electrodes for ablation in a sterile pericarditis canine atrial fibrillation model (138). By sliding the catheter forward over a guide wire with the tip constrained, a bowed shape was created, allowing the catheter to push outward against the atrial wall. Transmural lesions were created along the posterolateral and anterior right atrial wall in dogs. Atrial fibrillation inducibility was significantly reduced in the model. The same catheter design was later used to terminate atrial fibrillation in animals by creating linear lesions in the left atrium (139). Other investigators have proposed the creation of larger lesions using multiple panel electrodes on a catheter tip that are electrically isolated from each other (140, 141).

Several studies have examined the power requirements for radiofrequency ablation in the atrium (142, 143). Avitall's work with standard 4-mm tip electrodes suggests a maximum power of 15 to 20 W to avoid atrial tissue tearing and explosions. McRury's work with multielectrode catheters suggests that very high power levels (>100 W) are required to achieve adequate tissue heating for simultaneous energy delivery to four or five band or coil electrodes. In sequential unipolar mode, power requirements were slightly more than 30 W to achieve higher tissue temperatures using the same catheters.

Animal research by Haines and McRury (144) has shown that chronic, sustained atrial fibrillation can be terminated in an animal model by using multicoil electrode catheters. However, despite the use of temperature control, the extensive pattern of left and right atrial lesions that was created in these animals resulted in significant morbidity. Olgin and colleagues (145) have shown that multicoil ablation catheters using temperature control when positioned with intracardiac ultrasound guidance can create linear lesions in the right atria of animals that consistently show conduction block without associated morbidity. Animal data from Nakagawa and associates (146) suggest that the addition of saline cooling may permit the delivery of higher power through long coil electrodes with reduced incidence of impedance rise. Avitall and coworkers (147) demonstrated that noncontiguous lesions can be proarrythmic. Results from other animal series by Nakagawa and colleagues and Tondo and associates (148,149) suggested that a single large lesion at a location that is strategic to interatrial conduction (e.g., Bachmann's bundle, fossa ovalis) can terminate or prevent certain types of atrial fibrillation.

Catheter designs for atrial fibrillation ablation are at an early stage. Multielectrode ablation catheters are a popular means for generating long lesions, and delivery of radiofrequency energy to individual electrodes sequentially may be the most effective method of creating the lesions with a limit of 50 W. Inclusion of temperature sensors in each electrode can provide valuable information regarding tissue contact and likelihood of lesion success. The alternative, dragging standard ablation catheters through sheaths, may be more labor intensive. The advantages of sheaths in improving catheter-to-tissue contact and stability are proven, however. Perhaps a blending of the two technologies, multiple electrodes for easier creation of linear lesions and long sheaths that position these catheters at the optimal sites, can produce atrial fibrillation ablation tools that are effective and practical.

The multiarm spline or basket designs may also

have merit for atrial fibrillation ablation compared with individual steerable ablation catheters. The advantages of the spline or basket approach may include improved electrode-to-tissue contact, less catheter manipulation required, and quicker ablations. Disadvantages may include less flexibility in the selection of lesion locations and greater device complexity. It may be that the most appropriate device design for atrial fibrillation ablation will depend on which approach proves most effective: an extensive maze procedure or the creation of a few atrial "compartments." If specific lines need to be ablated between anatomic landmarks or the optimal line locations prove to be highly variable, a steerable catheter may be best. Steerable catheters that are used for atrial fibrillation ablation will likely have to use novel steering means or special curve shapes to achieve lesions in specific orientations and areas.

Left-Sided Atrial Ablation

Many researchers are focusing on the right atrium as an easier target for catheter-based ablation procedures. Concerns regarding ablation in the left atrium include the following:

1. If the procedure is attempted by a retrograde transaortic approach, there may be significant reduction in catheter steerability and the potential for mitral valve damage from bulky devices, long procedure duration, and extensive maneuvering.
2. If a transseptal approach is used, the liabilities include risks associated with the procedure (e.g., aortic perforation) and difficulties dealing with the Mullins sheath as a platform for ablation catheter maneuvering.
3. Concerns about thromboembolism from coagulum on ablation electrodes or lesions are amplified by the expectation that many more and larger lesions will be required for atrial fibrillation ablation than are needed for left-sided accessory pathways ablation.

Although right-side-only maze procedures may be effective for treating some paroxysmal atrial fibrillation patient groups (e.g., lone atrial fibrillation), it is likely that left-sided lesions may be necessary to treat chronic atrial fibrillation in which one or both atria have been abnormally dilated. Swartz's early experience seems to bear out the fact that right-sided lesions alone may not work for worst-case chronic atrial fibrillation, because he was not able to terminate atrial fibrillation until the left atrial lesions were performed even though the right atrium was ablated first. Data from Swartz suggest that left-sided lesions alone may be effective in treating some chronic atrial fibrillation patients. Regarding transaortic left-sided access, improvements in device maneuverability may open new doors. For transseptal procedures, training, more experience, improved sheaths, and better visualization may make the procedure more routine for many electrophysiologic laboratories. Intracardiac ultrasound may provide the needed confidence level. Temperature monitoring and control could address concerns about coagulum by increasing the safety margin. Intracardiac ultrasound may also prove useful for monitoring catheter contact, lesion growth, and thrombus formation.

Direct Ablation to Prevent Atrial Fibrillation

Perhaps most attractive is the prospect of placing a much smaller lesion or series of lesions in a strategic location designed to prevent atrial fibrillation initiation or sustenance. Some reports suggest that the right atrium may contain such regions (150–152). Early research into defining these critical areas is underway. Precise mapping may be required for the location of any atrial zones that are critical to the initiation or sustenance of atrial fibrillation. Devices that facilitate rapid mapping, such as basket arrays, may find application here. Pacing to prevent or terminate atrial fibrillation is an alternative or possibly complementary concept, and significant research continues in this field (153–155).

It is likely that hybrid therapies involving combinations of catheter ablation, pacing, defibrillation, and other options will prove valuable in treating atrial fibrillation. An example is the prospect of using linear lesions in the atria to reduce atrial defibrillation thresholds, as reported by Kalman and coworkers (156).

VENTRICULAR TACHYCARDIA

Mapping

For most idiopathic ventricular tachycardias that do not involve structural heart disease, pace mapping and activation mapping using available steerable catheters have been shown to be successful (157,158). These ventricular tachycardias tend to be hemodynamically stable and focal in nature, not unlike SVTs. Ventricular tachycardias related to a myocardial infarction and those that involve structural heart disease are more difficult to map and ablate. Ventricular tachycardias with structural heart disease can often be multifocal, and the location of the ventricular tachycardia focus or critical pathways can be midmyocardial or subepicardial (159). The zone of slow conduction that is critical to the maintenance of the ventricular tachycardia may occupy several square centimeters (160). Scarring can also prevent accurate mapping. Ventricular tachycardias that are not hemodynamically stable present a very limited time frame in which mapping can be accomplished. For these ventricular tachycardias, steerable catheters are not adequate for locating ablation targets rapidly and precisely.

Several researchers and industry partners have been developing multielectrode arrays as a possible solution. The array places a large number of electrodes over a region of the ventricle or the entire ventricle, allowing the simultaneous recording of electrograms from various sites of interest. After this electrogram information is collected, it must be presented in an easily comprehended form. Some of the array developers have also developed graphical display systems for two-dimensional (2-D) or three-dimensional (3-D) representation of electrical activation maps, using the array information.

Electrode arrays were first developed for ventricular tachycardia surgery. These arrays included epicardial plaques, socks, and endocardial balloons (161–163) (Fig. 4-46). Information from these devices was displayed in activation map form using custom-developed software. Intraoperative arrays have progressively improved, with greater electrode densities, better conformation to ventricular anatomy, and better computer-driven tools for representation of the electropotential data. Endocardial balloon arrays for

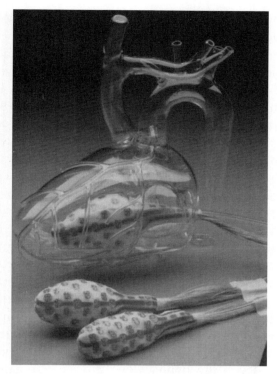

FIGURE 4-46. Examples of epicardial sock arrays and endocardial balloon arrays used for intraoperative mapping. These reusable devices are available in various sizes and electrode densities. (Courtesy of CR Bard, Inc., Tewksbury, MA.)

intraoperative mapping have become less invasive, and atriotomies and ventriculotomies are less frequently required for device placement (161). The treatment of simpler forms of ventricular tachycardia moved from the surgical suite to the electrophysiologic laboratory in the late 1980s. Since then, the intraoperative array mapping tools that are required for more complex ventricular tachycardias have been progressively adapted for endocardial deployment and percutaneous delivery, and mapping of these ventricular tachycardias with catheter-based tools is approaching clinical practicality.

Basket Arrays: Global

Davis and colleagues attempted to create a 60-electrode array covering a substantial portion of the left ventricle as evenly as possible using a number of decapolar catheters placed simultaneously in various locations (164). In their patient series, the technique was used to perform preoperative ventricular tachycardia mapping. Advantages of preoperative mapping over intraoperative mapping include frequent difficulty in inducing the clinical ventricular tachycardia in the intraoperative setting because of general anesthetic agents and surgical handling of the heart, as well as time limitations to minimize bypass duration. Left ventricular recordings were obtained by two or three decapolar catheters placed by a transaortic approach (i.e., against the anterior and posterior left ventricular walls), two or three decapolar catheters placed with a transseptal approach (i.e., against the lateral and septal walls), and one decapolar catheter in the coronary sinus. At least one additional catheter was placed in the right ventricle to obtain septal recordings. Overall, a spatial resolution of 1 to 2 cm was achieved. Simultaneous recording of up to 64 electrograms was accomplished by using a computerized mapping system. The preoperative maps obtained with the described technique correlated well with intraoperative maps. Limitations include complications related to insertion of the large number of catheters, including perforations, access site trauma, long procedure duration, long fluoroscopy time, and high equipment expense.

To simplify the mapping procedure and reduce the number of catheters required to map a substantial area, devices that place an array of electrodes against a substantial portion of ventricular endocardium, rather than a single line, have been developed. The most popular approach to area arrays for ventricular tachycardia mapping is the multielectrode basket. Basket arrays are generally intended to provide a global map of the ventricle—an activation map of the entire chamber. Several versions of basket arrays are being investigated. One such version, previously described in the section on atrial fibrillation mapping, is a five-armed basket containing 25 bipole electrode pairs. Triedman and associates used this device to map the right ventricles of lambs (165). In this study, right ventricular electrograms were obtained from 90% of the bipole pairs. Complications included endocardial abrasions that healed in about 4 to 8 weeks and one right ventricular apical puncture. Other research by Widman and coworkers centered on determining the best algorithm for localizing an area of activation using the array (166).

A second global basket array catheter consisting of 32 bipole pairs on eight self-expanding struts has been evaluated in the left ventricles of two different groups of swine. One group of 11 swine was subjected to anterior myocardial infarction (167). In this study, Smith and colleagues reported that electrode stability was present in 78% of the bipole pairs, and activation mapping, pace mapping, and entrainment techniques were used to locate the site of ventricular tachycardia origin. The basket did not show left ventricular injury. In a separate abstract, Smith and associates concluded that placement of the basket in the left ventricle of 15 swine 4 weeks after myocardial infarction did not significantly affect right and left heart size and performance parameters (168). Another multianimal study conducted by Fitzpatrick and coworkers demonstrated the utility of the same basket as a tool for rapidly developing ventricular activation maps (169).

A third multiarmed basket design with as many as 64 bipole pairs is also being used in animal investigations. This basket uses "flex circuit" technology for creating the electrode bipoles, shape-memory metal arms for flexibility and reliable deployment and retraction, and multiplexing technology to reduce the number of conductors required to carry signals from the large number of electrodes (170) (Fig. 4-47). A sophisticated software program has been developed to graphically represent activation maps produced by the array. In one embodiment, provision has been made for a roving ablation catheter to be deployed

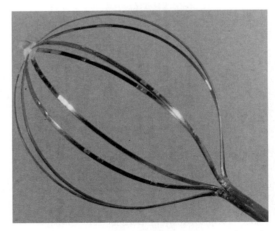

FIGURE 4-47. Left ventricular basket array with eight arms, each containing four bipole electrode pairs. Radiopaque markers facilitate fluoroscopic orientation. This device is part of a mapping system that includes a workstation with a monitor. The 32 channels of data can be viewed in real time or stored for generation of isochronal maps. (Courtesy of Cardiac Pathways, Inc., Sunnyvale, CA.)

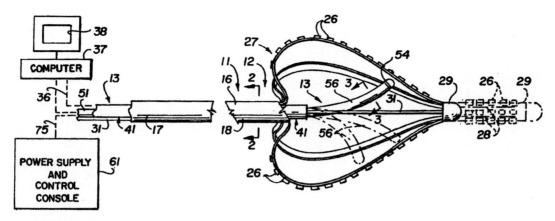

FIGURE 4-48. Drawing of a basket array with a central roving catheter. The array design is similar to that described in Figure 4-47, with the addition of a deflectable-tip ablation catheter that is deployed through a central lumen in the sheath. The deflectable catheter tip can be directed to most locations that are mappable by the array. (From Imran MA. Endocardial mapping and ablation system utilizing a separately controlled ablation catheter and method. US Patent No 5,324,284, 1994, with permission.)

through the same sheath that delivers the expandable array (171) (Fig. 4-48). Some of the array designs mentioned have exhibited reasonable mapping success in animals, but some studies have shown evidence of significant complications such as chamber wall trauma and clotting. Other initial fears that seem to have been allayed by good animal results, such as valve damage during deployment and hemodynamic compromise, could still become problems with use in treating diseased human hearts. Initial clinical studies using these mapping baskets have been reported (172). However, more experience with these devices in treating humans is needed before a definitive assessment of safety and clinical utility can be made.

Another family of multielectrode array concepts includes several catheter versions having multiple individual arms that splay outward, each of which contains one or more mapping electrodes (173–175) (Figs. 4-49 and 4-50). In most of these concepts, the arms can be individually deployed and adjusted for optimal contact with the ventricular wall. Most also have provisions to avoid trauma or puncture of the chamber wall, such as curved or bulbous ends.

A further iteration of the multielectrode array concept is the balloon idea, in which the surface of an inflatable, shape-conforming balloon is outfitted with electrodes. Advantages of this approach include probable improved electrode-to-tissue contact in difficult-to-reach areas of the ventricle. One disadvantage is blockage of blood flow through the chamber, which could possibly be addressed by gating the balloon inflation to the cardiac cycle. Continual inflation and deflation could make electrode stability and mapping accuracy suffer, however. A balloon design that permits blood flow while inflated is another alternative.

Another concept for a noncontact multielectrode array has been reduced to practice and extensively evaluated in animals (176). This concept involves the placement of an inflatable ellipsoid array of electrodes in the ventricle whose size is substantially smaller than the ventricle itself. A reference electrode can be placed in contact with the endocardial wall (Fig. 4-51). The volume and shape of the heart chamber can be calculated by using impedance information. The array position is determined relative to the reference electrode. Electrical potential fields measured by the array elements are used to generate a 3-D volumetric electric field distribution, and a 3-D activation map is graphically displayed (Fig. 4-52). Theoretical advantages of such a system include little effect on blood flow, no interference with ventricular activation by pressure from array elements, less risk of trauma to the ventricular wall or valves through array element contact, and less risk of coagulum formation, because

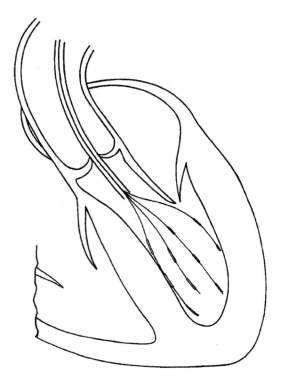

FIGURE 4-49. Drawing of a multielectrode mapping array that has three or more spring legs, each containing multiple electrodes. The legs spring out when deployed from a sheath, and each leg contains a unique combination of electrode size and number for easy fluoroscopic identification. Staggering the electrodes allows greater endocardial coverage and a lower collapsed profile. (From Gelinas SL. Endocardial electrode. U.S. Patent No 4,522,212, 1985, with permission.)

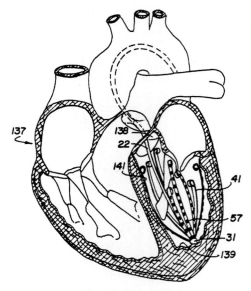

FIGURE 4-50. Multielectrode mapping array that has multiple individually adjustable arms attached only at their distal ends. Basket-type arrays, which have arms attached at the proximal and distal ends, can interfere with the mitral valve when deployed in the left ventricle and can fail to make good contact with the posterior wall. The open proximal end and individually movable arms are designed to reduce difficulties encountered with the mitral valve. (From Imran MA. Mapping and ablation catheter with individually deployable arms and method. US Patent No 5,327,889, 1994, with permission.)

the smaller array does not have to be an open, flow-through design. Potential issues include uncertain resolution and accuracy compared with contact array designs. Limited data from Peters and colleagues (177) on early clinical use of this device are encouraging, but improvements in data processing are required to permit more widespread clinical assessment.

Basket Arrays: Regional

A multielectrode array catheter concept that is somewhat different from the global approach is the regional array. With regional arrays, the idea is to map a several-square-centimeter portion of the endocardium, with a smaller array on the end of a steerable catheter. The assumption is that the electrophysiologist typically knows what general area of the heart is most

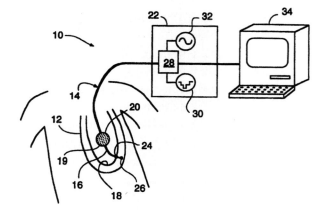

FIGURE 4-51. System for noncontact mapping of a heart chamber. An inflatable balloon array with an expanded dimension much smaller than that of the chamber includes a large number of electrodes on its surface. The electrode array is spatially referenced to a point on the endocardial surface by a reference electrode, which may or may not be part of the array. Because of the small array size and no wall contact requirement, some of the mechanical problems with basket arrays are avoided. The system includes an interface box comprising a signal generator and voltage acquisition equipment, as well as a workstation and monitor for data processing and display. (From Beatty GE, Kagan J, Budd JR. Endocardiol mapping system. US Patent No 5,297,549, 1944, with permission.)

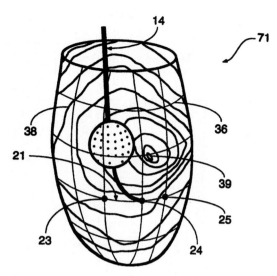

FIGURE 4-52. Drawing of a 3-D electrical activity map created from noncontact array information. Impedance signals from the array elements are used to measure the volumetric shape of the chamber, and a 3-D model of the chamber is constructed. Potentials measured by the array elements are processed (using the inverse solution) and superimposed on the dimensional model for a near real-time 3-D map of electrical activity. This map can be represented in a variety of 2-D graphic formats. Electrical and positional information is calibrated against the reference catheter information. (From Beatty GE, Kagan J, Budd JR. Endocardial mapping system. US Patent No 5,297,549, 1994, with permission.)

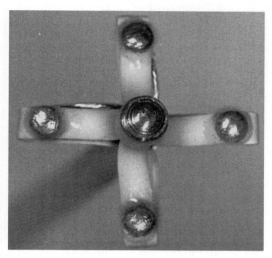

FIGURE 4-53. End-on view of a regional mapping and ablation array having a cross pattern of five electrodes when deployed. The design is a minibasket that flattens when deployed to place all five electrodes in endocardial contact. The dimension across the array is about 1 cm. One electrode has a radiopaque marker. All electrodes are capable of recording and ablation. (From Desai JM, Nyo H, Vera Z, et al. Orthogonal electrode catheter array for mapping of endocardial focal site of ventricular activation. *Pacing Clin Electrophysiol* 1991;14:557–576, with permission.)

interesting to map and that a global map of the entire ventricle is unnecessary. The regional array places a higher electrode density over an area of interest for better resolution. One design uses four electrodes on expandable arms forming a cross pattern, with a fifth electrode at the center (178) (Fig. 4-53). The four arms can be contracted to form a low profile for introduction into the heart.

In practice, deployment of this array against the endocardium creates an orthogonal arrangement of electrodes. Observing the relative timing of potentials recorded by each of the electrodes allows the determination of the direction of propagation of an activation wavefront. This information can be used to move the array in the direction of propagation until it is over the zone of earliest activation. Radiofrequency ablation can then be accomplished in unipolar or bipolar fashion from any electrode or combinations of electrodes to destroy the arrhythmogenic focus. In one study by Desai involving eight dogs, previously placed plunge electrodes that were used to activate the ventricle were accurately located in all eight dogs. The plunge electrode was within the 1 cm^2 area of ablation created by the array after mapping localization (179) (Fig. 4-54 and Table 4-5).

An alternative to the orthogonal regional mapping array described previously is a coil-shaped multielectrode array (Fig. 4-40). This array comprises eight or more bipole pairs on a shape-memory metal backbone. The array is deployed from a steerable lumen catheter, transforming from a straight configuration within the constraints of the lumen catheter into a 3-D coil shape outside the catheter. The lumen catheter provides a convenient sheath for the exchange of different arrays or ablation catheters. As with the orthogonal array, the mapping electrodes can also serve as multiple ablation electrodes that are powered individually or in combination for an area lesion. Potential advantages of the two-catheter system design include greater flexibility in array geometries and a simplified array catheter design. Potential disadvantages include

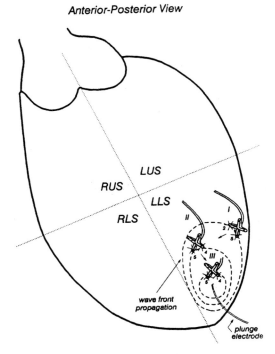

FIGURE 4-54. Schematic diagram shows movement of the array during pacing from a plunge electrode. After placement of the array at position I, unipolar electrograms show wavefront arrival first at electrodes 2 and 5. The array is then moved about 1 cm in the direction of the wavefront propagation to position II. At position II, the wavefront arrives first at electrodes 4 and 5, and the array is moved in that direction to position III. At position III, the wavefront arrives at electrodes 4 and 5 in $\geq$ −30 msec or more with reference to the surface electrocardiogram. This site is considered the point of earliest activation, and radiofrequency ablation is performed. (From Desai JM, Nyo H, Vera Z, et al. Orthogonal electrode catheter array for mapping of endocardial focal site of ventricular activation. *Pacing Clin Electrophysiol* 1991;14:557–576, with permission.)

TABLE 4-5 • RADIOFREQUENCY ABLATION: MORPHOMETRY OF ENDOCARDIAL LESIONS

Dog	Maximum Depth (mm)	Maximum Width (mm)	Technique
1	9.0[a]	3.0	b
2	1.5	10.0	b
3	4.0	8.0	c
4	9.0[a]	3.0	b
5	9.0[a]	3.0	b
6	2.0	10.5	d
7	1.5	11.0	c
8	1.0	10.5	c
Mean ± SD[e]	5 ± 3.5	7 ± 3.5	

[a] Plunge electrode site.
[b] All five electrodes to backplate.
[c] Central to four peripheral electrodes.
[d] Central electrode to backplate.
[e] Lesion sizes were achieved with various RF ablation patterns using the cross-pattern array. Lesions tended to be broad and shallow in ablating from central electrode to peripheral electrodes. Deeper lesions were usually created by ablating from one or more array electrodes to the indifferent electrode.
From Desai JM, Nyo H, Vera Z, et al. Orthogonal electrode catheter array for mapping of endocardial focal site of ventricular activation. PACE 1991; 14:557–576, with permission.

added complexity of maneuvering two devices, although the steerable delivery catheter may provide needed support. Either of the regional arrays described previously requires a switchbox for convenient electrode selection. The switchbox can be manual or programmable to automatically create desired mapping or ablation patterns.

Intravascular Mapping

A final approach to ventricular tachycardia mapping that is worth mentioning is the placement of multielectrode mapping catheters into coronary arteries and veins, with the goal of mapping epicardial breakthrough points of ventricular tachycardia reentrant circuits. Canine studies using these devices have been described by Arruda and colleagues and Littmann and associates (180,181). The catheter designs that are used for mapping in these small vessels are similar to coronary angioplasty catheters. Ranging from 2.5 to 3.6 Fr in diameter, they have 4 to 16 band electrodes on a slender, flexible shaft (Fig. 4-13). The catheters can be fixed-wire (i.e., incorporating a flexible coil spring tip that is steerable), over-the-wire (i.e., using a standard coronary guide wire), or rapid-exchange style (i.e., allowing exchange for a different catheter using a standard guide wire). Animal studies using multiple catheters placed simultaneously in coronary arteries and veins demonstrated that experimentally induced myocardial infarctions have been successfully mapped by using a computerized activation mapping system.

Thermal Mapping

Thermal mapping is an attractive method for reversibly stunning myocardium to determine whether a particular area is an arrhythmogenic focus. Long used in cryosurgical ablation for arrhythmias, low-temperature or "ice" mapping takes advantage of the fact that the temperature required to stun myocardium and that required to cause irreversible damage are reasonably far apart. Studies by Gessman and coworkers have shown that cooling myocardial tissue from 37°C to 27°C can create complete conduction block, but cooling tissue to 0°C is reversible, allowing conduction to resume on rewarming (182). It is possible to selectively test ablation targets within a wide range of low temperatures to determine probable ablation effectiveness without creating unnecessary damage. Application of cryoblation technology to small-diameter, flexible, steerable catheters has not yet been perfected, but research and product development continue. A number of different methods have been used to achieve cold catheter tips, including fluid-to-gas phase change, gas volume expansion, and the thermoelectric effect.

Elevated-temperature (e.g., radiofrequency) mapping is faced with a significant obstacle: the stun and kill temperatures are quite a bit closer together when myocardial tissue is heated than when it is cooled. According to Nath and colleagues, the reversible injury range for myocardium may be between 45°C and 50°C (42). This reversible injury range was confirmed in a separate *in vivo* series of AV junction ablation in 18 dogs by Hirao and associates (183). The irreversible kill temperature for canine myocardium has also been reported by Haines and coworkers to be 46°C to 49°C after 90 seconds' exposure (41). The ranges for reversible myocardial injury using elevated temperatures and the irreversible kill temperature are overlapping or very close at best. Elevated-temperature mapping may be challenging for this reason. Nonetheless, Nath and colleagues reported successful use of thermal mapping in clinical AV junction ablation (13). Cote and associates later demonstrated clinical success with elevated-temperature mapping of accessory pathways (14). Although animal and clinical research continues, it is not yet clear whether thermal mapping (hot or cold) will become a practical clinical reality.

Ablation

Most of the research and development into improvements in ablation for ventricular tachycardia center on the effort to create larger or deeper lesions for the following reasons:

1. Current ventricular tachycardia mapping techniques are imprecise, especially when poorly tolerated ventricular tachycardias severely limit the time allowed for mapping.
2. Ventricular tachycardias can be multifocal, involving multiple reentry circuits.
3. Critical ablation targets for ventricular tachycardias can be subendocardial or epicardial.
4. Ischemic ventricular tachycardias can require ablation through scar tissue.
5. Significantly higher wall motion than that seen in SVT ablation can make achieving good contact challenging.
6. Extreme endocardial surface irregularity can make achieving good contact challenging.

Some of the designs and technologies under investigation for creating large lesions include large-surface-area electrodes, high-power radiofrequency ablation, fluid-assisted radiofrequency ablation, high- and low-energy DC ablation, microwave ablation, laser ablation, cryoblation, and ultrasound ablation.

Large-Surface-Area Electrodes

The potential benefits of large-tip electrodes for SVT and atrial flutter ablation were previously mentioned. Animal studies by Langberg and coworkers and Chan and colleagues have shown that 7-Fr, 8- to 10-mm tips can create atrial or ventricular lesion volumes two to four times those of 7-Fr, 4-mm-tip electrodes (43, 44) (Fig. 4-22). These studies also demonstrate that longer-tip electrodes require more power to achieve necessary tissue temperatures and that tip lengths beyond 8 to 10 mm may result in smaller lesions. Rosenbaum and associates have shown in canine ventricles that 8-mm-long tip electrodes can double the lesion volume of 4-mm tips if 80 W are available but that 12-mm-long tips could not generate further increases (184) (Fig. 4-55). Rosenbaum also observed that larger ventricular lesions may result in a higher incidence of ventricular fibrillation (Fig. 4-56). Because heating peaks occur at the areas of highest curvature on tip electrodes, long electrodes, which have more straight length, have different heating patterns than shorter electrodes, including possible central cool spots (185) (Fig. 4-57). Another example of the "bigger is better" school of ventricular ablation is the 12-mm spherical electrode, which does not suffer from

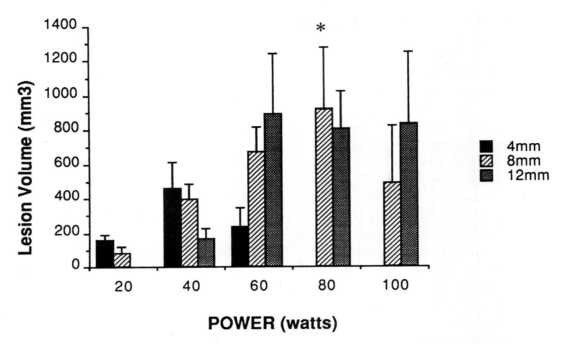

FIGURE 4-55. Effects of electrode size and radiofrequency power on lesion volume. For all three electrode lengths, lesion size increased with increasing power up to the point at which impedance rise occurred. This maximum lesion size was twice as large for 8-mm as for 4-mm tip electrodes, but 12-mm tips did not increase maximum lesion size further. Minimal lesions were observed with large tips at powers less than 40 W. Higher power (60 to 80 W) was required to optimize lesion volume with the 8- and 12-mm tips compared with the 4-mm tip (40 W). (From Rosenbaum R, Greenspon AJ, Smith M, Walinsky P. Advanced radiofrequency catheter ablation in canine myocardium. *Am Heart J* 1994;127:851–857, with permission.)

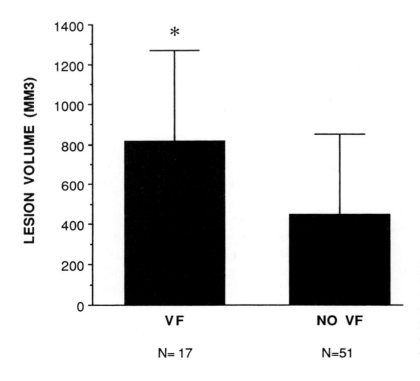

FIGURE 4-56. For animals in which ventricular fibrillation occurred, postmortem examination revealed that ventricular radiofrequency lesions were twice as large. (From Rosenbaum R, Greenspon AJ, Smith M, Walinsky P. Advanced radiofrequency catheter ablation in canine myocardium. *Am Heart J* 1994; 127:851–857, with permission.)

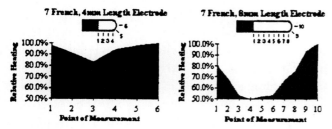

FIGURE 4-57. Graphs showing instantaneous heating maps for 4- and 8-mm-long, 7-Fr tip electrodes. The 8-mm-long electrodes had significantly longer and cooler cool zones during radiofrequency ablation at 30 W than the 4-mm-long tips. Heating peaks occur at points of curvature because of the higher current densities at these points. Temperature sensors should be placed at points of maximum electrode curvature, and noncylindrical shapes may prove useful for long electrodes. (From Chang I, Mirotznik MS, Schwartzman D, et al. Radiofrequency energy delivery results in non-uniform heating patterns [Abstract]. *J Am Coll Cardiol* 1994;1A–484A:836–2, with permission.)

the "cool spot" phenomenon. This design was used by Satake and coworkers in conjunction with a 100-W radiofrequency generator to create lesions 8.5 mm deep in animal studies. The same system was used to terminate seven of eight bundle branch ventricular tachycardias in human patients (186).

Special Electrode Designs

In an effort to create long, continuous lesions across the rough, trabeculated endocardial surface of the ventricle, rotating-tip electrodes have been proposed by Avitall and colleagues (20). Experiments in dogs have produced ventricular lesions up to 4 cm long, 12 mm wide, and 6 mm deep using this technique. Technical obstacles remain to be resolved with this approach, however. In an effort to create deeper lesions and to penetrate scar tissue associated with a myocardial infarction, several burrowing ablation electrode designs have been proposed. These include an electrode design that incorporates a retractable needle (187) (Fig. 4-58). In practice, the needle would penetrate the myocardium to a depth of several millimeters and then would deliver radiofrequency energy at that point below the surface, enabling the creation of lesions having an expected depth of 8 to 10 mm.

Ohtake and associates have evaluated the *in vivo* ablation performance of a needle electrode having a 3-mm exposed section (188). For a variety of radiofrequency power levels, the needle electrode created significantly deeper lesions than a control 2-mm dome electrode. Lesions created by needle electrodes had a smaller surface area than did the standard elec-

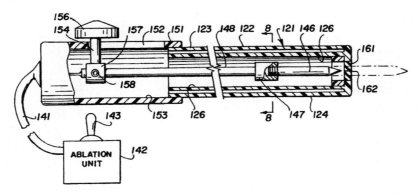

FIGURE 4-58. Concept for a deep lesion electrode capable of piercing the endocardial surface to deliver radiofrequency energy further into the myocardium than is achievable by current surface electrodes. The particular design shown incorporates a retractable needle. By puncturing the myocardium to approximately 2 to 3 mm, it should be possible to generate radiofrequency lesions having a depth of 8 to 10 mm and a width of 5 to 7 mm. Such a design may prove particularly useful for ablating through myocardial infarction–caused scar tissue, which may be more resistant than normal myocardium to penetration by radiofrequency energy from surface electrodes. (From Imran MA. Catheter having needle electrode for radiofrequency ablation. US Patent No 5,281,218, 1994, with permission.)

trode lesions, however, indicating that a deep but precise lesion could be achieved with such a device. Helical electrodes have been proposed for the same purpose by An and coworkers (189). Such electrodes could be screwed into the myocardium to maintain a stable position while radiofrequency energy is delivered. Theoretically, the screw could assist in maintaining tip position despite substantial wall movement or blood flow. Other concepts for improving electrode-to-wall contact have been tried, such as suction (190,191).

Multisite Ablation

As with atrial fibrillation ablation, the concept of ablating simultaneously or in rapid sequence from multiple electrodes has been proposed as a means to create large lesions for ventricular tachycardia ablation. In atrial fibrillation ablation, in which the objective seems to be creating of lines of block, orientation of multiple ablation electrodes along a catheter shaft may be appropriate. The same may be true for certain types of ventricular tachycardia, but most researchers and clinicians seem to be most interested in creating area lesions instead. Placement of multiple electrodes on a device that spreads out on the distal end of a catheter may be useful. Such a device has been proposed and evaluated by Desai and colleagues (179). Other versions, including a coil-shaped design, have also been tested. With many small electrodes, the problem remains that a limited amount of radiofrequency energy can be delivered to an individual electrode before it gets too hot and impedance rises. However, special techniques in the sequencing of radiofrequency application to the electrodes or the addition of fluid cooling may help to overcome this issue.

Fluid-Assisted Ablation

An area of substantial research focus is fluid-assisted radiofrequency ablation. Fluid-assisted radiofrequency ablation has several potential advantages over the use of large-tip electrodes. Large-tip electrodes may be less maneuverable *in vivo* because of the longer rigid section and may be more difficult to get into adequate tissue contact. Because they rely on convective cooling from the blood, large tips may be less effective at generating larger lesions in low flow areas, such as under valve leaflets, between trabeculations, or in vessels. Large-tip electrodes may also reduce mapping precision. In fluid-assisted ablation, the electrode cooling is determined by the externally supplied fluid flow and temperature; therefore, the electrode can be smaller. The smaller electrode size eliminates the disadvantages of larger electrodes (191).

At least three variations in catheter design have been proposed and evaluated in animal studies: saline infusion through holes in an ablation electrode (Fig. 4-59), closed-circuit fluid cooling of a tip electrode (Fig. 4-60), and saline infusion through a subsurface screw-in electrode (Fig. 4-61). For the design incorporating internally circulating fluid within the tip, the presumed mechanism for creation of larger lesions is allowing more power to be delivered to the tip electrode while keeping it cool to avoid coagulum formation. For the other two designs, in which fluid is emitted from the electrode, the saline medium provides a similar cooling function but may also serve to somewhat increase the effective surface area of the tip

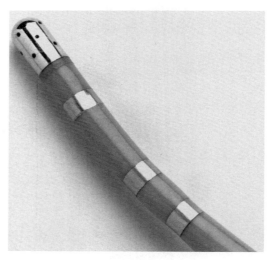

FIGURE 4-59. Open-system, saline-irrigated ablation electrode. This particular design has 13 holes arranged in an even pattern designed to prevent hot spots at the proximal edge of the electrode. A thermocouple is incorporated in the tip. Saline flow rates ranging from 2 to 20 mL/min have provided effective cooling with this design. The longer-duration, high-power radiofrequency ablations made possible by saline cooling have resulted in lesions that are typically four times the size of lesions from nonirrigated 4-mm tips. (Courtesy of Medtronic CardioRhythm, Inc., San Jose, CA.)

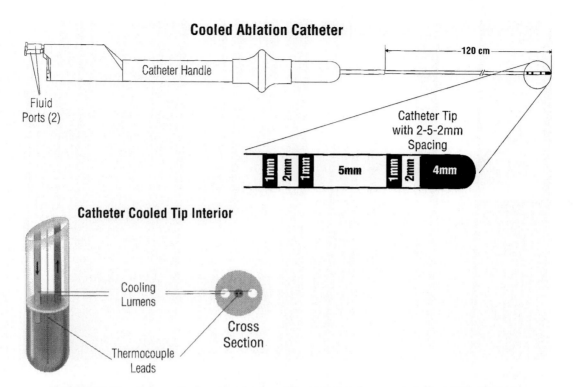

FIGURE 4-60. Schematic drawing of a closed-loop system for a cooled-tip ablation catheter. Two fluid channels circulate normal saline within the tip electrode. Patient volume loading concerns are not an issue with the closed-system approach. The electrode also incorporates a thermocouple. (Courtesy of Cardiac Pathways, Inc., Sunnyvale, CA.)

electrode. Because the saline is a conductive medium, it may create a "virtual electrode" composed of the electrode surrounded by a radiofrequency-charged saline cloud.

Open System

As an initial approach, saline infusion through holes in a tip electrode has been tried in several design variations. The simplest design has a large central hole at the distal end of the tip electrode. Although easier and less costly to manufacture, this design tends to focus most of the cooling at the distal end of the electrode. Another design incorporates multiple holes, smaller in size (0.010- to 0.016-inch diameter), spaced more evenly across the ablation electrode surface. This design is not overly complex or costly and permits a more even distribution of saline over the electrode surface. A third design uses a porous material for tip electrode construction. Although theoretically providing the most even cooling, this design may present problems in ensuring even flow from all pores, clogging, and maintaining electrode integrity (avoiding the loss of particles), and it may be more costly to produce.

An *in vitro* study by Adler and associates of a single-hole catheter design with a 30 mL/min saline flow showed substantially larger and deeper lesions with minimal thrombus and eschar (192). A ventricular ablation study by Mittleman and coworkers in 10 dogs comparing saline-cooled, three-hole, 2-mm electrodes with standard 2-mm electrodes showed a 2-mm average increase in any measured lesion dimension (length, width, or depth) for the saline-cooled electrode (193) (Fig. 4-62). This difference held true for two different radiofrequency power levels. The saline flow rate was a low 1.67 mL/min. Increased impedance caused by coagulum formation was dramatically reduced for the saline-cooled electrode.

In a study by Nakagawa and colleagues, a 5-mm-tip electrode with six 0.010-inch-diameter irrigation

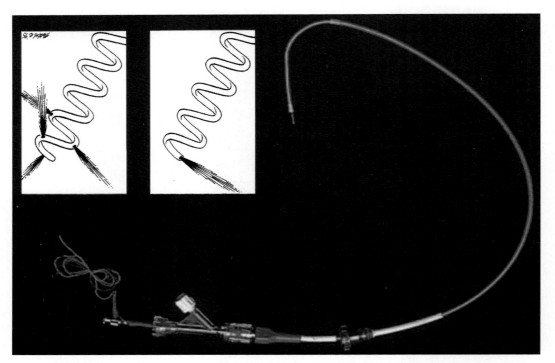

FIGURE 4-61. Helical screw-tip electrode catheter. Two styles of exit ports create a symmetric or an asymmetric lesion. In animal studies, saline has been infused at rates ranging from 0.5 to 4 mL/min for 50-W radiofrequency ablation durations as long as 4 minutes without producing impedance rise or coagulum. Mixing contrast medium with the saline allows fluoroscopic imaging of the "virtual electrode." The feasibility of performing reversible test ablations using cold saline has also been demonstrated. (Courtesy of Michael Hoey, University of Minnesota, Minneapolis, MN.)

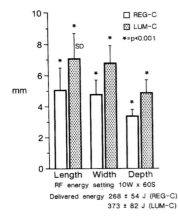
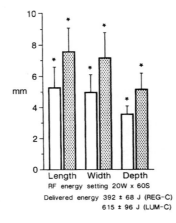

FIGURE 4-62. Graphs of lesion dimensions for saline-irrigated (<2 mL/min) and for nonirrigated radiofrequency ablation using 2-mm tip electrodes. The irrigated electrode was a three-hole design. At 10- and 20-W power levels, lesions were substantially larger for the saline-irrigated system. Delivered energy was also substantially higher with saline irrigation, based on longer radiofrequency duration before impedance rise. (From Mittleman RS, et al. Use of saline infusion electrode catheter for improved energy delivery and increased lesion size in radiofrequency catheter ablation. *Pacing Clin Electrophysiol* 1995;18:1022–1027, with permission.)

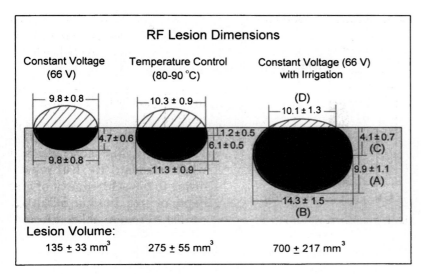

FIGURE 4-63. Diagram of the lesion dimensions for the three groups studied shows maximal lesion depth (A), maximal lesion diameter (B), lesion depth at maximum diameter (C), and lesion surface diameter (D). Lesions made with open-system, multihole, saline-irrigated tips were dramatically larger than those of the other two groups, with a larger portion of the lesion residing below the endocardial surface. (From Nakagawa H, Yamanashi WS, Pitha JV, et al. Comparison of in vivo tissue temperature profile and lesion geometry for radiofrequency ablation with a saline-irrigated electrode versus temperature control in canine thigh muscle preparation. *Circulation* 1995;91:2264–2273, with permission.)

holes spaced radially equidistant 1 mm from the tip was used for *in vivo* ablation on canine thigh muscle (191). Heparinized saline was infused through the tip at 20 mL/min. Ablation lesions with this system were compared with those created by using the temperature-control mode and voltage-control mode without the saline assist (Fig. 4-63). The voltage-control group experienced early impedance rise, which limited ablation time; therefore this group had the smallest lesions (135 mm^3). The temperature-control group did not have impedance rises, but voltage had to be substantially reduced to keep the tip temperature under 90°C. This resulted in intermediate-size lesions (275 mm^3). The saline-assisted ablations could be performed at a higher voltage, producing the largest lesions (700 mm^3). Lesion sizes were still growing rapidly at the end of the 60-second ablation, and tissue temperatures measured 3.5 and 7 mm below the surface were substantially higher than those in the other two groups (Fig. 4-64). The subsurface lesion was significantly larger than the surface lesion for the saline-cooled group, indicative of the high degree of surface convective cooling (Fig. 4-63).

Additional canine ablation studies with saline-irrigated tips conducted by Nakagawa and associates demonstrated that significant lesions could be created on myocardial infarct border zones (194).

Another *in vivo* study by Skrumeda and coworkers compared ventricular lesions in 10 dogs created by 7-Fr, 4-mm-tip electrodes with and without saline irrigation (195). The cooled electrode had nine 0.013-inch-diameter holes spaced evenly over the entire electrode, and saline flow was 2.5 mL/min. At 50 W for a maximum 2 minutes for both groups, the noncooled electrodes quickly experienced impedance rise, limiting lesion volume to about one fourth that of the saline-irrigated group (142 versus 753 mm^3). Further *in vivo* work by Nakagawa and colleagues suggests that saline-irrigated ablation with smaller electrodes (e.g., 2-mm length) may create larger lesions, because less radiofrequency current is shunted to the blood (196).

Although saline-irrigated ablation was developed primarily for ventricular tachycardia ablation applications, the initial clinical experience with this technology has been in SVT ablation. In the series reported by Nakagawa and associates and Arruda and coworkers, saline-irrigated accessory pathway ablation was successfully performed on more than 20 patients who had prior failed accessory pathway ablations (197, 198). Presumably, the saline electrode worked where standard radiofrequency had previously failed because of the achievement of greater lesion depth or area. In some of the patients, epicardial accessory pathways were ablated from the middle cardiac vein. At least one occurrence of distal right coronary artery narrowing related to saline ablation from the nearby coronary sinus is a cause for some caution with this technique (198). Additional early clinical data reported by Borggrefe and colleagues about the use of cooled-tip cath-

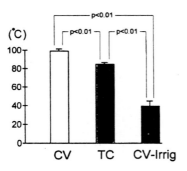
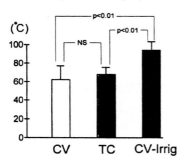
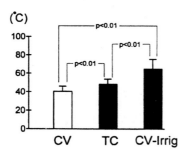

FIGURE 4-64. Bar graphs show the peak electrode temperature and tissue temperatures at 3.5 and 7.0 mm depths during radiofrequency ablations using constant voltage (CV), constant temperature (CT), and CV irrigation (CV-irrig) groups. In the CV-irrig group, the peak electrode temperature and the tissue temperature at each depth were significantly greater than those in the other groups. (From Nakagawa H, Yamanashi WS, Pitha JV, et al. Comparison of in vivo tissue temperature profile and lesion geometry for radiofrequency ablation with a saline-irrigated electrode versus temperature control in a canine thigh muscle preparation. *Circulation* 1995;91:2264–2273, with permission.)

eters for ventricular tachycardia ablation in humans also present cause for concern because of the postablation incidence of rapid ventricular tachycardia, ventricular fibrillation, and stroke.

Limitations and Improvements

Because of the apparently greater lesion depth that is achievable with saline-irrigated electrodes, a primary concern is control of lesion size. When ablating with saline-cooled electrodes from the coronary sinus in dogs, before the previously mentioned clinical series, Nakagawa and associates found evidence of thermal damage to nearby coronary arteries (199) (Fig. 4-65). Similar complications observed in early clinical trials emphasize the need to proceed cautiously in using this technique. One useful indicator of ablation efficacy, tip electrode temperature monitoring, seems to be somewhat less useful with saline irrigation because the tip is kept artificially cool. Other options for controlling lesion size could include precise impedance

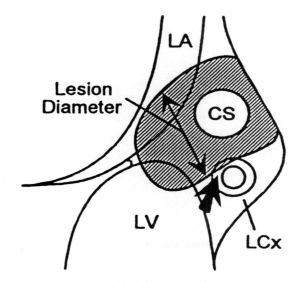

FIGURE 4-65. Schematic diagram of representative lesion size surrounding the coronary sinus after saline-irrigated radiofrequency ablation at 66 V for 60 seconds at 18 ablation sites in dogs. Seventeen of 18 radiofrequency sites at 66 V had epicardial lesions, but only 1 of 10 sites at 50 V had them. No endocardial lesions were observed. Segmental necrosis of the adventitia and media of the left circumflex coronary artery occurred in 8 of 18 lesions at 66 V and none of 10 at 50 V. (From Nakagawa H, Yamanashi WS, Pitha JV, et al. Effective delivery of radiofrequency energy through the coronary sinus without impedance rise using a saline irrigated electrode. *J Am Coll Cardiol* 1995; 7(6):777–781, with permission.)

measurement, subsurface temperature measurement, and monitoring of lesion growth with intracardiac ultrasound.

Another limitation of saline-irrigated ablation is the incidence of audible popping and resultant crater formation caused by localized boiling at or below the electrode-to-tissue interface. The problems associated with this phenomenon include possible electrode slippage, high-impedance shutdown, endocardial trauma, thrombus site creation, and perforation. Options for reducing the incidence of popping include methods for inducing a gradual release of steam from the tissue and possibilities in enhanced impedance or temperature monitoring to control power or fluid delivery.

Closed-Loop System
Another option for cooling the ablation electrode is to circulate a cool fluid within the tip rather than permitting it to exit through the tip into the blood (200). Theoretical advantages of this approach include the elimination of "volume loading" of the patient with infused saline and elimination of any reduction in tip-to-tissue contact that may be caused by fluid jets in an open-system tip. Because different pumps can be used on the inlet and outlet sides of a closed system, it is theoretically possible to have an internal catheter pressure that is substantially lower than that in an open system, which may improve system safety.

An *in vitro* study by Sykes and coworkers comparing closed-system cooled tips with standard 4-mm tips showed that substantially longer ablation times were possible with the cooled tip for power levels above 25 W, which produced lesions that were up to four times larger (201) (Fig. 4-66). *In vivo* animal studies with the closed-system method of tip cooling reported by Wharton and colleagues and Nibley and associates demonstrated increased power-handling

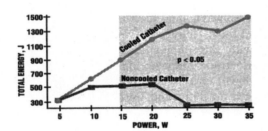

Cooled RF enabled more energy (Joules) delivery for a longer period of time than noncooled RF at powers greater than 15 W, resulting in larger lesions at powers greater than 25 W.

Mean Values of Lesion Size and Volume and Energy Delivery Time For Cooled (CRF) vs Noncooled (NCRF) RF Ablation

	POWER, W	5	10	15	20	25	30	35
CRF	Width, mm	6.5	7.8	9.2	10.8	10.4	12.3	12.0
	Depth, mm	4.3	3.7	4.7	5.4	5.4	5.9	5.7
	Volume, mm³	117	116	206	335	316	481	446
	Mean Time, sec	60	60	60	60	52	41.5	41.3
NCRF	Width, mm	6.0	8.8	9.5	9.9	8.2	9.3	7.2
	Depth, mm	2.5	4.8	4.8	5.1	3.7	4.3	3.5
	Volume, mm³	51	201	259	276	161	225	101
	Mean Time, sec	60	60	20.4	26.2	10.2	9.8	6.3

Data show that above 15 W, the cooled tip catheter results in significantly greater energy delivered for longer times, resulting in larger lesions than noncooled tip catheter.

$p < 0.05$

FIGURE 4-66. Graph and table show the energy delivered and lesion size for closed-loop, cooled-tip ablation versus standard radiofrequency (RF) ablation. The cooled tip enabled more radiofrequency energy delivery for a longer period at powers greater than 15 W, resulting in larger lesions at powers greater than 25 W. Lesions were more than four times larger for the cooled tip at 35-W RF power. (From Sykes C, Riley R, Pomeranz M, et al. Cooled tip ablation results in increased radiofrequency power delivery and lesion size [Abstract]. *Pacing Clin Electrophysiol* 1994;17:782, with permission.)

TABLE 4-6 • SUMMARY OF LESION VOLUME FOR 50-WATT RADIOFREQUENCY ABLATION USING SCREW-TIP ELECTRODE

Ablation Time (sec)	Saline Infusion (2 ML/min Before And During RF)	Lesion Volume (mm^3) (mean ± SEM)	Number Of Samples
240	Yes	6090 ± 335.8	5
180	Yes	5569.5 ± 326.9	10
120	Yes	2978.9 ± 324.8	10
60	Yes	836.22 ± 89.2	10
30	Yes	509.0 ± 48.1	10
20	Yes	329.9 ± 23.8	2
High impedance limited	No infusion	369.4 ± 54.5	10

capability, elimination or delay of impedance rise (depending on the power setting), and increased lesion volumes compared with standard radiofrequency ablation (202,203). Tip temperature monitoring by a thermocouple could predict impedance rise (204).

Screw-in Electrode

A needle electrode or helical screw-in electrode that is capable of infusing a conductive medium directly into the myocardium may have certain advantages over the surface contact cooled tips just mentioned. These advantages may include the creation of a virtual electrode composed of conductive saline, allowing a larger volume of tissue to be ablated; deeper or transmural lesions due to the subendocardial location of the electrode; reduced incidence of popping or cratering observed with surface contact cooled tips; and active fixation of the ablation electrode to tissue to prevent inadvertent movement. Hoey and co-workers reported an *in vivo* animal study of screw-in electrodes with saline infusion in 15 dogs that demonstrated the capability of producing lesions of almost unlimited size, depending on radiofrequency power and duration (205). A correlation of lesion volume with ablation parameters is shown in Table 4-6. No impedance rise was observed during these ablations. A contrast agent was mixed with the infused saline to permit fluoroscopic imaging of lesion size (Fig. 4-67).

Chemical Ablation

Although chemical ablation has not been a major area of research, animal and clinical research has been conducted using this technique. In one method, chemical ablation is performed through a needle electrode inserted into the endocardium from a steerable ablation catheter. An animal study by Hartung and colleagues using this technique demonstrated the capability of infusing lidocaine to reversibly stun intended ablation sites and infusing ethanol to create permanent lesions of predictable size (average volume = 1,250 mm^3) (206). Another animal study reported by Lu and associates, in which a preimplanted subepicardial ventricular tachycardia focus was successfully ablated in 18 of 18 dogs, showed controllable lesions, but 20% of the ventricular tachycardias were reinducible after 10 days (207).

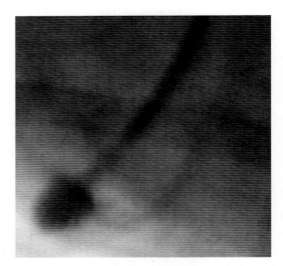

FIGURE 4-67. Fluoroscopic image of a virtual electrode created by intramyocardial infusion of a contrast-saline mixture using a helical screw-tip ablation catheter. (Courtesy of Michael Hoey, University of Minnesota, Minneapolis, MN.)

An alternative method for chemical ablation is to deliver the chemical agent epicardially from one of the coronary arteries. In this method, the delivery catheter is usually a very-low-profile (3-Fr), flexible infusion catheter (Fig. 4-13). The catheter can be delivered over a coronary guide wire, as with angioplasty balloons. Intracoronary ethanol was used in early preliminary clinical investigations by Brugada and coworkers for AV nodal ablation and ventricular tachycardia ablation (208,209). A potential advantage of using coronary arteries for ablation is that reversible test ablations can be performed using iced saline. Significant downsides to intracoronary ethanol ablation mentioned by Haines and colleagues include the possible migration of ethanol to myocardial tissue beyond the desired ablation target because of reflux of ethanol into another coronary artery (210). Other experimentally identified problems include a high degree of lesion size variability for a given ethanol dose and the possibility that these lesions could be arrhythmogenic (211).

Intravascular Radiofrequency Ablation

Somewhat related to the concept of intracoronary chemical ablation is radiofrequency ablation from coronary veins for termination of ventricular tachycardia. In a study of 11 dogs conducted by Arruda and associates, coronary venous anatomy was visualized by balloon occlusion of the coronary sinus and retrograde contrast infusion (180). The 2.5-to 3.6-Fr, over-the-wire catheters containing 4, 8, or 16 mapping electrodes were advanced to the distal end of various coronary veins. Epicardial electrograms were obtained, and the ventricle was paced. In some of the animals, a 4-Fr catheter with a 4-mm, saline-irrigated ablation electrode was advanced into the vein, and radiofrequency ablations were performed. Lesions with a 9.4-mm average depth and 13-mm diameter were created. Potential for late damage to nearby coronary arteries remains to be determined.

Alternative Energy Sources: Catheter Considerations

For microwave and cryoablation, significant obstacles are yet to be overcome in terms of catheter size, flexibility, and thermal characteristics.

Cryocatheters, which typically must carry relatively high-pressure fluid or gas, have tended to be stiff and larger than 7 Fr. Microwave catheters, because of the requirement for a coaxial cable, tend to have similar problems, although not to the same degree. Cryocatheters tend to have significant unintended cooling along the shaft because of heat exchange, and microwave catheters tend to have significant heating along the shaft caused by impedance matching and reflected power. These issues may be resolved for either or both technologies, given enough creative applied engineering, but they nonetheless currently pose significant hurdles. Catheters for delivering laser and ultrasound energy may not have these difficulties, but the fiberoptics or transducer electronics present flexibility, complexity, and cost challenges to incorporation into disposable steerable catheters. Efficient microwave antennas, ultrasound transducers, and lenses for focusing laser energy add further complication and cost to catheter designs for these technologies.

INTRACARDIAC IMAGING

Visual guidance during electrophysiologic mapping and ablation procedures is typically accomplished with biplane fluoroscopy. Fluoroscopic imaging of the cardiac chambers provides general positional information, but identification of specific anatomic detail can be challenging. Even finding a structure as large as the coronary sinus os can sometimes be challenging with fluoroscopy, although difficulties can as often be related to catheter maneuverability as to poor visualization. Although much of the electrophysiologic mapping for SVT involves the recording of electrograms, knowledge about catheter position relative to valves and other structures is also important. This is especially true for the more anatomically based SVT procedures (e.g., AV nodal modification, epicardial pathway ablation from the coronary sinus). New indications for radiofrequency ablation (e.g., direct ablation of atrial fibrillation using linear burns) may be even more anatomically based. Several imaging technologies are currently in clinical use or under investigation for electrophysiologic mapping and ablation.

These include ultrasound, electromagnetic position determination, and magnetic resonance imaging.

Ultrasound

Transesophageal Echo Ultrasound

Transesophageal echo (TEE) ultrasound has been available as a diagnostic tool for many years. Advantages of TEE over transthoracic echo (TTE) ultrasound for cardiac imaging in electrophysiology include improved resolution and penetration and easier location of intracardiac catheters. TTE also creates problems in terms of maintaining a sterile field. Disadvantages of TEE include a significantly more invasive procedure that requires general or significant local anesthesia. The TEE probe can also create shadows during fluoroscopic imaging.

TEE can be complementary to fluoroscopy because it can provide another imaging plane for more certainty in catheter tip positioning, and it can reduce reliance on fluoroscopy and therefore bring down fluoroscopic exposure time (e.g., as a means of monitoring catheter position during ablation to prevent inadvertent slippage). A number of studies have explored the potential utility of TEE for the guidance of ablation catheters. As reported by Saxon and coworkers, Gallais and colleagues, and Avitall and associates, TEE has shown utility in observing microcavitation bubbles indicative of impedance rise and coagulum formation (212–214). Omran and coworkers demonstrated the utility of TEE for imaging vascular structures such as coronary sinus diverticula and middle cardiac veins (215).

TEE is best suited for imaging the left atrium. TEE has also shown utility in imaging the transseptal puncture procedure for accessing the left atrium (214,216, 217). Septal "tenting" before puncture and thrombus on the puncture needle have been readily observed in these patient series. However, some experienced ultrasound investigators feel that TEE does not provide adequate resolution for imaging important intracardiac structures.

Intracardiac Echo Ultrasound

A later entry into the ultrasound imaging arena is intracardiac echo (ICE) ultrasound. ICE has the advantages over TEE of further enhanced resolution, no need for patient general anesthesia, and minimal probe shadowing of the fluoroscopic image. In early cardiac imaging research studies for electrophysiologic applications, ICE probes that were originally developed for intravascular use were used. These devices operated at frequencies of at least 20 MHz and could provide high-resolution images of structures adjacent to the transducer, but the depth of view was limited. To provide a penetration depth adequate to image most of the right atrium, frequencies less than 10 MHz are required. ICE probes operating at 12.5, 10, and 7.5 MHz have been made available for animal and human research.

Many of the ICE probes that have been used in animal and clinical research have been fairly large (e.g., 10 Fr) or have lacked adequate flexibility and steerability. Some researchers reported success using intracardiac imaging probes as small as 6 Fr, however. Some ultrasound systems that are under investigation for intracardiac imaging generate a thin 360-degree imaging plane perpendicular to the probe shaft (i.e., orthogonal imaging). Two alternative technologies are available for orthogonal imaging: the synthetic aperture arrays and mechanical systems. Current synthetic aperture arrays use up to 64 transducer elements electronically activated in sequence. Mechanical systems can consist of a rotating transducer or a stationary transducer with a rotating mirror. In addition to orthogonal imaging, array elements can also be oriented in a linear fashion (i.e., phased array) to provide a sector-shaped view parallel to the probe axis. The phased arrays (also used in TTE and TEE) have the potential for greater resolution, penetration depth, and flexibility than mechanical systems have.

Early animal studies by Chu and colleagues demonstrated that 10-MHz ICE (mechanical) could be used to assess specific anatomic landmarks (e.g., interatrial septum, right atrial appendage, coronary sinus, all valves) that were not adequately visible on fluoroscopy (218). It was also possible to determine catheter-to-endocardial wall contact with ICE, and lesion locations determined by using ICE were within 5 mm of actual targets 82% of the time. Microcavitation, thrombus formation, and actual lesion formation were observed in some cases. Another animal study by Chan and associates showed improved lesion location accuracy compared with fluoroscopy (219). Subsequent animal studies using 7.5-MHz phased array devices by Packer and coworkers demonstrated 7-cm imaging depth, combined with an ability to resolve ablation catheter orientation and evolving lesion formation (220). Similar results have been reported by Tardif and colleagues using a 20-MHz mechanical system to guide and assess microwave ablation in dogs (221). A comparison of ICE versus TEE for guidance of transseptal puncture conducted by Kyo and associates indicated greater ease in precise needle positioning with ICE (217).

Other animal work by Hummel and coworkers has shown that a 6-Fr, 20-MHz ICE probe can be used to accurately guide the placement of long lesions in the flutter isthmus area without the use of fluoroscopy (222). In clinical studies by Kalman and associates, 10-MHz ICE (mechanical) has been used to identify atrial anatomic landmarks such as the crista terminalis to aid in the mapping of atrial flutter and other atrial tachycardias (223,224). Chan and colleagues created 7.5-MHz (phased array) ICE-guided linear lesions in dogs at typical endocardial maze locations for atrial fibrillation ablation (e.g., inferior vena cava to superior vena cava, tricuspid valve annulus to inferior vena cava, along crista terminalis) (225). For these locations, ICE placed the lesions within 5 mm of the ablation target in 93% of cases, a significantly better rate than with fluoroscopy (52%). Limitations of the ICE technology that was used in most of these studies include the large sheath size required for the probe (usually 10 Fr or larger), limited probe maneuverability, and marginal ability to image the left atrium using 10-MHz or higher frequencies.

In summary, ICE may provide a valuable tool for accurately locating radiofrequency lesions relative to anatomic landmarks for anatomically based procedures such as atrial flutter and atrial fibrillation. ICE can increase accuracy of lesion location and significantly reduce exposure to ionizing radiation. Future areas for improvement of ICE catheters include significant reduction of catheter size and stiffness and the addition of steerability (tip deflection) so that difficult-to-access areas of the chamber are within reach. Probably even more important is a transition to lower frequencies (<10 MHz) for greater penetration. Combination of ICE with ablation capability on the same catheter could potentially reduce complexity by eliminating a separate imaging probe. This approach would provide an ultrasound "headlight" for the ablation catheter, rather than a global image of the chamber or area of interest. Another approach is the combined ultrasound probe and ablation catheter port described by Packer and coworkers (220). While reducing system complexity, this approach permits global imaging and independent ablation catheter movement.

Ultimately, an ideal global ICE catheter should be able to image all or most of the left and right atria from a position in the right atrium. In addition to greater penetration depth, an ability to scan the atrium and to use this information to create a 3-D volumetric image of the chamber may eventually obviate the need for fluoroscopy or at least significantly reduce its use. An experimental version of such a system has been developed and is under investigation (226). In this system of forward-looking ultrasound, a unique transducer radiates acoustic beams in a cone-shaped pattern from the tip of a catheter. The acoustic information is acquired and processed to generate a 3-D image shaped like a truncated cone.

Catheter Location with Ultrasound

Although ICE makes it easier to visualize catheters under ultrasound than does TEE or TTE, it can still be challenging to image catheters in a variety of orientations using ICE. To address this issue, device developers and researchers have developed markers that can locate any catheter position in the ultrasound image. One such passive marker consists of a spherical piezoelectric transducer that, when placed on a catheter, functions as an omnidirectional receiver for ultrasound pulses (227). When ultrasound pulses hit the transducer, it sends an electronic signal through wires in the catheter shaft to an interface box that is connected to the ultrasound equipment. The interface box determines which ultrasound ray from the scanning head has hit the transducer and measures the time delay of the pulse to determine a distance. This positional information is then used to generate a graphic on the ultrasound display indicating the catheter position. An alternative active marker for catheters also consists of a piezoelectric crystal that, when stimulated by ultrasound, sends a small voltage to a transponder (228). The transponder sends a stronger signal back to the piezoelectric crystal, causing it to vibrate and appear clearly on the ultrasound display screen.

Alternatives to Ultrasound

Ultrasound may be the imaging technology that is most familiar to electrophysiologists next to fluoroscopy, and as an alternative to ionizing radiation for electrophysiologic procedures, it is receiving substantial research and development attention. Other methods for enhanced imaging and catheter location are under development as well. One approach is to substantially reduce the patient's and physician's exposure to x-rays using a low-dose scanning beam digital x-ray system (229). The developer of this system claims that a 10-fold reduction in x-ray exposure is possible. A scintillator-tipped fiberoptic can be placed within a catheter to provide real-time 2-D positional information. By using two emitter-detector pairs oriented at 90 degrees, 3-D imaging and catheter location are feasible.

Another system that is under development uses multiple time-varying magnetic fields generated by devices positioned under the patient that are sensed by small orthogonally oriented coils in the catheter tip (230). As the catheter moves within these magnetic fields, currents are generated in the coils. This information is used to generate a 3-D model of the chamber to be mapped and to establish the real-time position of the catheter within the model. Electrogram information is also collected at a variety of sites within the chamber and is used to generate an activation map superimposed on the 3-D physical model. One of the most interesting potential capabilities of this system is to allow the operator to return to a previously located spot in space, which could greatly facilitate rapid mapping. Several alternative technologies for 3-D locations of intracardiac catheters are also under investigation.

CONCLUSIONS

For the imaging technologies and some of the sophisticated mapping and ablation technologies discussed, a key issue is cost. For many of these systems, the disposable element and the hardware plus software system probably add significant expense to an electrophysiologic mapping or ablation procedure. Whether the market will bear these additional costs depends on the degree to which they can make the current practice of catheter mapping and ablation simpler, safer, or easier. Some of these innovations in catheter design and ancillary systems may provide the key that unlocks the potential for a dramatic step forward in treating conditions such as atrial fibrillation and ischemic ventricular tachycardia.

REFERENCES

1. Haissaguerre M, Darliques IF, Warin JF, et al. Electrogram patterns predictive of successful catheter ablation of accessory pathways: value of unipolar recording mode. *Circulation* 1991; 84:188–202.
2. Grimm W, Hoffmann J, Josephson ME. Value of unipolar recordings for identification of appropriate target sites for RF-ablation of manifest accessory AVC-connections [Abstract]. *Pacing Clin Electrophysiol* 1994;17:845.
3. Simmers TA, Hauer RNW, Wever EFD, et al. Unipolar electrogram models for prediction of outcome in radiofrequency ablation of accessory pathways. *Pacing Clin Electrophysiol* 1994; 17:186–198.
4. Riccardi R, Richiardi E, Giustetto C, et al. Catheter ablation of WPW accessory pathways: usefulness of unipolar recording [Abstract]. *Eur J Card Pacing Electrophysiol* 1994;4:874.
5. Kadish AH, Schmaltz SJ, Morady F. A comparison of QRS complexes resulting from unipolar and bipolar pacing: implications for pace-mapping. *Pacing Clin Electrophysiol* 1991;14: 823–832.
6. Stevenson WG. Radiofrequency catheter ablation of atrial tachycardia. Advanced catheter ablation of cardiac arrhythmias [Program]. Bethesda, MD, April 1995.
7. Jackman WM, Friday KJ, Yeung-Lai-Wah JA, et al. New catheter technique for recording left free-wall accessory atrioventricular pathway activation: identification of pathway fiber orientation. *Circulation* 1988;78:598–611.
8. Goldreyer BN, Stephens K, Tobias SA. Junctional rhythms predictive of antegrade conduction delay during slow pathway ablation [Abstract]. *Circulation* 1994;90:I-125.
9. Kuck KH. The split-tip electrode catheter: improvements in AP potential recording [Abstract]. *J Am Coll Cardiol* 1993; 744–746.
10. Jackman WM, Friday KJ, Fitzgerald DM, et al. Localization of left free-wall and posteroseptal accessory atrioventricular pathways by direct recording of accessory pathway activation. *Pacing Clin Electrophysiol* 1989;12:204–214.
11. Fogel RI, Gest C, Evans JJ, Prystowsky EN. Oblique accessory pathway orientation: new observations and implications for mapping and successful ablation [Abstract]. *Circulation* 1993; 88:I-296.
12. Cappato R, Antz M, Weiss C. Radiofrequency current ablation of accessory pathways in Ebstein's anomaly [Abstract]. *Circulation* 1994;90:I-126.

13. Nath S, Mounsey JP, DiMarco JP, et al. Correlation of temperature and pathophysiological effect during radiofrequency catheter ablation of the atrioventricular junction: feasibility of thermal mapping [Abstract]. *Circulation* 1994;90:I-335.
14. Cote M, Epstein J, Treidman J, et al. Low temperature (T) mapping predicts site of successful ablation while minimizing myocardial damage [Abstract]. *J Am Coll Cardiol* 1996; 786–786.
15. Fitzpatrick AP, Fisher WG, Epstein LM, et al. Entrainment mapping and ablation of atrial flutter in patients facilitated by a 20-polar "halo" catheter in the right atrium [Abstract]. *J Am Coll Cardiol* 1994:341A.
16. Avitall B. A new catheter for mapping and RF ablation of AV node and right-sided APs [Abstract]. *J Am Coll Cardiol* 1993: 808–803.
17. Cappato R, Hebe J, Weib C, et al. Radiofrequency current ablation of accessory pathways in Ebstein's anomaly [Abstract]. *J Am Coll Cardiol* 1993;21:744–741.
18. Cappato R, Antz M, Weiss C. Radiofrequency current ablation of accessory pathways in Ebstein's anomaly [Abstract]. *Circulation* 1994:676.
19. Kuck KH, Schluter M, Siebels J, Hebe J. Right-sided epicardial accessory atrioventricular pathways: rare but there [Abstract]. *Circulation* 1994;90:I-127.
20. Avitall B, Hare J, Krum D, Dhala A. The anatomical determinants for the design of intracardiac mapping and ablation catheters. *Pacing Clin Electrophysiol* 1994;17:908–918.
21. Guiraudon GM, Guiraudon CM, Klein GJ, et al. Atrio-fascicular (Mahaim) fibres: surgical anatomy and pathology: experiment with 13 patients [Abstract]. *Pacing Clin Electrophysiol* 1994; 17:741.
22. Kuck K, Cappato R, Braun E, et al. Insights on the physiology of right-sided accessory fibers with Mahaim-type preexcitation [Abstract]. *Pacing Clin Electrophysiol* 1995;18:834.
23. Grogin HR, Lee RJ, Kwasman M, et al. Radiofrequency catheter ablation of atriofascicular and nodoventricular Mahaim tracts. *Circulation* 1994;90:272–281.
24. Brugada J, Martinez-Sanchez J, Kuzmicic B, et al. Radiofrequency catheter ablation of atriofascicular accessory pathways guided by discrete electrical potentials recorded at the tricuspid annulus. *Pacing Clin Electrophysiol* 1995;18:1388–1394.
25. Martinez-Alday J, Peinado R, Almendral J, et al. Evidence favoring that right accessory pathways with "Mahaim physiology" are a second "parallel" conduction system [Abstract]. *Eur Soc Cardiol* 1993:P1585.
26. Miles WM. Bundle branch and Mahaim fiber ablation: technique and results. Program of the Second International Symposium on Interventional Electrophysiology in the Management of Cardiac Arrhythmias. Newport, RI, July 1994.
27. Miller JM, Harper GR, Rothman SA, Hsia HH. Radiofrequency catheter ablation of an atriofascicular pathway during atrial fibrillation: a case report. *J Cardiovasc Electrophysiol* 1994; 5:846–853.
28. Haissaguerre M, Fischer B, Le Metayer P, Warin JF. Nature of the distal insertion site of Mahaim fibers as defined by catheter ablation [Abstract]. *Eur Soc Cardiol* 1993.
29. Chieng CE, Chen SA, Yang CR, et al. Incidence and significance of coronary sinus abnormalities in patients receiving radiofrequency ablation of supraventricular tachycardia [Abstract]. *Eur Soc Cardiol* 1993:P1398.
30. Giorgberidze I, Saksena S, Krol R, et al. Radiofrequency ablation of left-sided accessory pathways from coronary sinus [Abstract]. *J Am Coll Cardiol* 1995;1008:14.
31. Tebbenjohanns J, Pfeiffer D, Schumacher B, et al. Prospective angiography of the coronary sinus: impact for posteroseptal accessory pathway ablation [Abstract]. *Pacing Clin Electrophysiol* 1994;17:741.
32. Arruda M, Otomo K, Tondo C, et al. Coronary sinus angiography using an "occlusion" technique as an aid to RF ablation of epicardial accessory pathways [Abstract]. *Pacing Clin Electrophysiol* 1995;18:833.
33. Saul JP, Hulse E, Papagiannis J, et al. Late enlargement of radiofrequency lesions in infant lambs: implications for ablation procedures in small children. *Circulation* 1994;90:492–499.
34. Kottkamp H, Hindricks G, Chen X, et al. Temperature-controlled radiofrequency ablation of accessory pathways and atrioventricular nodal reentrant tachycardia: the 5-French approach [Abstract]. *Circulation* 1995;92:3822.
35. Kottkamp H, Hindricks G, Herold A, et al. Five-French or 7-French catheter for ablation of accessory pathways of modification of the AV node: a prospective, randomized study [Abstract]. *Pacing Clin Electrophysiol* 1996;19:431.
36. Langberg JJ, Hummel JD, Man DC, et al. Recognition and catheter ablation of epicardial accessory pathways. [Abstract] *J Am Coll Cardiol* 1993;21:173A.
37. Giorgberidze I, Pfeiffer D, Krol RB, et al. Primary or secondary ablation of left-sided accessory pathways via the coronary sinus [Abstract]. *Pacing Clin Electrophysiol* 1995;18:833.
38. Manolis AS, Wang PJ, Gadhoke A, et al. Transaortic and transseptal techniques for ablation of left-sided accessory pathways [Abstract]. *Pacing Clin Electrophysiol* 1994;17:814.
39. Mittleman RS, Huang SKS, Gillette PC, et al. Comparison of the trans-septal vs. retrograde aortic approach for left-sided accessory pathway radiofrequency ablation [Abstract]. *Pacing Clin Electrophysiol* 1994;17:833.
40. Ma C, Dong J, Yang X, et al. A randomized comparison between retrograde and transseptal approach for radiofrequency ablation of left-sided accessory pathways [Abstract]. *Pacing Clin Electrophysiol* 1995;18:915.
41. Haines DE, Watson DD, Verow AF. Electrode radius predicts lesion radius during radiofrequency energy heating: validation of a proposed thermodynamic model. *Circ Res* 1990;67: 124–129.
42. Nath S, DiMarco JP, Haines DE. Basic aspects of radiofrequency catheter ablation. *J Cardiovasc Electrophysiol* 1994;5: 863–876.
43. Langberg JJ, Gallagher M, Strickberger SA, Amirana O. Temperature-guided radiofrequency catheter ablation with very large distal electrodes. *Circulation* 1993;88:245–249.
44. Chan R, Johnson S, Packer D. The effect of ablation electrode length and catheter tip-endocardial orientation on radiofrequency lesion size in the canine right atrium [Abstract]. *Pacing Clin Electrophysiol* 1994;17:797.
45. Simmons WN, Mackey SC, He DS, Marcus FI. Comparison of maximum myocardial lesion depth using radiofrequency energy delivered with a gold or platinum electrode [Abstract]. *Circulation* 1994g:61456.
46. Nath S, Haines DE. Biophysics and pathology of catheter energy delivery systems. *Prog Cardiovasc Dis* 1995;37:185–204.
47. Pires LA, Huang SKS, Wagshal AB, et al. Temperature-guided radiofrequency catheter ablation of closed-chest ventricular myocardium with a novel thermistor-tipped catheter. *Am Heart J* 1994;127:1614–1618.
48. Chang I, Schwartzman D, Mirtoznik MS, et al. Does a thermistor provide useful information about electrode-tissue contact? [Abstract]. *Pacing Clin Electrophysiol* 1994;17:862.
49. Calkins H, Prystowsky E, Carlson M, et al, for the Atakr Multicenter Investigators Group. Temperature monitoring during RF catheter ablation procedures using closed loop control. *Circulation* 1994;90:1279–1285.

50. O'Connor BK, Case, CL, Balaji S, et al. Closed-loop temperature-controlled radiofrequency catheter ablation reduces impedance rise in children and adolescents [Abstract]. *J Am Coll Cardiol* 1994:304A.
51. Gillette PC, Case CL, Calkins HG. Closed loop temperature controlled radiofrequency catheter ablation [Abstract]. *Circulation* 1993;88:I-165.
52. Farre J, Asso A, Castro J, et al. Prevention of carbonization during radiofrequency catheter ablation [Abstract]. *Eur Heart J* 1994;15:286.
53. Calkins HG, Prystowsky EN, Carlson MD, et al. Site dependent variability of electrode temperature during radiofrequency catheter ablation procedures [Abstract]. *J Am Coll Cardiol* 1994: 1A–484A.
54. Calkins H, Prystowsky E, Klein L, et al. Electrode temperatures during radiofrequency catheter ablation procedures: relationship to ablation target and ablation result [Abstract]. *Pacing Clin Electrophysiol* 1994;17:813.
55. Choi YS, Sohn KS, Sohn DW, et al. Temperature-guided radiofrequency catheter ablation of slow pathway in atrioventricular nodal reentrant tachycardia. *Am Heart J* 1995;129: 392–399.
56. Stellbrink C, Haltern G, Ziegert K, et al. Different temperature curves observed during temperature-guided radiofrequency ablation of accessory pathways correlate with application success [Abstract]. *Pacing Clin Electrophysiol* 1994;17:788.
57. Carpinteiro LA, Cappato R, Schneider MAE, et al. Are local electrogram criteria predictive of catheter stability at the atrial tricuspid annulus? [Abstract]. *Pacing Clin Electrophysiol* 1995; 18:834.
58. Mackey S, Marcus FI, Simmons W. Tip temperature is not an indicator of intramyocardial temperatures during radiofrequency catheter ablation [Abstract]. *Pacing Clin Electrophysiol* 1995;18:801.
59. Kongsgaard E, Steen T, Amlie JP, et al. Temperature guided radiofrequency catheter ablation: catheter tip temperature underestimates tissue temperature [Abstract]. *Circulation* 1994; 90(4):1457.
60. Wittkampf FHM, Simmers TA, Hauer RNW, et al. Myocardial temperature response during radiofrequency catheter ablation. *Pacing Clin Electrophysiol* 1995;18:307–317.
61. Hoshino T, Sato T, Masai A, et al. Conduction system ablation using ferrite rod for cardiac arrhythmia. *IEEE Trans Magnetics* 1994;30:4689–4691.
62. Blouin, LT, Marcus FI, Lampe L. Assessment of effects of a radiofrequency energy field and thermistor location in an electrode catheter on the accuracy of temperature measurement. *Pacing Clin Electrophysiol* 1991;14:807–881.
63. Langberg JJ, Calkins H, El-Atassi R, et al. Temperature monitoring during radiofrequency catheter ablation of accessory pathways. *Circulation* 1992;86:1469–1474.
64. Wang PJ, Lenihan T, Guetersloh M, et al. Circumferential temperature monitoring versus single point monitoring during microwave ablation [Abstract]. *J Am Coll Cardiol* 1995:315A.
65. McRury ID, Whayne JG, Haines DE. Temperature measurement as a determinant of tissue heating during radiofrequency catheter ablation: an examination of electrode thermistor positioning for measurement accuracy. *J Cardiovasc Electrophysiol* 1995;6:268–278.
66. Remp T, Hoffmann E, Gerth A, et al. Drop in impedance and safety during catheter ablation: validation of a predictive marker for impedance rise [Abstract]. *Eur Heart J* 1994:P1541.
67. Strickberger SA, Ravi S, Daoud EG, et al. The relationship between impedance and temperature during radiofrequency ablation of accessory pathways. *J Am Coll Cardiol* 1995: 777–785.
68. Hartung W, McTeague K, Burton, et al. Estimation of temperature during radiofrequency catheter ablation using impedance measurement [Abstract]. *Pacing Clin Electrophysiol* 1994;17:741.
69. Hoffman E, Remp T, Gerth A, et al. Preablation 50 kHz impedance: a new parameter for assessing myocardial wall contact before radiofrequency catheter ablation [Abstract]. *J Am Coll Cardiol* 1993;21:49A.
70. Strickberger SA, Vorperian VR, Man KC, et al. Relation between impedance and endocardial contact during radiofrequency catheter ablation. *Am Heart J* 1994;128:226–229.
71. Hoffmann E, Remp T, Gerth A, et al. Does preablation impedance measurement improve the safety of radiofrequency catheter ablation [Abstract]. *Eur Soc Cardiol* 1993:P404.
72. Saul JP, Bergau D, Weindling SN, Rittman WJ. Determinants and usefulness of radiofrequency impedance: quantitative effects of tissue contact and frequency [Abstract]. *Pacing Clin Electrophysiol* 1994;17:846.
73. Cosio FG, Lopez-Gil M, Goicolea A, et al. Radiofrequency ablation of the inferior vena cava–tricuspid valve isthmus in common atrial flutter. *Am J Cardiol* 1993;71:705–709.
74. Feld GK, Fleck P, Chen PS, et al. Radiofrequency catheter ablation for the treatment of human type 1 atrial flutter. *Circulation* 1992;86:1233–1240.
75. Arenal A, Munoz R, Almendral J, et al. Is atrial flutter a circus movement around the tricuspid ring? Observations in the transplanted heart [Abstract]. *J Am Coll Cardiol* 1995:943–949.
76. Calkins H, Leon AR, Deam AG, et al. Catheter ablation of atrial flutter using radiofrequency energy. *Am J Cardiol* 1994; 73:353–356.
77. Fischer B, Haissaguerre M, Garrigues S, et al. Radiofrequency catheter ablation of common atrial flutter in 80 patients. *J Am Coll Cardiol* 1995;25:1365–1372.
78. Haissaguerre M, Saoudi N. Role of catheter ablation for supraventricular tachyarrhythmias, with emphasis on atrial flutter and atrial tachycardia. *Curr Opin Cardiol* 1994;9:40–52.
79. Rigden LB, Klein LS, Mitrani RD, et al. Improved success rate by ablating atrial flutter with anatomic posteroseptal linear lesions compared with discrete lesions guided by endocardial mapping techniques [Abstract]. *Pacing Clin Electrophysiol* 1995; 18:859.
80. Feld G, Fujimura O, Green U, Mazzola F. Radiofrequency catheter ablation of human type 1 atrial flutter—comparison of results with 8 mm versus 4 mm tip ablation catheter [Abstract]. *J Am Coll Cardiol* 1995:943–912.
81. Lesh MD, Van Hare GF, Fitzpatrick AP, et al. Curing reentrant atrial arrhythmias. *J Electrocardiol* 1993;26[Suppl]:194–203.
82. Baal T, Chen X, Kotikamp H, Borggrefe M. Radiofrequency catheter ablation: improving lesion size achieved with conventional catheters [Abstract]. *Circulation* 1994;90:I-272.
83. Cosio F, Arribas F, Lopez-Gill M, et al. New catheter design for ablation of the inferior vena cava–tricuspid isthmus in atrial flutter [Abstract]. *Pacing Clin Electrophysiol* 1996;19:335.
84. Poty H, Saoudi N, Anselme F, et al. Success of radiofrequency ablation of type I atrial flutter may be predicted using electrophysiological criteria [Abstract]. *Pacing Clin Electrophysiol* 1995; 18:242.
85. Nakagawa H, Khastgir T, Beckman K, et al. Rapid reliable identification of a line of block and successful ablation of atrial flutter [Abstract]. *Circulation* 1995;92:396.
86. Sarter B, Schwartzman D, Movsowitz C, et al. Atrial arrhythmias following successful ablation of atrial flutter associated with conduction block in the inferior vena cava–tricuspid valve isthmus [Abstract]. *Pacing Clin Electrophysiol* 1996;19:279.

87. Philippon F, Epstein AE, Plumb VJ, et al. Predictors of atrial fibrillation following catheter ablation of atrial flutter [Abstract]. *Pacing Clin Electrophysiol* 1994;17:758.
88. Fischer B, Haissaguerre M, Cauchemez B, et al. Frequency of recurrent atrial fibrillation after successful radiofrequency catheter ablation of common atrial flutter: results in 100 consecutive patients [Abstract]. *Pacing Clin Electrophysiol* 1995;18:856.
89. Walsh EP, Saul JP, Hulse JE, et al. Transcatheter ablation of ectopic atrial tachycardia in young patients using radiofrequency current. *Circulation* 1992;86:1138–1146.
90. Lesh MD, Van Hare GF, Kwasman MA, et al. Curative radiofrequency (RF) catheter ablation of atrial tachycardia and flutter [Abstract]. *J Am Coll Cardiol* 1993;21:798–801.
91. Kall J, Olshansky B, Baerman J, et al. Radiofrequency catheter ablation for atrial tachycardia [Abstract]. *J Am Coll Cardiol* 1993;21:856–848.
92. Shenasa H, Merrill JJ, Hamer ME, Wharton JM. Distribution of ectopic atrial tachycardias along the crista terminalis: an atrial ring of fire [Abstract]. *Circulation* 1993:141.
93. Poty H, Haissaguerre M, Warin JF, et al. Radiofrequency catheter ablation of atrial tachycardias [Abstract]. *Eur J Card Pacing Electrophysiol* 1994;4:820.
94. Weiss C, Hatala R, Cappato R, et al. The "encircling" mapping technique: a simplified approach to radio-frequency current ablation of ectopic atrial tachycardia [Abstract]. *J Am Coll Cardiol* 1994:1A-484A.
95. Brown JW, Porter CE, Plumb VJ, Kay GN. The double catheter mapping technique for radiofrequency ablation of atrial tachycardias: a new strategy [Abstract]. *Pacing Clin Electrophysiol* 1994;17:806.
96. Cox JL, Boineau JP, Schuessier RB, et al. Five-year experience with the maze procedure for atrial fibrillation [Abstract]. *Ann Thorac Surg* 1993;56:814–823.
97. Cox JL. The surgical treatment of atrial fibrillation [Abstract]. *Eur J Card Pacing Electrophysiol* 1994;4:70.
98. Swartz JF, Pellersels G, Silvers J, et al. A catheter-based curative approach to atrial fibrillation in humans [Abstract]. *Circulation* 1994;90:I-335.
99. Haissaguerre M, Gencel L, Fischer B, et al. Successful catheter ablation of atrial fibrillation. *J Cardiovasc Electrophysiol* 1994;5:1045–1052.
100. Jenkins KJ, Walsh, EP, Colan SD, et al. Multipolar endocardial mapping of the right atrium during cardiac catheterization: description of a new technique. *J Am Coll Cardiol* 1993;22:1105–1110.
101. Triedman JK, Jenkins KJ, Saul J, et al. Right atrial mapping in humans using a multielectrode basket catheter [Abstract]. *Pacing Clin Electrophysiol* 1995;18:800.
102. Harvey MN, Morady F. Radiofrequency catheter ablation for atrial fibrillation. *Coron Artery Dis* 1995;6:115–120.
103. Grogan M, Smith HC, Gersh B, et al. Left ventricular dysfunction due to atrial fibrillation in patients initially believed to have idiopathic dilated cardiomyopathy. *Am J Cardiol* 1992;69:1570–1573.
104. Heinz G, Siostrzonek P, Kreiner G, et al. Improvement in left ventricular function by ablation of atrioventricular conduction in selected patients with lone atrial fibrillation. *Am J Cardiol* 1992;69:489–492.
105. Rodriquez LM, Smeets JL, Xie B, et al. Reversible left ventricular dysfunction secondary to rapid atrial fibrillation. *Am J Cardiol* 1993;72:1137–1141.
106. Helguera ME, Pinski SL, Khoudeir Y, et al. Improvement in left ventricular systolic function after successful radiofrequency AV junctional ablation in patients with chronic atrial fibrillation and moderate ventricular response [Abstract]. *Pacing Clin Electrophysiol* 1994;17:799.
107. Clementy J, Lataste D, Poquet F, Cheradame I. Functional status of patients after AV junction catheter ablation for refractory atrial arrhythmias: experience of 50 patients with up to 6 years follow-up [Abstract]. *Eur J Card Pacing Electrophysiol* 1994;4:826.
108. Gianfranchi L, Brignole M, Menozzi C, et al. Effects on quality of life and cardiac performance of atrio-ventricular junction radiofrequency ablation in patients with chronic atrial fibrillation and flutter [Abstract]. *Eur J Card Pacing Electrophysiol* 1994;4:191.
109. Rosenqvist M, Lee MA, Moulinier L, et al. Long term follow up of patients after transcatheter direct current ablation of the atrioventricular junction. *J Am Coll Cardiol* 1990;16:1467–1474.
110. Williamson BD, Man KC, Daoud E, et al. Radiofrequency catheter modification of atrioventricular conduction to control the ventricular rate during atrial fibrillation. *N Engl J Med* 1994;331:910–917.
111. Tebbenjohanns J, Schumacher B, Pfeiffer D, et al. Reduction in ventricular response during atrial fibrillation after ablation of the slow pathway: acute results and follow-up [Abstract]. *J Am Coll Cardiol* 1995;65A:911–935.
112. Bella PD, Carbucicchio C, Tondo C, Riva S. Modulation of atrioventricular conduction by ablation of the "slow" atrioventricular node pathway in patients with drug-refractory atrial fibrillation or flutter. *J Am Coll Cardiol* 1995;25:39–46.
113. Blanck Z, Dhala A, Krum D, et al. Dramatic reduction in ventricular response during atrial fibrillation by ablating the atrioventricular nodal slow pathway: electrophysiologic and clinical implications [Abstract]. *Circulation* 1993;88:I-584.
114. Feld G. Radiofrequency catheter ablation versus modification of the AV node for control of rapid ventricular response in atrial fibrillation. *J Cardiovasc Electrophysiol* 1995;6:217–228.
115. Williamson BD, Strickberger SA, Hummel JD, et al. Radiofrequency modification of atrioventricular conduction for control of ventricular response in atrial fibrillation [Abstract]. *Pacing Clin Electrophysiol* 1994;17:775.
116. Menozzi C, Brignole M, Gianfranchi L, et al. Radiofrequency catheter ablation and modulation of atrioventricular conduction in patients with atrial fibrillation. *Pacing Clin Electrophysiol* 1994;17:2143–2149.
117. Shenasa M, Shenasa H. Distinct "bimodal distribution" in R-R interval histograms during atrial fibrillation: implications for radiofrequency current modification of the A-V node [Abstract]. *Pacing Clin Electrophysiol* 1995;18:843.
118. Cox JL, Boineau JP, Schuessler RB, et al. A review of surgery for atrial fibrillation. *J Cardiovasc Electrophysiol* 1991;2:541–561.
119. Kosakai Y, Kawaguchi A, Sasako Y, et al. Maze procedure modified to preserve the sinus node arteries [Abstract]. *Pacing Clin Electrophysiol* 1993;16:880.
120. Tsui S, Grace AA, Schofield PM, et al. Maze 3: two cuts too few? [Abstract]. *Eur J Card Pacing Electrophysiol* 1994;4:82.
121. Chiba N, Itoh M, Kubota M. Maze III procedure creates anatomical slow conduction zone as developing reentrant atrial tachycardia [Abstract]. *Circulation* 1994;90:I-595.
122. Jantene MB, Sosa E, Tarasoutchi F, et al. Atrial fibrillation and mitral valve disease: concomitant surgical treatment with "maze" procedures [Abstract]. *Circulation* 1994;90:I-595.
123. van Hemel NM, Defauw JJAMT, Kingma JH, et al. Long-term results of the corridor operation for atrial fibrillation. *Br Heart J* 1994;71:170–176.
124. van Hemel NM, Defauw JAM, Jaarsma W, et al. Efficacy of

"corridor" surgery to treat drug resistant paroxysmal atrial fibrillation [Abstract]. *J Am Coll Cardiol* 1994:1664.
125. Seifert MJ, Friedman MF, Sellke FW, Josephson ME. Radiofrequency maze ablation for atrial fibrillation [Abstract]. *Circulation* 1994;90:3203.
126. Elvan A, Pride HP, Zipes DP. Replication of the "maze" procedures by radiofrequency catheter ablation reduces the prevalence of atrial fibrillation [Abstract]. *Eur Heart J* 1994;15:329.
127. Kempler P, Littmann L, Chuang CH, et al. Radiofrequency ablation of the right atrium: acute and chronic effects [Abstract]. *Pacing Clin Electrophysiol* 1994;17:797.
128. Elvan A, Rigden LB, Kisanuki A, et al. Radiofrequency catheter ablation (RFCA) of the atria effectively abolishes pacing induced chronic atrial fibrillation [Abstract]. *Pacing Clin Electrophysiol* 1995;18:856.
129. Jancin B. Atrial fibrillation getting serious attention. *Int Med News Cardiol News* 1994; Nov 15.
130. Avitall B, Hare J, Helms R. Vagally mediated atrial fibrillation in a dog model can be ablated by placing linear radiofrequency lesions at the junction of the right atrial appendage and the superior vena cava [Abstract]. *Pacing Clin Electrophysiol* 1994; 17:857.
131. Allessie MA, Lammers WJEP, Bonke FIM, et al. Experimental evaluation of Moe's multiple wavelet hypothesis of atrial fibrillation. In: Zipes DP, Jalife J, eds. *Cardiac electrophysiology and arrhythmias.* Orlando, FL: Grune & Stratton, 1985:265–275.
132. Jaïs P, Haissaguerre M, Shah D, et al. Staged approach for paroxysmal atrial fibrillation [Abstract]. *Pacing Clin Electrophysiol* 1996;19:62.
133. Natale A, Tomassoni G, Kearney M, et al. Catheter ablation approach on the right side only for paroxysmal atrial fibrillation therapy [Abstract]. *Circulation* 1995;92:1265.
134. Avitall B, Hare J, Mughal K, et al. Ablation of atrial fibrillation in a dog model [Abstract]. *J Am Coll Cardiol* 1994:276A.
135. Haines DE, McRury IA, Whayne JG, Fleischman SD. Radiofrequency ablation at the tricuspid-inferior vena cava isthmus: unipolar vs. bipolar delivery [Abstract]. *Circulation* 1994;90:I-594.
136. Haines DE, McRury IA, Whayne JG, Fleishchman SD. Atrial radiofrequency ablation: the use of novel deploying loop catheter design to create long linear lesions [Abstract]. *Circulation* 1994;90:I-335.
137. Avitall B, Hare J, Mughal K, Silverstein E. Segmented ablation electrode: a system for flexible lesion size [Abstract]. *Circulation* 1994;90:I-126.
138. Avitall B, Hare J, Mughal K, et al. A catheter system to ablate atrial fibrillation in a sterile pericarditis dog model [Abstract]. *Pacing Clin Electrophysiol* 1994;17:774.
139. Avitall B, Helms R, Chiang W, Kotov A. Technology and method for the creation of left atrial endocardial linear lesions to ablate atrial fibrillation [Abstract]. *J Am Coll Cardiol* 1996; 27:1037–1032.
140. Groeneveld PW, Haugh C, Estes NAM III, Wang PJ. Panel electrode "pigtail" catheter using flexible electrically conductive material: a new design for increasing radiofrequency ablation lesion size? [Abstract]. *Pacing Clin Electrophysiol* 1993;16:923.
141. Wang PJ, Groeneveld PW, Gadhoke A, Estes NAM III. Electrode panels: a new design for radiofrequency ablation catheters [Abstract]. *J Am Coll Cardiol* 1993:765–766.
142. McRury IA, Whayne JG, Fleischman SD, Haines DE. What are the power requirements for radiofrequency ablation with multielectrode catheters in the atrium? [Abstract] *Circulation* 1994;90:I-336.
143. Avitall B, Hare J, Krum D, et al. Catheter ablation of supraventricular arrhythmias [Abstract]. *J Am Coll Cardiol* 1994:276A.
144. Haines D, McRury I. Primary atrial fibrillation ablation (PAFA) in a chronic atrial fibrillation model [Abstract]. 1995; 92:1261.
145. Olgin J, Kalman J, Maguire M, et al. Electrophysiologic effects of long linear atrial lesions placed under intracardiac echo guidance [Abstract]. *Pacing Clin Electrophysiol* 1996;19:64.
146. Nakagawa H, Yamanishi W, Pitha J, Imai S. Creation of long linear transmural radiofrequency lesions in atrium using a novel spiral ribbon–saline irrigated electrode catheter [Abstract]. *J Am Coll Cardiol* 1996;27:768–762.
147. Avitall B, Helms R, Chiang W, Periman B. Nonlinear atrial radiofrequency lesions are arrhythmogenic: a study of skipped lesions in the normal atria [Abstract]. *Circulation* 1995;92:1263.
148. Nakagawa H, Kumagai K, Imai S, et al. Catheter ablation from Bachmann's bundle from the right atrium eliminates atrial fibrillation in a canine sterile pericarditis model [Abstract]. *Pacing Clin Electrophysiol* 1996;19:61.
149. Tondo C, Otomo K, Antz M, et al. Successful radiofrequency ablation of atrial fibrillation by a single lesion to the inter-atrial septum [Abstract]. *Circulation* 1995;92:1260.
150. Carlson MD, Why KV, Wallick D, Martin P. Is the high right atrium the key to vagally mediated atrial fibrillation? [Abstract]. *Circulation* 1994;90:I-182.
151. Wolfe DA, Baker JH II, Philippon F, et al. Initiation and termination sites of spontaneous atrial fibrillation [Abstract]. *Circulation* 1994;90:I-376.
152. Papageorgiou P, Boyle N, Monahan K, et al. Site-dependent intra-atrial conduction delay: relationship to initiation of atrial flutter/fibrillation [Abstract]. *J Am Coll Cardiol* 1995;[Spec issue]:169A.
153. Prakash A, Saksena S, Krol RB, et al. Electrophysiology of acute prevention of atrial fibrillation and flutter with dual site right atrial pacing [Abstract]. *Pacing Clin Electrophysiol* 1995;18:803.
154. Haffajee C, Stevens S, Mongeon L, et al. High frequency atrial burst pacing for termination of atrial fibrillation [Abstract]. *Pacing Clin Electrophysiol* 1995;18:804.
155. Giorgberidze I, Saksena S, Krol RB, et al. Clinical efficacy and electrophysiologic effects of high frequency atrial pacing for type 2 atrial flutter and atrial fibrillation [Abstract]. *Pacing Clin Electrophysiol* 1995;18:804.
156. Kalman J, Olgin J, Karch M, et al. Effect of right atrial linear lesions on atrial defibrillation threshold: implications for "hybrid therapy" [Abstract]. *Pacing Clin Electrophysiol* 1996;19:237.
157. Klein LS, Shih H, Hackett K, et al. Radiofrequency catheter ablation of ventricular tachycardia in patients without structural heart disease. *Circulation* 1992;85:1666–1674.
158. Smeets JLRM, Rodriquez L, Metzger J, et al. Can ventricular tachycardia in the absence of structural heart disease be cured by radiofrequency catheter ablation? *Eur Soc Cardiol* 1993:P1400.
159. Littman L, Svenson RH, Gallagher JJ, et al. Functional role of the epicardium in postinfarction ventricular tachycardia: observations derived from computerized epicardial activation, mapping entrainment, and epicardial laser photoablation. *Circulation* 1991;83:1577–1591.
160. Downar E, Kimber S, Harris L, et al. Endocardial mapping of ventricular tachycardia in the intact human heart. II. Evidence for multiuse reentry in a function sheet of surviving myocardium. *J Am Coll Cardiol* 1992;20:869–878.
161. Harris L, Downar E, Mickleborough L, et al. Activation sequence of ventricular tachycardia: endocardial and epicardial mapping studies in the human ventricle. *J Am Coll Cardiol* 1987;10:1040–1047.

162. Kaltenbrunner W, Cardinal R, Dubuc M, et al. Epicardial and endocardial mapping of ventricular tachycardia in patients with myocardial infarction: is the origin of the tachycardia always subendocardially localized? *Circulation* 1991;84:1058–1071.
163. Chen, TCK, Parson ID, Downar E. The construction of endocardial balloon arrays for cardiac mapping. *Pacing Clin Electrophysiol* 1991;14:470–479.
164. Davis LM, Cooper M, Johnson DC, et al. Simultaneous 60-electrode mapping of ventricular tachycardia using percutaneous catheters. *J Am Coll Cardiol* 1994;24:709–719.
165. Triedman JK, Praagh RV, Lock JE, et al. Basket catheter mapping of atrial and ventricular activation: animal studies. *Circulation* 1994;90:I-595.
166. Widman LE, Jackman WM, Lazzara R. Localization of diastolic activation with multielectrode catheter arrays: mathematical algorithms for interpolation [Abstract]. *Pacing Clin Electrophysiol* 1994;17:781.
167. Smith MF, Guzzo JA, Buonocore RV, Greenspon AJ. Endocardial activation mapping of ventricular tachycardia in swine using a percutaneous multielectrode "basket" catheter. *Circulation* 1994;90:I-485.
168. Smith MF, Hsu S, Maniet A, et al. Hemodynamic evaluation of a multielectrode "basket" catheter for endocardial mapping [Abstract]. *Pacing Clin Electrophysiol* 1995;18:916.
169. Fitzpatrick AP, Chin MC, Stillson CA, et al. Successful percutaneous deployment, pacing and recording from a 64-polar, multi-strut "basket" catheter in the swine left ventricle [Abstract]. *Pacing Clin Electrophysiol* 1994;17:861.
170. Imran MA. Method of forming a flexible expandable member for use with a catheter probe. US Patent No 5,404,638, 1995.
171. Imran MA. Endocardial mapping and ablation system utilizing a separately controlled ablation catheter and method. US Patent No 5,324,284, 1994.
172. Triedman J, Jenkens K, Colan S, Saul P. High-density transcatheter mapping shows diverse mechanisms for atrial reentrant tachycardia after congenital heart surgery [Abstract]. *J Am Coll Cardiol* 1996;27:768–766.
173. Gelinas SL, Cerundolo DG, Concord EA. Endocardial electrode. US Patent No 4,522,212, 1985.
174. Waldman L, Chen PS. Endocardial electrical mapping catheter. US Patent No 5,237,996, 1993.
175. Imran MA. Mapping and ablation catheter with individually deployable arms and method. US Patent No 5,327,889, 1994.
176. Beatty GE, Kagan J, Budd JR. Encodardial mapping system. US Patent No 5,297,549, 1994.
177. Peters N, Jackman W, Schilling R, et al. Initial experience with mapping human endocardial activation using a novel non-contact catheter mapping system [Abstract]. *Pacing Clin Electrophysiol* 1996;19:138.
178. Desai, JM. Catheter for mapping and ablation and method therefor. US Patent No 4,940,064, 1990.
179. Desai JM, Nyo H, Vera Z, et al. Orthogonal electrode catheter array for mapping of endocardial focal site of ventricular activation. *Pacing Clin Electrophysiol* 1991;14:557–576.
180. Arruda M, Otomo K, Tondo C, et al. Epicardial left ventricular mapping and RF catheter ablation from the coronary veins: a potential approach for ventricular tachycardia [Abstract]. *Pacing Clin Electrophysiol* 1995;18:857.
181. Littmann L, Wu G, Amirana O, et al. Rapid localization of epicardial breakthrough sites using multielectrode intracoronary mapping catheters in dogs [Abstract]. *Pacing Clin Electrophysiol* 1994;17:862.
182. Gessman LJ, Agarwal JBN, Endo T, Helfant RH. Localization and mechanism of ventricular tachycardia by ice mapping 1 week after the onset of myocardial infarction in dogs. *Circulation* 1983;68:657–666.
183. Hirao K, Sato T, Otomo K, et al. The response of atrioventricular junctional tissue to temperature. *Jpn Circ J* 1994;58:351–361.
184. Rosenbaum R, Greenspon AJ, Smith M, Walinsky P. Advanced radiofrequency catheter ablation in canine myocardium. *Am Heart J* 1994;127:851–857.
185. Chang I, Mirotznik MS, Schwartzman D, et al. Radiofrequency energy delivery results in non-uniform heating patterns [Abstract]. *J Am Coll Cardiol* 1994;1A–484A:836–842.
186. Satake S, Ohira H, Okishige K, et al. Temperature guided radiofrequency ablation of ventricular tachycardia using 12 F sphere tip electrode [Abstract]. *Circulation* 1994;90:I-271.
187. Imran MA. Catheter having needle electrode for radiofrequency ablation. US Patent No 5,281,218, 1994.
188. Ohtake H, Misaki T, Matsunaga Y, et al. Development of a new intraoperative radiofrequency ablation technique using a needle electrode. *Ann Thorac Surg* 1994;58:750–753.
189. An H, Saksena S, Janssen M, Osypka P. Radiofrequency ablation of ventricular myocardium using active fixation and passive contact catheter delivery systems. *Am Heart J* 1989;118:69–77.
190. Lavergne T, Prunier L, Cuize L. Transcatheter radiofrequency ablation of atrial tissue using a suction catheter. *Pacing Clin Electrophysiol* 1989;12:177–186.
191. Nakagawa H, Yamanashi WS, Pitha JV, et al. Comparison of in vivo tissue temperature profile and lesion geometry for radiofrequency ablation with a saline-irrigated electrode versus temperature control in a canine thigh muscle preparation. *Circulation* 1995;91:2264–2273.
192. Adler SW, Lafontaine D, Hastings R, et al. Hydro-ablation: a new method for transcatheter radiofrequency ablation [Abstract]. *Eur J Card Pacing Electrophysiol* 1994;4:192.
193. Mittleman RS, Huang SKS, De Guzman WT, et al. Use of the saline infusion electrode catheter for improved energy delivery and increased lesion size in radiofrequency catheter ablation. *Pacing Clin Electrophysiol* 1995;18:1022–1027.
194. Nakagawa H, Yamanashi WS, Pitha JV, et al. Comparison of radiofrequency lesions in the canine left ventricle using a saline irrigated electrode versus temperature control [Abstract]. *J Am Coll Cardiol* 1995:42A.
195. Skrumeda LL, Maguire MA, Mehra R. Effect of delivering saline at a low flow rate on RF lesion size in the left ventricle [Abstract]. *Pacing Clin Electrophysiol* 1995;18:921.
196. Nakagawa H, Yamanashi W, Wittkampf F, et al. Comparison of tissue temperature and lesion size in radiofrequency ablation using saline irrigation with a small versus large tip electrode in a canine thigh muscle preparation [Abstract]. *Pacing Clin Electrophysiol* 1995;18:917.
197. Nakagawa H, Khastgir T, Arruda M, et al. Radiofrequency catheter ablation using a saline irrigated electrode in patients with prior failed accessory pathway ablation [Abstract]. *Pacing Clin Electrophysiol* 1995;18:832.
198. Arruda M, Nakagawa H, Khastgir T, et al. Facilitation of accessory pathway ablation from the middle cardiac vein by a saline irrigated catheter electrode [Abstract]. *Pacing Clin Electrophysiol* 1995;18:832.
199. Nakagawa H, Yamanashi WS, Pitha JV, et al. Effective delivery of radiofrequency energy through the coronary sinus without impedance rise using a saline irrigated electrode [Abstract]. *J Am Coll Cardiol* 1995;777:1.
200. Imran MA, Pomeranz ML. Catheter for RF ablation with cooled electrode. US Patent No 5,348,554, 1994.
201. Sykes C, Riley R, Pomeranz M, et al. Cooled tip ablation

results in increased radiofrequency power delivery and lesion size [Abstract]. *Pacing Clin Electrophysiol* 1994;17:782.
202. Wharton JM, Nibley C, Sykes CM, et al. Establishment of a dose-response relationship for high power chilled-tip radiofrequency current ablation in sheep [Abstract]. *J Am Coll Cardiol* 1995:293A.
203. Nibley C, Sykes DM, Chapman T, et al. Prevention of impedance rise during radiofrequency current catheter ablation by intra-electrode tip chilling [Abstract]. *Circulation* 1994;90:I-271.
204. Nibley C, Sykes CM, Rowan R, et al. Predictors of abrupt impedance rise during chilled-tip radiofrequency catheter ablation [Abstract]. *J Am Coll Cardiol* 1995:293A.
205. Hoey MF, Mulier PM, Shake JG. Intramural ablation using radiofrequency energy via screw-tip catheter and saline electrode [Abstract]. *Pacing Clin Electrophysiol* 1995;18:917.
206. Hartung WM, Lesh M, Hidden-Lucet F, et al. Transcatheter subendocardial infusion of ethanol: a new ablative technique for ventricular myocardium [Abstract]. *Circulation* 1994;90:I-487.
207. Lu C, Liu X, Jia G, Mao S. Experimental ventricular tachycardia treated by transcatheter intramyocardial chemical ablation [Abstract]. *Pacing Clin Electrophysiol* 1994;17:861.
208. Brugada P, de Swart H, Smeets J, et al. Transcoronary chemical ablation of atrioventricular conduction. *Circulation* 1990;81:757–761.
209. Brugada P, de Swart H, Smeets JL, et al. Transcoronary chemical ablation of ventricular tachycardia. *Circulation* 1989;79:475–482.
210. Haines DE, Verow AF, Sinusas AJ, et al. Intracoronary ethanol ablation in swine: characterization of myocardial injury in target and remote vascular beds. *J Cardiovasc Electrophysiol* 1994;5:41–49.
211. Haines DE, Whayne JG, DiMarco JP. Intracoronary ethanol ablation in swine: effects of ethanol concentration on lesion formation and response to programmed ventricular stimulation. *J Cardiovasc Electrophysiol* 1994;5:422–431.
212. Saxon LA, Stevenson WG, Fonarow GC, et al. Transesophageal echocardiography during radiofrequency catheter ablation of ventricular tachycardia. *Am J Cardiol* 1993;72:658–661.
213. Gallais Y, Lascault G, Tonet J, et al. Transoesophageal echocardiographic assessment of radio-frequency heating: an accurate method to detect thrombus during catheter ablation? [Abstract]. *Eur J Card Pacing Electrophysiol* 1994;4:803.
214. Avitall B, Hare J, Mughal K, Silverstein E. Transeophageal echocardiography: an important tool during the cardiac ablation procedure [Abstract]. *Pacing Clin Electrophysiol* 1994;17:788.
215. Omran H, Pfeiffer D, Tebbenjohanns J, et al. Echocardiographic imaging of coronary sinus diverticula and middle cardiac veins in patients with preexcitation syndrome: impact for catheter ablation [Abstract]. *Circulation* 1994;90:I-595.
216. Tucker KJ, Curtis AB, Conti JB, et al. Comparison of transesophageal echocardiographic guidance of transseptal left heart catheterization during mitral valvuloplasty and radiofrequency ablation of left-sided accessory pathways [Abstract]. *Pacing Clin Electrophysiol* 1994;17:813.
217. Kyo S, Miyamoto N, Matsumura M, et al. Brockenbrough transseptal puncture and left atrial cannulation with guidance of transesophageal and/or intracardiac echocardiography [Abstract]. *Circulation* 1994;90:I-596.
218. Chu E, Fitzpatrick AP, Chin MC, et al. Radiofrequency catheter ablation guided by intracardiac echocardiography. *Circulation* 1994;89:1301–1305.
219. Chan RC, Johnson SB, Seward JB, Packer DL. Initial experience with left ventricular endocardial catheter manipulation guided by intracardiac ultrasound visualization: improved accuracy over fluoroscopic imaging [Abstract]. *J Am Coll Cardiol* 1995:41A.
220. Packer DL, Chan R, Johnson SB, Seward JB. Ultrasound cardioscopy: initial experience with a new high resolution combined intracardiac ultrasound/ablation system [Abstract]. *Eur J Card Pacing Electrophysiol* 1994;4:833.
221. Tardif J, Groeneveld PW, Haugh CJ, et al. Intracardiac echocardiography can guide microwave ablation of arrhythmic foci: an in vitro study [Abstract]. *Circulation* 1994;90:I-595A.
222. Hummel J, Crowley R, Davis J, Bach DS. Radiofrequency ablation of the critical isthmus for atrial flutter can be guided by intracardiac echocardiography. *Circulation* 1994;90:I-336.
223. Olgin J, Kalman J, Fiztpatrick A, et al. Intracardiac echo identifies the crista terminalis and eustachian ridge as barriers during type I atrial flutter in man [Abstract]. *Pacing Clin Electrophysiol* 1995;18:857.
224. Kalman J, Olgin, J, Fitzpatrick A, et al. "Cristal tachycardia": relationship of right atrial tachycardias to the crista terminalis identified using intracardiac echocardiography [Abstract]. *Pacing Clin Electrophysiol* 1995;18:861.
225. Chan RC, Johnson SB, Seward JB, Packer DL. Utility of intracardiac ultrasound for guiding atrial ablation [Abstract]. *Pacing Clin Electrophysiol* 1995;18:856.
226. Current and developing clinical applications of intravascular ultrasound. In: Cavaye DM, White RA, eds. *Intravascular ultrasound imaging*. New York: Raven Press, :106–110.
227. Ferrara-Ryan M, Brener BJ, Cluley SR, et al. Ultrasound-guided balloon angioplasty: a new technique. *J Vasc Technol* 1992;16:28–34.
228. Landzberg JS, Franklin JO, Langberg JJ, et al. The transponder system: a new method of precise catheter placement in the right atrium under echocardiographic guidance. *J Am Coll Cardiol* 1988;12:753–756.
229. Moorman JW, Melen RE, Skillicorn B, et al. Three-dimensional endocardial mapping system utilizing a novel x-ray imager and locating catheter. *Proceedings of the 19th conference of the International Society for Computerized Electrocardiology.* 1994:1–9.
230. Ben-Haim S. Apparatus and method for treating cardiac arrhythmias. US Patent No 5,391,199, 1995.

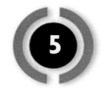

CARDIAC MAPPING SYSTEMS AND THEIR USE TO TREAT TACHYARRHYTHMIAS

• • •

GREGORY P. WALCOTT, RAYMOND E. IDEKER

The heart pumps blood through the circulatory system. Controlling this mechanical activity is an electrical system. For much of the 20th century, electrodes on or in the heart have been used to map the spread of electrical activity throughout the myocardium (1). Hundreds of mapping studies have supplied much information about normal and abnormal conduction and about the mechanisms of arrhythmias. Initially, recordings were made sequentially with a single electrode that was moved from point to point on the epicardium. In the past 20 years, computer-assisted cardiac mapping techniques have been developed to record from many sites simultaneously (2). This information has been used to develop a greater understanding of the cardiac electrical system and to develop techniques to control and cure abnormal cardiac rhythms.

◉ TECHNICAL CONSIDERATIONS IN CARDIAC MAPPING

The fundamental tasks involved in mapping cardiac activity have remained unchanged throughout this period. For most types of mapping, the electrodes must be placed on the heart to record an adequate electrogram without artifacts; the recorded potentials must be amplified; the presence and time of activation at each recording site must be determined from these recordings; the location of the recording electrodes on the heart must be ascertained; and the spread of activation throughout the mapped region must be displayed (3).

After the electrogram has been recorded, it is necessary to determine whether activation occurred at a particular electrode. Activation may be absent because of conduction block or because of the placement of the electrode on connective tissue instead of viable myocardium. Recording electrodes can be unipolar or bipolar, but determining whether activation occurred can be difficult for both types of recording electrodes. With unipolar electrode recordings, one electrode is in direct contact with the heart and the return electrode is located at a distance from the heart. For bipolar electrode recordings, both electrodes are placed close together touching the heart. With unipolar recordings, activation is indicated by a rapid downslope in the tracing, whereas in bipolar recordings, activation is represented by a rapidly changing complex of almost any morphology. Figure 5-1 shows three unipolar complexes, each of which exhibits a distinct downslope. The complexes in Figure 5-1A and 5-1C represent activations, but the slightly less rapid downslope in Figure 5-1B does not represent an activation.

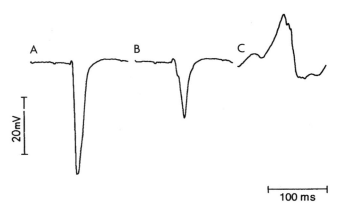

FIGURE 5-1. Examples of complexes recorded at unipolar electrodes, indicating the difficulty in detecting local activation. **A:** A complex with a large amplitude and rapid downslope, representing a normal activation front passing through the tissue surrounding the electrode. **B:** A smaller complex with a less rapid downslope recorded from the center of a region of necrosis created by freezing. The nearest viable muscle is about 1.5 mm away from the recording electrode. This complex does not represent local activation but rather a distant normal activation front that at its closest point is approximately 1.5 mm from the recording site. **C:** A small complex with a slow downslope that was generated by the passage of an activation front by a recording electrode during ventricular fibrillation. This complex does represent a local activation, albeit an abnormal one. (From Ideker RE, Smith WM, Blanchard SM, et al. The assumptions of isochronal cardiac mapping. *Pacing Clin Electrophysiol* 1989;12:456–478, with permission.)

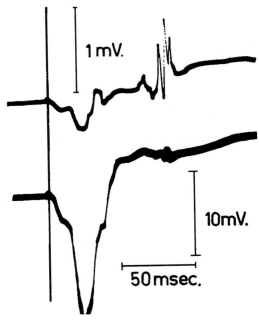

FIGURE 5-3. Durrer's original tracings of fractionated electrograms over a transmural canine infarct. Multiple small-amplitude deflections occur 75 msec after the beginning of the QRS complex and are recorded in the local bipolar *(top)* and unipolar *(bottom)* electrogram. (From Durrer D, Formione P, van Dam A, et al. The electrocardiogram in normal and some abnormal conditions in revived human fetal heart and in acute and chronic coronary occlusion. *Am Heart J* 1961;61:303–314, with permission.)

After an activation has been identified in a recording, the time at which the activation front passes the electrode must then be determined. This time can occasionally be ambiguous, as illustrated for unipolar and bipolar recordings in Figure 5-2. Abnormal late or fractionated recordings (Fig. 5-3) can arise from regions of patchy infarction or fibrosis interspersed with viable myocardium (Fig. 5-4A) or from subendocardial regions of normal or abnormal spared myocardium beneath an infarct (Fig. 5-4B). The regions where the proper interpretation of the electrode recordings is most difficult are also the regions from which arrhythmias frequently arise.

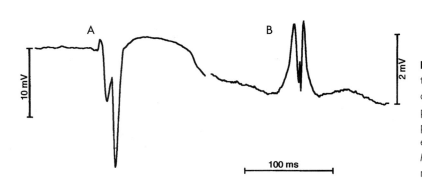

FIGURE 5-2. Examples of electrograms in which the time of activation is ambiguous. **A:** Unipolar recording with two regions of rapid downslope. **B:** Bipolar recording with more than one peak of absolute potential. (From Ideker RE, Smith WM, Blanchard SM, et al. The assumptions of isochronal cardiac mapping. *Pacing Clin Electrophysiol* 1989;12:456–478, with permission.)

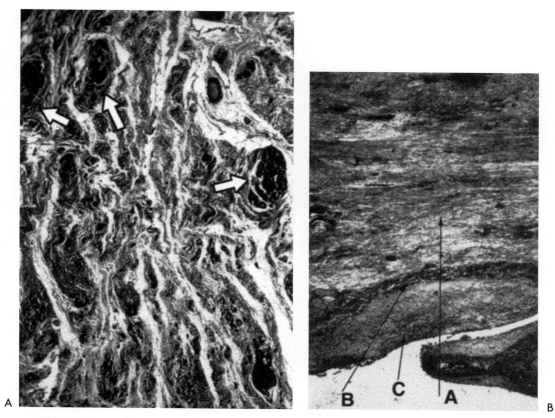

FIGURE 5-4. Photomicrographs of the types of spared myocardium associated with myocardial infarcts that may give rise to fractionated or late potentials. **A:** Photomicrograph of an old myocardial infarction scar on the left ventricle of a deceased patient. Small bundles of spared viable myocardium *(arrows)* traverse this scar and may serve as part of a reentrant pathway. Although in this two-dimensional cross section the surviving myocardium appears to be isolated islands of tissue, three-dimensional reconstruction of the tissue indicates that these spared regions form interconnecting strands of tissue. The strands may activate at different times, generating a fractionated, long-duration complex. Some strands may activate late because of the long, complex pathway needed to reach them, generating delayed potentials. **B:** A thin rim of spared myocardium (B) between the left ventricular cavity on the bottom and an old myocardial infarct scar (A) at the top. Between the thin layer of surviving subendocardial myocardium and the endocardial cavity is a thin layer of fibroelastic connective tissue (C) that is formed in response to stretching of the infarcted wall due to aneurysmal bulging during systole in the weeks to months after the infarction occurs. The thin layer of spared myocardium is frequently an important part of the reentrant pathway of ventricular arrhythmias and is the tissue removed by endocardial resection. Abnormalities within this spared myocardial layer and the separation of mapping electrodes on the endocardium from this layer by the fibroelastic tissue may also cause fractionated electrograms.

◉ RESEARCH AND CLINICAL MAPPING TECHNIQUES

Although mapping in the animal laboratory and in the human operating room has similar goals, mapping in the animal laboratory can use more invasive techniques. For example, needles with multiple electrodes along their length can be inserted through the myocardial wall of animals to obtain multiple intramural recordings to determine the transmural activation sequence (Fig. 5-5). In the animal laboratory, the hearts can be removed from the body at the end of the study to determine cardiac anatomy, cardiac pathology, and the location of the recording electrodes on or in the heart (Fig. 5-6).

Although plunge needles occasionally have been

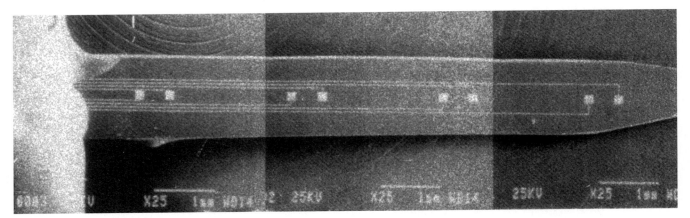

FIGURE 5-5. Scanning electron micrograph of a multielectrode needle for mapping intramural cardiac activation. The needle is constructed using microelectronic techniques. It contains six small electrode contacts spaced 1 mm apart. Traces from each electrode can be seen running from the electrodes to the left side of the needle, where wires are bonded to carry the signals to the mapping system. The needle is plunged through the ventricular wall with the right-most portion toward the endocardium and the left-most portion toward the epicardium.

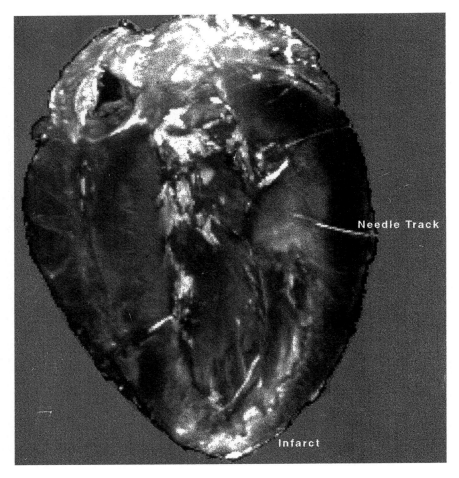

FIGURE 5-6. The left and right ventricular cavities are shown in a longitudinal section of a three-dimensional reconstruction of a magnetic resonance image of the heart. Several tracks made by plunge needles are visible *(asterisk)*, as is a myocardial infarct at the apex of the left ventricle. The image is T2-weighted.

inserted through the wall of the heart in the human operating room (4), most human recordings are confined to the epicardial and the endocardial surfaces of the heart. In the operating room, epicardial recordings are typically made from electrodes embedded in plaques, in elastic socks that are pulled over the epicardium from the apex, or in parallel strips that surround the heart. Human or animal endocardial recordings can be obtained from an everted sock placed over a balloon that is inserted into the left ventricular cavity and then inflated so that the electrodes on the sock are in contact with the endocardium (5).

Current clinical mapping systems record 32 to 128 electrograms simultaneously. Because clinical decisions are based on the recordings, it is not practical to review and analyze more data than this in "real time." Research mapping systems may acquire 500 to 2,000 electrograms simultaneously (6). Because much of the data analysis occurs well after the end of the experiment, much more data can be collected. Because more electrograms can be acquired simultaneously, electrodes can be placed closer together. Recording and analyzing ventricular fibrillation requires recording electrodes to be 1 to 2 mm apart (7). It is not yet possible to record from the entire epicardium of an animal with electrode spacing of 2 mm, but as technology improves, it is likely that such systems will be designed. Optical mapping systems already can record from almost the entire epicardium with a pixel spacing of much less than 2 mm (8). However, such recordings can only be made in an isolated, perfused heart, and intramural recordings are not possible.

Mapping in the Surgical Suite

During the past several years, operative mapping has been used less frequently for surgical procedures. Many of the conditions for which it was previously used, such as Wolff-Parkinson-White syndrome and ventricular tachycardia, are now treated more commonly by transvenous catheter ablation techniques than by cardiac surgery. Although the maze procedure for atrial fibrillation is still primarily a surgical rather than a catheter procedure, the locations of the incisions are determined primarily by anatomic landmarks instead of activation sequence data, so that operative mapping does not play a large part in this surgical procedure (9). It remains to be seen whether thoracoscopic surgery will play a major role in the treatment of arrhythmias and whether operative mapping can contribute to this new surgical technique.

Computer-Assisted Mapping in the Clinical Electrophysiology Laboratory

Although there has been a great decrease in the use of operative mapping, there has been an even greater increase in mapping in the electrophysiology laboratory. Techniques range from a single catheter moved along the endocardial surface to two electrodes on the endocardial surface to multiple electrode arrays that may or may not contact the endocardial surface. Most electrophysiology and ablation studies performed today use one or two steerable catheters, each with two bipolar pairs of electrodes that are steered over the endocardial surface using fluoroscopic guidance. A single catheter is most often used if the site to be ablated is relatively well localized. These sites include the right atrial isthmus for atrial flutter (10, 11) near the atrioventricular (AV) groove for Wolff-Parkinson-White disease and near the AV node for AV node reentrant tachycardia. Two catheters are often used for locating the origin of ectopic atrial or ventricular tachycardias. One catheter is used to find a relatively early activation site. After such a site is found, the second catheter is used to search for an even earlier activation site near the location of the first catheter. If an earlier site of activation is found, the second catheter is then left stationary while the first catheter is used to search for an even earlier site around the second catheter. This process is repeated until no earlier site can be found.

An improvement in single-catheter mapping is the development of systems that record the catheter position in three dimensions, as well as the electrogram and local activation time. Two systems have been described that perform this task. The BioSense system uses a location sensor in the tip of the catheter to detect three magnetic fields that are created by a pad underneath the patient and that vary in space to determine the catheter position (12). The LocalLisa system uses a standard electrophysiology catheter to measure the electric field produced by passing an approximately 30-kHz sinusoidal current through three sets of orthogonal electrodes on the body surface of the patient. From these voltage measurements, the x, y, and z coordinates of the catheter tip can be determined. The advantage of these systems is that they can integrate data from multiple catheter positions into a complete picture of cardiac activation in any chamber of the heart (Fig. 5-7). The catheter position can be determined in the heart without the need of fluoroscopy, lowering the radiation dose to the patient (13). A disadvantage of these systems is that they require a large number of measurements to be made sequentially, one point at a time, until an adequate activation map can be obtained. The arrhythmia must

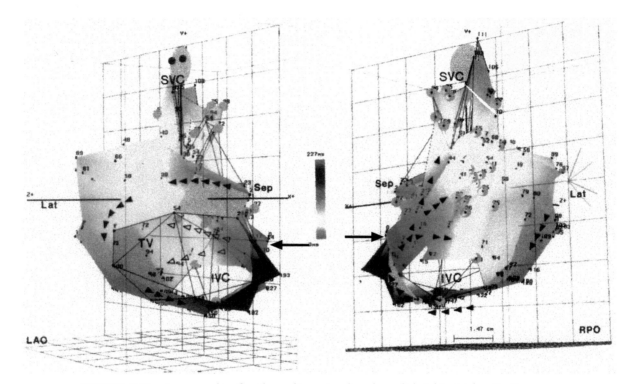

FIGURE 5-7. An example of a three-dimensional endocardial right atrial activation map during counterclockwise right atrial flutter (cycle length = 230 msec) reconstructed with 172 points covering 99% of the cycle length. The gray-scale reconstruction demonstrates the arbitrary zone of earliest activation *(arrow)*. The anatomic contours of the map are evident, with appropriately placed defects representing the inferior vena cava (IVC) and the tricuspid valve orifices. The superior vena cava (SVC) is recognizable as a "chimney." Each data point *(black dot)* is accompanied by its activation time. Some of the activation times are partly obscured because of the overlying three-dimensional structure of the map. Roundels indicate double potentials. The left panel depicts a left anterior oblique perspective of the three-dimensional map, and the right panel depicts a right posterior oblique perspective. Notice the relatively linear but ragged and wide localization of double potentials in the posterior right atrium (scale bar = 1.47 cm) and in the SVC. The lateral (Lat) right atrium and septal (Sep) right atrium activate craniocaudally and caudocranially, respectively, and activation proceeds lateromedially through the isthmus. Superiorly, a broad activation front proceeds between the SVC and the tricuspid valve annulus. However, posteriorly, a septally originating wavefront activates this region in a highly complex manner with oblique and horizontally traversing wavefronts, slowing and blocking in a rather wide and heterogenous zone centered on the double potentials marked by roundels. (From Shah DC, Jaïs P, Haïssaguerre M, et al. Three-dimensional mapping of the common atrial flutter circuit in the right atrium. *Circulation* 1997; 96:3904–3912, with permission.)

be unchanging and the patient hemodynamically stable for several minutes while the measurements are made.

The next step beyond recording from a single electrode is to record from multiple electrodes on the same catheter. A good example of such a catheter is a Halo catheter that is used to record the activation sequence of atrial flutter. This catheter has up to 20 electrodes along its length. It is positioned so that it is parallel with the plane of the tricuspid annulus. The first five bipole pairs are positioned to map activation along the anterolateral free wall of the right atrium, and the other five bipoles map activation along the interatrial septum. This catheter is used to diagnose common atrial flutter (Fig. 5-8) and to assess the efficacy of ablation therapy by showing bidirectional block across the flutter circuit (14,15). Linear catheters, such as the Halo, are useful in defining activation sequences of arrhythmias that follow well-defined one-dimensional pathways that can be reached by a linear catheter. Activation sequences are easily interpreted using a strip chart–type display.

An extension to catheters that record activation sequences in one dimension are catheter arrays such as basket catheters that record activation sequences in two dimensions (Fig. 5-9). These catheters are, in essence, a series of five to eight linear catheters that each have five to eight electrodes. The basket catheter is inserted collapsed into a chamber of the heart, usually the right atrium or the left ventricle, and allowed to expand until the struts are in contact with the endocardial surface. These catheters have been used to map ectopic atrial tachycardia and atrial flutter (16) and ventricular tachycardia in experimental animals (17,18). The advantage of these electrode arrays is that activations are recorded simultaneously from multiple locations, allowing an arrhythmia to be mapped from a single beat. Hemodynamically unstable arrhythmias and arrhythmias that are changing activation sequence from beat to beat can be mapped using these arrays.

A problem with two-dimensional arrays such as these basket catheters is that the spatial relationship between electrodes is no longer simple. For a linear catheter, a strip chart can be used to display elec-

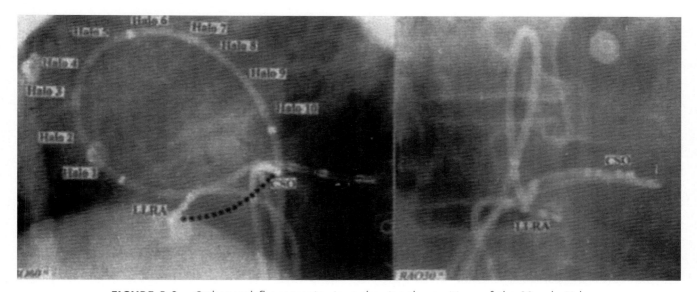

FIGURE 5-8. Orthogonal fluoroscopic views showing the positions of the 20-pole Halo catheter and the two pacing electrodes at the low lateral right atrium (LLRA) and coronary sinus ostium (CSO). On the left is the 60-degree left anterior oblique (LAO) view, and on the right is the 30-degree right anterior oblique (RAO) view. Halo 1 to Halo 5 bipoles are used to map the anterolateral free wall of right atrium, and Halo 6 to Halo 10 bipoles map the septum. Another coronary sinus catheter is in position for guiding in the area of the coronary sinus ostium and for mapping the interatrial conduction. (From Lin JL, Lai LP, Lin LJ, et al. Electrophysiological determinant for induction of isthmus dependent counterclockwise and clockwise atrial flutter in humans. *Heart* 1999;81:73–81, with permission.)

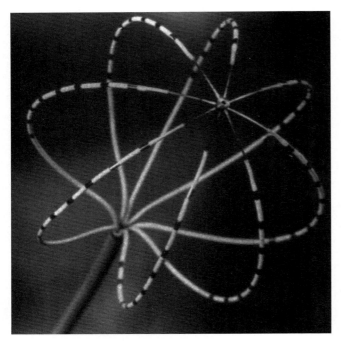

FIGURE 5-9. A basket catheter is used for endocardial mapping. The 8-Fr catheter is inserted into the desired cardiac chamber with the basket in the closed position. After the basket is in place, eight struts are distended at the distal end of the catheter. Each strut contains eight electrodes that are designed to contact the endocardium when the basket is deployed. At the end of the mapping procedure, the basket is collapsed, and the catheter is withdrawn. (Courtesy of EP Technologies, Sunnyvale, CA.)

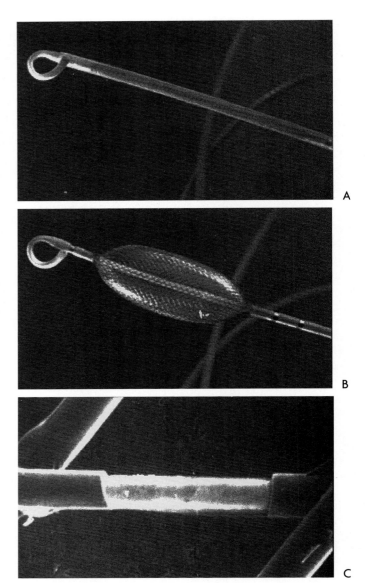

FIGURE 5-10. An endocardial balloon catheter is used for cardiac mapping. **A:** The 9-Fr catheter is inserted into the desired cardiac cavity with the balloon deflated. **B:** After the catheter is in place, the balloon is inflated with saline. **C:** The surface of the balloon contains 64 electrodes. Although a few of these electrodes may contact the endocardium when the balloon is inflated, most do not. A mathematical inverse procedure is performed to calculate the endocardial potentials from the recorded potentials on the surface of the balloon. At the end of the mapping procedure, the balloon is deflated and the catheter removed. (Courtesy of Endocardial Solutions, St. Paul, MN.)

trogram data because the electrograms for nearest neighbors to a particular electrode are always on adjacent traces. For a basket catheter, the nearest neighbors to a particular electrode are not only adjacent to it on the same strut, but are also on adjacent struts. One solution to this problem is to display activation times for all electrodes as an isochronal map. Such a display allows the more complex spatial relationships of the basket catheter electrodes to be simplified for the user (3).

So far, all of the mapping techniques described have electrodes physically touching cardiac tissue. Another method of mapping is to place a probe or balloon with 64 to 128 electrodes on it in a chamber of the heart and record far-field electrical activity (Fig. 5-10). What the electrogram would have looked like if an electrode had been recording from a particular location on the endocardium is then calculated from the far-field signals and a knowledge of heart chamber geometry. With the development of faster computers, these calculations can be done rapidly enough to make it possible to use these techniques in a clinical setting.

When using these noncontact mapping methods, the recording electrodes must be less than 3.4 cm (19) from the endocardial surface for the reconstructed electrograms to be accurate. An advantage of these systems is that an arrhythmia's activation sequence can be recorded from one beat.

● CONCLUSIONS

Catheter-based ablation for the treatment of ventricular tachyarrhythmias has focused on ventricular tachycardia (20–23). If ventricular tachycardia is monomorphic and stable, a single, catheter-based electrode can be moved sequentially from point to point on the endocardium to determine the activation sequence during the arrhythmia and the region to be ablated.

The ability to record from all electrodes simultaneously with an array of basket or balloon electrodes touching the endocardial surface or floating in the blood pool means that all recordings can be made in a single beat and raises the possibility that the site of ablation for unstable ventricular tachyarrhythmias, including ventricular fibrillation, can be determined. It may be possible to use catheter ablation to prevent ventricular fibrillation recurrence in a subset of patients who survive cardiac arrest (24).

Atrial fibrillation is a complex arrhythmia that is gaining the attention of the interventional electrophysiologist. A significant number of atrial fibrillation patients have a focal initiator for their arrhythmia. Most foci have been found at the junction of the left atrium and the ostia of the pulmonary veins. Because of the risk of pulmonary vein stenosis with the application of radiofrequency energy to the orifice of a pulmonary vein (25), techniques need to be developed that quickly and accurately identify the location of these foci so that they can be ablated with a minimum of applied energy. With the development of catheter-based ablation strategies that are based on the surgical maze procedure for stopping atrial fibrillation, mapping techniques will be needed to determine whether a lesion is continuous and transmural.

● ACKNOWLEDGMENTS

The authors gratefully acknowledge Kate Sreenan for her assistance in preparing this manuscript. This work was supported in part by the National Institutes of Health grant HL33637 and The Whitaker Foundation.

REFERENCES

1. Janse MJ. Some historical notes on the mapping of arrhythmias. In: Shenasa M, Borggrefe M, Breihardt G, et al, eds. *Cardiac mapping*. Mount Kisco, NY: Futura Publishing, 1993:3–10.
2. Ideker RE, Smith WM, Wallace AG, et al. A computerized method for the rapid display of ventricular activation during the intraoperative study of arrhythmias. *Circulation* 1979;59:449–458.
3. Ideker RE, Smith WM, Blanchard SM, et al. The assumptions of isochronal cardiac mapping. *Pacing Clin Electrophysiol* 1989;12:456–478.
4. Pogwizd SM, Hoyt RH, Saffitz JE, et al. Reentrant and focal mechanisms underlying ventricular tachycardia in the human heart. *Circulation* 1992;86:1872–1887.
5. Downar E, Harris L, Mickleborough LL, et al. Endocardial mapping of ventricular tachycardia in the intact human ventricle: evidence for reentrant mechanisms. *J Am Coll Cardiol* 1988;11:783–791.
6. Wolf PD, Rollins DL, Simpson EV, et al. A 528 channel system for the acquisition and display of defibrillation and electrocardiographic potentials. In: Murray A, Arzbaecher R, eds. *Computers in cardiology*. Los Alamitos, CA: IEEE Computer Society Press, 1993:125–128.
7. Bayly PV, Johnson EE, Idriss SF, et al. Efficient electrode spacing for examining spatial organization during ventricular fibrillation. *IEEE Trans Biomed Eng* 1993;40:1060–1066.
8. Gray RA, Jalife J. Video imaging of cardiac fibrillation. In: Rosenbaum DS, Jalife J, eds. *Optical mapping of cardiac excitation and arrhythmias*. Armonk, NY: Futura Publishing, 1998.
9. Cox JL. The surgical treatment of atrial fibrillation: IV. surgical technique. *J Thorac Cardiovasc Surg* 1991;101:584–592.
10. Kirkorian G, Moncada E, Chevalier P, et al. Radiofrequency ablation of atrial flutter: efficacy of an anatomically guided approach. *Circulation* 1994;90:2804–2814.
11. Feld GK, Fleck P, Chen P-S, et al. Radiofrequency catheter ablation for the treatment of human type 1 atrial flutter: identification of a critical zone in the reentrant circuit by endocardial mapping techniques. *Circulation* 1992;86:1233–1240.
12. Gepstein L, Hayam G, Ben-Haim SA. A novel method for nonfluoroscopic catheter-based electroanatomical mapping of the heart: in vitro and in vivo accuracy results. *Circulation* 1997;95:1611–1622.
13. Worley SJ. Use of a real-time three-dimensional magnetic navigation system for radiofrequency ablation of accessory pathways. *Pacing Clin Electrophysiol* 1998;21:1636–1645.

14. Lin JL, Lai LP, Lin LJ, et al. Electrophysiological determinant for induction of isthmus dependent counterclockwise and clockwise atrial flutter in humans. *Heart* 1999;81:73–81.
15. Poty H, Saoudi N, Abdel Aziz A, et al. Radiofrequency catheter ablation of type 1 atrial flutter: prediction of late success by electrophysiological criteria. *Circulation* 1995;92:1389–1392.
16. Schmitt C, Zrenner B, Schneider M, et al. Clinical experience with a novel multielectrode basket catheter in right atrial tachycardias. *Circulation* 1999;99:2414–2422.
17. Eldar M, Fitzpatrick AP, Ohad D, et al. Percutaneous multielectrode endocardial mapping during ventricular tachycardia in the swine model. *Circulation* 1996;94:1125–1130.
18. Hsu S, Smith MF, Ohad DG, et al. Insights into the mechanism of ventricular tachycardia in a closed-chest porcine model utilizing a multielectrode basket catheter. *Pacing Clin Electrophysiol* 1996;19:714.
19. Schilling RJ, Peters NS, Davies DW. Simultaneous endocardial mapping in the human left ventricle using a noncontact catheter: comparison of contact and reconstructed electrograms during sinus rhythm. *Circulation* 1998;98:887–898.
20. Morady F, Scheinman MM, Di Carlo LA Jr, et al. Catheter ablation of ventricular tachycardia with intracardiac shocks: results in 33 patients. *Circulation* 1987;75:1037–1049.
21. Evans GT Jr, Scheinman MM, Zipes DP, et al. The percutaneous cardiac mapping and ablation registry: final summary of results. *Pacing Clin Electrophysiol* 1988;11:1621–1626.
22. Fitzgerald DM, Friday KJ, Wah JAYL, et al. Electrogram patterns predicting successful catheter ablation of ventricular tachycardia. *Circulation* 1988;77:806–814.
23. Trappe H-J, Klein H, Frank G, et al. Role of mapping-guided surgery in patients with recurrent ventricular tachycardia. *Am Heart J* 1992;124:636–644.
24. Reek S, Klein HU, Ideker RE. Can catheter ablation in cardiac arrest survivors prevent ventricular fibrillation recurrence? *Pacing Clin Electrophysiol* 1997;20:1840–1859.
25. Robbins IM, Colvin EV, Doyle TP, et al. Pulmonary vein stenosis after catheter ablation of atrial fibrillation. *Circulation* 1998;98:1769–1775.
26. Shah DC, Jaïs P, Haïssaguerre M, et al. Three-dimensional mapping of the common atrial flutter circuit in the right atrium. *Circulation* 1997;96:3904–3912.

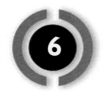

ABLATION OF LEFT-SIDED ACCESSORY PATHWAYS

THE RETROGRADE AORTIC VERSUS THE TRANSSEPTAL APPROACH

• • •

HUAGUI LI, ROBERT A. SCHWEIKERT, ANDREA NATALE

The left-sided accessory pathway is the most common type of atrioventricular connection. Because the true prevalence of patients with accessory pathways (overt and concealed) in the general population is unknown, the proportion of the left-sided accessory pathways in all patients with accessory pathways is uncertain. Based on several series of ablation studies, the percentage of the left-sided accessory pathway is 41% to 73% (1–4), which is more common than accessory pathways in posteroseptal, anteroseptal, or right free wall sites.

Left-sided accessory pathways may be manifest or concealed. Manifest pathways have a preexcited QRS demonstrated by the electrocardiogram and may show antegrade and retrograde conduction or only unidirectional conduction at the electrophysiologic study. By definition, a concealed accessory pathway has retrograde conduction only. The diagnosis of a left-sided accessory pathway is made by using electrocardiographic criteria, pacing from different sites such as the coronary sinus and the high right atrium (Fig. 6-1), examination of the activation sequence during orthodromic atrioventricular reentry tachycardia (Fig. 6-2), tachycardia cycle length prolongation with left bundle branch block (Fig. 6-3), and determination of the shortest atrioventricular or ventriculoatrial interval during mapping in sinus rhythm with preexcitation or in orthodromic atrioventricular reentry tachycardia. Typically, patients with manifest left-sided accessory pathway conduction have minimal preexcitation in sinus rhythm. In such cases, a small delta wave is generally more evident in the precordial leads V_3, V_4, and V_5. For patients showing a fully preexcited QRS, the delta wave is positive in lead V_1 and negative in lead aVL (Fig. 6-4). Multiple accessory pathways may represent a challenge and require meticulous analysis of the intracardiac tracings (Fig. 6-5) and thorough execution of diagnostic maneuvers during the electrophysiologic study (Fig. 6-6).

Treatment options for tachycardia mediated by an accessory pathway includes medical therapy (i.e., palliation) and ablation therapy (i.e., cure). The success rate of ablation for the left-sided accessory pathways is higher than for the other locations. The reasons for such a high success rate are probably the smaller mitral annulus compared with the tricuspid annulus and the more stable catheter position. There appears to be fewer epicardially located left-sided accessory pathways than at the other locations.

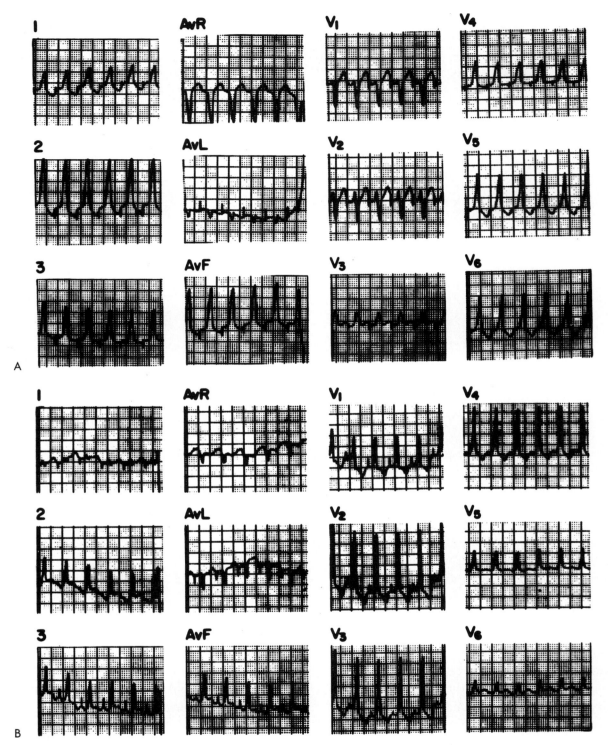

FIGURE 6-1. The site of pacing may affect the ability to demonstrate a left-sided accessory pathway. **A:** A 12-lead electrocardiogram during right atrial pacing reveals the presence of an anteroseptal accessory pathway. **B:** A 12-lead electrocardiogram during proximal coronary sinus pacing in the same patient reveals the presence of a left lateral accessory pathway.

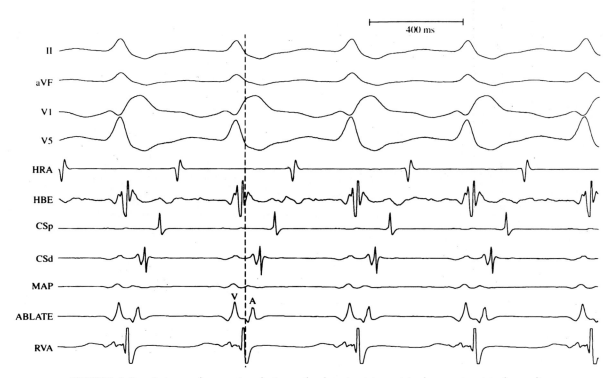

FIGURE 6-2. Retrograde mapping during orthodromic atrioventricular reentrant tachycardia. The patient had a rate-dependent right bundle branch block during the tachycardia. The earliest retrograde atrial activation is at the distal poles of the coronary sinus catheter. Mapping along the mitral valve annulus shows the shortest ventriculoatrial interval (ABLATE) in the posterolateral region. The recording was obtained from the transseptal approach. From top to bottom are the surface ECG leads II, aVF, V_1, and V_5 and intracardiac electrograms from the high right atrium (HRA), the His bundle region (HBE), the proximal (CSp) and distal (CSd) coronary sinus, the proximal (MAP) and distal (ABLATE) electrode pairs of the ablation catheter, and the right ventricular apex (RVA).

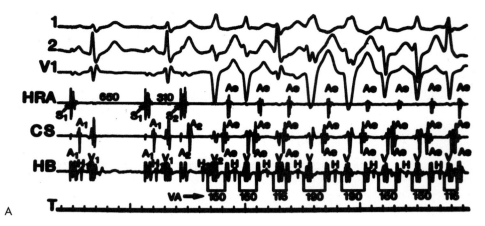

ORTHODROMIC TACHYCARDIA WITH LEFT BUNDLE BRANCH BLOCK
(Left sided AP)

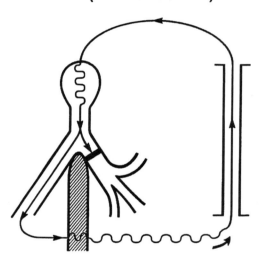

AH + HV + VA = CL

FIGURE 6-3. The diagnosis of left-sided accessory pathway is supported by tachycardia cycle length prolongation with left bundle branch block. **A:** Initiation of orthodromic atrioventricular reentrant tachycardia with right atrial pacing (S_1 to S_1) and a premature atrial extrastimulus (S_2). During tachycardia, there is spontaneous development of left anterior fascicular block, right bundle branch block, complete left bundle branch block,, and left posterior fascicular block. The site of block correlates with the extent of prolongation of the ventriculoatrial conduction time. During complete left bundle branch block, the longest ventriculoatrial conduction time (190 msec) is observed. During left anterior fascicular block, the ventriculoatrial conduction time (150 msec) is less prolonged. During left posterior fascicular block, the ventriculoatrial conduction time (115 msec) is the same as during right bundle branch block. This is consistent with a left lateral location of the accessory pathway. From top to bottom are the surface ECG leads I, II, and V_1; intracardiac electrograms from the high right atrium (HRA), coronary sinus (CS), and His bundle region (HB); and timeline (T) marked in 100-msec increments from left to right. A, atrial electrogram; Ae, atrial electrogram during tachycardia; H, His bundle electrogram; V, ventricular electrogram. **B:** Diagram illustrates orthodromic atrioventricular reentrant tachycardia using a left-sided accessory pathway and shows the mechanism of tachycardia cycle length prolongation with the development of left bundle branch block. AH, atrial-His conduction time; AP, accessory pathway; CL, tachycardia cycle length; HV, His-ventricle conduction time; VA, ventriculoatrial conduction time.

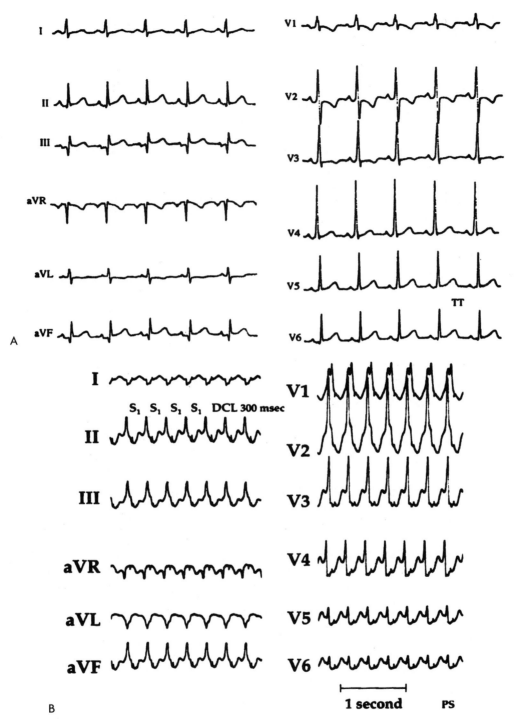

FIGURE 6-4. QRS morphology during different degrees of ventricular preexcitation with a left-sided accessory pathway. **A:** A 12-lead electrocardiogram during sinus rhythm with minimal preexcitation; a small delta wave is visible in the precordial leads V_3, V_4, and V_5. **B:** A 12-lead electrocardiogram during atrial pacing with maximal ventricular preexcitation from a left-sided accessory pathway. The delta wave is positive in lead V_1 and negative in lead aVL.

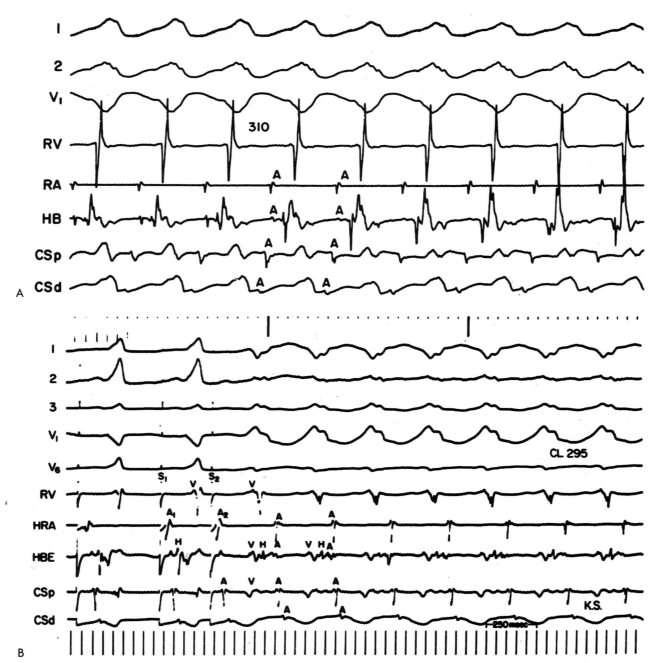

FIGURE 6-5. Intracardiac recordings from patients with multiple accessory pathways. **A:** Atrioventricular reentrant tachycardia using a right-sided accessory pathway as the antegrade limb and a left-sided accessory pathway as the retrograde limb. From top to bottom are the surface ECG leads I, II, and V_1 and the intracardiac electrograms from the right ventricle (RV), right atrium (RA), His bundle region (HB), and proximal (CSp) and distal (CSd) coronary sinus. **B:** The first two beats are atrial paced (S_1 to S_1) with a manifest right lateral accessory pathway. After a single atrial extrastimulus (S_2), antidromic atrioventricular reentrant tachycardia using a left-sided accessory pathway is induced. From top to bottom are the surface ECG leads I, II, III, and V_6 and the intracardiac electrograms from the right ventricle (RV), high right atrium (HRA), His bundle region (HBE), and proximal (CSp) and distal (CSd) coronary sinus. A, atrial electrogram; CL, tachycardia cycle length; H, His bundle electrogram; V, ventricular electrogram.

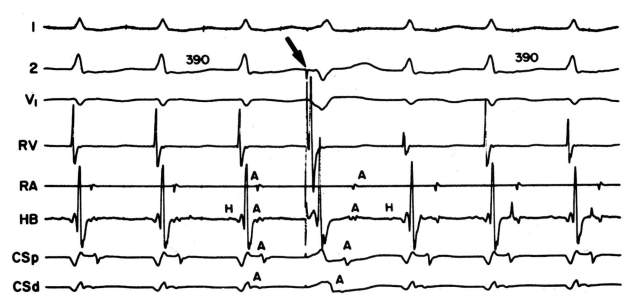

FIGURE 6-6. Orthodromic atrioventricular reentrant tachycardia at a cycle length (CL) of 390 msec. In the first three beats, the retrograde activation suggests fusion between a right- and a left-sided accessory pathway. Notice the early retrograde atrial activation in the distal coronary sinus poles and in the right atrium. A ventricular extrastimulus *(arrow)* is delivered during His refractoriness and results in block in the right-sided accessory pathway and retrograde conduction exclusively over the left-sided accessory pathway. Notice the earliest retrograde atrial activation in the distal coronary sinus poles. From top to bottom are the surface ECG leads I, II, and V_1 and the intracardiac electrograms from the right ventricle (RV), right atrium (RA), His bundle region (HB), and proximal (CSp) and distal (CSd) coronary sinus. A, atrial electrogram; H, His bundle electrogram; V, ventricular electrogram.

● CATHETER ABLATION FOR LEFT-SIDED ACCESSORY PATHWAYS

Preablation evaluation is important and should include a thorough history and physical examination. Special attention should be given to allergies or reactions to sedatives. A history of sleep apnea should alert the physician to the possibility of problems with airway management during sedation. Peripheral vascular disease should be identified. Consideration should be given to discontinuation of antiarrhythmic medications and AV nodal blocking agents. Instrumentation with multielectrode catheters for recording, pacing and internal defibrillation may be advantageous for patients with frequent episodes of atrial fibrillation. The practitioner should consider transesophageal echocardiography in the older patient to assess for large aortic atheromas, which could be dislodged during catheter manipulation and result in embolic complications.

Preliminary data from one institution appeared to advocate preablation administration of aspirin and ticlopidine to reduce the postprocedure risk of embolic stroke (5). This is not considered common practice in most of the large volume centers.

Ablation of left-sided accessory pathways can be effected by retrograde aortic, transseptal, and less commonly, coronary sinus approaches.

Technique of the Retrograde Aortic Approach

The retrograde aortic approach is probably the most commonly used method worldwide, probably because it does not require the equipment and expertise of the atrial transseptal puncture. The right femoral artery is generally used for catheter insertion, although the left femoral artery can also be considered in special conditions. The patient should be heparinized to prevent clot formation after the arterial access is established. To cross the aortic valve, the ablation catheter tip is deflected, and a clockwise torque is applied when the catheter is advanced. The deflected tip of the ablation catheter helps to avoid engaging the catheter in the orifice of a coronary artery or perforating the aortic valve (6). If the catheter enters the orifice of the coronary artery, the curve should be released and the catheter withdrawn immediately. Low-amplitude atrial and ventricular electrograms may be recorded at the aortic root or within a coronary artery. Such electrograms can be similar to those recorded from the mitral annulus and should never be misinterpreted as the ablation target.

After the ablation catheter enters the left ventricle, the tip of the ablation catheter is straightened to allow the tip to drop to the left ventricular cavity. Because the mitral annulus is posterolateral to the aortic valve, the ablation catheter needs to be pulled up gradually, with the tip deflected while a counterclockwise rotation is applied. Such a combined maneuver often facilitates the ablation catheter to enter the left ventricular inflow tract and is best performed in the right anterior oblique view. Sometimes, catheter-induced premature ventricular complexes can affect mapping and catheter stability.

Although successful ablation can be achieved with the single-catheter technique (7), a coronary sinus catheter can serve as an anatomic and activation reference. Unlike the transseptal approach, ablation is usually attempted from the ventricular side in the retrograde aortic approach. To visualize the full length of the posterolateral mitral annulus, the left anterior oblique view is usually the best. Because of the obstacles created by the papillary muscle or the chorda tendineae, a simple torque of the catheter may encounter difficulty in moving the tip of the ablation catheter medially or laterally on the mitral annulus. To map the mitral annulus systematically for locating the ablation target, it may be necessary to release the curve of the ablation catheter and let it drop back

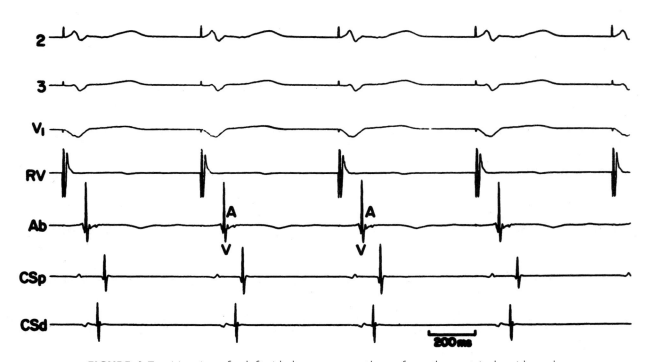

FIGURE 6-7. Mapping of a left-sided accessory pathway from the ventricular side under the mitral valve during ventricular pacing. Notice the relatively small atrial electrogram recorded from this location, which may make correct identification of the atrial electrogram difficult. From top to bottom are the surface ECG leads II, III, and V_1 and the intracardiac electrograms from the right ventricle (RV), ablation catheter (Ab), and proximal (CSp) and distal (CSd) coronary sinus. A, atrial electrogram; V, ventricular electrogram.

into the left ventricle before the next attempt to place the catheter at a different position on the mitral annulus. It is helpful to rotate the catheter during this process to place it at a different site. Because the ablation catheter has been bent twice (at the aortic arch and in the left ventricle), it can be difficult to orient and direct the catheter in the area of interest. In general, a counterclockwise torque of the catheter causes the catheter tip to move posteromedially, and a clockwise torque causes the tip of the catheter to move anterolaterally. When the ablation is attempted from the ventricular side under the mitral valve, the amplitude of the atrial electrogram is much smaller than that of the ventricular electrogram. This may create difficulties in correct identification of the atrial electrogram when mapping has to be performed during ventricular pacing or during orthodromic atrioventricular reentry tachycardia (Fig. 6-7).

Ablation from the atrial side may also be attempted with the retrograde aortic approach if the initial attempt from the ventricular side is unsuccessful (Fig. 6-8). In some centers, ablation from the atrial side with the retrograde aortic approach has been used as the first choice and excellent results have been reported (8,9).

Technique of the Transseptal Approach

The transseptal approach is probably less widely used than the retrograde aortic approach. However, as data from the Pediatric Registry have shown, the choice of the transseptal approach is directly related to the number of procedures performed (Table 6-1). The most critical step of the transseptal approach is the transseptal puncture. To cross the atrial septum without complications, particularly cardiac perforation, requires a skilled operator. Formal training on the transseptal procedure under the supervision of an experienced operator with at least 20 cases should be required before the transseptal procedure is attempted. In centers where the cardiac electrophysiologists are not trained in the transseptal technique, an interventional cardiologist with transseptal experience may assist in performing the transseptal puncture. Although such a "team effort" creates some inconvenience, it ensures the safety of the patient. An adjunc-

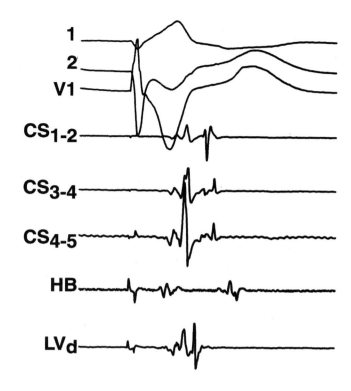

FIGURE 6-8. Mapping from the atrial side of the mitral valve with the retrograde aortic approach. Notice the relatively large amplitude of the atrial electrogram recorded from the ablation catheter (LVd). From top to bottom are the surface ECG leads I, II, and V_1 and the intracardiac electrograms from the distal (CS_{1-2}), middle (CS_{3-4}), and proximal (CS_{4-5}) coronary sinus, His bundle region (HB), and distal left ventricle (LVd).

tive approach includes the guidance of transseptal instrumentation with intracardiac or transesophageal echocardiography.

For patients with a patent foramen ovale, the ablation catheter can directly cross to the left atrium, and the transseptal puncture may not be required (10). It may be helpful to explore the foramen ovale by using the flexible ablation catheter before the transseptal puncture. Sometimes, it may be difficult to obtain a stable catheter position because of the lack of a sheath support. In these cases, the ablation catheter can be removed and then reintroduced with a Mullins sheath (11).

The standard approach to the transseptal puncture is through the right femoral vein. A J-tipped guide

TABLE 6-1 • CATHETER APPROACHES FOR RADIOFREQUENCY ABLATION OF LEFT ACCESSORY PATHWAYS: OBSERVATION FROM THE PEDIATRIC REGISTRY

Number Of Transatrial Procedures/Left Accessory Pathways[a]	Previous Experience: Number Of Procedures
92/216 (44%)	<10
102/177 (58%)	10–19
73/144 (51%)	20–29
136/261 (52%)	30–49
287/468 (61%)	50–99
486/680 (71%)	100+

[a] $p < 0.001$.

From Kugler JD, Danford DA, Silka MJ, et al. Ablation of left-sided accessory pathways: transatrial, retrograde, or coronary sinus approach? In: Singer I, Barold SS, Camm AJ, eds. *Nonpharmacological therapy of arrhythmias for the 21st century: the state of the art.* Armonk, NY: Futura Publishing, 1998:73–85, with permission.

wire (0.028- to 0.032-inch diameter, 145- to 150-cm length) is advanced through the right femoral vein and the tip is positioned into the superior vena cava. An 8-Fr Mullins sheath (50 to 67 cm long) with its dilator is introduced along the guide wire with the tip of the dilator positioned in the superior vena cava (12). After the guide wire is removed, a Brockenbrough needle (13) is inserted into the dilator. The tip of the needle should be kept about 1 cm inside the dilator. At this point, the needle can be connected with a pressure transducer. With the sheath-dilator-needle assembly aligned in the same direction and the needle hub arrow pointing at about 4 o'clock (viewing from the patient's feet) to the left posterior direction, the assembly as a single unit is withdrawn under continuous fluoroscopy. When the tip of the dilator brushes across the aorta, a jump is observed. Continued withdrawal of the unit encounters a second jump when the tip of the dilator falls into the fossa ovale. At this point, the cardiac movement can be felt when a slight advancement of the assembly is made. For patients with a patent foramen ovale, such a slight advancement may cross to the left atrium. If transesophageal or intracardiac echocardiographic guidance is used, the atrial septum can be observed to protrude (i.e., "tenting") toward the left atrium (14) (Fig. 6-9). The unit should be held stable, and multiple fluoroscopic views should be checked to ensure that the tip of the assembly is pointing posterior to the His bundle catheter and anterosuperior to the coronary sinus catheter. Some operators also position a 5-French pigtail catheter into the ascending aorta to serve as another anatomic reference (4,8).

After the proper position is confirmed, the needle is advanced. When the needle crosses the atrial septum, a "pop" can be felt, and the typical atrial pressure tracing should be recorded. Some operators also inject radiocontrast or measure the oxygen saturation to further confirm entry into the left atrium. After successful entry into the left atrium is confirmed, the needle is held steady. The dilator and the sheath as a unit are then advanced approximately 1 to 2 cm. Thereafter, the needle and the dilator are held steady, and the sheath is advanced to the lateral wall of the left atrium. A sheath with an x-ray marker at the tip helps to locate the exact position of the sheath in the left atrium. The sheath is held steady, and the needle and dilator are removed together. The sheath should be immediately flushed with heparinized saline with the subsequent slow drip through the side arm to prevent clot formation. The ablation catheter is then inserted into the left atrium through the Mullins sheath. We prefer to defer initiation of systemic heparinization until the typical electrogram of the mitral annulus is recorded from the ablation catheter. Such an approach may cause a delay of anticoagulation for a few minutes, but it further ensures absence of perforation before heparin is infused. After the removal of the dilator and Brockenbrough needle, the tip of the sheath may drop into one of the left pulmonary veins. In such cases, the tip of the ablation catheter can be advanced just beyond the tip of the sheath, and then the sheath is pulled back into the left atrium. A deflected tip of the ablation catheter often helps to enter the mitral annulus when the catheter is withdrawn from the pulmonary vein.

With the transseptal approach, it is relatively easy to map the mitral annulus systematically because of the absence of anatomic obstacles. Similar to the retrograde aortic approach, the mitral annulus is better visualized with the 40- to 45-degree left anterior oblique view. To position the tip of the ablation catheter on the mitral annulus requires clockwise or counterclockwise torque of the catheter. Counterclock-

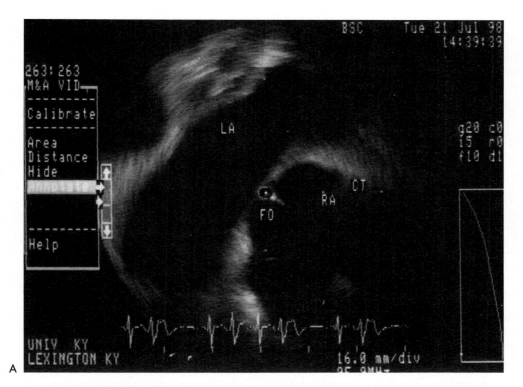

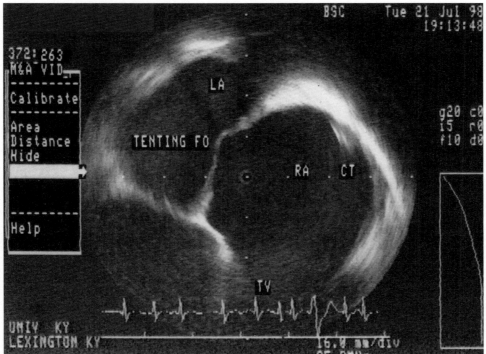

FIGURE 6-9. Intracardiac echocardiographic images during transseptal puncture. **A:** Cardiac structures before the procedure. **B:** Protrusion (i.e., tenting) of the atrial septum toward the left atrium as the sheath-dilator-needle assembly is advanced against the fossa ovalis. CT, crista terminalis; FO, fossa ovalis; LA, left atrium; RA, right atrium; TV, tricuspid valve.

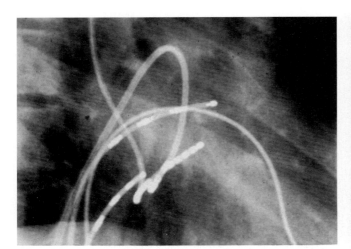 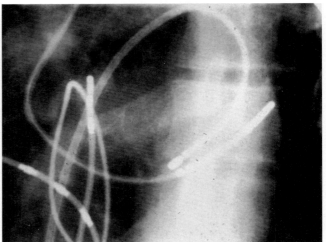

FIGURE 6-10. Fluoroscopic image shows the positions of the intracardiac catheters during an ablation procedure for a left-sided accessory pathway with the transseptal approach. The ablation catheter is deployed along the posterolateral region of the mitral valve annulus. Notice the position of the ablation catheter just above the coronary sinus catheter. A right anterior oblique projection *(left)* and a left anterior oblique projection *(right)* are shown.

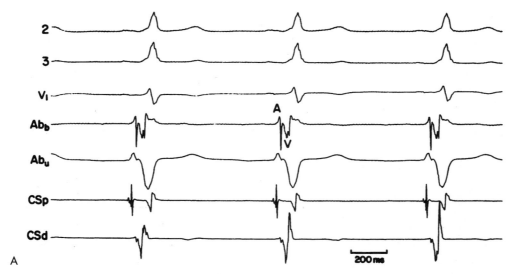

FIGURE 6-11. Electrocardiograms obtained during mapping of left-sided accessory pathways by the transseptal approach. **A:** Mapping during sinus rhythm. At the successful site, a short atrioventricular interval is recorded (Ab$_b$), and the ventricular electrogram precedes the onset of the delta wave. The atrial electrogram amplitude recorded from the ablation catheter is one third or more of the ventricular electrogram amplitude, and the unipolar ventricular electrogram from the ablation catheter (Ab$_u$) shows a large, negative signal. ***(continues)***

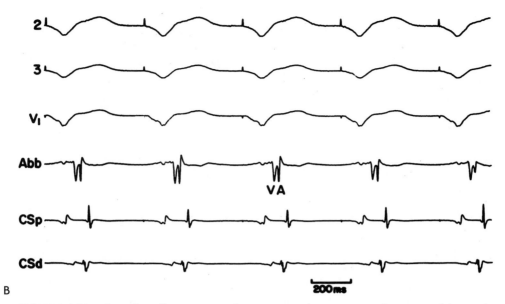

FIGURE 6-11. *(continued)* B: Mapping during ventricular pacing. At the successful site, the earliest and shortest retrograde atrial activation time during ventricular pacing is recorded at the ablation catheter. From top to bottom are the surface ECG leads 2, 3, and V$_1$ and the intracardiac electrograms from the bipolar (Ab$_b$) ablation catheter, proximal (CSp) and distal (CSd) coronary sinus.

wise torque helps to move the catheter toward the ventricular side, and clockwise rotation helps to move the catheter toward the atrial side. When the typical annulus electrogram of almost equal atrial and ventricular amplitude is recorded, bending the catheter moves its tip medially, and unbending moves the tip laterally. To position the catheter near the posteroseptal region, it often requires further withdrawal of the Mullins sheath. A large curve then is made at the tip of the ablation catheter. With clockwise rotation, slow release of the curve usually allows the tip of the ablation catheter to drop to the posteromedial mitral annulus (Fig. 6-10). However, ablation of the extremely lateral accessory pathway may require counterclockwise rotation of a relatively straight ablation catheter. When catheter stability becomes a problem, advancement or withdrawal of the Mullins sheath is often helpful. It is also helpful to rotate the catheter together with the Mullins sheath in the same direction. Long sheaths with different preformed curves are available to facilitate placement of the ablation catheter at more anterior sites along the annulus. When the mapping is performed on the atrial side, the tip of the ablation catheter usually appears superior to the coronary sinus catheter. The ideal ablation site should have an atrial electrogram amplitude of one third or more of the ventricular electrogram amplitude plus the earliest activation time with or without an accessory pathway potential (Fig. 6-11).

Similar to the retrograde aortic approach, ablation may also be attempted from the ventricular side with the transseptal approach if ablation from the atrial side is unsuccessful. However, it may be difficult to change the catheter to a different position with such a combination.

MAPPING THE ABLATION TARGET

Conventional mapping using the intracardiac electrogram can be performed in sinus rhythm or during atrial pacing for patients with manifest preexcitation. This anterograde mapping method involves searching for an ablation target where the local ventricular electrogram recorded from the ablation catheter is earlier than or at least simultaneous with the delta wave onset (Fig. 6-12). Anterograde mapping is the only method for patients with accessory pathways having only uni-

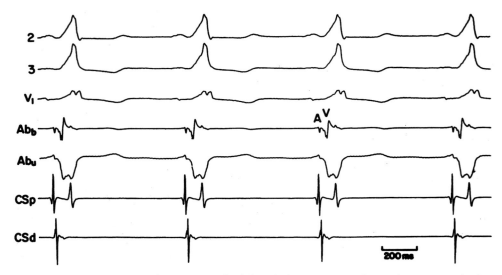

FIGURE 6-12. Anterograde mapping of a left-sided accessory pathway during sinus rhythm with the retrograde aortic approach. The ventricular electrogram recorded from the ablation catheter is earlier than or at least simultaneous with the delta wave onset in the surface ECG leads. The unipolar electrogram from the ablation catheter (Ab$_u$) shows a large, negative ventricular electrogram, suggesting a location near the accessory pathway. From top to bottom are the surface ECG leads 2, 3, and V$_1$ and the intracardiac electrograms from the bipolar (Ab$_b$) and unipolar (Ab$_u$) ablation catheters and the proximal (CSp) and distal (CSd) coronary sinus.

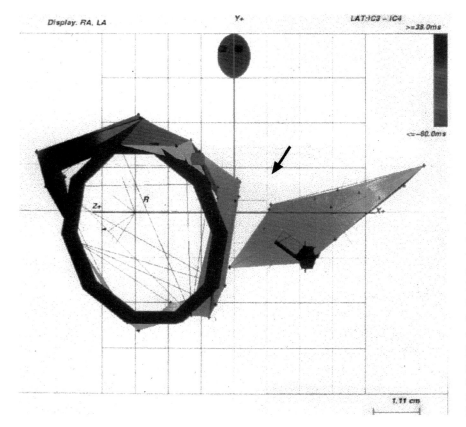

FIGURE 6-13. A gray-scale electroanatomic map of a left-sided accessory pathway using the Carto-Biosense Webster system. In this patient, ablation from the atrial and ventricular sides of the mitral annulus had previously failed, suggesting an epicardial location of the pathway. The ablation catheter was then advanced within the coronary sinus, where a single lesion in the left posterior region eliminated the accessory pathway conduction. The catheter tip is shown at the successful site within the coronary sinus *(arrow)*. The His bundle location is marked with a tag.

directional anterograde conduction. Mapping may also be performed during ventricular pacing or orthodromic atrioventricular reentrant tachycardia. This retrograde mapping method involves searching for a target where the local atrial electrogram recorded from the ablation catheter is earlier than or at least simultaneous with the earliest atrial activation recorded from the coronary sinus electrodes (Fig. 6-2). Retrograde mapping is the only method for patients with a concealed accessory pathway. When ablation is attempted during atrioventricular reentrant tachycardia, the catheter may dislodge as the result of tachycardia termination. Li and colleagues (15) found that entrainment of the tachycardia with ventricular pacing helped to maintain catheter stability when the tachycardia was terminated during the ablation. The accessory pathway potential may not always be recorded at the successful ablation site, but its presence usually increases the probability of successful ablation.

Computerized three-dimensional (3-D) nonfluoroscopic mapping has been reported to be an effective method for successful ablation of accessory pathways (16). Electroanatomic mapping using the Carto-Biosense Webster system provides the opportunity to tag ablation sites (Fig. 6-13). This feature is valuable in the case of catheter dislodgment during the ablation because it helps in repositioning the catheter at nearly the same location. This system may also reduce the fluoroscopy time and the number of unnecessary ablation current applications. This new technique may be particularly useful for repeat ablations.

COMPARISON OF RETROGRADE AORTIC AND TRANSSEPTAL APPROACHES

Only one small, randomized trial has compared the success rate and complications of the retrograde aortic and transseptal approaches for ablation of left-sided accessory pathways (Table 6-2). In this study, Ma and coworkers randomized 100 patients to the retrograde aortic approach or the transseptal approach. There was no significant difference in ablation success rate, fluoroscopy time, or complications for the two approaches (17). Adequate-size, prospective, randomized trials of the two methods may never be performed appropriately because individual electrophysiologists usually are trained predominantly in only one of the approaches. The training experience and subsequent practice often reflect a preference of one approach over the other. Such a difference makes it unfair to compare the outcome of the two approaches in a random fashion.

Several nonrandomized studies have compared the outcome of the two approaches. De Ponti and associates (11) compared the outcome of the retrograde aortic versus the transseptal approach in 33 patients undergoing left-sided accessory pathway ablation. The investigators attempted the retrograde aortic ap-

TABLE 6-2 • STUDIES OF TRANSSEPTAL VERSUS RETROAORTIC METHODS FOR ABLATION OF LEFT FREE WALL ACCESSORY PATHWAYS

Study	Number		Efficacy		Fluoroscopy Time (min)		Complications	
	Transseptal	Retroaortic	Transseptal	Retroaortic	Transseptal	Retroaortic	Transseptal	Retroaortic
De Ponti (11)	18	15	17 (94%)	6 (40%)	43 ± 27	68 ± 42	0	0
Lesh (19)	33	89	26 (85%)	76 (85%)	44.7 ± 5.1	44.1 ± 4.4	2 (6%)	6 (7%)
Natale (18)	31	49	31 (100%)	43 (88%)	34 ± 18	42 ± 29	0	2 (4%)
Manolis (10)	28	54	24 (86%)	47 (87%)	81 ± 57	121 ± 81	0	4 (7%)
Deshpande (8)	52	56	44 (85%)	54 (96%)	53 ± 22	51 ± 32	6 (10%)	0
Vora (9)	13	36	13 (100%)	36 (100%)	60.7 ± 45	38.4 ± 30.2	1 (8%)	1 (3%)
Pediatric Registry (20)	845	364	804 (95%)	336 (92%)	10	10	30/966 (3%)	13/462 (3%)
Ma[a] (17)	50	50	50 (100%)	48 (96%)	12 ± 7	13 ± 8	0	0

[a] Randomized study.

proach first in 15 patients and achieved successful ablation in only 6 (40%) patients. Seven of the failed patients subsequently underwent the transseptal approach, and all had successful ablation. The other 18 patients all had successful ablation using the transseptal approach as the initial approach, although 1 patient required two ablation sessions. The total procedure time was shorter with the transseptal approach than with the retrograde aortic approach (3.3 ± 0.9 versus 4.0 ± 1.3 hours, $p < 0.05$). No complications were encountered in any patient. These results might have been affected by the learning experience of the investigators at that time.

In another study by Natale and colleagues (18), the retrograde aortic approach was initially attempted as the first choice in 49 of 80 patients. Later, the transseptal approach was attempted as the first choice in the remaining 31 patients. The initial success rate was 88% for the retrograde aortic approach and 100% for the transseptal approach ($p < 0.03$). Although not statistically significant, there was a trend of shorter fluoroscopy time (34 ± 18 versus 42 ± 29 minutes) and fewer current applications (5.9 ± 4.2 versus 7.3 ± 0.6) with the transseptal approach than with the retrograde aortic approach. The effect of the operator learning experience might have played a role in this study.

In a similar study, Lesh and coworkers (19) compared the outcome of the retrograde aortic versus the transseptal approach in 106 patients. The initial 65 patients underwent ablation with the retrograde aortic approach as the first choice and had a success rate of 85%. The other 51 patients underwent ablation with the transseptal approach as the first choice and also had a success rate of 85%. Eleven patients undergoing the initial retrograde aortic approach subsequently crossed over to the transseptal approach because of unsuccessful ablation, and 10 had successful ablation with the transseptal approach. Four patients in the transseptal group subsequently crossed over to the retrograde aortic approach because of unsuccessful ablation, and all had successful ablation with the retrograde aortic approach. The total procedure time and the fluoroscopy time were not significantly different between the two approaches. However, the ablation time was significantly shorter for the transseptal approach than for the retrograde aortic approach (43.4 ± 9.3 versus 69.2 ± 10.5 minutes, $p < 0.01$). The results suggest that the time added by the transseptal puncture may be compensated by the shortened ablation time for the transseptal approach. The complication rates were comparable between the two approaches (6.7% for the retrograde aortic approach versus 6.1% for the transseptal approach). A case of coronary artery dissection with myocardial infarction caused by the retrograde aortic approach was reported. In addition to the operators' learning experience, this study might also have been affected by the availability of a physician trained in transseptal puncture.

Manolis and colleagues (10) reported that the initial success rate of the retrograde aortic and the transseptal approach was similar (87% versus 86%), but the fluoroscopy time was significantly shorter with the transseptal approach than with the retrograde aortic approach (81 ± 57 versus 121 ± 81 minutes, $p < 0.05$). Crossover to the other approach was needed in 4 (17%) of 24 patients of the transseptal approach and 5 (10%) of 50 patients of the retrograde aortic approach, suggesting that one approach alone may not be sufficient to achieve successful ablation in all cases.

In a study of 100 patients by Deshpande and associates (8), 14 of 58 patients undergoing the transseptal approach subsequently crossed over to the retrograde aortic approach, whereas only 1 of 42 patients undergoing the retrograde aortic approach subsequently crossed over to the transseptal approach. Although the final overall success rate was 100%, there was a case of ablation-related atrial perforation and another case of transseptal puncture related hemopericardium in the transseptal group. There were only two cases of mild mitral regurgitation in the retrograde aortic group. Six cases of inadvertent fallback of the ablation catheter from the left atrium were reported, suggesting that the operators might have been less experienced in the transseptal approach. In contrast, in a study of 49 pediatric patients, Vora and colleagues (9) found that the fluoroscopy time was significantly shorter with the retrograde aortic approach than with the transseptal approach (38.4 ± 30.2 versus 60.7 ± 45 minutes, $p < 0.05$).

Kugler and associates (20) reported observations from the Pediatric Radiofrequency Catheter Ablation Registry. Of 845 transatrial procedures, 804 (95%) were successful, and of 364 retrograde aortic procedures, 336 (92%) were successful. There was no significant difference in fluoroscopy time or complication rates.

The overall success rate for catheter ablation of left-sided accessory pathways is approximately 85% to 100%, with a recurrence rate of 4% to 7%. Operator experience and preference may have an important role in the outcome of an individual approach. On the other hand, competence with both techniques could be advantageous when the approach is dictated by specific situations such as the presence of severe aortic stenosis or a prosthetic valve, severe peripheral atherosclerosis, or congenital diseases.

◉ APPROACH-RELATED COMPLICATIONS

Transseptal Approach

Cardiac perforation is probably the most feared complication for the transseptal approach. Because the atrial wall is very thin and often cannot seal the perforation through myocardial contraction, perforation of the atrium can cause sustained intrapericardial bleeding and may require open heart surgery. Although some physicians have been fortunate enough to have no perforation even in large series of patients (21,22), a rate of cardiac perforation up to 4% has been reported (23). Even with guidance by the transesophageal echocardiography, cardiac perforation may not be completely eliminated (14,24). The data appear to suggest that operator experience may play a more important role than the guiding technique itself in the occurrence of cardiac perforation. However, cardiac perforation can also be directly caused by the ablation (8). Intracardiac shunting at the atrial level appears to be common shortly after the transseptal procedure (25), but hemodynamically significant shunting has not been observed during a short-term follow-up study with transesophageal echocardiography (26).

Retrograde Aortic Approach

Placement of an arterial sheath with prolonged catheter manipulation can cause femoral artery injury, including femoral arteriovenous fistula, pseudoaneurysm, thrombotic occlusion, or retroperitoneal hematoma. Coronary artery damage with occlusion or dissection of the coronary artery is a rare but serious complication of the retrograde aortic approach (19, 27,28). Aortic or mitral valve injury has been almost exclusively observed in patients undergoing the retrograde aortic approach. In an echocardiographic study of patients undergoing the retrograde aortic approach, the incidence of valvular injury was found to be 8.4%, including mitral (6.7%) and aortic (3.3%) regurgitation (29). One patient had hemodynamically significant valvular lesion. It appears that a mild valvular lesion causes only transient valvular dysfunction that disappeared during the follow-up (30). Valvular injury also has the potential to cause clot formation (31). Catheter entrapment in the mitral or aortic valve apparatus has been encountered only in patients undergoing the retrograde aortic approach and may require open heart surgery for removal in difficult cases (32). In this respect, catheters with a soft tip should be used with caution, avoiding looping around the mitral apparatus.

Transient atrioventricular conduction block or asystole has been reported in several patients undergoing ablation with the retrograde aortic approach. Some of these cases might have been the result of a vasovagal reaction induced by the ablation (33–35), but others were likely the result of injury to the atrioventricular junction (36). Permanent complete atrioventricular conduction block has been reported in a patient undergoing ablation of a left posteroseptal accessory pathway using the retrograde aortic approach (37). During the attempted ablation of a left posteroseptal accessory pathway, multiple fluoroscopic views may help avoid injury to the atrioventricular junction as this structure is located anteromedially at the base of the ventricular septum.

Air embolism or thromboembolism can happen with the transseptal and the retrograde aortic approaches (38,39). However, air embolism is observed more frequently after transseptal instrumentation and is more likely to occur with the use of larger size sheaths.

● SUGGESTIONS AND TIPS

In rare patients, ablation within the coronary sinus may be required for successful ablation (Fig. 6-13). Careful titration of the energy during ablation in the coronary sinus is important to prevent perforation.

Simple precautions during left-sided instrumentation may avoid or reduce complications. Strict attention to achieving and maintaining the activated coagulation time above 250 seconds is of paramount importance for reducing the risk of thromboembolism. Maintenance of a continuous high-pressure infusion of heparinized saline through the transseptal sheath may reduce the chance of air embolism. The transseptal sheath should also be flushed if the ablation catheter is removed and reinserted. Anticoagulant or antiplatelet therapy after ablation is a matter of debate. Most centers prefer to use aspirin therapy for a period of 4 to 6 weeks after ablation of a left-sided accessory pathway. The use of antiplatelet agents such as ticlopidine or clopidogrel or anticoagulants such as warfarin is more controversial.

● CONCLUSIONS

Successful and safe ablation of the left-sided accessory pathway can be achieved with the retrograde aortic or the transseptal approach in experienced hands. It appears that the total procedure time may be shorter with the transseptal approach than the retrograde aortic approach for operators with equivalent experience in both techniques. Although the transseptal puncture adds additional time, it may be compensated by the time saved during the mapping and ablation phase. It is fair to say that the retrograde aortic approach and the transseptal approach are complementary. The question is not which approach is better, but rather which approach should be used as the first choice. The transseptal puncture cannot be performed in a heparinized patient because of the risk of serious bleeding if perforation happens. For patients with a failed retrograde aortic approach, reversal of the heparin effect with protamine or prolonged waiting is required before the transseptal approach can be attempted. The transseptal approach may be attempted first in centers that have abundant experience in both approaches.

The decision to use a specific approach as the first choice should be mainly based on the physician's experience. However, every electrophysiologist should be trained in and be capable of using both approaches. Perhaps the two approaches should be alternatively performed as the first choice to maintain competence in both techniques. Such a strategy may be quite useful because the increasing number of mapping and ablation procedures in the left atrium mandates dexterity in the transseptal approach for any cardiac electrophysiologist.

Because of the high acute success rate, low incidence of complications, and low recurrence rate at follow-up, catheter ablation of left-sided accessory pathways provides an appealing and valid alternative to drug therapy.

REFERENCES

1. Jackman WM, Wang XZ, Friday KJ, et al. Catheter ablation of accessory atrioventricular pathways (Wolff-Parkinson-White syndrome) by radiofrequency current. *N Engl J Med* 1991;324:1605–1611.
2. Schluter M, Geiger M, Siebels J, et al. Catheter ablation using radiofrequency current to cure symptomatic patients with tachyarrhythmias related to an accessory atrioventricular pathway. *Circulation* 1991;84:1644–1661.
3. Calkins H, Langberg J, Sousa J, et al. Radiofrequency catheter ablation of accessory atrioventricular connections in 250 patients: abbreviated therapeutic approach to Wolff-Parkinson-White syndrome. *Circulation* 1992;85:1337–1346.
4. Lesh MD, Van Hare GF, Schamp DJ, et al. Curative percutaneous catheter ablation using radiofrequency energy for accessory pathways in all locations: results in 100 consecutive patients. *J Am Coll Cardiol* 1992;19:1303–1309.
5. Manolis AS, Maounis T, Vassilikos V, et al. Pretreatment with antithrombotic agents during radiofrequency catheter ablation: a randomized comparison of aspirin versus ticlopidine. *J Cardiovasc Electrophysiol* 1998;9:1144–1151.
6. Seifert MJ, Morady F, Calkins HG, Langberg JJ. Aortic leaflet perforation during radiofrequency ablation. *Pacing Clin Electrophysiol* 1991;14[Pt 1]:1582–1585.
7. Kuck KH, Schluter M. Single-catheter approach to radiofrequency current ablation of left-sided accessory pathways in patients with Wolff-Parkinson-White syndrome. *Circulation* 1991;84:2366–2375.
8. Deshpande SS, Bremner S, Sra JS, et al. Ablation of left free-wall accessory pathways using radiofrequency energy at the atrial

insertion site: transseptal versus transaortic approach. *J Cardiovasc Electrophysiol* 1994;5:219–231.
9. Vora AM, McMahon S, Jazayeri MR, Dhala A. Ablation of atrial insertion sites of left-sided accessory pathways in children: efficacy and safety of transseptal versus transaortic approach. *Pediatr Cardiol* 1997;18:332–338.
10. Manolis AS, Wang PJ, Estes NA 3rd. Radiofrequency ablation of left-sided accessory pathways: transaortic versus transseptal approach. *Am Heart J* 1994;128:896–902.
11. De Ponti R, Casari A, Salerno JA, et al. Radiofrequency transcatheter ablation of anomalous left atrioventricular pathways: the role of the transseptal approach. *G Ital Cardiol* 1992;22:1255–1264.
12. Mullins CE. Transseptal left heart catheterization: experience with a new technique in 520 pediatric and adult patients. *Pediatr Cardiol* 1983;4:239–245.
13. Brockenbrough EC, Braunwald E. A new technique for left ventricular angiography and transseptal left heart catheterization. *Am J Cardiol* 1960;6:1062–1064.
14. Tucker KJ, Curtis AB, Murphy J, et al. Transesophageal echocardiographic guidance of transseptal left heart catheterization during radiofrequency ablation of left-sided accessory pathways in humans. *Pacing Clin Electrophysiol* 1996;19:272–281.
15. Li HG, Klein GJ, Zardini M, et al. Radiofrequency catheter ablation of accessory pathways during entrainment of AV reentrant tachycardia. *Pacing Clin Electrophysiol* 1994;17[Pt 1]:590–594.
16. Fisher WG, Swartz JF. Catheter-based three-dimensional electrogram acquisition and analysis system. *J Electrocardiol* 1993;26[Suppl]:174–181.
17. Ma C, Dong J, Yang X, et al. A randomized comparison between retrograde and transseptal approach for radiofrequency ablation of left-sided accessory pathways. [Abstract] *Pacing Clin Electrophysiol* 1995;18:915.
18. Natale A, Wathen M, Yee R, et al. Atrial and ventricular approaches for radiofrequency catheter ablation of left-sided accessory pathways. *Am J Cardiol* 1992;70:114–116.
19. Lesh MD, Van Hare GF, Scheinman MM, et al. Comparison of the retrograde and transseptal methods for ablation of left free wall accessory pathways. *J Am Coll Cardiol* 1993;22:542–549.
20. Kugler JD, Danford DA, Silka MJ, et al. Ablation of left-sided accessory pathways: transatrial, retrograde, or coronary sinus approach? In: Singer I, Barold SS, Camm AJ, eds. *Nonpharmacological therapy of arrhythmias for the 21st century: the state of the art.* Armonk, NY: Futura Publishing, 1998:73–85.
21. Swartz JF, Tracy CM, Fletcher RD. Radiofrequency endocardial catheter ablation of accessory atrioventricular pathway atrial insertion sites. *Circulation* 1993;87:487–499.
22. De Ponti R, Zardini M, Storti C, et al. Trans-septal catheterization for radiofrequency catheter ablation of cardiac arrhythmias: results and safety of a simplified method. *Eur Heart J* 1998;19:943–950.
23. Yip AS, Chow WH, Yung TC, et al. Radiofrequency catheter ablation of left-sided accessory pathways using a transseptal technique and specialized long intravascular sheaths: efficacy, recurrence rate and complications. *Jpn Heart J* 1997;38:643–650.
24. Hahn K, Gal R, Sarnoski J, et al. Transesophageal echocardiographically guided atrial transseptal catheterization in patients with normal-sized atria: incidence of complications. *Clin Cardiol* 1995;18:217–220.
25. Kessler DJ, Pirwitz MJ, Horton RP, et al. Intracardiac shunts resulting from transseptal catheterization for ablation of accessory pathways in otherwise normal hearts. *Am J Cardiol* 1998;82:391–392.
26. Fitchet A, Turkie W, Fitzpatrick AP. Transseptal approach to ablation of left-sided arrhythmias does not lead to persisting interatrial shunt: a transesophageal echocardiographic study. *Pacing Clin Electrophysiol* 1998;21[Pt 1]:2070–2072.
27. Chatelain P, Zimmermann M, Weber R, et al. Acute coronary occlusion secondary to radiofrequency catheter ablation of a left lateral accessory pathway. *Eur Heart J* 1995;16:859–861.
28. Kosinski DJ, Burket MW, Durzinsky D. Occlusion of the left main coronary artery during radiofrequency ablation of the Wolff-Parkinson-White syndrome. *Eur J Card Pacing Electrophysiol* 1993;1:63–66.
29. Neuzner J, Faude I, Pitschner HF, Schlepper M. Incidence of intervention-related heart valve lesions after high-frequency catheter ablation of the left-side accessory atrioventricular conduction pathways [in German]. *Z Kardiol* 1995;84:1002–1008.
30. Olsson A, Darpo B, Bergfeldt L, Rosenqvist M. Frequency and long term follow up of valvar insufficiency caused by retrograde aortic radiofrequency catheter ablation procedures. *Heart* 1999;81:292–296.
31. Raitt MH, Schwaegler B, Pearlman AS, et al. Development of an aortic valve mass after radiofrequency catheter ablation. *Pacing Clin Electrophysiol* 1993;16:2064–2066.
32. Conti JB, Geiser E, Curtis AB. Catheter entrapment in the mitral valve apparatus during radiofrequency ablation. *Pacing Clin Electrophysiol* 1994;17:1681–1685.
33. Tsai CF, Chen SA, Chiang CE, et al. Radiofrequency ablation-induced asystole during transaortic approach for a left anterolateral accessory pathway: a Bezold-Jarisch–like phenomenon. *J Cardiovasc Electrophysiol* 1997;8:694–699.
34. Stamato NJ, Eddy SL, Whiting DJ. Transient complete heart block during radiofrequency ablation of a left lateral bypass tract. *Pacing Clin Electrophysiol* 1996;19:1351–1354.
35. Singh B, Sudan D, Kaul U. Transient complete atrioventricular block following radiofrequency ablation of left free wall accessory pathway. *J Interv Card Electrophysiol* 1998;2:305–307.
36. Seidl K, Hauer B, Zahn R, Senges J. Unexpected complete AV block following transcatheter ablation of a left posteroseptal accessory pathway. *Pacing Clin Electrophysiol* 1998;21[Pt 1]:2139–2142.
37. Liu J, Dole LR. Late complete atrioventricular block complicating radiofrequency catheter ablation of a left posteroseptal accessory pathway. *Pacing Clin Electrophysiol* 1998;21[Pt 1]:2136–2138.
38. Georgiadis D, Hill M, Kottkamp H, et al. Intracranial microembolic signals during radiofrequency ablation of accessory pathways. *Am J Cardiol* 1997;80:805–807.
39. Thakur RK, Klein GJ, Yee R, Zardini M. Embolic complications after radiofrequency catheter ablation. *Am J Cardiol* 1994;74:278–279.

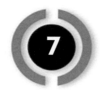

ABLATION OF RIGHT FREE WALL AND ATRIOFASCICULAR ACCESSORY PATHWAYS
• • •

GERY TOMASSONI, LOGAN KANAGARATNAM, WALID SALIBA, ROBERT A. SCHWEIKERT, ANDREA NATALE

Radiofrequency catheter ablation has emerged as a first-line therapy for most supraventricular tachycardias. In patients with tachycardias using an atrioventricular accessory pathway, radiofrequency catheter ablation has been demonstrated to be highly effective and safe (1–10), with a high (>90%) success rate, relatively few complications, low recurrence rates, and overall short procedural times (1–10). However, radiofrequency catheter ablation of right free wall accessory pathways has been associated with a lower initial success rate and a higher rate of recurrence (5–7). Although less common than left-sided and septal accessory pathways, right free wall accessory pathways represent an important subset of atrioventricular connections. As a result of unique anatomic differences between the tricuspid valve and the mitral valve annuli, radiofrequency catheter ablation of accessory pathways originating along the right free wall can be technically difficult and time consuming. Novel mapping and catheter ablation techniques however may improve the initial success and lower the rate of recurrence for accessory pathways originating along the right free wall.

The purpose of this chapter is to review the anatomic features, electrophysiologic evaluation, electrocardiographic manifestations, and new and old catheter techniques for mapping and ablation of right free wall accessory pathways. Catheter ablation of so-called Mahaim accessory pathways, which have decremental properties, long conduction times, and distal ventricular insertion sites is also reviewed because they represent a unique form of right-sided preexcitation.

● RIGHT FREE WALL ACCESSORY PATHWAYS

Anatomic Locations

Normally, the atrioventricular annulus is composed of fibrous tissue that is devoid of electrical conductive properties. The typical route of electrical activation travels along specialized electrical tissue from the sinoatrial node to the atrioventricular (AV) node and His bundle. Accessory pathways represent developmental abnormalities of the atrioventricular ring that contain myocardial fibers capable of electrical conduction (11–12). These accessory pathways can occur anywhere along the atrioventricular ring and have been described according to their location: left-sided accessory pathways along the mitral valve or right-sided accessory pathways along the tricuspid valve annulus. Left-sided accessory pathways are more common, and right-sided accessory pathways tend to be more frequently associated with congenital abnormalities (13). Accessory pathways originating along the anterior, anterolateral, lateral, posterolateral, and posterior wall of the tricuspid valve annulus have been defined as right free wall accessory pathways (Fig. 7-1). The reported incidence of right free wall accessory pathways is 10% to 15% in most of the larger published series (1–10).

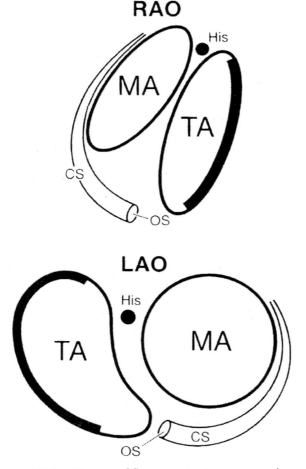

FIGURE 7-1. Diagram of fluoroscopic views commonly used for the right free wall accessory pathways. In the right anterior oblique (RAO) view, the tricuspid annulus (TA) is foreshortened. In the left anterior oblique (LAO) view, the TA is viewed like a clock face. The area darkened in black outlines the locations of right-sided accessory pathways. CS, coronary sinus; MA, mitral annulus. (Adapted from Zhu DWX. Ablation of right free wall and Mahaim accessory pathways. In: Singer I, Barold SS, Camm AJ, eds. *Nonpharmacological therapy of arrhythmias for the 21st century: the state of the art*. Armonk, NY: Futura Publishing, 1998, with permission.)

Important anatomic differences exist between the tricuspid valve annulus and mitral valve annulus (11, 12,14): significantly larger endocardial area is present along the tricuspid valve because of the greater circumference of its annulus and the lack of atrioventricular connections between the right and left fibrous trigones along the mitral valve annulus; more apical location on a slightly different horizontal plane of the tricuspid valve annulus compared with the mitral valve annulus; folding over of the right atrium onto the right ventricle near the tricuspid annulus, creating a more acute angle of attachment of the tricuspid valve to the annulus and resulting in less room available for manipulation of the catheter tip (Fig. 7-2); higher incidence of anatomic variations (e.g., Ebstein's anomaly) and multiple accessory atrioventricular connections along the tricuspid valve annulus compared with the mitral valve; and the lack of a nearby, easily accessible anatomic structure along the tricuspid valve annulus, such as the coronary sinus, that can serve as a guide for accessory pathway localization after cannulation with a multipolar catheter. As a result of the anatomic differences and the association of congenital abnormalities, radiofrequency catheter ablation of right free wall accessory pathways has yielded a lower success rate (7), produced a higher recurrence rate (9), and often requires more radiofrequency applications (10) for elimination.

The traditional location and structure of accessory muscular atrioventricular connections has been questioned (12). It was previously thought that accessory pathways traversed gaps in the fibrous plates, which subsequently gave rise to the tricuspid and mitral valve leaflets (15). However, initial reports (16,17) have described the course of the atrioventricular connections along the epicardial tissue planes of the fibrofatty atrioventricular groove, typically at the site of attachment of the valvular leaflets (Fig. 7-3). Most septal accessory pathways have been shown by surgical dissection to be extensions of the fibrofatty atrioventricular grooves and therefore part of the epicardial tissues of the heart (12). Several case reports of atypical accessory atrioventricular connections have confirmed the epicardial nature of accessory pathways (18–20). Accessory atrioventricular connections extending from the undersurface of the right atrial appendage, crossing the right fibrofatty atrioventricular groove, and inserting into the supraventricular crest of the right

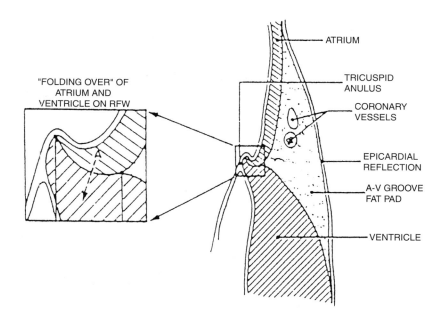

FIGURE 7-2. Sketch shows folding over of the atrial free wall on the right ventricle, creating an acute angle of attachment of the tricuspid valve. A-V, atrioventricular. (Adapted from Cox JL, Ferguson TB Jr. Surgery for the Wolff-Parkinson-White syndrome: the endocardial approach. *Semin Thorac Cardiovasc Surg* 1989;1: 34–46, with permission.)

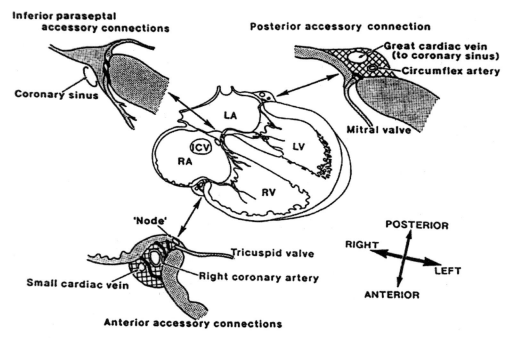

FIGURE 7-3. Four-chamber, long-axis view of the heart shows potential locations of the accessory pathways. Unlike the left-sided accessory pathways, right-sided accessory pathways can be located "deep" or further away from the AV groove. ICV, inferior caval vein; LA, left atrium; LV, left ventricle; RA, right atrium; RV, right ventricle. (Adapted from Anderson RH, Yen Ho S. Structure and location of accessory muscular AV connections. *J Cardiovasc Electrophysiol* 1999;10:1119–1123, with permission.)

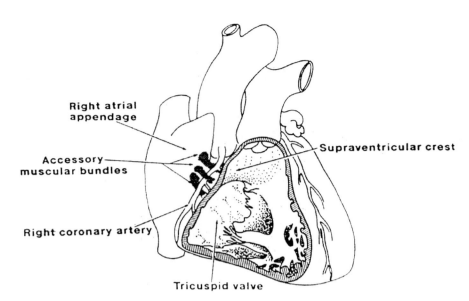

FIGURE 7-4. Potential anatomic locations of accessory pathways connecting the right atrial appendage to the right ventricle. They traverse the AV groove epicardially in front or behind the right coronary artery. (From Anderson RH, Yen Ho S. Structure and location of accessory muscular AV connections. *J Cardiovasc Electrophysiol* 1999;10:1119–1123, with permission.)

ventricle have been recognized (Fig. 7-4). It appears that accessory atrioventricular connections can originate and insert at multiple sites, including close to and far away from the atrioventricular groove with a significant number of connections being epicardial in nature.

Historical Perspectives

Possible tachycardias using an atrioventricular accessory pathway had been recorded in early 1900s, but it was not until 1966 that the first epicardial maps were created for patients with Wolff-Parkinson-White syndrome, which demonstrated the less common right-sided accessory pathway (21,22). The first successful surgical procedure was performed in 1968 after an epicardial map during preexcitation demonstrated the location of a right lateral accessory pathway (23, 24). Preexcitation was eliminated, and the tachycardia abolished with a surgical incision at the right ventricular atrioventricular groove. Despite this initial surgical success, the procedure was limited to refractory cases because of its associated morbidity.

During the early 1980s, techniques and catheters were developed to record accessory pathway potentials and to map pathway localization with greater precision. Successful catheter ablation using direct current (DC) energy was reported in 1984 (25), which was soon followed by the first successful radiofrequency ablation of an accessory pathway in 1987 (26). By the early 1990s, a series of publications were released showing high success rates with very few complications (1–10). Radiofrequency catheter ablation of accessory pathways is now widespread and constitutes first-line therapy for patients with tachycardias using an atrioventricular accessory pathway.

Electrocardiographic Manifestations

With antegrade function of an accessory pathway, fusion of antegrade conduction through the AV node and accessory pathway can occur, resulting in ventricular preexcitation. Because the polarity of the delta wave and the QRS morphology on the surface 12-lead electrocardiogram (ECG) reflects the relative position of the accessory pathway, several algorithms have been developed to determine the accessory pathway localization on the atrioventricular ring (27–29). Earlier localization criteria were developed by using surgical or intraoperative mapping as the reference or gold standard for accessory pathway localization (30). The sensitivity and specificity of the proposed algorithms ranged from 57% to 89% and 66% to 70%, respectively (27–29). The location of the accessory pathway is the right free wall if the following patterns are present: frontal plane main deflection QRS axis is leftward at 30 to −60 degrees (28); QRS deflection in leads V_1-V_3 is negative, resulting in a left bundle

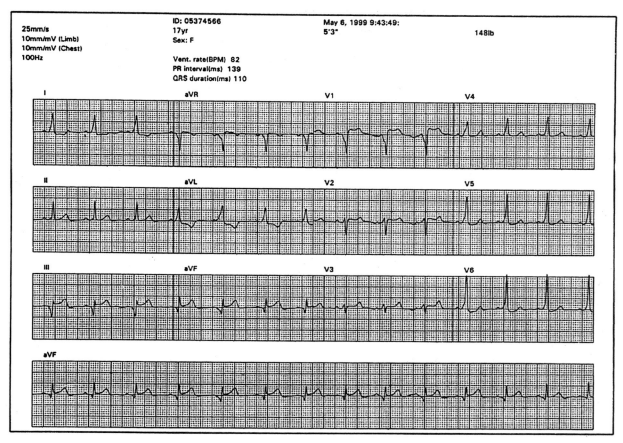

FIGURE 7-5. Electrocardiogram from a patient with a right-sided accessory pathway. Notice the negative QRS in lead V_1, negative delta waves in leads III and aVF, and frontal plane QRS axis of 0 degrees.

branch block (LBBB) pattern (29); frontal plane delta wave axis of −30 to −60 degrees (28); and negative delta waves in leads III and aVF, with positive delta waves in I and aVL (28) (Fig. 7-5).

Newer algorithms have been created using the site of successful catheter ablation as the reference standard for accessory pathway localization (31–33). The newer algorithms use variables, including precordial QRS lead transition, delta wave frontal axis and amplitude, and R wave amplitude (32). The ECG criteria based on the newer algorithms have improved overall sensitivity and specificity.

Unfortunately, no single algorithm is totally reliable in predicting the accessory pathway location accurately because multiple factors can affect the degree of preexcitation present. These factors include the position of the heart, thoracic configuration, and coexisting anomalies such as hypertrophy, infarction, dilatation, and congenital defects (34,35). There may be a significant degree of overlap in the preexcitation patterns, especially with right anteroseptal, midseptal, and right free wall accessory pathways (31), making it extremely difficult to define the precise location. To pinpoint the accessory pathway location, electrophysiologic study with fluoroscopic or nonfluoroscopic mapping techniques are usually needed.

Electrophysiologic Testing

For patients undergoing radiofrequency catheter ablation, a diagnostic electrophysiologic study is mandatory. The objectives of the electrophysiologic evaluation are to diagnose the presence, functional characteristics, and location of a single or multiple accessory pathways; to characterize the induction and termination of the clinical tachycardia; to determine whether the accessory pathway is a integral part of the tachycardia circuit; and to aid and facilitate accessory pathway localization for catheter ablation.

Before the electrophysiologic study, all antiarrhythmic medications should be discontinued for at least five half-lives, and AV nodal blocking agents should be held for a minimum of 48 hours. The patient is brought to the clinical electrophysiologic laboratory in a fasting state. After sedation is achieved under local anesthesia, 6-Fr quadripolar catheters are advanced from the femoral vein to the high right atrium, right ventricular apex, and His bundle area for recording and pacing. A 6-Fr decapolar catheter is typically advanced in the coronary sinus from the internal jugular, right subclavian, or femoral vein. The decapolar catheter is typically positioned with its most proximal pair of electrodes located at the coronary sinus ostium. If a left-sided accessory pathway exists, the catheter can be advanced further into the coronary sinus in an attempt to "bracket" the location of the accessory pathway.

After diagnostic catheter insertion, right ventricular stimulation conduction studies usually are performed first because they are particularly useful in the diagnosis of concealed (no antegrade function) accessory pathways. During right ventricular pacing, the absence of decremental conduction can suggest the presence of an accessory pathway. Decremental right ventricular pacing and ventricular extrastimulus testing is then performed to determine the pattern of retrograde atrial activation, retrograde effective refractory period of the AV node and accessory pathway, and the manner of induction of the clinical tachycardia. To identify an antegrade conducting accessory pathway, ventricular preexcitation must be demonstrated. If not already present in the baseline state, decremental atrial pacing or atrial extrastimulus testing can be used to unmask ventricular preexcitation. At faster pacing rates, the degree of preexcitation generally increases as more ventricular myocardium is activated by the nondecremental accessory pathway compared with the slower decremental conduction down the AV node. The sequence of atrial activation and the antegrade conduction properties of the accessory pathway can also be assessed.

If a tachycardia arises spontaneously or is induced by pacing, the protocol is interrupted, and the characteristics of the arrhythmia are then investigated. The most common tachycardia in patients with accessory pathways is orthodromic reciprocating tachycardia (34) (Fig. 7-6). During this tachycardia, antegrade conduction to the ventricle occurs through the normal AV node, whereas retrograde conduction to the atria occurs by means of the accessory pathway. The QRS width is usually narrow unless preexisting or functional bundle branch block is present. To differentiate a right-sided accessory pathway from AV nodal reentrant tachycardia (AVNRT), ventricular stimuli are delivered at the time of His bundle refractoriness. If the timing of the atrial signal is advanced, retrograde conduction must have occurred by means of the accessory pathway. If the tachycardia is reset, the accessory pathway is an active participant in the arrhythmia mechanism. Functional right bundle branch block (RBBB) during the tachycardia can also provide an important diagnostic clue and demonstrate active participation of the accessory pathway in the tachycardia. If the ventriculoatrial (VA) interval or the tachycardia cycle length prolongs, the active participation of a right-sided accessory pathway in the tachycardia is confirmed. The location of the right-sided accessory pathway can also be ascertained by the degree of VA interval prolongation (31). If the VA interval prolongation is greater than 40 msec, the accessory pathway is more likely to have a free wall location, but minimal VA prolongation favors a more septal location. A 2:1 AV block excludes the diagnosis of orthodromic reciprocating tachycardia because the atria and ventricles are integral parts of the tachycardia.

Several types of tachyarrhythmias can occur if antegrade conduction over the accessory pathway exists. Antidromic reciprocating tachycardia is seen clinically in 5% to 15% of patients with Wolff-Parkinson-White syndrome (35). During this tachycardia, antegrade conduction through the accessory pathway occurs with retrograde conduction up the AV node. Because ventricular activation occurs exclusively through the accessory pathway, the width of the surface QRS complex is broad, demonstrating maximal preexcitation. Atrial fibrillation, atrial flutter, atrial tachycardia, and AVNRT can also occur in patients

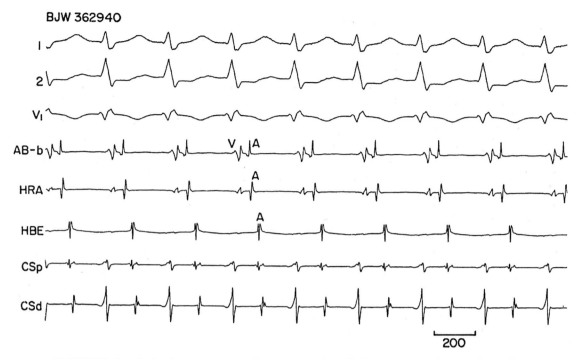

FIGURE 7-6. Orthodromic tachycardia using a right-sided accessory pathway. The earliest atrial activation (retrograde) occurs close to the ablation catheter. From top to bottom are surface leads 1, 2, and V_1. AB-b, recording from the ablation catheter that is positioned along the right AV groove; HBE, His bundle electrogram; CSp and CSd, proximal and distal coronary sinus recordings.

with an accessory pathway. With these arrhythmias, the accessory pathway may not participate in the tachycardia but instead acts as an innocent bystander. Further electrophysiologic evaluation is needed to distinguish antidromic reciprocating tachycardia from atrial tachycardia or AVNRT with bystander accessory pathway conduction. The most useful pacing maneuver is the introduction of premature atrial extrastimuli. Atrial extrastimuli should be delivered close to the annulus, near the atrial insertion site of the accessory pathway. Delivery of atrial extrastimuli should be performed when the atrium near the His bundle area is refractory. If preexcitation occurs with the same sequence of ventricular activation, antero-grade conduction over the accessory pathway is present. If ventricular activation is advanced and the tachycardia is reset, accessory pathway participation in the tachycardia is confirmed. If the tachycardia is not reset, only bystander participation of accessory pathway is present. The use of certain medications such as adenosine or procainamide and their effects on the tachycardia can also help arrive at the correct diagnosis.

Intracardiac Mapping

Technique

Electrical mapping of right free wall accessory pathways usually is performed from the femoral venous approach. In certain accessory pathway locations (i.e., right anterior and anterolateral), catheter manipulation from the right internal jugular or left subclavian vein can facilitate tissue contact (Fig. 7-7). Typically, a 7-Fr, 4- to 6-mm-long, deflectable-tip catheter suitable for the delivery of radiofrequency energy is used for mapping and ablation. In most cases, mapping of the accessory pathway is performed by positioning the catheter on the atrial side. Catheter stability may be enhanced with the use of long intravascular

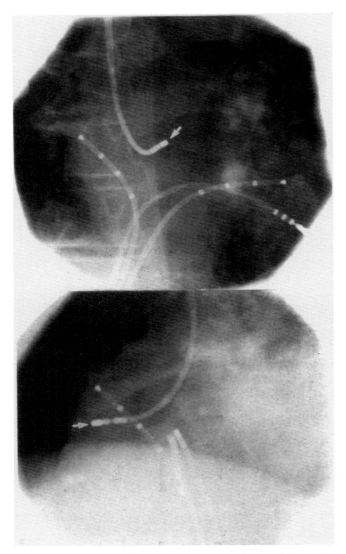

FIGURE 7-7. The ablation catheter is advanced from the right internal jugular vein to achieve better contact in a patient with right anterolateral accessory pathway. Right anterior oblique *(top)* and left anterior oblique *(bottom)* projections are shown.

sheaths. The long sheaths have different distal curves to aid in obtaining catheter tip positioning at different locations along the tricuspid annulus. In rare circumstances, catheter stability may be better suited on the ventricular side of the tricuspid annulus. The mapping catheter is placed across the tricuspid valve annulus and looped back under the tricuspid valve. Positioning of the tip is then adjusted according to the local atrial and ventricular intracardiac signals.

Mapping catheter placement is guided by the use of fluoroscopy in conjunction with intracardiac electrogram criteria. Typically, mapping is performed in the left anterior oblique view, and the tricuspid annulus is depicted as a face of a clock: His bundle area (2 o'clock), coronary sinus os (5 o'clock), right posterior wall (6 o'clock), right lateral wall (9 o'clock), and the right anterior wall (12 o'clock). Using this technique for localization is limited by high radiation exposure, a lack of precise catheter localization, the inability to view the endocardial anatomic structures of the heart, and the failure to recreate the heart in a three-dimensional manner. A novel mapping technique may improve the precision of target site localization and reduce radiation exposure. The CARTO system acquires, analyzes, and displays electroanatomic maps of the heart chambers with minimal use of fluoroscopy (36) (Fig. 7-8). With the aid of a magnetic field, it is possible to reconstruct the anatomy of the cardiac chambers with superimposed electrical activation. The ability to return the catheter to a specific target site in a precise manner and the ability to define the location of the AV node–His bundle system makes this technique an attractive alternative to fluoroscopy for mapping and ablation of right free wall accessory pathways (37). The CARTO system is also useful in locating unusual accessory pathways such as the right atrial appendage to right ventricular connections (Fig. 7-9).

Electrophysiologic Criteria of Catheter Ablation Target Site

Electrogram patterns predictive of successful catheter ablation of accessory pathways have been reported extensively in the literature (38–42). During preexcitation, the site of earliest ventricular activation should be localized. Characteristics of bipolar electrograms at the successful site for right free wall accessory pathways include a short local AV interval (<50 msec), local ventricular activation preceding the onset of the surface ECG delta wave, and the presence of electrical accessory pathway potentials (40,41) between the atrial and ventricular electrograms. Accessory pathway potentials represent electrical signals measured directly from the accessory pathway and should precede the onset of the delta wave. Some accessory pathways may have widely separated atrial and ven-

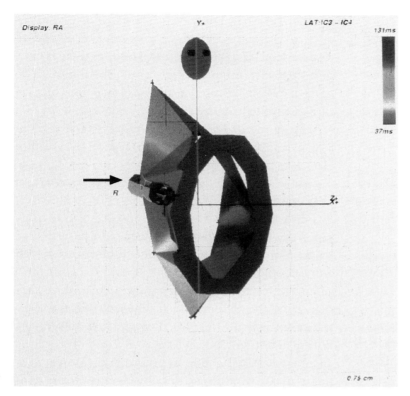

FIGURE 7-8. Electroanatomic (CARTO) map (gray scale) in a patient with right free wall accessory pathway. The map is displayed in the right anterior oblique view. The atrial activation was mapped along the right AV groove during right ventricular pacing. The tricuspid annulus is shown as a ring. The earliest activation area *(arrow)* is shown. With this system, the catheter tip is visualized on the map, facilitating navigation to the target area.

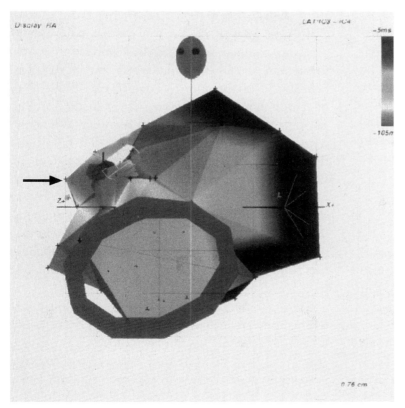

FIGURE 7-9. Electroanatomic map (gray scale) of a patient with an accessory pathway between the right atrial appendage and right ventricle. The map is shown in left anterior oblique view, with the tricuspid annulus marked as a ring. During right ventricular pacing, the earliest atrial activation was recorded in the right atrial appendage *(arrow)*, and ablation at this site eliminated the accessory pathway.

tricular insertion sites. The accessory pathway potential may represent the ideal target site. This is less of an issue for right free wall accessory pathways because they do not usually traverse the annulus in an oblique manner. The unipolar electrogram demonstrating a QS morphology of the local ventricular signal has also been associated with a high success rate (42). Caution is advised if using the shortest AV interval criteria alone. If the local ventricular activation time compared with the delta wave onset is late, it most likely represents an unsuccessful site for ablation, especially for right anteroseptal and right lateral accessory pathways.

If no antegrade conduction is present, mapping of the earliest atrial activation can be performed during orthodromic reciprocating tachycardia or ventricular pacing using a rate at which conduction occurs exclusively over the accessory pathway. Target sites are identified by a short local VA interval and the presence of an accessory pathway potential. Continuous electrical activity involving the local atrial and ventricular electrograms can also serve as a reasonable site of ablation. The continuous activity is generated by fragmentation of atrial or ventricular signals, fusion of the atrial and ventricular signals, or localization of an accessory pathway potential. However, fragmentation of local electrograms at target sites where previously failed ablation attempts have been performed can appear to possess some of the electrogram criteria for successful ablation. Detailed mapping should be performed along the entire annulus before the delivery of radiofrequency energy at a specific site is initiated. Close review of the local electrograms should be done during tachycardia and in sinus rhythm to ensure adequate atrial-ventricular (A/V) ratios.

Radiofrequency Catheter Ablation

Radiofrequency catheter ablation can be performed after the precise location of the accessory pathway has been determined and catheter stability has been achieved. Catheter stability can be assessed by the stability of the fluoroscopic position, stability of the electrogram signals, or by performing pacing thresholds from the electrode tip. The electrogram morphology reflects catheter stability when there is less than 10% variation in the atrial or ventricular electrogram amplitudes between consecutive beats (39). Radiofrequency current is delivered between the tip of the catheter and a patch electrode placed on the patient's skin, typically along the right posterior thorax. The current can be delivered in a fixed-power or temperature-controlled mode.

During the delivery of radiofrequency current, in a small rim of adjacent tissue surrounding the ablation electrode the temperature increases by volume heating with all further tissue heating being the result of heat conduction into the tissue and convective heat loss into the blood. To provide adequate tissue heating, a significant amount of power must be delivered over a period of time to the tissue. Unfortunately, the amount of power is limited by coagulum formation, a sudden impedance rise, and interruption of current delivery if the temperature at the electrode-tissue interface exceeds 100°C (43). Temperature monitoring during radiofrequency delivery can avoid overheating and coagulum formation by adjusting the power output to maintain adequate but not excessive tissue temperatures (44). The use of temperature-controlled ablation is also helpful because the temperature at the electrode tissue interface can predict radiofrequency tissue injury and lesion volume. Although irreversible tissue damage occurs at a temperature of 50°C (43), a mean of 62°C is required to permanently destroy accessory pathway function (44). Temperature monitoring can also assess catheter stability. If a sudden decrease in temperature occurs during the delivery of radiofrequency current, a change in the catheter position is the most likely explanation. When the temperature during radiofrequency delivery is less than 50°C, catheter tip contact may be inadequate. In this situation, switching to a higher power output or repositioning of the catheter is necessary to ensure adequate lesion formation. Conversely, if a temperature greater than 60°C is achieved without elimination of accessory pathway function, repeated applications of radiofrequency current at that site are unlikely to succeed.

During temperature-controlled ablation, the target temperature is usually set at 65°C to 70°C. Coagulum formation generally has not been observed at temperatures of 70°C (45). The time required for the temperature to reach 90% of steady state is 2.2 ± 3 seconds (44). If accessory pathway conduction persists or if the tachycardia does not terminate after the delivery of radiofrequency current for 10 to 15 seconds, the delivery of current is stopped. Additional mapping is then required to find an effective target site. If tachycardia terminates or accessory pathway block occurs, the delivery of radiofrequency current should be continued for approximately 30 to 60 seconds at that site. It is not uncommon to see transient accessory pathway block during radiofrequency current delivery, especially with right free wall accessory pathways. Remapping of the area should be performed to ensure adequate tissue contact and stable catheter positioning. After successful ablation, the patient is generally monitored for 30 to 60 minutes to determine whether the accessory pathway function recurs and additional radiofrequency applications are needed. Patients are usually ambulatory 4 to 6 hours after the procedure. Depending on the level of sedation used, patients are discharged the same day or admitted for overnight observation.

Results

The initial success, recurrence, and complication rates from nine trials are summarized in Table 7-1. The success rates of ablation for left free wall accessory pathways are higher (97%) compared with right free wall accessory pathways (92%). The recurrence rate after ablation for left free wall accessory pathways (5%) is lower than for right free wall accessory pathways (14%). Although the complications were not subdivided among the different accessory pathways locations, complication rates were very low (0% to 5%). The incidence of right free wall accessory pathways (16%) was much lower than septal (27%) and left free wall accessory pathways (57%). The success rate of a second ablation after initial recurrence was high (90% to 93%) (40–42).

Previous studies have identified factors associated with initial failure and recurrence of accessory pathway function (46–48). Reasons for initial failure of ablation include the inability to position the ablation catheter at the effective target site, instability of the ablation catheter at the target site, errors in accessory pathway localization, and the presence of an epicardial accessory pathway. Problems of maintaining catheter stability during initial procedural failure were much more common with accessory pathways located in the right free wall compared with other locations. Unstable local atrial and ventricular electrograms and prolonged time (>12 seconds) for accessory pathway conduction block during delivery of radiofrequency current were independent predictors of recurrence. Recurrence of conduction also occurred more commonly with right-sided accessory pathways. In patients undergoing a second or third radiofrequency procedure, errors in accessory pathway localization can be caused by the previously failed, ineffective tar-

TABLE 7-1 • INITIAL SUCCESS, RECURRENCE, AND COMPLICATION RATES WITH RADIOFREQUENCY CATHETER ABLATION OF ACCESSORY PATHWAYS

Study	Initial Success			Recurrence			Complication Rate (%)
	RFW	Septal	LFW	RFW	Septal	LFW	
Jackman (3)	15/15	53/56	106/106	2/15	8/56	5/105	1.8
Schluter (2)	9/11	24/28	49/57	3/11	0/28	0/57	3.3
Leather (7)	8/16	10/18	45/47	8/16	8/18	12/47	5.3
Lesh (5)	17/21	36/43	44/45	2/17	4/36	2/44	4
Calkins (4)	46/47	54/59	152/161	NA	NA	NA	4
Chen (8)	25/27	40/43	63/69	2/27	3/43	6/69	NA
Kay (6)	57/62	114/123	186/187	5/57	10/123	4/186	1.1
Wang (9)	41/41	34/34	164/164	7/41	2/34	6/164	0.01
Iesaka (10)	23/23	26/28	84/84	1/23	0/28	0/84	0
Total	241/263 (92%)	391/432 (91%)	893/920 (97%)	27/207 (14%)	35/366 (10%)	35/756 (5%)	

RFW, right free wall; LFW, left free wall; NA, data not available.

get sites appearing as fractionated signals. The fractionated signals can masquerade as accessory pathway potentials.

When the primary reason for recurrence or primary failure is a result of unstable catheter positioning, stability can be improved with the use of long intravascular sheaths or switching to a different venous approach. The use of the CARTO system can aid the electrophysiologist in defining the precise accessory pathway localization and positioning the catheter at the effective target site (37). Using this system, mapping and reconstruction of the entire tricuspid valve annulus with delineation of the earliest sites of activation can be performed. The system allows visualization of the catheter movement during ablation and the ability to return the catheter to a specific site. Catheter position at the beginning and the end of the ablation can be confirmed. Repeated applications of energy at a previously unsuccessful ablation site can be avoided. If the catheter is dislodged during ablation and there is loss of accessory pathway function, the catheter can be returned to the same precise location for additional deliveries of energy.

Associated Congenital Anomalies

Certain types of congenital heart disease are commonly associated with accessory pathways. L-transposition of the great arteries, hypertrophic cardiomyopathy, and Ebstein's anomaly have been associated with the presence of accessory pathways. Of the three, Ebstein's anomaly is by far the most common. Tachycardias using an accessory pathway have been reported in 25% to 30% of patients with Ebstein's anomaly with ventricular preexcitation present on the surface ECG in approximately 10% to 25% (49). In patients with Ebstein's anomaly, absence of RBBB pattern should alert the physician to the possible presence of accessory pathway. In patients with Ebstein's anomaly, the accessory pathways are often multiple (reported as high as 50%) and are typically right sided (50). The most common accessory pathway location in patients with Ebstein's anomaly is right posteroseptal. However, the combination of a right free wall and posteroseptal accessory pathways is also common.

Ebstein's anomaly is a congenital malformation characterized by the downward displacement of the tricuspid valve leaflets into the right ventricle (51). The septal and posterior tricuspid leaflets are usually deformed and attach to the right ventricular wall rather than to the atrioventricular ring. The anterosuperior leaflet is usually larger than normal. A portion of the right ventricle therefore lies between the displaced atrioventricular ring and the origin of the valve at the level of the tricuspid annulus (Fig. 7-10). This segment is "atrialized," resulting in only a small distal

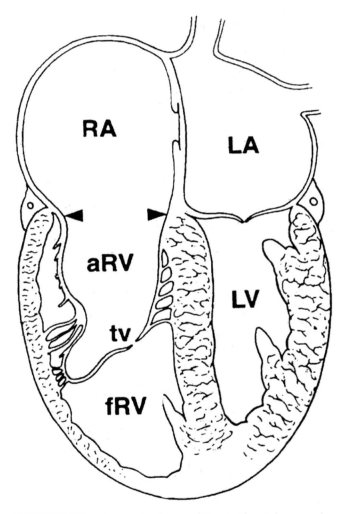

FIGURE 7-10. Anatomic abnormalities in Ebstein's anomaly. Notice the downward displacement of the tricuspid valve into the right ventricle, creating an "atrialized portion of the right ventricle" (aRV) and a smaller distal functional right ventricle (fRV). LA, left atrium; LV, left ventricle; RA, right atrium; TV, tricuspid valve annulus. (From Armstrong WF. Congenital heart disease. In: Feigenbaum H, ed. *Echocardiography*, 4th ed. Malvern, PA: Lea & Febiger, 1986:365–461, with permission.)

functional right ventricular chamber. Significant tricuspid regurgitation, right atrial enlargement, and other coexisting anomalies such as an atrial septal defect and pulmonic atresia or stenosis may also be present.

From a catheter ablation standpoint, successful elimination of accessory pathway function can be quite challenging. The accessory pathway traverses the anatomic annulus irrespective of the right ventricular location of the tricuspid valve. Unfortunately, mapping of the dysplastic tricuspid valve tissue can produce highly fractionated electrograms, resulting in difficulty discerning atrial from ventricular electrograms and isolating effective ablation target sites (53). The combination of the downward displacement of the tricuspid valve and the presence of significant tricuspid regurgitation can result in tenuous catheter stability along the atrioventricular groove. The fluoroscopic identification of the atrioventricular groove can also be challenging. The inability to achieve adequate catheter tip temperature during radiofrequency ablation despite maximum power can occur as a result of the atrialized right ventricle (54). Patients with Ebstein's anomaly can have multiple accessory pathways and have a tendency for developing recurrent atrial fibrillation during the electrophysiologic study.

Long intravascular sheaths, temperature-controlled ablation catheters, multiple venous approaches, and special 2-Fr mapping catheters for deployment in the right coronary artery (Fig. 7-11) to aid atrioventricular groove mapping and localization have been employed during catheter ablative procedures for patients with Ebstein's anomaly (53). Several groups of investigators have reported their experience with catheter ablation of accessory pathways in Ebstein's anomaly (Table 7-2). Cappato and associates (53) studied 21 patients with a total of 34 right-sided accessory pathways. Eleven (52%) of the 21 patients had multiple accessory pathways. In 10 patients (14 accessory pathways), normal endocardial electrograms with distinct atrial and ventricular deflections were present

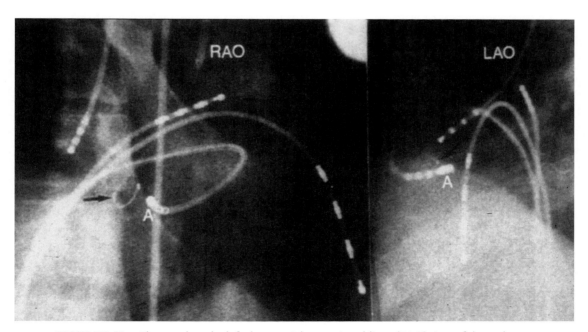

FIGURE 7-11. The panel on the left shows a right anterior oblique (RAO) view of the catheters during a right-sided accessory pathway ablation. Catheters are placed in the right ventricular apex, His bundle position, high right atrium, and the ablation catheter at the right AV groove. The arrow shows a guide wire in the right coronary artery, which helps with identification of the AV groove. To achieve better contact, the ablation catheter is advanced into the right ventricle and then retroflexed. The panel on the right shows the same image in the left anterior oblique (LAO) projection.

TABLE 7-2 • EBSTEIN'S ANOMALY: RESULTS OF RADIOFREQUENCY ABLATION

Study	Patients (n)	No. Of AP	Multiple AP	Initial Success			Recurrence		
				RFW	Septal	LFW	RFW	Septal	LFW
Cappato et al. (53)	21	34	11/21	86% (11/22)	83% (10/12)	0	25% (4/16)		0
Pediatric Registry (81)	65	82	21/65	79% (41/52)	89% (24/27)	75% (5/20)	25%	26%	20%
Okishige et al. (55)	4	7	3/4	100% (7/7)		0	0	0	0

AP, accessory pathways; RFW, right free wall; LFW, left free wall.

at all sites along the tricuspid valve annulus. Successful elimination of accessory pathway function was achieved in all 10 patients. In the remaining 11 patients (20 accessory pathways), abnormal fractionated electrograms could only be identified along the atrialized right ventricle. Atrial stimulation techniques and right coronary artery mapping were helpful in identifying successful target sites. Fourteen of the 20 accessory pathways with abnormal electrograms were successfully ablated for a total of 28 (82%) of 34 accessory pathways. At 22 ± 12 months, 4 (25%) of 16 patients with initial ablative success had recurrence. Factors accountable for failure included accessory pathways located along the atrialized right ventricle and the presence of abnormal fractionated endocardial signals. Okishige and colleagues (55) reported successful radiofrequency catheter ablation of eight accessory pathways (one Mahaim) in four patients with Ebstein's anomaly. All accessory pathways were right sided and successfully ablated at the atrioventricular annulus and not along the atrialized right ventricular. At 14 ± 4 months, no arrhythmias had recurred. As shown in Table 7-2, similar results were reported in the Pediatric Registry.

ATRIOFASCICULAR OR MAHAIM ACCESSORY PATHWAYS

Historical Perspectives and Definition

Mahaim first described fibers of conductive tissue serving as discrete anatomic connections between the normal AV node and the ventricles (56). Patients with Mahaim fibers represented a unique and rare form of preexcitation syndrome, exhibiting slow and decremental antegrade conduction with minimal preexcitation during sinus rhythm and no retrograde conduction across the accessory pathway. During tachycardia however, full preexcitation with a left bundle branch morphology occurs (Fig. 7-12). In 1971, Wellens proposed the concept of a nodoventricular connection to explain the electrophysiologic properties associated with this preexcitation syndrome (57). In 1975, Anderson and coworkers subsequently proposed a classification of the Mahaim fibers based on their anatomic and functional properties with nodoventricular pathways connecting the AV node to the ventricle, nodofascicular pathways connecting the AV node to the fascicle, and fasciculoventricular fibers connecting the fascicles to the ventricle (58).

It was not until 1982 that the true location of these fibers was delineated. Gillette and associates reported a series of patients with clinical and electrophysiologic characteristics suggesting a nodoventricular fiber (59). However, successful surgical ablation of the accessory connection occurred along the right anterior epicardial tricuspid valve annulus. Subsequent intraoperative and surgical ablative studies demonstrated that patients who were clinically diagnosed with a Mahaim fiber usually had atriofascicular pathways connecting the right atrium to the distal right bundle branch or, less commonly, an atrioventricular connection with decremental conduction at the level of the tricuspid valve (60,61). With the development of catheter ablative procedures and the need for precise accessory pathway localization, it became clear that the clinical and electrophysiologic presentation previously ascribed to nodoventricular Mahaim fibers were instead mainly atriofascicular connections. The anatomic course of these pathways was generally long, with the atrial insertion at variable locations along the tricuspid atrioventricular ring and the ventricular

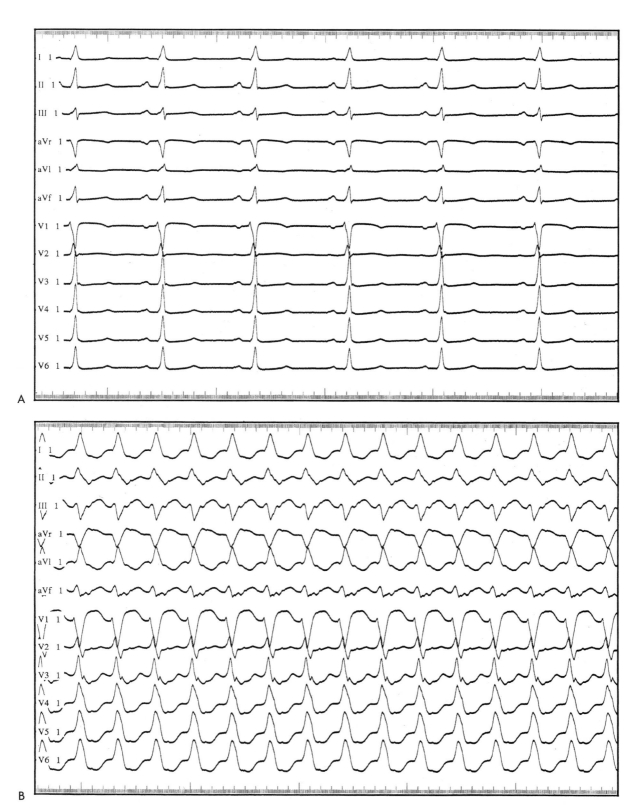

FIGURE 7-12. Electrocardiograms recorded during normal sinus rhythm **(A)** and antidromic AV reentrant tachycardia (AVRT) using a right atriofascicular pathway **(B)**. Notice the minimal ventricular preexcitation during normal sinus rhythm. During AVRT, the QRS has typical left bundle branch block morphology, with short RP (160 msec) and long PR (200 msec) intervals.

insertion at the apical right ventricular region near or at the distal right bundle branch (62–68). A smaller number of Mahaim fibers inserted into the basal right ventricle near the tricuspid valve annulus (Fig. 7-13). Not much evidence supports the existence of functional nodoventricular or nodofascicular fibers (66,69,70). The term Mahaim fibers is replaced in the remaining portions of this chapter with the term atriofascicular pathways or atrioventricular pathways with decremental antegrade conduction.

Clinical and Electrocardiographic Features

Atriofascicular pathways are not common, representing less than 3% of all accessory pathways (71). Patients with atriofascicular pathways tend to be young, with and without structurally normal hearts. There is an association with Ebstein's anomaly of the tricuspid valve (72,73). Dual AV nodal pathways and other accessory pathways have also been reported (67).

Preexcitation on the surface 12-lead ECG during sinus rhythm is typically minimal or absent, with preferential activation of the ventricle through the AV node. However, the surface 12-lead ECG in a patient with an atriofascicular pathway and antidromic AV reentrant tachycardia (AVRT) has several distinctive features: left bundle branch block (LBBB) morphology with a QRS duration generally equal to or less than 150 msec, superior axis or axis between 0 and 75 degrees, presence of an R wave in lead I, presence of an rS in lead V_1, and a QRS transition at or after V_4 (74) (Fig. 7-12).

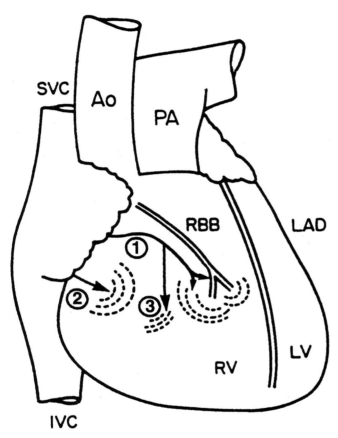

FIGURE 7-13. Right atriofascicular accessory pathway. In most patients, the distal end inserts into the apical region of the right ventricle (RV) free wall, close to the distal component of the right bundle branch (RBB) (1). However, even in such cases, mapping along the tricuspid annulus identifies a region with a shorter AV interval, suggesting the existence of branches proximal to the distal insertion into the right bundle (3). In rare cases, the decremental accessory pathway travels only a short distance and inserts at the base of the RV at the level of the annulus (2). (Adapted from Klein GJ, Guiraudon GM, Kerr CR, et al. "Nodoventricular" accessory pathway: evidence for a distinct accessory atrioventricular pathway with AV node–like properties. *J Am Coll Cardiol* 1988;11:1035–1040, with permission.)

Electrophysiologic Testing

Several unique features of atriofascicular pathways have been demonstrated during electrophysiologic studies. Usually, only antegrade conduction occurs. Conduction over the accessory pathway demonstrates AV node–like decremental properties. Prolongation of the A-to-delta interval can be demonstrated with atrial extrastimuli or incremental atrial pacing (Fig. 7-14). A preexcited pattern consisting of a LBBB morphology can be elicited by right atrial pacing. The preexcited QRS pattern during atrial pacing is similar to the preexcitation present during antidromic AVRT. A more marked degree of preexcitation typically occurs with right atrial pacing compared with left atrial pacing at similar pacing rates, which is consistent with the usual location of these accessory pathways along the anterolateral aspect of the tricuspid valve annulus.

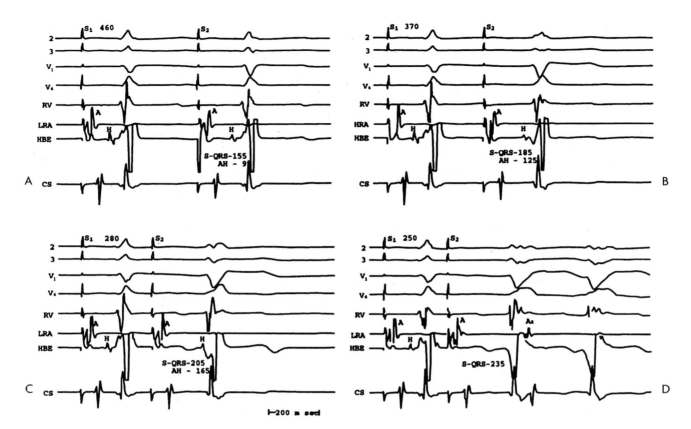

FIGURE 7-14. Intracavitary recordings during premature atrial stimuli (S$_2$) introduced at progressively shorter coupling intervals in a patient with atriofascicular pathway. As the atrial extrastimulus becomes more premature, there is prolongation of the AH interval and merging of the His deflection into the QRS complex, which becomes progressively more preexcited. The S-QRS interval is prolonged, indicating the decremental properties of the pathway **(A, B, and C)**. At a critical CI, a reentrant atrial echo beat (A$_E$) is induced, with the QRS being fully preexcited. The anterograde limb of this reentrant cycle is the accessory pathway, and the retrograde limb is the normal AV conduction system **(D)**. CS, coronary sinus; HBE, His bundle electrogram; LRA, low right atrium; RV, right ventricle; 2, 3, V$_1$, V$_6$, electrocardiographic leads. (From Reich J, Auld D, Hulse E, et al. The pediatric radiofrequency ablation registry's experience with Ebstein's Anomaly. *J Cardiovasc Electrophysiol* 1998;9:1370–1377, with permission.)

At a critical coupling interval, antidromic AVRT with a LBBB pattern can be induced. Earliest ventricular activation from intracardiac recordings during antidromic AVRT occurs at the right ventricular apical catheter with activation at or before the onset of the surface ECG QRS. RBB activation precedes the His bundle activation as antegrade conduction occurs over the atriofascicular pathway with retrograde conduction over the normal AV node conduction system. A short VA interval usually occurs as retrograde atrial activation begins near the end of the QRS complex. A shift in the His bundle activation from the onset of the surface QRS to late in the QRS may be seen if transient retrograde right bundle branch block develops during the tachycardia (Fig. 7-15).

Because of the association between atriofascicular pathways and dual AV nodal pathways as well as other accessory pathways, antidromic AVRT should be distinguished from AVNRT or atrial tachycardia with bystander accessory pathway activation (Fig. 7-16). An electrical activation sequence showing the RBB activation preceding the His bundle activation during

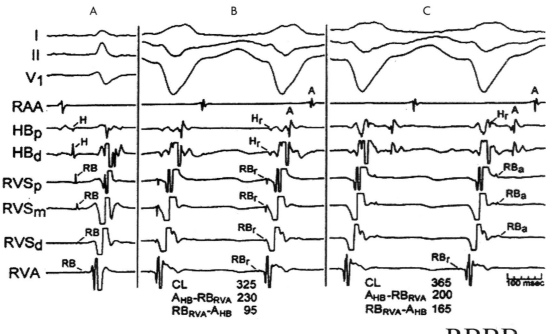

FIGURE 7-15. Intracardiac electrograms during sinus rhythm (**A**), antidromic atrioventricular (AV) reentrant tachycardia using an atriofascicular pathway without right bundle branch block (**B**), and after development of right bundle branch block (**C**). RVS, right ventricular septum; p, proximal; m, middle; d, distal. During sinus rhythm, there is antegrade activation from the His to the right bundle (RB). In antidromic AV reentrant tachycardia, there is retrograde activation from the distal RB (RB_r) to the His (H_r) and AV node. The earliest atrial activation is seen in HB_p and occurs before the end of the QRS complex, producing a short VA interval. With the development of right bundle branch block from catheter trauma, the antegrade conduction across the accessory pathway is not interrupted. There is retrograde block in the distal right bundle at the level of RVS_d. The impulse activates the right ventricular apex (RVA), propagates across the interventricular septum, and moves retrogradely over the left bundle branch up to the His bundle and then activates antegradely the right bundle down to the site of the block. This resulted in a 70-msec increase in the RB_{RVA}-A_{HB} interval to 165 msec. This delay in atrial activation resulted in a 30-msec shortening of the conduction time over the right atriofascicular pathway. The overall tachycardia CL was increased by 40 msec to 365 msec. (Adapted from McClelland JH, Wang X, Beckman KJ, et al. Radiofrequency catheter ablation of right atriofascicular [Mahaim] accessory pathways guided by accessory pathway activation potentials. *Circulation* 1994;89:2655–2666, with permission.)

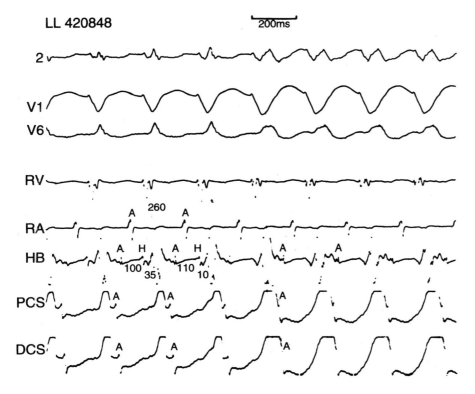

FIGURE 7-16. Intracardiac recordings during reentrant tachycardia with a cycle length of 260 msec. The QRS on the surface ECG tracings becomes more preexcited as the AH interval prolongs and the His recording merges into the QRS complex. The earliest retrograde activation is at the proximal coronary sinus (PCS) recording, suggesting an orthodromic AV reentrant tachycardia using a posteroseptal pathway as the retrograde limb with a bystander atriofascicular connection. HB, His bundle recording; PCS and DCS, proximal and distal coronary sinus recordings; V_2, V_1, V_6, electrocardiographic leads; RA, right atrial electrogram; RV, right ventricular electrogram. (From Natale A, Klein G, Yee R. Preexcitation update. In: Fisch C, Surawicz B, eds. *Current topics in cardiology*. New York: Elsevier Science Publishing, 1991, with permission.)

tachycardia favors antidromic AVRT (Fig. 7-17). Introduction of an atrial extrastimulus that does not advance the atrial activation and terminates the tachycardia excludes the possibility of an atrial tachycardia with bystander accessory pathway activation. An atrial extrastimulus that does not advance septal atrial activation but preexcites the ventricle with the same activation sequence is diagnostic of the presence of an atriofascicular accessory pathway. Moreover, if the tachycardia is reset, the accessory pathway is involved in the reentrant circuit (Fig. 7-18). Adenosine can induce conduction block in the accessory pathway, suggesting AV node–like properties for these atriofascicular connections (Fig. 7-19). This has also been confirmed in histopathologic analysis of specimens obtained from surgical cases, demonstrating the presence of AV node–like cells along the tricuspid atrioventricular groove.

Atrioventricular accessory pathways with decremental properties along the tricuspid valve region may have electrophysiologic features similar to an atriofascicular pathway. The major difference is the insertion of the accessory pathway into the right ventricle at the level of the annulus. During atrial pacing or antidromic AVRT, the earliest ventricular activation occurs near the tricuspid valve annulus. Right ventricular apical and His bundle activation occurs late after the onset of the surface QRS complex. The development of RBBB during the tachycardia increases the cycle length and the local VA interval with an atrioventricular and atriofascicular accessory pathway.

Intracardiac Mapping and Radiofrequency Catheter Ablation

Technique

For the most part, the technique of ablation of right free wall accessory pathways summarized in the Intracardiac Mapping section is the same technique used for ablation of atriofascicular pathways. The ablation catheter is advanced to the tricuspid valve annulus typically from a femoral vein approach. Long intravascular sheaths are recommended to aid in catheter stability. Delivery of radiofrequency energy would be performed during atrial pacing or tachycardia.

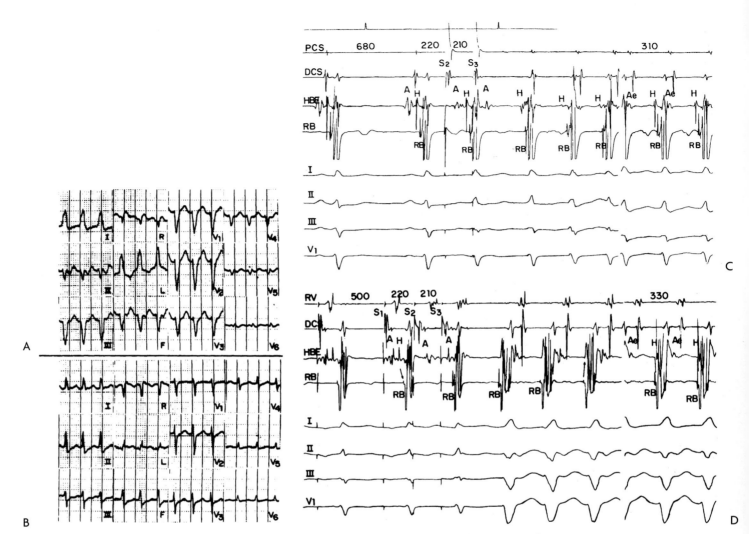

FIGURE 7-17. Electrocardiographic (left) and intracardiac (right) tracings from a patient exhibiting wide (A, top) and narrow (B, bottom) QRS tachycardias. The narrow QRS tachycardia appeared to be AV node reentry (C). During tachycardia, the His bundle electrogram (H) preceded the right bundle electrogram (RB). In the same patient, during wide QRS tachycardia (D) with left bundle branch block and left axis QRS morphology, the RB activation occurred before the His bundle recording. This is consistent with an antidromic tachycardia using an atriofascicular pathway. RV, right ventricular electrogram; DCS, distal coronary sinus; HBE, His bundle electrogram; A, atrial electrogram; PCS, proximal coronary sinus; surface lead I, II, III, V_1.

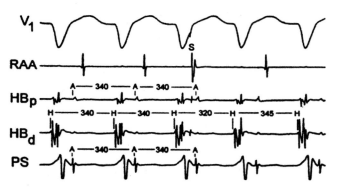

FIGURE 7-18. A right atrial extrastimulus delivered during antidromic AV reentrant tachycardia (AVRT) preexcited the ventricle by 20 msec without advancing the septal atrial electrogram (HB_p) (i.e., without penetrating the AV node). This is consistent with an accessory pathway with a right atrial connection (i.e., right atriofascicular accessory pathway) and excludes a nodoventricular pathway. (From Tchou P, Lehman MH, Jazayeri M, Akhtar M. Atriofascicular connection or a nodoventricular Mahaim fiber? Electrophysiologic elucidation of the pathway and associated reentrant circuit. *Circulation* 1988;77:837–848, with permission.)

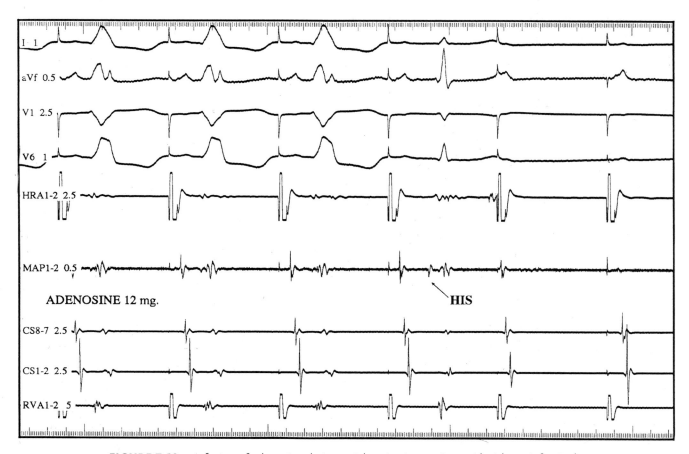

FIGURE 7-19. Infusion of adenosine during atrial pacing in a patient with right atriofascicular bypass tract. The MAP catheter is in the HIS position. There is antegrade block in the accessory pathway (4th complex) followed by a block in the AV node (5th complex). Right atriofascicular bypass tracts have AV node–like behavior and exhibit conduction block in response to adenosine.

Electrophysiologic Criteria of Catheter Ablation Site

The absence of retrograde conduction through the atriofascicular pathway mandates that mapping be performed during atrial pacing or antidromic AVRT. Because the distal insertion site of the atriofascicular pathway is located near the RBB in most patients, mapping for earliest ventricular activation at the level of the tricuspid annulus is futile. However, mapping for the shortest AV interval may help in confining the area of interest to a region of the tricuspid annulus. This finding could be consistent with branching of the atriofascicular pathway at sites proximal to the distal insertion (Fig. 7-13).

Other mapping techniques have aided the identification of an effective target site for ablation. Atrial pace mapping at the level of the tricuspid valve annulus has been used in an attempt to locate the atrial insertion site of the atriofascicular pathway (75). This is achieved by measuring the stimulus to delta wave interval at multiple right atrial sites until the shortest interval is found. The introduction of a late premature atrial stimulus from the ablation catheter during tachycardia to determine the site that results in the greatest advance in the timing of the next QRS complex has also been used in the past (64). Unfortunately, both strategies are technically difficult, relatively imprecise, and tedious. Cappato and colleagues described induction of mechanical conduction block by bumping the ablation catheter tip against the atrial insertion site of the atriofascicular pathway (68). Radiofrequency energy was delivered at the site of mechanical block after preexcitation returned. The possibility of causing significant trauma to the target site, resulting in loss of preexcitation for an extended period and loss of catheter stability while waiting for the resumption of preexcitation limits the usefulness of the technique. Localization of the atrial insertion site by mapping for the presence of accessory pathway or Kent potentials has been the most effective strategy for identifying an effective target site (65–67) (Figs. 7-20 and 7-21). Mapping of these potentials is performed along the tricuspid valve annulus of the right free wall. At the atrial insertion site, distinct atrial, accessory pathway, and ventricular potentials are present, usually separated by long isoelectric intervals.

Results

The results of radiofrequency catheter ablation of accessory pathways with decremental antegrade conduction from eight series of patients are shown in Table 7-3. The overall success rate approaches 95%, with no reported complications and a 2% chance of recurrence. Most accessory pathways (83 [83%] of 99) appear to be atriofascicular. The accessory pathways were right sided, with most present along the free wall

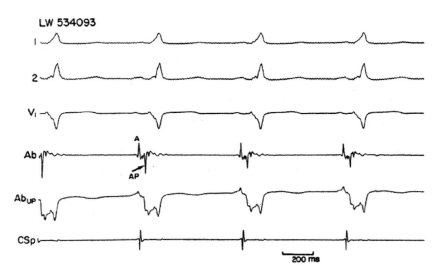

FIGURE 7-20. Recording of accessory pathway potential in a patient with a right-sided pathway with decremental properties (Mahaim-like) and distal insertion close to the tricuspid annulus. The ablation catheter is positioned along the lateral border of the tricuspid annulus. Unipolar (Ab_{up}) and bipolar (Ab) recordings are displayed. There is a distinct His-like accessory pathway potential that precedes the QRS onset and coincides with the negative deflection on the unipolar recording. Application of radiofrequency energy at this site eliminated accessory pathway conduction. (From Li HG, Klein GJ, Yee R, et al. Radiofrequency ablation of decremental accessory pathways mimicking "nodoventricular" conduction. *Am J Cardiol* 1994;74:829–833, with permission.)

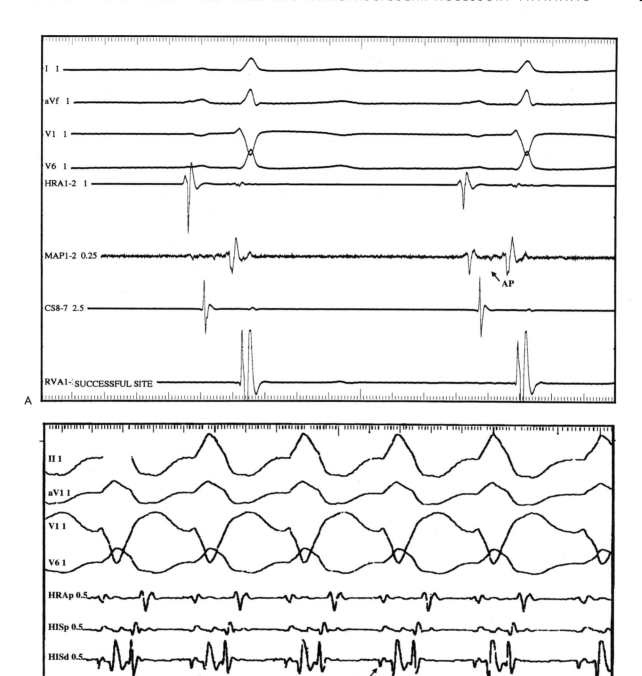

FIGURE 7-21. Recordings during sinus rhythm (A) and wide QRS antidromic tachycardia using an atriofascicular pathway (B). The mapping catheter (MAP 1-2) is at 9 o'clock along the tricuspid annulus. A distinct accessory pathway potential is observed 50 msec before onset of the QRS (A). The same potential (AP) is observed during antidromic tachycardia (ABL 1-2) and appeared to precede the HIS bundle recording (B). Radiofrequency ablation at this site eliminated accessory pathway conduction.

TABLE 7-3 • OUTCOME OF RADIOFREQUENCY CATHETER ABLATION OF RIGHT-SIDED ACCESSORY PATHWAYS WITH ANTEGRADE DECREMENTAL CONDUCTION

Study	Date	Patients (n)	AF	AV	Success (%)	Complications	Recurrence (%)	Mapping Techniques
Klein (64)	1993	4	3	1	4 (100%)	0	0	Stim to Δ interval
McClelland (65)	1994	26	23	3	26 (100%)	0	0	Mahaim potentials
Grogin (66)	1994	6	4	2	6 (100%)	0	0	Mahaim potentials
Cappato (68)	1994	11	11	—	9 (82%)	0	1 (10%)	Mechanical block
Heald (67)	1995	20	16	4	18 (90%)	0	1 (5%)	Mahaim potentials
Li (78)	1994	4	3	1	4 (100%)	0	0	Mahaim potentials
Haissaguerre (62)	1995	21	17[a]	4	21 (100%)	0	0	Mahaim potentials/V side
Okishige (63)	1997	7	6	1	6 (85%)	0	0	Mahaim potentials/stim to Δ interval
Total		99	83	16	94 (95%)	0	2 (2%)	

AF, atriofascicular accessory pathways; AV, atrioventricular accessory pathways.
[a] Seven patients demonstrated distal accessory pathway insertion in the anterior right ventricle several centimeters below the tricuspid valve annulus and away from the right bundle branch system.

(Fig. 7-22). No left-sided, decrementally antegrade-conducting accessory pathways were identified. However, isolated case reports of successful radiofrequency ablation of left free wall, decrementally conducting atrioventricular accessory pathways have been published (76). Rare atriofascicular pathways with the atrial insertion in the posterior and posteroseptal region of the right atrium can also be encountered (Fig. 7-23).

CONCLUSIONS

Right free wall accessory pathways represent an important subset of atrioventricular connections. Although less common than left-sided and septal accessory pathways, radiofrequency catheter ablation of right free wall accessory pathways generally have lower success and higher recurrence rates compared with ablation of other accessory pathways. Because of anatomic differences between the tricuspid valve and mitral valve annulus, a higher incidence of multiple accessory pathways, and the association with congenital heart disease such as Ebstein's anomaly, radiofrequency catheter ablation of right free wall accessory pathways can sometimes represent a technical challenge. With improved catheter technology and a better understanding of the pathophysiologic features associated with right free wall accessory pathways, success rates will continue to improve. Newer mapping techniques allowing three-dimensional reconstruction of the tricuspid valve annulus and precise catheter localization can facilitate procedural success and reduce radiation exposure.

Patients with atriofascicular pathways or atrioventricular accessory pathways with antegrade decremental conduction only represent a rare form of ventricu-

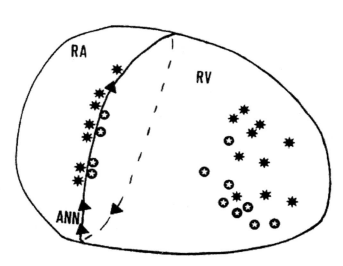

FIGURE 7-22. Right anterior oblique view of types of anterograde, decrementally conducting accessory pathways. Black stars and white stars on a black background represent the long AV accessory pathways. Triangles indicate the short AV accessory pathways. ANN, annulus; RA, right atrium; RV, right ventricle. (From Haissaguerre M, Cauchemez B, Marcus F, et al. Characteristics of the ventricular insertion sites of accessory pathways with anterograde decremental conduction properties. *Circulation* 1995;91:1077–1085, with permission.)

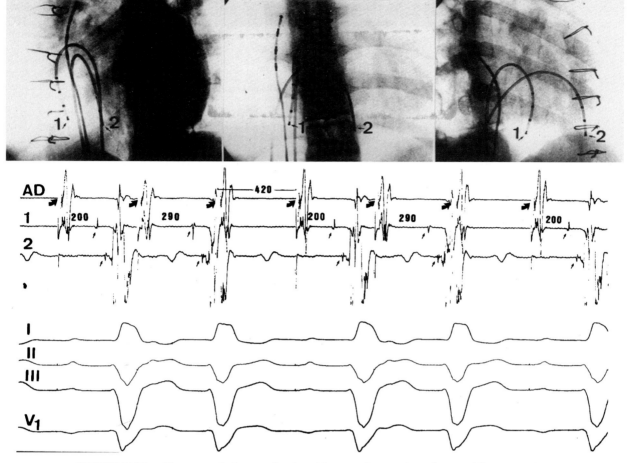

FIGURE 7-23. Fluoroscopic images *(top)* and intracardiac tracings *(bottom)* from a patient with an atriofascicular pathway. Catheters are placed in the high right atrium (RA), right bundle branch recording (2), and in the posterior region of the tricuspid annulus (1). Recordings from the distal electrode pair of catheter number 1 show a His-like accessory pathway potential. During atrial pacing with preexcited QRS, the His-like potential (1) preceded the right bundle recording (2). Progressive prolongation of the RA/His-like potential interval was followed by block above the accessory pathway.

lar preexcitation. In most cases, the accessory pathway inserts proximally along the right atrial free wall, with its distal insertion site at the low right ventricle or in the right bundle branch system. Radiofrequency catheter ablation guided by identification of a Mahaim potential at the level of the tricuspid valve annulus is safe, is highly effective, and offers definitive treatment.

REFERENCES

1. Warin JF, Haissaguerre M, D'ivernois C, et al. Catheter ablation of accessory pathways: technique and results in 248 patients. *Pacing Clin Electrophysiol* 1990;13:1609–1614.
2. Schluter M, Geiger M, Siebels J, et al. Catheter ablation using radiofrequency current to cure symptomatic patients with tachyarrhythmias related to an accessory atrioventricular pathway *Circulation* 1991;84:1644–1661.
3. Jackman WM, Wang X, Friday KJ, et al. Catheter ablation of accessory AV pathways (Wolff-Parkinson-White syndrome) by radiofrequency current. *N Engl J Med* 1991;324:1605–1611.
4. Calkins H, Langberg J, Sousa J, et al. Radiofrequency catheter ablation of accessory atrioventricular connections in 250 patients. *Circulation* 1992;85:1337–1346.
5. Lesh MD, Van Hare G, Schamp DJ, et al. Curative percutaneous catheter ablation using radiofrequency energy for accessory pathways in all locations: results in 100 consecutive patients. *J Am Coll Cardiol* 1992;19:1303–1309.
6. Kay GN, Epstein AE, Dailey SM, et al. Role of radiofrequency ablation in the management of supraventricular arrhythmias: experience in 760 consecutive patients. *J Clin Electrophysiol* 1993;4:372–389.
7. Leather RA, Leitch JW, Klein GJ, et al. Radiofrequency cathe-

ter ablation of accessory pathways: a learning experience. *Am J Cardiol* 1991;68:1651–1655.
8. Chen SA, Chiang CE, Chiou CW, et al. Serial electrophysiologic studies in the late outcome of radiofrequency ablation for accessory atrioventricular pathway mediated tachyarrhythmias. *Eur Heart J* 1993;14:734–743.
9. Wang L, Hu D, Ding Y, et al. Predictors of early and late recurrence of atrioventricular accessory pathway conduction after apparently successful radiofrequency catheter ablation. *Int J Cardiol* 1994;46:61–65.
10. Iesaka Y, Takahashi A, Chun Y, et al. Radiofrequency catheter ablation of atrioventricular accessory pathways in Wolff-Parkinson-White syndrome with drug-refractory and symptomatic supraventricular tachycardia—its high effectiveness irrespective of accessory pathway location and properties. *Jpn Circ J* 1994;58:767–777.
11. Becker AE, Anderson RH. The Wolff-Parkinson-White syndrome and its anatomical substrates. *Anat Rec* 1981;201:169–177.
12. Anderson RH, Yen Ho S. Structure and location of accessory muscular atrioventricular connections. *J Cardiovasc Electrophysiol* 1999;10:1119–1123.
13. Deal BJ, Keana JF, Gillette PC, et al. Wolff-Parkinson-White syndrome and supraventricular tachycardia during infancy: management and follow-up. *J Am Coll Cardiol* 1985;5:130–135.
14. Cox JL, Ferguson TB Jr. Surgery for the Wolff-Parkinson-White syndrome: the endocardial approach. *Semin Thorac Cardiovasc Surg* 1989;1:34–46.
15. Verduyn LAA. Significance of annulus fibrosus of heart in relation to atrioventricular conduction and ventricular activation in cases of Wolff-Parkinson-White syndrome. *Br Heart J* 1972;34:1267–1271.
16. Wood FC, Wolferth CG, Geckler GD. Histologic demonstration of accessory muscular connections between auricle and ventricle in a case of short P-R interval and prolonged QRS complex. *Am Heart J* 1943;25:454–462.
17. Ohnell RF. Preexcitation, a cardiac abnormality. Pathophysiological, patho-anatomical and clinical studies of an excitatory spread phenomenon. *Acta Med Scand* 1944;152[Suppl 1]:167.
18. Gotlieb AI, Chan M, Palmer WH, et al. Ventricular preexcitation syndrome. Accessory left atrioventricular connection and rhabdomyomatous myocardial fibers. *Arch Pathol Lab Med* 1977;101:486–489.
19. Ho SY, Russell G, Rowland E. Coronary venous aneurysms and accessory atrioventricular connections. *Br Heart J* 1988;60:348–351.
20. Goya M, Takahashi A, Nakagawa H, et al. A case of catheter ablation of accessory atrioventricular connection between the right atrial appendage and right ventricle guided by a three-dimensional electroanatomical mapping system. *J Clin Electrophysiol* 1999;10:1112–1118.
21. Durrer D, Roos JP. Epicardial excitation of the ventricles in a patient with a Wolff-Parkinson-White syndrome (type B). *Circulation* 1967;35:15–21.
22. Burchell HB, Frye RL, Anderson MW, et al. Atrioventricular and ventriculoatrial excitation in Wolff-Parkinson-White syndrome (type B): temporary ablation at surgery. *Circulation* 1967;36:663–672.
23. Cobb FR, Blumenschein SD, Sealy WC, et al. Successful surgical interruption of the Bundle of Kent in a patient with Wolff-Parkinson-White syndrome. *Circulation* 1986;38:1018–1029.
24. Gallagher JJ, Selle JG, Svenson RH, et al. Surgical treatment of arrhythmia. *Am J Cardiol* 1988;61:27A–44A.
25. Morady F, Scheinman MM. Transvenous catheter ablation of a posteroseptal accessory pathway in a patient with the Wolff-Parkinson-White syndrome. *N Engl J Med* 1984;310:705–707.
26. Borggrefe M, Budde T, Podczeck A, et al. High frequency alternating current ablation of an accessory pathway in humans. *J Am Coll Cardiol* 1987;10:576–582.
27. Tonkin AM, Wagner GS, Gallagher JJ, et al. Initial forces of ventricular depolarization in the Wolff-Parkinson-White syndrome: analysis based upon localization of the accessory pathway by epicardial mapping. *Circulation* 1975;52:1030–1036.
28. Reddy GV, Schamroth L. The localization of bypass tracts in the Wolff-Parkinson-White syndrome from the surface electrogram. *Am Heart J* 1987;113:984–993.
29. Milstein S, Sharma A, Guiraudon GM, et al. An algorithm for the electrocardiographic localization of accessory pathways in the Wolff-Parkinson-White syndrome. *Pacing Clin Electrophysiol* 1987;10:555–563.
30. Gallagher JJ. Localization of accessory atrioventricular pathways: what's the "gold standard"? *Pacing Clin Electrophysiol* 1987;10:583–584.
31. Scheinman MM, Wang YS, Van Hare GF, Lesh MD. Electrocardiographic and electrophysiologic characteristics of anterior, midseptal, and right anterior free wall accessory pathways. *J Am Coll Cardiol* 1992;20:1220–1229.
32. Fitzpatrick AP, Gonzales RP, Lesh MD, et al. New algorithm for the localization of accessory atrioventricular connections using a baseline electrocardiogram. *J Am Coll Cardiol* 1994;23:107–116.
33. Xie B, Heald SC, Bashir Y, et al. Localization of accessory pathways from the 12-lead electrocardiogram using a new algorithm. *Am J Cardiol* 1994;74:161–165.
34. Obel OA, Camm AJ. Accessory pathway reciprocating tachycardia. *Eur Heart J* 1998:19G3–E24.
35. Bardy GH, Packer DL, German LD, et al. Pre-excited reciprocating tachycardias in patients with Wolff-Parkinson-White syndrome: incidence and mechanisms. *Circulation* 1984;70:377–391.
36. Gepstein L, Evans SJ. Electroanatomical mapping of the heart: basic concepts and implications for the treatment of cardiac arrhythmias. *Pacing Clin Electrophysiol* 1998;21:1268–1278.
37. Worley S. Use of a real-time three-dimensional magnetic navigation system for radiofrequency ablation of accessory pathways. *Pacing Clin Electrophysiol* 1998;21:1636–1645.
38. Haissaguerre M, Dartigues JF, Warin JF, et al. Electrogram patterns predictive of successful catheter ablation of accessory pathways. *Circulation* 1991;84:188–202.
39. Calkins H, Kim YN, Schmaltz S, et al. Electrogram criteria for identification of appropriate target sites for radiofrequency catheter ablation of accessory atrioventricular connections. *Circulation* 1992;85:565–573.
40. Jackman WM, Friday KJ, Wah YL, et al. New catheter technique for recording left free-wall accessory atrioventricular pathway activation: identification of pathway fiber orientation. *Circulation* 1988;78:598–611.
41. Jackman WM, Friday KJ, Fitzgerald DM, et al. Localization of left free-wall and posteroseptal accessory atrioventricular pathways by direct recording of accessory pathway activation. *Pacing Clin Electrophysiol* 1989;12:204–214.
42. Haissaguerre M, Dartigues JF, Warin JF, et al. Electrogram patterns predictive of successful catheter ablation of accessory pathways: value of unipolar recording mode. *Circulation* 1991;84:188–202.
43. Nath S, Lynch C, Whayne JG, et al. Cellular electrophysiological effects of hyperthermia on isolated guinea pig papillary muscle: implications for catheter ablation. *Circulation* 1993;88:1826–1831.

44. Langberg JL, Calkins H, El-Atassi R, et al. Temperature monitoring during catheter ablation of accessory pathways. *Circulation* 1992;86:1469–1474.
45. Calkins H, Prystowsky E, Carlson M, et al. Temperature monitoring during RF catheter ablation procedures using closed loop control. *Circulation* 1994;90:1279–1286.
46. Morady F, Strickberger A, Man KC, et al. Reasons for prolonged or failed attempts at radiofrequency catheter ablation of accessory pathways. *J Am Coll Cardiol* 1996;27:683–689.
47. Xie B, Heald SC, Camm AJ, et al. Radiofrequency catheter ablation of accessory atrioventricular pathways: primary failure and recurrence of conduction. *Heart* 1997;77:363–368.
48. Langberg JJ, Calkins H, Kim YN, et al. Recurrence of conduction in accessory atrioventricular connections after initially successful radiofrequency catheter ablation. *J Am Coll Cardiol* 1992; 19:1588–1592.
49. Smith WM, Gallagher JJ, Kerr CR, et al. The electrophysiologic basis and management of symptomatic recurrent tachycardia in patients with Ebstein's anomaly of the tricuspid valve. *Am J Cardiol* 1982;49:1223–1234.
50. Colavita PG, Packer DL, Pressley JC, et al. Frequency, diagnosis, and clinical characteristics of patients with multiple accessory atrioventricular pathways. *Am J Cardiol* 1987;59:601–606.
51. Scheibler GL, Adams P, Anderson RC, et al. Clinical study of twenty-three cases of Ebstein's anomaly of the tricuspid valve. *Circulation* 1959;19:165–187.
52. Armstrong WF. Congenital heart disease. In: Feigenbaum H, ed. *Echocardiography*, 4th ed. Malvern, PA: Lea & Febiger, 1986: 365–461.
53. Cappato R, Schluter M, Weib C, et al. Radiofrequency current catheter ablation of accessory atrioventricular pathways in Epstein's anomaly. *Circulation* 1996;94:376–383.
54. Van Hare GF. Radiofrequency ablation of accessory pathways associated with congenital heart disease. *Pacing Clin Electrophysiol* 1997;20:2077–2081.
55. Okishige K, Azegami K, Goseki Y, et al. Radiofrequency of tachyarrhythmias in patients with Ebstein's anomaly. *Int J Cardiol* 1997;60:171–180.
56. Mahaim I, Benatt A. Nouvelles recherches sur les connexions superiieures de la branche gauche du faisceau de His-Tawara avec cloison interventriculaire. *Cardiologia* 1938;1:61–76.
57. Wellens HJJ. The preexcitation syndrome. In: Wellens HJJ, ed. *Electrical stimulation of the heart in the study and treatment of tachycardias*. Baltimore, MD: University Park Press, 1971:97–109.
58. Anderson RH, Becker AE, Brechenmacher C, et al. Ventricular preexcitation: a proposed nomenclature for its substrates. *Eur J Cardiol* 1975;3:27–36.
59. Gillette PC, Garsoh A Jr, Cooley DA, et al. Prolonged and decremental antegrade conduction properties in right anterior accessory connections: wide QRS antidromic tachycardia of left bundle branch block pattern without Wolff-Parkinson-White configuration in sinus rhythm. *Am Heart J* 1982;103:66–74.
60. Klein GJ, Guiraudon GM, Kerr CR, et al. "Nodoventricular" accessory pathway: evidence for a distinct accessory atrioventricular pathway with AV node–like properties. *J Am Coll Cardiol* 1988;11:1035–1040.
61. Leitch JW, Klein GJ, Yee R, et al. New concepts on nodoventricular accessory pathways. *J Clin Electrophysiol* 1990;1: 220–230.
62. Haissaguerre M, Cauchemez B, Marcus F, et al. Characteristics of the ventricular insertion sites of accessory pathways with anterograde decremental conduction properties. *Circulation* 1995; 91:1077–1085.
63. Okishige K, Goseki Y, Itoh A, et al. New electrophysiologic features and catheter ablation of atrioventricular and atriofascicular accessory pathways: evidence of decremental conduction and the anatomic structure of the Mahaim pathway. *J Clin Electrophysiol* 1998;9:22–33.
64. Klein LS, Hackett FK, Zipes DP, et al. Radiofrequency catheter ablation of Mahaim fibers at the tricuspid annulus. *Circulation* 1993;87:738–747.
65. McClelland JH, Wang X, Beckman KJ, et al. Radiofrequency catheter ablation of right atriofascicular (Mahaim) accessory pathways guided by accessory pathway activation potentials. *Circulation* 1994;89:2655–2666.
66. Grogin HR, Lee RJ, Kwasman M, et al. Radiofrequency catheter ablation of atriofascicular and nodoventricular Mahaim tracts. *Circulation* 1994;90:272–281.
67. Heald SC, Davies DW, Ward DE, et al. Radiofrequency catheter ablation of Mahaim potentials at the tricuspid annulus. *Br Heart J* 1995;73:250–257.
68. Cappato R, Schluter M, Weiss C, et al. Catheter induced mechanical conduction block of right-sided accessory fibers with Mahaim-type preexcitation to guide radiofrequency ablation. *Circulation* 1994;90:282–290.
69. Benditt DG, Epstein ML, Benson DW Jr. Dual accessory nodoventricular pathways: role in paroxysmal wide QRS reciprocating tachycardia. *Pacing Clin Electrophysiol* 1983;6:577–586.
70. Klein GJ, Guiraudon G, Guiraudon C, et al. The nodoventricular Mahaim pathway: an endangered concept? *Circulation* 1994; 90:636–638.
71. Murdock C, Leitch J, Klein G, et al. Epicardial mapping in patients with "nodoventricular" accessory pathways. *Am J Cardiol* 1991;68:208–214.
72. Gallagher JJ, Smith WM, Kasell JH, et al. Role of Mahaim fibers in cardiac arrhythmias in man. *Circulation* 1981;64:176–189.
73. Ellenbogen KA, Ramirez MN, Packer DL, et al. Accessory nodoventricular (Mahaim) fibres: a clinical review. *Pacing Clin Electrophysiol* 1986;9:868–884.
74. Bardy GH, Fedor JM, German LD, et al. Surface electrocardiographic clues suggesting presence of a nodo-fascicular Mahaim fibre. *J Am Coll Cardiol* 1984;3:1161–1168.
75. Okishige K, Strickberger SA, Walsh EP, et al. Catheter ablation of the atrial origin of a decrementally conducting atriofascicular accessory pathway by radio-frequency current. *J Clin Electrophysiol* 1991;2:465–475.
76. Johnson CT, Brooks C, Jaramillo J, et al. A left free-wall, decrementally conducting, atrioventricular (Mahaim) fiber: diagnosis at electrophysiological study and radiofrequency catheter ablation guided by direct recording of a Mahaim potential. *Pacing Clin Electrophysiol* 1997;20:2486–2488.
77. Zhu DWX. Ablation of right free wall accessory and Mahaim accessory pathways. In: Singer I, Barold SS, Camm AJ, eds. *Nonpharmacological therapy of arrhythmias for the 21st century: the state of the art*. Armonk, NY: Futura Publishing, 1998:98–116.
78. Li HG, Klein GJ, Yee R, et al. Radiofrequency ablation of decremental accessory pathways mimicking "nodoventricular" conduction. *Am J Cardiol* 1994;74:829–833.
79. Tchou P, Lehman MH, Jazayeri M, Akhtar M. Atriofascicular connection or a nodoventricular Mahaim fiber? Electrophysiologic elucidation of the pathway and associated reentrant circuit. *Circulation* 1988;77:837–848.
80. Natale A, Klein G, Yee R. Preexcitation update. In: Fisch C, Surawicz B, eds. *Current topics in cardiology*. New York: Elsevier Science Publishing, 1991.
81. Reich J, Auld D, Hulse E, et al. The pediatric radiofrequency ablation registry's experience with Ebstein's Anomaly. *J Cardiovasc Electrophysiol* 1998;9:1370–1377.

CATHETER ABLATION OF POSTEROSEPTAL ACCESSORY PATHWAYS

• • •

FRED MORADY

The first report of successful catheter ablation of a posteroseptal accessory pathway using a direct current shock delivered near the ostium of the coronary sinus was in 1984 (1). In a subsequent series of 48 patients with a posteroseptal accessory pathway published in 1989, direct current ablation was found to have a success rate of approximately 70%, with a small risk of cardiac tamponade and atrioventricular (AV) block (2). Because of the potential for complications related to barotrauma, direct current ablation of posteroseptal accessory pathways generally was limited to patients with severe symptoms who could not be adequately managed with pharmacologic therapy.

With the advent of radiofrequency catheter ablation in the late 1980s, the efficacy and safety of catheter ablation of accessory pathways dramatically improved and catheter ablation quickly became the preferred therapy for patients symptomatic from arrhythmias involving an accessory pathway. This chapter reviews various aspects of the identification and ablation of posteroseptal accessory pathways.

⊙ ANATOMIC CONSIDERATIONS

The anatomy of the posteroseptal space was best described by Dr. Will Sealy, a pioneer in the development of surgical techniques for the ablation of accessory pathways (3). The posteroseptal space has the configuration of a trihedral pyramid with unequal faces that is lying on its side (Fig. 8-1). The epicardium of the crux serves as the base of the pyramid, and the right fibrous trigone (i.e., junction of the mitral and tricuspid annuli, the aortic annulus, the membranous septum, and the atrial septum) serves as its apex. The right side of the pyramid is the septal portion of the right atrium, the left side is the left atrium, and the third side, which also is the floor, consists of the posterior superior process of the left ventricle and the muscular ventricular septum. The ostium of the coronary sinus is located at the posterior superior aspect of the right face of the pyramid. The pyramidal space contains adipose tissue, the AV nodal artery, and the anterior portion of the coronary sinus.

In the electrophysiology laboratory, the ostium of the coronary sinus provides a convenient landmark for identification of the posteroseptal region, and posteroseptal accessory pathways generally are found in proximity to this landmark. However, there are no fluoroscopic indicators of the lateral boundaries of the posteroseptal space, and this has led to different definitions of what constitutes a posteroseptal accessory pathway.

In conventional practice, accessory pathways that

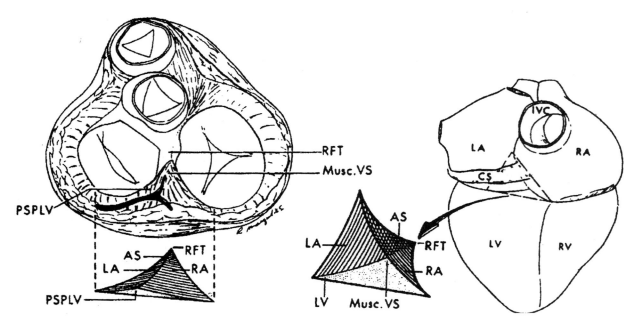

FIGURE 8-1. Schematic representation of the posteroseptal space. AS, anterior septum; CS, coronary sinus; IVC, inferior vena cava; LA, left atrium; LV, left ventricle; Musc. VS, muscular ventricular septum; PSPLV, posteroseptal process of the left ventricle; RA, right atrium; RFT, right fibrous trigone; RV, right ventricle. (From Sealy WC, Gallagher JJ. The surgical approach to the septal area of the heart based on experiences with 45 patients with Kent bundles. *J Thorac Cardiovasc Surg* 1980;79:542–551, with permission.)

are localized to within 1 to 2 cm of the ostium of the coronary sinus are considered to be posteroseptal in location, and those that are localized to beyond 1 to 2 cm from the ostium are considered to lie within the left free wall. The validity of these criteria for identification of accessory pathway location was brought into question by a study that measured the dimensions of the posteroseptal space in 48 human cadaver hearts (4). The mean distance from the coronary sinus ostium to the left border of the posteroseptal space was 2.3 ± 0.4 cm (± standard deviation). The proximal 1.5 cm of the coronary sinus was usually within the posteroseptal space, and the left free wall was located more than 1.75 cm to the left of the coronary sinus ostium in all adults with a body weight of 60 kg or more (4). Depending on age and body weight, there was up to a 27% probability that a site within the coronary sinus 3 cm from the ostium was located within the posteroseptal space. These data suggest that many accessory pathways that are diagnosed as being left free wall in location may actually be posteroseptal. However, although electrophysiologists underestimate the true frequency of posteroseptal accessory pathways, this probably has little or no clinical impact on the results of catheter ablation. In practice, when accessory pathways are localized within the coronary sinus beyond 1 to 2 cm from the ostium, a left-sided endocardial approach is almost always effective, regardless of whether the accessory pathway is in the left free wall or within the posteroseptal space.

SURGICAL DELINEATION OF POSTEROSEPTAL ACCESSORY PATHWAYS

In a study of 31 patients who underwent surgical ablation of a posteroseptal accessory pathway, Sealy and Gallagher reported that approximately 40% of the accessory pathways were located between the right fibrous trigone and the coronary sinus, approximately 20% were near the bundle of His, and another 20% were located underneath the coronary sinus at the crux of the heart (3). Successful surgical interruption of these accessory pathways usually was achieved through a right or a left and right atriotomy. In later reports involving larger numbers of patients, posteroseptal accessory pathways often were found to connect the right atrium and the left ventricle (5,6).

In 1988, Guiraudon and coworkers reported that 6 of 65 patients with a posteroseptal accessory pathway were found in the operating room to have a coronary sinus diverticulum in the posteroseptal region (7). The coronary sinus diverticula consisted of a venous pouch 2 to 5 cm in diameter within the left ventricular wall, proximal to the midcardiac vein, with a 5- to 10-mm neck opening into the coronary sinus (Fig. 8-2). Successful ablation of the accessory pathway in these six patients required separation of the neck of the coronary sinus diverticulum from the left ventricle. This important study demonstrated that the target site for successful radiofrequency ablation of a posteroseptal accessory pathway occasionally may lie within a coronary sinus diverticulum.

● ELECTROCARDIOGRAPHIC FINDINGS

The electrocardiogram of a patient with a manifest posteroseptal accessory pathway often demonstrates inverted delta waves in the inferior leads that may be mistaken as evidence of an inferior myocardial infarction. The prevalence of inverted delta waves is 100% in lead III, 90% in aVF, and 50% in lead II (8). The delta waves are uniformly positive in leads I and aVL, and the QRS frontal plane axis is between +30 and −60 degrees. There is an R : S ratio of more than 1 in V_2, and tall R waves are present in V_3 through V_6 (8). The configuration of the delta wave and of the QRS complex in V_1 is variable, with right posteroseptal accessory pathways usually having a negative or isoelectric delta wave in V_1 (Fig. 8-3) and left posteroseptal accessory pathways usually having a positive delta wave and an R : S ratio of more than 1 in V_1 (Fig. 8-4). However, because exceptions occur, the accurate differentiation of right and left posteroseptal accessory pathways is not always possible based on the electrocardiogram.

● DIAGNOSIS IN THE ELECTROPHYSIOLOGY LABORATORY

For a manifest posteroseptal accessory pathway, the site of earliest ventricular activation often is at or near the ostium of the coronary sinus or inside the coronary sinus within 1 to 2 cm of the ostium. Because accessory pathways may have an oblique course, the site of earliest atrial activation during retrograde accessory pathway conduction does not always correspond with the site of earliest ventricular activation. Mapping of retrograde atrial activation through the accessory pathway is best performed during orthodromic reciprocating tachycardia to avoid the confounding effects of retrograde AV nodal conduction.

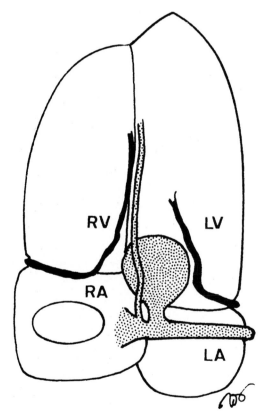

FIGURE 8-2. Schematic representation of a coronary sinus diverticulum. LA, left atrium; LV, left ventricle; RA, right atrium; RV, right ventricle. (From Guiraudon GM, Guiraudon CM, Klein GJ, et al. The coronary sinus diverticulum: a pathologic entity associated with the Wolff-Parkinson-White syndrome. *Am J Cardiol* 1988;62:733–735, with permission.)

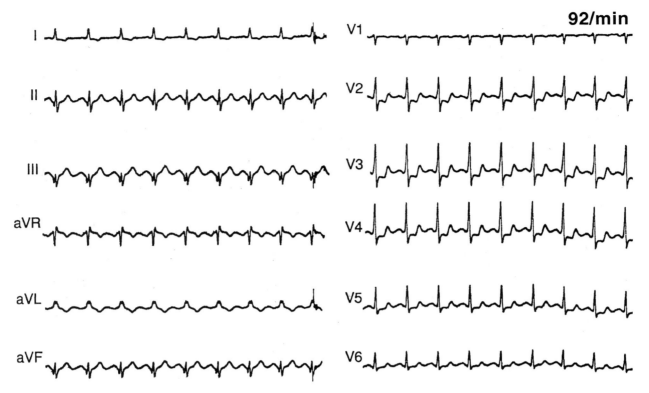

FIGURE 8-3. Typical electrocardiogram of a patient with a manifest right posteroseptal accessory pathway. The negative delta waves in the inferior leads may mimic the pattern of an inferior myocardial infarction.

In orthodromic reciprocating tachycardia using a posteroseptal accessory pathway, left bundle branch block usually prolongs the ventriculoatrial interval, although by less than 25 msec, as opposed to an increase of more than 30 msec when the accessory pathway lies in the left free wall (9). Right bundle branch block does not affect the ventriculoatrial interval.

If orthodromic reciprocating tachycardia is not inducible, retrograde conduction through a posteroseptal accessory pathway can be distinguished from retrograde conduction through a rapidly conducting AV nodal pathway by comparing the ventriculoatrial intervals during ventricular pacing at the right ventricular apex and at a posterobasal right ventricular site (10). If a posteroseptal accessory pathway is present, the ventriculoatrial interval during right ventricular pacing at a basal site is shorter than when pacing at the apex; if retrograde conduction occurs through the AV node–His–Purkinje axis, the opposite is observed. Martinez-Alday and associates reported that the difference between the ventriculoatrial intervals measured during apical and posterobasal pacing ranged between +10 and +70 msec in the presence of a posteroseptal accessory pathway, compared with values between −50 and +50 msec when retrograde conduction was through the AV node (10).

Another useful maneuver for distinguishing retrograde conduction through a posteroseptal accessory pathway from retrograde conduction through a rapidly conducting AV nodal pathway is para-Hisian pacing (11). When the stimulus-atrial electrogram intervals during ventricular capture and during ventricular plus His bundle capture are equal, it indicates retrograde conduction over an accessory pathway (Fig. 8-5A). In contrast, when retrograde conduction occurs through the AV node, the stimulus-atrial electrogram interval when there is ventricular plus His bundle capture is shorter than when there is ventricu-

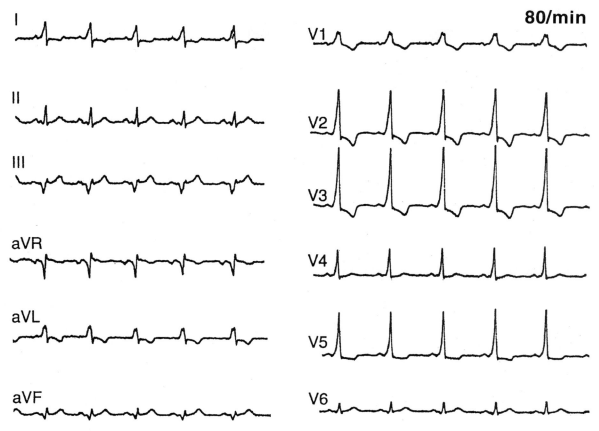

FIGURE 8-4. Electrocardiogram of a patient with a left posteroseptal accessory pathway. The delta waves are positive in I, II, and aVL and negative in III and aVF, as is typical of right posteroseptal accessory pathways. The feature that distinguishes a left posteroseptal accessory pathway from a right posteroseptal accessory pathway is the positive delta wave and monophasic R wave configuration in V_1.

lar capture alone (Fig. 8-5B). Hirao and colleagues found an accessory pathway response to para-Hisian pacing in each of 56 patients with a posteroseptal accessory pathway, compared with an AV nodal response in each of 53 patients who had AV nodal reentrant tachycardia and no accessory pathway (11).

Ventriculoatrial block in response to adenosine has been proposed to be useful in distinguishing ventriculoatrial conduction over the AV node from ventriculoatrial conduction over an accessory pathway, because adenosine typically has no effect on accessory pathways. However, retrograde conduction through fast AV nodal pathways often is not blocked by adenosine, impairing the diagnostic value of an adenosine challenge (12).

Right Versus Left Posteroseptal Accessory Pathways

In patients with a posteroseptal accessory pathway, a positive delta wave in V_1 and ventriculoatrial interval prolongation of 10 to 25 msec associated with a functional left bundle branch block during orthodromic tachycardia indicate that the accessory pathway is left sided. However, categorization of posteroseptal accessory pathways as right sided or left sided does not necessarily predict where the effective target site for ablation will be. In a study of 50 consecutive patients with a posteroseptal accessory pathway, Dhala and colleagues found that 10 patients had a left posteroseptal accessory pathway, but only 1 of these 10 pa-

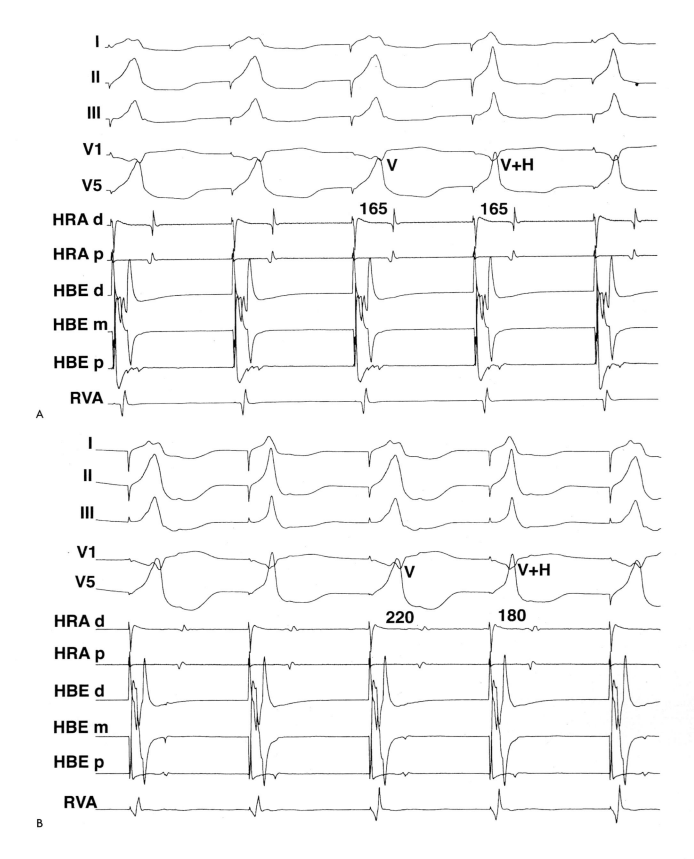

tients required a left-sided approach for ablation (13). In the other 9 patients with a left-sided posteroseptal accessory pathway, the successful target site for ablation was at the coronary sinus ostium or within the first 1 cm of the coronary sinus in 5 patients, at the posteroseptal aspect of the tricuspid annulus in 2 patients, and at the inferomedial right atrium posterior to the coronary sinus ostium in 2 patients. Among the 40 other patients who had a right-sided posteroseptal accessory pathway, the accessory pathway was successfully ablated using a right-sided approach in 39. The results of this study suggest that most posteroseptal accessory pathways can be ablated using a right-sided approach, even when an accessory pathway is classified as left sided based on electrocardiographic or electrophysiologic criteria.

A left-sided approach for ablation may be necessary even when a posteroseptal accessory pathway does not have the typical electrocardiographic pattern of a left-sided posteroseptal accessory pathway. In a series of patients in whom lengthy or multiple procedures were needed for successful ablation, several patients had a posteroseptal accessory pathway thought to be right-sided based on the absence of a positive delta wave in V_1, the presence of an R : S ratio of less than 1 in V_1, and because right-sided applications often resulted in transient accessory pathway block (14). After multiple ineffective applications of radiofrequency energy at or near the ostium of the coronary sinus, successful ablation was achieved by targeting the posteroseptal aspect of the mitral annulus. A left ventricular or left atrial approach should be considered if several right-sided applications of radiofrequency energy are ineffective in ablating a posteroseptal accessory pathway.

The delta wave configuration in lead II may be helpful in identifying whether a right-sided approach will be effective for ablating a posteroseptal accessory pathway. Two studies have demonstrated that ablation at the right posteroseptal region is effective in 80% to 82% of patients who have a positive or biphasic delta wave in lead II (13,15).

Analysis of atrial activation during orthodromic tachycardia also may be helpful in predicting whether a right- or left-sided approach is necessary in patients with a posteroseptal accessory pathway. Among 89 consecutive patients with a concealed posteroseptal accessory pathway, 36 patients (39%) required a left atrial or left ventricular endocardial approach for ablation (16). The ΔVA was defined as the ventriculoatrial interval recorded with the His bundle catheter during orthodromic tachycardia or ventricular pacing minus the shortest ventriculoatrial interval recorded within the proximal coronary sinus (16). When the ΔVA was 25 msec or more, a left endocardial approach was necessary, and when the ΔVA was less than 25 msec, successful ablation usually was achieved on the right side, at or near the ostium of the coronary sinus (Fig. 8-6). The use of a left ventricular endocardial approach early in the procedure when the ΔVA is 25 msec or more may significantly reduce the procedure duration, the amount of radiation exposure, and the number of radiofrequency energy applications needed for successful ablation (16).

Identification of Epicardial Posteroseptal Accessory Pathways

Some posteroseptal accessory pathways cannot be ablated using a right- or left-sided endocardial approach

FIGURE 8-5. Examples of para-Hisian pacing. Pacing was performed at a cycle length of 500 msec using the distal pair of electrodes of the His bundle catheter (HBE d). There is ventricular capture (V) and ventricular plus His bundle capture (V + H), and the QRS complexes are wider with the former than with the latter. **A:** In a patient with a concealed posteroseptal accessory pathway, the stimulus-atrial interval is constant at 165 msec during ventricular and ventricular plus His bundle capture. **B:** After radiofrequency ablation of the posteroseptal accessory pathway, para-Hisian pacing demonstrates a longer stimulus-atrial interval during ventricular (V) capture (220 msec) than during ventricular plus His bundle (V + H) capture (180 msec). d, m, and p, distal, medial, and proximal pair of electrodes, respectively; HRA, high right atrium; RVA, right ventricular apex.

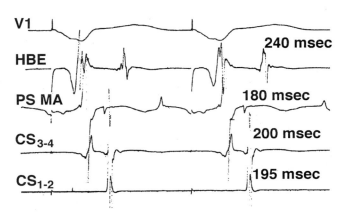

FIGURE 8-6. Measurement of the ΔVA during ventricular pacing at a cycle length of 500 msec. The ΔVA is the difference between the ventriculoatrial interval measured at the His bundle position (240 msec) and the shortest ventriculoatrial interval (VA) recorded within the coronary sinus (195 msec). When the ΔVA is less than 25 msec, a posteroseptal accessory pathway usually can be ablated using a right-sided approach. The ΔVA in this case was 45 msec, indicating the need for a left endocardial approach. The accessory pathway was ablated at the posteroseptal mitral annulus (PS MA), where the ventriculoatrial interval was 180 msec. CS_{1-2}, distal pair of electrodes of the coronary sinus catheter; CS_{3-4}, proximal pair of electrodes of the coronary sinus catheter (positioned at the ostium); HBE, His bundle electrogram.

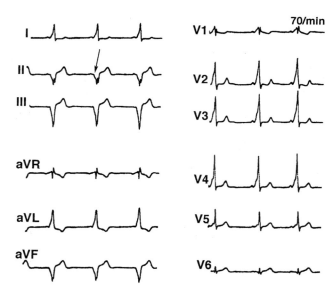

FIGURE 8-7. Electrocardiogram of a patient with an epicardial posteroseptal accessory pathway. The steeply negative delta wave in lead II (arrow) is characteristic of posteroseptal accessory pathways requiring ablation within the coronary sinus or one of its branches.

and may be epicardial in location. Delivery of radiofrequency energy within the coronary sinus or one of its branches may be necessary for ablation of these epicardial accessory pathways. An electrocardiographic finding that may be useful in predicting the need for delivery of energy within the coronary sinus is the presence of a steeply negative delta wave in lead II (Fig. 8-7). In a study of 121 consecutive patients with a single manifest accessory pathway, Arruda and coworkers found that 14 patients required ablation within the coronary venous system (17). A negative delta wave in lead II was highly accurate in predicting the need for ablation within the coronary venous system, with the sensitivity, specificity, and positive- and negative-predictive values all being 100% (17).

In another study that examined the electrocardiographic features of posteroseptal accessory pathways (18), a steeply negative delta wave in lead II was not as accurate in predicting the need for ablation within the coronary sinus or one of its branches as in the study by Arruda and coworkers (17). Takahashi and colleagues found that a negative delta wave in lead II during sinus rhythm had a sensitivity of 87% for identifying a posteroseptal accessory pathway requiring ablation within the coronary venous system, with a specificity of 79% and a positive predictive value of only 50% (18). The different findings of the two studies may be attributable to different measurement or mapping techniques. Nevertheless, the study by Takahashi and colleagues (18) indicates that a steeply negative delta wave in lead II is not necessarily pathognomonic of an epicardial posteroseptal accessory pathway.

The other electrocardiographic clues that a posteroseptal accessory pathway may be epicardial are a steeply positive delta wave in aVR and a deep S wave in V_6 (Fig. 8-8). The combination of a steeply positive delta wave in aVR and a deep S wave in V_6 were reported to have a sensitivity of 43% to 78%, a specificity of 99%, a positive predictive value of 91%, and a negative predictive value of 88% to 97% in identifying posteroseptal accessory pathways requiring ablation within the coronary sinus or one of its branches (18).

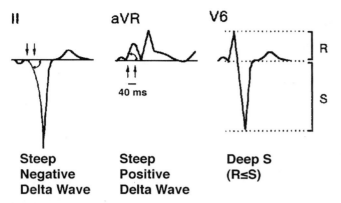

FIGURE 8-8. Characteristics during atrial pacing of leads II, aVR, and V$_6$ that are associated with an epicardial accessory pathway. (Adapted from Takahashi A, Shah DC, Jais P, et al. Specific electrocardiographic features of manifest coronary vein posteroseptal accessory pathways. *J Cardiovasc Electrophysiol* 1998;9:1015–1025, with permission.)

Visualization of the Coronary Sinus

If the electrocardiogram and results of initial endocardial and coronary sinus mapping suggest the presence of a posteroseptal accessory pathway that may require ablation within the coronary sinus, it is often helpful to visualize the coronary sinus by injection of contrast to determine the location and size of branches of the coronary sinus and to look for venous anomalies such as a diverticulum (19) (Fig. 8-9).

A transesophageal echocardiogram is useful for patients with posteroseptal accessory pathways because it allows visualization of the middle cardiac vein and coronary sinus diverticula. In 18 consecutive patients with a posteroseptal accessory pathway who underwent a transesophageal echocardiogram and coronary sinus angiogram, 5 of 5 coronary sinus diverticula and 22 of 22 middle cardiac veins were correctly identified with the transesophageal echocardiogram (20). In the 5 patients who had a coronary sinus diverticulum, the accessory pathway was successfully ablated in each by delivery of radiofrequency energy at the neck of the diverticulum (20). Whether by transesophageal echocardiography or coronary sinus angiography, it may be useful to visualize the anatomy of the coronary venous system.

ELECTROGRAM CRITERIA FOR SELECTION OF ABLATION SITES

The electrogram criteria for selecting sites for ablation of posteroseptal accessory pathways are the same as for accessory pathways in other locations. When the accessory pathway is manifest, the highest probability of success occurs at sites that have stable electrograms, a presumed accessory pathway potential, and where local ventricular activation occurs before the onset of the delta wave (21). When the accessory pathway is concealed, the best predictors of successful ablation are electrogram stability, a presumed retrograde accessory pathway potential, and retrograde continuous electrical activity during ventricular pacing or orthodromic tachycardia (21).

When searching for the site of earliest atrial activation in a patient with a concealed posteroseptal accessory pathway, mapping is best performed during orthodromic reciprocating tachycardia, because this guarantees that retrograde activation of the atria is occurring only through the accessory pathway. If mapping during orthodromic reciprocating tachycardia is not feasible, mapping must be performed during ventricular pacing, in which case the results may be confounded by retrograde conduction through the AV node. A rapid pacing rate or the administration of verapamil may be necessary to eliminate atrial fusion and allow the accurate identification of the atrial insertion of the accessory pathway.

During mapping in the electrophysiology laboratory, the characteristic features of posteroseptal accessory pathways that require ablation from within the coronary sinus include the absence of a clear-cut earliest site of endocardial activation during anterograde or retrograde accessory pathway conduction; a diminutive or absent endocardial accessory pathway potential; an accessory pathway potential within the coronary sinus or one of its branches that is larger than the largest amplitude accessory pathway potential that can be found at the endocardial surface; and a presumed accessory pathway potential recorded within the coronary sinus that is larger in amplitude than the atrial and ventricular electrograms (22) (Fig. 8-10).

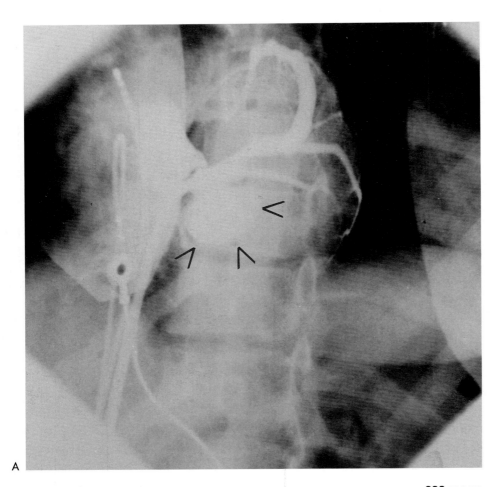

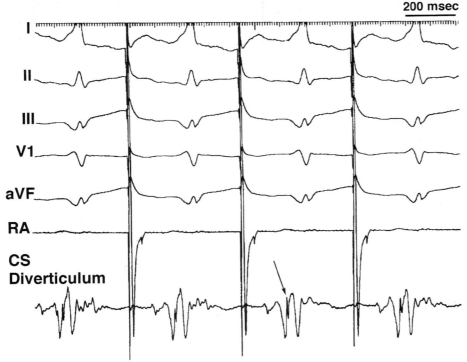

FIGURE 8-9. **A:** Left anterior oblique view of a coronary sinus venogram demonstrates a diverticulum *(arrowheads)* in a patient who had a posteroseptal accessory pathway. **B:** Mapping during atrial pacing at a cycle length of 450 msec demonstrated early ventricular activation and a presumed accessory pathway potential *(arrow)* at the neck of the diverticulum. The accessory pathway was successfully ablated at this site. The delta wave in lead II is isoelectric or slightly negative, demonstrating that posteroseptal accessory pathways that require ablation within the coronary sinus (CS) are not always associated with a steeply negative delta wave in lead II. RA, right atrial electrogram.

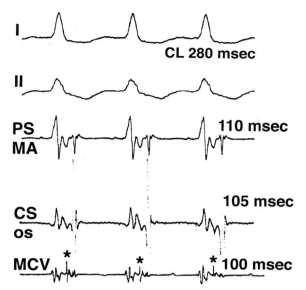

FIGURE 8-10. Electrogram characteristics of a concealed, epicardial, posteroseptal accessory pathway. Mapping was performed during orthodromic reciprocating tachycardia at a cycle length of 280 msec. There is a presumed accessory pathway potential *(asterisk)* recorded within the middle cardiac vein (MCV), which is larger in amplitude than the ventricular (V) and atrial (A) electrograms. The ventriculoatrial interval in the middle cardiac vein is 100 msec, which was shorter than the shortest ventriculoatrial intervals recorded at the posteroseptal mitral annulus (PS MA, 110 msec) and coronary sinus (CS) ostium (105 msec).

◉ PERMANENT JUNCTIONAL RECIPROCATING TACHYCARDIA

Permanent junctional reciprocating tachycardia (PJRT) is an incessant form of orthodromic reciprocating tachycardia that uses a slowly conducting accessory pathway as the retrograde limb of the reentry circuit. The accessory pathway is concealed and has decremental conduction properties (23). The incessant nature of the tachycardia often results in a tachycardia-induced cardiomyopathy, which is largely reversible after restoration of sinus rhythm (24,25). Although the accessory pathway sometimes may be located in the left or right free wall or in the midseptum, it most often has a right posteroseptal location (24,25). The electrocardiogram demonstrates a long RP tachycardia and inverted P waves in leads II, III, aVF, and V_4 through V_6 (Fig. 8-11). When the P wave during tachycardia is upright in lead I, catheter ablation usually can be accomplished at the ostium of the coronary sinus or in the right posteroseptal region (24).

Because the accessory pathway is concealed and because of possible retrograde activation of the atria through the AV node during ventricular pacing, mapping usually is possible only during the tachycardia. Target sites for ablation are identified by searching for

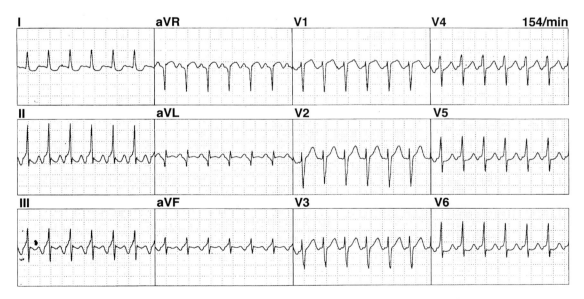

FIGURE 8-11. The electrocardiogram recorded during permanent junctional reciprocating tachycardia. The tachycardia has a rate of 154 bpm. The long RP interval and the inverted P waves in leads II, III, aVF, and V_4 through V_6 are characteristic of this type of tachycardia.

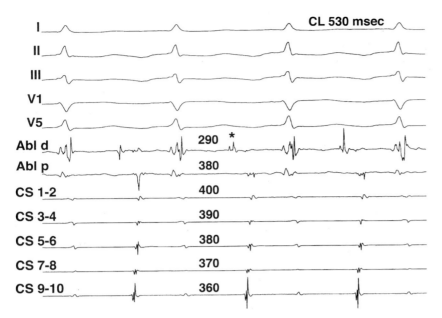

FIGURE 8-12. The permanent junctional reciprocating tachycardia has a cycle length 530 msec. The ablation catheter (ABL d) is positioned at the site of earliest retrograde atrial activation *(asterisk)*, which was in the right posterior septum adjacent to the ostium of the coronary sinus. Although the ventriculoatrial interval at this site is long (290 msec), it was the shortest ventriculoatrial interval that could be identified, and ablation at this site was successful. The ventriculoatrial interval at each recording site is indicated in milliseconds. The coronary sinus catheter had 10 electrodes, and the five pairs of electrodes used for bipolar recordings are indicated; CS 9-10 was positioned at the ostium, and CS 1-2 was positioned adjacent to the lateral aspect of the mitral annulus. ABL p, proximal pair of electrodes of the ablation catheter; CS, coronary sinus.

the site of earliest retrograde activation of the atrium. Because the accessory pathway conducts slowly, the ventriculoatrial at the effective ablation site is long, and the site of earliest activation is identified only by comparison with ventriculoatrial intervals at adjacent areas (Fig. 8-12).

◉ TECHNIQUES FOR DELIVERY OF RADIOFREQUENCY ENERGY

When posteroseptal accessory pathways are ablated using a right- or left-sided endocardial approach, an electrode-tissue interface temperature of at least 60°C should be attained to minimize the possibility of a recurrence of accessory pathway conduction (26). Temperatures greater than 90°C should be avoided to prevent coagulum formation (26). Ablation catheters that have a thermistor embedded in the distal electrode are widely available, and these catheters allow manual or automatic titration of power to maintain an electrode-tissue interface temperature between 60°C and 80°C.

For ablation of epicardial posteroseptal accessory pathways, the results of experimental and clinical studies have suggested that the application of radiofrequency energy within the coronary sinus generally is safe. Delivery of approximately 25 W of radiofrequency energy inside the coronary sinus of dogs resulted in well-circumscribed areas of necrosis and fibrosis in the fat of the AV sulcus, with no involvement of the circumflex coronary artery and no instances of coronary sinus perforation (27).

In a clinical study, nine patients were found to have a left posteroseptal accessory pathway based on the presence of a prominent accessory pathway potential within the proximal coronary sinus (28). Radiofrequency energy was delivered for 5 to 30 seconds at a power of 5 to 30 W inside the coronary sinus or within the middle cardiac vein or a venous anomaly. Seven (78%) of the nine accessory pathways were successfully ablated, and the only complication was transient coronary sinus spasm not associated with any clinical sequelae. Although this study demonstrated that ablation of posteroseptal accessory pathways within the coronary sinus or one of its branches can be accomplished safely, it is noteworthy that energy levels greater than 30 W and applications within small branches of the coronary sinus where the vessel lumen was occluded by the ablation catheter were avoided (28). Hemopericardium and cardiac tamponade may occur if radiofrequency energy is delivered within a small venous branch of the coronary sinus (29).

A cautious approach is warranted when ablating posteroseptal accessory pathway from within the coronary venous system. To minimize the possibility of perforation and cardiac tamponade, pericarditis, or injury to a coronary artery, the goal during energy application is to identify the lowest effective electrode-tissue interface temperature. A target temperature of 45°C is initially used, with gradual titration upward until accessory pathway conduction is eliminated. The application is then continued for 20 to 30 seconds at the temperature that first resulted in accessory pathway block. If the ablation catheter appears to be occluding the vein, an attempt at ablation may not be advisable unless a smaller caliber ablation catheter that does not occlude the vein is available.

Delivery of radiofrequency energy between the distal electrodes of two catheters positioned at the posteroseptal aspects of the tricuspid and mitral annuli has been reported to be effective in ablating a posteroseptal accessory pathway when conventional unipolar applications at these locations individually have been ineffective (30). Bipolar applications may result in necrosis that extends from one electrode tip to the other, thereby interrupting accessory pathways that are deep within the septum (30).

Compared with conventional radiofrequency catheter ablation, larger lesions also can be created using a saline-cooled radiofrequency ablation catheter (31). However, the larger lesion size, although more efficacious in ablating accessory pathways that are deep within the septum or epicardial (32,33), may also significantly increase the risk of serious complications. In a preliminary report, radiofrequency ablation within the coronary venous system was found to be associated with a risk of coronary artery injury (34). This risk was minimized by visualizing the coronary artery that was adjacent to the ablation site with intravascular ultrasound and by terminating applications of radiofrequency energy at the onset of echocardiographic changes in the vessel wall (34).

Efficacy of Catheter Ablation of Posteroseptal Accessory Pathways

In the earliest reports of patients undergoing radiofrequency ablation of accessory pathways, the success rates for posteroseptal accessory pathways ranged from 81% to 98% (29,35–38). Some investigators observed that posteroseptal accessory pathways were more difficult to ablate compared with accessory pathways in other locations (35,37). The recurrence rate of posteroseptal accessory pathway conduction ranged from 7% to 10%, similar to the recurrence rate for accessory pathways in other locations (29,36–38). In later studies, refined mapping and ablation techniques resulted in success rates of 97% to 100% and recurrence rates as low as zero (13,16,18).

At the University of Michigan, radiofrequency ablation of 199 posteroseptal accessory pathways was attempted between 1990 and June of 1999, and 190 (95%) of these accessory pathways were successfully ablated (unpublished data). A recurrence of accessory pathway conduction occurred in 3% of patients, and all but one of these patients had a successful long-term outcome after a second procedure.

Distribution of Effective Ablation Sites

In two studies that consisted of 74 and 117 consecutive patients who underwent successful radiofrequency ablation of a posteroseptal accessory pathway, the ablation site was right-sided in 51% to 69% of patients, left-sided in 20% to 29% of patients, and within the coronary sinus or one of its branches in 11% to 20% (18,39).

At the University of Michigan Medical Center, 199 (17%) of 1,165 accessory pathways in 1,100 patients who underwent catheter ablation of an accessory pathway were found to be posteroseptal (unpublished data, 1999). Among the 190 posteroseptal accessory pathways that were successfully ablated, 67% were ablated in the posteroseptal region of the right atrium, 28% were ablated at the posteroseptal aspect of the mitral annulus, and the remaining 5% were ablated in the coronary sinus or one of its branches (unpublished data, 1999).

In comparing the distribution of ablation sites between different centers, the reason for the wide range in the percentage of posteroseptal accessory pathways (5% to 20%) that are epicardial is unclear but may be attributable to different referral patterns.

Although the pooled experience at high-volume centers indicates that approximately 25% of posteroseptal accessory pathways require a left ventricular approach for ablation, the results from other centers have been widely divergent, with the percentage of posteroseptal accessory pathways requiring a left ventricular approach varying from only 4% (13) to as high as 39% (16). This variability in the need for a left ventricular approach may be a reflection of the different criteria that have been used to identify posteroseptal accessory pathways. For example, Dhala and coworkers (13) defined an accessory pathway as posteroseptal when the earliest site of atrial or ventricular activation was within the proximal 1 cm of the coronary sinus, whereas Chiang and associates (16) used a 2-cm criterion. The use of a 1-cm criterion probably excludes posteroseptal accessory pathways that are most likely to require a left ventricular approach, explaining why only 4% of pathways required a left-sided approach in the study of Dhala and colleagues, compared with 39% when the 2-cm criterion was used. It also is possible that some posteroseptal accessory pathways are ablatable from the right or left side of the septum, depending on how persistently a given approach is attempted.

COMPLICATIONS

Radiofrequency catheter ablation of posteroseptal accessory pathways is associated with a small risk of the complications that may result from any invasive electrophysiologic procedure, including thrombophlebitis, damage to the femoral artery, or right ventricular perforation. The only complication that has been reported with the endocardial approach to radiofrequency ablation of posteroseptal accessory pathways has been high-degree AV block. As is the case with radiofrequency ablation of the slow pathway in patients with AV nodal reentrant tachycardia, ablation sites in the posterior septum occasionally may be close enough to the AV node to cause high-degree AV block. The incidence of this complication has been reported to be approximately 2% (29,36). However, in the updated University of Michigan series of 199 patients who underwent radiofrequency ablation of a posteroseptal accessory pathway, only 1 patient (0.5%) developed persistent AV block and required implantation of a pacemaker (unpublished data, 1999). The risk of AV block as a complication of posteroseptal accessory pathway ablation should be less than 1%.

During slow pathway ablation, delivery of radiofrequency energy in the posterior septum often results in junctional ectopy, and the occurrence of ventriculoatrial block during the junctional ectopy is a warning of impending AV block (40). When ablating right-sided posteroseptal accessory pathways, delivery of radiofrequency energy in the posterior septum also may provoke junctional ectopy. However, in this situation, ventriculoatrial block cannot be used as an indicator of impending AV block, because ventriculoatrial conduction over the posteroseptal accessory pathway may persist despite injury to the AV node. To minimize the risk of AV block, it is prudent to discontinue an application of radiofrequency energy that provokes junctional ectopy. If provocation of junctional ectopy cannot be avoided at the optimal target sites for ablation of a posteroseptal accessory pathway, radiofrequency energy should be delivered during atrial pacing at a cycle length shorter than the cycle length of the junctional ectopy. If the accessory pathway is concealed, the application of radiofrequency energy should be discontinued immediately if the PR interval lengthens. If the accessory pathway is manifest, an increase in the degree of preexcitation is an indicator of slowing of conduction through the AV node and should lead to immediate interruption of the energy application. With these techniques for delivery of radiofrequency energy in the posterior septum, the risk of AV block can be minimized.

Other complications have been associated with ablation of epicardial posteroseptal accessory pathways from within the coronary sinus or one of its branches. These include pericarditis (29), pericardial effusion (13), cardiac tamponade (29), and coronary sinus spasm (28). The risk of these complications probably is minimal if radiofrequency energy delivery is avoided within small branches of the coronary sinus that are completely occluded by the ablation electrode.

CONCLUSIONS

Although posteroseptal accessory pathways may be more challenging to ablate than free wall accessory pathways, a high success rate is achievable if mapping is approached in a systematic fashion. If there is manifest preexcitation, the electrocardiogram can provide clues for determining whether a right-sided, left-sided, or coronary sinus approach is needed for ablation. The ΔVA during orthodromic tachycardia also may provide information helpful in determining whether a right- or left-sided approach is needed. For example, if the delta wave is positive in lead II and the ΔVA during orthodromic tachycardia is less than 25 msec, detailed right-sided mapping in the region of the coronary sinus ostium is warranted. However, if coronary sinus mapping demonstrates that the earliest site of atrial or ventricular activation is more than 2 cm into the coronary sinus and if the ΔVA during orthodromic tachycardia is greater than 25 msec, a left-sided endocardial approach is appropriate using transseptal catheterization or a retrograde aortic approach into the left ventricle. When there is a markedly negative delta wave in lead II, particularly when there also is a steeply positive delta wave in aVR and a deep S wave in V_6, the accessory pathway probably is epicardial, and the coronary sinus and its branches should be thoroughly mapped.

In some patients, the clues available from the electrocardiogram, the ΔVA, and preliminary mapping in the posterior septum and coronary sinus may be contradictory. For example, a positive delta wave in lead II (pointing to a right posteroseptal accessory pathway) may coexist with a ΔVA that is greater than 25 msec (pointing to a left posteroseptal accessory pathway). In other patients, such as the patient with a concealed accessory pathway in whom orthodromic reciprocating tachycardia is not readily inducible, clues from the electrocardiogram or the ΔVA may not be available. In such cases, the following stepwise approach to mapping and ablation of a posteroseptal accessory pathway may be appropriate:

1. Map the right posterior septum and coronary sinus within 1 cm of the ostium to look for a presumed accessory pathway potential or for the site of earliest atrial or ventricular activation through the accessory pathway. Application of radiofrequency energy is warranted at sites where local ventricular activation precedes the onset of the delta wave or where an accessory pathway potential is recorded. If the accessory pathway is concealed, an application of energy is appropriate at the site of earliest retrograde atrial activation through the accessory pathway.
2. Transseptal catheterization or cannulation of the femoral artery allows mapping of the posteroseptal region of the mitral annulus. Application of radiofrequency energy is warranted at sites where local ventricular activation precedes the onset of the delta wave, where an accessory pathway potential is recorded, or if the accessory pathway is concealed where there is earliest retrograde atrial activation through the accessory pathway.
3. Injection of contrast into the coronary sinus is used to determine the location and caliber of the middle cardiac vein and to look for a coronary sinus diverticulum, followed by detailed mapping within the coronary sinus and its branches. Careful delivery of radiofrequency energy within the coronary sinus, middle cardiac vein, or coronary sinus diverticulum may be appropriate if mapping demonstrates a site that is more attractive than the right- and left-sided endocardial sites and if the ablation catheter does not appear to be completely occluding the venous structure.

This systematic approach to mapping and ablation of posteroseptal accessory pathways should result in a successful outcome. In exceptional cases in which successful ablation is not achieved with conventional radiofrequency ablation, one of the following options may be appropriate, depending on the particular clinical circumstances: pharmacologic treatment, radiofrequency ablation using a saline-cooled catheter, or surgical ablation of the accessory pathway.

REFERENCES

1. Morady F, Scheinman MM. Transvenous catheter ablation of a posteroseptal accessory pathway in a patient with the Wolff-Parkinson-White syndrome. *N Engl J Med* 1984;310:705–707.
2. Morady F, Scheinman MM, Kou WH, et al. Long-term results of catheter ablation of a posteroseptal accessory AV connection in 48 patients. *Circulation* 1989;79:1160–1170.
3. Sealy WC, Gallagher JJ. The surgical approach to the septal area of the heart based on experiences with 45 patients with Kent bundles. *J Thorac Cardiovasc Surg* 1980;79:542–551.
4. Davies LM, Byth K, Ellis P, et al. Dimensions of the posterior septal space and coronary sinus. *Am J Cardiol* 1991;68:621–625.
5. Sealy WC, Mikat EM. Anatomical problems with identification and interruption of posterior septal Kent bundles. *Ann Thorac Surg* 1983;36:584–595.
6. Guiraudon GM, Klein GJ, Sharma AD, et al. Surgical ablation of posterior septal accessory pathways in the Wolff-Parkinson-White syndrome by a closed heart technique. *J Thorac Cardiovasc Surg* 1986;92:406–413.

7. Guiraudon GM, Guiraudon CM, Klein GJ, et al. The coronary sinus diverticulum: a pathologic entity associated with the Wolff-Parkinson-White syndrome. Am J Cardiol 1988;62:733–735.
8. Rodriguez LM, Smeets JL, de Chillou C, et al. The 12-lead electrocardiogram in midseptal, anteroseptal, posteroseptal and right free wall accessory pathways. Am J Cardiol 1993;72:1274–1280.
9. Kerr CR, Gallagher JJ, German LD. Changes in ventriculoatrial intervals with bundle branch block aberration during reciprocating tachycardia in patients with accessory AV pathways. Circulation 1982;66:196–201.
10. Martinez-Alday JD, Almendral J, Arenal A, et al. Identification of concealed posteroseptal Kent pathways by comparison of ventriculoatrial intervals from apical and posterobasal right ventricular sites. Circulation 1994;89:1060–1067.
11. Hirao K, Otomo K, Wang X, et al. Para-Hisian pacing: a new method for differentiating retrograde conduction over a accessory AV pathway from conduction over the AV node. Circulation 1996;94:1027–1035.
12. Souza JJ, Zivin A, Flemming M, et al. Differential effect of adenosine on anterograde and retrograde fast pathway conduction in patients with AV nodal reentrant tachycardia. J Cardiovasc Electrophysiol 1998;9:820–824.
13. Dhala AA, Deshpande SS, Bremner S, et al. Transcatheter ablation of posteroseptal accessory pathways using a venous approach and radiofrequency energy. Circulation 1994;90:1799–1810.
14. Morady F, Strickberger SA, Man KC, et al. Reasons for prolonged or failed attempts at radiofrequency catheter ablation of accessory pathways. J Am Coll Cardiol 1996;27:683–689.
15. Arruda M, Wang X, McClelland J, et al. ECG algorithm for predicting radiofrequency ablation site in posteroseptal accessory pathways [Abstract]. Pacing Clin Electrophysiol 1992;15:535.
16. Chiang CE, Chen SA, Tai CT, et al. Prediction of successful ablation site of concealed posteroseptal accessory pathways by a novel algorithm using baseline electrophysiologic parameters: implication for an abbreviated ablation procedure. Circulation 1996;93:982–991.
17. Arruda MS, McClelland JM, Wang X, et al. Development and validation of an ECG algorithm for identifying accessory pathway ablation site in Wolff-Parkinson-White syndrome. J Cardiovasc Electrophysiol 1998;9:2–12.
18. Takahashi A, Shah DC, Jais P, et al. Specific electrocardiographic features of manifest coronary vein posteroseptal accessory pathways. J Cardiovasc Electrophysiol 1998;9:1015–1025.
19. Lesh MD, Van Hare G, Kao AD, Scheinman MM. Radiofrequency catheter ablation for Wolff-Parkinson-White syndrome associated with a coronary sinus diverticulum. Pacing Clin Electrophysiol 1991;110:1479–84.
20. Omran H, Pfeiffer, Tebbenjohanns J, et al. Echocardiographic imaging of coronary sinus diverticula and middle cardiac veins in patients with preexcitation syndrome: impact on radiofrequency catheter ablation of posteroseptal accessory pathways. Pacing Clin Electrophysiol 1995;18:1236–1243.
21. Calkins H, Kim YN, Schmaltz S, et al. Electrogram criteria for identification of appropriate target sites for radiofrequency catheter ablation of accessory atrioventricular connections. Circulation 1992;85:565–573.
22. Langberg JJ, Man KC, Vorperian VR, et al. Recognition and catheter ablation of subepicardial accessory pathways. J Am Coll Cardiol 1993;22:1100–1004.
23. Critelli G, Gallagher JJ, Monda V, et al. Anatomic and electrophysiologic substrate of the permanent form of junctional reciprocating tachycardia. J Am Coll Cardiol 1984;4:601–610.
24. Gaita F, Haissaguerre M, Giustetto C, et al. Catheter ablation of permanent junctional reciprocating tachycardia with radiofrequency current. J Am Coll Cardiol 1995;25:648–654.
25. Dorostkar PC, Silka MJ, Morady F, Dick M. Clinical course of persistent junctional reciprocating tachycardia. J Am Coll Cardiol 1999;33:366–375.
26. Langberg JJ, Calkins H, Atassi R, et al. Temperature monitoring during radiofrequency catheter ablation of accessory pathways. Circulation 1992;86:1469–1474.
27. Langberg J, Griffin JC, Herre JM, et al. Catheter ablation of accessory pathways using radiofrequency energy in the canine coronary sinus. J Am Coll Cardiol 1989;13:491–496.
28. Giorgberidze I, Saksena S, Krol RB, et al. Efficacy and safety of radiofrequency catheter ablation of left-sided accessory pathways through the coronary sinus. Am J Cardiol 1995;76:359–365.
29. Jackman WM, Wang X, Friday KJ, et al. Catheter ablation of accessory AV pathways (Wolff-Parkinson-White syndrome) by radiofrequency current. N Engl J Med 1991;324:1605–1611.
30. Bashir Y, Heald SC, O'Nunain S, et al. Radiofrequency current delivery by way of a bipolar tricuspid annulus-mitral electrode configuration for ablation of posteroseptal accessory pathways. J Am Coll Cardiol 1993;22:550–556.
31. Nakagawa H, Yamanashi WS, Pitha JV, et al. Comparison of in vivo tissue temperature profile and lesion geometry for radiofrequency ablation with a saline-irrigated electrode versus temperature control in a canine thigh muscle preparation. Circulation 1995;91:2264–2273.
32. Nakagawa H, Khastgir T, Arruda M, et al. Radiofrequency catheter ablation using a saline irrigated electrode in patients with prior failed accessory pathway ablation [Abstract]. Pacing Clin Electrophysiol 1995;18:832.
33. Arruda M, Nakagawa H, Khastgir T, et al. Facilitation of accessory pathway ablation from the middle cardiac vein by a saline irrigated catheter electrode [Abstract]. Pacing Clin Electrophysiol 1995;18:832.
34. Arruda M, Nakagawa H, Chandrasekaran K, et al. Radiofrequency ablation in the coronary venous system is associated with risk of coronary artery injury which may be prevented by use of intravascular ultrasound [Abstract]. J Am Coll Cardiol 1996;27:160A.
35. Schluter M, Geiger M, Siebels J, et al. Catheter ablation using radiofrequency current to cure symptomatic patients with tachyarrhythmia related to an accessory atrioventricular pathway. Circulation 1991;84:1644–1661.
36. Calkins H, Langberg J, Sousa J, et al. Radiofrequency catheter ablation of accessory AV connections in 250 patients: abbreviated therapeutic approach to Wolff-Parkinson-White syndrome. Circulation 1992;85:1337–1346.
37. Lesh MD, Van Hare GF, Schamp DJ, et al. Curative percutaneous catheter ablation using radiofrequency energy for accessory pathways in all locations: results in 100 consecutive patients. J Am Coll Cardiol 1992;19:1303–1309.
38. Swartz JF, Tracy CM, Fletcher RD. Radiofrequency endocardial catheter ablation of accessory atrioventricular pathway atrial insertion sites. Circulation 1993;87:487–499.
39. Wang X, Jackman WM, McClelland J, et al. Sites of successful radiofrequency ablation of posteroseptal accessory pathways [Abstract]. Pacing Clin Electrophysiol 1992;15:535.
40. Jentzer JH, Goyal R, Williamson BD, et al. Analysis of junctional ectopy during radiofrequency ablation of the slow pathway in patients with atrioventricular nodal reentrant tachycardia. Circulation 1994;90:2820–2826.

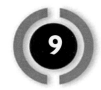

CATHETER ABLATION OF ANTEROSEPTAL AND MIDSEPTAL ACCESSORY PATHWAYS
• • •
HUGH CALKINS, RONALD D. BERGER

During the past two decades, catheter ablation has emerged from being a highly experimental technique to its current role as first-line therapy for the treatment of many cardiac arrhythmias, including the Wolff-Parkinson-White syndrome and paroxysmal supraventricular tachycardia involving an accessory pathway (1–3). Accessory pathways can be classified according to their location, direction of conduction (i.e., manifest or concealed), and rate of conduction (i.e., decremental or nondecremental and rapid or slow conduction). This chapter reviews the current state of knowledge concerning the technique, results, and complications associated with radiofrequency catheter ablation of anteroseptal and midseptal accessory pathways. Anteroseptal and midseptal accessory pathways are uncommon, accounting for less than 10% of accessory pathways (4–17) (Tables 9-1 and 9-2). Their importance rests primarily on the increased risk of developing atrioventricular block as a complication of catheter ablation as a result of the proximity of these accessory pathways to the specialized conduction system.

⊙ ANATOMY OF THE ANTEROSEPTAL AND MIDSEPTAL SPACE

In the most general sense, the location of accessory pathways can be subdivided into four regions of the heart: right free wall, left free wall, anteroseptal, and posteroseptal (18,19). A somewhat more detailed classification scheme that subdivides the location of accessory pathways into 14 separate regions is commonly used by interventional electrophysiologists (Fig. 9-1). Although this simplified scheme is widely used, it fails to highlight the anatomic complexity of the midseptal and anteroseptal space (20,21). Figure 9-2 is an anatomic view of the heart viewed from above with the atria removed. It can be appreciated that the aortic valve is wedged between the mitral and tricuspid valves. The leaflets of the mitral and aortic valves are in fibrous continuity, with the fibrous tissue at each end thickened to form the right and left fibrous trigones. The aortic outflow tract itself extends posteriorly in the left ventricle such that only a small part of the annulus of the mitral valve abuts the ventricular septum. In this area, the septal leaflet of the tricuspid valve is displaced apically relative to the attachments of the mitral valve so that there is a muscular atrioventricular septum between the attachments of the mitral and tricuspid valves. The muscular interventricular septum is replaced in its anterior portion by a membranous septum that is located immediately below the right and posterior aortic valve cusps. The membranous septum is divided into two parts by the septal leaflet of the tricuspid valve, which inserts more api-

TABLE 9-1 • CATHETER ABLATION OF ANTEROSEPTAL ACCESSORY PATHWAYS

Study	Patients (n)	Incidence	Approach (IVC/SVC)	Approach (A/V)	Success (n)	AV Block (n)	Other AV Block (n)	RBBB (n)	Recurrence (n)
Jackman (5)	13	8%	SVC	V	13 (100%)	0	0	5	2 (15%)
Lesh (6)	7	6%	IVC	V	7 (100%)	0	0	3	0 (0%)
Calkins (4)	10	4%	IVC		8 (80%)	2	0	0	
Swartz (7)	10	8%	IVC	A	9 (90%)	0	0		0
Kay (8)	19	5%	IVC or SVC	V	19 (100%)	0	0		0
Yeh (14)	11	4%	IVC		9 (82%)	0	3	4	
Haissaguerre (9)	8	1%	IVC or SVC	V	8 (100%)	0	0	1	0
Satake (10)	10		IVC	V	10 (100%)	0	0	0	0
Xie (11)	6	NA	IVC		5 (83%)	0	0	0	
Schluter (13)	12	8%	SVC	A	12 (100%)	0	0	2	1 (10%)
Brugada (16)	60	13%	IVC	V	56 (93%)	1			3 (5%)
Total	166				156 (94%)	3 (2%)	3 (2%)	15 (10%)	6 (5%)

A, atrial; AV, atrioventricular; IVC, inferior vena cava; RBBB, right bundle branch block; SVC, superior vena cava; V, ventricular; NA, not available.

cally than the septal attachments of the mitral valve. There is a membranous interventricular septum and a membranous atrioventricular septum. The central fibrous body, which is the keystone of the cardiac fibrous skeleton, is formed by this membranous septum and the right fibrous trigone. The muscular atrioventricular septum is located immediately posterior to the membranous septum.

When considered from this anatomic perspective, it can be appreciated that the midseptum is in reality the only true area of muscular septal contiguity in the atrioventricular junction and represents the area between the offset attachments of the leaflets of the mitral and tricuspid valves (Fig. 9-2). The anteroseptal and posteroseptal areas could be more accurately described as the areas anterior and posterior to the true septum.

The term *atrioventricular junction* refers to the atrioventricular myocardial continuity that allows atrial impulses to be transmitted to the ventricular myocardium through the normal atrioventricular (AV) node and His bundle system. The compact AV node lies

TABLE 9-2 • CATHETER ABLATION OF MIDSEPTAL ACCESSORY PATHWAYS

Study	Patients (n)	Incidence	Approach (IVC/SVC)	Approach (A/V)	Success (n)	AV Block (n)	Other AV Block (n)	RBBB (n)	Recurrence (n)
Lesh (6)	6	6%	IVC	V	6 (100%)	0	0	0	2 (33%)
Calkins (4)	5	2%	IVC		5 (100%)	0	0	0	0
Swartz (7)	11	9%	IVC	A	11 (100%)	1		0	
Kay (8)	12	3%	IVC or SVC	V	11 (92%)	0	1	np	
Yeh (14)	3	1%	IVC		1 (33%)	1	1	0	
Satake (10)	7		IVC	V	7 (100%)	0	0	0	0
Xie (11)	20		IVC		17 (85%)	2	0	0	
Kuck (15)	6	4%	SVC	A	6 (100%)	0	0	0	1 (17%)
Lorga (12)	15		IVC		15 (100%)	0	0	0	3 (20%)
Brugada (16)	37	8%	IVC	V	33 (89%)	1			1 (3%)
Total	122				112 (92%)	5 (4%)	2 (3%)		7 (10%)

A, atrial; AV, atrioventricular; IVC, inferior vena cava; RBBB, right bundle branch block; SVC, superior vena cava; V, ventricular.

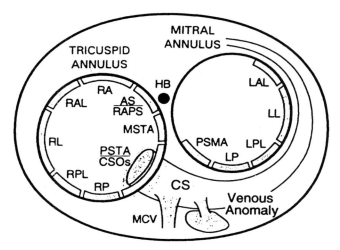

at the apex of the triangle of Koch and rests on the atrial aspect of the muscular atrioventricular septum. The triangle of Koch is bordered superiorly by the tendon of Todaro and inferiorly by the annular extent of the septal tricuspid leaflet; it contains the ostium of the coronary sinus in its posterior part (Fig. 9-3). The tendon of Todaro merges with the central fibrous body at the anterior tip of Koch's triangle. In humans, it has been estimated that the compact AV node is

FIGURE 9-1. The the tricuspid and mitral annuli as viewed from a left anterior oblique projection. The standard classification of the location of accessory pathways into 13 distinct anatomic regions is shown. AS, anterospetal; CS, coronary sinus; CSO, coronary sinus ostium; HB, His bundle; LAL, left anterolateral; LL, left lateral; LP, left posterior; LPL, left posterolateral; MCV, middle cardiac vein; MSTA, midseptal tricuspid annulus; PSMA, posteroseptal mitral annulus; PSTA, posteroseptal tricuspid annulus; RA, right anterior; RAL, right anterolateral; RAPS, right anterior paraseptal; RL, right lateral; RP, right posterior; RPL, right posterolateral. (From Arruda MS, McClelland JH, Wang X, et al. Development and validation of an ECG algorithm for identifying accessory pathway ablation site in Wolff-Parkinson-White syndrome. *J Cardiovasc Electrophysiol* 1998;9:2–12, with permission.)

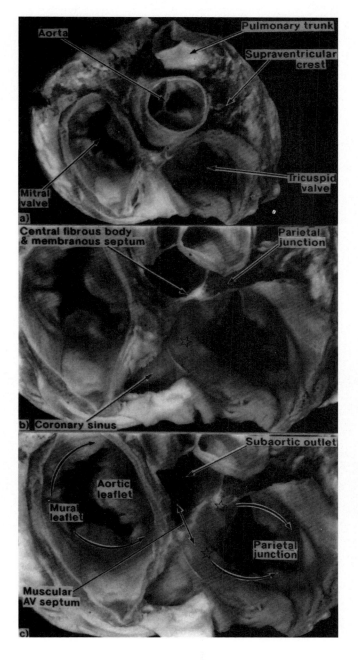

FIGURE 9-2. **A:** Series of dissections created by removing the segment of the heart where the atrial musculature inserts into the ventricular mass. **B:** Removal of the noncoronary (posterior) sinus of the aortic valve reveals the central fibrous body and atrioventricular (AV) component of the membranous septum. Part of the roof of the coronary sinus is removed. The star marks the position of the muscular component of the AV septum. **C:** Further excavation in a direction posterior to the central fibrous body exposes the muscular AV septum. The double-headed arrow shows its position between the right atrium and the left ventricular outlet. The musculature between the two stars is the true extent of the septal component of the AV junction. Curved arrows around the tricuspid valve indicate the nonseptal AV junction. On the left, the AV junction surrounds the two leaflets of the mitral valve, but because of the fibrous continuity between the aortic leaflet of the mitral valve and the aortic valve itself, only the atrial myocardium around the mural leaflet has the potential for communication with the ventricular myocardium. (From Dean JW, Ho SY, Rowland E, et al. Clinical anatomy of the atrioventricular junctions. *J Am Coll Cardiol* 1994;24:1725–1731, with permission.)

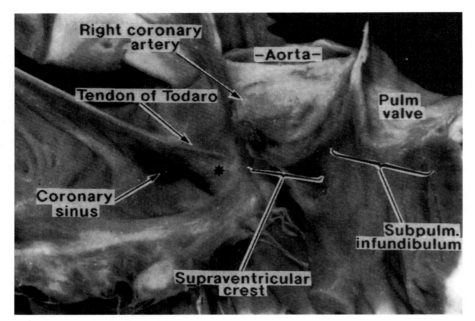

FIGURE 9-3. Dissection reveals the relation of the triangle of Koch to the anterior area of the septum. The position of the AV node is marked by an asterisk. (From Dean JW, Ho SY, Rowland E, et al. Clinical anatomy of the atrioventricular junctions. *J Am Coll Cardiol* 1994; 24:1725–1731, with permission.)

1.7 to 3 mm long (19). More anteriorly, the conduction axis becomes surrounded by a fibrous collar as it penetrates the central fibrous body to become the bundle of His, which is 1 to 1.5 cm long. The His bundle travels along the posterior edge of the membranous septum to the apex of the muscular interventricular septum, where it divides into the right and left bundle branches. The proximal portions of the ventricular bundle branches are encased by a thin sheath of fibrous tissue. The Wolff-Parkinson-White syndrome is associated with myocardial atrioventricular connections distinct from the normal AV node–His bundle system that allow the atrial or ventricular impulses to bypass the normal atrioventricular junction. Accessory pathways cannot lie in the region of the fibrous connection between the mitral and aortic valves because there is no potential continuity between the atrium and ventricle in this region.

⦿ ELECTROPHYSIOLOGIC CLASSIFICATION OF ANTEROSEPTAL AND MIDSEPTAL ACCESSORY PATHWAYS

In the electrophysiology laboratory, midseptal accessory pathways are defined as those that lie anterior to the coronary sinus os and posterior to a catheter positioned to record a His bundle potential. Anteroseptal accessory pathways are defined as those that lie in proximity to or immediately anterior to the His bundle. The term *anteroseptal accessory pathways* should be reserved for the subset of accessory pathways that have a His potential associated with the atrial or ventricular insertion of the accessory pathway (as evidenced by the presence of an accessory pathway potential or earliest activation) (Fig. 9-4). Haissaguerre and colleagues proposed that the term *para-Hisian accessory pathway* be reserved for the small subset of anteroseptal accessory pathways whose atrial and ventricular insertions are associated with a large His bundle (>0.1 mV), with virtually no distance between tip electrode of the ablation catheter and the His bundle catheter in any fluoroscopic view (9).

⦿ ELECTROCARDIOGRAPHIC CHARACTERISTICS OF ANTEROSEPTAL AND MIDSEPTAL ACCESSORY PATHWAYS

The characteristics of the 12-lead electrocardiogram (ECG) can be useful in the localization of manifest accessory pathways, which represented three fourths of the middle and anteroseptal accessory pathways in one large ablation series (16). This method of evalua-

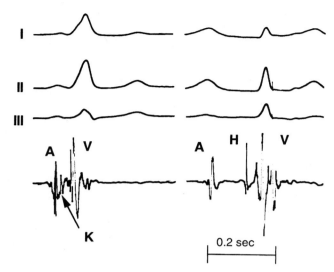

FIGURE 9-4. Local electrogram recorded at the successful ablation site of an anteroseptal accessory pathway. Notice the presence of an accessory pathway potential during preexcited rhythm and a large His potential, which can be observed after spontaneous block in the accessory pathway. Whenever possible, the size of the His potential should be less than 0.1 mV at sites of radiofrequency energy delivery.

tion is of particular value among patients with midseptal and anteroseptal accessory pathways. If the 12-lead ECG suggests the presence of an accessory pathway in this location, discussions regarding the potential risk of complete heart block can be initiated with the patient and patient's family before proceeding with electrophysiology testing and catheter ablation. Representative 12-lead ECGs obtained from a patients with an anteroseptal and midseptal accessory pathway are shown in Figures 9-5 and 9-6, respectively.

The normal sequence of ventricular depolarization begins with activation of the midportion of the interventricular septum. This occurs in a left-to-right direction on the surface ECG, resulting in a septal q waves in ECG leads I, V_5, and V_6 and r waves in leads V_1 and V_2. In contrast, in the presence of an antegrade conducting accessory pathway, atrioventricular conduction occurs through the specialized His-Purkinje system and by means of the accessory pathway, resulting in preexcitation of the portion of the right ventricle at the site where insertion of the accessory pathway occurs. With manifest anteroseptal and midseptal accessory pathways, premature activation of the summit of the right ventricle, with relatively unopposed left free wall forces, results in a left bundle branch block pattern.

Several studies have reported on the accuracy of various algorithms in determining the location of an accessory pathway based on the 12-lead ECG (11, 22,23). Arruda and colleagues (22) developed their algorithm by correlating a resting 12-lead ECG with a successful ablation site in 135 consecutive patients with a single, antegradely conducting accessory pathway and subsequently testing 121 consecutive patients. The ECG parameters that were evaluated included the polarity of the initial 20 msec of the delta wave in leads 1, 2, aVF, and V_1 (classified as positive, negative, or isoelectric) and the ratio of the R and S wave amplitudes in leads 3 and V_1 (classified as R ≥

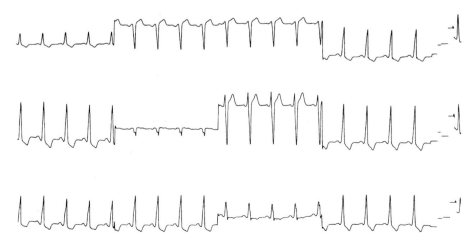

FIGURE 9-5. Twelve-lead electrocardiogram during normal sinus rhythm from a patient with an anteroseptal accessory pathway.

242   I. INTERVENTIONAL TECHNIQUES FOR ABLATION OF TACHYCARDIAS

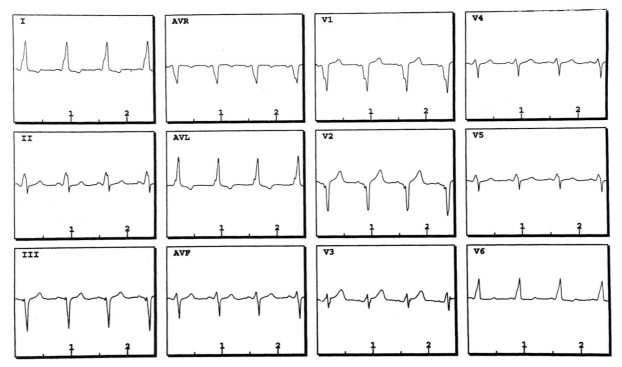

FIGURE 9-6. Twelve-lead electrocardiogram during normal sinus rhythm from a patient with a midseptal accessory pathway.

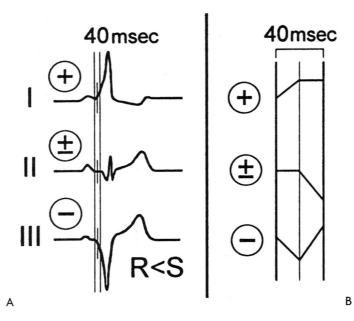

FIGURE 9-7. Delta wave polarity was determined by examining the initial 20 msec after the earliest delta wave onset in the limb leads. **A:** ECG leads 1, 2, and 3 of a patient with an accessory pathway located at the anteroseptal tricuspid annulus region. **B:** Determination of delta wave polarity (using the initial 20 msec) in the event of changes within 40 msec. (From Arruda MS, McClelland JH, Wang X, et al. Development and validation of an ECG algorithm for identifying accessory pathway ablation site in Wolff-Parkinson-White syndrome. *J Cardiovasc Electrophysiol* 1998;9:2–12, with permission.)

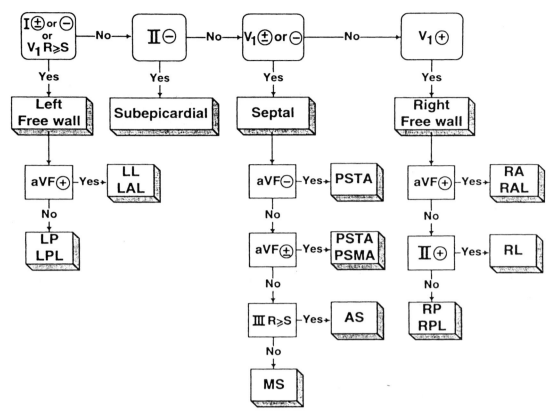

FIGURE 9-8. Stepwise ECG algorithm for determination of accessory pathway location. AS, anteroseptal; LAL, left anterolateral; LL, left lateral; LP, left posterior; LPL, left posterolateral; MSTA, midseptal tricuspid annulus; PSMA, posteroseptal mitral annulus; PSTA, posteroseptal tricuspid annulus; RA, right anterior; RAL, right anterolateral; RL, right lateral; RP, right posterior; RPL, right posterolateral. (From Arruda MS, McClelland JH, Wang X, et al. Development and validation of an ECG algorithm for identifying accessory pathway ablation site in Wolff-Parkinson-White syndrome. *J Cardiovasc Electrophysiol* 1998;9:2–12; with permission.)

S or R < S in Figs. 9-7 and 9-8). Septal accessory pathways were distinguished from right free wall accessory pathways by the presence of an isoelectric or negative delta wave in V_1 and a positive delta wave in aVF. Anteroseptal accessory pathways were characterized by an R ≥ S in lead 3, whereas midseptal accessory pathways were characterized by an R < S in lead 3 (Fig. 9-8). Prospective testing revealed that this algorithm was particularly useful in correctly localizing anteroseptal accessory pathways (sensitivity of 75%, specificity of 99%) and midseptal accessory pathways (sensitivity of 100%, specificity of 98%).

Fitzpatrick and colleagues (23) developed a somewhat different algorithm that relied in part on the QRS transition zone across the precordium. Right-sided septal accessory pathways (anteroseptal, midseptal, and posteroseptal) could be distinguished from right free wall accessory pathways based on the presence of a QRS transition (from negative to positive) at or before lead V_3 or a QRS transition in V_4 combined with a delta wave in lead 2 of 1.0 mV or more. The sum of the delta wave polarities in the inferior leads 2, 3, and aVF was the most important variable for distinguishing among accessory pathways located in the septal area. If this sum was greater than +1, the accessory pathway was anteroseptal. If the sum was less than −1, it was posteroseptal, and if it was −1, 0, or +1, it was midseptal.

Several other studies have focused on the ECG characteristics of specific subsets of anteroseptal and midseptal accessory pathways. Lorga and colleagues subdivided the location of midseptal accessory pathways into three zones spanning the region between the His bundle catheter and the coronary sinus os (zones 1 through 3, with zone 1 being most anterior) (12). Each patient had a positive delta wave in 1, 2, aVL, and V_3 through V_6 and a negative delta wave in 3 and aVR. The delta wave polarity in aVF was the only ECG parameter that predicted the accessory pathway location. Six of eight ablated in zone 3 had a negative delta wave in aVF, and six of seven ablated in zones 1 and 2 had positive or isoelectric delta waves in aVF. Haissaguerre analyzed the ECG patterns from eight patients with what was called a para-Hisian accessory pathway (9). This subset of anteroseptal accessory pathways were defined as present when its atrial and ventricular insertions were associated with a large His bundle of more than 0.1 mV, with virtually no distance between tip electrode of the ablation catheter and the His bundle catheter in any fluoroscopic view. The ECG characteristics of para-Hisian accessory pathways are similar to anterospetal accessory pathways, including positive delta waves in 1, 2, and aVF. However, the para-Hisian accessory pathway can be differentiated from anteroseptal accessory pathways by the presence of negative delta waves in V_1 and V_2, with a positive and negative predictive accuracy of 86% and 93%, respectively .

In summary, the results of these studies suggest that in the presence of significant preexcitation physicians should be alert to the presence of an anteroseptal or midseptal accessory pathway in a patient who presents with an a 12-lead ECG characterized by a left bundle pattern in lead V_1, an isoelectric or negative delta wave in V_1, and a positive delta wave in aVF. Anteroseptal accessory pathways were characterized by an R $\geq$ S in lead 3, whereas midseptal accessory pathways were characterized by an R $<$ S in lead 3.

⦿ ABLATION OF ANTEROSEPTAL AND MIDSEPTAL ACCESSORY PATHWAYS

A diagnostic electrophysiologic study is performed before or in conjunction with the catheter ablation procedure. The study can confirm the presence of an accessory pathway and determine the number and conduction characteristics of the accessory pathways, as well as define the role of the accessory pathway in the patient's clinical tachycardia. Standard quadripolar electrode catheters are introduced through the inferior vena cava and positioned in the high right atrium, the His-bundle position, and at the apex of the right ventricle. Typically, a multielectrode catheter is also positioned in the coronary sinus by way of the superior vena cava or inferior vena cava. Atrial and ventricular pacing and programmed stimulation is then performed using standard techniques. Orthodromic atrioventricular reciprocating tachycardia is the most commonly induced sustained arrhythmia. The presence of an accessory pathway with retrograde conduction can be determined by delivering a late ventricular extrastimulus during orthodromic tachycardia in an attempt to advance the timing of atrial activation when the His bundle is refractory. For anteroseptal accessory pathways, the preexcitation index is usually less than 25 msec (24). When functional left or right bundle branch block occurs spontaneously during orthodromic reciprocating tachycardia involving a midseptal or anteroseptal accessory pathway, the ventriculoatrial interval does not change or lengthens by less than 30 msec (25). The development of ipsilateral functional bundle branch block during orthodromic reciprocating tachycardia results in a ventriculoatrial conduction interval prolongation of 35 msec or more in the presence of a free wall accessory pathway (26).

When an accessory pathway participates in the antegrade direction during the reentrant tachycardia, the resulting tachycardia is called antidromic atrioventricular reentrant tachycardia (AVRT). Antidromic AVRT occurs rarely in the presence of a single midseptal or anteroseptal accessory pathway (27). When supraventricular tachycardia cannot be induced (particularly in the presence of an anteroseptal or midseptal accessory pathway), it may be difficult to differentiate retrograde accessory pathway conduction from retrograde AV nodal conduction. Several techniques may be useful in this setting. First, the administration of intravenous adenosine to selectively block retrograde AV node conduction can help in mapping and ablating anteroseptal and midseptal accessory pathways. Demonstration of ventriculoatrial conduction block with adenosine after, but not before, catheter ablation can provide a useful end point for catheter ablation (28,29).

A second approach involves repositioning the right ventricular pacing catheter from the right ventricular apex toward the site of earliest retrograde activation (30–32). The stimulus-atrial interval shortens with retrograde accessory pathway conduction, whereas it increases in patients with only retrograde AV nodal conduction.

A third approach involves the use of para-Hisian pacing (32). This approach involves positioning an electrode catheter with close interelectrode spacing close to the His bundle or proximal right bundle branch. The pacing output is altered to produce ventricular capture with intermittent His bundle capture to selectively alter the timing of His bundle activation without changing the timing of local ventricular activation. In the presence of an accessory pathway with retrograde conduction, the loss of His bundle capture should not change the timing or the activation sequence of retrograde atrial activation. In the setting of retrograde AV nodal conduction, the delay in timing of retrograde His bundle activation should produce an equal delay in the timing of retrograde atrial activation without changing the retrograde atrial activation sequence. Hirao and colleagues (32) reported that para-Hisian pacing correctly identified retrograde accessory pathway conduction in 132 of 147 accessory pathway patients, including all septal and right free wall accessory pathways. Accessory pathways that were not correctly identified using this technique included those in 9 of 34 patients with left free wall accessory pathways and 6 of 9 patients with PJRT (Figs. 9-9 through 9-11).

After the diagnostic electrophysiology study has been performed, confirming the indication for catheter ablation, efforts are focused on localization of the accessory pathway. In patients with a manifest accessory pathway, regional localization is accomplished with analysis of a maximally preexcited electrocardiogram as described previously. In patients with a concealed accessory pathway, localization of the accessory pathway is performed by mapping the sequence of retrograde atrial activation during orthodromic atrioventricular reciprocating tachycardia or during ventricular pacing. Whenever possible, mapping of the retrograde activation sequence should be performed

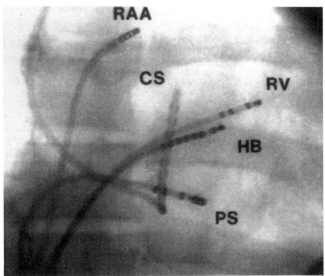

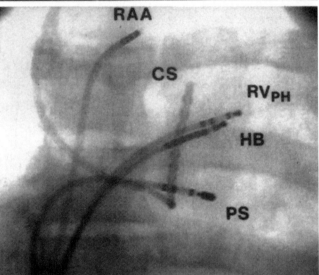

FIGURE 9-9. Radiographs using the right anterior oblique projection illustrate the catheter position used for para-Hisian pacing. (From Hirao K, Otomo K, Wang X, et al. Para-hisian pacing: a new method for differentiating retrograde conduction over an accessory AV pathway from conduction over the node. *Circulation* 1996;94:1027–1035, with permission.)

during orthodromic atrioventricular reciprocating tachycardia, because this eliminates the confounding factor of fusion of atrial activation due to retrograde ventriculoatrial conduction across the accessory pathway and AV node.

Mapping is typically performed with a steerable quadripolar electrode catheter with a 4-mm distal electrode that is initially positioned in the right ventricle and withdrawn to position the electrode pairs

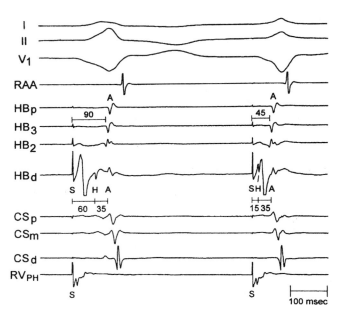

FIGURE 9-10. Para-Hisian pacing, demonstrating retrograde conduction over the fast AV nodal pathway. The pacing stimulus in the left complex did not produce His bundle (HB) capture, reflected by the wide QRS complex and relatively late His bundle activation (S-H interval = 60 msec). HB capture was achieved on the right complex, reflected by narrowing of the QRS complex and shortening of the S-H interval to 15 msec. The 45-msec shortening in the S-H interval was matched by a 45-msec shortening in the sinoatrial (S-A) interval from 90 to 45 msec, without a change in the atrial activation sequence. The constant atrial-His bundle (A-H) interval (35 msec) and atrial activation sequence indicate that retrograde conduction depended on activation of the His bundle and not on the local ventricular myocardium (From Hirao K, Otomo K, Wang X, et al. Para-hisian pacing: a new method for differentiating retrograde conduction over an accessory AV pathway from conduction over the node. *Circulation* 1996;94:1027–1035, with permission.)

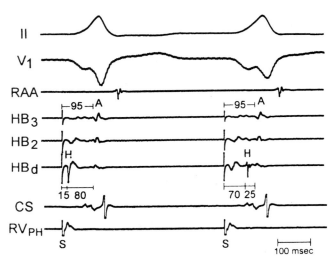

FIGURE 9-11. Para-Hisian pacing demonstrating retrograde conduction over an anteroseptal accessory pathway. The pacing stimulus in the left complex produced HB capture, reflected by the His bundle activation (S-H) interval of 15 msec. Loss of His bundle (HB) capture in the right complex resulted in a 55 msec increase in the S-H interval to 70 msec. The sinoatrial (S-A) interval remained fixed at 95 msec, and the atrial activation sequence remained identical, indicating that retrograde conduction depended on the timing of ventricular activation and not on the timing of the retrograde His bundle activation. (From Hirao K, Otomo K, Wang X, et al. Para-hisian pacing: a new method for differentiating retrograde conduction over an accessory AV pathway from conduction over the node. *Circulation* 1996;94:1027–1035, with permission.)

along the tricuspid annulus. Bipolar intracardiac electrograms (2- or 5-mm interelectrode spacing) from the distal and proximal electrode pairs are recorded. In this manner, the electrophysiologist can establish a prominent ventricular signal distally and a smaller atrial signal proximally along the ablation catheter. The electrograms are recorded using a bandpass filter of 50 to 500 Hz, amplified at a low gain (20 mm/mV) and recorded at paper speeds of 100 or 200 mm/sec. Mapping of accessory pathways, including anteroseptal and midseptal accessory pathways, is most readily accomplished by viewing the position of the intracardiac electrode catheters in the left anterior oblique (LAO) and right anterior oblique (RAO) projections. The LAO projection allows the tricuspid annulus to be viewed as a clock face, with His bundle position at 1 o'clock and the coronary sinus os at 5 o'clock. In the LAO fluoroscopic projection, the catheter can be manipulated with clockwise or counterclockwise rotation and moved along the tricuspid annulus. In the RAO view, the position of the tricuspid valve can be identified as a relative lucency because of the presence of the fat pad located along the atrioventricular groove.

We have found several tools useful in mapping right-sided accessory pathways. The first is the use of long, preshaped sheaths (Daig SR0) to deliver the ablation catheter. We may also use 24-pole halo catheters (Figs. 9-12 and 9-13). These catheters can be delivered through a long sheath and positioned along

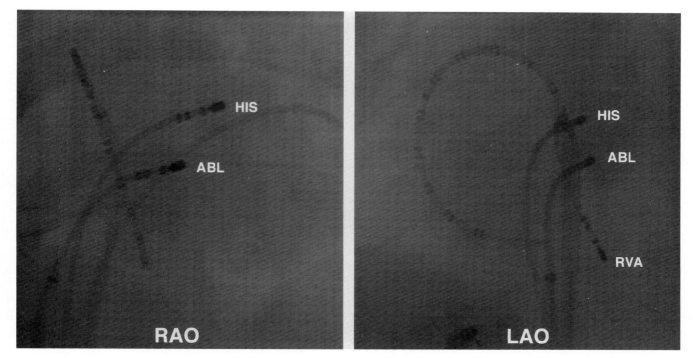

FIGURE 9-12. Representative right and left anterior oblique fluoroscopic images show a site for ablation of an anteroseptal accessory pathway. The ablation catheter has been stabilized with a sheath. A halo catheter was placed to rapidly map the retrograde atrial activation sequence along the tricuspid annulus.

the tricuspid annulus. Sites of early retrograde atrial activation can be rapidly identified with this method. Although these catheters typically do not encompass the midseptal and anteroseptal space, they may be useful in rapidly excluding right free wall accessory pathways.

After the accessory pathway has been localized to a precise region of the tricuspid annulus, the ablation catheter is manipulated until the local electrogram recorded from the distal electrode pair demonstrates "optimal" electrogram characteristics for ablation. Particular attention should be focused on identifying a deflection consistent with an accessory pathway potential. After electrogram stability has been established, radiofrequency energy is delivered. Generally, between 30 and 50 W of radiofrequency energy is delivered for 30 to 60 seconds in the temperature-control mode, with a target temperature set to between 60°C and 70°C (33,34). With right-sided accessory pathways outside the posteroseptal space, the targeted temperature is rarely achieved because of catheter instability and convective cooling by the blood pool. The average electrode temperature at successful ablation sites of right-sided and septal accessory pathways has been reported to be 58°C ± 10°C and 57°C, respectively, compared with 60°C ± 16°C for left free wall accessory pathways (33,34). These target dependent differences may reflect important differences in electrode-tissue contact, catheter stability, and convective heat loss to the blood pool during catheter ablation at these anatomic sites. Catheter positions used during ablation of posteroseptal and left free wall accessory pathways generally result in more stable catheter contact with less exposure to high velocity blood flow compared with those used for right free wall accessory pathways. If no effect is observed after 10 to 15 seconds, the application of radiofrequency energy is generally aborted and the catheter repositioned. After a successful application of radiofrequency energy, the patient is monitored for 30 minutes for recurrence. Electrophysiology testing and administration of adenosine is performed before with-

Ablation of Para-Hisian Accessory Pathway

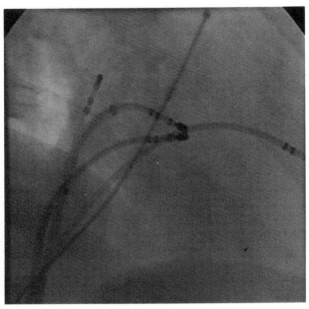
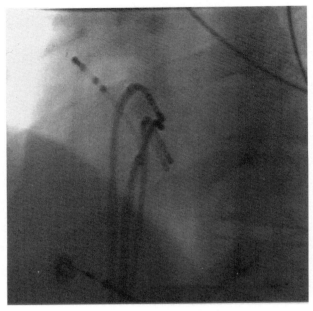

RAO LAO

FIGURE 9-13. Representative right and left anterior oblique fluoroscopic images show a site for ablation of a para-Hisian anteroseptal accessory pathway. The His catheter and the ablation catheter have been stabilized with a sheath. In both projections, the His catheter and ablation catheter are very close to one another.

drawal of the electrode catheters to confirm the absence of early recurrence.

At the conclusion of the ablation procedure, sheaths are removed, and the patient is monitored for a minimum of 3 hours. Catheter ablation of accessory pathways is routinely performed on an outpatient basis (35). However, postprocedure hospitalization for 24 hours should be strongly considered, particularly if any evidence of transient atrioventricular block was observed during the ablation procedure. Although the benefit of aspirin has not been proven, particularly among those patients undergoing catheter ablation on the right side of the heart, we recommend that patients take aspirin for 4 weeks after the ablation procedure. Because of the low risk of recurrence after a successful ablation procedure, follow-up electrophysiology studies usually are not performed on a routine basis (17,36,37).

● ELECTROGRAM CRITERIA FOR SELECTION OF TARGET SITES

Criteria have been developed to identify appropriate target sites for radiofrequency ablation of accessory pathways, which can generally be applied during catheter ablation of accessory pathways in all locations (38). During the ablation of manifest accessory pathways, electrogram characteristics that are independent predictors of success include electrogram stability, the interval between activation of the ventricular component of the local ventricular electrogram and the onset of the delta wave, and the presence of a probable or possible accessory pathway potential. It is important to note that ablation sites should be identified by bracketing the site of earliest activation rather than merely targeting sites with a short or even the shortest atrioventricular interval (38,39). During the ablation of concealed accessory pathways, electrogram characteristics that are predictors of success include electrogram stability, the presence of retrograde continuous electrical activity, and the presence of a probable or possible accessory pathway potential (38).

● POWER DELIVERY AND REDUCING THE RISK OF ATRIOVENTRICULAR BLOCK

The increased risk of complete heart block associated with radiofrequency catheter ablation of anteroseptal accessory pathways was first emphasized in 1992 (4). In this study, complete heart block occurred during catheter ablation in 3 (1%) of 250 patients undergoing catheter ablation of one or more accessory pathways. Two (20%) of 10 patients who underwent catheter ablation of an anteroseptal accessory pathway developed complete heart block. These findings have subsequently been confirmed by others. Chen and colleagues reported two instances of complete heart block among 191 patients undergoing catheter ablation of an accessory pathway (40). Both patients who developed complete heart block were undergoing catheter ablation of an "anteromidseptal" accessory pathway. Yeh and colleagues reported a 33% incidence of complete heart block among patients undergoing catheter ablation of a midseptal accessory pathway (14). Similarly, the Pediatric Catheter Ablation Registry reported the development of second- or third-degree atrioventricular block among 11 (10%) of 106 children who underwent catheter ablation of a midseptal accessory pathway (with four children developing complete heart block) and in 3 (3%) of 111 children undergoing catheter ablation of an anteroseptal accessory pathway (with two children developing complete heart block) (41) (Fig. 9-14). Convincing evidence exists to demonstrate the importance of this complication during catheter ablation of midseptal and anteroseptal accessory pathways.

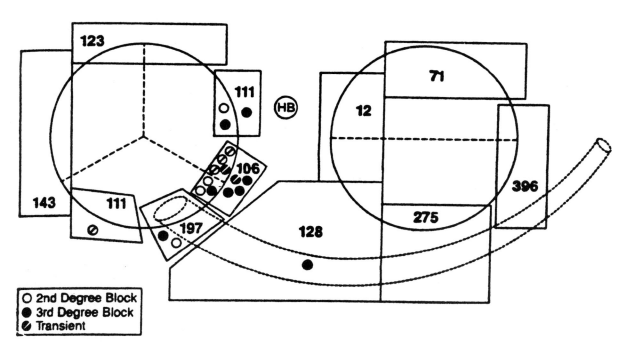

FIGURE 9-14. Sites of atrioventricular block that occurred during catheter ablation in children based on the Pediatric Radiofrequency Ablation Registry. The increased risk of atrioventricular block during ablation in the anteroseptal and especially in the midseptal area can be appreciated. (From Schaffer MS, Silka MJ, Ross BA, Kugler JD. Inadvertent atrioventricular block during radiofrequency catheter ablation: results of the Pediatric Radiofrequency Ablation Registry. *Circulation* 1996;94:3214–3220, with permission.)

Several techniques have been proposed to minimize the risk of complete heart block in this area. The first involves the use of low power output, low temperatures, and short applications of radiofrequency energy. We typically perform catheter ablation in this region using low power (i.e., 10 W) that can gradually be increased while carefully monitoring for the development of a junctional rhythm or atrioventricular block. If temperature-controlled radiofrequency ablation is used, we set the initial target temperature to 50°C. Applications of energy are interrupted if accessory pathway block does not occur within 10 seconds or if a sustained junctional rhythm of more than five consecutive beats develops. In rare cases, overdrive atrial pacing during radiofrequency delivery is required to assess whether preexcitation has resolved because of the development of a junctional rhythm during the radiofrequency application. During current delivery, the catheter position should be continuously monitored fluoroscopically in the LAO projection to verify catheter position stability. The second technique involves maximizing the distance between the ablation catheter and the catheter positioned to record the His bundle. If possible, catheter ablation should be performed at sites at which no His bundle potential is present or, if necessary, a site at which the His potential is less than 0.1 mV. The third technique concerns the selective delivery of radiofrequency energy on the atrial or ventricular side of the annulus. Advocates of delivering radiofrequency energy on the ventricular side of the annulus claim that the fibrous tissue that surrounds the penetrating His bundle, combined with its location deep to the endocardium, renders it less susceptible to thermal injury (5,6,8–10,16). Others have advocated that delivering energy on the atrial side of the annulus reduces the risk of atrioventricular block (7,13,15). These investigators propose that the atrial approach is preferable based on the observation that conduction block typically occurs between the atrial electrogram and the accessory pathway potential during radiofrequency catheter ablation procedures (42). Warin and colleagues reported no instances of complete heart block among 25 patients who underwent catheter ablation of an anteroseptal accessory pathway using direct current energy delivered on the atrial side of the annulus just anterior to the His bundle (43). Advocates exist for the atrial and ventricular approaches. It is unlikely that a prospective study will ever be performed to determine which approach is associated with a lower risk of complete heart block.

We prefer approaching anteroseptal and midseptal accessory pathways from the inferior vena cava and delivering radiofrequency energy at sites with an atrioventricular (A/V) ratio of less than 1. When catheter stability is a problem, we rapidly move to using a long sheath to stabilize the ablation catheter (Fig. 9-12). Regardless of which strategies are employed, the risk of atrioventricular block remains, and it is critical for the electrophysiologist to evaluate the risks of atrioventricular block in light of the severity and potential risks of the accessory pathway that is being ablated. Whereas a 3% risk of complete atrioventricular block may be acceptable for highly symptomatic patients who has failed conventional medical therapy or patients who presented with atrial fibrillation and a rapid ventricular response. This risk of atrioventricular block is not acceptable for asymptomatic or minimally symptomatic patients in whom the accessory pathway refractory period is long.

Catheter ablation of an anteroseptal or midseptal accessory pathway may initially fail because of inaccurate mapping, inadequate tissue heating, or rarely, the presence of a left midseptal accessory pathway. When initial attempts at catheter ablation fail, it is important to consider each of these three factors. In our experience, the most common reason for failure is inadequate tissue heating, often because of catheter instability. Awareness of this problem is readily apparent when temperature monitoring is employed. Approaches to remedy this problem include the use of different ablation catheters with different handling characteristics, an alternative approach to ablation (superior vena cava versus inferior vena cava), or the use of intravascular sheaths. Less common causes for failure are inaccurate mapping or the presence of a left-sided midseptal accessory pathway (11).

EFFICACY AND COMPLICATIONS

Catheter Ablation of Anteroseptal Accessory Pathways

Despite the challenges associated with catheter ablation of anteroseptal accessory pathways, radiofre-

TABLE 9-3 • REVIEW OF CATHETER ABLATION SERIES

Study	Patients (*n*)	AP (*n*)	AP Location					Success (%)
			LFW	PS	MS	AS	RFW	
Calkins (4)	250	267	161	44	5	10	47	94
Jackman (5)	166	177	106	43	0	13	15	99
Lesh (6)	100	109	45	30	6	7	21	89
Swarz (7)	114	122	76	13	11	10	12	95
Haissaguerre (39)	408	436	286	77	0	41	32	97
Kay (18)	363	384	187	92	12	19	62	96
Calkins (17)	500	541	270	90	40[a]		92	93
Total	1901	2036	1131	397	54	120	281	1799/1901 (95%)

AP, accessory pathway; AS, anterospetal; LFW, left free wall; MS, midseptal; PS, posteroseptal; RFW, right free wall.
[a] AS and MS APs not broken down according to location.

quency catheter ablation can be accomplished with a high success rate, approaching that of accessory pathways in other locations, and with only a small risk of complete atrioventricular block. The overall results of catheter ablation of accessory pathways in all locations that have been reported in large series are summarized in Table 9-3. The overall success rate for ablation of accessory pathways in all locations ranged from 89% to 99%. Overall, catheter ablation was successful in 1,799 (95%) of 1,901 patients. Conduction recurred in 10% of patients. A prospective, multicenter clinical trial enrolling 1,050 patients undergoing ablation of an accessory pathway, AV nodal reentrant tachycardia, or the atrioventricular junction, examined the relationship between the success and recurrence rates of catheter ablation and accessory pathway location (17). Among the 536 patients who underwent ablation of one or more accessory pathways in this series, success rates were lower among patients undergoing ablation of a right free wall and posteroseptal accessory pathways (90% and 88%, respectively) than ablation of left free wall accessory pathways (95%). Among the 40 patients who underwent ablation of an anterior or midseptal accessory pathway, the immediate success rate was 98%. Heart block occurred in 1 (2.5%) of these 40 patients, which was similar to the incidence of heart block associated with ablation of posteroseptal accessory pathways (3 [3%] of 98) but higher than the incidence of heart block associated with ablation of left free wall accessory pathways (1 [0.3%] of 270). The incidence of complete atrioventricular block associated with ablation of AV nodal reentrant tachycardia was 1.3% (5 of 373 patients). The incidence of conduction recurrence after successful ablation of an accessory pathway was higher among patients undergoing ablation of a right free wall, septal, or posterospetal accessory pathway than those with left free wall accessory pathways (Fig. 9-15).

The technique and results of catheter ablation of anteroseptal accessory pathways that have been reported in 11 published series are summarized on Table 9-1. Among a total of 166 accessory pathways, catheter ablation was successful in 156 (94%). Complications included complete atrioventricular block in 3 patients (2%), transient or second-degree atrioventricular block in an additional 3 patients (2%), and a new right bundle branch block in 15 patients (10%). Recurrence of accessory pathway conduction occurred in 6 patients (5%). Among 522 patients who have undergone radiofrequency catheter ablation of an accessory pathway at Johns Hopkins Hospital during the past 7 years, an anteroseptal accessory pathway was present in 10. Among these 10 patients, 9 were sufficiently symptomatic to justify the potential risk of complete atrioventricular block. The inferior vena cava approach was used in each with delivery of radiofrequency energy at sites with an atrioventricular ratio (A/V) of less than 1. Catheter ablation was successful in 8 of these 9 patients. Catheter ablation was prematurely terminated in the final patient with a para-Hisian accessory pathway who developed tran-

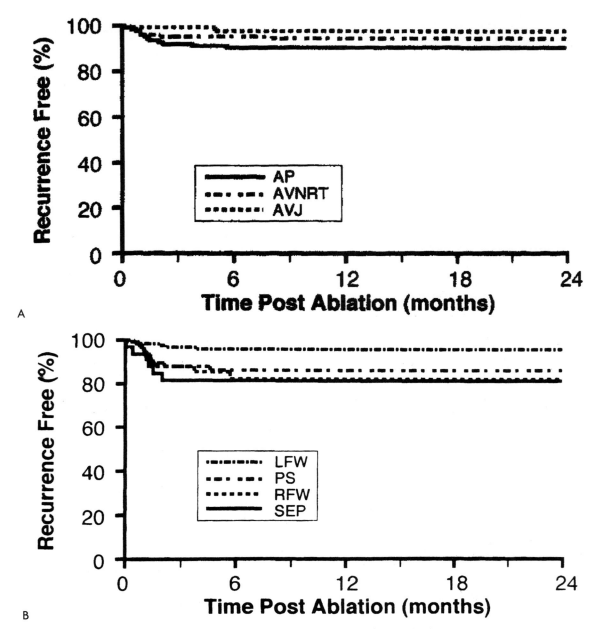

FIGURE 9-15. **A:** The Kaplan-Meier curve shows freedom from arrhythmia recurrence among patients who underwent successful ablation of an accessory pathway, AV nodal reentrant tachycardia, or the atrioventricular junction. This analysis was confined to patients in whom successful ablation was achieved with the investigation ablation system. **B:** The Kaplan-Meier curve shows freedom from arrhythmia recurrence among patients who underwent successful ablation of an accessory pathway subclassified by the location of the accessory pathway. This analysis was confined to patients in whom successful ablation was achieved with the investigation ablation system. LFW, left free wall; PS, posteroseptal; RFW, right free wall; SEP, septal. (From Calkins H, Mann C, Kalbfleisch S, et al. Site of accessory pathway block after radiofrequency catheter ablation in patients with the Wolff-Parkinson-White syndrome. *J Cardiovasc Electrophysiol* 1994;5:20–27, with permission.)

sient complete heart block with radiofrequency energy delivery.

Catheter Ablation of Midseptal Accessory Pathways

The technique and results of catheter ablation of midseptal accessory pathways that have reported in 10 published series are summarized in Table 9-2. Among a total of 122 accessory pathways, catheter ablation was successful in 112 (92%). Complications included complete atrioventricular block in 5 patients (4%) and transient or second degree atrioventricular block in 2 patients. Recurrence of conduction occurred in 7 patients (10%). Among 522 patients who have undergone radiofrequency catheter ablation of an accessory pathway at Johns Hopkins Hospital during the past 7 years, 9 underwent catheter ablation of a midseptal accessory pathway. The inferior vena cava approach was used in each, with delivery of radiofrequency energy at sites with an atrioventricular ratio (A/V) of less than 1. Catheter ablation was successfully accomplished in each patient.

● CONCLUSIONS

In summary, accessory pathways located in the anteroseptal and midseptal region represent an important subset of accessory pathways because of the increased risk of atrioventricular block that is associated with delivery of radiofrequency energy in this region. Catheter ablation of accessory pathways located in this region can be successfully accomplished in more than 90% of patients with a risk of complete heart block of approximately 2%. Because of this increased risk of atrioventricular block, catheter ablation of accessory pathways in this region must be approached cautiously and particular attention should be focused on analyzing the risk benefit ratio of proceeding with catheter ablation when an accessory pathway localized to the this region has been identified.

REFERENCES

1. Weber H, Schmidt L. Catheter technique for closed-chest ablation of an accessory pathway. *N Engl J Med* 1983;308:653–654.
2. Morady F, Scheinman MM. Transvenous catheter ablation of a posteroseptal accessory pathway in a patient with the Wolff-Parkinson-White syndrome. *N Engl J Med* 1984;310:705–707.
3. Zipes DP, DiMarco JP, Gillette PC, et al. Guidelines for clinical intracardiac electrophysiology study and catheter ablation procedures: a report of the American College of Cardiology/American Heart Association Task Force on Practice Guidelines. *Circulation* 1995;92:673–691.
4. Calkins H, Langberg J, Sousa J, et al. Radiofrequency catheter ablation of accessory atrioventricular connections in 250 patients. *Circulation* 1992;85:1337–1346.
5. Jackman WM, Xunzhang W, Friday KJ, et al. Catheter ablation of accessory atrioventricular pathways (Wolff-Parkinson-White syndrome) by radiofrequency current. *N Engl J Med* 1991;324:1605–1611.
6. Lesh MD, Van Hare GF, Schamp DJ, et al. Curative percutaneous catheter ablation using radiofrequency energy for accessory pathways in all locations: results in 100 consecutive patients. *J Am Coll Cardiol* 1992;19:1303–1309.
7. Swartz JF, Tracy CM, Fletcher RD. Radiofrequency endocardial catheter ablation of accessory atrioventricular pathway atrial insertion sites. *Circulation* 1993;87:487–499.
8. Kay GN, Epstein AE, Dailey SM, Plumb VJ. Role of radiofrequency ablation in the management of supraventricular arrhythmias: experience in 760 consecutive patients *J Cardiovasc Electrophysiol* 1993;4:371–389.
9. Haissaguerre M, Marcus F, Poquet F, et al. Electrocardiographic characteristics and catheter ablation of parahissian accessory pathways. *Circulation* 1994;90:1124–1128.
10. Satake S, Okishige K, Azegami K, et al. Radiofrequency ablation for WPW syndrome with monitoring the local electrogram at the ablation site. *Jpn Heart J* 1996;37:741–750.
11. Xie B, Herald SC, Bashir Y, et al. Localization of accessory pathways from the 12-lead electrocardiogram using a new algorithm. *Am J Cardiol* 1994;74:161–165.
12. Lorga FA, Sosa E, Scanavacca M, et al. Electrocardiographic identification of mid-septal accessory pathways in close proximity to the atrioventricular conduction system. *Pacing Clin Electrophysiol* 1996;10[Pt II]α84–1987.
13. Schluter M, Kuck KH. Catheter ablation from the right atrium of anteroseptal accessory pathways using radiofrequency current. *J Am Coll Cardiol* 1992;19:663–670.
14. Yeh SJ, Wang CC, Wen MS, et al. Characteristics and radiofrequency ablation therapy of intermediate septal accessory pathway. *Am J Cardiol* 1994;73:50–56.
15. Kuck KH, Schluter M, Gursoy S. Preservation of AV nodal conduction during radiofrequency current catheter ablation of midseptal accessory pathways. *Circulation* 1992;86:1743–1752.
16. Brugada J, Puigfel M, Mont L et al. Radiofrequency catheter ablation of anteroseptal, para-Hisian, and mid-septal accessory pathways using a simplified femoral approach. *Pacing Clin Electrophysiol* 1998;21[Pt 1]:735–741.
17. Calkins H, Yong P, Miller JM, et al. Catheter ablation of accessory pathways, AV nodal reentrant tachycardia, and the atrioventricular junction: final results of a prospective clinical trial. *Circulation* 1999;99:262–270.
18. Sealy WC, Gallagher JJ. The surgical approach to the septal area of the heart based on experiences with 45 patients with Kent bundles. *J Thorac Cardiovasc Surg* 1980;79:542–551.
19. Sealy WC. Kent bundles in the anterior septal space. *Ann Thorac Surg* 1983;36:180–186.
20. Dean JW, Ho SY, Rowland E, et al. Clinical anatomy of the atrioventricular junctions. *J Am Coll Cardiol* 1994;24:1725–1731.
21. Ho SY, Kilpatrick L, Kanai T, et al. The architecture of the

atrioventricular conduction axis in dog compared to man: its significance to ablation of the AV nodal approaches. *Cardiovasc Electrophysiol* 1995;6:26–39.
22. Arruda MS, McClelland JH, Wang X, et al. Development and validation of an ECG algorithm for identifying accessory pathway ablation site in Wolff-Parkinson-White syndrome. *J Cardiovasc Electrophysiol* 1998;9:2–12.
23. Fitzpatrick AP, Gonzales RP, Lesh MD, et al. New algorithm for the localization of accessory atrioventricular connections using a baseline electrocardiogram. *J Am Coll Cardiol* 1994;23:107–116.
24. Miles WM, Yee R, Klein G, et al. The preexcitation index: an aid in determining the mechanism of supraventricular tachycardia and localizing accessory pathways. *Circulation* 1986;74:493–500.
25. Scheinman MM, Wang YS, Van Hare GF, Lesh MD. Electrocardiographic and electrophysiologic characteristics of anterior, midseptal and right anterior free wall accessory pathways. *J Am Coll Cardiol* 1992;20:1220–1229.
26. Kerr CR, Gallagher JJ, German LD. Changes in ventriculoatrial intervals with bundle branch block aberration during reciprocating tachycardia in patients with accessory atrioventricular pathways. *Circulation* 1982;66:196–201.
27. Bardy GH, Packer DL, German LD, Gallagher JJ. Preexcited reciprocating tachycardia in patients with Wolff-Parkinson-White syndrome incidence and mechanism. *Circulation* 1984;70:377–391.
28. Keim S, Curtis AB, Belardinelli L, et al.. Adenosine-induced atrioventricular block: a rapid and reliable method to assess surgical and radiofrequency catheter ablation of accessory atrioventricular pathways. *J Am Coll Cardiol* 1992;19:1005–1012.
29. Engelstein ED, Wilber D, Wadas M, et al. Limitations of adenosine in assessing the efficacy of radiofrequency catheter ablation of accessory pathways. *Am J Cardiol* 1994;73:774–779.
30. Benditt DG, Benson DW, Dunnigan A, et al. Role of extrastimulus site and tachycardia cycle length in inducibility of atrial pre-excitation by premature ventricular stimulation during reciprocating tachycardia. *Am J Cardiol* 1987;60:811–819.
31. Martinez-Alday JD, Almendral J, Arenal A, et al. Identification of concealed posteroseptal Kent pathways by comparison of ventriculoatrial intervals from apical and posterobasal right ventricular sites. *Circulation* 1994;89:1060–1067.
32. Hirao K, Otomo K, Wang X, et al. Para-hisian pacing: a new method for differentiating retrograde conduction over an accessory AV pathway from conduction over the node. *Circulation* 1996;94:1027–1035.
33. Calkins H, Prystowsky E, Carlson M, et al, for the Atakar Multicenter Investigators Group. Temperature monitoring during radiofrequency catheter ablation procedures using closed loop control. *Circulation* 1994;90:1279–1286.
34. Dinerman JL, Berger RD, Calkins H. Temperature monitoring during radiofrequency ablation. *J Cardiovasc Electrophysiol* 1996;7:163–173.
35. Kalbfleisch SJ, El-Atassi R, Calkins H, et al. Safety, feasibility and cost of outpatient radiofrequency catheter ablation of accessory atrioventricular connections. *J Am Coll Cardiol* 1993;21:567–570.
36. Chen SA, Chiang CE, Yang CJ, et al. Usefulness of serial follow-up electrophysiologic studies in predicting late outcome of radiofrequency ablation for accessory pathways and AV nodal reentrant tachycardia. *Am Heart J* 1993;126:619–625.
37. Calkins H, Prystowsky E, Berger RD, et al, for the Atakr Multicenter investigators group. Recurrence of conduction following radiofrequency catheter ablation procedures: relationship to ablation target and electrode temperature. *J Cardiovasc Electrophysiol* 1996;7:704–712.
38. Calkins H, Kim YN, Schmaltz S, et al. Electrogram criteria for identification of appropriate target sites for radiofrequency catheter ablation of accessory atrioventricular connections. *Circulation* 1992;85:565–573.
39. Haissaguerre M, Gaita F, Marcus FI, Clementy J. Radiofrequency catheter ablation of accessory pathways: a contemporary review. *J Cardiovasc Electrophysiol* 1994;5:532–552.
40. Chen SA, Chiang CE, Tai CT, et al. Complications of diagnostic electrophysiologic studies and radiofrequency catheter ablation in patients with tachyarrhythmias: an eight year survey of 3,996 consecutive procedures in a tertiary referral center. *Am J Cardiol* 1996;77:41–46.
41. Schaffer MS, Silka MJ, Ross BA, Kugler JD. Inadvertent atrioventricular block during radiofrequency catheter ablation: results of the Pediatric Radiofrequency Ablation Registry. *Circulation* 1996;94:3214–3220.
42. Calkins H, Mann C, Kalbfleisch S, et al. Site of accessory pathway block after radiofrequency catheter ablation in patients with the Wolff-Parkinson-White syndrome. *J Cardiovasc Electrophysiol* 1994;5:20–27.
43. Warin J, Haissaguerre M, Divernois C, et al. Catheter ablation of accessory pathways: technique and results in 248 patients *Pacing Clin Electrophysiol* 1990;13:1609–1614.

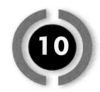

MODIFICATION OF THE ATRIOVENTRICULAR NODE FOR MANAGEMENT OF ATRIOVENTRICULAR NODAL REENTRANT TACHYCARDIA
• • •

DENNIS W.X. ZHU

Atrioventricular nodal reentrant tachycardia (AVNRT) is the most common type of paroxysmal supraventricular tachycardia in adults (1,2). It accounts for about 60% of adult patients with paroxysmal supraventricular tachycardia referred to an electrophysiology laboratory. During the last decade, radiofrequency catheter modification of atrioventricular (AV) node has revolutionized management of patients with AVNRT (3–24). The success rate at most centers exceeds 95% (11–24). The incidence of complications and rate of recurrence are low. The catheter therapy is also highly cost effective for the long term (25,26). As a result, catheter modification has been recommended as the first-line therapy for symptomatic AVNRT that is drug resistant or the patient who is drug intolerant or does not desire long-term drug therapy (27).

◉ CLINICAL PRESENTATION AND ELECTROCARDIOGRAPHIC FINDINGS

AVNRT can occur at any age, but it commonly manifests in young to middle-aged adults and is more common in women than in men. In a prospective, multicenter ablation catheter trial, the mean age of patients with AVNRT was 44 ± 18 years, and 70% of the patients were female (24). Depending on the patient's age at presentation, concomitant heart disease may or may not be present. AVNRT has also occurred in a transplanted heart (28). The literature does not suggest any particular relation to a specific form of organic heart disease. After initial presentation, recurrent episodes vary in frequency and duration and usually persist for years. There are generally no precipitating factors, although a relationship of posture or exercise to initiation of tachycardia is noticed by some patients. Typically, the onset and termination of the tachycardia occur abruptly. Palpitations or the feeling of a rapid heart beat is the most common symptom. This can be accompanied by dyspnea, chest tightness, and dizziness. Occasionally, syncope may be the presenting symptom with the patient not having any awareness of a rapid heart beat. In the absence of structural heart disease, the prognosis is usually excellent.

Documentation of the tachycardia is mandatory. Usually, a regular, narrow QRS complex tachycardia is observed, with rates ranging from 130 to 240 bpm.

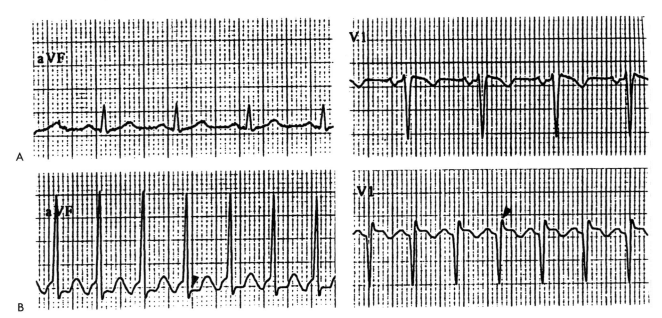

FIGURE 10-1. Electrocardiographic clues to typical AV nodal reentrant tachycardia (AVNRT). **A:** Sinus rhythm in leads aVF and V_1. **B:** During typical AVNRT, the retrograde P waves are observed at the terminal portion of the QRS complex in lead aVF, mimicking terminal delay *(arrow)*, and as a pseudo-r′ wave *(arrow)* in lead V_1. (From Zhu DWX, Maloney JD. Radiofrequency catheter ablative therapy for AV nodal reentrant tachycardia. In: Singer I, ed. *Interventional electrophysiology.* Baltimore: Williams & Wilkins, 1997:275–316, with permission.)

The rate of tachycardia may vary from episode to episode. In a typical AVNRT (slow/fast), the P wave occurs in proximity to the QRS complex. Commonly, the P wave is obscured by the QRS complex or may be seen slightly before or after the QRS complex. The presence of a pseudo-r′ wave in lead V_1 or a pseudo-s wave in leads II, III, and aVF suggests typical AVNRT (Fig. 10-1). In atypical AVNRT (fast/slow or slow/slow), the RP interval often equals or is greater than the PR interval. The P wave is inverted in leads II, III, and aVF. ST-T change of considerable magnitude is often observed and is a nonspecific phenomenon generally unrelated to structural heart disease. Functional bundle branch block may develop, rendering a wide QRS complex tachycardia (Fig. 10-2). However, functional bundle branch block should not affect the rate of tachycardia because the bundle branches are not part of the reentrant circuit. The onset of tachycardia is commonly preceded by a premature atrial beat that results in a sudden prolongation of the PR interval. During sinus rhythm, dual AV nodal pathways may manifest occasionally as a sudden and persistent prolongation of PR interval, PR alternans, and dual QRS complexes to a single P wave (29). Administration of adenosine during sinus rhythm may be useful for identifying patients with dual AV nodal pathways who are prone to AVNRT (30–31) (Fig. 10-3).

● EVOLVING CONCEPT OF AV NODAL REENTRANT TACHYCARDIA

Despite extensive investigation for nearly a century, understanding of the complex architecture of the AV node and the reentrant substrate of AVNRT continues to evolve.

AV Node

Since the pioneering work of Tawara around the turn of the last century (32,33), it has been recognized that

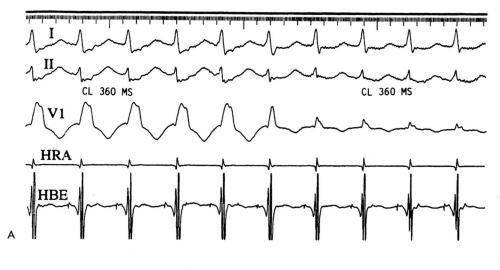

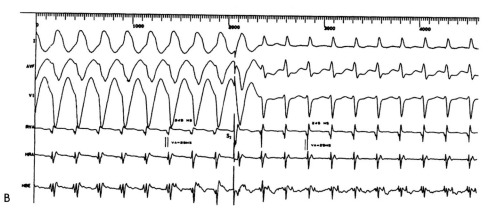

FIGURE 10-2. Surface electrocardiograms and intracardiac recordings during typical AV nodal reentrant tachycardia. **A:** The right bundle branch block aberration spontaneously resolves. **B:** The left bundle branch block aberration resolves with a single ventricular extrastimulus (S_2). The functional right or left bundle branch block does not affect the rate or the ventriculoatrial (VA) interval of the tachycardia, because the bundle branches are not part of the reentrant circuit. HRA, high right atrium; HBE, His bundle electrogram; RVA, right ventricular apex. (From Zhu DWX, Maloney JD. Radiofrequency catheter ablative therapy for AV nodal reentrant tachycardia. In: Singer I, ed. *Interventional electrophysiology.* Baltimore: Williams & Wilkins, 1997:275–316, with permission.)

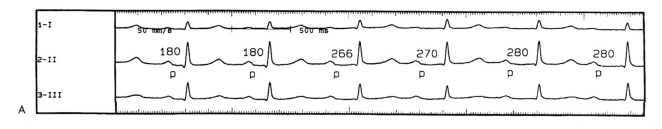

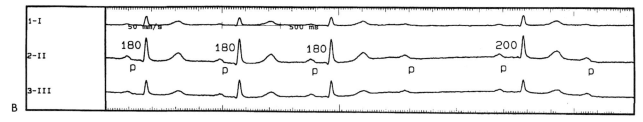

FIGURE 10-3. Response to adenosine during sinus rhythm in a patient with dual AV nodal physiology and inducible AV nodal reentrant tachycardia. **A:** A surface electrocardiogram at baseline shows a sudden prolongation of the PR interval from 180 to 266 msec (third beat) after a 6-mg intravenous bolus of adenosine, suggesting block of antegrade fast pathway conduction and the presence of dual AV nodal physiology. **B:** After slow pathway ablation, a sudden onset of second-degree AV block occurs after a 6-mg intravenous bolus of adenosine.

the AV node is the only conduction pathway between the atria and ventricles in a normal heart. The AV node can be identified as a distinct structure made up of three different components of specialized tissues: a transitional cell zone connecting the atrial myocardium and the compact AV node; the compact node; and the His bundle traveling through the membranous septum (34). Becker and Anderson divided the atrial nodal transitional cells into three groups: superficial, posterior, and deep (35). The superficial group was continuous with the anterior and superior aspect of the compact node, the posterior group joined the inferior and posterior aspect of the compact node, and the deep group linked the left atrium to the deep portion of the compact node. The AV node is traditionally considered to be contained within the triangle of Koch (36) (Fig. 10-4A). The superior border of the triangle is formed by the tendon of Todaro, a

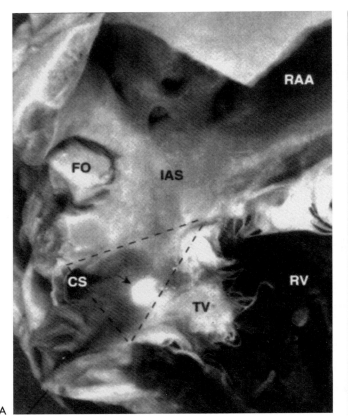
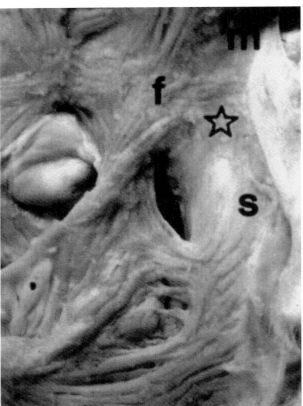

FIGURE 10-4. A: Heart specimen from a patient with typical AV nodal reentrant tachycardia who underwent a successful AV nodal slow pathway modification with a single radiofrequency application and died 5 months later from spontaneous intracranial hemorrhage. Koch's triangle *(dashed lines)* is delimited by the tendon of Todaro, coronary sinus (CS) ostium, and septal attachment of the tricuspid valve. The lesion is seen as a pale circular area *(arrow)* adjacent to the tricuspid annulus, just anterior to the CS ostium, and lies 11.5 mm from the apex of the triangle where the compact AV node is located. FO, fossa ovalis; IAS, intraatrial septum; RAA, right atrial appendage; RV, right ventricle; TV, tricuspid valve. (From Olgin JE, Ursell P, Kao AK, et al. Pathological findings following slow pathway ablation for AV nodal reentrant tachycardia. *J Cardiovasc Electrophysiol* 1996;7:625–631, with permission.) **B:** Close-up view of the arrangement of the subendocardial fibers in and around the triangle of Koch. *Star,* location of compact AV node; f, site of the fast pathway; s, site of the slow pathway. (From Anderson RH, Ho SY, Becker AE, Lang M. *Living anatomy: the CARTO and NOGA systems in the clinical arena.* Baldwin Park, Calif.: Biosense Inc., 1999:21. with permission.)

continuation of the commissure between the eustachian and thebesian valves into the musculature of the atrial septum. The inferior border of the triangle is the hinge of the septal leaflet of the tricuspid valve. The base of the triangle is marked by the ostium of the coronary sinus. The compact AV node is situated in the apex of the triangle anteriorly at the membranous septum, where it penetrates the central fibrous body to become the His bundle. The areas of the so-called fast and slow pathways into the AV node are composed histologically of ordinary atrial myocardium, with the orientation of the fibers possibly being a mechanism for preferential conduction (37) (Fig. 10-4B).

In adults, the compact AV node is relatively uniform in size, with a length of 5 to 7 mm and a width of 2 to 5 mm (38). A greater variability in the size of Koch's triangle was observed in the intraoperative and postmortem studies (39,40). Fluoroscopic measurement with coronary sinus angiography also found a marked variation in the triangle's dimensions (41). In the right oblique (RAO) view, the distance between the His potential recording site and the floor of coronary sinus ostium was 25.9 ± 7.9 mm. The size variations of Koch's triangle may be implicated in the risk of atrioventricular block during catheter modification for AVNRT. Marked differences in the arrangement of the superficial atrial muscle fibers in the area of the triangle of Koch have been reported in the normal hearts (42). Systematic anatomic investigation of the AV node in patients with AVNRT is lacking (43). No obvious histologic abnormalities have been identified (44). In a few available autopsy studies, the sites of successful slow pathway ablation were clearly distant from the histologic compact AV node (42,45,46) (Fig. 10-4A).

Dual AV Nodal Physiology

The concept of dual AV nodal physiology was introduced in 1950s by Moe and colleagues in an effort to explain the underlying mechanism of AVNRT (47). These early investigators proposed that AVNRT resulted from reentry confined within the compact AV node because of functional longitudinal dissociation of the AV node into a fast and a slow pathway. Dual AV nodal physiology is typically demonstrated by atrial extrastimulation pacing (Fig. 10-5A). With increasing prematurity of the atrial extrastimulus, there is a gradual and progressive conduction delay in the AV node. At a critical atrial coupling interval, a 10- to 20-msec decrement in A_1A_2 results in a marked prolongation (>50 msec) in A_2H_2. This sudden increase in conduction time (i.e., jump) has been defined as dual AV nodal physiology. Further 10- to 20-msec decrements in A_1A_2 result in relatively smaller additional prolongations (<50 msec) in A_2H_2. It has been suggested that the fast pathway has a shorter conduction time and a longer refractory period and that the slow pathway has a longer conduction time and a shorter refractory period. The abrupt rise in AV nodal conduction time is thought to represent conduction block in the fast pathway with selective conduction over the slow pathway. Using a single atrial extrastimulus, dual AV nodal physiology has been identified in 50% to 90% of patients with documented AVNRT (48) and in only 5% to 10% of subjects without a history of AVNRT (49).

Dual AV nodal physiology can also be demonstrated during decremental atrial pacing by a more than 50-msec increase in the atrial-His (AH) conduction interval after a 10- to 20-msec decrease in atrial pacing cycle length (48). Rosen and associates extended Moe's concept of dual AV nodal physiology to clinical AVNRT. They suggested unidirectional block in one of the pathways, with conduction over the alternate route leading to retrograde conduction over the previously blocked pathway allowing reentry (50–51). Although most investigators consider this concept is fundamentally correct, the specific anatomic circuit underlying the physiologic phenomenon remains controversial (48,52–54).

Because both pathways of the reentrant circuit were initially assumed to reside entirely within the compact AV node, the condition was considered incurable without causing atrioventricular block. This view was altered by a case report of Pritchett and coworkers, who described inadvertent cure of AVNRT after a failed attempt at surgical cryoablation of the AV node (55). This case demonstrated that at least part of the circuit critical to reentry could be ablated without significant functional damage to the AV node, which was a turning point in our under-

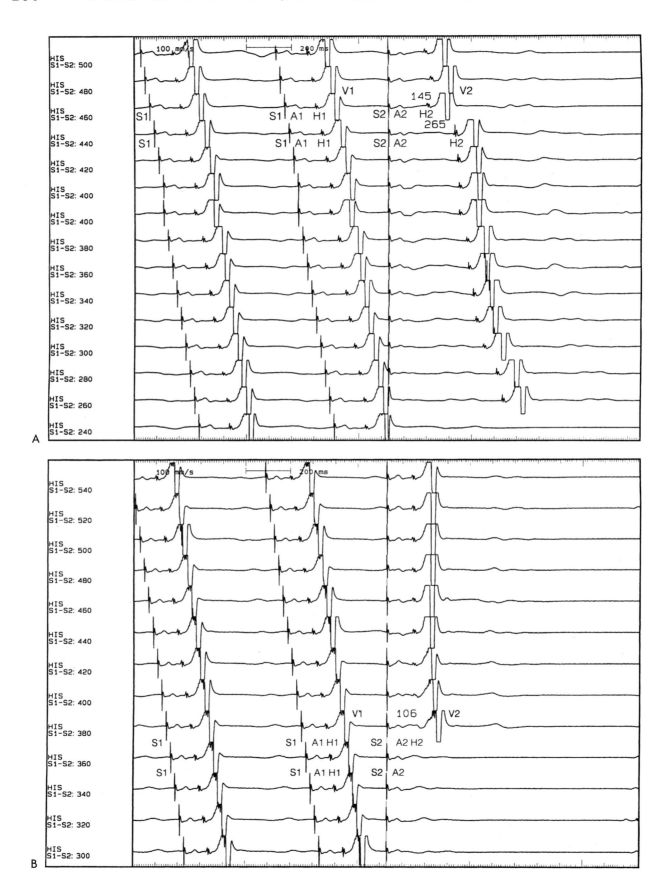

standing of AV nodal reentry. After this, surgical procedures developed to cure AVNRT had the rationale of disrupting the circuit by ablating "perinodal" tissue (56–59), and the suggestion of anatomically separate fast and slow pathways arose. The era of catheter ablation has refined our understanding of AV node reentry. Early attempts at AV nodal modification by fast pathway ablation were beset by a high incidence of atrioventricular block (4–10). This approach was rapidly replaced by the slow pathway technique, in which electrogram guidance was used to target a small area in the isthmus between the coronary sinus ostium and the tricuspid annulus at the base of the triangle of Koch. This procedure proved to be extremely reliable, and clinical cure can be achieved using a variety of approaches (12–24).

Despite some clinical success, we are only part way toward a better understanding of the reentrant circuit of a fascinating arrhythmia. Many aspects remain unclear, particularly the anatomic correlates of the two pathways and the two turnarounds of the circuit. It has been shown that the sites of earliest atrial activation during retrograde conduction over the fast and slow pathways are different (60). When retrograde conduction proceeds over the fast pathway, the site of earliest atrial activation is recorded at anterior septum superior to the tendon of Todaro (about 5 to 8 mm posterior and superior to the site recording the proximal His bundle potential). In contrast, the retrograde slow pathway conduction first activates the posterior septum between the tricuspid annulus and the coronary sinus ostium (Fig. 10-6). Early ablation experience led to the fast pathway being equated with an anatomically distinct region of atrial tissue anteroseptal to the compact node. However, activation of this part of the right atrium can be advanced by local extrastimuli without affecting the rest of the circuit (61). The fast retrograde limb of the tachycardia has a posterior exit site in some patients (62), and atrioventricular block can occasionally result from ablation in a posterior location (12,13,63). The slow pathway seems to correspond to the posterior extension of AV nodal tissue (usually to the right, but occasionally leftward) (64). AVNRT may be reset when late atrial extrastimuli are delivered outside the compact AV node to the posteroseptal right atrium and coronary sinus.

There is strong evidence that the slow pathway is not a single entity. Multiple slow pathways have been demonstrable in the AV nodal conduction curve in some patients with AVNRT (65–68) (Fig. 10-7). During ventricular extrastimulation pacing, it is not unusual to observe multiple ranges of the VA conduction interval, each with the earliest atrial activation recorded at a different site around the coronary sinus (60). Animal studies showed additional slow pathways entered the triangle of Koch anterior to the coronary sinus ostium (69). In patients with AVNRT and three or even more functionally defined AV nodal pathways, any of which can be involved in tachycardia initiation, a single radiofrequency energy delivery may eliminate these pathways singly or multiply (70). The antegrade fast and slow pathways may not always be identical to their retrograde counterparts. The lower turnaround point of the circuit appears to be within the compact AV node, although is not clear whether a lower common pathway exists between it and the His bundle. A lower common pathway is

FIGURE 10-5. Antegrade AV nodal conduction curves represented by His bundle electrograms during single atrial extrastimulation at a drive cycle length (S_1S_1) of 600 msec in a patient with dual AV nodal physiology and typical AVNRT. **A:** At baseline, a 20-msec decrement in S_1S_2 (A_1A_2) results in a relatively small prolongation (<50 msec) in A_2H_2 intervals until a critical coupling interval (S_1S_2 = 440 msec) is reached, when 20-msec decrement in S_1S_2 (A_1A_2) results in a marked lengthening in A_2H_2 interval from 145 to 265 msec. Further 20-msec decrements in S_1S_2 (A_1A_2) result in smaller additional prolongations in A_2H_2. Here, the AV nodal fast pathway effective refractory period is 440 msec, and the slow pathway effective refractory period is 240 msec or less. **B:** After ablation of the slow pathway, the discontinuous AV nodal conduction pattern is no longer present. The fast pathway effective refractory period has shortened to 360 msec.

Sites of Earliest Retrograde Atrial Activation

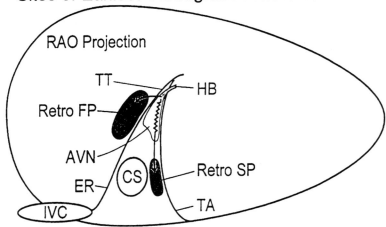

FIGURE 10-6. Sites of earliest atrial activation during retrograde conduction over the fast pathway (Retro FP) and the slow pathway (Retro SP). TT, tendon of Todaro; ER, eustachian ridge; AVN, compact AV node. (From Otomo K, Wang Z, Lazzara R, Jackman WM. AV nodal reentrant tachycardia: electrophysiological characteristics of four forms and implications for the reentrant circuit. In: Zipes DP, Jalife J, eds. *Cardiac electrophysiology: from cell to bedside*, 3rd edition. Philadelphia: WB Saunders, 2000, with permission.)

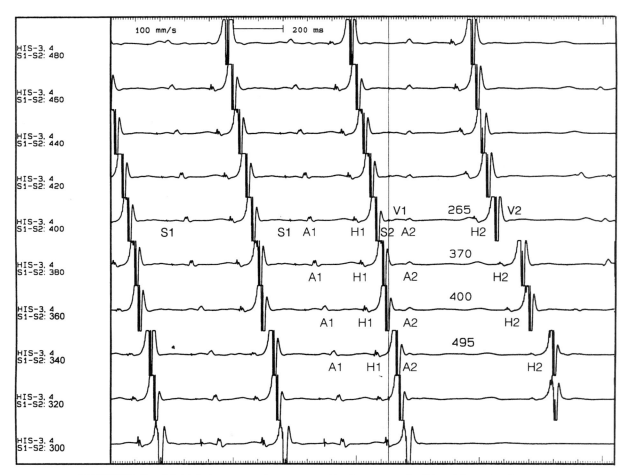

FIGURE 10-7. Multiple jumps are demonstrated in the antegrade AV nodal conduction curve as represented by His bundle electrograms during single atrial extrastimulation in a patient with atypical AV nodal reentrant tachycardia, suggesting the presence of multiple slow pathways. The A_2H_2 interval prolongs markedly from 265 to 370 msec and from 400 to 495 msec at S_1S_2 coupling intervals of 380 and 340 msec, respectively.

suggested by the occasional dissociation between the tachycardia and the His potential. However, comparison of the AH interval during tachycardia and ventricular pacing suggests that the His bundle is activated before the retrograde fast pathway (71). The upper portion of the circuit remains unclear. Although an excitable gap demonstrates that the posterior right atrial septum is involved in the circuit, it is not clear how the impulse travels from a retrograde fast pathway to this region, possibly by deeper layers of the septum, part of the coronary sinus, or even the left atrium. These findings, along with the lack of consistent structural differences at the histologic level in patients with dual AV nodal physiology, suggest that the functional properties and the spatial orientation of the existing atrionodal connections may ultimately determine the expression of dual AV nodal pathways and the development of AVNRT.

Types of AV Nodal Reentrant Tachycardia

Three types of AVNRT have been identified. Typical, or slow/fast AVNRT, is the most prevalent type, accounting for 85% to 90% of cases. Between 10% and 15% of patients present with atypical AVNRT that can be further differentiated into fast/slow or slow/slow AVNRT. Induction of typical and atypical AVNRT in the same patient is possible but unusual.

Slow/Fast AV Nodal Reentrant Tachycardia

Slow/fast AVNRT is thought to use the slow pathway for antegrade conduction and the fast pathway for retrograde conduction. When an atrial premature beat blocks in the fast pathway and proceeds slowly along the slow pathway, the fast pathway has enough time to recover from its refractoriness. This allows the impulse to activate the fast pathway retrogradely and return to the atrium, giving rise to an AV nodal reentrant echo beat. The impulse then travels down along the slow pathway again. Continuation of this process leads to development of AVNRT (Fig. 10-8,A, B). The AH interval during slow/fast AVNRT is usually longer than 200 msec. Because the retrograde AV conduction is through the fast pathway, the retrograde atrial activation sequence during tachycardia is concentric, with the earliest atrial activation recorded superior to the tendon of Todaro. The ventriculoatrial (VA) interval during tachycardia is usually less than 50 msec if atrial activation is measured at the His potential recording site, and it is usually less than 90 msec if measured at high right atrium (72) (Fig. 10-2). The short VA interval usually results in superimposition of the P wave onto the QRS complex in the electrocardiogram, obscuring most of the P wave. The terminal portion of the P wave may be distinguishable at the end of QRS complex, producing a characteristic late positive component in lead V_1 (pseudo-r'), a negative component in the inferior leads (pseudo-S wave), or both (Fig. 10-1). Premature ventricular stimulation during tachycardia should not preexcite the atrium when delivered at a time that the His bundle is refractory. When an earlier coupled premature ventricular stimulation advances the timing of the His bundle activation, the timing of atrial activation may also be advanced. However, the atrial activation sequence should remain unaltered. The evidence for an upper common pathway remains controversial. The distance between the atrial connections of the fast and slow pathways suggests that the reentrant circuit in slow/fast AVNRT may contain a relatively large atrial component in which the reentrant impulse propagates from the atrial end of the fast pathway to the atrial end of the slow pathway. The exact location of the atrial component remains unsolved.

Based on the data from resetting mapping with a late atrial extrastimulus delivered during tachycardia, a new hypothesis for the reentrant circuit in slow/fast AVNRT was proposed (60) (Fig. 10-9). In this hypothesis, retrograde activation over the fast pathway activates the right and left sides of the interatrial septum, but it is the left-sided activation that participates in the reentrant circuit. Propagation from the left atrial septum activates the coronary sinus musculature, approximately 1 to 3 cm from the ostium. The impulse travels through the coronary sinus musculature toward the ostium and right atrium, and it activates fibers that comprise the atrial connection to the slow pathway, followed by activation of the slow pathway itself. The lower common pathway is considered to be very short or minimal in slow/fast

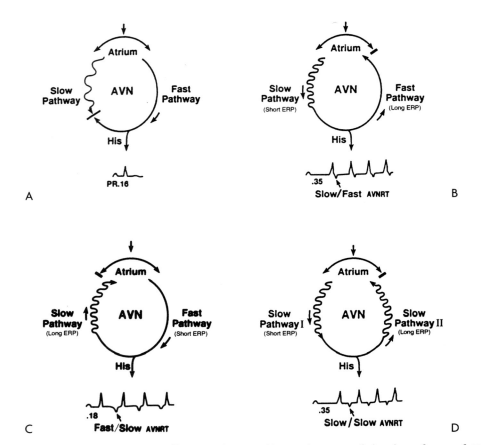

FIGURE 10-8. The diagrams illustrate the possible mechanisms of the three forms of AV nodal reentrant tachycardia (AVNRT). **A:** During sinus rhythm, the impulse antegradely penetrates the fast and slow pathways simultaneously. Because the impulse reaches the His bundle by means of the fast pathway, the PR interval is normal. The impulse conducting down the distal fast pathway may continue to activate the slow pathway retrogradely and collide with the incoming antegrade impulse in the slow pathway. **B:** In slow/fast AVNRT, the effective refractory period (ERP) of the fast pathway is longer than the slow pathway. An atrial premature beat may block in the fast pathway and conduct down the slow pathway to activate the His bundle. The PR interval is prolonged. Because the antegrade conduction along the slow pathway is slow, the fast pathway has enough time to regain its excitability. The impulse that has reached distal slow pathway may continue to activate the fast pathway retrogradely and return to the atrium, giving rise to a typical AV nodal reentrant echo beat. The impulse continues to conduct down the slow pathway to have repetitive antegrade reentrance. The continuation of this process leads to the development of slow/fast AVNRT. **C:** In fast/slow AVNRT, the fast pathway has a relatively shorter antegrade refractory period than the slow pathway. An atrial premature beat blocks in the slow pathway antegradely and conducts down the fast pathway with minimal prolongation in PR interval. As the impulse reenters the distal slow pathway, conduction through the slow pathway proceeds so slowly that the site of block has time to recover excitability and repetitive reentrance occurs, with the development of fast/slow AVNRT. **D:** In slow/slow AVNRT, the ERP of the fast pathway is longer than that of the slow pathways. Slow pathway II has a longer antegrade refractory period than slow pathway I. An atrial premature beat can block in the fast pathway and slow pathway II and then conduct down slow pathway I to activate the His bundle. The PR interval therefore is prolonged. Because the antegrade conduction along slow pathway I proceeds slowly, slow pathway II has enough time to regain its excitability. The impulse that has reached distal slow pathway I may continue to activate slow pathway II retrogradely and return to the atrium, giving rise to an atypical AV nodal reentrant echo beat. The impulse continues to conduct down the slow pathway I to have repetitive antegrade reentrance. Continuation of this process leads to the development of slow/slow AVNRT.

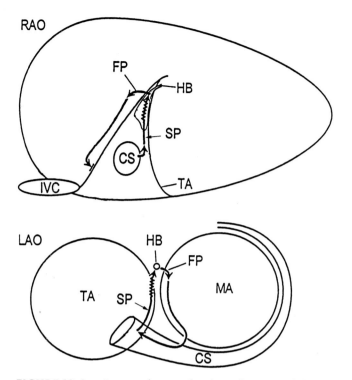

FIGURE 10-9. Proposed circuit for slow/fast AV nodal reentrant tachycardia. The retrograde activation over the fast pathway activates the right and left sides of the interatrial septum. The left-sided activation participates in the reentrant circuit. Propagation from the left atrial septum activates the coronary sinus musculature approximately 1 to 3 cm from the ostium. The impulse propagates through the coronary sinus musculature toward the ostium and right atrium, and it activates fibers that comprise the atrial connection to the slow pathway, followed by conduction over the slow pathway antegradely to activate the His bundle. The impulse that reaches the distal slow pathway may continue to activate the fast pathway retrogradely and return to the atrium, giving rise to slow/fast AVNRT. (Modified from Otomo K, Wang Z, Lazzara R, Jackman WR. AV nodal reentrant tachycardia: electrophysiological characteristics of four forms and implications for the reentrant circuit. In: Zipes DP, Jalife J, eds. *Cardiac electrophysiology: from cell to bedside, 3rd edition*. Philadelphia: WB Saunders, 2000:504–521, with permission.)

AVNRT. There is almost invariably a 1:1 atrioventricular relationship during AVNRT. Occasionally, tachycardia may continue without changing the cycle length in the presence of intermittent 2:1 block (73,74). A rapid reentrant circuit rather than impaired distal AV nodal or infranodal conduction may account for the phenomenon (74).

A rare left variant of slow/fast AVNRT has been described (75,76). The reentrant circuit of this variant of tachycardia may be situated entirely in the left heart. A very short HA interval (<15 msec) may occur during tachycardia. These patients often have the "2 for 1" phenomenon during atrial extrastimulation, in which an atrial extrastimulus produces two His bundle potentials, probably resulting from conduction over the fast and slow pathways. Although the earliest site of retrograde atrial activation is recorded above the tendon of Todaro, the slow pathway participating in the reentrant circuit cannot be ablated from the posteroseptal tricuspid annulus or coronary sinus ostium. Energy application at the posterior mitral annulus or in the middle coronary sinus initiates accelerated junctional rhythm and eliminates the tachycardia.

Fast/Slow AV Nodal Reentrant Tachycardia

Fast/slow AVNRT has been proposed to use the fast pathway for antegrade conduction and the slow pathway for the retrograde conduction (77,78) (Fig. 10-8C). Patients with fast/slow AVNRT frequently have a different electrophysiologic substrate. The effective refractory period of the fast pathway is longer than that of the slow pathway in the retrograde but not in the antegrade direction. These patients do not have discontinuous AV nodal conduction curve as those with slow/fast AVNRT do. Fast/slow AVNRT has a short AH interval and a long VA interval with the earliest atrial activation recorded at the posteroseptal right atrium or within the coronary sinus (78–80) (Fig. 10-10). This results in a RP interval longer than PR interval with an inverted P wave in the inferior leads. Tachycardia is easier to induce with ventricular pacing. Premature ventricular stimulation during tachycardia should not reset the atrium if delivered when the His bundle is refractory. When an earlier coupled premature ventricular stimulation advances the timing of the His bundle activation, the timing of atrial activation may also be advanced. However, the atrial activation sequence should remain unchanged. Ventricular extrastimulus must advance the timing of His bundle activation by at least 30 to 60 msec before advancing the timing of the next atrial

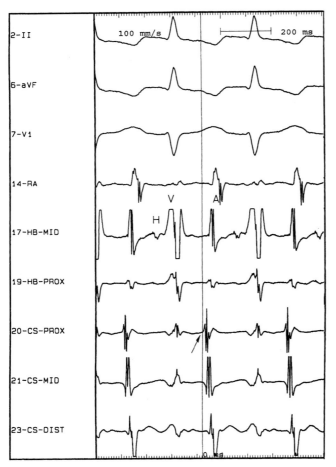

FIGURE 10-10. Surface electrocardiograms and intracardiac recordings during fast/slow AV nodal reentrant tachycardia (AVNRT). Fast/slow AVNRT has a short AH interval and a long VA interval, with earliest atrial activation recorded around the coronary sinus ostium. As a result, RP interval is longer than PR interval. CS, coronary sinus; HB, His bundle electrogram; RA, right atrium.

activation and resetting the tachycardia, suggesting a relatively long lower common pathway.

Slow/Slow AV Nodal Reentrant Tachycardia

Slow/slow AVNRT theoretically requires the presence of two or more slow pathways with different conduction properties and refractory periods. In slow/slow AVNRT, one slow pathway is used for antegrade conduction, and the other slow pathway is used for retrograde conduction (Fig. 10-8D). Similar to slow/fast AVNRT, the induction of slow/slow AVNRT by atrial pacing occurs with an abrupt (>50 msec) increase in the AH interval. The AH interval during slow/slow AVNRT is relatively long, usually more than 200 msec. These patients often exhibit multiple jumps in the A_2H_2 interval during atrial extrastimulation, consistent with multiple slow pathways (Fig. 10-7). Slow/slow AVNRT can be differentiated from slow/fast AVNRT by mapping the right atrium and coronary sinus during tachycardia, which reveals an atrial activation sequence typical of retrograde conduction over the slow pathway and the earliest atrial activation recorded at the posteroseptal right atrium between the tricuspid annulus and the coronary sinus ostium or within the coronary sinus, 30 to 60 msec earlier than atrial activation in the His bundle region. The VA interval is often very short with simultaneous atrial and ventricular activation, mimicking slow/fast AVNRT.

This tachycardia was previously considered to be a variant of slow/fast AVNRT with a posterior exit for the retrograde fast pathway (81) (Fig. 10-11). However, about one half of the patients with slow/slow AVNRT also have retrograde conduction over the fast pathway, and initiation of the tachycardia by ventricular extrastimulation is associated with block in the retrograde fast pathway and conduction over the retrograde slow pathway demonstrated by a shift in the retrograde atrial activation sequence. In patients with simultaneous atrial and ventricular activation during tachycardia, identification of retrograde atrial activation sequence may be facilitated by the insertion of a late ventricular extrastimulus that separates the atrial and ventricular potentials. Similar to fast/slow AVNRT, ventricular extrastimulus must advance the timing of His bundle activation by at least 30 to 60 msec before advancing the timing of the next atrial activation and resetting the tachycardia, suggesting a relatively long lower common pathway. Differentiation of slow/slow AVNRT with a short VA interval from slow/fast AVNRT is important because fast pathway ablation does not eliminate slow/slow AVNRT (82). Occasionally, patients with fast/slow or slow/slow AVNRT demonstrate eccentric retrograde atrial activation masquerading as tachycardia using a left-sided accessory pathway (83). Ablation of the slow pathway in the posterior right atrial septum eliminates tachycardia in these patients.

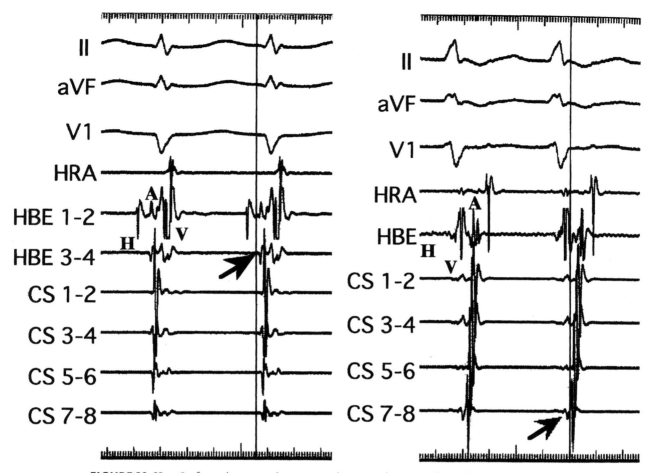

FIGURE 10-11. Surface electrocardiograms and intracardiac recordings during slow/slow AV nodal reentrant tachycardia (AVNRT) *(right)*. The earliest site of atrial activation during the tachycardia is at the coronary sinus ostium *(arrow)*. The His-atrial (HA) interval, which could have a wide range, is often very short with simultaneous atrial and ventricular activation, mimicking slow/fast AVNRT *(left)* in which the site of earliest atrial activation is recorded in the His region *(arrow)*. Slow/slow AVNRT was previously considered to be a variant of slow/fast AVNRT with a posterior exit for the retrograde fast pathway. CS, coronary sinus; HBE, His bundle electrogram; HRA, high right atrium. (From Fujii E, Kasai A, Omichi C, et al. Electrophysiological characteristics during slow pathway ablation of posterior atrioventricular junctional reentrant tachycardia. *Pacing Clin Electrophysiol* 1998;21[Pt II]:2510–2516, with permission.)

⦿ ELECTROPHYSIOLOGIC STUDY

Because the clinical presentation and electrocardiographic findings are often nonspecific, a comprehensive electrophysiologic study is essential for the diagnosis and differential diagnosis of AVNRT. Ideally, all antiarrhythmic drugs should be discontinued for at least five half-lives in advance of the study for accurate assessment of conduction properties and for facilitating tachycardia induction.

Placement of Catheters

With the patient under sedation and local anesthesia, 5- or 6-Fr, multipolar catheters are introduced into one of the femoral veins and advanced into the apex of the right ventricle, right atrium, and across the tricuspid valve for recording the His bundle potential. Recording the His bundle electrogram from closely spaced bipolar electrodes (2-mm interelectrode distance) minimizes the duration of the local ventricular electrogram and its overlapping with the His bundle potential, allowing better verification of antegrade and retrograde His bundle activation. Although coronary sinus recording is not critical for the diagnosis of typical AVNRT, placement of the coronary sinus catheter helps the diagnosis of atypical AVNRT and the differential diagnosis of other induced tachycardias. It is also useful for anatomic recognition of the ostium of the coronary sinus as a marker for slow pathway modification. Venous access for coronary sinus cannulation depends on operator's preference and may use the internal jugular, subclavian, or femoral veins. The coronary sinus catheter is positioned with the most proximal pair of electrodes in the vicinity of the ostium.

Decremental Ventricular Pacing

Decremental ventricular pacing is performed to evaluate the sequence of retrograde atrial activation and to measure the VA and HA intervals. Pacing is started at a cycle length slightly shorter than that of the sinus rhythm. The cycle length is then shortened gradually (by 10 or 20 msec) until a VA conduction block is observed. Four patterns of response have been encountered:

1. The usual response seen in patients with typical AVNRT is a rapid VA conduction by means of the fast pathway. Usually, no incremental conduction is observed down to the cycle length of VA block. Slow/Fast AVNRT may be induced infrequently.
2. The VA conduction occurs predominantly by means of the fast pathway at relatively long cycle lengths, and a sudden shift of conduction to the slow pathway is associated with an abrupt VA conduction prolongation and a corresponding change in the atrial activation sequence at a critical cycle length. After this shift occurs, further VA conduction prolongation may occur, with pacing cycle length shortening until retrograde conduction block occurs. Atypical AVNRT is often induced in this manner.
3. In some patients, retrograde conduction occurs predominantly over the slow pathway. These patients are prone to atypical AVNRT and may manifest typical AVNRT only after improvement of the retrograde fast pathway conduction with isoproterenol infusion.
4. Occasionally, VA conduction may be absent in the baseline recording and present only during isoproterenol infusion.

Ventricular Extrastimulation

Ventricular extrastimulation is performed using an eight-beat drive train followed by the introduction of single ventricular extrastimuli with decrements of 10 or 20 msec. The cycle length of the drive train is slightly shorter than that of the sinus rhythm. One of the following patterns may be observed:

1. A short VA interval is associated with the earliest atrial activation at the His bundle recording site. With progressive shortening of the coupling interval between V_1 and V_2, gradual VA prolongation is observed in some individuals that results primarily from a conduction delay in the His-Purkinje system.
2. In other patients, a sudden VA prolongation develops at a critical coupling interval because of a retrograde block in the right bundle and shift of the retrograde conduction to the left bundle–His axis or because of a shift of retrograde conduction from the fast to slow atrioventricular pathway with a corresponding change in the retrograde atrial activation sequence.

Decremental Atrial Pacing

Decremental atrial pacing is started at a cycle length slightly shorter than that of the sinus rhythm and decreased gradually by 10 or 20 msec until an atrioventricular conduction block is observed. The following patterns may be observed:

1. In most patients, the gradual increase in the AH interval is followed by an abrupt and marked AH prolongation (>50 msec), frequently resulting in the initiation of AVNRT. Continued decremental pacing during AVNRT leads to tachycardia en-

trainment and identifies the shortest pacing cycle length with 1 : 1 atrioventricular conduction.
2. For the remaining patients, a gradual and smooth AH interval prolongation is seen until antegrade block occurs. A PR interval that exceeds the RR interval during rapid atrial pacing with stable 1 : 1 atrioventricular conduction indicates the presence of antegrade slow pathway conduction and may lead to the induction of AVNRT (84).

Atrial Extrastimulation

Atrial extrastimulation is performed using an eight-beat drive train followed by the introduction of a single atrial extrastimulus that is decreased by 10 or 20 msec. The cycle length of the drive train should be slightly shorter than that of the sinus rhythm. One of three patterns may be encountered:

1. Dual AV nodal physiology with initiation of an AV nodal reentrant echo beat or AVNRT occurs in 70% of patients. Failure to induce tachycardia often results from poor retrograde fast pathway conduction that improves with isoproterenol infusion.
2. Multiple jumps are demonstrable in some patients (68,70). These patients may have multiple slow pathways and a more complex reentrant tissue mass. Slow/slow and fast/slow AVNRTs are often induced in patients with multiple jumps.
3. A smooth AV nodal conduction curve is associated with initiation of AVNRT at a critical coupling interval (85,86). This occurs when the conduction times of the two pathways are not markedly different, but the effective refractory period of the fast pathway is longer than the slow pathway. Introducing two atrial extrastimuli could reveal discontinuity of the A_2A_3/A_3H_3 curve in most of these patients (87).

Induction of AV Nodal Reentrant Tachycardia

To have a reliable end point for assessing catheter modification of AV node, it is essential to establish the reproducibility of tachycardia induction before the procedure. Typical AVNRT is usually induced when a critical degree of AV nodal conduction delay is achieved with decremental atrial pacing or delivery of a critically timed atrial extrastimulus. Addition of a second extrastimulus or use of short bursts of rapid atrial pacing at or slightly above 1 : 1 atrioventricular conduction may alter the conduction and refractoriness to allow expression of the dual AV nodal physiology and initiation of AVNRT (87). These maneuvers sometimes may also increase the risk of inducing atrial fibrillation. Retrograde His-Purkinje system conduction delay during ventricular extrastimulation prevents significant conduction delay or block in the AV node; therefore, the initiation of typical AVNRT is uncommon with this approach. Atypical AVNRT can be initiated with atrial or ventricular stimulation. The induction of AVNRT is poorly reproducible in approximately 10% of patients (88). Common mechanisms for the inability to induce AVNRT are the inability to achieve critical AH prolongation, fast pathway block, and slow pathway block. Isoproterenol may be required for initiation of AVNRT in about 35% to 50% of patients, especially those with poorer conduction properties over the antegrade slow pathway or retrograde fast pathway (89). Isoproterenol infusion is started at 1 μg/min and gradually titrated to increase the sinus rate by 20% to 30%. This improves conduction and shortens refractory periods of fast and slow pathways in antegrade and retrograde directions. Occasionally, simultaneous administration of isoproterenol and atropine is needed for the induction of AVNRT (90).

Differential Diagnosis of AV Nodal Reentrant Tachycardia

Typical AVNRT (slow/fast) has a distinct electrophysiologic appearance and can be differentiated from other forms of supraventricular tachycardia without much difficulty. It can be challenging to differentiate the atrial activation sequence of atypical AVNRT (fast/slow and slow/slow) from the atrial activation sequence of atrial tachycardia originating from the atrial septum or proximal coronary sinus or from orthodromic atrioventricular reciprocating tachycardia using a septal or left posterior accessory pathway. By accurately measuring the timing of atrial activation during tachycardia and applying critically timed ventricular extrastimulation, AVNRT can be differentiated from other forms of supraventricular tachycardias.

Orthodromic Atrioventricular Reciprocating Tachycardia

Orthodromic atrioventricular reciprocating tachycardia using an accessory pathway can be excluded if atrial activation during tachycardia occurs before or simultaneously with ventricular activation (VA interval ≤50 msec) and if the timing and sequence of retrograde atrial activation is unchanged by a ventricular extrastimulation that advances the timing of ventricular activation adjacent to the site of earliest atrial activation by 30 msec or more. This is best achieved by delivering ventricular extrastimulus to the posterobasal right ventricular septum for tachycardia with earliest atrial activation at the posteroseptal tricuspid annulus or proximal coronary sinus and to the site adjacent to (but not capturing) the proximal right bundle branch for tachycardia with earliest atrial activation in the anterior septum. Measuring the difference between the VA interval during ventricular pacing at the right ventricular apex and base may also be helpful. The VA interval shortens when the ventricular stimulation is moved from the apex to the base in the presence of a posteroseptal accessory pathway, whereas the VA interval tends to lengthen in patients with normal conduction or AVNRT because the impulse must propagate toward the apex of the heart before it can reach the His-Purkinje system. Para-Hisian pacing during sinus rhythm with intermittent His bundle capture can be used to differentiate retrograde conduction over a posteroseptal accessory pathway from retrograde conduction over the AV node (91). If an accessory pathway does coexist with AVNRT, the former should be targeted first before proceeding to selective modification of the AV node.

Atrial Tachycardia

Atrial tachycardia is unlikely if there is an identical sequence of retrograde atrial activation during tachycardia and ventricular pacing. Ventricular extrastimulation that retrogradely advances the timing of His bundle activation by 30 msec or more advances the timing of atrial activation or produces VA block and terminates tachycardia in AVNRT, but it should not alter the timing of atrial activation in atrial tachycardia. In typical AVNRT, retrograde atrial activation is usually advanced as soon as the timing of His bundle activation is altered. In atypical AVNRT (fast/slow or slow/slow), a ventricular extrastimulus must advance the timing of His bundle activation by 30 to 60 msec before advancing the timing of retrograde atrial activation. Atrial tachycardia is established if ventricular stimulation during tachycardia advances His bundle activation by more than 60 msec without changing the timing of atrial activation. Entrainment of the tachycardia by ventricular pacing at a cycle length 10 to 20 msec shorter than the tachycardia cycle length with an identical atrial activation sequence distinguishes AVNRT from atrial tachycardia. Termination of the tachycardia by a premature ventricular stimulation that did not conduct to the atrium definitely excludes atrial tachycardia. When adenosine is injected during tachycardia, development of complete atrioventricular block without altering the timing of atrial activation strongly suggests atrial tachycardia. Knight and colleagues developed a simple technique for the rapid differential diagnosis of atrial tachycardia (92). During supraventricular tachycardia, right ventricular pacing was initiated at a cycle length 10 to 60 msec shorter than the tachycardia cycle length until 1:1 ventriculoatrial conduction occured, at which point pacing was discontinued. If ventricular pacing did not terminate the tachycardia, the atrial electrogram sequence immediately after the last ventricular paced complex was analyzed. Two patterns of sequence were identified: atrial-atrial-ventricular (A-A-V) and atrial-ventricular (A-V). The A-A-V response was observed in all 19 cases of atrial tachycardia. In contrast, the A-V response was observed in all 145 cases of AVNRT and orthodromic reciprocating tachycardia.

CATHETER MODIFICATION OF THE AV NODE

Historical Background

Drug therapy was the earliest available management for AVNRT. Although drug therapy was effective in reducing the frequency and severity of recurrence in most patients, it was limited by side effects, proarrhythmic risk, expense, and patient compliance. For drug-resistant patients, the only available nonpharmacologic therapy was a surgically created complete atrioventricular block followed by implantation of a permanent pacemaker. The advent of surgical modification of the AV node provided high cure rates for AVNRT (56–59), but the procedure was associated with operative morbidity, prolonged hospital stay, and limited availability. Early application of catheter management of AVNRT involved the use of direct current shocks for creation of a complete heart block and later for selective ablation of the fast or slow pathway (93,94). These techniques are now only of historical interest.

Introduction of the radiofrequency catheter modification revolutionized the treatment for AVNRT. The lesions generated by radiofrequency energy are small, discrete, and more homogenous than earlier results. Radiofrequency ablation also eliminates the need for general anesthesia. The radiofrequency energy output can be temperature controlled or manually titrated to achieve the desired effects. Although newer energy sources and tools are emerging (95), radiofrequency catheter ablation is superior to any other currently available technique. Initial attempts that targeted the fast pathway were followed by preferential modification of the slow pathway because of a lower incidence of inadvertent atrioventricular block, a greater likelihood of maintaining a normal PR interval during sinus rhythm, and efficacy in treating typical and atypical AVNRT.

Slow Pathway Modification

In the development process of slow pathway modification, two principal approaches for modifying slow pathway have been introduced. In the first approach, the local atrial electrogram configuration is used to identify the target sites (13). In the second approach, target sites are localized primarily on the basis of fluoroscopically identified anatomic landmarks (18). Other approaches have been proposed. Nonfluoroscopic electroanatomic mapping and intracardiac echocardiography may facilitate slow pathway ablation in patients with unusual cardiac or intrathoracic anatomy.

Basic Techniques

Catheter modification of AV node is usually performed after a diagnostic electrophysiologic study during the same session. A 7-Fr, quadripolar catheter (spacing of 2-5-2 mm) with a deflectable segment and a 4-mm-long tip electrode has been most commonly used. The ablation catheter is usually inserted into the right femoral vein. The venous access sheath should be one French size bigger than the ablation catheter to allow for convenient manipulation. The radiofrequency energy is delivered between the catheter tip electrode and an adhesive electrosurgical pad attached on the right posterior chest. Compared with power guided energy delivery, temperature-controlled energy delivery allows for safe delivery of more power, achieves a higher primary success rate, and is generally preferred (96–98). Temperature, impedance, and power should be continuously monitored. The fluoroscopic right anterior oblique (RAO) view at 15 to 30 degrees and the left anterior oblique view (LAO) at 40 to 60 degrees are commonly used for mapping and ablation. Monoplane fluoroscopy is usually adequate. The RAO view is initially used for catheter placement because it best displays Koch's triangle in profile.

After an appropriate target site is identified, radiofrequency energy is usually delivered at a preselected temperature of 50°C to 60°C (99,100) or a power output of 20 to 30 W for up to 60 seconds. Higher temperature is associated with a higher success rate but also a higher risk of atrioventricular block. If the target site is close to the His potential, it is prudent to start with a lower temperature or power output and to titrate upward, using the onset of accelerated junctional rhythm as the end point. Successful ablation of AVNRT is usually achieved at an electrode-tissue interface temperature of 48°C (range, 42°C to 56°C) (101,102). Energy is usually applied during sinus rhythm. Occasionally, current may be delivered during atrial pacing or tachycardia. Accelerated junctional rhythm during radiofrequency energy application occurs in most of the effective sites (Fig. 10-12). However, it also occurs in up to two thirds of ineffective applications (103). Autonomic blockade

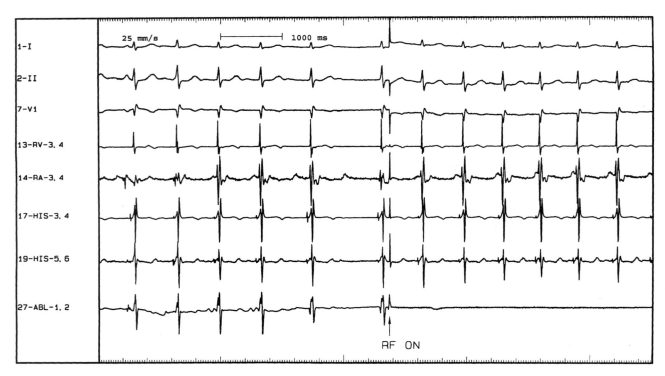

FIGURE 10-12. Accelerated junctional rhythm initiated by catheter-induced mechanical pressure at the slow pathway region and continued during radiofrequency (RF) application. There is a 1:1 ventriculoatrial (VA) conduction with a short VA interval during accelerated junctional rhythm. This is the desired response during radiofrequency ablation of the slow pathway. The appearance of VA block during accelerated junctional rhythm may herald the onset of atrioventricular block, and radiofrequency delivery should be discontinued immediately. His, His bundle electrogram; HRA, high right atrium; RVA, right ventricular apex.

does not affect the occurrence of accelerated junctional rhythm (104). The absence of junctional rhythm generally predicts inefficacy of the application, and the radiofrequency energy delivery should not be continued for more than 15 seconds at the same site. Rarely, successful slow pathway modification has been achieved in the absence of junctional rhythm (105). Intact VA conduction is expected during the accelerated junctional rhythm that accompanies slow pathway ablation, even when there is poor VA conduction during baseline ventricular pacing. The appearance of VA block during accelerated junctional rhythm may herald the onset of atrioventricular block (positive predictive value of about 20%), and the energy application should be discontinued immediately (103,106,107). Energy delivery is also immediately terminated at first sight of a nonconducted P wave and in the event of an impedance rise or displacement of the catheter tip.

Inducibility of AVNRT is tested after each likely successful energy application to determine whether the end point of the procedure has been achieved. It has been shown that catheter modification of the slow pathway on an outpatient basis is safe (26). At our center, over 95% of the patients were discharged home on the same day of the procedure.

Electrogram-Guided Approach

Positioning of the ablation catheter is best performed during sinus rhythm, because the atrial and ventricular electrograms on the tricuspid valve are more easily distinguishable. After the ablation catheter has been manipulated to cross the tricuspid valve and record the His bundle potential, an inferoposterior deflection of the distal segment is made, and the catheter is slowly withdrawn with gentle clockwise torque applied so that the tip of the catheter lies along the

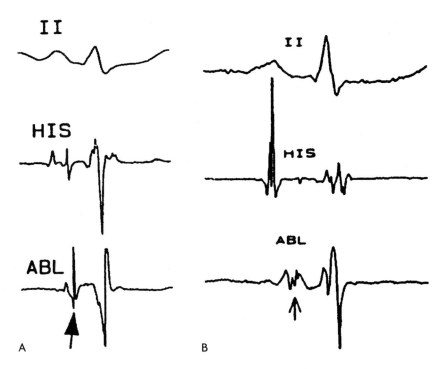

FIGURE 10-13. Two types of probable slow pathway potentials were identified at successful sites of ablation. **A:** The discrete, sharp, high-frequency deflection resembling a His potential occurs 10 to 40 msec after the local atrial electrogram. **B:** An atrial electrogram with multiple low-amplitude components. (From Zhu DWX, Maloney JD. Radiofrequency catheter ablative therapy for AV nodal reentrant tachycardia. In: Singer I, ed. *Interventional electrophysiology.* Baltimore: Williams & Wilkins, 1997:275–316, with permission.)

tricuspid annulus near the ostium of the coronary sinus but not in or posterior to the coronary sinus ostium. During sinus rhythm, the area along the posteromedial tricuspid annulus in proximity to the coronary sinus ostium is carefully mapped with bipolar recordings from the distal pair of electrodes of the ablation catheter. The electrogram criteria used to identify the target site are an atrial-to-ventricular electrogram ratio of less than 0.5 and the presence of a probable slow pathway potential.

Two types of slow pathway potentials have been identified (Fig. 10-13). Jackman and colleagues targeted a sharp, discrete, high-frequency potential after the initial atrial electrogram by 10 to 40 msec during sinus rhythm (13). This sequence reverses during atypical AVNRT. This type of slow pathway potential may represent activation of the atrial connection with the slow pathway and is frequently located in the area adjacent to the ostium of the coronary sinus. Energy was usually applied at sites where the largest, sharpest, and latest potentials were recorded during sinus rhythm or occasionally at sites where the largest, sharpest, and earliest potentials were recorded during retrograde slow pathway conduction. Successful modification eliminated the potentials and the inducibility of AVNRT. In Jackman's series, only a median of two applications of radiofrequency energy was required to eliminate AVNRT in 78 (97.5%) of 80 patients. Haissaguerre and colleagues identified a multicomponent, low-frequency atrial electrogram usually recorded in the middle to posterior right atrial septum near tricuspid annulus and anterior to the coronary sinus ostium (12). A median of two radiofrequency energy applications rendered AVNRT noninducible in all 64 patients without inadvertent atrioventricular block. Successful ablation of AVNRT did not necessarily eliminate these potentials. Such potentials were also recorded in most individuals without AVNRT (108).

Occasionally, slow pathway potentials have been recorded posterior to or within the ostium of coronary sinus. If the characteristic electrograms are recorded from multiple sites, the most posterior area should be attempted first. The inducibility of AVNRT is assessed after each likely successful application of radiofrequency energy.

Stepwise Anatomic Approach

In the stepwise anatomic approach, target sites are selected mainly on the basis of fluoroscopic landmarks. The only electrogram criteria used was an atrial-to-ventricular electrogram ratio of less than 0.5. No effort is made in particular to search for a slow pathway potential to target catheter modification. Jazayeri and colleagues reported the initial series of patients who underwent slow pathway modification guided by an anatomic approach (7). In the RAO view, the posteromedial tricuspid annulus between the level of the coronary sinus ostium and the His potential recording site was divided anatomically into posterior, medial, and anterior zones. Energy was delivered along the tricuspid annulus, starting at the most posterior site, the floor of the coronary sinus ostium, and progressing to the most anterior site, just inferior to the His potential recording site. The inducibility of AVNRT was assessed after each likely successful application. If the tachycardia was still inducible after two radiofrequency energy applications within each of the anatomic zones, the process was repeated. With this approach, the slow pathway was successfully ablated in 188 (97%) of 193 patients (18). No patient developed atrioventricular block. Other anatomically based approaches have been described (14–17).

Comparison of the Electrogram-Guided and Stepwise Anatomic Approaches

A prospective, randomized study compared the outcome of the anatomic and electrogram-guided approaches for modification of the slow pathway (109). The anatomic approach was effective in 21 (84%) of 25 patients, and the electrogram-guided approach was effective in all 25 (100%) patients. The four patients for whom the anatomic approach was ineffective had a successful outcome with the electrogram-guided approach. There was no significant difference with respect to the time required for modification, duration of fluoroscopic exposure, or mean number of radiofrequency energy applications. Although both methods are comparable in efficacy for modification of the slow pathway, the target sites may be outside the region of the anatomic approach in some patients, and the electrogram-guided approach may be required.

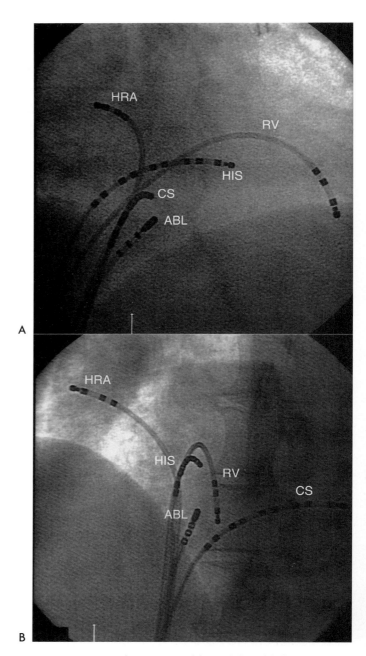

FIGURE 10-14. Right anterior oblique **(A)** and left anterior oblique **(B)** radiographs of a successful site of catheter ablation of slow pathway in a patient with typical AV nodal reentrant tachycardia (AVNRT). The ablation catheter (ABL) was positioned at right atrial septum near the posteromedial tricuspid annulus, between the coronary sinus ostium and the His potential recording site. A slow pathway potential was recorded on the distal pair of electrodes. The application of radiofrequency energy led to the development of accelerated junctional rhythm. Slow pathway conduction and AVNRT were eliminated. CS, coronary sinus catheter; HIS, His potential catheter; HRA, high right atrium; RV, right ventricular catheter.

Integrated Approach

Although the electrogram-guided and the stepwise anatomic approaches have been developed independently, a combined approach was adopted by many practicing electrophysiologists in which fluoroscopic landmarks and intracardiac electrograms are used complementarily in determining the target site for modification. We developed an approach in which the target site was initially identified by an atrial-to-ventricular electrogram ratio of less than 0.5 and as having a probable slow pathway potential. Mapping is usually performed in the RAO view, and the ablation catheter tip position is confirmed in the LAO view (Fig. 10-14). Mapping is started in the posterior septum near the coronary sinus ostium and proceeds into the midseptal region if necessary (Fig. 10-15). If the characteristic atrial electrogram is not identified in the described regions, the area posterior to or within the coronary sinus ostium is mapped. Under continuous electrocardiographic monitoring, the radiofrequency energy was delivered during sinus rhythm. Bursts of accelerated junctional rhythm should develop and then subside after 10 to 20 seconds. The ablation catheter tip is then carefully withdrawn 3 to 4 mm from its initial site until accelerated junctional rhythm occurs again. When bursts of junctional rhythm persist at one location, further pullback should be held until the junctional rhythm subsides. Guided by slow pathway potentials and fluoroscopic landmarks, several such linear lesions may be generated within the triangle of Koch if necessary to eliminate AVNRT and interrupt slow pathway conduction.

The protocol should be adjusted depending on the size of coronary sinus ostium, the geometry of the triangle of Koch, the ease of identifying a slow path-

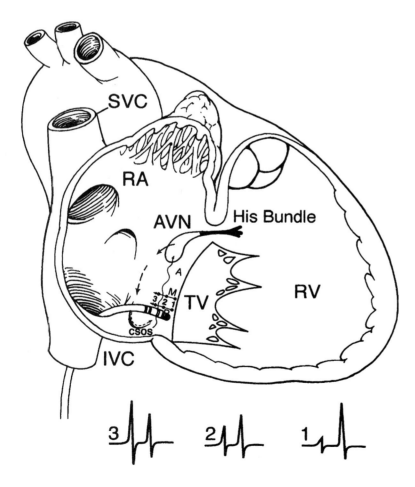

FIGURE 10-15. Determination of catheter position in AV nodal slow pathway ablation uses the integrated approach in the right anterior oblique view. The tricuspid annulus between the coronary sinus ostium and the His potential recording site is divided into posterior (P), medial (M), and anterior (A) zones. The mapping is started in the M and P zones and may proceed to the A zone to search for the possible slow pathway potentials. If the characteristic atrial electrogram is not identifiable in these areas, the areas posterior to or within the coronary sinus ostium should be mapped. Positions 1, 2, and 3 on the right atrium represent three consecutive sites during a single ablation catheter pullback with intermittent or continuous radiofrequency application. The corresponding electrograms of positions 1, 2, and 3 demonstrate the increasing size of the atrial electrogram relative to the ventricular electrogram. Position 1 is identified on the basis of the atrial electrogram to ventricular electrogram ratio of less than 0.5 and the presence of a probable slow pathway potential. Additional linear lesions may be created until the AV nodal reentrant tachycardia is eliminated. AVN, compact AV node; CSOS, coronary sinus ostium; IVC, inferior vena cava; RA, right atrium; RV, right ventricle; SVC, superior vena cava; TV, septal leaflet of tricuspid valve. (From Zhu DWX. Modification of AV node for management of AV nodal reentrant tachycardia. In: Singer I, Barold SS, Camm AJ, eds. *Nonpharmacological therapy of arrhythmias for the 21st century: the state of the art.* Armonk, NY: Futura Publishing, 1998:157–195, with permission.)

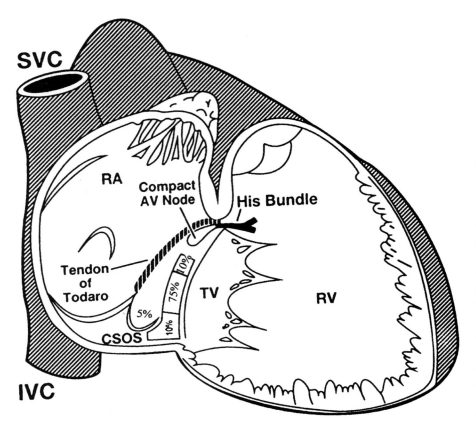

FIGURE 10-16. The schematic distribution of successful sites of slow pathway ablation in the right anterior oblique view. Most sites are located near the tricuspid annulus at the level of or superior to the coronary sinus ostium. The remaining 5% to 10% of sites are located posterior to or within the coronary sinus ostium. CSOS, coronary sinus ostium; IVC, inferior vena cava; RA, right atrium; RV, right ventricle; SVC, superior vena cava; TV, septal leaflet of tricuspid valve. (From Zhu DWX, Maloney JD. Radiofrequency catheter ablative therapy for AV nodal reentrant tachycardia. In: Singer I, ed. *Interventional electrophysiology.* Baltimore: Williams & Wilkins, 1997:275–316, with permission.)

way potential, and the stability of the ablation catheter. Using this approach in 156 consecutive patients with AVNRT, we achieved a success rate of 99.5%. Eighty-eight percent of the patients had slow/fast AVNRT, 7% had fast/slow AVNRT, and 5% had slow/slow AVNRT. Ten percent of the patients had two types of inducible AVNRT. Two patients experienced transient atrioventricular block, and both completely recovered. AVNRT recurred in two patients within 3 months and was successfully eliminated during a second procedure. Distribution of successful sites for slow pathway ablation in these patients is shown in Fig. 10-16. Most successful sites were near the tricuspid annulus at the roof of or superior to the coronary sinus ostium. The slow pathway was successfully modified in a patient with slow/fast AVNRT in the transplanted heart (28).

Yamane and associates limited the mapping area for slow pathway potential along the tricuspid annulus around the upper margin of the coronary sinus ostium in 59 patients with typical AVNRT (110). Detailed analysis of the fluoroscopic images with coronary sinus angiography showed that the distance between His potential recording site and successful ablation site varied according to the length of Koch's triangle, but the distance between successful ablation site and upper margin of coronary sinus ostium was relatively constant. Most successful sites were within 5 mm above and below the level of the upper margin of coronary sinus ostium. All patients were successfully treated by a mean of 1.4 ± 0.7 applications of radiofrequency energy. Only a single application of energy was needed to eliminate the tachycardia in 78% of these patients.

Left-Sided Approach

Rarely, the slow pathway participating in the slow/fast AVNRT cannot be ablated from the posteroseptal right atrium or the coronary sinus ostium. The tachycardia can be reset by atrial extrastimuli delivered to the posterior aspect of the mitral annulus. Energy delivery at the posterior aspect of the mitral annulus or coronary sinus more than 2 cm from the ostium initiated accelerated junctional rhythm and elimination of the slow pathway conduction and AVNRT (75–76).

Other Approaches

Retrograde conduction by the slow pathway may be demonstrated in about one third of patients with AVNRT (11,17). The target site is identified on the basis of the earliest atrial activation during retrograde slow pathway conduction. Radiofrequency energy can be delivered during sinus rhythm, atypical AVNRT, or ventricular pacing. The end points are noninducibility of AVNRT, selective loss of retrograde slow pathway conduction, or both. This approach has been used successfully in patients with atypical AVNRT.

The response of typical AVNRT to subthreshold stimulation (111) or a single atrial extrastimulus (112) delivered from the ablation catheter has been used to identify a target site for slow pathway modification. Theoretically, these techniques may reduce the number of ineffective radiofrequency energy deliveries. These approaches have not been compared with others.

Newer Mapping and Imaging Techniques

A recently introduced technique uses an electroanatomic mapping system (CARTO, Biosense, Baldwin Park, Calif.) and a magnetic field sensing catheter to create a three-dimensional endocardial map with a spatial resolution of less than 1 mm (113). This system can be used in patients undergoing catheter modification for AVNRT to generate accurate maps of the triangle of Koch and to guide application of radiofrequency energy (114). The magnetic field emitter is attached to the underside of the procedure table. Electroanatomic maps are usually created using a single mapping and ablation catheter and a posteriorly positioned external reference catheter. The initial mapping of right atrium is obtained with fluoroscopic guidance to outline the junctions with superior vena cava and inferior vena cava and the ostium of coronary sinus. The remainder of the mapping can be achieved without fluoroscopy. Typically, the catheter is dragged across the endocardium, and a global map of the right atrium is generated. The major landmarks of the triangle of Koch are identified by sampling points from the sites where a His potential is present and from the ostium of coronary sinus, with care taken to delineate the roof and floor of the ostium. The annular border of the triangle of Koch is defined by serial acquisition of points recording a low-amplitude atrial electrogram and a high-amplitude ventricular electrogram (ratio <0.5) from the His region to the level of the floor of the coronary sinus ostium. The triangle of Koch is best revealed in the right lateral and LAO views (Fig. 10-17). In the right lateral view, the tip of the sensing and ablation catheter is positioned anterior and just superior to the roof of the coronary sinus ostium. The initial site of modification is a few millimeters from the annular border of the triangle and, if possible, is guided by a slow pathway potential. The site is tagged before radiofrequency energy delivery. If junctional rhythm is not initiated or AVNRT remains inducible, a site more proximally located along the His region–coronary sinus ostium axis is attempted. Such sites should always be kept at least 1 cm from the most inferoposterior His recording site.

With experienced operators, a limited map of the septal right atrium may provide sufficient guidance to perform a successful slow pathway ablation. Cooke and Wilber reported their initial experience in 14 patients with AVNRT (114). A median of two radiofrequency applications eliminated the inducibility of AVNRT without causing atrioventricular block. The availability of multiple simultaneous projections not accessible by conventional fluoroscopy and the ability to construct accurate maps of critical structures may be particularly useful in patients with unusual anatomic features, minimizing the risk of atrioventricular block and potentially reducing procedure time and radiation exposure. Controlled comparison of this new technique with those traditional approaches are not available.

Intracardiac echocardiography has been used adjunctively with conventional fluoroscopy and electrogram guidance to identify the anatomic sites of successful slow pathway ablation in patients with typical AVNRT (115). Fisher and colleagues reported that radiofrequency energy application directed by intracardiac echocardiography to atrial tissue 2 to 7 mm

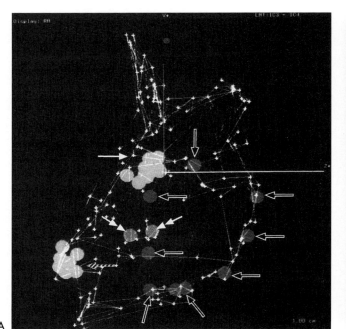 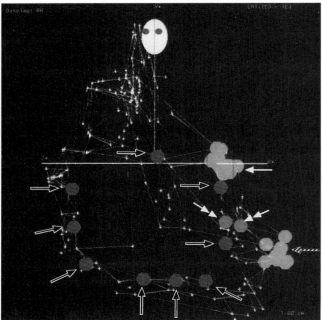

FIGURE 10-17. Nonfluoroscopic electroanatomic mapping in a patient with typical AV nodal reentrant tachycardia undergoing successful slow pathway modification (reproduced in gray scale). Right lateral view **(A)** and left anterior oblique view **(B)** open up the triangle of Koch and are considered the most useful projections for mapping. The His potentials recorded on the intracardiac electrogram are indicated *(white arrow)*, as are the borders of the coronary sinus *(striped arrow)*, sites along the tricuspid annulus *(dark arrows)*, and ablation sites *(double arrowheads)*. (Modified from Cooke PA, Wilber DJ. Radiofrequency catheter ablation of AV nodal reentry tachycardia utilizing nonfluoroscopic electroanatomical mapping. *Pacing Clin Electrophysiol* 1998;21:1802–1809, with permission.)

posterior to the insertion of the tricuspid valve into the atrioventricular muscular septum eliminated antegrade slow pathway conduction in all 25 patients. In contrast, radiofrequency energy applications delivered more posteriorly between the coronary sinus ostium and tricuspid annulus resulted in accelerated junctional rhythm but failed to ablate the slow pathway. This suggests the presence of a critical portion of the slow pathway adjacent to the tricuspid valve overlying the atrioventricular muscular septum. Adjunctive intracardiac echocardiography may facilitate slow pathway ablation in patients with complicated cardiac or intrathoracic anatomy.

Therapeutic End Points

The end point of slow pathway modification is the elimination of AVNRT inducibility before and during infusion of isoproterenol that is sufficient to increase the sinus rate to between 120 and 130 bpm. It remains controversial whether the risk of recurrent AVNRT is higher when residual slow pathway conduction persists after elimination of AVNRT (116–123). Some investigators reported that the recurrence rate was substantially higher in patients with residual slow pathway conduction (116–119). Others found that residual slow pathway conduction with or without inducible single echo beat does not correlate with clinical tachycardia recurrence (120–123). Because evidence of residual slow pathway conduction may persist in approximately 40% of patients after successful elimination of AVNRT (12,13,15,18), it is not a specific predictor for recurrence. The risk of causing complete atrioventricular block may increase substantially by continuing attempts to eliminate the residual slow pathway conduction.

The outcome of repeat modification for recurrent tachycardia has been excellent. The persistence of residual dual AV nodal physiology and inducible single AV nodal reentrant echo beat should not be considered as an indication for continuing the ablation effort as long as isoproterenol infusion is administered and AVNRT is no longer inducible. Some investigators reported that the recurrence rate is greater for slow/slow AVNRT than for slow/fast AVNRT, and more ablation efforts in the right posteroseptal tricuspid annulus and coronary sinus ostium may be justifiable in these patients (60). Persistence of residual slow pathway conduction with two or more inducible echo beats indicates modification failure, and the chance of recurrent AVNRT in these patients is substantial. Ablation attempts should be continued until the end point of noninducibility has been achieved.

Changes in Electrophysiologic Parameters

After successful slow pathway ablation, the PR and AH intervals remained unchanged. The atrioventricular block cycle length and the AV nodal effective refractory period are lengthened, while the VA conduction and effective refractory period are not affected. During atrial extrastimulation, the jump in the A_2H_2 interval that previously initiated AVNRT is no longer demonstrable (Fig. 10-5B). These changes occur because the slow pathway has a shorter antegrade block cycle length and effective refractory period than the fast pathway. In patients with a smooth AV nodal conduction curve at baseline, slow pathway ablation may lengthen the AV nodal effective refractory period and shorten the maximal A_2H_2 and A_3H_3 intervals significantly (85–87) (Fig. 10-18). The pre-ablation PR/RR ratio of more than 1 during rapid atrial pacing may be reduced to a PR/RR ratio of less than 1 after slow pathway ablation (84). Slow pathway conduction may persist as residual dual AV nodal physiology and an inducible single echo beat in some patients after elimination of AVNRT. This phenomenon may be explained by a modified slow pathway that is unable to sustain AVNRT or the presence of another slow pathway that is not evident before ablation and is incapable of sustaining AVNRT. In most of these patients, the atrioventricular block cycle length and the AV nodal effective refractory period may not prolong after ablation (119). Although some have reported that the fast pathway's effective refractory period may shorten after slow pathway modification, these observations are not consistent, and the underlying mechanisms remain uncertain (124–126). No evidence suggests that radiofrequency catheter modification of slow pathway alters autonomic modulation of the sinus node or the AV node (127).

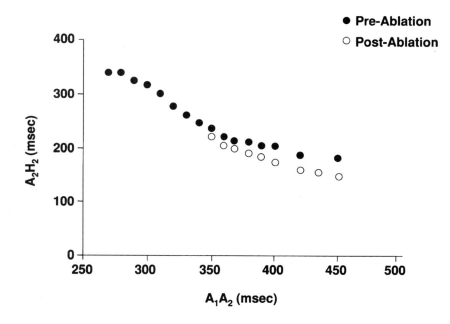

FIGURE 10-18. AV nodal conduction curves before and after ablation of a slow pathway in a patient with typical AV nodal reentrant tachycardia. Before ablation, a smooth curve shows no evidence of dual AV nodal physiology. Tachycardia is inducible after a critical atrial-His (A_2H_2) conduction time delay. Slow pathway ablation markedly shortens maximal A_2H_2 from 340 to 230 msec and eliminates the tail of the curve.

Ablation directed posteriorly in an attempt to modify slow pathway may occasionally result in fast pathway ablation. In a study using a posterior approach aimed at the slow pathway, unintentional ablation of the fast pathway occurred in 14% of cases (62). The retrograde fast pathway may be present posteriorly near the coronary sinus ostium in some patients, as shown in an intraoperative mapping study (128,129). Distortion of spatial relationship in the triangle of Koch by an enlarged coronary sinus ostium or altered orientation of the heart relative to fluoroscopic projection also may account for such observations rather than the displacement of the fast pathway. It is therefore essential to precisely map and localize the pathway targeted for modification along with the reciprocal pathway.

Outcome

Table 10-1 summarizes the results of radiofrequency catheter modification of the slow pathway using a variety of techniques. Overall, primary success rates ranged from 96% to 100%, and the incidence of inadvertent complete atrioventricular block was less than 2% (130,131). Other complications of slow pathway ablation, including vascular damage, deep venous thrombosis, pulmonary emboli, and cardiac tamponade, are rare (<1%) and are similar to the complications associated with any invasive electrophysiology study. No procedure-related deaths were reported.

The rate of recurrence of AVNRT after an initially successful slow pathway modification is 1% to 6%. It remains controversial whether the presence of residual slow pathway conduction with or without a single echo beat increases the risk of recurrent AVNRT. Outcomes for repeat procedures for recurrent AVNRT have been excellent, just as the initial attempts were (132).

Fast Pathway Modification

Early experience with catheter-based AV nodal modification principally targeted the fast pathway. However, the variable success rates, inadvertent atrioventricular block, postablation PR interval prolongation, and inefficacy for atypical AVNRT led to the development of selective slow pathway modification as an alternate method (133,134). Selective slow pathway modification has become the recommended approach, even in institutions that originally developed the technique for fast pathway ablation (135). Rarely, fast pathway ablation may be attempted when the slow pathway approach has failed (63).

Technique

For fast pathway modification, the ablation catheter is initially positioned along the His bundle catheter to record the maximal amplitude of the His potential from the distal pair of the electrodes. The catheter is then carefully withdrawn for several millimeters and manipulated slightly superior from the site where the maximal His potential is recorded until the amplitude

TABLE 10-1 • OUTCOME OF RADIOFREQUENCY CATHETER MODIFICATION OF AV NODAL SLOW PATHWAY

Study	Date	Patients (n)	Success Rate (%)	Heart Block (%)	Recurrence (%)	Technique
Haissaguerre et al. (12)	1992	64	64 (100%)	0	0	Electrogram
Jackman et al. (13)	1992	80	79 (99%)	1 (1%)	0	Electrogram
Akhtar et al. (18)	1993	193	188 (97%)	3 (3%)	0	Anatomic
Kay et al. (15)	1993	242	239 (98%)	2 (1%)	16 (6%)	Anatomic
Wu et al. (17)	1993	100	97 (97%)	3 (3%)	1 (1%)	Anatomic
Zhu et al. (22)	1996	78	78 (100%)	0	1 (1%)	Integrated
Chen et al. (130)	1996	580	580 (100%)	3 (0.5%)	11 (2%)	Integrated
Yamane et al. (110)	1999	119	119 (100%)	0	1 (1%)	Integrated
Calkins et al. (24)	1999	373	362 (97%)	5 (1%)	16 (5%)	Unspecified

of the local atrial potential is at least twice as high as the local ventricular potential and the proximal His potential is small or minimal (<0.1 mV). A gentle clockwise torque is applied to direct the catheter tip toward the atrial septum. The electrogram at the ablation site may be evaluated for retrograde atrial activation by means of the fast pathway during ventricular pacing or AVNRT to ensure that it occurs earlier than that recorded by the His catheter. Although the RAO view is generally used for positioning the ablation catheter, the LAO view is always used to confirm the position of the ablation catheter tip at the anterior atrial septum. Radiofrequency energy is initially delivered at 50°C for 15 seconds, usually during sinus rhythm. The surface electrocardiogram is continuously monitored, and energy delivery is stopped immediately if PR prolongation exceeds 50% or if a nonconducted P wave is observed.

Radiofrequency application at an effective site invariably results in the occurrence of an accelerated junctional rhythm. However, accelerated junctional rhythm may also occur at 25% of the ineffective sites (103). Ventriculoatrial dissociation is expected during the accelerated junctional rhythm when fast pathway modification is attempted. When accelerated junctional rhythm develops, it is advisable to pace the atrium at a faster rate to allow for continuous monitoring of the integrity of antegrade atrioventricular conduction. If AVNRT remains inducible or retrograde fast pathway conduction persists, the temperature is titrated up in increments of 5°C to 10°C up to 80°C, the ablation catheter is moved stepwise slightly inferiorly toward the midseptum, and modification is attempted again. When accelerated junctional rhythm occurs or a less than 50% prolongation of the PR interval develops, energy delivery should be held constant for an additional 10 to 20 seconds. Titration of temperature and a stepwise approach may reduce the risk of atrioventricular block (136).

Therapeutic End Points

The end points of the fast pathway modification are a PR or AH interval prolongation by up to 50% over baseline, elimination or marked attenuation of conduction over the retrograde fast pathway, and noninducibility of AVNRT before and during isoproterenol infusion (137). Dual AV nodal physiology was eliminated in 85% to 100% of the patients in whom it was present before the ablation. Because the slow pathway usually has a shorter antegrade block cycle length and effective refractory period than the fast pathway, the change in the shortest 1 : 1 atrioventricular conduction cycle length and AV nodal effective refractory period after the fast pathway ablation is minimal. Occasionally, patients who underwent fast pathway modification had only the retrograde fast pathway modified. This resulted in elimination of retrograde fast pathway conduction without a change in the PR or AH interval. This observation implies that, at least in some patients, the antegrade and retrograde fast pathways may be anatomically separate.

Outcome and Limitations

Because of the proximity of the ablation catheter to the compact AV node and His bundle, the most significant complication associated with modification of the fast pathway is the development of inadvertent complete heart block, which necessitated permanent pacemaker implantation in up to 20% of the patients in the early reports (5–8,10). Data from several large series showed that fast pathway ablation had a lower success rate (87% to 90% versus 96% to 99%) and a higher incidence of atrioventricular block (4% to 5.3% versus 0.4% to 2%) than slow pathway modification (134,138). Because a significant PR interval prolongation develops after successful ablation of the fast pathway, the suboptimal atrioventricular synchrony may result in adverse hemodynamic consequences in patients with heart failure. Selective modification of the fast pathway does not eliminate slow/slow AVNRT. Up to 13% of patients developed atypical AVNRT after fast pathway ablation for typical AVNRT, and they required slow pathway modification subsequently (133). Because of these inherent disadvantages in fast pathway modification, the technique is no longer used by most of the electrophysiologists. It may be attempted in patients in whom slow pathway modification is unsuccessful. Retrograde fast pathway ablation has been used in patients with typical AVNRT and a very prolonged PR interval during sinus rhythm (139–141).

Modification of the AV Node for AV Nodal Reentrant Tachycardia with Unusual Features

Despite the fact that modification of AV node constitutes well-established management for most patients with symptomatic AVNRT, many issues remain uncertain for patients with unusual electrophysiologic features.

AV Nodal Reentrant Tachycardia with Continuous AV Nodal Conduction Curves

Some patients with AVNRT do not manifest discontinuous AV nodal conduction curves. This may be explained by several possible mechanisms. First, if the difference between the conduction times over the slow and fast pathways are minimal (<50 msec), a typical jump may not be demonstrable even when there is a shift of antegrade conduction from the fast pathway to the slow pathway followed by the onset of typical AVNRT during atrial extrastimulation. Second, the functional refractory period of the atrium makes the refractory period of the fast pathway unobtainable, and it is therefore not possible to dissociate the fast and slow pathways. Third, the refractory periods of the fast and slow pathways may be similar. Using rapid atrial pacing, additional atrial extrastimuli, and administration of isoproterenol or propranolol may change the electrophysiologic properties of the fast and slow pathways such that dual AV nodal physiology becomes manifest. Successful ablation of the slow pathway in these patients resulted in a significant shortening of the maximal AH interval and prolongation of the AV nodal effective refractory period (85–87).

AV Nodal Reentrant Tachycardia with Multiple Discontinuities in AV Nodal Conduction Curves

The reported incidence of multiple jumps in the AV nodal conduction curves varied from 5% to 25% in patients with AVNRT (65–70). Patients with multiple AH jumps had a longer tachycardia cycle length, longer effective refractory period of the antegrade fast pathway, poor retrograde conduction, and a higher incidence of multiple types of AVNRT. Whether multiple jumps originate from anatomically different pathways is unclear. Among 78 patients with AVNRT undergoing slow pathway modification, multiple jumps were identified in 25% of the patients. When comparing the number of radiofrequency energy applications required to eliminate AVNRT, it became obvious that many more energy applications were needed in patients with multiple jumps than in those with no jump or only a single jump (68). The former group required a total of 5 ± 4 radiofrequency applications associated with accelerated junctional rhythm, and the latter group needed only 2 ± 1 radiofrequency applications ($p < 0.0001$). Multiple jumps in the antegrade AV nodal conduction curve may represent the presence of a more complex reentrant tissue mass. More radiofrequency energy deliveries are necessary to eliminate AVNRT in these patients.

AV Nodal Reentrant Tachycardia with Prolonged PR Interval during Sinus Rhythm

Sra and associates reported a 2.6% incidence of first-degree heart block for 268 patients with AVNRT, whereas Natale and colleagues found prolonged PR intervals in 2.7% of 259 patients (142,143). There is concern that slow pathway ablation in these patients may impair subsequent atrioventricular conduction. In most of these patients, antegrade AV nodal function was only modestly impaired (PR interval <300 msec). Slow pathway ablation was performed successfully with a low risk of early or late heart block. After slow pathway ablation, the AV nodal refractory period increased, but the fast pathway effective refractory period shortened (144). For patients with markedly prolonged PR intervals (>300 msec) and no demonstrable antegrade fast pathway function, the risk of heart block may be substantial after slow pathway ablation. Retrograde fast pathway ablation was attempted in such patients. None of these patients had dual AV nodal physiology at baseline or with isoproterenol infusion. Tachycardia was successfully eliminated in each patient without causing heart block or the need for permanent pacing (139–141).

Patients with Dual AV Nodal Pathways and Documented but Noninducible Supraventricular Tachycardia

Despite extensive efforts, tachycardia occasionally cannot be induced in some patients with dual AV nodal physiology and documented clinical episodes of supraventricular tachycardia with electrocardiographic features suggesting AVNRT. The incidence of noninducibility appears to be about 2% to 10%. The mechanisms for failure to reproducibly induce AVNRT are an inability to achieve critical AH prolongation, fast pathway block, and slow pathway block (145). The American College of Cardiology and the American Heart Association Committee on Clinical Intracardiac Electrophysiology and Catheter Ablation Procedures considered slow pathway modification in such patients to be a class II indication, reflecting the uncertainty and divided opinion on this issue (27,146–148). The decision to proceed with catheter modification in these patients is difficult and should be based on individual situations. Because of the lack of a valid end point, initiation of accelerated junctional rhythm during radiofrequency energy application at slow pathway region, prolongation of antegrade atrioventricular block cycle length, lengthening of AV nodal refractory period, and loss of dual AV nodal physiology may be used as surrogates in the laboratory for a successful outcome.

CONCLUSIONS

Radiofrequency catheter modification provides a safe, efficacious, and cost-effective treatment for AVNRT. The preferred technique for curing typical and atypical AVNRT is modification of the slow pathway. An integrated approach guided by intracardiac electrograms and fluoroscopically based anatomic landmarks is recommended. The nonfluoroscopic electroanatomic approach provides unique electrical activation mapping and may reduce procedure time and radiation exposure. Noninducibility of AVNRT is an acceptable end point for AV nodal modification. The outcome of the procedure is excellent by experienced operators, with success rates exceeding 95% and incidence of complications and recurrence less than 2%. Catheter modification of the slow pathway should be the treatment of choice in most patients with symptomatic AVNRT.

REFERENCES

1. Josephson ME. Paroxysmal supraventricular tachycardia: an electrophysiologic approach. *Am J Cardiol* 1978;41:1123–1126.
2. Wu D, Denes P, Amat-y-Leon F, et al. Clinical, electrocardiographic and electrophysiologic observations in patients with paroxysmal supraventricular tachycardia. *Am J Cardiol* 1978;41:1045–1051.
3. Scheinman MM. Patterns of catheter ablation practice in the United States: results of the 1992 NASPE survey. *Pacing Clin Electrophysiol* 1994;17:873–875.
4. Goy JJ, Fromer M, Schlaepfer J, et al. Clinical efficacy of radiofrequency current in the treatment of patients with AV node reentrant tachycardia. *J Am Coll Cardiol* 1990;16:418–423.
5. Lee MA, Morady F, Kadish A, et al. Catheter modification of the atrioventricular junction with radiofrequency energy for control of atrioventricular nodal reentry tachycardia. *Circulation* 1991;83:827–835.
6. Calkins H, Sousa J, El-Atassi R, et al. Diagnosis and cure of the Wolff-Parkinson-White syndrome or paroxysmal supraventricular tachycardias during a single electrophysiologic test. *N Engl J Med* 1991;324:1612–1618.
7. Jazayeri M, Hempe S, Sra J, et al. Selective transcatheter ablation of the slow pathway for the treatment of atrioventricular nodal reentrant tachycardia. *Circulation* 1992;85:1318–1328.
8. Langberg J, Harvey M, Calkins H, et al. Titration of power during radiofrequency catheter ablation of atrioventricular nodal reentrant tachycardia. *Pacing Clin Electrophysiol* 1993;16:465–470.
9. Mitrani RD, Klein LS, Hackett FK, et al. Radiofrequency ablation for atrioventricular node reentrant tachycardia: comparison between fast (anterior) and slow (posterior) pathway ablation. *J Am Coll Cardiol* 1993;21:432–441.
10. Chen S, Chiang C, Tsang W, et al. Selective radiofrequency catheter ablation of fast and slow pathways in 100 patients with atrioventricular nodal reentrant tachycardia. *Am Heart J* 1993;125:1–10.
11. Kottkamp H, Hindricks G, Willems S, et al. An anatomically and electrogram-guided stepwise approach for effective and safe catheter ablation of the fast pathway for elimination of atrioventricular node reentrant tachycardia. *J Am Coll Cardiol* 1995;22:974–981.
12. Haissaguerre M, Gaita F, Fischer B, et al. Elimination of atrioventricular nodal reentrant tachycardia using discrete slow potentials to guide application of radiofrequency energy. *Circulation* 1992;85:2162–2175.
13. Jackman W, Beckman K, McClelland J, et al. Treatment of supraventricular tachycardia due to atrioventricular nodal reentry by radiofrequency catheter ablation of slow pathway conduction. *N Engl J Med* 1992;327:313–318.
14. Wathen M, Natale A, Wolfe K, et al. An anatomically guided approach to atrioventricular node slow pathway ablation. *Am J Cardiol* 1992;70:886–889.
15. Kay G, Epstein A, Dailey S, et al. Selective radiofrequency

ablation of the slow pathway for the treatment of atrioventricular nodal reentrant tachycardia. *Circulation* 1992;85:1675–1688.
16. Moulton K, Miller B, Scott J, et al. Radiofrequency catheter ablation for AV nodal reentry: a technique for rapid transection of the slow AV nodal pathway. *Pacing Clin Electrophysiol* 1993;16:760–768.
17. Wu D, Yeh S, Wang C, et al. A simple technique for selective radiofrequency ablation of the slow pathway in atrioventricular node reentrant tachycardia. *J Am Coll Cardiol* 1993;21:1612–1621.
18. Akhtar M, Jazayeri MR, Sra J, et al. Atrioventricular nodal reentry: clinical, electrophysiological, and therapeutic considerations. *Circulation* 1993;88:282–295.
19. Trohman RG, Pinski SL, Sterba R, et al. Evolving concepts in radiofrequency catheter ablation of atrioventricular nodal reentry tachycardia. *Am Heart J* 1994;128:586–595.
20. Epstein LM, Lesh MD, Griffin JC, et al. A direct midseptal approach to slow atrioventricular nodal pathway ablation. *Pacing Clin Electrophysiol* 1995;18:57–64.
21. Strickberger S, Kalbfleisch S, Williamson B, et al. Radiofrequency catheter ablation of atypical atrioventricular nodal reentrant tachycardia. *J Cardiovasc Electrophysiol* 1993;4:526–532.
22. Zhu DWX, Maloney JD. Radiofrequency catheter ablative therapy for AV nodal reentrant tachycardia. In: Singer I, ed. *Interventional electrophysiology*. Baltimore: Williams & Wilkins, 1997:275–316.
23. Zhu DWX. Modification of AV node for management of AV nodal reentrant tachycardia. In: Singer I, Barold SS, Camm AJ, eds. *Nonpharmacological therapy of arrhythmias for the 21st century: the state of the art.* Armonk, NY: Futura Publishing, 1998:157–195.
24. Calkins H, Yong P, Miller JM, et al, for the Atakr Multicenter Investigator Group. Catheter ablation of accessory pathways, AV nodal reentrant tachycardia, and the atrioventricular junction: final results of a prospective, multicenter clinical trial. *Circulation* 1999;99:262–270.
25. Kalbfleisch SJ, Calkins H, Langberg JJ, et al. Comparison of the cost of radiofrequency catheter modification of the atrioventricular nodal and medical therapy for drug-refractory atrioventricular node reentrant tachycardia. *J Am Coll Cardiol* 1992;19:1583–1587.
26. Man KC, Kalbfleisch SJ, Hummel JD, et al. The safety and cost of outpatient radiofrequency ablation of the slow pathway in patients with atrioventricular nodal reentrant tachycardia. *Am J Cardiol* 1993;72:1323–1324.
27. Guidelines for clinical intracardiac electrophysiological and catheter ablation procedures: a report of the American College of Cardiology/American Heart Association Task Force on Practice Guidelines (Committee on Clinical Intracardiac Electrophysiological and Catheter Ablation Procedures). *Circulation* 1995;92:673–691.
28. Zhu DWX, Sun H. Radiofrequency catheter ablation of atrioventricular nodal reentrant tachycardia in a patient with heart transplantation. *J Interv Card Electrophysiol* 1998;2:87–89.
29. Fisch C, Mandrola JM, Rardon DR. Electrocardiographic manifestations of dual atrioventricular node conduction during sinus rhythm. *J Am Coll Cardiol* 1997;29:1015–1022.
30. Belhassen B, Fish R, Glikson M, et al. Noninvasive diagnosis of dual AV node physiology in patients with AV nodal reentrant tachycardia by administration of adenosine-5′-triphosphate during sinus rhythm. *Circulation* 1998;98:47–53.
31. Tebbenjohanns J, Niehaus M, Korte T, Drexler H. Noninvasive diagnosis in patients with undocumented tachycardia: value of the adenosine test to predict AV nodal reentrant tachycardia. *J Cardiovasc Electrophysiol* 1999;10:916–923.
32. Tawara K. Die topographie und histologie der bruckenfasern: ein beitrag zur lehre von der bedeutung der purkinjeschen faden. *Zentralbl Physiol* 1906;19:70–76.
33. Suma K, Shimada M. *The conduction system of the mammalian heart* (translated from German by Sunao Tawara). London: Imperial College Press, 1998.
34. Zipes DP. Genesis of cardiac arrhythmias: electrophysiological considerations. In: Braunwald E, ed. *Heart disease: a textbook of cardiovascular medicine,* 5th edition. Philadelphia: WB Saunders, 1997:548–592.
35. Becker A, Anderson R. Morphology of the human atrioventricular junctional area. In: Wellens H, Lie K, Janse M, eds. *The conduction system of the heart: structure, function and clinical implications.* Philadelphia: Lea & Febiger, 1976:263–286.
36. Koch WL. Weitere mitteilunger ueber den sinus-knoten des herzens. *Verh Dtsch Ges Pathol* 1909;13:85–92.
37. Anderson RH, Ho SY, Becker AE, Lang M. *Living anatomy: the CARTO and NOGA systems in the clinical arena.* Baldwin Park, Calif.: Biosense Inc., 1999:21.
38. Widran J, Lev M. The dissection of the atrioventricular node, bundle branches in the human heart. *Circulation* 1951;4:863–867.
39. McGuire MA, Johnson DC, Robotin M, et al. Dimensions of the triangle of Koch in humans. *Am J Cardiol* 1992;70:829–830.
40. Inoue S, Becker AE. Koch's triangle sized up: anatomical landmarks in perspective of catheter ablation procedures. *Pacing Clin Electrophysiol* 1998;21:1553–1558.
41. Ueng KC, Chen SA, Chiang CE, et al. Dimension and related anatomical distance of Koch's triangle in patients with atrioventricular nodal reentrant tachycardia. *J Cardiovasc Electrophysiol* 1996;7:1017–1023.
42. Sanchez-Quintana D, Davies DW, Ho SY, et al. Architecture of the atrial musculature in and around the triangle of Koch: its potential relevance to atrioventricular nodal reentry. *J Cardiovasc Electrophysiol* 1997;8:1396–1407.
43. Doig JC, Saito J, Harris L, et al. Coronary sinus morphology in patients with atrioventricular junctional reentry tachycardia and other supraventricular tachyarrhythmias. *Circulation* 1995;92:436–441.
44. Ho SW, McComb JM, Scott CD, et al. Morphology of the cardiac conduction system in patients with electrophysiologically proven dual atrioventricular nodal pathways. *J Cardiovasc Electrophysiol* 1993;4:504–512.
45. Gamache MC, Bharati S, Lev M, et al. Histopathological study following catheter guided radiofrequency current ablation of the slow pathway in a patient with atrioventricular nodal reentrant tachycardia. *Pacing Clin Electrophysiol* 1994;17:247–251.
46. Olgin JE, Ursell P, Kao AK, et al. Pathological findings following slow pathway ablation for AV nodal reentrant tachycardia. *J Cardiovasc Electrophysiol* 1996;7:625–631.
47. Moe GK, Preston JB, Burlington H. Physiologic evidence for a dual AV transmission system. *Circulation Res* 1956;4:357–375.
48. Jackman WM, Nakagawa H, Heidbuchel H, et al. Three forms of atrioventricular nodal (junctional) reentrant tachycardia: differential diagnosis, electrophysiological characteristics, and implications for anatomy of the reentrant circuit. In: Zipes DP, Jalife J, eds. *Cardiac electrophysiology: from cell to bedside,* 2nd edition. Philadelphia: WB Saunders, 1995:620–637.
49. Denes P, Wu D, Dhingra R, et al. Dual atrioventricular nodal pathways: a common electrophysiologic response. *Br Heart J* 1975;37:1069–1076.
50. Rosen KM, Mehta A, Miller RA. Demonstration of dual atrio-

ventricular nodal pathways in man. *Am J Cardiol* 1974;33: 291–294.
51. Denes P, Deleon W, Dhingra RC, et al. Demonstration of dual AN nodal pathways in patients with paroxysmal supraventricular tachycardia. *Circulation* 1973;48:549–555.
52. Josephson ME, Miller JM. Atrioventricular nodal reentry: evidence supporting an intranodal location. *Pacing Clin Electrophysiol* 1993;16:599–614.
53. McGuire MA, Robotin M, Yip ASB, et al. Electrophysiologic and histologic effects of dissection of the connections between the atrium and posterior part of the AV node. *J Am Coll Cardiol* 1994;23:693–701.
54. Josephson ME, Miller JM. Atrioventricular node reentry tachycardias: is the atrium a necessary link? In: Touboul P, Waldo A, eds. *Atrial arrhythmias: current concepts and management.* St. Louis: Mosby–Year Book, 1990:311–329.
55. Pritchett EL, Anderson RW, Benditt DG, et al. Reentry within the atrioventricular node: surgical cure with preservation of atrioventricular conduction. *Circulation* 1979;60: 440–446.
56. Holman VVL, Ikeshita M, Lease JG, et al. Alteration of antegrade atrioventricular conduction by cryoablation of peri-AV nodal tissue. *J Thorac Cardiovasc Surg* 1984;88:67–75.
57. Ross DL, Johnson DC, Denniss AR, et al. Curative surgery for atrioventricular junctional (AV nodal) reentrant tachycardia. *J Am Coll Cardiol* 1985;6:1383–1392.
58. Cox JL, Holman WL, Cain ME. Cryosurgical treatment of atricventricular node reentrant tachycardia. *Circulation* 1987; 76:1329–1336.
59. Fujimura O, Guiraudon GM, Yee R, et al. Operative therapy of atrioventricular node reentry and results of an anatomically guided procedure. *Am J Cardiol* 1989;64:1327–1332.
60. Otomo K, Wang Z, Lazzara R, Jackman WM. Atrioventricular nodal reentrant tachycardia: electrophysiological characteristics of four forms and implications for the reentrant circuit. In: Zipes DP, Jalife J, eds. *Cardiac electrophysiology: from cell to bedside,* 3rd edition. Philadelphia: WB Saunders, 2000:504–521.
61. Josephson ME, Kastor JA. Paroxysmal supraventricular tachycardias: is the atrium a necessary link? *Circulation* 1976;54: 430–435.
62. Englestein ED, Stein KM, Markowitz SM, et al. Posterior fast atrioventricular node pathways: implications for radiofrequency catheter ablation of atrioventricular node reentrant tachycardia. *J Am Coll Cardiol* 1996;27:1098–1105.
63. Langberg J, Leon A, Borganelli M, et al. A randomized comparison of anterior and posterior approaches to radiofrequency catheter ablation of atrioventricular nodal reentry tachycardia. *Circulation* 1993;87:1551–1556.
64. Inoue S, Becker AE. Posterior extensions of the human compact atrioventricular node: a neglected anatomic feature of potential clinical significance. *Circulation* 1998;97:188–193.
65. Dopirak MR, Schaal SF, Leier CV. Triple AV nodal pathways in man. *J Electrocardiol* 1980;13:185–188.
66. Kuck KH, Kuch B, Bleifeld W. Multiple antegrade and retrograde AV nodal pathways: demonstration by multiple discontinuities in the AV nodal conduction curves and echo time intervals. *Pacing Clin Electrophysiol* 1984;7:656–662.
67. Lee KL, Chun HM, Liem LB, et al. Multiple atrioventricular nodal pathways in humans: electrophysiologic demonstration and characterization. *J Cardiovasc Electrophysiol* 1998;9: 129–140.
68. Zhu DWX, Sun H, Arnold DJ, et al. The implication of multiple slow pathways on catheter ablation of atrioventricular nodal reentrant tachycardia [Abstract]. *Eur Heart J* 1997;18:465.
69. Antz M, Scherlag BJ, Otomo K, et al. Evidence for multiple atrio-AV nodal inputs in the normal dog heart. *J Cardiovasc Electrophysiol* 1998;9:395–408.
70. Tai CT, Chen SA, Chiang CE, et al. Multiple anterograde atrioventricular node pathways in patients with atrioventricular node reentrant tachycardia. *J Am Coll Cardiol* 1996;28: 725–731.
71. Heidbuchel H, Ector H, DeWare FV. Prospective evaluation of the length of the lower common pathway in the differential diagnosis of various forms of AV nodal reentrant tachycardia. *Pacing Clin Electrophysiol* 1998;21:209–216.
72. Benditt DG, Pritchett ELC, Smith WM, et al. Ventriculoatrial intervals: diagnostic use in paroxysmal supraventricular tachycardia. *Ann Intern Med* 1979;91:161–166.
73. Man KC, Brinkman K, Bogun F, et al. 2 : 1 atrioventricular block during atrioventricular node reentrant tachycardia. *J Am Coll Cardiol* 1996;28:1770–1774.
74. Lee SH, Chen SA, Tai CT, et al. Electrophysiologic characteristics and radiofrequency catheter ablation in atrioventricular node reentrant tachycardia with second-degree atrioventricular block. *J Cardiovasc Electrophysiol* 1997;8:502–511.
75. Tondo C, Otomo K, McClelland JH, et al. Atrioventricular nodal reentrant tachycardia: is the reentrant circuit always confined in the right atrium? [Abstract]. *J Am Coll Cardiol* 1996;27: 159A.
76. Tondo C, Beckman KJ, McClelland JH, et al. Response to radiofrequency catheter ablation suggests that the coronary sinus forms part of the reentrant circuit in some patients with atrioventricular nodal reentrant tachycardia [Abstract]. *Circulation* 1996;94:I-380.
77. Sung RJ, Styperek JL, Myerburg RJ, et al. Initiation of two distinct forms of atrioventricular nodal reentrant tachycardia during programmed ventricular stimulation in man. *Am J Cardiol* 1978;42:404–415.
78. Wu D, Denes P, Leon F, et al. An unusual variety of atrioventricular nodal re-entry due to retrograde dual atrioventricular nodal pathways. *Circulation* 1977;56:50–59.
79. McGuire MA, Alex SB, Yip SB, et al. Posterior (atypical) atrioventricular junctional reentrant tachycardia. *Am J Cardiol* 1994;73:469–477.
80. McGuire MA, Lau KC, Johnson DC, et al. Patients with two types of atrioventricular junctional (AV nodal) reentrant tachycardia: evidence that a common pathway of nodal tissue is not present above the reentrant circuit. *Circulation* 1991;83: 1232–1246.
81. Fujii E, Kasai A, Omichi C, et al. Electrophysiological characteristics during slow pathway ablation of posterior atrioventricular junctional reentrant tachycardia. *Pacing Clin Electrophysiol* 1998;21[Pt II]:2510–2516.
82. Goldberger J, Brooks R, Kadish A. Physiology of "atypical" atrioventricular junctional reentrant tachycardia occurring following radiofrequency catheter modification of the AV node. *Pacing Clin Electrophysiol* 1992;15:2270–2282.
83. Hwang C, Martin DJ, Goodman JS, et al. Atypical AV node reciprocating tachycardia masquerading as tachycardia using a left-sided accessory pathway. *J Am Coll Cardiol* 1997;30: 218–225.
84. Baker JH, Plumb VJ, Epstein AE, Kay GN. PR/RR interval ratio during rapid atrial pacing: a simple method for confirming the presence of slow AV nodal pathway conduction. *J Cardiovasc Electrophysiol* 1996;7:287–294.
85. Sheahan RG, Klein GJ, Yee R, et al. Atrioventricular node reentry with "smooth" AV node function curves: a different arrhythmia substrate? *Circulation* 1996;93:969–972.
86. Tai CT, Chen SA, Chiang CE, et al. Complex electrophysiological characteristics in atrioventricular nodal reentrant tachy-

87. Kuo CT, Lin KH, Cheng NJ, et al. Characterization of atrioventricular nodal reentry with continuous atrioventricular node conduction curve by double atrial extrastimulation. *Circulation* 1999;99:659–665.
88. Strickberger SA, Daoud EG, Niebauer MJ, et al. The mechanisms responsible for lack of reproducible induction of atrioventricular nodal reentrant tachycardia. *J Cardiovasc Electrophysiol* 1996;7:494–502.
89. Huycke EC, Lai WT, Nguyen NX, et al. Role of intravenous isoproterenol in the electrophysiologic induction of atrioventricular node reentrant tachycardia in patients with dual AV node pathways. *Am J Cardiol* 1989;64:1131–1137.
90. Yu WC, Chen SA, Chiang CE, et al. Effects of isoproterenol in facilitating induction of slow-fast atrioventricular nodal reentrant tachycardia. *Am J Cardiol* 1996;78:1299–1302.
91. Hirao K, Otomo K, Wang X, et al. Para-Hisian pacing: a new method for differentiating retrograde conduction over an accessory AV pathway from conduction over the AV node. *Circulation* 1996;94:1027–1035.
92. Knight BP, Zivin A, Souza J, et al. A technique for the rapid diagnosis of atrial tachycardia in the electrophysiology laboratory. *J Am Coll Cardiol* 1999;33:775–781.
93. Haissaguerre M, Warin JF, Lemetayer P, et al. Closed chest ablation of retrograde conduction in patients with atrioventricular nodal reentrant tachycardia. *N Engl J Med* 1989;320:426–433.
94. Epstein LM, Scheirunan MM, Langberg JJ, et al. Percutaneous catheter modification of the atrioventricular node: a potential cure for atrioventricular nodal reentrant tachycardia. *Circulation* 1989;80:757–768.
95. Weber HP, Kaltenbrunner W, Heinze A, et al. Laser catheter coagulation of atrial myocardium of ablation of atrioventricular nodal reentrant tachycardia: first clinical experience. *Eur Heart J* 1997;18:487–495.
96. Kavesh NG, Gosnell MR, Shorofsky SR, Gold MR, for the Polaris Investigator Group. Comparison of power- and temperature-guided radiofrequency modification of the atrioventricular node. *Am J Cardiol* 1997;80:1444–1447.
97. Strickberger SA, Daoud EG, Weiss R. A randomized comparison of fixed power and temperature monitoring during slow pathway ablation in patients with atrioventricular nodal reentrant tachycardia. *J Interv Card Electrophysiol* 1997;1:299–303.
98. Stellbrink C, Ziegert K, Schauerte P, Hanrath P. A prospective, randomized comparison of temperature-controlled vs manually delivered radiofrequency catheter ablation in patients undergoing atrioventricular nodal modification or accessory pathway ablation. *Eur Heart J* 1997;18:1780–1786.
99. Strickberger SA, Zivin A, Daoud EG, et al. Temperature and impedance monitoring during slow pathway ablation in patients with atrioventricular nodal reentrant tachycardia. *J Cardiovasc Electrophysiol* 1996;7:295–300.
100. Willems S, Shenasa H, Kottkamp H, et al. Temperature-controlled slow pathway ablation for treatment of atrioventricular nodal reentrant tachycardia using a combined anatomical and electrogram guided strategy. *Eur Heart J* 1996;17:1092–1102.
101. Strickberger SA, Tokano T, Tse HF, et al. Target temperature of 48°C versus 60°C during slow pathway ablation: a randomized comparison. *J Cardiovasc Electrophysiol* 1999;10:799–803.
102. Nath S, DiMarco P, Mounsey P, et al. Correlation of temperature and pathophysiological effect during radiofrequency catheter ablation of the AV junction. *Circulation* 1995;92:1188–1192.
103. Jentzer JH, Goyal R, Williamson BD, et al. Analysis of junctional ectopy during radiofrequency ablation for atrioventricular node reentrant tachycardia. *J Am Coll Cardiol* 1993;22:1706–1710.
104. Chen MC, Guo GB. Junctional tachycardia during radiofrequency ablation of the slow pathway in patients with AV nodal reentrant tachycardia: effects of autonomic blockade. *J Cardiovasc Electrophysiol* 1999;10:56–60.
105. Hsieh MH, Chen SA, Tai CT, et al. Absence of junctional rhythm during successful slow pathway ablation in patients with atrioventricular nodal reentrant tachycardia. *Circulation* 1998;98:2296–2300.
106. Thakur R, Klein G, Yee R, et al. Junctional tachycardia: a useful marker during radiofrequency ablation for atrioventricular node reentrant tachycardia. *J Am Coll Cardiol* 1993;22:1706–1710.
107. Hintringer F, Hartikainen J, Davies W, et al. Prediction of atrioventricular block during radiofrequency ablation of the slow pathway of the atrioventricular node. *Circulation* 1995;92:3491–3496.
108. Niebauer Mj, Daoud E, Williamson B, et al. Atrial electrogram characteristics in patients with and without atrioventricular nodal reentrant tachycardia. *Circulation* 1995;92:77–81.
109. Kalbfleisch S, Strickberger S, Williamson B. Randomized comparison of anatomic and electrogram mapping approaches to ablation of the slow pathway of atrioventricular node reentrant tachycardia. *J Am Coll Cardiol* 1994;23:716–723.
110. Yamane T, Iesaka Y, Goya M, et al. Optimal target site for slow AV nodal pathway ablation: possibility of predetermined focal mapping approach using anatomic reference in the Koch's triangle. *J Cardiovasc Electrophysiol* 1999;10:529–537.
111. Willems S, Weiss C, Hofmann T, et al. Subthreshold stimulation in the region of the slow pathway during atrioventricular node reentrant tachycardia: correlation with effect of radiofrequency catheter ablation. *J Am Coll Cardiol* 1997;29:408–415.
112. Sra J, Jazayeri M, Natale A, et al. Termination of atrioventricular nodal reentrant tachycardia by premature stimulation from ablating catheter. *Circulation* 1995;91:1095–1100.
113. Gepstein L, Hayam G, Ben-Haim SA. A novel method for nonfluoroscopic catheter-based electroanatomical mapping of the heart. *Circulation* 1997;95:1611–1622.
114. Cooke PA, Wilber DJ. Radiofrequency catheter ablation of atrioventricular nodal reentry tachycardia utilizing nonfluoroscopic electroanatomical mapping. *Pacing Clin Electrophysiol* 1998;21:1802–1809.
115. Fisher WG, Pelini MA, Bacon M. Adjunctive intracardiac echocardiography to guide slow pathway ablation in human atrioventricular nodal reentrant tachycardia: anatomic insights. *Circulation* 1997;96:3021–3029.
116. Li H, Klein G, Stites H, et al. Elimination of slow pathway conduction: an accurate indicator of clinical success after radiofrequency atrioventricular node modification. *J Am Coll Cardiol* 1993;22:1849–1853.
117. Baker J, Plumb V, Epstein A, et al. Predictors of recurrent atrioventricular nodal reentry after selective slow pathway ablation. *Am J Cardiol* 1994;73:765–769.
118. Tebbenjohanns J, Pfeiffer D, Schumacher B, et al. Impact of the local atrial electrogram in AV nodal reentrant tachycardia: ablation versus modification of the slow pathway. *J Cardiovasc Electrophysiol* 1995;6:245–251.
119. Tondo C, Bella PD, Carbuchicchio C, et al. Persistence of single echo beat inducibility after selective ablation of the slow pathway in patients with atrioventricular nodal reentrant tachycardia: relationship to the functional properties of the atrioventricular node and clinical implications. *J Cardiovasc Electrophysiol* 1996;7:689–696.

120. Lindsay B, Chung M, Gamache M, et al. Therapeutic end points for the treatment of atrioventricular node reentrant tachycardia by catheter guided radiofrequency current. *J Am Coll Cardiol* 1993;22:733–740.
121. Manolis AS, Wang PJ, Estes M III. Radiofrequency ablation of slow pathway in patients with atrioventricular nodal reentrant tachycardia: do arrhythmia recurrences correlate with persistent slow pathway conduction or site of successful ablation? *Circulation* 1994;90:2815–2819.
122. Chen SA, Wu TJ, Chiang CE, et al. Recurrent tachycardia after selective ablation of slow pathway in patients with AV nodal reentrant tachycardia. *Am J Cardiol* 1995;76:131–137.
123. Hummel JD, Strickberger SA, Williamson BD, et al. The course of recurrences of atrioventricular nodal reentrant tachycardia after radiofrequency ablation of the slow pathway. *Am J Cardiol* 1995;75:628–630.
124. Geller JC, Biblo LA, Carlson MD. New evidence that AV node slow conduction directly influences fast pathway function. *J Cardiovasc Electrophysiol* 1998;9:1026–1035.
125. Shen WK, Munger TM, Stanton MS, et al. Effects of slow pathway ablation on fast pathway function in patients with atrioventricular nodal reentrant tachycardia. *J Cardiovasc Electrophysiol* 1997;8:627–638.
126. Natale A, Klein G, Yee R, et al. Shortening of fast pathway refractoriness after slow pathway ablation: effects of autonomic blockade. *Circulation* 1994;89:1103–1108.
127. Kowallik P, Escher S, Peters W, Braun C, Meesmann M. Preserved autonomic modulation of the sinus and atrioventricular nodes following posteroseptal ablation for treatment of atrioventricular nodal reentrant tachycardia. *J Cardiovasc Electrophysio!* 1998;9:567–573.
128. Keim S, Werner P, Jazayeri M, et al. Localization of the fast and slow pathways in atrioventricular nodal reentrant tachycardia by intraoperative ice mapping. *Circulation* 1992;86:919–925.
129. McGuire MA, Bourke JP, Robotin MC, et al. High resolution mapping of Koch's triangle using sixty electrodes in humans with atrioventricular junctional (AV nodal) reentrant tachycardia. *Circulation* 1993;88:2315–2328.
130. Chen SA, Chiang CE, Tai CT, et al. Transient complete atrioventricular block during radiofrequency ablation of slow pathway for atrioventricular nodal reentrant tachycardia. *Am J Cardiol* 1996;77:1367–1370.
131. Fenelon G, d'Avila A, Malacky T, et al. Prognostic significance of transient complete atrioventricular block during radiofrequency ablation of atrioventricular node reentrant tachycardia. *Am J Cardiol* 1995;75:698–702.
132. Chen SA, Wu TJ, Chiang CE, et al. Recurrent tachycardia after selective ablation of slow pathway in patients with atrioventricular nodal reentrant tachycardia. *Am J Cardiol* 1995;76:131–137.
133. Langberg JJ, Kim YN, Goyal R, et al. Conversion of typical to "atypical" atrioventricular nodal reentrant tachycardia after radiofrequency catheter modification of the atrioventricular junction. *Am J Cardiol* 1992;69:503–508.
134. Hindricks G, for the Multicenter European Radiofrequency Survey (MERFS) Investigators. Incidence of complete atrioventricular block following attempted radiofrequency catheter modification of the atrioventricular node in 880 patients: results of the Multicenter European Radiofrequency Survey (MERFS). *Eur Heart J* 1996;17:82–88.
135. Kottkamp H, Hindricks G, Borggrefe M, Breithardt G. Radiofrequency catheter ablation of the anterosuperior and posteroinferior atrial approaches to the AV node for treatment of AV nodal reentrant tachycardia: techniques for selective ablation of "fast" and "slow" AV node pathways. *J Cardiovasc Electrophysiol*;8:451–468.
136. Langberg JJ. Radiofrequency catheter ablation of AVN nodal reentry: the anterior approach. *Pacing Clin Electrophysiol* 1993;16:615–622.
137. Deshpande S, Akhtar M, Panotopoulos P. Catheter ablation for atrioventricular nodal reentrant tachycardia. *Cardiol Clin* 1997;15:623–645.
138. Kalbfleisch SJ, Morady F. Catheter ablation of atrioventricular nodal reentrant tachycardia. In: Zipes DP, Jalife J, eds. *Cardiac electrophysiology: from cell to bedside*. Philadelphia: WB Saunders, 1995:1477–1487.
139. Reithmann C, Hoffmann E, Grunewald A, et al. Fast pathway ablation in patients with common atrioventricular nodal reentrant tachycardia and prolonged PR interval during sinus rhythm. *Eur Heart J* 1998;6:929–935.
140. Verdino RJ, Burke MC, Kall JG, et al. Retrograde fast pathway ablation for atrioventricular nodal reentry associated with markedly prolonged PR intervals. *Am J Cardiol* 1998;83:455–458.
141. Lee SH, Chen SA, Tai CT, et al. Atrioventricular node reentrant tachycardia in patients with a prolonged AH interval during sinus rhythm: clinical features, electrophysiologic characteristics and results of radiofrequency ablation. *J Interv Card Electrophysiol* 1997;1:305–310.
142. Sra JS, Jazayeri MR, Blanck Z, et al. Slow pathway ablation in patients with atrioventricular node reentrant tachycardia, and a prolonged PR interval. *J Am Coll Cardiol* 1994;24:1064–1068.
143. Natale A, Greenfield RA, Geiger MJ. Safety of slow pathway ablation in patients with long PR interval: further evidence of fast and slow pathway interaction. *Pacing Clin Electrophysiol* 1997;20:1698–1703.
144. Basta MN, Krahn AD, Klein GJ, et al. Safety of slow pathway ablation in patients with atrioventricular node reentrant tachycardia and a long fast pathway effective refractory period. *Am J Cardiol* 1997;80:155–159.
145. Strickberger SA, Daoud EG, Niebauer MJ, et al. The mechanisms responsible for lack of reproducible induction of atrioventricular nodal reentrant tachycardia. *J Cardiovasc Electrophysiol* 1996;7:494–502.
146. Bogun F, Knight B, Weiss R, et al. Slow pathway ablation in patients with documented but noninducible paroxysmal supraventricular tachycardia. *J Am Coll Cardiol* 1996;28:1000–1004.
147. Lee SH, Chen SA, Chiang CE, et al. Results of radiofrequency ablation in patients with clinically documented, but noninducible, atrioventricular node reentrant tachycardia and orthodromic atrioventricular reciprocating tachycardia. *Am J Cardiol* 1997;79:974–978.
148. Lin JL, Huang SSK, Lai LP, et al. Clinical and electrophysiologic characteristics and long-term efficacy of slow pathway catheter ablation in patients with spontaneous supraventricular tachycardia and dual atrioventricular node pathways without inducible tachycardia. *J Am Coll Cardiol* 1998;31:855–860.

ABLATION OF ATRIAL TACHYCARDIAS

JEFFREY E. OLGIN

The invasive electrophysiology era has led to a better understanding of the mechanism, substrate, and varieties of atrial tachycardias that has led to specific curative catheter ablation approaches. Many of these tachycardias can now be successfully eliminated with radiofrequency ablation. However, some atrial arrhythmias, such as atypical atrial flutter and atrial fibrillation remain somewhat elusive to cure. Over the past several years, advances in ablation of atrial tachycardias have been applied toward developing curative ablation techniques for atypical atrial flutters and atrial fibrillation.

Atrial tachycardias have been classified by a variety of schemes based variously on mechanism, substrate, surface electrocardiographic (ECG) pattern, or clinical presentation. The specific mechanism of an atrial tachycardia (i.e., reentrant, automatic, or triggered) often is difficult to define in a given individual, and ambiguous results are common during the search for a mechanism. The use of the surface ECG or clinical presentation alone is inadequate in classifying atrial tachycardias. For example, a macro-reentrant atrial tachycardia resulting from a surgical scar in the atrium may have an ECG appearance similar to that of a typical atrial flutter. Likewise, patients with repaired congenital heart disease may develop typical atrial flutter. The division of atrial flutter into subtypes based on a variety of criteria is not uniform in the literature.

This chapter adopts a general classification of atrial tachycardia based on a combination of the described features. The general techniques for mapping and ablation are common to each group of tachycardias. As we learn more about specific mechanisms and anatomic substrates, this scheme will likely become more sophisticated and refined.

Macro-reentrant atrial tachycardias use large circuits in the atria; examples are atrial flutter and atrial tachycardias due to surgical scars. Entrainment can be easily demonstrated by pacing during these tachycardias and is useful in localizing the tachycardia circuit. Mapping involves identifying conduction barriers and isthmuses, and ablation is accomplished by transecting the isthmus. Focal atrial tachycardias arise from a localized area of abnormal atrium and may result from micro-reentrant, automatic, or triggered mechanisms. Mapping is largely based on identifying the earliest site of activation, and these tachycardias can be eliminated by a focal ablation lesion. Examples include sinus node reentry, ectopic atrial tachycardias, and automatic atrial tachycardias. Atrial fibrillation remains largely an ECG diagnosis. In some patients with paroxysmal atrial fibrillation, a so-called focal mechanism may be responsible for initiating the atrial fibrillation, whereas in others, because the mechanism is different or the atria have remodeled, the maintenance substrate has become more important than focal trigger.

Atrial fibrillation is curable with ablation techniques in some patients. Although knowledge about the mechanism underlying atrial fibrillation has grown rapidly during the past few years, it remains a heterogeneous entity and will likely be further categorized into different types as we learn more about underlying mechanisms.

◉ MACRO-REENTRANT ATRIAL TACHYCARDIAS

The common feature of these tachycardias is that they use a macro-reentrant circuit somewhere in the atria and usually involve structural barriers that define the reentrant path. What varies is the specific nature and location of the barriers. Given a potential reentrant circuit, actual reentrant excitation can revolve in one of two possible directions. Atrial flutter is the prototypic macro-reentrant atrial tachycardia.

Definitions

Before the era of catheter ablation, the nomenclature used to define *atrial flutter* was somewhat confusing. However, because the only therapy was drugs, the distinction between various types of atrial flutter had little clinical applicability. The term atrial flutter had been used to describe a variety of different atrial tachycardias. What is sometimes referred to as atrial flutter after reparative surgery for congenital heart disease (e.g., Mustard, Senning, or Fontan operations; atrial septal defect repair) has a different reentrant circuit than what is called *the typical, classic, common, usual, type I, type A,* or *orthodromic atrial flutter* involving counterclockwise reentry (in the frontal plane) through an isthmus in the low right atrium (1–3). Such "typical atrial flutter" does not require prior surgical incisions in the atrium. Although typical atrial flutter had been defined by electrocardiographers as a regular atrial tachycardia with an atrial rate between 250 and 350 bpm and an ECG sawtooth pattern, flutter can be considerably slower in some patients, particularly those on antiarrhythmic drugs or with abnormal atria. Even more confusing is the division of atrial flutter into subtypes (3,4) based variously on rate, surface ECG morphology, ability to terminate with overdrive pacing from the high right atrium, and endocardial activation sequence, producing a variety of terms such as *atypical, uncommon, rare, antidromic, clockwise, type II, type B, unusual, fast, slow, left atrial,* and *reverse atrial flutter*. This chapter uses the definitions in Table 11-1, which classifies macro-reentrant atrial tachycardias largely based on known substrates.

The prototypic macro-reentrant atrial tachycardia is typical atrial flutter. The principles of mechanism, mapping, and ablation of all these arrhythmias are exemplified by typical atrial flutter.

Typical Atrial Flutter

Animal Models

Much of our understanding of the role of barriers in macro-reentrant atrial tachycardias has originated from animal models. Rosenblueth and Garcia-Ramos developed a canine model of atrial flutter by creating a crush lesion between the orifices of the venae cavae (5). This lesion produced an atrial tachycardia that was identical to atrial flutter in rate and morphology (5). Frame and colleagues employed a similar model of atrial flutter with a Y-shaped lesion in the right atrium between the venae cavae and a connecting lesion extending toward the right atrial appendage (6, 7). Mapping revealed that reentry occurred around the tricuspid annulus, not around the lesion itself (6, 7). The Y-shaped lesion served as a barrier to conduction, protecting the tissue between the lesion and the tricuspid annulus from being excited from an inferiorly spreading wavefront and remaining excitable when the reentrant wavefront arrived. These studies demonstrated the importance of two barriers between which reentry can occur, with a second barrier to "protect" the circuit from excitation by wavefronts other than the reentrant wavefront (i.e., short circuit). Other animal models have emphasized the importance of barriers in atrial flutter (8–12).

TABLE 11-1 • CLASSIFICATION OF ATRIAL FLUTTER

Type	ECG	Characteristic	Circuit	Mapping Techniques	Ablation Site
Typical atrial flutter					
Counter-clockwise	Negative Fl waves II, III, aVF; predominantly negative V$_6$	Macroreentrant in right atrium with regular rate (usually 250–350 bpm)	Around tricuspid annulus anterior to CT and ER	Anatomic, activation and entrainment to confirm critical isthmus	TA to IVC (ER)
Clockwise	Positive/notched Fl waves in II, III, aVF; predominantly positive in V$_6$	Rate, regularity and circuit same as counterlockwise but opposite rotation around TA	Around tricuspid annulus anterior to CT and ER	Anatomic, activation and entrainment to confirm critical isthmus	TA to IVC (ER)
Atypical flutter	Variable	Rate usually faster than typical, often more irregular	Unknown (pulmonary veins, portion of CT, functional barriers)	Activation sequence inconsistent with typical flutter; often difficult to entrain	?
Incisional reentry (atrial tachycardia in repaired congenital heart disease)	Variable	After surgical repair of congenital heart disease; rates variable depending on barriers, atrial disease, and length of circuit	Repair of congenital defects; circuit often involves surgical scars or prosthetic material; may also involve subeustachian isthmus	Identify lines of block with split potentials; activation mapping to identify early sites; entrainment mapping to identify critical isthmus	Variable, but must sever an isthmus from one barrier (surgical or anatomic) to another

CT, crista terminalis; ER, eustachian ridge; TA, tricuspid annulus; IVC, inferior vena cava; Fl, flutter.

Substrate for Typical Atrial Flutter

Typical atrial flutter has a characteristic pattern on 12-lead ECG, with superiorly directed flutter waves and rates in the range of 200 to 350 bpm (Fig. 11-1). The uniformity of these characteristics among patients with varied cardiac pathology suggests a common substrate for the arrhythmia. As hypothesized since early in the 20th century (13), it is established that atrial flutter is a reentrant arrhythmia confined to the right atrium (1,3,14). The unique endocardial anatomy of the right atrium, with its many orifices and distinct structures around which reentry could occur, probably explains the consistency of atrial flutter from patient to patient.

As was shown in the animal models of flutter, anatomic barriers are essential in typical atrial flutter to establish a circuit large enough that the circulating wavefront does not impinge on its own tail of refractoriness (15,16). Several studies have demonstrated that the crista terminalis and eustachian ridge form the posterior barriers of the typical flutter circuit and that the tricuspid annulus forms the anterior barrier (17–19). A critical isthmus has been identified in the low right atrium, bordered by the tricuspid annulus and the eustachian ridge between the inferior vena cava and the coronary sinus os (3,17–21). Reentry may occur in a counterclockwise or clockwise rotation in the frontal plane around the tricuspid annulus (19,22–24).

Mapping

Electrophysiologic evaluation of the patient with atrial flutter begins by identifying the type of atrial flutter, which then helps establish the appropriate site for ablation. This is accomplished by examining the morphology of the flutter wave on surface ECG, activation mapping, and entrainment mapping to identify a critical isthmus.

The surface ECG provides strong clues about the type of flutter. Typical counterclockwise atrial flutter produces the classic atrial flutter described by early electrocardiographers, with predominantly negative flutter waves in leads II, III, and aVF and predominantly positive flutter waves in lead V$_1$ (Fig. 11-1). When the flutter waves are recorded during sufficient atrioventricular block such that they are not distorted by the QRS or T waves, there is often a positive

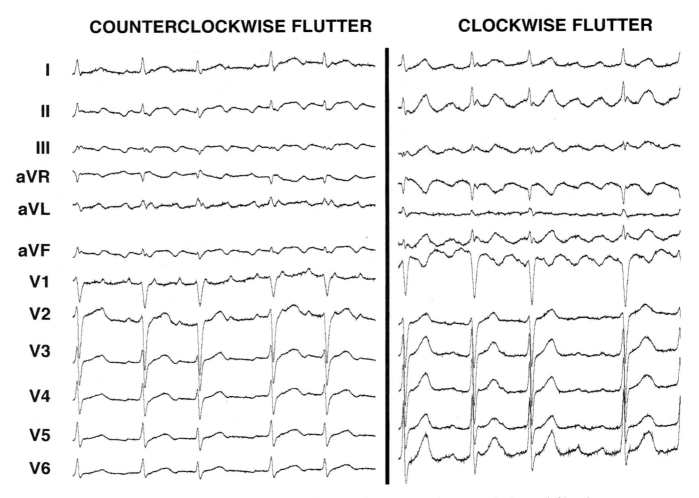

FIGURE 11-1. The 12-lead electrocardiogram of a patient with counterclockwise (left) and clockwise (right) atrial flutter. Counterclockwise flutter has the characteristic negative flutter waves in leads II, III, aVF, and V_1. Clockwise flutter produces the upright and notched flutter waves in leads II, III, and aVF along with the positive flutter wave in V_6.

portion (probably resulting from craniocaudal activation on the right atrial free wall and left atrium) after the predominant negative component that results from caudocranial activation up the septum and posterior atrial wall. Clockwise atrial flutter also produces characteristic flutter waves that are positive in leads II, III, and aVF; usually notched; and predominantly negative in lead V_1 (23,25) (Fig. 11-1). Because the circuit is identical, atrial rates for clockwise and counterclockwise flutter are nearly the same in a given patient (22,23).

Atypical flutter has variable characteristics on 12-lead ECG, and the flutter morphology may mimic that of typical flutter (23,26). By careful use of activation and entrainment mapping, it is possible to differentiate these arrhythmias from typical atrial flutter (23). The rates of atypical flutters are often faster than those of typical flutter, although there is a large overlap, and rate alone cannot be used as a distinguishing feature (23). Correctly identifying the type of atrial flutter is essential because ablation in the subeustachian isthmus has no effect on atypical flutter.

Activation Mapping

Multipolar mapping catheters such as a 20-pole halo catheter (Cordis-Webster, Miami, Fla.) are useful for

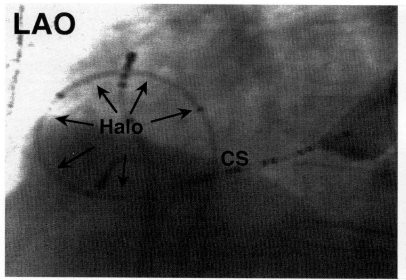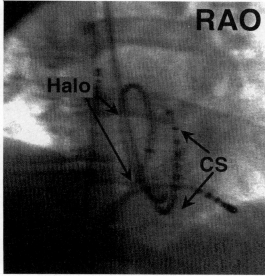

FIGURE 11-2. Fluoroscopic images of a halo catheter (Halo) positioned along the tricuspid annulus. Catheters are shown in the left anterior oblique (LAO) view and right anterior oblique (RAO) view. CS, coronary sinus. (Adapted from Olgin J, Kalman J, Saxon L, et al. Induction of atrial flutter in man: site dependence and site of unidirectional block. *J Am Coll Cardiol* 1997; 29:376–384, with permission.)

identifying the type of atrial flutter and for evaluating the ablation. The halo catheter is placed around the tricuspid annulus such that the distal pole is located near the coronary sinus os; the activation sequence around most of the tricuspid annulus can thus be recorded (Fig. 11-2). Care should be taken that the catheter is positioned along the tricuspid annulus anterior to the crista terminalis, because the atrium posterior to this structure is not part of the reentrant circuit in typical atrial flutter (17). Using these catheters, typical atrial flutter is identified by its counterclockwise or clockwise sequence (Fig. 11-3). Atypical flutter and incisional reentry are often inconsistent with either of these sequences.

A multipolar catheter placed in the coronary sinus such that the proximal pole is at the os is useful in mapping atrial flutter and in evaluating the success of ablation. In counterclockwise, typical flutter, this site is near the exit from the isthmus and usually corresponds to the onset of the flutter wave (17,19–21). Atrial activation recorded from the coronary sinus during typical atrial flutter travels from the os toward the distal pole near the lateral left atrium. Many atypical atrial flutters do not exhibit this sequence; a left-sided electrode is activated before the coronary sinus os. In this way, a coronary sinus catheter can be used to distinguish typical from atypical flutter.

Although halo catheters are used at many institutions for most patients with atrial flutter because they are relatively easy to place, any multipolar catheter or series of catheters placed within the typical atrial flutter circuit to map as much of the complete circuit as possible can be used.

Split Potentials

During activation mapping of atrial flutter, split potentials, defined as discrete electrograms separated by an isoelectric phase, frequently have been recorded during atrial flutter (3,17,19,27–29). Although controversy exists about whether isolated split potentials may indicate disparate endocardial and epicardial activation or merely slowed conduction, in many cases, they undoubtedly indicate activation on either side of a line of block (11,17,19,28,29). The finding of split potentials therefore may be a useful adjunct in defining boundaries of the reentrant circuit.

These split potentials have been recorded over the length of the crista terminalis and eustachian ridge

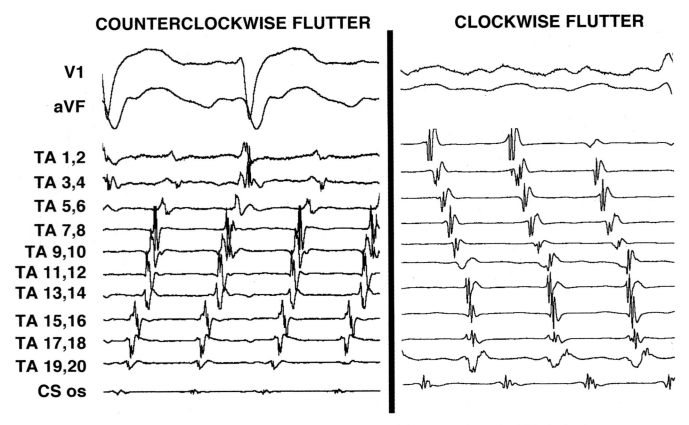

FIGURE 11-3. Endocardial activation sequence around the tricuspid annulus (TA) obtained from a halo catheter in a patient with counterclockwise and clockwise atrial flutter. Halo distal poles tricuspid annulus 1 and 2 (TA 1,2) are positioned in the low lateral right atrium, and the proximal poles (TA 19,20) are positioned on the septum near the His position. In counterclockwise flutter, the activation proceeds from the coronary sinus (CS) os up the septum to TA 19,20 in a counterclockwise fashion to TA 1,2. For clockwise flutter, the activation sequence is the opposite, with activation from the coronary sinus os proceeding first to TA 1,2 on the low lateral right atrium and then in a clockwise fashion toward TA 19,20. In both cases, the tricuspid annulus is activated in a sequential manner.

during typical flutter—the known barriers in typical flutter (16,17,19,23) (Fig. 11-4). Because the circuit for typical flutter is constant and well defined, a lengthy search for these barriers is unnecessary in each case. However, in incisional reentry or atypical flutter, in which the circuit is variable, identification of split potentials helps to define the barriers of the reentrant circuit and to guide the ablation (30).

Entrainment Mapping

Transient entrainment was first described in 1977 to demonstrate that atrial flutter was a reentrant arrhythmia (31). Subsequently, concealed entrainment was described, demonstrating the importance of the pacing site on the characteristics of entrainment (32). Multielectrode endocardial recordings of entrainment from the subeustachian isthmus during atrial flutter demonstrated that endocardial fusion is not present on the surface ECG because it occurs in a protected isthmus. The work by Stevenson and coworkers in ventricular tachycardia further contributed to our understanding of entrainment and provided techniques for mapping atrial reentrant circuits to identify critical components suitable for ablation (17,18,30,33,34).

A detailed discussion of entrainment is beyond the scope of this chapter, but several reviews on this topic

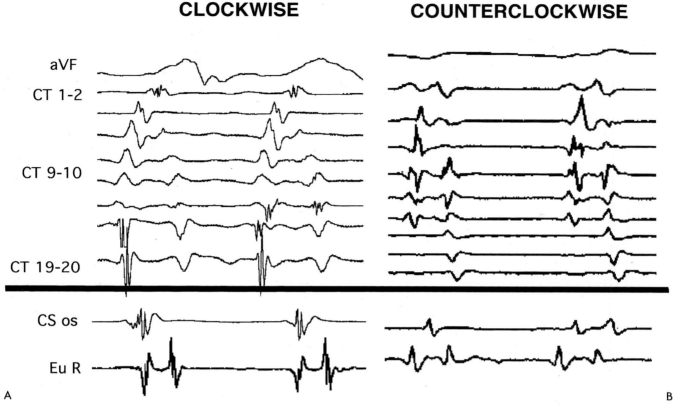

FIGURE 11-4. Split potentials recorded along the crista terminalis (**A**) and eustachian ridge (**B**) in counterclockwise and clockwise (typical) flutter. These structures were mapped with intracardiac echocardiography guidance to ensure catheter location. Each component of the split potentials along the crista is activated in opposite sequence. (Adapted from Olgin J, Kalman J, Fitzpatrick A, Lesh M. The role of right atrial endocardial structures as barriers to conduction during human type I atrial flutter: activation and entrainment mapping guided by intracardiac echocardiography. *Circulation* 1995;92:1893–1848, with permission.)

have been published (16,17,33). *Entrainment* is the acceleration of a reentrant tachycardia by pacing into the circuit. Entrainment does not affect the reentrant circuit, and when pacing ceases, the tachycardia continues unchanged. This allows identification of critical components of the reentrant circuit. Entrainment is accomplished by pacing slightly faster (10 to 30 msec) than the tachycardia cycle length to minimize possible decrement within the circuit (35). Comparing the *postpacing interval* (i.e., interval from the last entrained beat to the first spontaneous beat measured at the pacing site) with the spontaneous tachycardia cycle length indicates whether a site is inside or outside the reentrant circuit (17,30,33,34) (Fig. 11-5). Sites within the reentrant circuit have postpacing intervals equal to the tachycardia cycle length, whereas those outside the circuit have postpacing intervals longer than the tachycardia cycle length. *Concealed fusion* (i.e., entrainment without fusion on the surface ECG) indicates that the pacing site is within a protected isthmus (16,17,33,34). With atrial flutter, P-wave fusion on the surface ECG can often be difficult to determine, especially if atrioventricular conduction is good. The use of multielectrode catheters such as a halo catheter can be useful to identify parts of the circuit that are antidromically and orthodromically captured. Entrainment mapping can also be useful to identify the extent of a protected isthmus by examin-

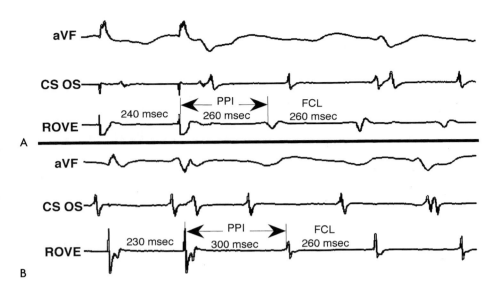

FIGURE 11-5. Entrainment of atrial flutter from two different sites. **A:** Pacing is accomplished from a site on the inferior aspect of the tricuspid annulus in the subeustachian isthmus. The postpacing interval (PPI) is equal to the flutter cycle length (FCL). This site is within the reentrant circuit. **B:** Pacing is performed from the right atrial appendage. The PPI is longer than the FCL. This site is not within the reentrant circuit. (Adapted from Olgin J, Kalman J, Fitzpatrick A, Lesh M. The role of right atrial endocardial structures as barriers to conduction during human type I atrial flutter: activation and entrainment mapping guided by intracardiac echocardiography. *Circulation* 1995;92:1848–1893, with permission.)

ing the activation time from pacing stimulus to the flutter wave on the last entrained beat (17,20,30,33). Entrainment from the entrance produces a long stimulus to flutter wave interval, whereas entrainment from the exit produces a short interval.

In a patient with atrial flutter, entrainment mapping is useful to confirm that the flutter is typical (i.e., involves the subeustachian isthmus) and to define the extent of the isthmus (17). Limited and targeted entrainment mapping is usually sufficient in typical flutter. For other macro-reentrant arrhythmias, in which the location of a critical isthmus is more variable, entrainment techniques are invaluable in targeting sites for ablation (30,33,34).

Induction of Flutter

Patients who are referred for atrial flutter often present to the laboratory in sinus rhythm. Although ablation can be performed during sinus rhythm, it is useful to confirm the diagnosis of typical atrial flutter and perform limited endocardial mapping to guide ablation. Several studies have shown that the induction of atrial flutter with programmed stimulation is highly specific (36,37). In large groups of patients undergoing programmed stimulation, only in those with a clinical history of or risk factors for flutter could atrial flutter be induced (36,37). However, in a given patient, atrial flutter is difficult to induce, with only 6.2% of 838 induction attempts in 10 patients with clinical atrial flutter producing atrial flutter (22).

Because the circuits for counterclockwise and clockwise flutter are the same, the site from which flutter is induced with programmed stimulation determines which direction the flutter rotates (22). Pacing from the smooth right atrium posterior to the crista terminalis and eustachian ridge induces counterclockwise flutter, whereas pacing from the trabeculated right atrium anterior to these structures produces clockwise flutter (22). This site dependence exists because the initiating unidirectional block occurs in the subeustachian isthmus (22).

In the laboratory, flutter is induced before attempted ablation to confirm the presence of typical flutter and electrophysiologically guide the ablation by confirming which sites lie within the critical isthmus. However, after this is done, the ablation and confirmation of success can be performed in sinus rhythm as detailed later.

Ablation

In the laboratory, limited electrophysiologic mapping is performed to confirm that typical flutter is present (i.e., the subeustachian isthmus is critical to the reentrant circuit and roughly determines the extent of the isthmus), and then an anatomic approach is employed.

The ablation line can be drawn anywhere in the

isthmus from the lateral border of the inferior vena cava and tricuspid annulus to the septal border between tricuspid annulus and coronary sinus os. In some instances, the eustachian ridge does not form a complete line of block from the inferior vena cava to the coronary sinus os, as shown electrophysiologically and with pathologic examination of human hearts (17,38). Olgin and associates, using intracardiac echocardiography to identify the eustachian ridge, demonstrated that the exit to the isthmus is posterior to the coronary sinus os in some patients (17). Adachi and colleagues performed autopsy examinations of the flutter isthmus and found that the eustachian ridge was "incomplete" in some individuals (38). Nakagawa and coworkers demonstrated that an ablation lesion from the tricuspid annulus to the coronary sinus os was insufficient to eliminate typical flutter in 13 of 27 patients (19). An additional line of ablation from the coronary sinus os to the eustachian ridge was successful in 12 of the patients (19). Several other factors are important in determining where in the isthmus (e.g., lateral, middle, medial) to create the ablation line in typical flutter. The subeustachian isthmus can be very wide, particularly in patients with dilated atria, and is usually narrowest at the septal aspect. The subeustachian isthmus is not a smooth endocardial surface but has many peaks and valleys, making creation of long ablation lines difficult. Most importantly, the line must be complete from the tricuspid annulus to the inferior vena cava or eustachian ridge. The ablation lesion should be made wherever in the isthmus optimal catheter tissue contact is best over the entire distance from tricuspid annulus to inferior vena cava.

End Point testing

Although high immediate success rates for terminating typical atrial flutter with ablation can be achieved, the recurrence rate for flutter was high (up to 25%) in earlier studies (39–43). In these studies, immediate success was defined as the termination of flutter with the ablation and the inability to reinduce the flutter after ablation. However, atrial flutter is not easily or repeatedly inducible in a given patient, even before ablation (22). Repeat inducibility is therefore an inadequate end point for ablation and may explain the high recurrence rate in these early studies.

Demonstration of whether the ablation lesion has electrically severed the subeustachian isthmus with pacing techniques is the accepted end point for flutter ablation. Several studies have confirmed that the demonstration of complete, bidirectional block in the subeustachian isthmus is a more reliable indicator of long-term success, with recurrence rates near 0% (19, 24,44–46). This assessment is accomplished by initiating pacing during sinus rhythm on one side of the ablation lesion and demonstrating that activation does not proceed across the isthmus lesion (Figs. 11-6 and 11-7). For example, during pacing from the coronary sinus os before ablation, activation proceeds through the subeustachian isthmus to activate the low lateral right atrium (Fig. 11-6). After successful ablation, activation cannot proceed through the isthmus, and the low lateral right atrium is activated late, after the high lateral right atrium. A halo catheter can demonstrate this change in activation after successful ablation. Because patients in whom only unidirectional or rate-dependent block was achieved have a significantly higher recurrence rate, it is important to pace at slower rates and on both sides (i.e., low lateral right atrium and coronary sinus os) of the lesion to establish the presence of bidirectional, rate-independent conduction block (44,45).

This technique of confirming conduction block provides a better end point for ablation and allows ablation of the flutter in sinus rhythm (44). In our laboratory, this is preferred because the development of conduction block can more readily be identified.

Atypical Atrial Flutters

Atypical atrial flutters do not use the same circuit as typical atrial flutter. The rates and endocardial activation are inconsistent with clockwise or counterclockwise flutter and can be varied. The rate of these tachycardias can be very fast (180 to 220 msec), and entrainment may be difficult because pacing may accelerate or change the activation sequence. My colleagues and I have observed several reentrant circuits responsible for these tachycardias, including reentry around a portion of the crista terminalis (23), reentry

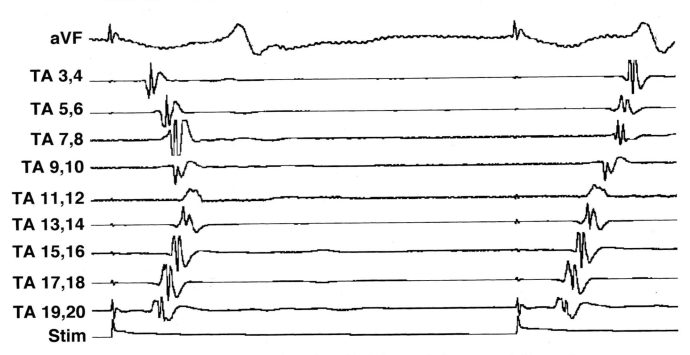

FIGURE 11-6. Demonstration of an isthmus block during radiofrequency (RF) ablation of a patient with atrial flutter. After the flutter was terminated, pacing from the coronary sinus (CS) os was performed during RF ablation. Two paced beats are shown during RF energy application. On the left, activation of the halo catheter proceeds in the clockwise and counter-clockwise directions, with fusion of the wavefronts near tricuspid annulus (TA) poles 11 and 12 (TA 1,2). On the next beat, a conduction block in the isthmus was completed as evidenced by activation of the halo catheter in a counterclockwise direction only.

involving the myocardium of the coronary sinus (47), and reentry around idiopathic scarring in the posterior right atrium. In patients with reentry around the crista terminalis, the area of slow conduction appears to be functional, and ablation of the this area results in a change in the tachycardia cycle length and point of breakthrough across the crista. Ablation over a segment of the crista is required as the "functional gap" is chased. We have described one form of atypical flutter that involves reentry in the myocardium of the coronary sinus, separated from the myocardium of the left atrium (47). Figure 11-8 shows the circuit mapped by activation and entrainment mapping. During this tachycardia, split potentials can be recorded in the coronary sinus (Fig. 11-9), and ablation within the coronary sinus terminates the tachycardia (47).

Other forms of atypical flutter may be caused by macro-reentry in the left atrium, in which the role of anatomic barriers such as the pulmonary veins or mitral annulus still must be explored. Because the circuits for these flutters are unknown, there is no specific ablation for atypical flutter. Mapping with activation and entrainment mapping and identification of split potentials are often required. With three-dimensional (3-D) mapping technology, the entire circuit of some of these tachycardias can be more readily mapped.

Incisional Reentry

Animal Models and Substrate

Canine models of incisional reentry have been developed, simulating the Mustard and the Fontan proce-

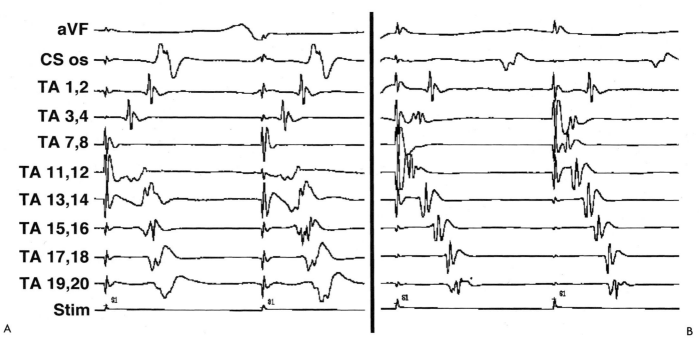

FIGURE 11-7. Demonstration of a bidirectional block in the patient shown in Figure 11-5. **A:** Pacing from the low lateral right atrium in the region of tricuspid annulus (TA) poles 5 and 6 (TA 5,6) before ablation demonstrates activation of the coronary sinus (CS) os through the flutter isthmus; TA 3,4 is activated before TA 1,2, which is activated before the coronary sinus os. **B:** After ablation, pacing from the low lateral right atrium demonstrates that the coronary sinus os is activated after TA 19,20, confirming the block in the flutter isthmus.

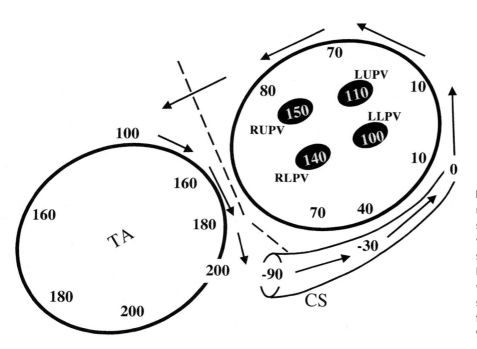

FIGURE 11-8. Activation times in the right atrium, left atrium, and coronary sinus during an atypical atrial flutter involving the myocardium of the coronary sinus. (From Olgin JE, Jayachandran JV, Engelstein E, et al. Atrial macroreentry involving the myocardium of the coronary sinus—a unique mechanism for atypical flutter. *J Cardiovasc Electrophysiol* 1998; 9:1094–1099, with permission.)

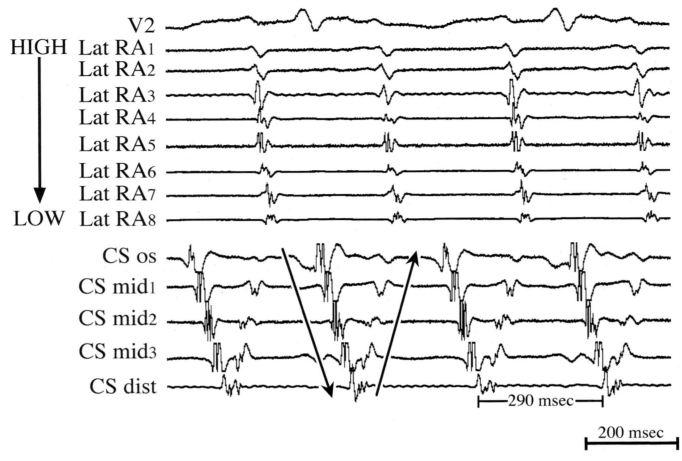

FIGURE 11-9. Electrograms from a coronary sinus catheter during the atypical flutter shown in Figure 11-8. Split potentials can be observed over the length of the coronary sinus. (From Olgin JE, Jayachandran JV, Engelstein E, et al. Atrial macroreentry involving the myocardium of the coronary sinus—a unique mechanism for atypical flutter. *J Cardiovasc Electrophysiol* 1998;9:1094–1099, with permission.)

dures (48,49). In the canine model of the Mustard procedure, suture lines were placed, mimicking those positioned during placement of the baffle, including an atriotomy, a septectomy, and the usual baffle location (48). Most of the tachycardias revolved around the tricuspid annulus or around the atriotomy incision (48). Rarely, the tachycardias involved both atria or revolved around the mitral annulus (48). In the canine model of the Fontan operation, a suture line simulating a cavopulmonary connection suture line is placed through an atriotomy (49). In this model, all induced atrial tachycardias involved an isthmus created by the lateral margin of the cavopulmonary suture line (49).

These arrhythmias can occur in any patient who has undergone an atriotomy, usually as part of a surgical repair of congenital heart disease. The atriotomy scar and any other suture lines may be a potential substrate for macro-reentry. Reentrant arrhythmias have been reported in patients after atrial septal defect repair, Mustard procedure, Fontan repair, Senning procedure, and Rastelli procedure (30,50). The substrate for this group of arrhythmias is variable and is determined by the surgical scars as well as artificial and natural obstacles in the atrium. The reentrant circuit can involve one or more of these artificial obstacles and anatomic obstacles such as those involved in typical flutter (e.g., crista terminalis, subeustachian isthmus); in these patients reentrant arrhythmias involving the typical flutter isthmus may have different activation sequences and surface P waves because of the distorted atrial anatomy. Because the substrate for reentry is so variable and isthmuses can be wide at points, extensive mapping is necessary in each case to identify appropriate ablation targets. A given patient may have several different circuits. The principles of mapping atrial flutter (i.e., split potentials and entrainment mapping) are applicable to this patient population. Mapping and ablation are further complicated by the potential for multiple tachycardias in a patient.

Mapping and Ablation

Several series have demonstrated the effectiveness of ablation of reentrant atrial tachycardias after repair of congenital heart disease (30,50–52). Mapping techniques are similar to those described for atrial flutter. Because the barriers are variable among patients and isthmuses can be wide, entrainment mapping and recording of split potentials are particularly useful for defining barriers in patients (30,50–52). Ablation is targeted to isthmuses that are demonstrated to be critical to the reentrant circuit using entrainment techniques (30,50,52). Patients may have multiple atrial reentrant circuits (53), and in general, studies have involved ablation of "clinical" arrhythmias only (30, 50–52). Using this approach, radiofrequency ablation has an 80% to 93% immediate success rate. However, the long-term success rate appears to be less, with a recurrence rate of about 40% (30,50–52). Because these patients may have multiple circuits for atrial reentry, it is unclear whether these recurrences are new tachycardias or true recurrences (53). Many patients who have ablation of incisional reentry involving an atriotomy return with atrial flutter using the subeustachian isthmus.

Unlike atrial flutter, the end point for ablation of these tachycardias may be inadequate, because it is difficult to confirm conduction block produced by the ablation lesion. *Successful ablation* is defined as termination of the tachycardia and inability to reinduce the same tachycardia. Other tachycardias, however, may remain inducible. Newer technologies that provide 3-D or higher-resolution mapping will likely improve the techniques for mapping, ablation, and end point testing in this population.

⦿ FOCAL ATRIAL TACHYCARDIAS

Substrate

The mechanism of "ectopic" or focal atrial tachycardia is heterogeneous and may include enhanced automaticity, triggered activity, or micro-reentry (54–56). However, these arrhythmias, including atrial tachycardias and sinus node reentry, originate from a single discrete focus. It is this focal nature (rather than the electrophysiologic mechanism) that directs the mapping and ablation technique.

Several studies have shown that focal atrial tachycardias have a highly characteristic anatomic distribution (57–60). In the left atrium, common sites include the ostia of the pulmonary veins and the left atrial appendage. For right atrial tachycardias, the atrial tachycardia foci cluster along the crista terminalis, within the right atrial appendage, and near the region of the coronary sinus ostium (51,57–60). This distribution in the right atrium has been confirmed with electrophysiologic-anatomic mapping using intracardiac echocardiography (61). Mallavarapu and associates reported left atrial tachycardias arising from near the mitral annulus (62). In rare instances, atrial tachycardias may arise from abnormal atrial structures such as tumors or abnormal trabeculations (63).

Mapping and Ablation

The 12-lead ECG often provides information about the anatomic location of the atrial tachycardia focus (64). The P-wave vector in leads aVL and V_1 is useful in differentiating right from left atrial foci, and leads II, III, and aVF are useful in differentiating superior from inferior foci (64). There are, however, some problems with and exceptions to this approach. In many focal atrial tachycardias, atrioventricular conduction is usually 1 : 1, and identification of a "pure" P wave isolated from the T wave is usually difficult. The use of adenosine is useful for differentiating atrial tachycardias from atrioventricular reentrant tachycardias and often useful for identifying pure P waves. Left atrial tachycardias arising from the right pulmonary veins often have P-wave vectors suggestive of right atrial foci or are ambiguous. This occurs because the right pulmonary veins lie directly behind the right atrium and are anatomically rightward structures (63).

Several methods for mapping atrial tachycardias have been reported (51,57,58,65,66). Activation mapping is the most useful means of mapping atrial tachycardias. Sites with local activation before the onset of the surface P wave (15 to 60 msec) have been demonstrated to be good targets for ablation (51,57, 58). Fragmented electrograms have been recorded from areas near successful ablation sites in some patients (51). Because atrial tachycardias may not be sustained during the electrophysiology study, mapping of monomorphic premature atrial contractions (PACs) or nonsustained atrial tachycardia is occasionally necessary. When high-degree atrioventricular block is not present and the P-wave morphology and onset not apparent, the use of intracardiac surrogate markers for P-wave onset is often useful.

Unlike mapping of accessory pathways, where mapping is limited to the two-dimensional structure of the atrioventricular valves, mapping of focal atrial tachycardias involves mapping in the complex 3-D structure of the atria. Mapping techniques for atrial tachycardias have included leapfrogging two mapping catheters in an attempt to localize the sites of earliest activation (51,57). Other investigators have proposed using pace mapping to match the P-wave morphology or endocardial activation sequence (65). Pace mapping using P-wave morphology is frequently difficult in the absence of a high-degree atrioventricular block. Pace mapping using an endocardial activation sequence is limited by the number of intracardiac recording sites.

Knowledge of the characteristic distribution (along the crista terminalis and pulmonary veins) of atrial tachycardias can expedite mapping. Kalman and colleagues have described a mapping technique whereby a multipolar catheter is placed along the crista terminalis under intracardiac echocardiography to guide initial mapping (61). Intracardiac echocardiography is used to identify the crista terminalis and guide place-

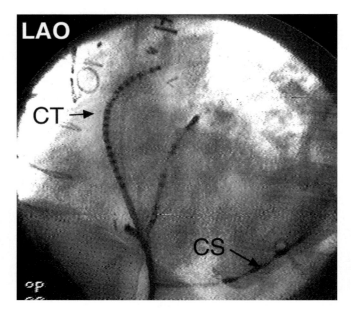 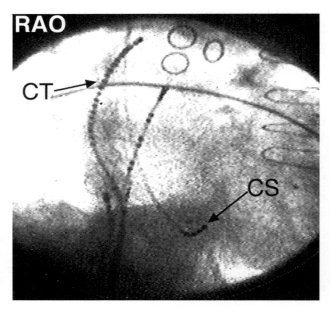

FIGURE 11-10. Fluoroscopy of a 20-pole catheter positioned along the crista terminalis using intracardiac echocardiography. Catheters are shown in the left anterior oblique (LAO) and right anterior oblique (RAO) views. CS, coronary sinus. (Adapted from Olgin J, Kalman J, Fitzpatrick A, Lesh M. The role of right atrial endocardial structures as barriers to conduction during human type I atrial flutter: activation and entrainment mapping guided by intracardiac echocardiography. *Circulation* 1995;92:1848–1893, with permission.)

ment of this 20-pole catheter along its entire extent (Fig. 11-10). Intracardiac echocardiography is necessary because the course of the crista terminalis can be quite variable (67). This provides an initial "road map" for guiding the mapping (61). For tachycardias arising from the crista terminalis, the earliest site of activation along the multipolar crista terminalis catheter facilitates mapping with the ablation catheter (Fig. 11-11). For tachycardias arising away from the crista terminalis, activation of this multipolar crista terminalis catheter lacks dispersion of activation times and is relatively late in relation to the surface P wave. This technique is useful for mapping sustained tachycardias and a single PAC.

The use of intracardiac echocardiography is useful in demonstrating the complex anatomy of the atria and is especially helpful in guiding mapping to distinguish right pulmonary vein tachycardias from right

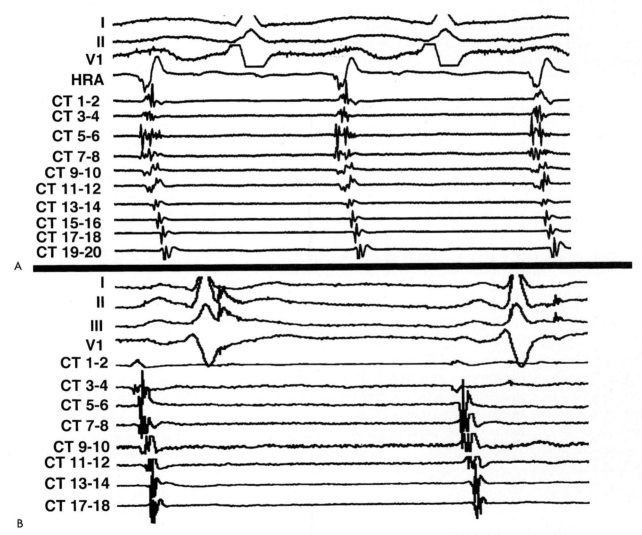

FIGURE 11-11. Intracardiac recordings from a 20-pole catheter placed along the crista terminalis (CT) during atrial tachycardia **(A)** and during sinus rhythm **(B)**. During atrial tachycardia, the earliest activation is in the middle crista terminalis, near poles 7 and 8. This information guides initial mapping in the region of these bipoles along the crista. HRA, high right atrium; CT 1,2, distal poles positioned superiorly on the crista terminalis; CT 19,20, proximal poles positioned inferiorly on the crista terminalis.

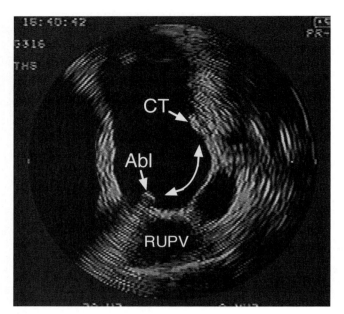

FIGURE 11-12. Intracardiac echocardiography demonstrating fine mapping between the crista terminalis (CT) and the right atrial wall opposite the right upper pulmonary vein (PUPV). This technique is useful in differentiating tachycardias arising near the CT from those arising from the right pulmonary vein. Abl, ablation catheter.

atrial tachycardias arising from the high crista terminalis (61). The right upper pulmonary vein lies directly posterior to the crista terminalis and is a rightward structure. Using intracardiac echocardiography to guide fine mapping between the crista terminalis and the posterior right atrium opposite the pulmonary vein, one can distinguish between tachycardias originating from these sites (61) (Fig. 11-12). This region is often small and requires mapping in relation to anatomy of 1 cm or less. Intracardiac echocardiography is useful for anatomically based electrophysiologic mapping of focal atrial tachycardias. Mapping with technology that provides detailed 3-D maps can also facilitate ablation of these tachycardias.

● INAPPROPRIATE SINUS TACHYCARDIA

The syndrome of inappropriate sinus tachycardia is characterized by an increased resting sinus rate and exaggerated increase in sinus rate with minor exertion (68–70). The precise mechanism is not well understood, but this syndrome is distinct from focal atrial tachycardias originating from the crista terminalis, such as sinus node reentry (68,69,71). The anatomic substrate for this tachycardia appears to be based on the electrophysiology of the sinus mechanism, which lies within the crista terminalis. Several studies have demonstrated that the entire crista terminalis is responsible for the sinus mechanism, with faster rates arising from the superior portion and slower rates arising from the lower portions (70,72–75). The relationship between heart rate and the site of impulse origin within the crista terminalis in response to autonomic inputs has been well documented (72,73,75, 76). Vagal stimulation produces sinus slowing associated with an inferior shift in the dominant pacemaker (Fig. 11-13). Sympathetic activation produces a faster sinus rate associated with a cranial and anterior shift in the dominant pacemaker (72–76) (Fig. 11-13).

For patients who are symptomatic and unresponsive to medical therapy, radiofrequency modification of the sinus pacemaker can be performed. The feasibility of modifying the rapid sinus rates arising from the superior portions of the crista terminalis has been described for animals and humans (70,74). A combined anatomic and electrophysiologic approach was used. Mapping is performed much as described for focal atrial tachycardias, with a multipolar catheter placed along the crista terminalis under intracardiac echocardiography guidance. Ablation is targeted at the superior sites along the crista terminalis under maximal autonomic stimulation (i.e., isoproterenol and atropine), with ablation gradually progressing inferiorly until a 25% to 30% reduction in rate is achieved (70,74). Care must be taken not to damage the right phrenic nerve; ablation pulses should not be delivered if pacing from the ablation catheter stimulates the diaphragm.

Although this approach has had good immediate results, with few permanent pacemakers required, the long-term results appear to be poor, with a 68% recurrence rate of symptoms (77). It is unclear whether sinus tachycardia exists in all patients with symptomatic recurrences. In some patients, a more extensive sinus node ablation may be needed.

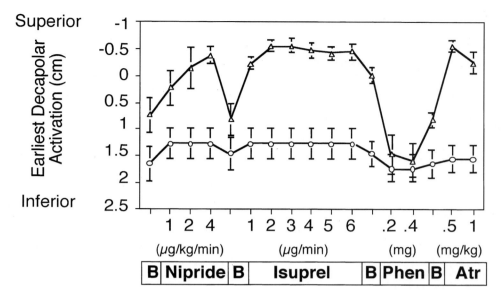

FIGURE 11-13. A shift in the sinus focus along the crista terminalis with autonomic manipulation is demonstrated with a 20-pole catheter placed along the crista terminalis with intracardiac echocardiography guidance. Earliest activation at the second bipole was taken as the 0-cm reference point, and distances from this location were calculated according to the bipole distance along the catheter. Before sinus node modification *(triangles)*, the sinus focus shifted over a distance of up to 2 cm, moving superiorly with sympathetic stimulation (i.e., Nipride and isoproterenol) and inferiorly with parasympathetic stimulation (i.e., atropine). After sinus node modification *(circles)*, the earliest activation site was shifted inferiorly, and no significant movement occurred in response to sympathetic stimulation. At, atropine; B, baseline; Phen, phenylephrine. (Adapted from Kalman JM, Lee RJ, Fisher WG, et al. Radiofrequency catheter modification of sinus pacemaker function guided by intracardiac echocardiography. *Circulation* 1995;92:3070–3081, with permission.)

● ATRIAL FIBRILLATION

There has been an intensive research effort to develop a catheter-based procedure to cure atrial fibrillation. The principles of catheter ablation to cure atrial fibrillation have been demonstrated in the surgical maze procedure (78)—the creation of lines of conduction block in the atria to prevent atrial fibrillation. Two reports suggest that this is feasible in humans (79,80). In these studies, standard ablation catheters were used to create linear ablation lesions by dragging the catheter over the endocardial surface during radiofrequency energy application (79,80). These procedures were moderately effective (60% to 80%) at reducing symptomatic atrial fibrillation but were complicated by macro-reentrant atrial tachycardias and required very long procedures (79,80). Technology must evolve to enable the ablationist to create continuous linear lesions more effectively and efficiently. Newer catheters with multiple ablation coils have been developed that enable creation of linear, transmural linear lesions that produce conduction block (81,82). Specially designed long vascular sheaths have been developed to improve catheter stability during drag lesions (79). Because the linear lesions may be in part anatomically determined, intracardiac echocardiography, electrospatial mapping, or both may be useful to guide lesion placement and confirm lesion contiguity (81,82).

Some patients with paroxysmal atrial fibrillation have focal mechanisms for their atrial fibrillation. These focal mechanisms include focal initiators (i.e., PACs) or rapid, irregular atrial tachycardias that are required for the maintenance of the atrial fibrillation.

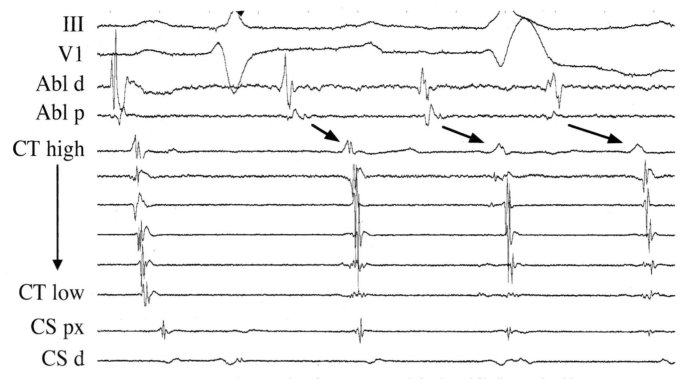

FIGURE 11-14. Intracardiac recordings from a patient with focal atrial fibrillation. The ablation catheter (Abl) is at the focus in the left upper pulmonary vein. A Wenckebach pattern of conduction is out of the focus compared with the rest of the atrium, as demonstrated by the prolonged conduction time from the ablation catheter to the rest of the atrial signals.

Several reports of ablation of these foci in patients with atrial fibrillation have demonstrated an impressive cure rate (83–85). It appears that these foci are anatomically distributed in the pulmonary veins and along the crista terminalis in the right atrium, similar to those of atrial tachycardias. My colleagues and I have found similar patients at our institution. Mapping of these foci can be complicated by several factors:

1. The events that are mapped (often PACs) can be difficult to initiate and are often transient.
2. Conduction properties around the foci can be complex, occasionally producing Wenckebach-like conduction (Fig. 11-14) or exit block from the focus to the atrium (Fig. 11-15).
3. The regular rhythm or PAC can frequently degenerate (Fig. 11-16) or initiate atrial fibrillation.
4. End point testing after ablation can be difficult to determine, and a clinical end point often is required.

Three-dimensional (3-D) systems mapping can be useful in mapping these foci. Technology is being developed to take a more anatomic approach of encircling the pulmonary vein orifices. Currently, there are no clinical data on this approach.

THREE-DIMENSIONAL MAPPING

Given the complexity of mapping of focal atrial tachycardias, atypical flutter, incisional reentry, and focal atrial fibrillation, systems that provide more detailed activation mapping and electrospatial maps are desirable. Multipolar basket catheters have been used for mapping atrial tachycardias (53). These multipolar catheters (64 poles) can provide an activation se-

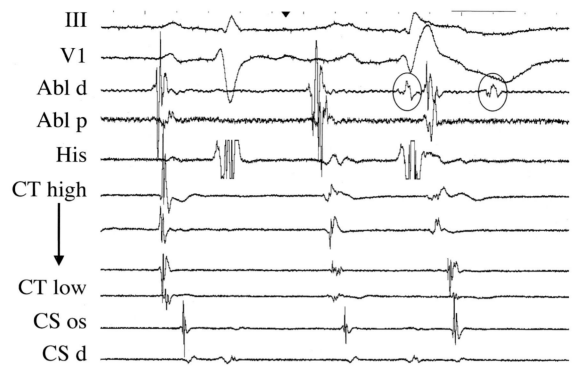

FIGURE 11-15. Intracardiac recordings from a patient with focal atrial fibrillation. The focus exhibits exit block, with the first premature atrial contraction (PAC) *(circled)* conducting to the rest of the atrium and the second PAC (from the same focus in the right upper pulmonary vein) demonstrating exit block. Notice the two components of the local electrogram during the PACs, which are fused during sinus rhythm.

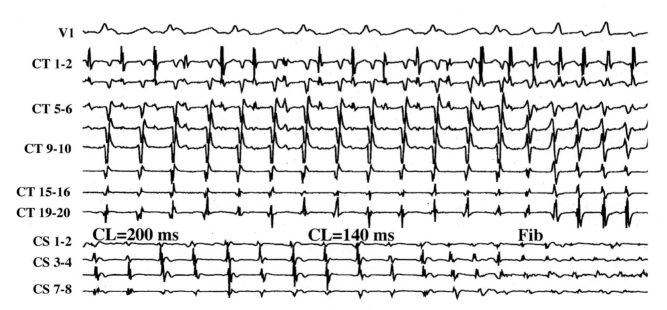

FIGURE 11-16. Intracardiac recordings from a patient with focal atrial fibrillation. On the left part of the tracing, a regular, rapid atrial tachycardia has a cycle length of 200 msec. It was a stable rhythm for 20 minutes before this tracing. The tachycardia suddenly speeds to a cycle length of 140 msec and then results in atrial fibrillation.

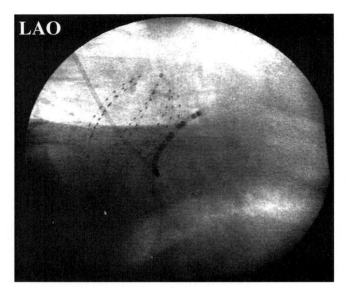

FIGURE 11-17. Right anterior oblique view of a 64-pole basket catheter (EP Technologies, San Jose, Calif.) deployed in the right atrium for mapping of a right atrial tachycardia. The other catheter is in the coronary sinus.

quence in a chamber with a higher degree of resolution than standard mapping catheters (Fig. 11-17). However, the electrogram quality can be poor in many electrodes because the baskets do not easily conform to the complex shape of the atrium and localization of individual electrodes can be challenging. Moreover, resolution of 64 electrodes is insufficient for most difficult atrial tachycardias and focal atrial fibrillation.

Another technique uses electrospatial mapping with a computer based system to localize a mapping catheter in 3-D space (CARTO) (85) (Fig. 11-18). The system involves a special mapping and ablation catheter capable of registering location, and tachycardias are sequentially mapped. Facilitation of ablation of typical flutter, other macro-reentrant atrial tachycardias, and focal atrial tachycardias and creation of linear atrial lesions using this system have been described (87–90). This technique is limited to mapping regular, sustained tachycardias and can only be used with special catheters. However, in addition to creat-

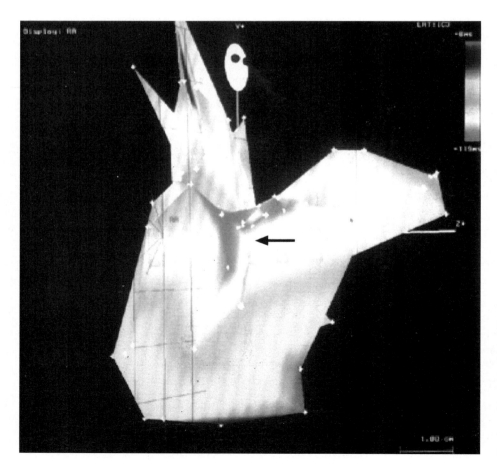

FIGURE 11-18. Three-dimensional activation map (displayed in gray scale) of a patient with a focal right atrial tachycardia created by the CARTO system (Biosense, Johnson & Johnson, Diamond Bar, Calif.). The earliest activation is located on the crista terminalis *(arrow),* and activation emanates from there.

ing activation maps, the system can create voltage maps, which can identify scarred areas. Another system (LocaLisa) uses a similar approach; however, instead of magnetic fields to localize the catheter, it uses radiofrequency energy (91). This system can use any catheter and can localize many catheters at once. However, so far there is only a limited experience with LocaLisa system.

The major limitation to the sequential 3-D mapping systems are that transient tachycardias cannot be efficiently mapped. Another 3-D mapping system uses a noncontact balloon catheter (Fig. 11-19) to determine calculated endocardial virtual electrograms (92,93). This system has the advantage of collecting 3,000 points simultaneously and providing a detailed activation map on a beat-by-beat basis. This system enables rapid mapping of transient tachycardias or isolated PACs (Fig. 11-20). The system also provides electrospatial information, using technology similar to that of LocaLisa, and it therefore allows location of standard ablation and multipolar catheters. Although this technology appears to be promising, there has been only limited experience with this system.

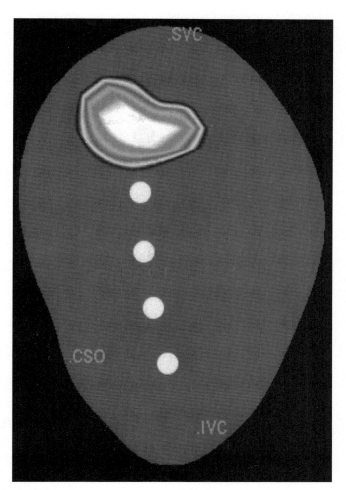

FIGURE 11-20. Three-dimensional activation map (displayed in gray scale) of a right atrial focus in a patient with focal atrial fibrillation obtained with a noncontact balloon catheter (Endocardial Solutions, Inc., St. Paul, Minn.). In this patient, induction of only rare premature atrial contractions (PACs) (same morphology) was possible, which induced atrial fibrillation. This system allowed mapping from 3,000 virtual electrodes of a single PAC, which emanated from the superior portion of the crista terminalis. This area was ablated with a catheter guided by the system.

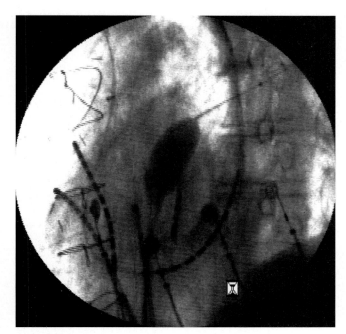

FIGURE 11-19. Left anterior oblique fluoroscopic view of a noncontact balloon mapping catheter (Endocardial Solutions, Inc., St. Paul, Minn.) placed transseptally into the left atrium to map a focal atrial fibrillation. Another ablation catheter is in the left atrium, placed by means of a second transseptal puncture.

Each of these systems has advantages and disadvantages unique to the mapping system. The major disadvantage of each of these systems (albeit to different degrees) is the cost of the system and special catheter requirements. Although many tachycardias can be successfully ablated with standard mapping and ablation techniques (e.g., typical flutter, incessant atrial tachycardias), the advantages of these systems are their ability to map complex reentrant circuits (as in atypical flutter or incisional reentry) or to map very transient events such as atypical flutters, PACs, or focal atrial fibrillation. These systems also may be used for targeting and confirming the creation of linear lesions for the treatment of atrial fibrillation.

REFERENCES

1. Klein G, Guiraudon G, Sharma A, Milstein S. Demonstration of macroreentry and feasibility of operative therapy in the common type of atrial flutter. *Am J Cardiol* 1986;57:587–591.
2. Saoudi N, Atallah G, Kirkorian G, Touboul P. Catheter ablation of the atrial myocardium in human type I atrial flutter. *Circulation* 1990;81:762–771.
3. Cosio FG, Lopez GM, Goicolea A, Arribas F. Electrophysiologic studies in atrial flutter. *Clin Cardiol* 1992;15:667–673.
4. Waldo AL, Wells JL Jr, Plumb VJ, et al. Studies of atrial flutter following open heart surgery. *Annu Rev Med* 1979;30:259–268.
5. Rosenblueth A, Garcia-Ramos J. The influence of artificial obstacles on experimental auricular flutter. *Am Heart J* 1947;33:677–684.
6. Frame L, Page R, Hoffman B. Atrial reentry around an anatomic barrier with a partially refractory excitable gap: a canine model of atrial flutter. *Circ Res* 1986;58:495–511.
7. Frame LH, Page RL, Boyden PA, et al. Circus movement in the canine atrium around the tricuspid ring during experimental atrial flutter and during reentry in vitro. *Circulation* 1987;76:1155–1175.
8. Boineau JP, Schuessler RB, Mooney CR, et al. Natural and evoked atrial flutter due to circus movement in dogs: role of abnormal atrial pathways, slow conduction, nonuniform refractory period distribution and premature beats. *Am J Cardiol* 1980;45:1167–1181.
9. Inoue H, Toda I, Saihara S, Sugimoto T. Further observations on entrainment of atrial flutter in the dog. *Am Heart J* 1989;118:467–474.
10. Yamashita T, Inoue H, Nozaki A, Sugimoto T. Role of anatomic architecture in sustained atrial reentry and double potentials. *Am Heart J* 1992;124:938–946.
11. Feld GK, Shahandeh RF. Mechanism of double potentials recorded during sustained atrial flutter in the canine right atrial crush-injury model. *Circulation* 1992;86:628–641.
12. Feld GK, Shahandeh RF. Activation patterns in experimental canine atrial flutter produced by right atrial crush injury. *J Am Coll Cardiol* 1992;20:441–451.
13. Lewis T. Observations upon flutter and fibrillation as it occurs in patients. *Heart* 1921;8:193.
14. Olshansky B, Wilber DJ, Hariman RJ. Atrial flutter—update on the mechanism and treatment. *Pacing Clin Electrophysiol* 1992;15:2308–2335.
15. Boyden P. Models of atrial reentry. *J Cardiovasc Electrophysiol* 1995;6:313–324.
16. Olgin J, Kalman J, Lesh M. Conduction barriers in atrial flutter—correlation of electrophysiology and anatomy. *J Cardiovasc Electrophysiol* 1996;7:1112–1126.
17. Olgin J, Kalman J, Fitzpatrick A, Lesh M. The role of right atrial endocardial structures as barriers to conduction during human type I atrial flutter: activation and entrainment mapping guided by intracardiac echocardiography. *Circulation* 1995;92:1848–1893.
18. Kalman J, Olgin J, Saxon L, et al. Activation and entrainment mapping defines the tricuspid annulus as the anterior barrier in typical atrial flutter. *Circulation* 1996;94:398–406.
19. Nakagawa H, Lazzara R, Khastgir T, et al. Role of the tricuspid annulus and the eustachian valve/ridge on atrial flutter: relevance to catheter ablation of the septal isthmus and a new technique for rapid identification of ablation success. *Circulation* 1996;94:407–424.
20. Feld GK, Fleck RP, Chen PS, et al. Radiofrequency catheter ablation for the treatment of human type 1 atrial flutter: identification of a critical zone in the reentrant circuit by endocardial mapping techniques. *Circulation* 1992;86:1233–1240.
21. Olshansky B, Okumura K, Hess PG, Waldo AL. Demonstration of an area of slow conduction in human atrial flutter. *J Am Coll Cardiol* 1990;16:1639–1648.
22. Olgin J, Kalman J, Saxon L, et al. Induction of atrial flutter in man: site dependence and site of unidirectional block. *J Am Coll Cardiol* 1997;29:376–384.
23. Kalman J, Olgin J, Saxon L, et al. Electrocardiographic and electrophysiologic characterization of atypical atrial flutter in man: Use of activation and entrainment mapping and implications for catheter ablation. *J Cardiovasc Electrophysiol* 1997;8:121–144.
24. Poty H, Saoudi N, Abdel Aziz A, et al. Radiofrequency catheter ablation of type 1 atrial flutter: prediction of late success by electrophysiological criteria. *Circulation* 1995;92:1389–1392.
25. Kall J, Glascock D, Kopp D, et al. Characterization and catheter ablation of the antidromic form of typical atrial flutter [Abstract]. *Circulation* 1995;92:I-84.
26. Lesh M, Kalman J. To fumble flutter or tackle tach? Toward updated classifiers for atrial tachyarrhythmias. *J Cardiovasc Electrophysiol* 1996;7:460–466.
27. Puech P, Latour H, Grolleau R. Le flutter et ses limites. *Arch Mal Coeur* 1970;63:116–144.
28. Olshansky B, Okumura K, Henthorn RW, Waldo AL. Characterization of double potentials in human atrial flutter: studies during transient entrainment. *J Am Coll Cardiol* 1990;15:833–841.
29. Cosio F, Arribas F, Barbero J, et al. Validation of double spike electrograms as markers of conduction delay or block in atrial flutter. *Am J Cardiol* 1988;61:775–780.
30. Kalman JM, VanHare GF, Olgin JE, et al. Ablation of "incisional" reentrant atrial tachycardia complicating surgery for congenital heart disease: use of entrainment to define a critical isthmus of conduction. *Circulation* 1996;93:502–512.
31. Waldo AL, McLean WAH, Karp RB, et al. Entrainment and interruption of atrial flutter with atrial pacing: studies in man following open heart surgery. *Circulation* 1977;56:737–745.
32. Okumura K, Henthorn RW, Epstein AE, et al. Further observations on transient entrainment: importance of pacing site and properties of the components of the reentry circuit. *Circulation* 1985;72:1293–1307.
33. Stevenson W, Sager P, Friedman P. Entrainment techniques for mapping atrial and ventricular tachycardias. *J Cardiovasc Electrophysiol* 1995;6:201–216.
34. Stevenson W, Khan H, Sager P, et al. Identification of reentry circuit sites during catheter mapping and radiofrequency ablation of ventricular tachycardia late after myocardial infarction. *Circulation* 1993;88:1647–1670.
35. Waldo A, Carlson M, Biblo L, Henthorn R. The role of transient entrainment in atrial flutter. In: Waldo, ed. *Atrial arrhythmias*. 1993:210–228.
36. Watson RM, Josephson ME. Atrial flutter. I. Electrophysiologic substrates and modes of initiation and termination. *Am J Cardiol* 1980;45:732–741.
37. Brignole M, Menozzi C, Sartore B, et al. The use of atrial pacing to induce atrial fibrillation and flutter. *Int J Cardiol* 1986;12:45–54.

38. Adachi M, Igawa O, Tomokuni A, et al. Anatomic characteristics of the eustachian ridge, a barrier to conduction during common type atrial flutter [Abstract]. *Circulation* 1996;94:I-380.
39. Lesh M, Van Hare G, Epstein L, et al. Radiofrequency catheter ablation of atrial arrhythmias: results and mechanisms. *Circulation* 1994;89:1074–1089.
40. Calkins H, Leon AR, Deam AG, et al. Catheter ablation of atrial flutter using radiofrequency energy. *Am J Cardiol* 1994; 73:353–356.
41. Kirkorian G, Moncada E, Chevalier P, et al. Radiofrequency ablation of atrial flutter: efficacy of an anatomically guided approach. *Circulation* 1994;90:2804–2814.
42. Fischer B, Haissaguerre M, Garrigues S, et al. Radiofrequency catheter ablation of common atrial flutter in 80 patients. *J Am Coll Cardiol* 1995;25:1365–1372.
43. Saxon LA, Kalman JM, Olgin JE, et al. Results of radiofrequency catheter ablation for atrial flutter. *Am J Cardiol* 1996;77: 1014–1016.
44. Poty H, Saouidi N, Nair M, et al. Radiofrequency catheter ablation of atrial flutter—further insights into the various types of isthmus block: application to ablation during sinus rhythm. *Circulation* 1996;94:3204–3213.
45. Cauchemez B, Haissaguerre M, Fischer B, et al. Electrophysiological effects of catheter ablation of inferior vena cava–tricuspid annulus isthmus in common atrial flutter. *Circulation* 1996;93: 284–294.
46. Fischer B, Jais P, Shah D, et al. Radiofrequency catheter ablation of common atrial flutter in 200 patients. *J Cardiovasc Electrophysiol* 1996;7:1225–1233.
47. Olgin JE, Jayachandran JV, Engelstein E, et al. Atrial macroreentry involving the myocardium of the coronary sinus—a unique mechanism for atypical flutter. *J Cardiovasc Electrophysiol* 1998; 9:1094–1099.
48. Cronin CS, Nitta T, Mitsuno M, et al. Characterization and surgical ablation of acute atrial flutter following the Mustard procedure: a canine model. *Circulation* 1993;88:II461–II471.
49. Rodefeld M, Bromberg B, Schuessler R, et al. Atrial flutter after lateral tunnel construction in the modified Fontan operation: a canine model. *J Thorac Cardiovasc Surg* 1996;111:514–526.
50. Triedman J, Saul J, Weindling S, Walsh E. Radiofrequency ablation of intra-atrial reentrant tachycardia after surgical palliation of congenital heart disease. *Circulation* 1995;91:707–714.
51. Lesh MD, Van Hare GF, Epstein LM, et al. Radiofrequency catheter ablation of atrial arrhythmias: results and mechanisms. *Circulation* 1994;89:1074–1089.
52. Baker B, Lindsay B, Bromberg B, et al. Catheter ablation of clinical intraatrial reentrant tachycardias resulting from previous atrial surgery: Localizing and transecting the critical isthmus. *J Am Coll Cardiol* 1996;28:411–417.
53. Triedman J, Jenkins K, Colan S, et al. Intra-atrial reentrant tachycardia after palliation of congenital heart disease: characterization of multiple macroreentrant circuits using fluoroscopically based three-dimensional endocardial mapping. *J Cardiovasc Electrophysiol* 1997;8:259–270.
54. Chen S, Chiang C, Yang C, et al. Sustained atrial tachycardia in adult patients: electrophysiological characteristics, pharmacological response, possible mechanisms and effects of radiofrequency ablation. *Circulation* 1994;90:1262–1278.
55. Engelstein E, Lippman N, Stein K, Lerman B. Mechanism-specific effects of adenosine on atrial tachycardia. *Circulation* 1994;89:2645–2654.
56. Haines D, DiMarco J. Sustained intraatrial reentrant tachycardia: clinical, electrocardiographic and electrophysiologic characteristics and long-term follow-up. *J Am Coll Cardiol* 1990;15: 1345–1354.
57. Kay G, Chong F, Epstein A, et al. Radiofrequency ablation for treatment of primary atrial tachycardias. *J Am Coll Cardiol* 1993; 21:901–909.
58. Walsh E, Saul J, Hulse J, et al. Transcatheter ablation of ectopic atrial tachycardia in young patients using radiofrequency current. *Circulation* 1992;86:1138–1146.
59. Sanders W, Sorrentino R, Greenfield R, et al. Catheter ablation of sinoatrial node reentrant tachycardia. *J Am Coll Cardiol* 1994; 23:926–934.
60. Shenasa H, Merrill J, Hamer M, Wharton J. Distribution of ectopic atrial tachycardias along the crista terminalis: an atrial ring of fire? [Abstract]. *Circulation* 1993;88:I-29.
61. Kalman J, Olgin J, Fitzpatrick A, et al. "Cristal tachycardia"—relationship of right atrial tachycardias to the crista terminalis identified using intracardiac echocardiography [Abstract]. *Pacing Clin Electrophysiol* 1995;18:861.
62. Mallavarapu C, Schwartzman D, Callans DJ, et al. Radiofrequency catheter ablation of atrial tachycardia with unusual left atrial sites of origin: report of two cases. *Pacing Clin Electrophysiol* 1996;19:988–992.
63. Kalman J, Olgin J, Karch M, Lesh M. Use of intracardiac echocardiography in interventional electrophysiology. *Pacing Clin Electrophysiol (in press)*.
64. Tang CW, Scheinman MM, Van Hare GF, et al. Use of P wave configuration during atrial tachycardia to predict site of origin. *J Am Coll Cardiol* 1995;26:1315–1324.
65. Tracy C, Swartz J, Fletcher R, et al. Radiofrequency catheter ablation of ectopic atrial tachycardia using paced activation sequence mapping. *J Am Coll Cardiol* 1993;21:910–917.
66. Poty H, Saoudi N, Haissaguerre M, et al. Radiofrequency catheter ablation of atrial tachycardias. *Am Heart J* 1996;131:481–489.
67. Weiss C, Hatala R, Carpinteiro L, et al. Topographic anatomy and in vitro fluoroscopic imaging of the crista terminalis: an attempt to more precisely localize the origin of ectopic atrial tachycardia [Abstract]. *Circulation* 1994:I-595.
68. Morillo CA, Klein GJ, Thakur RK, et al. Mechanism of "inappropriate" sinus tachycardia: role of sympathovagal balance. *Circulation* 1994;90:873–877.
69. Krahn A, Yee R, Klein G, Morillo C. Inappropriate sinus tachycardia: evaluation and therapy. *J Cardiovasc Electrophysiol* 1995; 6:1124–1128.
70. Lee RJ, Kalman JM, Fitzpatrick AP, et al. Radiofrequency catheter modification of the sinus node for "inappropriate" sinus tachycardia. *Circulation* 1995;92:2919–2928.
71. Bauernfeind R, Amat-y-Leon F, Dhingra R, et al. Chronic nonparoxysmal sinus tachycardia in otherwise healthy persons. *Ann Intern Med* 1979;91:702–710.
72. Boineau J, Schuessler R, Hackel D, et al. Widespread distribution and rate differentiation of the atrial pacemaker complex. *Am J Physiol* 1980;239:H406–H415.
73. Boineau J, Schuessler R, Roeske W, et al. Quantitative relation between sites of atrial impulse origin and cycle length. *Am J Physiol* 1983;245:H781–H789.
74. Kalman JM, Lee RJ, Fisher WG, et al. Radiofrequency catheter modification of sinus pacemaker function guided by intracardiac echocardiography. *Circulation* 1995;92:3070–3081.
75. Kalman J, Olgin J, Saxon L, et al. Electrophysiologic of the crista terminalis in normal human atria. *Pacing Clin Electrophysiol* 1996;19:578.
76. Jones S, Euler D, Hardie E, et al. Comparison of SA nodal and subsidiary atrial pacemaker function and location in the dog. *Am J Physiol* 1978;234:H471–H476.
77. Shinbane J, Lesh M, Scheinman M, et al. Long-term follow-up after radiofrequency sinus node modification for inappro-

priate sinus tachycardia [Abstract]. *J Am Coll Cardiol* 1997;29: 199A.
78. Cox J, Schuessler R, D'Agostino J, et al. The surgical treatment of atrial fibrillation. III. Development of a definitive surgical procedure. *J Thorac Cardiovasc Surg* 1991;101:569–583.
79. Swartz J, Pellersels G, Silvers J, et al. A catheter-based curative approach to atrial fibrillation in humans [Abstract]. *Circulation* 1994;90:I-335.
80. Haissaguerre M, Jais P, Shah D, et al. Right and left atrial radiofrequency catheter therapy of paroxysmal atrial fibrillation. *J Cardiovasc Electrophysiol* 1996;7:1132–1144.
81. Olgin JE, Strickberger SA, Lesh M, et al. Right atrial ablation of lone atrial fibrillation with multi-electrode coil catheters. *Pacing Clin Electrophysiol* 1999;22:904.
82. Olgin JE, Kalman JM, Chin M, et al. Electrophysiological effects of long, linear atrial lesions placed under intracardiac ultrasound guidance. *Circulation* 1997;96:2715–2721.
83. Chen SA, Tai CT, Yu WC, et al. Right atrial focal atrial fibrillation: electrophysiologic characteristics and radiofrequency catheter ablation. *J Cardiovasc Electrophysiol* 1999;10:328–335.
84. Haissaguerre M, Jais P, Shah DC, et al. Spontaneous initiation of atrial fibrillation by ectopic beats originating in the pulmonary veins. *N Engl J Med* 1998;339:659–666.
85. Hsieh MH, Chen SA, Tai CT, et al. Double multielectrode mapping catheters facilitate radiofrequency catheter ablation of focal atrial fibrillation originating from pulmonary veins. *J Cardiovasc Electrophysiol* 1999;10:136–144.
86. Gepstein L, Hayam G, Ben-Haim SA. A novel method for nonfluoroscopic catheter-based electroanatomical mapping of the heart: in vitro and in vivo accuracy results. *Circulation* 1997; 95:1611–1622.
87. Dorostkar PC, Cheng J, Scheinman MM. Electroanatomical mapping and ablation of the substrate supporting intraatrial reentrant tachycardia after palliation for complex congenital heart disease. *Pacing Clin Electrophysiol* 1998;21:1810–1819.
88. Marchlinski F, Callans D, Gottlieb C, et al. Magnetic electroanatomical mapping for ablation of focal atrial tachycardias. *Pacing Clin Electrophysiol* 1998;21:1621–1635.
89. Nakagawa H, Jackman WM. Use of a three-dimensional, nonfluoroscopic mapping system for catheter ablation of typical atrial flutter. *Pacing Clin Electrophysiol* 1998;21:1279–1286.
90. Schwartzman D, Kuck KH. Anatomy-guided linear atrial lesions for radiofrequency catheter ablation of atrial fibrillation. *Pacing Clin Electrophysiol* 1998;21:1959–1978.
91. Wittkampf FH, Wever EF, Derksen R, et al. LocaLisa: new technique for real-time 3-dimensional localization of regular intracardiac electrodes. *Circulation* 1999;99:1312–1317.
92. Kadish A, Hauck J, Pederson B, et al. Mapping of atrial activation with a noncontact, multielectrode catheter in dogs. *Circulation* 1999;99:1906–1913.
93. Khoury DS, Taccardi B, Lux RL, et al. Reconstruction of endocardial potentials and activation sequences from intracavitary probe measurements: localization of pacing sites and effects of myocardial structure. *Circulation* 1995;91:845–863.

ATRIAL FIBRILLATION ABLATION: PRESENT AND FUTURE
• • •

BOAZ AVITALL, VINAY MALHOTRA, ARVYDAS URBONAS, DALIA URBONIENE,
SCOTT C. MILLARD

Atrial fibrillation is the most common cardiac arrhythmia. The prevalence of atrial fibrillation increases with age (1–4). The incidence of atrial fibrillation is about 2 to 3 cases per 1,000 persons between the ages of 25 and 35 years, increasing to 30 to 40 cases per 1,000 of those between the ages of 55 and 60 years. The prevalence increases to about 8% to 10% by age 80 (5,6). At least 4% of the population has atrial fibrillation, and more than 70% of patients are older than 65 years (4).

Patients with atrial fibrillation have a fivefold increased risk of stroke compared with normal individuals (7). In the past, pharmacologic approach has involved using class 1A, class 1C, and class 3 agents. At 1 year, the efficacy of these agents is a little better than 50%. The use of these agents, especially class 1A and class 1C drugs, is associated with proarrhythmias and increased mortality in patients with impaired left ventricular systolic function (8–10). Amiodarone, a class III agent is associated with long-term, serious side effects (11,12).

The maze III operation is the most effective treatment of atrial fibrillation and has the highest long-term success rate. The maze procedure, pioneered by Cox and colleagues, is used to create lines of conduction block that interrupt all potential macro-reentrant circuits and thereby cure atrial fibrillation (13–17).

The maze III procedure involves the excision of appendages, isolation of pulmonary veins, and fragmentation of the atrium (15). Cox and colleagues have performed the maze procedure in 190 patients, 58% of whom had paroxysmal atrial fibrillation. Ninety percent of patients followed for more than 3 months were in normal sinus rhythm (NSR). Moreover, 29% of patients received a pacemaker for underlying sick sinus syndrome ($n = 28$) or for other complications ($n = 2$) (18). The maze procedure demonstrated that, to cure atrial fibrillation, it was important to reduce the surface area of the atria to the regions that would not allow the formation of the reentrant circuits (19).

INITIATION OF ATRIAL FIBRILLATION

Tissue fibrosis is a result of aging, coronary artery disease, hypertension, valvular disease, inflammation, and tissue injury caused by toxins. These changes in the atrial tissues may lead to electrophysiologic changes that further promote the induction of atrial fibrillation. Although these factors permanently affect the atria, the autonomic nervous system tone modulates the electrophysiologic properties of the atria. This may further contribute to the induction of

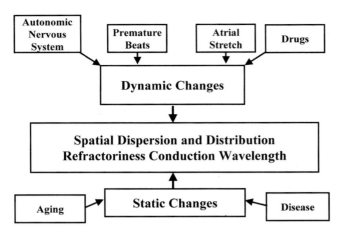

FIGURE 12-1. Factors that influence spatial dispersion and distribution of refractoriness and conduction. (From Michelucci A, Padeletti L, Porciani MC, et al. Dispersion of refractoriness and atrial fibrillation. In: Olsson SB, Allessie MA, Campbell RWF, eds. *Atrial fibrillation: mechanisms and therapeutic strategies.* Armonk, NY: Futura Publishing, 1994:81–107, with permission.)

ectopic activity (20) (Figs. 12-1 and 12-2). Ectopic activity by itself causes electrical remodeling, which leads to global electrical remodeling and the degeneration of the electrical synchrony, producing atrial fibrillation (21).

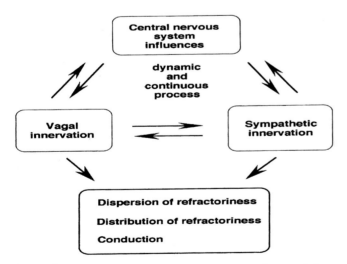

FIGURE 12-2. Autonomic nervous system regulation of electrophysiological properties. (From Michelucci A, Padeletti L, Porciani MC, et al. Dispersion of refractoriness and atrial fibrillation. In: Olsson SB, Allessie MA, Campbell RWF, eds. *Atrial fibrillation: mechanisms and therapeutic strategies.* Armonk, NY: Futura Publishing, 1994:81–107, with permission.)

MECHANISM OF ATRIAL FIBRILLATION

Automatic Foci

Scherf described the effect of application of aconitine to the right atrial appendage (22). Atrial fibrillation occurred when the single, rapidly firing automatic focus could be conducted to the atrium. He also demonstrated that ligation of the appendage terminated the atrial fibrillation (22). Haissaguerre and colleagues described three patients who underwent successful ablation of atrial fibrillation in 1994. In this report, the notion of focal atrial fibrillation was reinforced (23). Kuck and colleagues also reported patients with rapid irregular focal tachycardia that rapidly degenerated into atrial fibrillation (24). These studies provide the basis for the assumption that single, rapidly depolarizing ectopic foci can lead to atrial electrical remodeling that establishes the substrate for the initiation of atrial fibrillation.

In a subset of patients with paroxysmal atrial fibrillation, one or several foci that initiate premature atrial contractions or recurrent runs of atrial tachycardia result in paroxysmal atrial fibrillation (25). The most intriguing aspect of this arrhythmia is that the foci were often identified to be within the pulmonary veins, specifically the superior left and right pulmonary veins. It is hypothesized that bursts of atrial tachycardia, or even premature atrial contractions, may lead to atrial electrical remodeling, which leads to persistent and eventually chronic atrial fibrillation (25). Clinical experience with the ablation of paroxysmal atrial fibrillation points to a single or multiple triggering foci that initiate the rapid runs of atrial tachycardia. Additional support for the hypothesis that focal activity may be the cause of chronic atrial fibrillation was provided by a paper on the ablation of chronic atrial fibrillation in humans (26). In this investigation, linear lesions in the left atrium were directed at the regions of maximal electrical fractionated activity, which resulted in termination of the atrial fibrillation and unmasking of focal atrial tachycardia originating from the pulmonary vein ostium, trabeculated portions of the atrium, and left atrial appendage. However, it is possible that the atrial tachy-

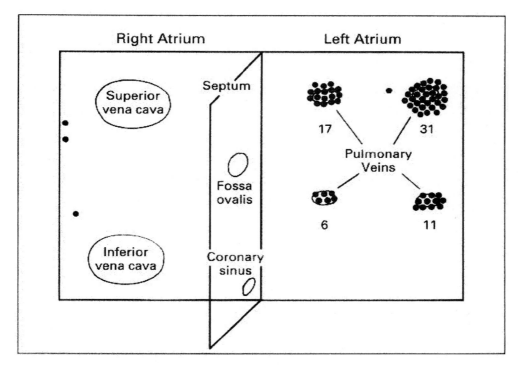

FIGURE 12-3. Sites of 69 foci triggering atrial fibrillation in 45 patients. Numbers indicate the distribution of foci in the pulmonary veins. (From Haissaguerre M, Jais P, Shah DC, et al. Spontaneous initiation of atrial fibrillation by ectopic beats originating in the pulmonary veins. *N Engl J Med* 1998;339:659–666, with permission.)

cardia is a result of noncontiguous or nontransmural linear lesions.

Paroxysmal atrial fibrillation ablation is becoming a common procedure in clinical cardiac electrophysiology practice. The pulmonary veins have become an important site for lesion location, leading clinicians to direct the atrial mapping exclusively to the pulmonary veins (27). As shown in Figures 12-3 through 12-5, the trigger points of atrial fibrillation were found at the left superior pulmonary vein in 12 patients, right superior pulmonary vein in 8 patients, and both superior pulmonary veins in 19 patients (25). From the 61 trigger points found at the pulmonary veins, 18 (30%) were in the ostia of pulmonary veins, and 43 (70%) were inside the pulmonary veins (9 to 40 mm into the vein). After 6 ± 3 applications of radiofrequency energy, 57 of 61 triggers were completely eliminated, and the other 4 triggers were partially eliminated. During a follow-up period of 8 ± 2 months, 37 (88%) patients were free of symptomatic atrial fibrillation without any antiarrhythmic drugs.

Further support for the role of the pulmonary veins in the initiation and inhibition of atrial fibrillation induction after pulmonary vein isolation has been reported in an acute atrial fibrillation induction protocol. Whereas atrial fibrillation before pulmonary vein isolation could be induced in eight sheep, none could be induced after surgical isolation of the pulmonary veins (21).

The unique structural anatomy of the pulmonary vein insertion into the left atrium (Fig. 12-6) strongly supports the argument that the left atrial tissues spiraling deep into the pulmonary vein, especially the superior pulmonary veins, may provide the substrate for atrial reentry arrhythmia (28,29). Muscle fibers form spirals around the pulmonary veins, and pacemaker-type cells were found within these structures (30), supporting the hypothesis of the ectopic activity and one or multiple reentry circuits leading to the forma-

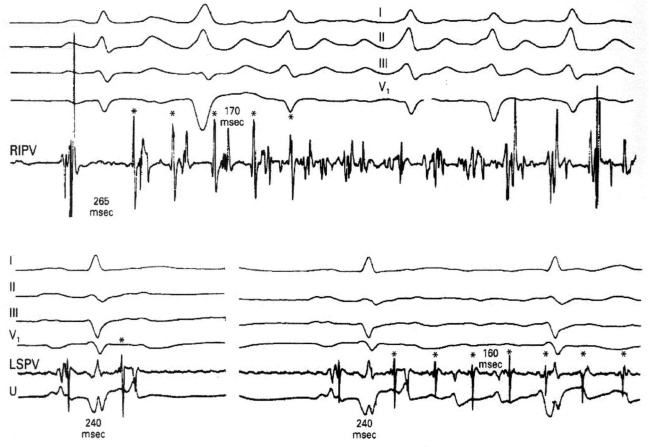

FIGURE 12-4. Two examples of the onset of atrial fibrillation from foci in a right inferior pulmonary vein (RIPV) and a left superior pulmonary vein (LSPV). Numbers indicate the distribution of foci in the pulmonary veins. (From Haissaguerre M, Jais P, Shah DC, et al. Spontaneous initiation of atrial fibrillation by ectopic beats originating in the pulmonary veins. *N Engl J Med* 1998;339:659–666, with permission.)

tion of atrial tachycardia. If atrial tachycardia is persistent, it will cause atrial electrical remodeling and the initiation of atrial fibrillation.

Experimental Technology for the Creation of Pulmonary Vein Isolation Lesions

In an effort to develop technologies for the isolation of the pulmonary vein insertion into the left atrium, several concepts are being tested. The hot balloon technology (Fig. 12-7) demonstrates the flexibility of this technology to adapt to various pulmonary vein sizes. Tissue heating is enhanced by the temporary obstruction of blood flow. The balloon is filled with saline and contrast medium, which allows the balloon size and location to be visualized fluoroscopically. The saline is heated internally by radiofrequency power, which is applied to two ring electrodes located on the catheter shaft within the balloon. This technology, although simple, is perhaps adequate for small vessels, in which the size of the heating chamber is only 0.5 to 1 cm in diameter. It is likely that the human pulmonary vein is too large for this technology to create adequate heating at the pulmonary vein–atrial junction.

The virtual electrode chamber is a catheter that has distal and proximal balloons. After the balloons are inflated, the space between the balloons is cleared of blood by flushing the chamber with saline. The radio-

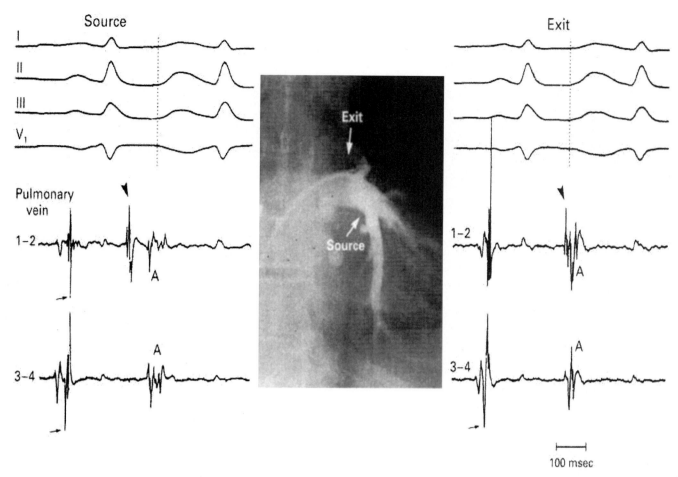

FIGURE 12-5. Angiogram of a left inferior pulmonary vein shows the source and exit of ectopic activity. The dotted lines indicate the onset of ectopic P wave, and 1-2 and 3-4 are bipolar recordings from the distal and proximal poles of the mapping catheter. Numbers indicate the distribution of foci in the pulmonary veins. (From Haissaguerre M, Jais P, Shah DC, et al. Spontaneous initiation of atrial fibrillation by ectopic beats originating in the pulmonary veins. *N Engl J Med* 1998;339:659–666, with permission.)

frequency power is applied to a ring electrode on the catheter shaft between the balloons, and a reference patch electrode is on the body. The radiofrequency power transverses the saline, with the maximal current density located at the tissue interface resulting in tissue heating. It is yet to be shown that this technology is capable of electrically isolating the pulmonary veins from the left atrium.

Another ablation concept is the use of ultrasound technology to focus the heat dissipation caused by the sound waves in the surrounding atrial tissues. An ultrasound transducer is mounted on a catheter shaft within an expandable balloon.

The most attractive means for mapping and ablating the pulmonary vein source of atrial fibrillation is cryoablative technology. By controlling the temperature, the catheter can be used to create localized stunning of tissues, called cold mapping, without creating permanent tissue injury, and if the electrical activity causing the arrhythmia is suppressed, the probe temperature can be lowered to temperature of less than $-40°C$ to create permanent tissue injury. Unlike tissue heating, tissue freezing does not interrupt the tissue's architecture, and it is regarded as a much more desirable means of tissue destruction.

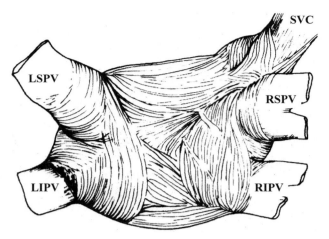

FIGURE 12-6. Atrial muscle tissues spiraling up the pulmonary veins. LIPV, left inferior pulmonary vein; LSPV, left superior pulmonary vein; RIPV, right inferior pulmonary vein; RSPV, right superior pulmonary vein; SVC, superior vena cava. (From Nathan H, Eliakim M. The junction between the left atrium and the pulmonary veins: an anatomic study of the human heart. *Circulation* 1966;34:412–422, with permission.)

Persistent and Chronic Atrial Fibrillation: Multiple Wavelet Reentry

Moe and colleagues (31,32), using a computer-generated model, suggested that atrial fibrillation is multiple, randomly wandering, macro-reentrant circuits. To initiate atrial fibrillation, an area of conduction block must be developed. The wavelength of the circuit must be short enough to allow the reentry (33). This hypothesis has since been confirmed by epicardial mapping of canine and human hearts (13,34). Allessie and coworkers estimated that an average of four to six wandering wavelets must be present to maintain atrial fibrillation. Allessie also defined wavelength as a product of the conduction velocity and refractory period. To set up a reentry, the wavelength of the premature beat must be short (35,36). He also suggested that the reentry pathways in atrial fibrillation were essentially functionally determined.

Tse and colleagues demonstrated that there was a regional heterogeneity in the changes of atrial electrophysiology in different parts of the atrium and that the spatial distribution of atrial refractoriness was increased in patients with chronic atrial fibrillation. Patients with paroxysmal atrial fibrillation showed intermediate changes in atrial conduction times and atrial refractoriness compared with patients with chronic atrial fibrillation, suggesting that paroxysmal atrial fibrillation was a transition state from the control state to chronic atrial fibrillation (37). Using animal models, it has been shown that atrial fibrillation induces a vicious cycle of electrophysiologic and structural changes that inevitably lead to domestication of

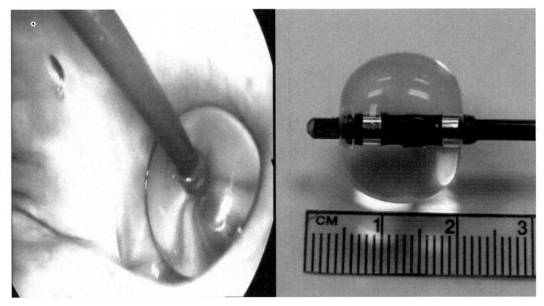

FIGURE 12-7. Hot balloon for pulmonary vein ablation.

the arrhythmia (i.e., atrial fibrillation begets atrial fibrillation) (38).

Apart from shortening of the refractory period, the properties of atrial conduction may also play an important role in the substrate of atrial fibrillation (39). An inhomogeneous downregulation of gap junctions may provide the necessary atrial conduction block, serving as turning points for wondering multiple wavelengths or circuits. Remodeling of these gap junctions could be part of the vicious cycle of remodeling that leads to permanent atrial fibrillation (40–43).

Narayan and coworkers demonstrated that the chronicity of atrial fibrillation is favored by increased atrial size and a shorter wavelength (44). Several factors increase the susceptibility to the development of atrial fibrillation: increased intraatrial pressure as a result of mitral regurgitation, hypertension or congestive heart failure resulting in increased atrial stretch, higher oxygen consumption creating relative ischemia, and progressive fibrosis.

Anatomic obstacles, including the pulmonary veins (i.e., interdigitations from vascular to atrial tissue), superior vena cava and inferior vena cava, ostium of the coronary sinus, and the eustachian valves have all been shown to be involved in macro-reentrant circuits (45).

CATHETER ABLATION OF ATRIAL FIBRILLATION

In 1994, Haissaguerre and colleagues described successful radiofrequency catheter ablation of atrial fibrillation in three patients with drug-resistant atrial arrhythmias. The first two patients had incessant atrial tachycardia or atrial fibrillation. In both patients, ablation of the atrial focus near the sinus node (first patient) and in the mid-lateral right atrial wall (second patient) led to the clinical disappearance of atrial fibrillation. In the third patient, ablation of type 1 atrial flutter resulted in elimination of atrial fibrillation (23). They also demonstrated successful ablation of paroxysmal atrial fibrillation by creating three linear lesions—two longitudinal and one transverse—in the right atrium. These lesions were created using 30 radiofrequency applications of 10 to 40 W. At 3 months, the patients were free of atrial fibrillation and were not on any medication (46). While describing the focal origin of atrial fibrillation, these investigators studied 45 patients with frequent episodes of atrial fibrillation (mean duration, 344 ± 326 minutes/24 hours) using multielectrode catheters. A single point of origin of atrial ectopy was identified in 29 patients; two points were identified in 9 patients, and three or four points of origin were identified in 7 patients. Ninety-four percent of the foci were found in the pulmonary veins. The earliest activation occurred 2 to 4 cm inside the veins. These were marked by a local depolarization preceding the atrial ectopy. During a follow-up period of 8 ± 6 months after ablation, 28 patients were free of atrial fibrillation (25).

Jais and associates described nine patients with paroxysmal atrial fibrillation or focal atrial fibrillation. Radiofrequency ablation in the right atrium and left atrium resulted in 100% immediate and long-term success, with no complications at 10 months' follow-up (47). Haissaguerre and colleagues described ablation for paroxysmal atrial fibrillation in 55 patients. Of these patients, 45 underwent ablation in the right atrium and 10 in the left atrium. In the first group (right atrial ablation only), 18 (40%) of 45 were free of atrial fibrillation right after the procedure, and 13% were free of atrial fibrillation after mean follow-up of 11 months. In the second group, 8 (80%) of 10 were free of atrial fibrillation immediately after ablation, and 60% were free of atrial fibrillation at the end of 11 months. Two patients had transient sinus node dysfunction, and one had hemopericardium (48).

Jais and coworkers reported long-term follow-up results after right atrial radiofrequency catheter treatment of paroxysmal atrial fibrillation. Thirty-six men and nine women with symptomatic daily episodes of atrial fibrillation were studied. The mean age of the patients was 51 ± 12 years. Progressively longer ablation lines were performed in three groups of 15 consecutive patients using a 14-electrode catheter or a single-electrode dragging technique. After 11 months of follow-up, 24 patients had favorable results from the ablation procedure with or without additional antiarrhythmic drug therapy. After 26 ± 5 months of follow-up, the success rate was reduced to 37% (17 patients) (49).

Man and associates described 12 patients with paroxysmal atrial fibrillation after ablation in the right atrium (50). The immediate success rate was 33%, and at a mean follow-up of 52 days, the success rate was as low as 8%. Garg and colleagues described 12 patients with atrial fibrillation ablation in the right atrium (51). During the 21-month follow-up period, 66% of patients were in normal sinus rhythm. Hwang and coworkers reported 14 patients with paroxysmal atrial fibrillation who underwent ablation in the left atrium, with a 94% immediate success rate and 93% success rate at 6 months (52). An update presented by Hwang included 40 patients (53). In 1999, Chen and colleagues described 8 patients with focal atrial fibrillation. The immediate and long-term results at 14 months were excellent: a 100% success rate without any complications (54). Maloney and associates described 15 patients with refractory chronic atrial fibrillation or focal atrial fibrillation, who underwent a two-stage biatrial linear and focal ablation to restore sinus rhythm. Of the 11 patients who were evaluated for a mean period of 21 months, 9 had normal sinus rhythm, 2 had pericardial tamponade, 1 had an inadvertent ablation-induced heart block, and 1 had a permanent pacemaker for troublesome bradycardia (55). Hsieh and colleagues reported 42 patients with focal atrial fibrillation. After 8 months, 88% of patients were free of arrhythmia (27).

Kuck and coworkers described 27 patients with idiopathic atrial fibrillation who, after atrial fibrillation ablation in both atria using the CARTO system, had a 59% success rate at 8 weeks after ablation (56). Gaita and associates reported 16 patients with idiopathic vagal atrial fibrillation with a 56% success rate at 11 months after ablation in the right atrium (57).

In 1994, Swartz reported that the creation of linear lesions in the right and left atria resulted in organization of atrial activity, ultimately restoring sinus rhythm in 29 patients (58). Sixteen (55%) of 29 required a second ablation procedure. The mean procedure duration and fluoroscopy times were 12 hours and 118 minutes, respectively. After 2 years of follow-up, 23 patients had normal sinus rhythm (on no medications), 3 patients had paroxysmal atrial flutter, 2 patients had incessant atrial flutter, and 3 patients had atrial fibrillation (59). Associated complications included two strokes, one case of pericardial effusion, one episode of pericarditis, one case of acute respiratory distress syndrome (ARDS), two episodes of gastrointestinal bleeding, and two urinary tract infections. Table 12-1 summarizes atrial fibrillation ablation efforts in humans.

Experimental Studies of Atrial Fibrillation Ablation

Atrial Fibrillation Models

Three animal models of atrial fibrillation are used by investigators: vagal stimulation, sterile pericarditis, and rapid atrial pacing. Vagal stimulation and sterile pericarditis have been shown to increase susceptibility to acute atrial fibrillation (60–63). To improve the clinical applicability of atrial fibrillation research, the rapid atrial pacing model was developed by Morillo and colleagues (64). With this technique, 82% of dogs have spontaneous atrial fibrillation within 6 weeks. Another chronic model involves the creation of mitral regurgitation by cutting some of the mitral valve's chordae tendineae. This model requires at least 3 months, after which 75% of the dogs have sustained atrial fibrillation. However, animal mortality using this model may approach 40% (13).

We introduced a variation to the Morillo technique by rapidly pacing the atria from two sites. The right atrial appendage was paced at 400 bpm, and a premature beat was introduced at every fourth beat to the low right atrial free wall. This technique resulted in atrial fibrillation initiation in 100% of the dogs studied ($n = 13$) within 41 ± 19 days and with no increase in mortality. Echocardiography showed that the development of atrial fibrillation in this model correlated with severe atrial enlargement and ventricular dysfunction. The right atrial size increased from 20 ± 2 to 27 ± 5 mm; left atrial size increased from 32 ± 3 to 43 ± 9 mm; and the left ventricular ejection fraction decreased from $50 \pm 10\%$ to $24 \pm 7\%$ (65).

Technology for the Segmentation of Atrial Tissues with Linear Lesions

Ablation of Atrial Fibrillation in the Animal Model Using Discrete Lesions

Elvan and colleagues assessed the effects of radiofrequency catheter ablation in the atria on pacing-in-

TABLE 12-1 • CATHETER ABLATION OF ATRIAL FIBRILLATION: CLINICAL RESULTS

Study	Patients (n)	Atrial Fibrillation	Ablation Site	Ablation System	Acute Success (%)	Chronic Success (%)	Mean Follow-up	Complications
Peer-Reviewed Manuscripts								
Haissaguerre et al. (25)	45	PAF/focal AF	RA & LA	Multiple	84	62	8 mo	None
Jais et al. (47)	9	PAF/focal AF	RA & LA	Multiple	100	100	10 mo	None
Haissaguerre et al. (48)	45	PAF	RA	Multiple	40	33	11 mo	2 transient SN dysfunction
	10	PAF	LA	Multiple	80	60	11 mo	1 hemopericardium
Jais et al. (49)	45	PAF				57	11 mo	
Garg et al. (51)	12		RA			66	21 mo	1 pacemaker implantation
Chen et al. (54)	8	Focal AF	RA		100	100	14 mo	None
Hsieh et al. (27)	42	Focal AF	LA			88	8 mo	19 small ASD, which closed spontaneously 1 mo later in 15 patients
Gaita et al. (57)	16	Idiopathic vagal AF	RA	NA		56	11 mo	None
Abstracts and Other Reports								
Man et al. (50)	12	PAF	RA	Standard	33	8	52 d	
Hwang et al. (52,53)	14	PAF/focal AF	LA	NA	94	93	6 mo	
Maloney et al. (26,55)	15[a]	CAF/focal AF	RA & LA	NA		82	21 mo	1 heart block, 1 pacemaker implant, 2 PE
Swartz et al. (59)	29	CAF	RA & LA	NA		79		2 CVAs, 1 PE, 1 ARDS
Kuck et al. (56)	27	Idiopathic AF	RA & LA	CARTO		59	8 wk	1 CVA, 1 pericardial tamponade
Haines et al. (90)	8	PAF	RA	EPT MECA		0		2 transient phrenic nerve injuries
	3	PAF	LA	EPT MECA		66		1 air embolism

AF, atrial fibrillation; PAF, paroxysmal AF; CAF, chronic AF; LA, left atrium; RA, right atrium; CARTO, CARTO Biosense mapping system; EPT MECA, EP Technologies MECA ablation system; SN, sinus node; ASD, atrial septal defect; ARDS, acute respiratory distress syndrome; CVA, cerebrovascular accident; PE, pericardial effusion; NA, not available; NS, not significant; RA, right atrium; LA, left atrium.

[a] Eleven of 15 patients were followed for 21 months.

duced, sustained atrial fibrillation. In each of 12 mongrel dogs, after ablation of the atrioventricular node, a VVI pacemaker was inserted. A high-rate pulse generator (20 to 30 Hz to induce atrial fibrillation) was connected to the right atrial endocardial lead. In group 1, atrial fibrillation was eliminated in 5 of 9 dogs with radiofrequency catheter ablation in the right side, and in 4 dogs, right and left atrial radiofrequency catheter ablation was required. In all these dogs, the sinus node recovery time and P-wave duration were prolonged. The intrinsic heart rate and maximal heart rate were decreased (66–68).

These investigators also showed in an open-chest canine model that, in the presence of continuous discrete transmural lesions at five atrial epicardial sites and in the coronary sinus wall, resulted in a reduction of inducibility of atrial fibrillation along with partial denervation of the vagus nerve (69). Kempler and colleagues demonstrated suppression of conduction across epicardially created radiofrequency linear lesions in dogs (70). Morillo and colleagues demonstrated that atrial fibrillation was readily inducible in 82% of dogs after rapid atrial pacing. They also showed that an area in the posterior left atrium had the shortest atrial fibrillatory cycle length and that cryoablation of this area resulted in restoration of sinus rhythm and prevention of inducibility of atrial fibrillation (64). Increased atrial area (by 40%) and shortening of effective refractory period were highly predictive for the induction of atrial fibrillation (35).

Attempts have been made to create linear lesions with the use of nonfluoroscopic electroanatomic guiding system. These efforts have been made in humans and experimentally, proving the feasibility of creating transmural contiguous linear lesions. The primary drawback of these efforts has been prolonged procedure time, which makes this technique not as useful as the primary method for the creation of linear lesions (71,72).

Atrial Fibrillation Ablation Using the Loop Catheter Design

We tested a catheter system with 24 4-mm ring electrodes that can create loops in the atria (Figs. 12-8 and

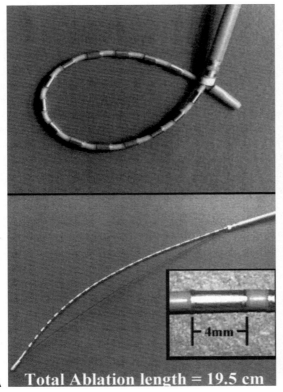
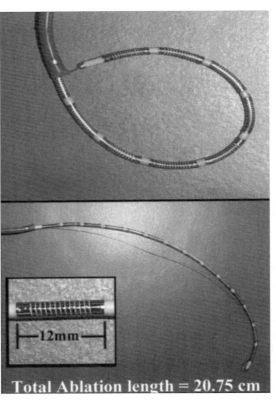

FIGURE 12-8. Ring and coil electrode ablation catheters. **A:** Ring electrode ablation catheter. **B:** Coil electrode ablation catheter.

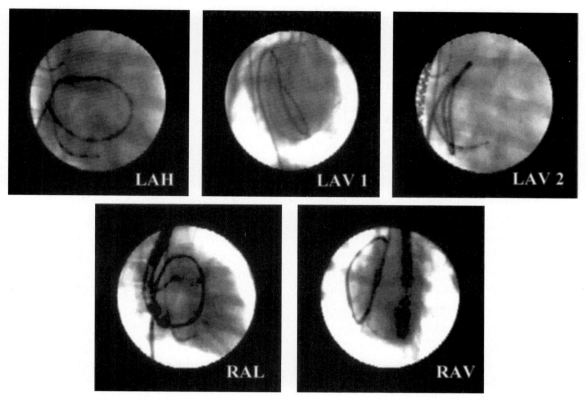

FIGURE 12-9. Loop catheter positions. LAH, circular left atrial lesion above the mitral valve identified as "left atrial horizontal"; LAV 1 and LAV 2, vertical left atrial lesions connecting the mitral valve and the top of left atria, bisecting the pulmonary veins laterally and medially; RAL, right anteromedial loop connecting the tricuspid ring superior vena cava (SVC) and inferior vena cava (IVC); RAV, right atrial vertical loop, connecting the SVC, IVC, and lateral right atrial wall.

12-9). The electrodes can be used to record electrical activity and deliver radiofrequency power for ablation. In 33 dogs, 82 linear lesions were generated using three power titration protocols: fixed levels, manual titration guided by local electrogram activity, and temperature control. Bipolar activity was recorded from the 24 electrodes before, during, and after lesion generation. The lesions were created principally in five loop catheter positions (Fig. 12-9). Data were gathered regarding lesion contiguity, transmurality, and dimensions; the changes in local electrical activity amplitude; the incidence rate of rapid impedance rise and desiccation or char formation; and rhythm outcomes. Catheter deployment usually requires less than 60 seconds. Linear lesions (12 to 16 cm long and 6 ± 2 mm wide) can be generated in 24 to 48 minutes without moving the catheter. Effective lesion formation can be predicted by a marked decrease in the amplitude of bipolar recordings (67 ± 34%). Splitting or fragmentation of the electrogram and increasing pacing threshold (3.1 ± 3.3 mV to 7.1 ± 3.8 mV, $p < 0.01$) are indicative of effective lesion formation. Impedance rises and char formation occurred at 91 ± 12°C. Linear lesion creation did not result in the initiation of atrial fibrillation, but atrial tachycardia was recorded after the completion of the final lesion in 3 of 12 hearts. When using temperature control, no char was seen in the left atrium, whereas 8% of the right atrial burns had char. Based on these results, we concluded that the adjustable loop catheter, which forces the atria to conform around the catheter, is capable of producing linear, contiguous lesions up to 16 cm long with minimal effort and radiation exposure.

Pacing thresholds and electrogram amplitude and character are markers of effective lesion formation.

Although atrial fibrillation could not be induced after the completion of the lesion set, sustained atrial tachycardia could be induced in 25% of the hearts. In an effort to increase the efficiency of the ablation system, we evaluated and reported the use of a loop catheter with 14 12-mm long coil electrodes 2 mm apart (Fig. 12-8) equipped with two thermistors, which were positioned at the two edges of each coil. The power is regulated to the maximal temperature measured between the two thermistors (73).

This catheter system was found to be effective and efficient when compared with the twenty-four 4-mm ring-type electrodes that were used in an earlier version of the technology (74). Although temperature monitoring has been essential for the prevention of overheating and char formation (75,76), we reported the use of local electrogram amplitude reduction as a marker for transmural lesion creation with the 12-mm-long coil electrodes (77). In this study, the P-wave reduction of greater than 50% was a marker of transmural lesion formation (Fig. 12-10), an example of which is shown in Figure 12-11. In several instances, regional tissue isolation or marked decremental conduction was recorded after the creation of several linear lesions in the left atrium. An example of such tissue isolation is shown in Figure 12-12, in which a segment of the left atrium has been isolated from the rest of the atria, which was still in atrial fibrillation. Distal coronary sinus isolation is shown in Figure 12-13.

Linear Lesion Efficacy and Outcomes

The creation of incomplete linear lesions promotes the initiation of atrial tachycardia in every case in which skipped lesions were created (78). Although skipped lesions do not result in the induction of atrial fibrillation in normal dog atria, these lesions placed in the right atrium result in induction of an incessant type of atrial tachycardia that could not always be terminated with overdrive pacing. In dogs with chronic atrial fibrillation induced by rapid pacing, linear lesions in both atria resulted in 83% conversion of the atrial fibrillation. However, in 33% of the dogs, sustained atrial tachycardia, which could be terminated by overdrive pacing (Fig. 12-14), was induced with burst pacing (79,80). These results imply that lesions creation for the ablation of atrial fibrillation must be kept to a minimum and that the lesions must be contiguous and transmural, terminating at a nonconductive barrier. Although noncontiguous and transmural lesions have been shown to promote atrial

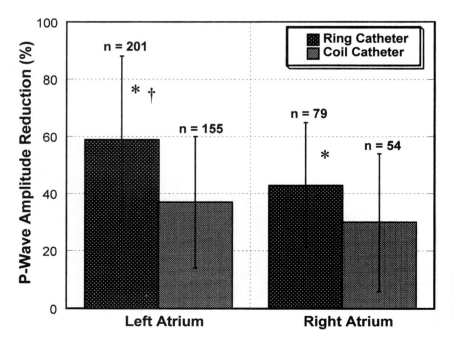

FIGURE 12-10. Left (LA) and right atrial (RA) P-wave reduction after radiofrequency lesions (*$p < 0.05$ for ring versus coil electrodes; †$p < 0.01$ for LA versus RA ring electrodes).

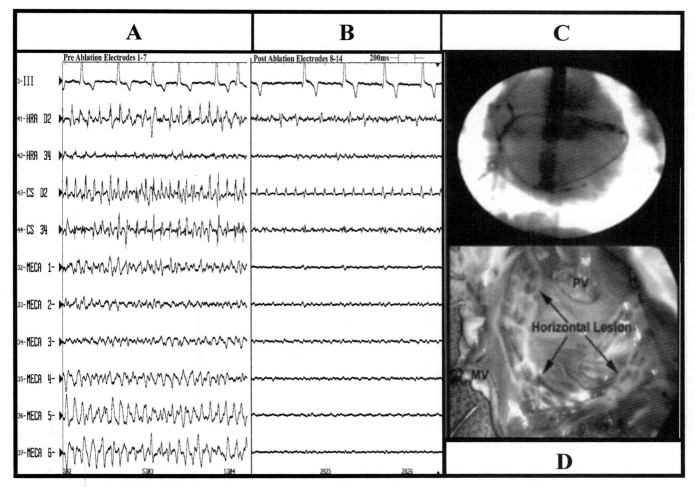

FIGURE 12-11. Before and after ablation 12-mm P-wave reduction for lesion 1. **A:** Preablation electrodes 1 through 7. **B:** Postablation electrodes 8 through 14. **C:** Radiographic position of the loop catheter. **D:** Gross pathology of the lesion.

tachycardia, the ablation of atrial fibrillation does not require contiguous and transmural lesions (81).

When identifying the atrial tissues that promote atrial fibrillation in the rapid-pacing dog model, we hypothesized that linear lesions placed at regions of maximal fractionated electrical activity would cause generalized changes in the rate and character of the atrial fibrillation. These lesions would eventually lead to the termination of atrial fibrillation, implying localized dominance of these regions. In dogs with chronic atrial fibrillation, induced by the rapid-pacing dog model, atrial mapping and linear contiguous lesions were placed in the regions of maximal fractionated activity. The heterogenicity of localized electrical activity was divided into four types: type 0, normal sinus rhythm or atrial tachycardia; type 1, atrial flutter or atrial tachycardia; type 2, high-voltage atrial fibrillation with no baseline fractionation; and type 3, atrial fibrillation with baseline fractionation (Fig. 12-15). In these dogs, left atrial lesions connecting the pulmonary vein and the mitral valve were associated with sudden termination of local electrical activity of types 3 to 1 or 0 and were regionalized to the pulmonary vein.

Results of this study indicate that regionalized linear lesions targeted at fractionated localized recorded activity cause global changes in atrial fibrillation electrical activity, which lead to the termination of atrial fibrillation. An example of atrial fibrillation activity and termination during left atrial linear lesion is

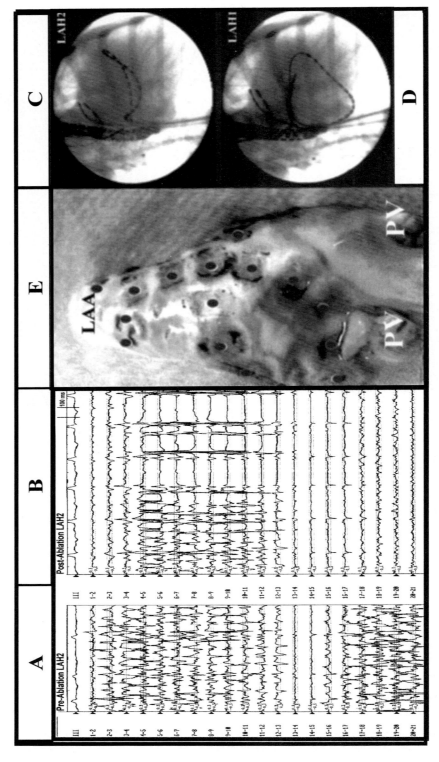

FIGURE 12-12. Local electrogram activity before and after ablation, showing the left atrial horizontal (LAH) 2 position (lesion 2). The high-level conduction block occurs in isolated left atrial tissue. **A:** Before ablation of LAH 2. **B:** After ablation of LAH 2. **C:** Radiographic image of the loop catheter in the LAH 2 position. **D:** Radiographic image of the loop catheter in the LAH 1 position. **E:** Gross anatomy of the lesion in the left atrial appendage (LAA). PV, pulmonary vein.

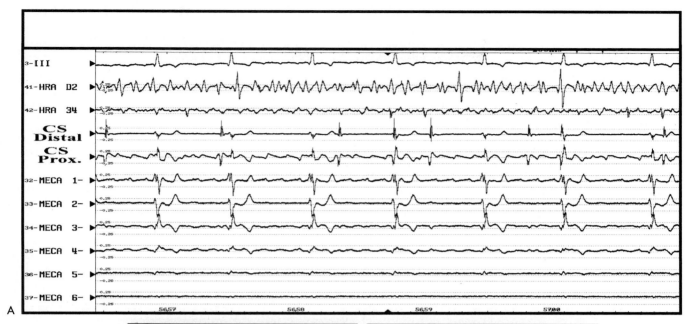
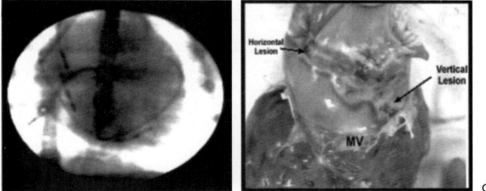

FIGURE 12-13. Example of the coronary sinus disconnection from the rest of the atria after ablation. **A:** The electrogram indicates distal coronary sinus isolation from the rest of the right atrium. **B:** Radiographic image of the loop catheter in left atrial horizontal (LAH) lesion position. **C:** Gross anatomy of the left atrium, showing horizontal and vertical lesions.

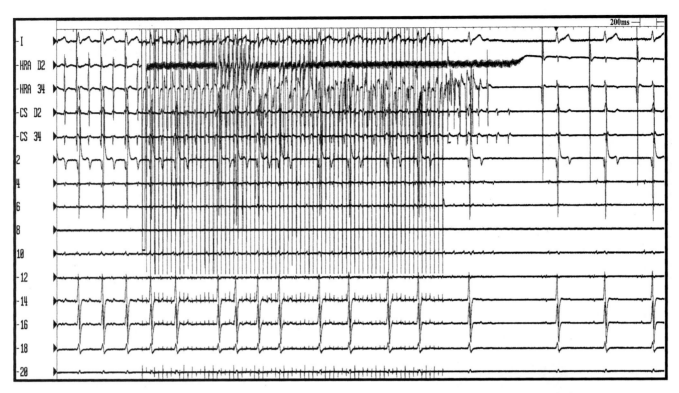

FIGURE 12-14. Conversion after burst pacing from was achieved with placement of the quadripolar distal tip in the high right atrium (HRA D2).

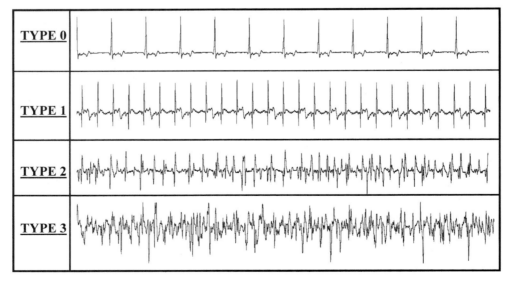

FIGURE 12-15. Grading of atrial electrical activity: type 0, normal sinus rhythm or atrial tachycardia; type 1, atrial flutter or atrial tachycardia; type 2, high-voltage atrial fibrillation with no baseline fractionation; and type 3, atrial fibrillation with baseline fractionation.

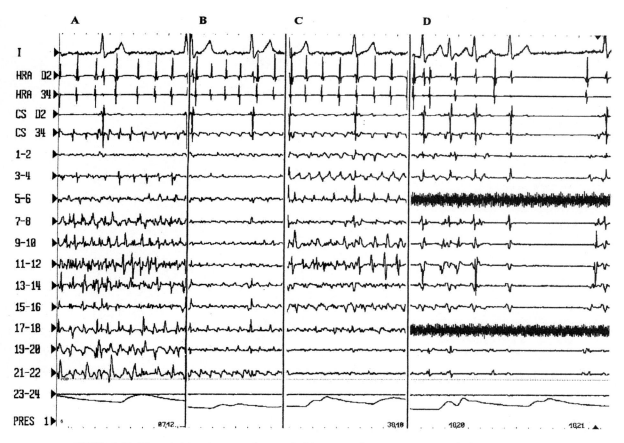

FIGURE 12-16. A 24-pole recording and ablation catheter is positioned above the mitral valve and under the pulmonary veins (PVs). **A:** Electrical activity is continuous and fractionated, especially in electrodes 7 through 14, which are under the left superior PV; activity in the coronary sinus (CS) and the high right atrium (HRA) is organized. **B:** After completion of left atrial sub-PV lesion ablation, the amplitude of the electrical activity decreased. **C:** The catheter was then placed in a vertical position, bisecting the roof of the atria and showing highly fractionated activity in electrodes 13 through 18. **D:** Atrial fibrillation fractionation decreased and converted to discrete electrogram activity followed by normal sinus rhythm during radiofrequency delivery to electrode 17.

shown in Figure 12-16 and the localized depolarization organization that it is often a prelude to conversion is shown in Figure 12-17. This finding implies localized dominance for these regions in driving the atrial fibrillation. The common characteristic of these regions in 66% of cases was type 3 atrial fibrillation. Identification of highly maximal fractionated local electrical activity provides a mappable target for regionalized ablation, most of which is under the pulmonary veins (82). The fractionated activity that was recorded in the dog model was found to be similar to the activity that was mapped in humans with atrial fibrillation whose local atrial electrical activity was mapped in the operating room before mitral valve replacement and the maze operation for the treatment of chronic atrial fibrillation (83,84).

We further hypothesized that nonlinear analysis of the local electrogram activity in the coronary sinus and right atrial appendage could predict the efficacy of linear lesions placed in either atrium to ablate atrial fibrillation. Two nonlinear dynamic measurements were calculated; the Lyapunov exponent (LE) and

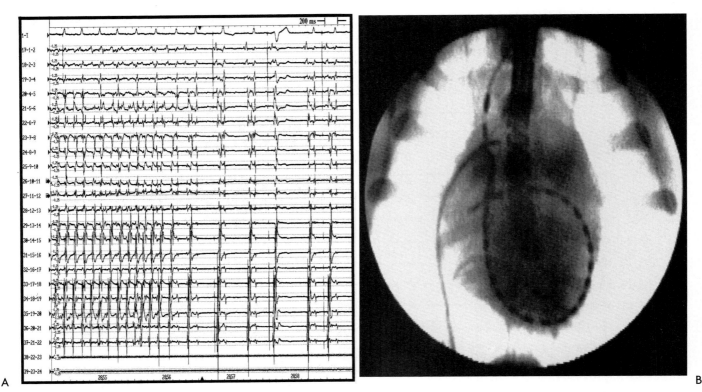

FIGURE 12-17. Spontaneous conversion from atrial fibrillation to normal sinus rhythm with a 24-ring electrode during ablation at electrode 10 at the left atrial horizontal (LAH) position as shown in the fluoroscopic image. **A:** Electrograms. **B:** Fluoroscopic image of the catheter position.

the correlation dimension (CD) on 5-second notch-filtered signals from a catheter in the coronary sinus and the high right atrium before and after ablation. The CD was calculated using the Grassberger-Procaccia algorithm. The CD, which is a predictor of the complexity of a system, steadily decreased after ablation of each lesion. Initially, the CD was 1.63 ± 0.65, and the LE was 0.121 ± 0.05. After ablation of each lesion, the CD decreased by 0.255 ± 0.19, and the LE decreased by 0.025 ± 0.014. On achieving normal sinus rhythm, the CD was 0.281 ± 0.033, and the LE was 0.006 ± 0.006. There is evidence that nonlinear dynamic measurements are good predictors of the organization of atrial electrograms from atrial fibrillation to normal sinus rhythm after consecutive generation of linear lesions. CD and LE may be used to define the efficacy of each linear lesion (85).

Long-Term Outcome of Atrial Fibrillation Ablation in the Rapid-Pacing Dog Model

Twenty-nine dogs were in spontaneous atrial fibrillation for 6 months before ablation and were monitored for 6 months after the ablation. In 7 (24%) of 29, the atrial fibrillation was converted to normal sinus rhythm with lesions that were placed in only the left atrium or right atrium. In 6 of 7 dogs, the lesions were placed in the left atrium, and in 1 dog, the lesions were placed in the right atrium. In 4 of 7, the rhythm was converted to atrial tachycardia, and in 2 of 7 dogs, only one lesion was needed to convert the atrial fibrillation. In 26 of 29 dogs, the atrial fibrillation was converted to normal sinus rhythm or to atrial tachycardia, which could have been converted with overdrive pacing. Only 3 (7%) dogs could not be converted with linear lesions in both atria. Conversion of atrial fibrillation to normal sinus rhythm or atrial tachycardia required placement of 5 ± 2 lesions. In 15 (73%) of 21 dogs, left linear lesions resulted in atrial fibrillation conversion to atrial tachycardia, and in only 6 (27%) of 21 dogs, right atrial lesions resulted in the conversion of the atrial fibrillation to atrial tachycardia. The conversion rate to normal sinus rhythm or atrial tachycardia was similar with the use of 4-mm rings (92%) and 12-mm coil electrodes (87%). However, in the short term, the 12-mm coil electrode multielectrode loop catheter design is more likely to convert the atrial fibrillation to atrial tachycardia (60% versus 42%), and similar differences were observed for nonconversion. Only 5 dogs after 4-mm multielectrode loop catheter ablations were followed for 6 months, and all of these dogs had normal sinus rhythm at the terminal study. Seven (70%) of 10 dogs after 12-mm multielectrode loop catheter ablation had normal sinus rhythm, 1 (10%) of 7 had overdriveable atrial tachycardia, 1 (10%) of 7 had sustained atrial tachycardia, and 1 (10%) of 7 had atrial fibrillation. The 6-month combined chronic rhythm outcome was 80% in normal sinus rhythm and 7% (1 dog) in each of the other rhythm states (Table 12-2).

Of the 26 dogs in which the atrial fibrillation was converted, 12 had left atrial vertical and sub-pulmonary vein lesions that connected the mitral valve ring to the dome of the atria in the anterior posterior position, 5 had only left atrial horizontal-type lesions encircling the pulmonary veins above the mitral ring, 9 had right atrial lesions that resulted in conversions (i.e., 1 right atrial isthmus and 8 right atrial loops connecting the tricuspid valve anteriorly to the right atrial appendage, to the superior vena cava, and to the inferior vena cava).

Atrial Fibrillation Prevention by Linear Lesions

We investigated whether linear atrial lesions provide protection from atrial fibrillation in two sets of dogs. One group (7 dogs weighing 35 ± 3 kg) previously had chronic atrial fibrillation caused by rapid atrial pacing, but atrial fibrillation was converted to normal sinus rhythm after the creation of linear lesions. This group is referred to as the atrial fibrillation dogs. The other group (5 dogs weighing 30 ± 4 kg) included normal dogs in normal sinus rhythm in which linear lesions were created. Rapid-pacing pacemakers were implanted in the 7 mongrel dogs. Rapid atrial pacing was maintained for 56 ± 9 days. Spontaneous, sustained atrial fibrillation was recorded after 21 ± 8 days. The dogs maintained spontaneous atrial fibrillation for 178 ± 64 days as verified by weekly rhythm evaluations by surface ECG and telemetry from the intracardiac leads. Linear lesions were made in both groups of dogs using a loop catheter capable of creating expanding loops in both atria. The catheter has fourteen 12-mm coil electrodes. Radiofrequency energy was delivered through each electrode, and power was titrated with automatic temperature control to attain an average target temperature of 70°C for 60 seconds. In the 7 atrial fibrillation dogs, normal sinus rhythm was attained after 5 ± 2 lesions were placed in the left atrium and 2 ± 1 in the right atrium. In the 5 normal dogs, linear lesions were placed in the left atrium (3 ± 1) and right atrium (2 ± 1) using the loop catheter. Rhythm status after creating of the linear lesions was monitored weekly by surface ECG and telemetry from the intracardiac pacing leads.

After 6 months of recovery, arrhythmia inducibil-

TABLE 12-2 • ACUTE AND CHRONIC HEART RHYTHM OUTCOME USING 4- TO 6-mm RING AND 12-mm COIL MULTIELECTRODE LOOP CATHETERS

Rhythm	4- To 6-mm Ring		12-mm Coil		Combined	
	Acute	Chronic	Acute	Chronic	Acute	Chronic
NSR	7/14 (50%)	5/5 (100%)	4/15 (27%)	7/10 (70%)	11/29 (38%)	12/15 (80%)
OdrAfltr	3/14 (21%)		4/15 (27%)	1/10 (10%)	7/29 (24%)	1/15 (7%)
NSR/Afltr	3/14 (21%)		5/15 (33%)	1/10 (10%)	8/29 (28%)	1/15 (7%)
AF	1/14 (7%)		2/15 (13%)	1/10 (10%)	3/29 (10%)	1/15 (7%)

NSR, normal sinus rhythm; OdrAfltr, overdrivable atrial flutter; Afltr, atrial flutter; AF, atrial fibrillation.

TABLE 12-3 • REINDUCTION OF ATRIAL FIBRILLATION WITH RAPID PACING 6 MONTHS AFTER LINEAR LESIONS

Subjects	Rhythm	Post Burst	1 Week	2 Weeks	3 Weeks	1 Month
AF dogs (paced 31 ± 8 days)	NSR	2	0	1	0	0
	Afltr	4	0	1	4	1
	AF	1	7	5	3	6
NSR dogs (paced 34 ± 5 days)	NSR	4	2	0	0	0
	Afltr	1	2	3	3	2
	AF	0	1	2	2	3

NSR, normal sinus rhythm; Afltr, atrial flutter; AF, atrial fibrillation; Burst, burst pacing (10 times at 50 msec cycle length for 5 sec).

ity was tested with burst pacing (10 times at a 50-msec cycle length for 5 seconds). In the atrial fibrillation group, after the termination of burst pacing, 2 dogs remained in normal sinus rhythm, 4 dogs exhibited atrial tachycardia, and 1 dog had nonsustained atrial fibrillation. Among the normal dogs, a run of nonsustained atrial tachycardia was induced in 1 dog (Table 12-3). Right atrial rapid pacing at 400 bpm was initiated in both groups for 33 ± 7 days. Rhythm was evaluated daily during rapid pacing and 2 weeks after the pacemaker was turned off. After the creation of linear lesions and 5 ± 1 weeks of repacing rapidly, atrial fibrillation and atrial tachycardia were induced in all the dogs. As shown in Table 12-4, within 3 days of cessation of pacing, none of the normal dogs were in atrial fibrillation, and 2 of the atrial fibrillation group remained in atrial fibrillation. Within 2 weeks, all of the normal dogs returned to normal sinus rhythm, and 1 dog from the atrial fibrillation group remained in atrial fibrillation (Figs. 12-18 through 12-20).

Based on this preliminary study, it was concluded that rapid pacing induced sustained atrial fibrillation in all paced dogs within 1 month of rapid pacing without the linear lesions. The linear lesions were highly effective in ablating the atrial fibrillation in this model. During the 6 months of recovery after the linear lesions were created, no atrial fibrillation was recorded in either group. In the atrial fibrillation group, after burst pacing for 5 seconds (10 times), normal sinus rhythm returned immediately in 2 of 7 dogs, atrial tachycardia was induced in 4 of 7, and only 1 of 7 had sustained atrial fibrillation. After 4 weeks of rapid repacing, only 2 of 7 atrial fibrillation dogs had sustained atrial fibrillation after linear lesion placement. Linear lesions in the left atrium and right atrium prevented the reinitiation of sustained atrial fibrillation in all of the normal sinus rhythm dogs. Only one normal sinus rhythm dog had nonsustained atrial tachycardia. Linear lesions did not prevent induction of atrial fibrillation in both sets of dogs as a result of rapid pacing. Constant rapid repacing re-

TABLE 12-4 • RHYTHM OUTCOMES AFTER STOPPING RAPID ATRIAL PACING POST LINEAR LESIONS

Subjects (n)	Rhythm	15 Min After Repacing Termination	3 Days After Repacing Termination	1 Week After Repacing Termination	2 Weeks After Repacing Termination
AF dogs (7)	NSR	2	4	4	4
	Afltr	2	1	1	2
	AF	3	2	2	1
NSR dogs (5)	NSR	0	2	4	5
	Afltr	2	3	1	0
	AF	3	0	0	0

NSR, normal sinus rhythm; Afltr, atrial flutter; AF, atrial fibrillation.

12. ATRIAL FIBRILLATION ABLATION

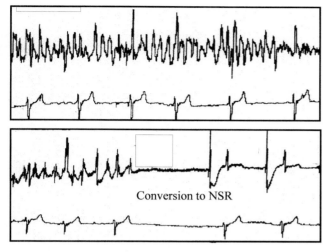

FIGURE 12-18. Examples of atrial fibrillation (AF) conversion to normal sinus rhythm (NSR). **A:** AF dog 24 weeks after AF ablation and 4 weeks of rapid pacing. **B:** In the same dog, AF was converted to NSR immediately after cessation of rapid pacing.

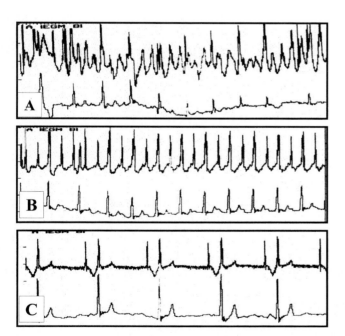

FIGURE 12-19. Sequential conversion to atrial flutter (Afltr) and normal sinus rhythm (NSR). **A:** Dog with NSR 6 months after linear lesion ablation and after 4 weeks of rapid pacing, which caused atrial fibrillation. **B:** The same NSR dog 3 days after cessation of rapid pacing that was converted to Afltr. **C:** The same NSR dog 1 week after cessation of rapid pacing that was converted to NSR.

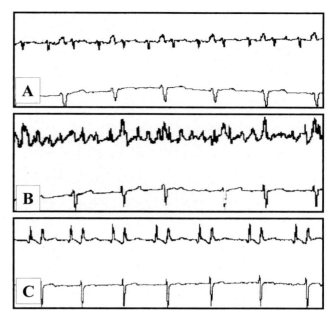

FIGURE 12-20. Conversion from atrial flutter to atrial fibrillation (AF) and normal sinus rhythm (NSR). **A:** Dog with AF 24 weeks after AF ablation with linear lesions. Atrial flutter was induced after 2 weeks of rapid repacing. **B:** In the same AF dog after 3 weeks of rapid repacing, the atrial flutter had degenerated to AF. **C:** After 3 days of cessation of rapid pacing in the same dog, spontaneous conversion to NSR occurred.

sulted in short-lived (1 to 2 weeks) atrial fibrillation and atrial tachycardia in both groups. The evidence indicates that linear lesions protect the atria from the induction of sustained atrial fibrillation (86).

Studies of Left Atrium Mechanical Function

Although the primary goal of radiofrequency ablation of atrial fibrillation is to achieve normal sinus rhythm, restoration of left atrial mechanical function is an important secondary goal. We evaluated left atrial mechanical function before and after linear lesion creation using standard transthoracic echocardiography and pulsed Doppler techniques. Two groups of 6 dogs were studied. The normal group comprised healthy dogs in normal sinus rhythm, and the atrial fibrillation group comprised dogs with chronic atrial fibrillation for 6 months due to rapid atrial pacing for 57 ± 14 days. In both groups, long linear lesions were created in the left atrium and right atrium with an expanding loop catheter.

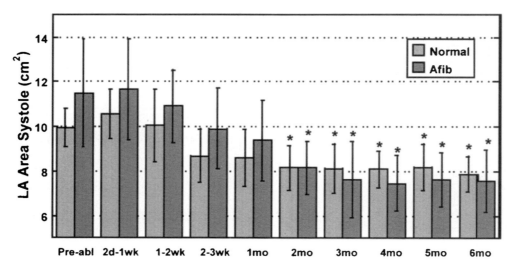

FIGURE 12-21. Changes of the left atrial (LA) systolic area from before ablation to up to 6 months after ablation in dogs with normal sinus rhythm or atrial fibrillation (*$p < 0.05$ versus atrial fibrillation before ablation and 2 days to 1 week after ablation).

Normal sinus rhythm was restored with linear lesions in the 6 atrial fibrillation dogs. In 10 of 12 dogs, overdriveable reentry-type atrial tachycardia was inducible after ablation; however, all dogs maintained normal sinus rhythm 6 months after ablation. Left ventricular function was preserved in both sets of dogs. Moderate mitral regurgitation was present in 50% of the atrial fibrillation dogs before ablation. At 6 months after ablation, 2 of 5 atrial fibrillation dogs had only mild mitral regurgitation. The left atrial systolic area was significantly larger before ablation in the atrial fibrillation group compared with the normal sinus rhythm group (12 ± 1.7 versus 10 ± 1.3 cm^2, $p < 0.032$). The atria decreased in size and reached a plateau within 2 months after ablation. The atrial size was similar in both groups and was significantly

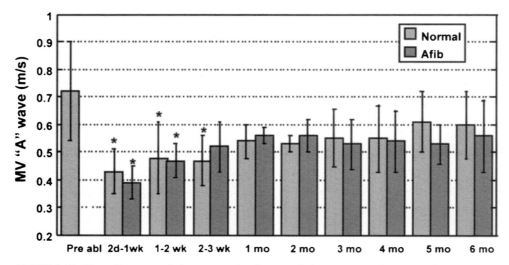

FIGURE 12-22. Changes of the maximal velocity of the transmitral A wave from before ablation to up to 6 months after ablation in dogs with normal sinus rhythm or atrial fibrillation (*$p < 0.05$ versus normal before ablation).

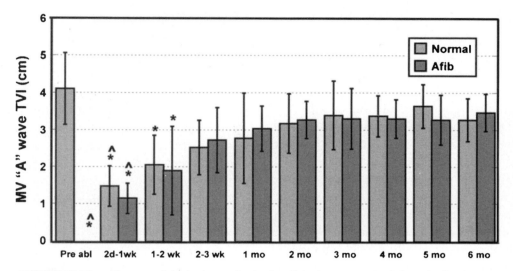

FIGURE 12-23. Changes of the integrated velocity of the late transmitral diastolic flow–time velocity integral (TVI) of the A wave from before ablation to up to 6 months after ablation in dogs with normal sinus rhythm or atrial fibrillation (*$p < 0.05$ versus normal before ablation; †$p < 0.05$ versus normal and atrial fibrillation at 2, 3, 4, 5, and 6 months).

smaller than before ablation (Fig. 12-21). Using Doppler echocardiography, no active left atrial contraction was identified in the atrial fibrillation group of dogs before conversion to normal sinus rhythm, but within 2 days after ablation, there was recorded left atrial active contraction with the maximal velocity of the transmitral A wave of 0.21 ± 0.24 m/sec. The A wave amplitude was reduced by 43% from 0.7 ± 0.2 to 0.4 ± 0.08 m/sec in the normal dogs 2 days after ablation. Atrial mechanical function was recorded within 2 months after ablation, and the difference between the two groups was not statistically significant (87–89) (Figs. 12-22 through 12-24). The equal recovery suggests that the chronic atrial fibrilla-

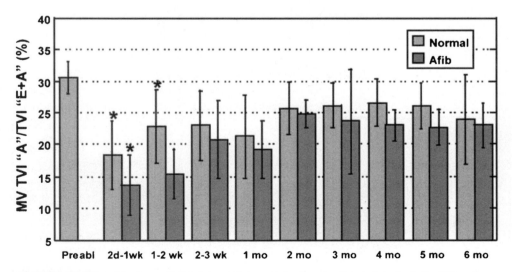

FIGURE 12-24. Changes of the late atrial contribution to the total diastolic filling from before ablation to up to 6 months after ablation in dogs with normal sinus rhythm or atrial fibrillation (*$p < 0.05$ versus normal before ablation).

tion in this rapid-pacing dog model is not from pathologic injury to the atria, but rather caused by electrical remodeling. After 6 months of recovery, there was no evidence of thrombus or changes of the heart valves.

Based on these data, significant acute reduction in left atrial mechanical activity was identified in the first week after ablation in all dogs. This finding supports the postablation need for anticoagulation to prevent strokes. For the lesion set described here, left atrial mechanical activity recovery was completed 2 months after ablation, reaching 71% to 80% of the preablation state (89). These results occurred despite the lesion endocardial surface area of 12 to 15 cm^2, suggesting that the left atrial appendage, which was not ablated, may be the principal factor in the preservation of atrial contribution to transmitral flow.

RESULTS AND PROJECTIONS

Gross and Histologic Findings

Evaluation of atrial fibrillation ablation in this model was further extended into the histopathologic characteristics of the lesions and chronic atrial function with the use of the 4-mm ring-type ablation catheter. The linear lesions were composed of thin, dense, beadlike individual lesions protruding from the endocardial and epicardial surfaces (Fig. 12-25). The individual lesions fused into one contiguous rigid cord, which was sharply different from the surrounding tissue. The average size of each bead was 6 × 7 mm, with the maximal length of the lesion up to 16 cm (i.e., left atrial circular lesion around the pulmonary veins). The lesions transected the atria, dividing them into distinct regions, some of which were completely isolated. Histologically, the lesions were characterized by extensive cartilage formation, proliferation of connective tissue, fibrosis, and the presence of chronic inflammatory cells on the epicardial site. Among these changes, some interrupted areas of relatively healthy myocardium were observed. From the endocardial side, lesions were totally covered with endothelium, and there was no sign of clot formation.

The linear lesions that were created with the 12-mm coil electrodes are shown in Figures 12-26 and 12-27. The lesions were contiguous, and unlike the

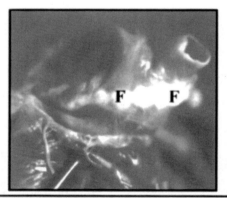
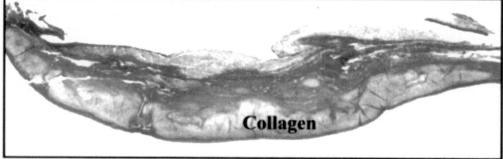

FIGURE 12-25. Histopathology of the atrial fibrillation ablation linear lesions created with the 4-mm ring-type ablation catheter. F, fibrous tissue.

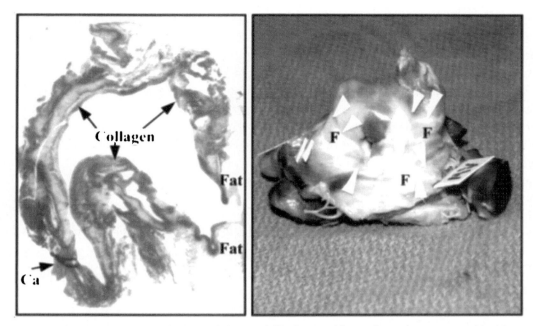

FIGURE 12-26. Histopathology of the atrial fibrillation ablation linear lesions created with the 12-mm coil electrodes. Ca, calcium, F, fibrous tissue.

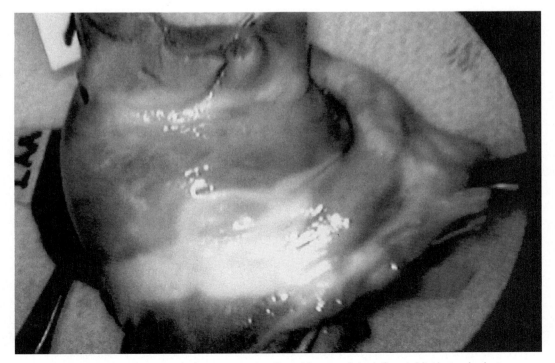

FIGURE 12-27. Gross pathology 6 months after ablation of the left atrial (LA) circular lesions created with the 12-mm coil electrodes.

lesions that were created with the 4-mm ring electrode, the lesions were flat and less calcified. The long-term organization of the radiofrequency lesion includes fibrosis, extensive formation of cartilage, and proliferation of connective tissue resulting in the formation of rigid transmural structures within the atria. Such structures have the potential to restrict atrial mechanical function. Complete endothelialization of lesions reduces the danger of thrombogenesis (81). Left atrial lesion dimensions in the atrial fibrillation and normal groups were, respectively, 19 ± 4 and 17 ± 4 cm long; 8 ± 0.9 and 7 ± 1 mm in diameter, and 15 ± 4 and 12 ± 3 cm^2 total lesion area (p was not significant between groups). Calcification was palpable in $30 \pm 24\%$ versus $53 \pm 37\%$ of lesions in the atrial fibrillation and normal groups, respectively. On histologic examination, the lesions consisted primarily of fibrous tissue, but calcium was observed in 30% to 50% of the linear lesions (86). Microscopic evaluation of the linear lesions was performed after 6 months of recovery from linear lesions. Four dogs were in normal sinus rhythm and 3 in atrial fibrillation. Histologic analysis showed that all lesions in the 4 normal sinus rhythm dogs were transmural and contiguous, and all 3 atrial fibrillation dogs had at least one non-contiguous and non-transmural lesion (1, 2, and 3 lesion gaps in each dog) (91).

What We Have Learned

Maze Operation

With the appropriate schema of surgical cuts and cryoablative lesions, atrial fibrillation can be ablated with a high long-term cure rate. Other variations of the maze, such as the compartment operation, have proven that pulmonary vein isolation is not mandatory for curing atrial fibrillation. Despite the extensive left atrial cuts, atrial mechanical function can be documented by Doppler echocardiography.

Focal Atrial Fibrillation Ablation

Paroxysmal atrial fibrillation can be mapped to ectopic foci, mostly in the superior pulmonary veins. Ablation of these foci can result in long-term cure in these patients and has a reported success rate of 100%. Identification of the ectopic foci may be difficult during the procedure because the initiation of these foci can be unpredictable. In preliminary work with pulmonary vein local electrical activity recordings and balloon catheter ablation, we found the pulmonary veins contained highly fractionated activity during atrial fibrillation, marked heterogeneity of local activity, and split potentials.

Catheter Approach to the Creation of Linear Lesions for the Ablation of Atrial Fibrillation

Initial experience has shown that atrial fibrillation ablation in the right atrium is possible but has a success rate of only 13% to 42%. Greater success can be achieved with linear lesions in both atria in patients with paroxysmal atrial fibrillation, with reported success rates between 62% and 100% (47–63). No long-term success data are available for chronic atrial fibrillation. Most of the procedures were done with the use of the catheter drag technique and were associated with considerable complication rates.

We have learned that the current ablation technology is not suitable for the creation of transmural contiguous linear lesions and that such technology is subjecting the patient to the prolonged procedures with considerable risk of complications. The loop catheter design and perhaps other designs of ablation technology, which is specifically targeted for the creation of linear lesions, should be developed if the catheter approach for the ablation of atrial fibrillation is to succeed.

Where We Are Going

Ongoing Trials

The Boston Scientific EP Technology (EPT)/multielectrode catheter ablation (MECA) phase II trial uses an array of tools, including the standard 4-mm ablation catheter, loop catheter with 12-mm coil electrodes that are 2 mm apart, and deflectable catheters with 12-mm coil electrodes that are 2 mm apart, to create linear lesions in both atria. The target population has paroxysmal and persistent atrial fibrillation. In

1998, Haines and colleagues described three patients with paroxysmal atrial fibrillation who underwent EPT/MECA ablation in the left atrium. Two of the three procedures were successful, but ablation using the same ablation system in the right atrium (8 patients) had no success (90).

Guidant's Heart Rhythm Technology (HRT) phase I clinical trial uses deflectable multielectrode ablation catheters. The Cardima Feasibility Study for microcatheter multielectrodes uses ablation catheters.

Technologic Needs: Loop Catheter Design Evaluation

For lesion generation, the loop catheter design is an effective tool to create long, contiguous, transmural linear lesions. The design was modified to 12-mm coils, which increased the efficiency of the system. In multiple studies using the acute and chronic dog model in normal sinus rhythm and chronic atrial fibrillation, we have proven that this catheter technology is capable of creating long (16 to 19 cm) linear lesions and ablating atrial fibrillation with 83% to 90% efficacy rate.

For confirmation of lesion adequacy, more than 50% reduction in the amplitude of bipolar recordings of local electrical activity and a temperature of 70°C provides a measure of lesion contiguity and transmurality. Incomplete lesions that are nontransmural, noncontiguous, or both, result in atrial tachycardia. The most important lesions to ablate (causing rapid pacing–induced atrial fibrillation) were the set of left atrial lesions, for which the total conversion to normal sinus rhythm or atrial tachycardia occurred in 15 (73%) of 21 the dogs, whereas for only 6 (27%) of 21 of right atrial lesions, ablation resulted in conversion. Linear lesion sets placed in both atria after the ablation of atrial fibrillation or atrial ablation in the normal sinus rhythm dogs was found to prevent sustained, rapid pacing–induced atrial fibrillation in 92% of the dogs.

The tissue constituting the site of ablation must be localized. Identification of highly fractionated local electrical activity provides a mappable target for regionalized ablation, most of which is under the pulmonary veins.

Histopathologic analysis of the linear lesions 6 months later revealed that the lesions were completely endothelialized and included fibrosis, extensive formation of cartilage, and proliferation of connecting tissue, resulting in the formation of rigid transmural structures within the atria.

Assessment of left atrial mechanical function revealed a 43% reduction in left atrial mechanical activity in the first week after ablation in all dogs. Left atrial mechanical activity recovery was completed 2 months after ablation, reaching 71% to 80% of the preablation state, despite the lesion endocardial surface area being 12 to 15 cm^2.

Future Techniques for the Ablation of Atrial Fibrillation

The goal of catheter-based ablation of atrial fibrillation should be safe minimal tissue destruction that allows restoration of normal sinus rhythm under autonomic nervous system control combined with recovery of atrial mechanical transport to prevent thromboembolic events and provide hemodynamic benefits for the patient.

The amount of tissue ablated should be the minimum necessary to convert and maintain the atria in normal sinus rhythm while allowing for effective recovery of atrial transport. To justify exposing the patient to this procedure, a high safety margin and the recovery of atrial mechanical function after the procedure are imperative. Theoretically, ablating most of the atrial tissues can terminate atrial fibrillation; however, if mechanical function is not restored, the risk of thromboembolic stroke remains, requiring continuous anticoagulation. Other than rate control, no mechanical benefit can be provided to the patient. If this is the outcome of a catheter-based atrial fibrillation intervention, AV node modification or AV node or His ablation, followed by permanent pacer insertion and continued anticoagulation, may be a more appropriate therapy for highly symptomatic patients form whom medical therapy has failed. Such an approach provides minimal, short-term risks and often is rewarding (91).

CONCLUSIONS

Much effort has been made in the design and testing of catheter systems and the development of methodology for the effective ablation of atrial fibrillation in humans and in experimental models. However, other than the ablation of a focal source of atrial fibrillation, which appears feasible, the ablation of persistent and chronic atrial fibrillation has been associated with mixed results and numerous complications. It is thought that the initial source of chronic atrial fibrillation is ectopic focal atrial depolarization, and the ablation of such foci can prevent the induction of chronic atrial fibrillation. Although no data support this hypothesis, in patients with paroxysmal atrial fibrillation, the attempt to map and ablate the source of arrhythmia could be rewarding for a follow-up period of 11 months. We believe that, with appropriate ablation catheter technology coupled with rapid electroanatomic mapping systems (i.e., three-dimensional intracardiac echocardiography and electrical mapping and three-dimensional guidance systems), it may be possible to reproduce maze-type atrial lesions. This goal does not exclude the use of other energy forms to create the desired lesions such as laser, cryoablation, ultrasound, and others. However, it remains to be seen whether linear lesions in the human atria provide the long-term protection from reinitiation of atrial fibrillation in the face of continued cellular degeneration and decoupling.

REFERENCES

1. Kannel WB, Abbott RD, Savage DD, McNamara PM. Coronary heart disease and atrial fibrillation: the Framingham Study. *Am Heart J* 1983;106:386–396.
2. Kannel WB, Abbott RD, Savage DD, McNamara PM. Epidemiologic features of chronic atrial fibrillation: the Framingham Study. *N Engl J Med* 1982;306:1018–1022.
3. Krahn AD, Manfreda J, Tate RB, et al. The natural history of atrial fibrillation: incidence, risk factors, and prognosis in the Manitoba follow-up study. *Am J Med* 1995;98:476–484.
4. Podrid JP. Atrial fibrillation in the elderly. *Cardiol Clin* 1999;17:173–188.
5. Furberg CD, Psaty BM, Manolio TA, et al. Prevalence of atrial fibrillation in elderly subjects (The Cardiovascular Health Study). *Am J Cardiol* 1994;74:236–241.
6. Psaty BM, Manolio TA, Kuller LH, et al. Incidence of and risk factors of atrial fibrillation in older adults. *Circulation* 1997;96:2455–2461.
7. Wolf PA, Abbott RD, Kannel WB. Atrial fibrillation as an independent risk factor for stroke: the Framingham Heart Study. *Stroke* 1991;22:983–988.
8. Coplen SE, Antman EM, Berlin JA, et al. Efficacy and safety of Quinidine therapy for maintenance of sinus rhythm after cardioversion: a meta-analysis of randomized control trials. *Circulation* 1990;82:1106–1116.
9. Flaker GC, Blackshear JL, McBride R, et al. Antiarrhythmic drug therapy and cardiac mortality in atrial fibrillation. The stroke prevention in atrial fibrillation investigators. *J Am Coll Cardiol* 1992;20:527–532.
10. Cardiac Arrhythmia Suppression Trial (CAST) Investigators. Preliminary report: effects of encainide and flecainide on mortality in a randomized trial of arrhythmia suppression after myocardial infarction. *N Engl J Med* 1989;321:406–412.
11. Vrobel TR, Miller PE, Mostow ND, Rakita L. A general overview of amiodarone toxicity: its prevention, detection, and management. *Cardiovasc Dis* 1989;31:393–426.
12. Sanoski CA, Schoen MD, Gonzalez RC, et al. Rationale, development, and clinical outcomes of a multidisciplinary amiodarone clinic. *Pharmacotherapy* 1998;18[Pt 2]:146S–151S.
13. Cox JL, Canavan TE, Schuessler RB, et al. The surgical treatment of atrial fibrillation, II: intraoperative electrophysiologic mapping and description of the electrophysiologic basis of atrial flutter and atrial fibrillation. *J Thorac Cardiovasc Surg* 1991;101:406–426.
14. Cox JL. Evoking applications of the maze procedure for atrial fibrillation [Editorial]. *Ann Thorac Surg* 1993;55:578–580.
15. Cox JL, Boineau JP, Schuessler RB, et al. Five-year experience in the maze procedure for atrial fibrillation. *Ann Thorac Surg* 1993;56:814–824.
16. Cox JL, Boineau JP, Schuessler RB, et al. Surgical interruption of atrial re-entry as a cure for atrial fibrillation. In: Olsson SB, Allessie MA, Campbell RWF, eds. *Atrial fibrillation: mechanisms and therapeutic strategies*. Armonk, NY: Futura Publishing, 1994: 373–404.
17. Cox JL, Jaquiss RDB, Schuessler RB, Boineau JP. Modification of the maze procedure for atrial flutter and atrial fibrillation. *J Thorac Cardiovasc Surg* 1995;110:485–495.
18. Sundt TM, Camillo CJ, Cox JL. The maze procedure for cure of atrial fibrillation. *Cardiol Clin* 1997;15:739–748.
19. Cox JL, Boineau JP, Schuessler RB, et al. Operation for atrial fibrillation. *Cardiol Clin* 1991;14:827–834.
20. Michelucci A, Padeletti L, Porciani MC, et al. Dispersion of refractoriness and atrial fibrillation. In: Olsson SB, Allessie MA, Campbell RWF, eds. *Atrial fibrillation: mechanisms and therapeutic strategies*. Armonk, NY: Futura Publishing, 1994:81–107.
21. Fieguth HG, Wahlers T, Borst HG. Inhibition of atrial fibrillation by pulmonary vein isolation and auricular resection—experimental study in a sheep model. *Eur J Cardiothorac Surg* 1997;11:714–721.
22. Scherf D. Studies on auricular tachycardia cured by aconitine administration. *Proc Soc Exp Biol Med* 1947;4:233–239.
23. Haissaguerre M, Marcus FI, Fischer B, Clementy J. Radiofrequency catheter ablation in unusual mechanisms of atrial fibrillation: report of 3 cases. *J Cardiovasc Electrophysiol* 1994;5:743–751.
24. Kuck KH, Hebe J, Schulter M, et al. Irregular atrial tachycardia: complex ECG pattern caused by as single focus [Abstract]. *Pacing Clin Electrophysiol* 1992;20:1106A.
25. Haissaguerre M, Jais P, Shah DC, et al. Spontaneous initiation of atrial fibrillation by ectopic beats originating in the pulmonary veins. *N Engl J Med* 1998;339:659–666.
26. Maloney JD, Milner L, Barold S, Czerska B. Two-staged biatrial linear and focal ablation to restore sinus rhythm in patients with refractory chronic atrial fibrillation: procedure experience and follow-up beyond 1 year. *Pacing Clin Electrophysiol* 1998;21[Pt 2]:2527–2532.
27. Hsieh MH, Chen SA, Tai CT, et al. Double multielectrode mapping catheters facilitate radiofrequency catheter ablation of focal atrial fibrillation originating from pulmonary veins. *J Cardiovasc Electrophysiol* 1999;10:136–144.
28. Nathan H, Eliakim M. The junction between the left atrium

and the pulmonary veins: an anatomic study of the human heart. *Circulation* 1966;34:412–422.
29. Rexford C, Calhoun LM. The extent of cardiac muscle in the great veins of the dog. *Anat Rec* 1964;150:249–256.
30. Masani F. Node-like cells in the myocardial layer of the pulmonary vein of rats: an ultrastructural study. *J Anat* 1986;145:133–142.
31. Moe GK. On the multiple wavelet hypothesis of atrial fibrillation. *Arch Int Pharmacodyn Ther* 1962;140:183–188.
32. Moe GK, Rheinholdt WC, Abildshov J. A computer model of atrial fibrillation. *Am Heart J* 1964;67:200–220.
33. Lammen WJ, Allessie MA. Pathophysiology of atrial fibrillation: current aspects. *Hertz* 1993;18:1–8.
34. Konings KTS, Kirchhof CJHJ, Smeets JRLM, et al. Arrhythmias/innervation/pacing: high density mapping of electrically induced atrial fibrillation in humans. *Circulation* 1994;89:1665–1680.
35. Allessie MA, Rensma PL, Brugada J, et al. Pathophysiology of atrial fibrillation. In: Zipes D, Jaliffe J, eds. *Cardiac electrophysiology: from cell to bedside.* Philadelphia: WB Saunders, 1995:548–559.
36. Allessie M, Lammen WJ, Bonke F, et al. Experimental evaluation of Moe's multiple wavelet hypothesis of atrial fibrillation. In: Zipes D, Jaliffe J, eds. *Cardiac electrophysiology and arrhythmia.* New York: Grune & Stratton, 1985:265–275.
37. Tse H-F, Lau C-P, Ayers GM. Heterogeneous changes in electrophysiologic properties in the paroxysmal and chronically fibrillating human atrium. *J Cardiovasc Electrophysiol* 1999;10:125–135.
38. Allessie MA. Atrial electrophysiologic remodelling. *J Cardiovasc Electrophysiol* 1998;9:1378–1393.
39. Cosio FG. Intra-atrial conduction and atrial fibrillation. In: Olsson SB, Allessie MA, Campbell RWF, eds. *Atrial fibrillation: mechanisms and therapeutic strategies.* Armonk, NY: Futura Publishing, 1994:51–65.
40. Wijffels MCEF, Kirchhof CJHJ, Dorland R, Allessie MA. Atrial fibrillation begets atrial fibrillation: a study in awake chronically instrumented goats. *Circulation* 1995;92:1954–1968.
41. Zipes DP. Electrophysiological remodeling of the heart owing to rate. *Circulation* 1997;95:1745–1748.
42. Zipes D. Atrial fibrillation: a tachycardia induced atrial cardiomyopathy. *Circulation* 1997;95:562–564.
43. Gallaghar MM, Obel OA, Camm AJ. Tachycardia induced atrial myopathy: an important mechanism in the pathophysiology of atrial fibrillation. *J Cardiovasc Electrophysiol* 1997;8:1065–1074.
44. Narayan SM, Cain ME, Smith JM. Atrial fibrillation. *Lancet* 1997;350:943–950.
45. Kalman JM, Scheinman MM. Radiofrequency catheter ablation for atrial fibrillation. *Cardiol Clin* 1997;15:721–737.
46. Haissaguerre M, Gencel L, Fischer B, et al. Successful catheter ablation of atrial fibrillation. *J Cardiovasc Electrophysiol* 1994;5:1045–1052.
47. Jais P, Haissaguerre M, Shah DC, et al. A focal source of atrial fibrillation treated by discrete radiofrequency ablation. *Circulation* 1997;95:572–576.
48. Haisssaguerre M, Jais P, Shah DC, et al. Right and left atrial radiofrequency catheter of therapy of paroxysmal atrial fibrillation. *J Cardiovasc Electrophysiol* 1996;7:1132–1144.
49. Jais P, Shah DC, Takahashi A, Haissaguerre M, Clementy J. Long-term follow-up after right atrial radiofrequency catheter treatment of paroxysmal atrial fibrillation. *Pacing Clin Electrophysiol* 1998;21[Pt 2]:2533–2538.
50. Man KC, Daoud E, Knight B, et al. Right atrial radiofrequency catheter ablation of paroxysmal atrial fibrillation. *J Am Coll Cardiol* 1996;27[Suppl A]:188A.
51. Garg A, Finneran W, Mollerus M, et al. Right atrial compartmentalization using radiofrequency catheter ablation for management of patients with refractory atrial fibrillation. *J Cardiovasc Electrophysiol* 1999;10:763–771.
52. Hwang C, Karaguezian HS, Chen PS. The left atrial tract within the ligament of Marshall as the source for focal atrial fibrillation. *Pacing Clin Electrophysiol* 1998;21[Pt 2]:804A.
53. Hwang C, Karaguezian HS, Chen PS. Idiopathic paroxysmal atrial fibrillation induced by focal discharge mechanism in the left superior pulmonary veins: possible roles of the ligament of Marshall. *J Cardiovasc Electrophysiol* 1999;10:636–648.
54. Chen SA, Tai CT, Yu WC, et al. Right atrial focal atrial fibrillation: electrophysiologic characteristics and radiofrequency catheter ablation. *J Cardiovasc Electrophysiol* 1999;10:328–335.
55. Maloney JD, Milner L, Markel M, et al. Biatrial linear and focal ablation to restore sinus rhythm in patients with refractory atrial fibrillation, procedure experience and follow-up beyond one year. *Pacing Clin Electrophysiol* 1998;21[Pt 2]:922A.
56. Kuck KH, Ernst S, Khanedani A, et al. Clinical follow-up after primary catheter based ablation of atrial fibrillation using the CARTO system. *Pacing Clin Electrophysiol* 1998;21[Pt 2]:868A.
57. Gaita F, Riccardi R, Calo L, et al. Atrial mapping and radiofrequency catheter in patients with idiopathic atrial fibrillation. *Circulation* 1998;97:2136–2145.
58. Swartz JF, Pellersels G, Silvers J, et al. A catheter based curative approach to atrial fibrillation in humans. *Circulation* 1994;90[Suppl 1]:335A.
59. Swartz JF III. Ablation of atrial fibrillation. Presented at the the 17th annual scientific sessions of the North American Society of Pacing and Electrophysiology [Audiotape SY4]. Seattle, Wash., May 15, 1996.
60. Avitall B, Hare J, Mughal K, et al. Ablation of atrial fibrillation in a dog model. *J Am Coll Cardiol* 1994;[Suppl]:276A.
61. Avitall B, Hare J, Mughal K, et al. A catheter system to ablate atrial fibrillation in a sterile pericarditis dog model. *Pacing Clin Electrophysiol* 1994;17[Pt 2]:774A.
62. Avitall B, Hare J, Mughal K, et al. Right-sided driven atrial fibrillation in a sterile pericarditis dog model. *Pacing Clin Electrophysiol* 1994;17[Pt 2]:774A.
63. Avitall B, Hare J, Helms R. Vagally mediated atrial fibrillation in a dog model can be ablated by placing linear radiofrequency lesions at the junction of the right atrial appendage and the superior vena cava. *Pacing Clin Electrophysiol* 1995;18[Pt 2]:857A.
64. Morillo CA, Klein GJ, Jones DL, Guiraudon CM. Electrophysiology/arrhythmias: chronic rapid atrial pacing: structural, functional and electrophysiological characteristics of a new model of sustained atrial fibrillation. *Circulation* 1995;91:1588–1595.
65. Kotov A, Bharati S, Helms RW, et al. The chronic atrial fibrillation canine model: a new approach to increase yield and efficiency. *J Am Coll Cardiol* 1997;29[Suppl A]:471A.
66. Elvan A, Huang X, Pressler ML, Zipes DP. Radiofrequency catheter ablation of atria eliminates pacing-induced sustained atrial fibrillation and reduces connexin 43 in dogs. *Circulation* 1997;96:1675–1685.
67. Elvan A, Rigden LB, Kisanuki A, et al. Radiofrequency catheter ablation of the atria effectively abolishes pacing induced chronic atrial fibrillation. *Pacing Clin Electrophysiol* 1995;18[Pt 2]:856A.
68. Elvan A, Wylie K, Zipes DP. Pacing-induced chronic atrial fibrillation impairs sinus node function in dogs. Electrophysiologic remodeling. *Circulation* 1996;94:2953–2960.
69. Elvan A, Pride HP, Eble JN, Zipes DP. Radiofrequency catheter ablation of the atria reduces inducibility and duration of atrial fibrillation in dogs. *Circulation* 1995;91:2235–2244.
70. Kempler P, Littman L, Chuang CH, et al. Radiofrequency abla-

tion of the right atrium: acute and chronic effects. *Pacing Clin Electrophysiol* 1994;17[Pt 2]:797A.
71. Pappone C, Oreto G, Lamberti F, et al. Catheter ablation of paroxysmal atrial fibrillation using a 3D mapping system. *Circulation* 1999;100:1203–1208.
72. Gepstein L, Hayam G, Shpun S, et al. Atrial linear ablations in pigs: chronic effects on atrial electrophysiology and pathology. *Circulation* 1999;100:419–426.
73. Avitall B, Helms R, Koblish J, et al. The creation of linear contiguous lesions in the atria with an expandable loop catheter. *J Am Coll Cardiol* 1999;33:972–984.
74. Gupta G, Millard S, Urbonas A, et al. The creation of linear lesions to ablate atrial fibrillation: 12-mm coil electrodes vs. 4-mm ring electrodes. *Pacing Clin Electrophysiol* 1998;21[Pt 2]:804A.
75. Haines D. The biophysics of radiofrequency catheter ablation in the heart: the importance of temperature monitoring. *Pacing Clin Electrophysiol* 1993;16:587–591.
76. Avitall B, Kotov A, Helms R. New monitoring criteria for transmural ablation of atrial tissues. *Circulation* 1996;94:I-904A.
77. Avitall B, Helms R, Kotov A, et al. The use of temperature versus local depolarization amplitude to monitor atrial lesion maturation during the creation of linear lesions in both atria. *Circulation* 1996;94:I-904A.
78. Avitall B, Helms R, Chiang W, Perlman B. Nonlinear atrial radiofrequency lesions are arrhythmogenic: a study of skipped lesions in the normal atria. *Circulation* 1995;92:I-265A.
79. Avitall B, Gupta G, Bharati S, et al. Atrial fibrillation in the chronic dog model: the long term success and failure. *Circulation* 1997;96:I-382A.
80. Avitall B, Kotov A, Helms RW, et al. Transcatheter ablation of chronic atrial fibrillation in the canine rapid atrial pacing model: is the cure worse than the disease? *J Am Coll Cardiol* 1997;29[Suppl A]:32A.
81. Avitall B, Gupta G, Bharati S, et al. Are transmural contiguous lesions essential? Postatrial fibrillation ablation: lesion morphology vs. outcome. *J Am Coll Cardiol* 1998;31[Pt 2]:367A.
82. Avitall B, Kotov A, Bharati S, et al. Mapping of atrial fibrillation: directed localized ablation of fractionated local electrical activity confers conversion. *Circulation* 1997;96:I-382A.
83. Avitall B, Hartz R, Bharati S, et al. The correlation of local histology with fractionated local electrical activity during atrial fibrillation in patients undergoing the maze procedure and mitral valve replacement. *Pacing Clin Electrophysiol* 1996;19[Pt 2]:725A.
84. Avitall B, Bharati S, Kotov A, et al. Histopathologic similarities between the human mitral disease chronic atrial fibrillation and the canine rapid pacing model of chronic atrial fibrillation. *Pacing Clin Electrophysiol* 1997;20:1139A.
85. Gupta G, Helms R, Kotov A, et al. Chaos analysis predicts stepwise changes in the character of atrial fibrillation prior to termination by the creation of linear lesions. *Circulation* 1997;96:I-259A.
86. Avitall B, Urbonas A, Millard S, Helms R. Do linear lesion provide protection from induction of atrial fibrillation? *Pacing Clin Electrophysiol* 1999;22[Pt 2]:893A.
87. Avitall B, Helms R, Chiang W, Kotov A. The impact of transcatheter generated atrial linear radiofrequency lesions on atrial function and contractility. *Pacing Clin Electrophysiol* 1996;19[Pt 2]:698A.
88. Avitall B, Urbonas A, Gupta G, et al. Intra-atrial ultrasound pre and post linear lesions: alterations in atrial mechanical function. *Circulation* 1998;98:I-643A.
89. Urbonas A, Urboniene D, Gupta G, et al. Time course of atrial rhythm and mechanical recovery following the creation of linear lesions in the left and right atria in normal dogs vs. chronic atrial fibrillation model dogs. *Pacing Clin Electrophysiol* 1998;21[Pt 2]:963A.
90. Haines DE, Langberg JJ, Lesh MD, et al. Catheter ablation of atrial fibrillation using the multiple electrode catheter ablation (MECA) system: preliminary clinical results. *Pacing Clin Electrophysiol* 1998;21[Pt 2]:832A.
91. Feld GK, Fleck RP, Fujimura OP, et al. Electrophysiology/pacing: control of rapid ventricular response by radiofrequency catheter modification of the atrioventricular node in patients with medically refractory atrial fibrillation. *Circulation* 1994;90:2299–2307.

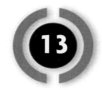

ABLATION OF IDIOPATHIC LEFT VENTRICULAR TACHYCARDIA, RIGHT VENTRICULAR OUTFLOW TACHYCARDIA, AND BUNDLE BRANCH REENTRY TACHYCARDIA

• • •

WILLIAM M. MILES, RAUL D. MITRANI

The purpose of this chapter is to delineate the characteristics, mechanisms, and ablation techniques for the two varieties of ventricular tachycardia most amenable to radiofrequency ablation: idiopathic ventricular tachycardia and bundle branch reentrant ventricular tachycardia (Table 13-1). Ventricular tachycardia is most commonly associated with coronary artery disease. The efficacy of ablation for ventricular tachycardia associated with coronary artery disease has been limited by several factors: (1) difficulty in the radiofrequency energy penetrating scarred endocardium or clot; (2) intramyocardial or epicardial origin of the ventricular tachycardia; (3) difficulty identifying an appropriate ablation site to eliminate the complex ventricular tachycardia circuit; (4) the existence of multiple ventricular tachycardia morphologies or sites in a single patient; (5) the hemodynamic instability of ventricular tachycardia in many patients, precluding adequate mapping; and (6) the progressive nature of the underlying disease, leading to the emergence of new ventricular tachycardias over time. Although ablation techniques continue to improve, ablation is usually not considered the first-line therapy in patients with ventricular tachycardia due to coronary artery disease (1–4); antiarrhythmic drug therapy or implantable cardioverter-defibrillator (ICD) therapy is more commonly used. Ventricular tachycardia in patients with no apparent structural heart disease (i.e., idiopathic ventricular tachycardia) (5–8), although not as frequently encountered as ventricular tachycardia in patients with coronary artery disease, can be eliminated by radiofrequency ablation in a high percentage of patients (9–10). Idiopathic ventricular tachycardias usually are uniform, hemodynamically stable, and focal in origin, and are not associated with underlying cardiac pathology, which can interfere with delivery of ablation energy to the site of the ventricular tachycardia origin. Ablation may be considered as the first-line therapy for patients with symptomatic idiopathic ventricular tachycardia.

The only other ventricular tachycardia for which ablation is considered as the first-line therapy is bundle branch reentrant ventricular tachycardia (11,12). This ventricular tachycardia usually occurs in the setting of significant myocardial disease but is characterized by a well-defined macro-reentrant circuit involving the bundle branches and intervening myocardium. After the diagnosis is established and the macro-reentrant circuit defined, it is relatively easy to ablate a bundle branch to eliminate the arrhythmia,

TABLE 13-1 • CATHETER ABLATION FOR VENTRICULAR TACHYCARDIAS (VTs)

Arrhythmia	Ablation Efficacy
Idiopathic VT	+++
Bundle branch reentry	+++
Sustained VT (incessant)	++
Sustained VT (inducible/stable)	+
Sustained VT (unstable)	−
Polymorphic VT	−
Ventricular fibrillation	−

+++, consider as first-line therapy; ++, reasonable success if drugs fail; +, acceptable therapy for particularly refractory or recurrent cases; −, catheter ablation not indicated.

although patient survival is limited by the underlying myocardial pathology.

IDIOPATHIC VENTRICULAR TACHYCARDIA

Characteristics

Idiopathic ventricular tachycardia (5–8) accounts for up to 10% of patients with ventricular tachycardia referred to specialized electrophysiology centers. Related but not synonymous terms include right ventricular tachycardia, repetitive monomorphic ventricular tachycardia, catecholamine-sensitive ventricular tachycardia, exercise-induced ventricular tachycardia, adenosine-sensitive ventricular tachycardia, and verapamil-sensitive ventricular tachycardia. Buxton and colleagues (13) reported that 27% of their patients with idiopathic ventricular tachycardia were asymptomatic, 40% presented with palpitations, 43% had dizziness, and 23% had syncope. Cardiac arrest has been reported, but is rare (14). Because of incomplete understanding of tachycardia mechanisms, a universally accepted classification of these tachycardias has not yet been developed. The ventricular tachycardia may be classified by the clinical pattern such as repetitive monomorphic ventricular tachycardia (i.e., multiple episodes of mostly nonsustained and self-terminating ventricular tachycardia interrupted by occasional sinus beats) or paroxysmal sustained ventricular tachycardia (i.e., episodes of sustained ventricular tachycardia separated by periods of sinus rhythm). The site of ventricular tachycardia origin can be used for classification. Approximately 70% of ventricular tachycardia cases arise from the right ventricle (mostly the right ventricular outflow tract) and have a QRS morphology resembling a left bundle branch block. Idiopathic ventricular tachycardia arising from the left ventricle usually has a right bundle branch block QRS morphology. Idiopathic ventricular tachycardia may also be classified by its response to pharmacologic or physiologic manipulations, such as exercise, or response to catecholamines, verapamil, and adenosine.

Potential mechanisms include reentry, abnormal automaticity, and triggered activity due to afterdepolarizations. Abnormalities of autonomic innervation have been reported (15): in nine patients with a structurally normal heart and ventricular tachycardia, five patients (55%) had regional left ventricular sympathetic denervation demonstrated with ^{123}I-labeled *meta*-iodobenzylguanidine (^{123}I-MIBG) scintigraphy, compared with none of nine control patients with a structurally normal heart ($p = 0.029$) (Fig. 13-1). Five patients underwent right ventricular radiofrequency ablation of ventricular tachycardia, and sympathetic denervation occurred adjacent to the ablation site in one of these patients. The role of regional cardiac sympathetic denervation in arrhythmogenesis has not been determined, but it could be related to the frequent provocation of idiopathic ventricular tachycardia by exercise or catecholamines. Regional abnormalities of left ventricular sympathetic innervation have been reported in 83% of patients with arrhythmogenic right ventricular dysplasia (16).

Results of the patient evaluation, including physical examination, electrocardiogram (ECG), and echocardiogram, are normal. In selected patients, left and right ventriculography, coronary angiography, magnetic resonance imaging (MRI), and endomyocardial biopsy may be performed to exclude structural heart disease. Carlson and coworkers (17) reported right ventricular abnormalities in 21 of 22 patients with right ventricular outflow ventricular tachycardia using cine-MRI. These abnormalities included fixed focal wall thinning, excavation, and decreased systolic thickening localized to the right ventricular outflow tract. Echocardiography showed abnormalities in only 2 of 21 patients. Similar right ventricular MRI

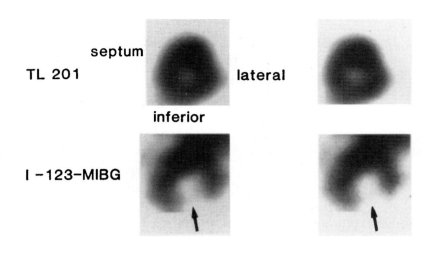

FIGURE 13-1. Short-axis thallium-201 (TL 201) and iodine-123-metaiodobenzylguanidine (I-123-MIBG) images from a patient with a structurally normal heart and nonsustained ventricular tachycardia. Notice the decreased inferior uptake *(arrows)* of I-123-MIBG imaging compared with normal uptake on thallium-201 imaging, consistent with sympathetic denervation. (From Mitrani R, Klein LS, Miles WM, et al. Regional cardiac sympathetic denervation in patients with ventricular tachycardia in the absence of coronary artery disease. *J Am Coll Cardiol* 1993; 22:1344–1353, with permission.)

abnormalities have been reported by others (18–20), although the relationship between the location of these abnormalities and the tachycardia ablation site is inconsistent. Right ventricular outflow ventricular tachycardia may arise from a diverticulum in the interventricular septum at the right ventricular outflow tract that is demonstrable by angiography (21). Right ventricular outflow tract ventricular tachycardia has also been reported after blunt chest trauma (22).

Repetitive monomorphic ventricular tachycardia (23,24) usually occurs in young or middle-aged patients. These patients may present with dizziness or (rarely) syncope but are frequently asymptomatic. The arrhythmias are often associated with physical or emotional stress, but exercise may suppress the arrhythmia in some patients. ECG features include repetitive runs of nonsustained ventricular tachycardia interspersed with normal sinus rhythm (Fig. 13-2).

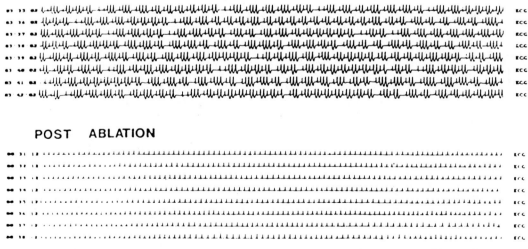

FIGURE 13-2. Electrocardiographic tracings from a patient with no structural heart disease who presented with repetitive monomorphic ventricular tachycardia. The spontaneous arrhythmia *(top)* is illustrated before ablation. After ablation *(bottom)*, all spontaneous ventricular arrhythmia was eliminated. (From Klein LS, Shih H-T, Hackett FK, et al. Radiofrequency catheter ablation of ventricular tachycardia in patients without structural heart disease. *Circulation* 1992;85:1666–1671, with permission.)

Premature ventricular contractions (PVCs) and couplets are common. Ventricular tachycardia usually has the morphology of a left bundle branch block with a normal or right axis (i.e., right ventricular outflow tract ventricular tachycardia). These patients usually do not have inducible ventricular tachycardia with programmed ventricular stimulation. Rarely, tachycardia-induced cardiomyopathy may occur because of repetitive monomorphic ventricular tachycardia and may improve after ventricular tachycardia ablation (25).

Patients with paroxysmal sustained monomorphic ventricular tachycardia (26) present with symptoms similar to those of repetitive monomorphic ventricular tachycardia, but in the former group, ventricular tachycardia tends to be episodic and sustained and therefore more symptomatic. This type of ventricular tachycardia is more often inducible with programmed stimulation, often during isoproterenol infusion. Lerman and associates (26) demonstrated that these patients frequently have ventricular tachycardia initiated and terminated by programmed stimulation. Ventricular tachycardia induction is often facilitated by isoproterenol (Fig. 13-3), and can be terminated with

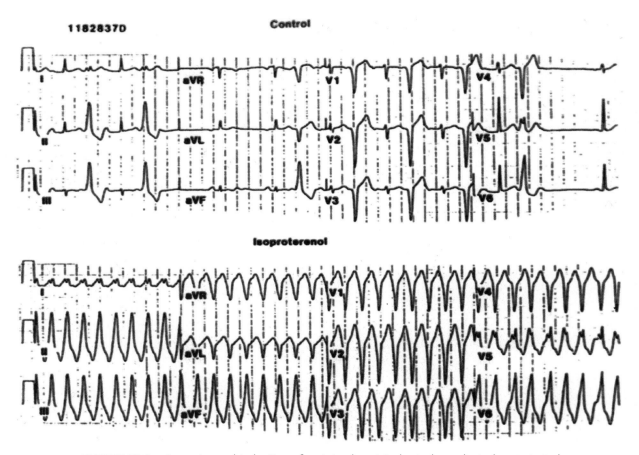

FIGURE 13-3. Isoproterenol induction of sustained ventricular tachycardia is demonstrated by the two scalar 12-lead electrocardiograms from a patient with exercise-induced ventricular tachycardia (VT). The top tracing is taken at rest, when the patient is having only ventricular extrasystoles. The bottom tracing shows sustained VT that occurred spontaneously during isoproterenol infusion. The QRS morphology of the VT is typical for right ventricular outflow tract VT. Notice that the premature ventricular contractions (PVCs) that occurred at rest are morphologically identical to the VT. Often, PVCs are all that can be induced during an electrophysiology study, and they can be used successfully as a target to ablate VT. (From Klein LS, Miles WM. Ventricular tachycardia in patients with normal hearts. *Cardiol Rev* 1993; 1:336–339, with permission.)

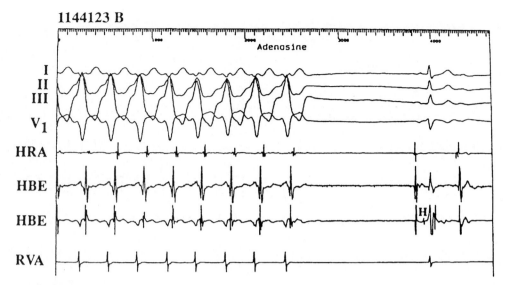

FIGURE 13-4. Termination of ventricular tachycardia (VT) with intravenous adenosine. Sustained VT arising from the right ventricular outflow tract is demonstrated on the left. Fourteen seconds after the administration of intravenous adenosine, VT stops, and sinus rhythm is restored, consistent with adenosine-sensitive VT. HRA, high right atrium; HBE, His bundle electrogram; RVA, right ventricular apex. (From Miles WM, Klein LS. Radiofrequency ablation of idiopathic ventricular tachycardia and bundle branch reentrant tachycardia. In: Singer I, ed. *Interventional cardiology*. Baltimore: Williams & Wilkins, 1996:383–412, with permission.)

adenosine (Fig. 13-4), verapamil, the Valsalva maneuver, or carotid massage. Beta blockade either terminates ventricular tachycardia or prevents ventricular tachycardia induction in these patients. The mechanism is therefore thought to be triggered activity mediated by cyclic AMP (cAMP). The prognosis usually is good for these patients, but occasionally, syncope and rare deaths have been reported.

Idiopathic Left Ventricular Tachycardia

Lerman and colleagues (27) postulated three distinct subgroups of idiopathic left ventricular tachycardia based on mechanism and pharmacologic sensitivity. The most prevalent form is a verapamil-sensitive intrafascicular tachycardia that originates in the region of the left posterior fascicle (28–34). It is adenosine insensitive, can be entrained by pacing techniques, and is thought to be caused by reentry. The second subgroup is analogous to adenosine-sensitive right ventricular outflow ventricular tachycardia. It may originate from deep within the interventricular septum and exit from the left side of the septum (left ventricular outflow tachycardia is discussed later). It also is verapamil sensitive and is thought to result from cAMP-mediated triggered activity. The third subgroup is propranolol sensitive. It is neither initiated nor terminated by programmed electrical stimulation, nor is it sensitive to verapamil, but it is transiently suppressed by adenosine. This subgroup is most consistent with an automatic mechanism.

Patients with verapamil-sensitive left septal ventricular tachycardia (28–34) are generally young and usually symptomatic with sustained ventricular tachycardia. The ventricular tachycardia has the morphology of a right bundle branch block with a leftward axis (Fig. 13-5) and is usually inducible with programmed ventricular stimulation. The ventricular tachycardia origin is usually at the inferior left ventricular midseptum or apex in the region of the posterior fascicle, although occasionally, it may originate from the anterior septum and have a rightward axis (35–40). Ventricular tachycardia is unresponsive to beta blockers or adenosine. The prognosis usually is good, but these patients may be highly symptomatic. Syncope may

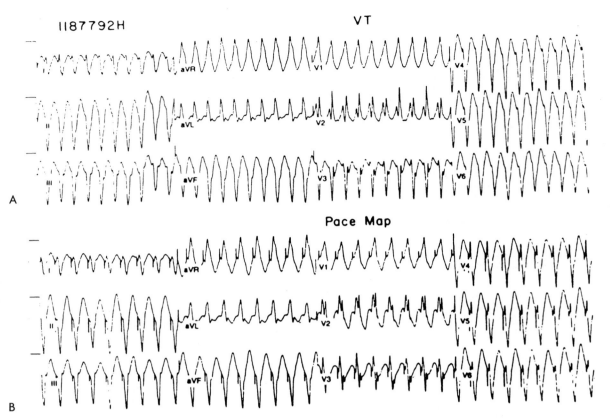

FIGURE 13-5. Scalar electrocardiogram of a patient with verapamil-sensitive left ventricular tachycardia (VT). The QRS morphology is that of a right bundle branch block with extreme left axis deviation. This patient did not have structural heart disease. **A:** The spontaneous episode of VT. **B:** Pace map made at during the electrophysiology study shows a QRS morphology during pacing from the successful ablation site similar to that of VT. (From Klein LS, Miles WM. Ablative therapy for ventricular arrhythmias. *Progr Cardiovasc Dis* 1995;37:225–242, with permission.)

occur and, rare sudden deaths have been reported. Although the mechanism of this tachycardia may not always be uniform, investigators have found that idiopathic left ventricular tachycardia can be entrained, suggesting reentry as a mechanism (41). The reentrant circuit may involve the distal left specialized conduction system, because ablation experience has shown that distinct fascicular potentials are often recorded before ventricular activation at successful sites (42). Detailed anatomy of the reentrant circuit in this arrhythmia has not been defined. However, ablation of the midseptum at locations 2 to 4 cm from the more apical tachycardia exit site can eliminate the tachycardia, suggesting that the mechanism is probably macroreentry encompassing the middle and apical interventricular septum (43,44).

Idiopathic Ventricular Tachycardia in Children

Idiopathic ventricular tachycardia in infancy and childhood is rare and has not been as extensively studied. The Association for European Pediatric Cardiology reported a retrospective multicenter study of 98 pediatric patients with monomorphic ventricular tachycardia and no structural heart disease (45). The mean age was 5.4 years (range, 0.1 to 15.1 years), and 27% of patients had ventricular tachycardia as infants. Clinical symptoms were present in 36% of patients, of which one third (12% of the whole population) were severe (i.e., heart failure or syncope). There were no deaths after a mean follow-up of 47 months (range, 12 to 182 months). Sixty-four percent of patients were free of ventricular tachycardia at final follow-up without antiarrhythmic drug therapy (7 patients were successfully ablated). The prognosis was significantly better when ventricular tachycardia occurred in the first year of life (ventricular tachycardia resolution in 87% of patients) than when ventricular tachycardia occurred after the first year of life (ventricular tachycardia resolution in 56%). Ventricular tachycardia presumably arising from the right ventricle was associated with significantly fewer symptoms than ventricular tachycardia arising from the left ventricle (25% versus 67% of patients) and a higher rate of ventricular tachycardia resolution (76% versus 37%).

The safety and efficacy of ventricular tachycardia ablation in the right ventricular outflow tract of children older than 6 years of age is probably comparable to that in adults (46). However, studies of radiofrequency lesions in the ventricles of infant lambs have suggested that these lesions enlarge over time (47). The long-term safety of ventricular tachycardia ablation in very young children is unknown.

Management and Differential Diagnosis of Idiopathic Ventricular Tachycardia

Pharmacologic management for idiopathic ventricular tachycardia usually involves beta blockers or calcium blockers, depending on which has been demonstrated to be more effective in any particular patient. Membrane-active antiarrhythmic drugs (class I or class III) are often effective, but the risk-benefit ratio may not warrant use of these medications since these varieties of ventricular tachycardia are rarely life threatening, and effective ablation techniques are available. Catheter ablation is indicated for patients in whom antiarrhythmic drugs have been ineffective or are not tolerated. Catheter ablation may be the therapy of choice in patients who wish to avoid long-term drug therapy. Ablation has been effective in patients for eliminating frequent, severely symptomatic, monomorphic, drug-refractory ventricular ectopy (48–51), but should not be considered for most patients with benign ventricular ectopy (52).

Patients with idiopathic ventricular tachycardia provide potentially the simplest substrate for ventricular tachycardia ablation. They have a stable monomorphic ventricular tachycardia that is usually tolerated long enough for mapping, in absence of scar, fibrosis, hypertrophy, or other abnormality of cardiac muscle to interfere with adequate delivery of the ablation energy to the ventricular tachycardia focus. Most of these patients do not have progressive myocardial disease that would be associated with subsequent appearance of new ventricular tachycardia foci. However, an occasional patient thought to have idiopathic ventricular tachycardia arising from the right ventricle, especially if ventricular tachycardia is not arising from the right ventricular outflow tract, may instead have an early form of arrhythmogenic right ventricular dysplasia (53) (Table 13-2). In these patients, electrophysiologic study may reveal more than one form of ventricular tachycardia. Ablative therapy, although still possibly effective, has a lower success rate because of the multiple ventricular tachycardia morphologies and because progressive myocardial disease may allow appearance of new ventricular tachycardia foci in the future. Thinning of the right ventricular wall in arrhythmogenic right ventricular dysplasia may pose an increased risk of cardiac perforation during the ablation procedure. Studies have shown that ventricular tachycardia in arrhythmogenic right ventricular dysplasia shows many of the characteristics of ventricular tachycardia due to myocardial infarction, and entrainment techniques can be used to characterize reentry circuits and guide ablation, with 8 of 19 ventricular tachycardias rendered noninducible in one study (54–56). Although ablation has been clinically suc-

TABLE 13-2 • ARRHYTHMOGENIC RIGHT VENTRICULAR DYSPLASIA VERSUS IDIOPATHIC RIGHT VENTRICULAR TACHYCARDIA

The following features favor ARVD:
1. Family history of VT
2. History of resuscitation
3. ECG
   a. Terminal rightward conduction delay in V_1 (epsilon wave)
   b. Anterior T-wave inversions
4. Late potentials on signal-averaged ECG or abnormal body surface QRST integral maps
5. Multiple VT morphologies
6. Right ventricular dilatation or wall motion abnormalities
7. Entrainment of VT

ARVD, arrhythmogenic right ventricular dysplasia; VT, ventricular tachycardia.

cessful in selected patients with arrhythmogenic right ventricular dysplasia, it is not considered a primary therapy if this diagnosis is entertained. Ablation is often more a palliative than curative procedure.

Idiopathic ventricular fibrillation is distinct from idiopathic ventricular tachycardia and has a much different prognosis (57). It is defined as cardiac arrest in the absence of structural heart disease and other identifiable causes of ventricular fibrillation. It accounts for 1% to 9% of survivors of out-of-hospital cardiac arrest. The mean age is 35 to 40 years, and 70% to 75% are men. Between 20% and 30% of patients have recurrent cardiac arrest, and an ICD is the treatment of choice. Brugada syndrome is a variant of idiopathic ventricular fibrillation with characteristic ECG findings (i.e., right bundle branch block and ST elevation in leads V_1 through V_3) (58,59). The ECG findings may be intermittent and are thought to result from abnormal electrophysiologic activity in the right ventricular epicardium.

Ablation Techniques for Idiopathic Ventricular Tachycardia Arising from the Right Ventricle

In patients with no apparent structural heart disease who present with ventricular tachycardia having a left bundle branch block morphology, the origin of the ventricular tachycardia and subsequent ablation site are usually the right ventricle (10,60,61). An exception is idiopathic ventricular tachycardia that originates presumably from deep in the interventricular septum and may have a left or right bundle branch block QRS morphology (62). In patients who have coronary artery disease and previous infarction (particularly inferior infarction), ventricular tachycardias arising from the left ventricle may also have a left bundle branch block morphology because of a septal origin of the tachycardia with initial exit of the circuit toward the right side of the septum.

Ventricular tachycardia arising from the right ventricular outflow tract usually has a relatively narrow QRS duration (approximately 140 msec). There is a typical left bundle branch block configuration in lead V_1, with the precordial transition in the middle to lateral precordial leads (usually V_4 to V_5). The frontal plane QRS axis is close to 90 degrees (or occasionally

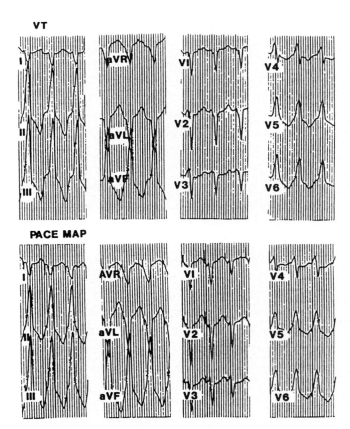

FIGURE 13-6. Electrocardiograms of ventricular tachycardia (VT) *(top)* and a pace map from the successful ablation site *(bottom)* are shown in a patient whose VT arose from the right ventricular outflow tract. The site of the best pace map was the successful ablation site. This was the same site at which earliest endocardial activation was recorded during VT. (From Klein LS, Shih H-T, Hackett FK, et al. Radiofrequency catheter ablation of ventricular tachycardia in patients without structural heart disease. *Circulation* 1992;85:1666–1671, with permission.)

rightward) with very tall upright QRS complexes in leads II, III, and aVF and low-amplitude (or negative) QRS complexes in lead I (Fig. 13-6). In ventricular tachycardia arising from the right ventricular inflow region close to the bundle of His, the precordial QRS complexes are similar to those previously described, and the QRS complexes in the inferior leads are also positive but not as tall as those in right ventricular outflow ventricular tachycardia (10).

Induction of Ventricular Tachycardia

Idiopathic right ventricular tachycardias may be difficult to induce consistently in the electrophysiology

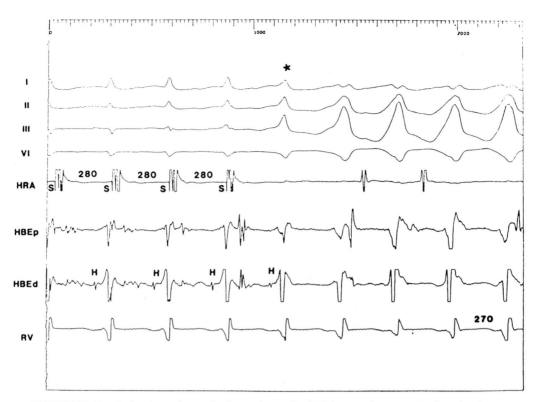

FIGURE 13-7. Induction of ventricular tachycardia (VT) by atrial pacing. Surface leads I, II, III, and V_1 are displayed along with intracardiac leads from the high right atrium (HRA), proximal His bundle region (HBEp), distal His bundle region (HBEd), and right ventricle (RV). Rapid atrial pacing at a cycle length of 280 msec results in induction of VT after a fusion beat *(asterisk)*. (From Klein LS, Miles WM. Ventricular tachycardia in patients with normal hearts. *Cardiol Rev* 1993;1:336–339, with permission.)

laboratory. An occasional patient may have very frequent episodes of ventricular tachycardia just before or after the procedure, but ventricular tachycardia is unable to be induced in the laboratory. In some patients, atrial or ventricular drive trains or burst pacing may induce ventricular tachycardia, whereas premature ventricular extrastimuli do not (Fig. 13-7), suggesting the possibility of a triggered mechanism (29). Many of these ventricular tachycardias—those inducible by programmed ventricular stimulation and those that are not—are sensitive to adrenergic stimulation. Isoproterenol in doses of 1 to 6 μg/min is commonly used to facilitate the occurrence of spontaneous ventricular tachycardia or its induction by programmed ventricular stimulation. In patients in whom ventricular tachycardia is infrequent or nonsustained, infusion of isoproterenol may produce sustained ventricular tachycardia, frequent runs of nonsustained ventricular tachycardia, or PVCs that can be used for mapping and as target arrhythmias for ablation. In a few patients, adrenergic stimulation may increase the sinus rate and decrease the frequency of ventricular tachycardia. If isoproterenol does not increase the ventricular tachycardia frequency or duration, infusion of epinephrine (0.01 to 0.03 μg/kg/min) may increase the ventricular tachycardia, implying that alpha-adrenergic stimulation may be important in some patients. Many patients have more spontaneous ventricular tachycardias when they are awake and alert (and probably anxious) rather than after sedation. In these patients, it may be useful to reverse sedation with narcotic or benzodiazepine antagonists if ventricular tachycardia is difficult to induce after sedation. After a dose of isoproterenol or epinephrine has been demonstrated to facilitate spontaneous or inducible ventricular tachycardia, the infusion is usually maintained throughout the procedure to provide as much arrhythmia as possible so that activation mapping can be performed efficiently and the efficacy of ablation can be quickly assessed. In some patients, only uniform PVCs with a morphology identical to that of their ventricular tachycardia are present at the time of study. If frequent, these can be used effectively for mapping and assessment of ablation efficacy for ventricular tachycardia.

Activation Mapping

The two techniques commonly used for localization of an appropriate site for ablation are activation mapping and pace mapping. Unlike the electrograms in patients with ventricular tachycardia associated with coronary artery disease, the local electrograms at successful sites in patients with idiopathic right ventricular tachycardia are usually not fractionated. Fractionated potentials or mid-diastolic potentials are not useful for mapping. However, because these tachycardias appear to be focal rather than macro-reentrant in origin, searching for the site of earliest ventricular activation during sustained ventricular tachycardia, nonsustained ventricular tachycardia, or frequent isolated PVCs (having the same morphology as ventricular tachycardia) is effective (i.e., activation mapping) (Fig. 13-8). Local ventricular activation during ventricular tachycardia occurs 20 to 50 msec before the onset of the QRS complex at the successful ablation site. In most patients, the final successful ablation site is the site recording earliest endocardial activation. It is difficult in many patients to define precisely the onset of the QRS in the surface leads. It is important

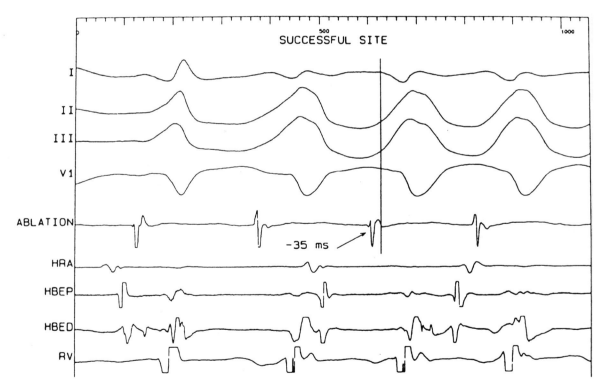

FIGURE 13-8. Examples of activation mapping in a patient with right ventricular outflow tachycardia. The site of successful ablation corresponds to the site of earliest ventricular activation that occurs in the ablation catheter electrogram and precedes the QRS complex by 35 msec. The first QRS complex is a fusion between sinus and ventricular tachycardia. Surface leads: I, II, III, and V_1. Electrogram leads: ABLATION, ablation catheter; HRA, high right atrium; HBEP, proximal His bundle; HBED, distal His bundle; RV, right ventricle. (From Miles WM, Klein LS. Radiofrequency ablation of idiopathic ventricular tachycardia and bundle branch reentrant tachycardia. In: Singer I, ed. *Interventional cardiology.* Baltimore: Williams & Wilkins, 1996:383–412, with permission.)

to display many surface leads simultaneously to ascertain the onset of ventricular activation relative to the surface QRS. A subtle deviation from the isoelectric baseline may occur 20 to 30 msec before the onset of the first sharp QRS deflection. This may be because when ventricular tachycardia originates in the right ventricular outflow tract where there are no specialized conduction fibers, initial conduction of the impulse from the ventricular tachycardia focus is from ventricular cell to cell, giving rise to a slow initial QRS deviation before the more rapid QRS deflection after the Purkinje system is activated. In any patient, the eventual successful ablation site is that with the earliest activation, although how early this needs to be varies from patient to patient and depends on operator selection of the QRS onset during ventricular tachycardia.

Pace Mapping

Pace mapping is more useful for guiding ablation of idiopathic ventricular tachycardia than it is in patients with ventricular tachycardia associated with coronary artery disease (1–4). Because the right ventricular wall is thin and these tachycardias are focal in origin, pacing from the endocardium at the site of tachycardia origin results in QRS complexes on a 12-lead ECG that almost exactly mimic those of the ventricular tachycardia (Figs. 13-6 and 13-9). Pace mapping is distinct from entrainment mapping of reentrant tachycardia, for which pacing must be initiated during tachycardia, and the QRS morphology during entrainment pacing is different from that during pacing from the same site when tachycardia has terminated (2). Pace mapping may be performed as an adjunct

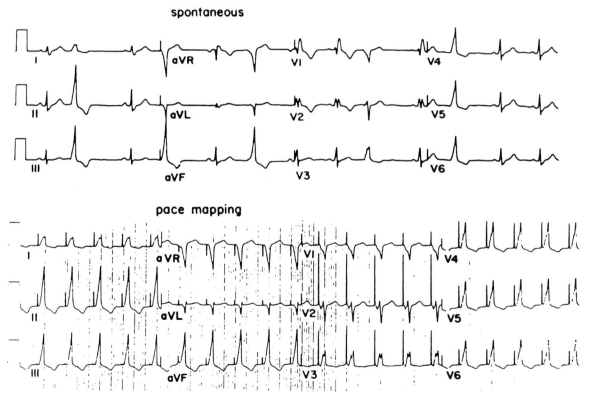

FIGURE 13-9. A 12-lead electrocardiogram of premature ventricular contractions (PVCs) *(top)* is compared with a pace map from the successful ventricular tachycardia (VT) ablation site *(bottom)*. The paced QRS complexes and the PVCs have nearly identical morphology. VT gradually subsided during the study, but PVCs having the same morphology as the VT occurred repeatedly and were used for mapping. (From Klein LS, Shih H-T, Hackett FK, et al. Radiofrequency catheter ablation of ventricular tachycardia in patients without structural heart disease. *Circulation* 1992;85:1666–1671, with permission.)

to activation mapping or may be used as the primary mapping technique in patients whose arrhythmia frequency is low at the beginning of the procedure or diminishes as the procedure progresses. In an occasional patient, if only a single run of ventricular tachycardia or a PVC having the tachycardia morphology occurs, the procedure can be guided wholly by pace mapping. However, pace mapping using only reference ECGs of ventricular tachycardia recorded at a previous setting (e.g., in the emergency room) is not adequate for ablation mapping because of the differences in lead placement. Pace mapping is relatively tedious, but computerized electrophysiologic recording systems decrease the time required for pace mapping by allowing stored ventricular tachycardia reference ECGs to be compared quickly with paced QRS complexes.

In patients with right ventricular tachycardia, the pace map at the successful site is an almost exact match with that during ventricular tachycardia, including the frontal plane axis, the precordial transition, and subtle notches on the QRS complexes. Any pace map that fails to resemble the ventricular tachycardia to this extent probably reflects an inadequate ablation location. Pace mapping should be performed at a cycle length near that of the ventricular tachycardia so that rate-related changes in the QRS morphology are minimized between the ventricular tachycardia and the pace map (63). Care must be taken during pace mapping so that the pacing does not induce a run of ventricular tachycardia that is then mistaken for an excellent pace map. An advantage of pace mapping is that the existence of ventricular capture during pacing from the ablation catheter confirms adequate catheter-tissue contact for ablation and confirms that the catheter is located below the pulmonic valve.

We have performed pace mapping using a pacing amplitude of 10 mA and a pulse width of 2 msec delivered in a bipolar fashion between the 4-mm distal ablating electrode and a ring electrode located 2 mm or more proximally on the ablating catheter (10). In theory, it may be advantageous to use unipolar rather than bipolar pacing and to use lower pacing outputs to minimize the volume of tissue depolarized directly by the pacing current and therefore, to obtain a more precise pace map (2). However, possibly because the distal ablation electrode is so large, we have found that bipolar pacing is adequate.

Catheter Positioning

Appropriate catheter position to ablate right ventricular outflow tachycardia can usually be established using the anteroposterior fluoroscopic view, although the right and left anterior oblique views may also be useful (Fig. 13-10). A deflectable catheter is introduced into the femoral vein and advanced across the tricuspid valve. Using catheter deflection and torque, the catheter can be advanced to the right ventricular outflow tract just under the pulmonic valve. If the catheter crosses the pulmonic valve, the ventricular electrogram suddenly diminishes in amplitude. The catheter usually points toward the patient's left, just below the pulmonic valve, although the exact position of the catheter within the outflow tract may vary from patient to patient. This region of the right ventricle is very smooth, and it is often difficult to stabilize the catheter just under the pulmonic valve, although this can usually be accomplished from the femoral approach. Occasionally, the superior vena caval approach or stabilization with a long sheath may help. Temperature monitoring during radiofrequency ablation is advantageous to confirm adequate catheter-tissue contact and to prevent an impedance rise. Excessive heating in this thin-walled region can rarely result in cardiac perforation. Repetitive ventricular responses with QRS morphology identical to the clinical ventricular tachycardia sometimes occur during radiofrequency energy delivery to the right ventricular outflow tract (64). The repetitive responses usually slow and then disappear with continued radiofrequency application and presumably result from heating of the arrhythmogenic myocardium.

Advanced computer mapping systems may be useful for localization of idiopathic ventricular tachycardia. These include body surface mapping (65–67) and nonfluoroscopic electroanatomic mapping (68,69) (Fig. 13-11), and noncontact multielectrode array endocardial mapping (70). These modalities are under intense investigation and may be particularly helpful when precise localization of the ventricular tachycardia site of origin is unclear or induction of ventricular tachycardia is poorly reproducible. Electroanatomic mapping systems may also be useful for ventricular tachycardia arising near the atrioventricular conduction system; sites where a His bundle potential is

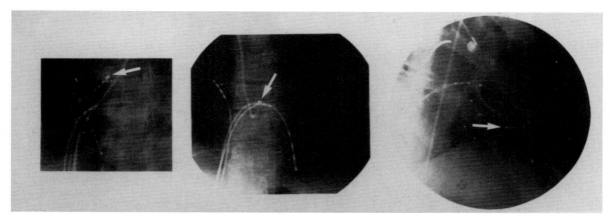

FIGURE 13-10. Radiographs of typical catheter positions. **A:** Left anterior oblique radiograph of catheter position in a patient whose ventricular tachycardia (VT) arose from the right ventricular outflow tract. The electrode *(arrow)* was used for successful ablation. **B:** Right anterior oblique radiograph of catheter position at the successful ablation site in a patient whose VT arose from an anteroseptal region just across the tricuspid valve and adjacent to the His bundle. The tip of the ablation catheter is shown *(arrow)* with a distal loop adjacent to the His bundle catheter. The tip of this catheter was across the tricuspid valve and in the right ventricle. **C:** Right anterior oblique radiograph of an ablation catheter in the left ventricle to ablate a posterior fascicular tachycardia. The ablating tip *(arrow)* is in the posteroseptal region at the middle left ventricular level; this was the successful ablation site. (From Klein LS, Shih H-T, Hackett FK, et al. Radiofrequency catheter ablation of ventricular tachycardia in patients without structural heart disease. *Circulation* 1992;85:1666–1671, with permission.)

recorded are tagged, and ablation energy is not delivered at those sites (71).

Ablation Techniques for Idiopathic Left Septal Ventricular Tachycardia

Idiopathic left septal ventricular tachycardia is usually sensitive to verapamil and arises in the region of the left posterior fascicle (i.e., left posterior fascicular ventricular tachycardia or verapamil-sensitive ventricular tachycardia) (28–36,41,42,72). Idiopathic left septal ventricular tachycardia usually has the QRS morphology of a right bundle branch block and left axis deviation. Rodriguez and coworkers described two distinct groups of idiopathic left septal ventricular tachycardia (73). Ventricular tachycardia in one group had a left axis and more narrow QRS. It originated from the inferoposterior left ventricle, and mapping revealed activation of a Purkinje potential before ventricular activation in most cases. Ventricular tachycardia in the other group had a left superior axis and a wider QRS. It originated from the inferoapical left ventricle, and no Purkinje activity was recorded at the successful ablation site. Our experience is that the former variety is more common. Because these ventricular tachycardias are often able to be entrained by ventricular pacing (41), they are probably caused by reentry using His-Purkinje fibers for at least part of the circuit. The exact circuit is unknown but may involve several centimeters of the left ventricular septum (74), and ablation guided by an early Purkinje potential may be successful with or without a perfect pace map (35, 75).

Suwa and associates described a false tendon in the left ventricle of a patient with idiopathic left ventricular tachycardia in whom ventricular tachycardia was eliminated by surgical resection of the tendon (76). Using transthoracic and transesophageal echocardiography, Thakur and colleagues found false tendons extending from the posteroinferior left ventricle to the left ventricular septum in 15 of 15 patients with idiopathic left ventricular tachycardia but in only 5% of control patients (77). They speculated that the false

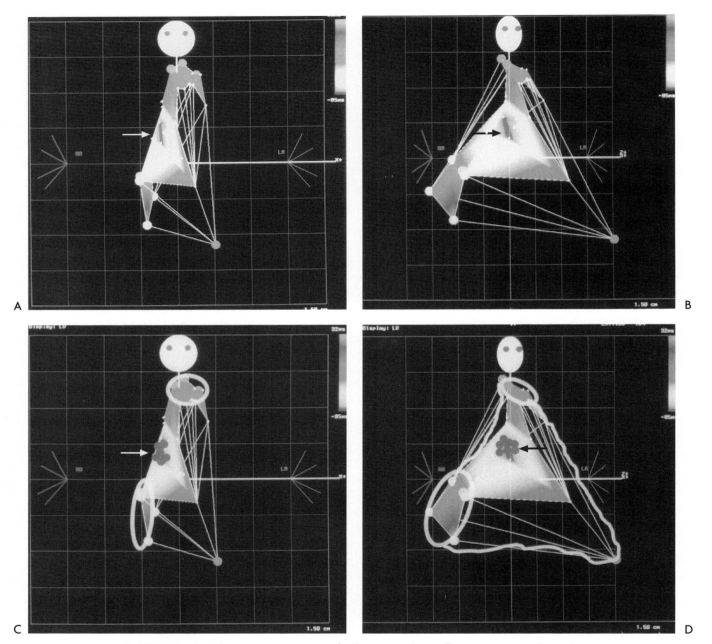

FIGURE 13-11. Electroanatomic maps of right ventricular outflow tract ventricular tachycardia (VT) reproduced in gray scale. Anteroposterior **(A)** and right anterior oblique **(B)** projections of the right ventricle. Detailed activation mapping has been performed in only a portion of the overall right ventricular chamber. Earliest activation during VT *(arrow)* arises from the right ventricular outflow tract medially between the pulmonic valve and the superior aspect of the tricuspid annulus. The anteroposterior **(C)** and right anterior oblique **(D)** views during VT in the same patient with more anatomic detail in the electroanatomic maps, including the location *(arrow)* of radiofrequency ablation pulses *(dots)*. The pulmonic valve is represented by the superior ring and the tricuspid valve by the inferior ring. **D:** The general shape of the right ventricular chamber has been outlined.

tendon may be involved with tachycardia by providing a conduction pathway or producing stretch in the Purkinje fiber network on the septum. Lin and coworkers (78) also found that 17 of 18 patients with idiopathic left ventricular tachycardia had this fibromuscular band, but they also found it in 35 of 40 control patients. They concluded that the band was a common echocardiographic finding and was not a specific anatomic substrate for idiopathic left ventricular tachycardia, although they could not exclude the possibility that the band was a potential substrate for ventricular tachycardia.

Ablation is performed by introducing a catheter by means of the retrograde transaortic approach across the aortic valve into the left ventricle. Left ventricular endocardial mapping during tachycardia is performed in the posteroapical left ventricular septal region (35, 42). The left anterior oblique fluoroscopic view is used to guide the catheter toward the septum, and the right anterior oblique view to guide the catheter posteriorly and toward the apical third of the septum. While mapping the distal left ventricular septum, the earliest ventricular activation during ventricular tachycardia is usually preceded by a distinct fascicular potential, preceding the QRS by 15 to 40 msec (Fig. 13-12). A fascicular potential can be recorded during sinus rhythm at this site and at sites near fascicles that are not associated with the ventricular tachycardia focus. The successful ablation site usually has the earliest fascicular potential during ventricular tachycardia, not necessarily that with earliest ventricular activation. This is because the site of ventricular tachycardia origin within the fascicle may be different from where the impulse "exits" or activates ventricular tissue (QRS onset) (Fig. 13-13). Pace mapping at this site may result in QRS complexes that closely resemble those of ventricular tachycardia but an exact match is not always obtained, probably because pacing in the region of the early fascicular potential may also activate local ventricular myocardium. A pace map having a QRS complex identical to that of ventricular tachycardia may not necessarily represent a successful ablation site because of the possibility of capture of the Purkinje fiber network at a site remote from the origin of the tachycardia. Another mapping technique is to use entrainment mapping to target a site within the ventricular tachycardia circuit distant from the "exit" site, usually the middle of the left ventricular septum (43,44).

Ablation Results for Idiopathic Ventricular Tachycardia

We performed radiofrequency ablation in 73 consecutive patients with idiopathic ventricular tachycardia referred to Indiana University Hospital between March 1990 and May 1995 (79). Ventricular tachycardias were mapped to the right ventricle in 55 (75%) and to the left ventricle in 18 (25%) of the 73 patients. Of the right ventricular tachycardias, 46 originated from the right ventricular outflow tract, 7 from the right ventricular inflow region, and 2 from the right ventricular free wall. Of the left ventricular tachycardias, 13 mapped to the left ventricular posterior septum in the region of the posterior fascicle, and 5 mapped to other left ventricular sites, including 3 anterolateral basal, 1 anteroseptal, and 1 apical. No patient had more than one ventricular tachycardia focus targeted for ablation.

Overall, idiopathic ventricular tachycardia was successfully eliminated in 61 (84%) of the 73 patients. There was a higher ablation success rate with ventricular tachycardia arising from the right ventricular outflow tract than any other site: 45 (98%) of 46 patients. Ventricular tachycardia was successfully ablated in only 3 (33%) of 9 patients in whom ventricular tachycardia arose from right ventricular sites other than the outflow tract (right ventricular inflow tract in 2, right ventricular free wall in 1). This difference in success rate depending on right ventricular site of origin has been reflected by other investigators (80) and may represent site specific technical differences, a nonendocardial site of origin, or patients with an early form of arrhythmogenic right ventricular dysplasia.

Ventricular tachycardia arising from the left ventricle was eliminated in 13 (72%) of 18 patients. Ten (77%) of 13 patients with left ventricular septal tachycardia had ventricular tachycardia successfully ablated, whereas 3 of 5 patients with ventricular tachycardia arising from other left ventricular sites were successfully ablated (1 of 3 from the anterolateral base, 1 of 1 from the anteroseptal region, and 1 of 1 from the apex). Ablation in patients with idiopathic ventricular

358   I. INTERVENTIONAL TECHNIQUES FOR ABLATION OF TACHYCARDIAS

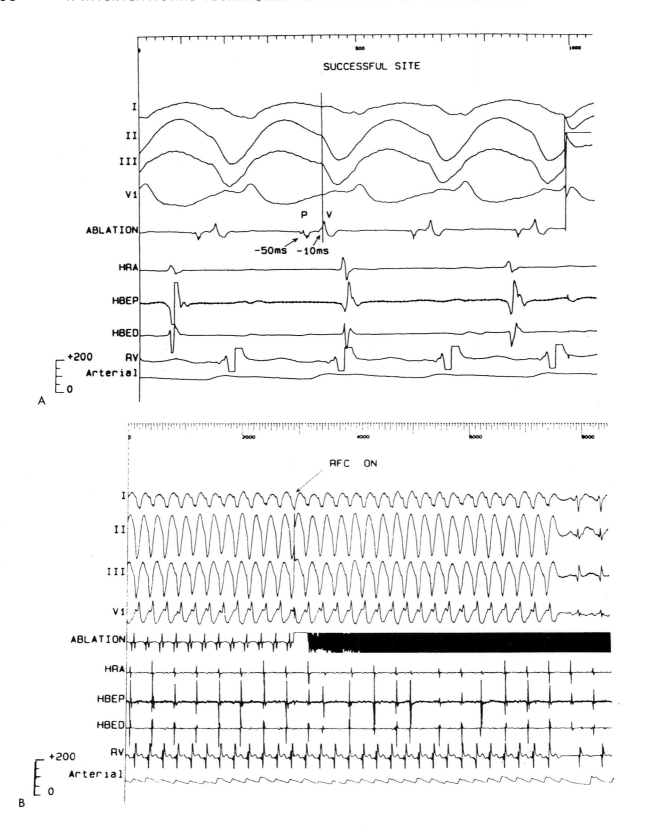

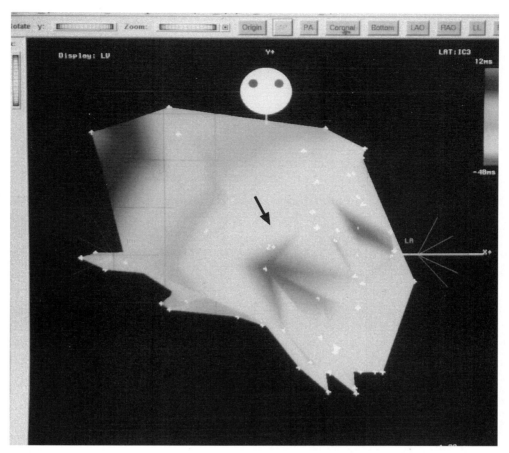

FIGURE 13-13. Electroanatomic map (gray scale) of the left ventricle during left septal ventricular tachycardia indicates earliest activation *(arrow)*. The anteroposterior projection shows the left ventricular septum with the apex to the bottom right of the figure and the base of the septum to the top left. There are two simultaneous sites of early activation during ventricular tachycardia corresponding to the approximate exit of the left posterior fascicle and the left anterior fascicle. The second, dark site is not labeled. Presumably, this tachycardia originates from within the fascicles and exits at approximately the same time from both major fascicles. Ablation was performed in this patient by targeting an early Purkinje potential that occurred before any ventricular activation.

◀──

FIGURE 13-12. Left posterior fascicular tachycardia. Surface leads I, II, III, and V_1 are displayed along with ablation (ABLATION), high right atrium (HRA), proximal His bundle (HBEP), distal His bundle (HBED), and right ventricular (RV) electrograms. An arterial pressure recording (Arterial) is also shown. **A:** The ablation catheter is positioned in the left posteroseptal region two thirds of the way toward the apex. A fascicular potential (P) is recorded before the ventricular (V) electrogram. The ventricular electrogram precedes the QRS complex by 10 msec, and the fascicular potential precedes it by 50 msec. **B:** Elimination of the fascicular tachycardia. Radiofrequency (RF) current is turned on in the middle of the figure, and the left posterior fascicular tachycardia terminates abruptly. The tachycardia was no longer inducible in this patient after delivery of this RF pulse. Surface leads I, II, III, and V_1 are displayed along with ablation (ABLATION), high right atrium (HRA), proximal His bundle (HBEP), distal His bundle (HBED), and right ventricular (RV) electrograms. (From Klein LS, Miles WM. Ablative therapy for ventricular arrhythmias. *Progr Cardiovasc Dis* 1995;37:225–242, with permission.)

tachycardia is most successful in patients in whom the ventricular tachycardia arises from the right ventricular outflow tract or, less often, from the left ventricular septum.

Nine (14%) of 61 patients who had initially successful ventricular tachycardia ablations had recurrent arrhythmia and required two ablation sessions for elimination of ventricular tachycardia. Four (5%) of the 73 patients had a procedure-related complication. Three patients developed pericardial effusions due to cardiac perforation; two of the three patients required emergent pericardiocentesis. Other investigators have reported a death from pericardial tamponade during attempted ablation of a right ventricular outflow tract tachycardia (61). One patient who underwent successful ablation of a left posterior fascicular ventricular tachycardia had an asymptomatic inferior wall motion abnormality identified on a two-dimensional echocardiogram 24 hours after the procedure. The wall motion abnormality resolved within 6 weeks and might have been caused by myocardial "stunning" from the ablation pulses.

Ventricular Tachycardias Mimicking Those Arising from the Right Ventricular Outflow Tract

As investigators confirmed that ablation of ventricular tachycardia arising from the right ventricular outflow tract was highly successful, it became apparent that ventricular tachycardias with similar ECG features may originate outside the right ventricular outflow tract. Krebs and associates (62) reviewed 29 consecutive patients referred for ablation of monomorphic ventricular tachycardia having a left bundle branch block pattern in lead V_1 and tall monophasic R waves inferiorly. Nineteen patients (group A) had ventricular tachycardias ablated from the right ventricular outflow tract, and 10 patients (group B) had ventricular tachycardias that could not be ablated from the right ventricular outflow tract. The QRS morphology during ventricular tachycardia was the only variable that distinguished the two groups (Fig. 13-14). During ventricular tachycardia or target PVCs, ECGs of group B patients displayed significantly earlier precordial transition zones (median V_3 versus V_5) and more commonly had small R waves in V_1 (10 of 10 versus 9 of 19 patients) (Fig. 13-15). Radiofrequency ablation from the right ventricular outflow tract failed to eliminate ventricular tachycardia in any group B patient, but ablation from the left ventricular outflow tract eliminated ventricular tachycardia in 2 of 6 patients in whom left ventricular ablation was attempted. The absence of an R wave in lead V_1 and a late precordial transition zone suggest a right ventricular outflow tract origin of ventricular tachycardia, whereas an early precordial transition zone characterizes ventricular tachycardias that mimic a right ventricular outflow tract origin. The latter ventricular tachycardias occasionally can be ablated from the left ventricular outflow tract; the others may arise from deep within the ventricular septum or from the epicardium in the outflow region. Recognition of these ECG variations may help the physician advise patients concerning the likelihood of ablation success and direct the approach to ventricular tachycardia mapping and radiofrequency ablation.

Arruda and colleagues (81) reported subepicardial ventricular tachycardias arising from the ventricular outflow tracts. Endocardial ablation of these ventricular tachycardias proved unsuccessful, and their elimination required mapping and ablation in the great cardiac or anterior interventricular vein. These ventricular tachycardias had tall R waves across the precordium and did not resemble the ECG of right ventricular outflow tract ventricular tachycardia. Similarly, the two ventricular tachycardias ablated by Callans and coworkers (82) from the left ventricular outflow tract did not have a left bundle branch block pattern in lead V_1. The other two ventricular tachycardias that they described had a left bundle branch block pattern in lead V_1 and mimicked right ventricular outflow tract ventricular tachycardia, but ablation was not attempted because pace maps of similar configuration to that of the spontaneous ventricular tachycardia localized these ventricular tachycardias to the basal aspect of the superior left ventricular septum, adjacent to a His recording in sinus rhythm. Coronary venous mapping has been used more extensively to define epicardial or deep intramural origins of outflow tract ventricular tachycardia (83,84). Epicardial mapping and ablation through a pericardial needle puncture has also been performed in patients with ventric-

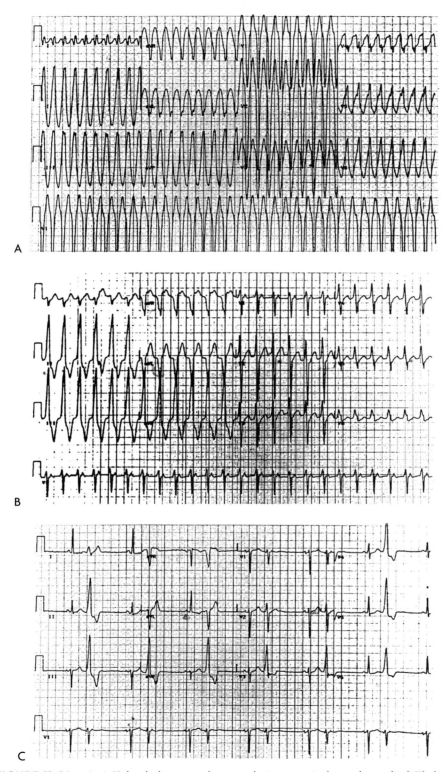

FIGURE 13-14. **A:** A 12-lead electrocardiogram during ventricular tachycardia (VT) that was ablated successfully from the right ventricular outflow (RVOT) tract. **B:** Electrocardiogram during VT that could not be ablated from the RVOT. **C:** Ventricular premature complexes ablated successfully from the anterior base of the left ventricle. (From Krebs ME, Krause PC, Engelstein ED, et al. Ventricular tachycardias mimicking those arising from the right ventricular outflow tract. *J Cardiovasc Electrophysiol* 2000;11:45–51, with permission.)

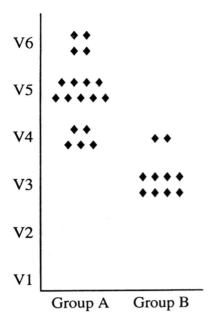

FIGURE 13-15. Location of the electrocardiographic precordial transition zone during ventricular tachycardia in patients in groups A (ablated from the RVOT) and B (not ablatable from the RVOT). (From Krebs ME, Krause PC, Engelstein ED, et al. Ventricular tachycardias mimicking those arising from the right ventricular outflow tract. *J Cardiovasc Electrophysiol* 2000; 11:45–51, with permission.)

ular tachycardia due to Chagas' disease (85,86) and could be applicable in the future to patients with idiopathic ventricular tachycardia arising from the epicardium.

Only a minority of left ventricular outflow ventricular tachycardias can be ablated from the endocardium (62,87,88). The mechanism of many of these tachycardias is analogous to that of the adenosine-sensitive right ventricular outflow tract ventricular tachycardias (i.e., nonreentrant, probably cAMP-mediated triggered activity) (24,27,87), but success is limited by possible nonendocardial sites of origin and the proximity to the left main and left anterior descending coronary arteries (89). Preliminary reports have described ablation of selected left ventricular outflow tract ventricular tachycardias from the supravalvular region of the aortic cusp (90). Saline-cooled radiofrequency electrode catheters may be useful to generate deeper lesions (91) but also have the potential to increase complications (e.g., perforation, valve damage, conduction block, coronary vascular injury).

Conclusions about Ablation of Idiopathic Ventricular Tachycardias

Idiopathic ventricular tachycardia can be ablated safely using radiofrequency energy, and in many cases, ablation may be used as a primary therapy. Adrenergic stimulation is often required to provide adequate frequency of arrhythmia for an ablation target. The site of origin of the ventricular tachycardia correlates with the success of ablation, with right ventricular outflow tract ventricular tachycardia having the highest success rates. Endocardial activation mapping and pace mapping are useful for right ventricular tachycardias, and recording of an early Purkinje potential is useful in the left posteroseptal ventricular tachycardias. If ablation is acutely successful and clinical follow-up at 4 to 6 weeks is negative, a long-term success is likely.

● BUNDLE BRANCH REENTRANT TACHYCARDIA

Mechanism of Tachycardia

In normal human hearts, the introduction of single ventricular extrasystoles in the electrophysiology laboratory commonly results in single nonstimulated bundle branch reentrant QRS complexes (92–94). Typically, a tightly coupled ventricular extrastimulus introduced from the right ventricle may block retrogradely in the right bundle branch but travel across the septum and activate the left bundle branch and His bundle retrogradely. If the right bundle branch has recovered excitability, it may then be reentered anterogradely and generate a ventricular depolarization with a left bundle branch block morphology. Because of the rapid conduction in normal His-Purkinje tissue and the relatively short length of the reentrant circuit, bundle branch reentry is extinguished after one or two revolutions in normal hearts. However, in patients with abnormal His-Purkinje conduction (i.e., slowed conduction time) and dilated left ventricles (i.e., longer circuit), sustained ventricular tachycardia can occur because of macro-reentry within the bundle branches (11,95–98).

Bundle branch reentrant tachycardia was initially thought to be rare, but it has become apparent that this mechanism is frequently responsible for ventricular tachycardia in patients with dilated cardiomyopathy. It accounted for 6% of all ventricular tachycardias encountered in an active electrophysiology laboratory and up to 40% of ventricular tachycardias in patients with idiopathic dilated cardiomyopathy (12). It is usually rapid and is often associated with syncope and hemodynamic collapse. It may occur in patients with myotonic dystrophy due to severe conduction system delay even in the absence of myocardial dysfunction (99,100). Narasimhan and associates (101) found that 9 (29%) of 31 patients who had inducible ventricular tachycardia after valve surgery had bundle branch reentry as the ventricular tachycardia mechanism. Bundle branch reentrant ventricular tachycardia tended to occur early after surgery (median of 10 days after surgery compared with 72 months for postmyocardial infarction ventricular tachycardia), and 4 of the 9 patients with bundle branch reentrant ventricular tachycardia had normal left ventricular function.

For reentry to perpetuate within the bundle branches, there must be bundle branch conduction delay (usually with a prolonged His-ventricular [HV] interval). Ventricular dilation is usually present, the importance of which may be twofold: dilated cardiomyopathy is commonly associated with His-Purkinje conduction delay, and the dilated ventricle may provide a longer distance between the right and left bundle branches, enlarging the tachycardia circuit and enhancing the ability of the tachycardia to sustain. The most common form of bundle branch reentrant tachycardia has a left bundle branch block QRS morphology; its circuit consists of anterograde conduction down the right bundle branch, transseptal conduction to the left bundle branch, retrograde conduction up the left bundle branch, and subsequent reactivation of the right bundle branch anterogradely. Each QRS complex during bundle branch reentrant tachycardia is preceded by a His bundle potential with the same HV interval as during sinus rhythm, a longer HV interval if anterograde conduction in the right bundle branch is further delayed during tachycardia, or a slightly shorter HV interval if the recording site of the His bundle potential is proximal to its bifurcation into the bundle branches.

Ventriculoatrial dissociation is usually present during bundle branch reentrant tachycardia and, if present, helps to distinguish it from supraventricular tachycardia with aberrancy. Characteristically, any irregularity of the ventricular cycle length at the initiation of bundle branch reentry is *preceded* by changes in the H-H intervals, whereas in an intramyocardial ventricular tachycardia with retrograde activation of the bundle branches without their integral participation in the tachycardia, H-H cycle length changes would be expected to *follow* each respective change in the V-V interval (Figs. 13-16 and 13-17). This pattern occurs because variations in conduction intervals tend to occur in transseptal or retrograde left bundle branch conduction rather than in anterograde right bundle branch conduction. Such irregularity is common in the first few seconds after tachycardia induction. It is important to differentiate bundle branch reentrant tachycardia from supraventricular tachycardia with aberration, both of which have HV intervals equal to or longer than those during sinus rhythm. Intraventricular reentrant ventricular tachycardia, fascicular tachycardia, and antidromic atrioventricular reentry using an atriofascicular (Mahaim) fiber must also be excluded.

In a few patients, the direction of the tachycardia circuit may be reversed, giving rise to tachycardia with a right bundle branch block QRS morphology. The HV interval is equal to, longer than, or (if the His recording site is proximal) slightly shorter than the HV interval during sinus rhythm. However, the right bundle branch is activated before the His bundle during tachycardia. Even more unusual cases may involve reentry within the left anterior and left posterior fascicles (i.e., interfascicular reentry) (12,102,103). In this arrhythmia, anterograde conduction occurs by means of the left anterior or posterior fascicle with retrograde conduction through the opposite fascicle.

Recording of right or left bundle branch in addition to His bundle potentials may help to define the mechanism of bundle branch reentrant ventricular tachycardia (102–105). For example, during sinus rhythm, the His bundle potential should occur before the right bundle branch potential, and this same relationship should persist during supraventricular tachycardia with aberration. However, during typical bundle branch reentrant ventricular tachycardia with anterograde conduction through the right bundle branch and retrograde conduction through the left

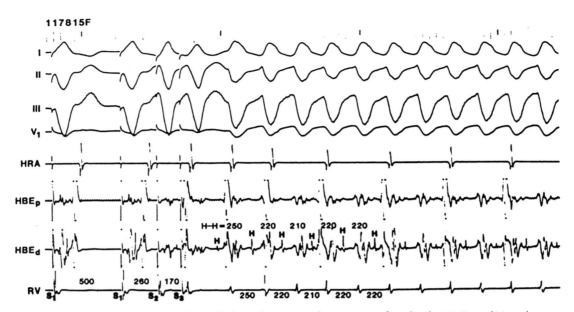

FIGURE 13-16. Sustained bundle branch reentry. Shown are surface leads I, II, III, and V_1 and intracardiac recordings from the high right atrium (HRA), proximal His bundle (HBE_p), distal His bundle (HBE_d), and right ventricle (RV). Two right ventricular extrastimuli (S_2, S_3) are introduced into the right ventricle after a pacing drive train. There is retrograde right bundle branch block with subsequent delay in the ventricular-His (VH) interval. Sustained bundle branch reentrant tachycardia ensues with a His depolarization identifiable before each QRS complex. During cycle length variation at the beginning of the tachycardia, alterations in the H-H intervals precede alterations in the V-V intervals, consistent with bundle branch reentry rather than bystander participation of the His-Purkinje system from retrograde penetration during intramyocardial ventricular tachycardia. (From Klein LS, Zipes DP, Miles WM. Ablation of ventricular tachycardia in patients without coronary artery disease and ventricular tachycardia due to bundle branch reentry. In: Huang SKS, ed. *Radiofrequency catheter ablation of cardiac arrhythmias: basic concepts and clinical applications.* Armonk, NY: Futura Publishing, 1994:479–490, with permission.)

bundle branch, the interval between His bundle and right bundle branch activation is shorter than that during sinus rhythm or supraventricular tachycardia, with the degree of shortening depending on the location (proximal or distal) of the His bundle recording site. If the unusual "reversed" variety of bundle branch reentry occurs, consisting of anterograde conduction through the left bundle branch and retrograde conduction through the right bundle branch, activation of the His bundle and right bundle branch is reversed compared with sinus rhythm or supraventricular tachycardia with aberration. In patients with bundle branch reentrant tachycardia having a right bundle branch block QRS morphology, recording of the left and right bundle branch potentials may be necessary to fully define the tachycardia mechanism.

If the tachycardia uses the left anterior or posterior fascicles for anterograde conduction but requires the right bundle branch for retrograde conduction, ablation of the right bundle branch can eliminate the tachycardia. If, however, the tachycardia involves anterograde conduction through one left fascicle and retrograde conduction through the other, with the right bundle branch being a bystander (i.e., interfascicular reentry), ablation of the right bundle branch is not sufficient to eliminate tachycardia, and ablation of a left fascicle is necessary.

It is important to delineate the anterograde limb of the reentrant pathway, because it represents the final common pathway, the ablation of which eliminates ventricular tachycardia (103). The QRS morphology of the ventricular tachycardia gives an im-

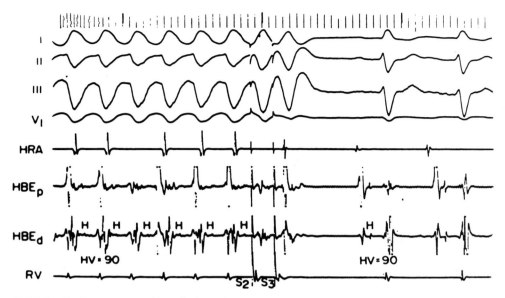

FIGURE 13-17. Sustained bundle branch reentry terminated by two ventricular prematures. This is the same patient as in Figure 13-16. Each QRS complex is preceded by a His (H) pattern, and the His-ventricular (HV) interval during tachycardia (90 msec) is identical to that recorded during sinus rhythm. (From Klein LS, Miles WM. Ablative therapy for ventricular arrhythmias. *Progr Cardiovasc Dis* 1995;37:225–242, with permission.)

portant clue about where to look for that final common pathway. Bundle branch reentry with left bundle branch block morphology suggests the right bundle branch as the final common pathway. Bundle branch reentry with a right bundle branch block, right axis morphology suggests the left anterior fascicle as the final common pathway and may require ablation of that fascicle for definitive elimination of interfascicular reentry. After a left fascicle has been ablated in an interfascicular tachycardia, the right bundle branch may also need to be ablated if typical bundle branch reentrant tachycardia is still inducible. Although interfascicular reentry is thought to be rare, the true incidence and clinical significance are unknown, because it may be difficult to induce and accurately diagnose.

Even a patient who has complete anterograde left bundle branch block may maintain retrograde left bundle branch conduction and be susceptible to bundle branch reentrant tachycardia. Blanck and colleagues (104) described such a patient, in whom there was complete anterograde left bundle branch block on the surface ECG. Typical bundle branch reentrant tachycardia having a left bundle branch block morphology was inducible (i.e., anterograde conduction through the right bundle branch and retrograde through the left bundle branch). Complete anterograde left bundle branch block during sinus rhythm was confirmed by demonstrating retrograde activation of the left bundle branch during sinus rhythm by recording a left bundle branch potential. In this patient, elimination of bundle branch reentrant ventricular tachycardia through right bundle branch ablation could be expected to result in complete heart block. The ventricular tachycardia was interrupted by delivering radiofrequency energy to the proximal left bundle branch, preserving conduction through the right bundle branch and avoiding atrioventricular block.

Ablation Techniques for Bundle Branch Reentrant Ventricular Tachycardia

In susceptible patients, bundle branch reentrant tachycardia is inducible by premature ventricular stimuli. However, in up to one half of patients, special pacing drive train cadences, left ventricular pacing, and drug infusion (i.e., isoproterenol or procainamide) are necessary to induce the tachycardia. Ventricular pacing drive trains consisting of eight complexes followed by a longer pacing interval before introduction of premature ventricular stimuli are particularly effective at producing His-Purkinje delay and inducing bundle branch reentrant tachycardia (106,107).

It is useful to record His bundle, right bundle branch, and occasionally left bundle branch potentials to make the diagnosis of bundle branch reentrant tachycardia or interfascicular reentrant tachycardia. Recording of His bundle and right bundle branch potentials can often be accomplished by using one multipolar electrode catheter positioned across the anterior leaflet of the tricuspid valve. The catheter is advanced such that the distal electrodes are beyond the usual His bundle recording site; a right bundle branch potential may then be recorded on the more distal electrodes and a His bundle potential on the more proximal electrodes. It is sometimes useful to display proximal and distal His bundle recordings. Alternatively, separate catheters can be introduced to optimize recording of each potential. It is more difficult to record left bundle branch potentials, and the process introduces the additional risk of an arterial catheter. Therefore, we do not routinely record a left bundle branch potential unless it is needed for diagnostic purposes. An electrode catheter is introduced into the left ventricle by means of the retrograde transaortic approach. The catheter is manipulated to the septum just under the aortic valve until a sharp fascicular potential is recorded. The left bundle to ventricular interval is at least 20 msec shorter than the HV interval.

After the diagnosis of bundle branch reentry has been confirmed, ablation of the right bundle branch eliminates the tachycardia, unless the tachycardia is interfascicular, in which case the right bundle branch is a bystander (98,108–111). To ablate the right bundle branch, an ablating electrode is positioned across the anterior leaflet of the tricuspid valve to record a typical His bundle potential. The catheter is then advanced further across the valve until a large ventricular potential is recorded, little or no atrial potential is recorded, and a right bundle branch potential is identified. The interval between the right bundle branch potential and ventricular activation is at least 20 msec shorter than the HV interval measured from the distal His bundle recording electrodes (Fig. 13-18). When radiofrequency energy is delivered to the area, complete right bundle branch block occurs, after which attempts at reinducing the tachycardia should be unsuccessful (Fig. 13-19). The right bundle branch can be successfully ablated in virtually all patients (12).

It is more difficult to ablate the left bundle branch than the right bundle branch. Left bundle branch ablation is indicated only if interfascicular reentry is present or if complete anterograde left bundle branch block is thought to exist. The technique of positioning the catheter to ablate the left bundle branch is the same as described for recording a left bundle branch potential.

Ablation Results for Bundle Branch Reentrant Ventricular Tachycardia

Long-term survival of most patients with bundle branch reentrant ventricular tachycardia is limited by left ventricular dysfunction. Although ablation of the right bundle branch eliminates the bundle branch reentrant tachycardia, these patients may be at risk for other serious ventricular arrhythmias, which may necessitate additional antiarrhythmic drug or ICD therapy for selected patients (12,112–117).

In the past, we performed electrophysiology studies in all patients with dilated cardiomyopathy who presented with sustained ventricular tachycardia or cardiac arrest to look for bundle branch reentrant ventricular tachycardia. However, these patients are probably still at risk of sudden cardiac death even after ablation to eliminate bundle branch reentrant ventricular tachycardia. With the advent of reliable pectoral ICDs, it is reasonable to manage these patients with an ICD no matter what the ventricular tachycardia mechanism may be. Subsequently, if bundle branch reentrant ventricular tachycardia results in ICD shocks, bundle branch ablation can be performed. An exception to this approach may be the patient with muscular dystrophy who has bundle branch reentrant ventricular tachycardia without left ventricular dysfunction. Bundle branch ablation alone may be sufficient in this type of patient.

Although patients with bundle branch reentry have

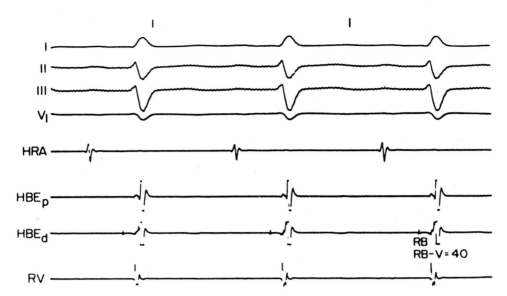

FIGURE 13-18. Recordings of a right bundle branch potential in the same patient as in Figures 13-16 and 13-17. The catheter recording the His potential is advanced slightly into the ventricle so that there is no atrial recording on the catheter. At this point, a sharp potential representing right bundle branch activation (RB) is present and precedes QRS by 40 msec, whereas the His-ventricular (HV) interval (Fig. 13-17) was 90 msec in this patient. The difference between the His recording and the right bundle recording is the shorter RB-V interval compared with the HV interval and the absence of atrial activation recorded from the electrode pair recording the right bundle branch potential. (From Klein LS, Miles WM. Ablative therapy for ventricular arrhythmias. *Progr Cardiovasc Dis* 1995;37:225–242, with permission.)

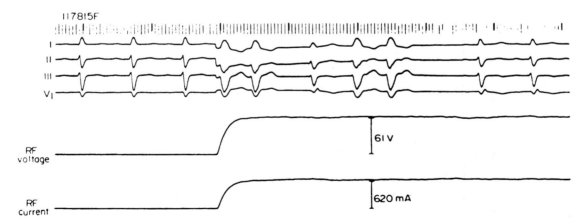

FIGURE 13-19. Delivery of radiofrequency (RF) energy in the same patient as in Figures 13-16 through 13-18. RF energy is delivered during sinus rhythm. After several premature complexes, right bundle branch block occurs. This RF pulse eliminated right bundle branch conduction and inducible bundle branch reentry tachycardia. (From Klein LS, Zipes DP, Miles WM. Ablation of ventricular tachycardia in patients without coronary artery disease and ventricular tachycardia due to bundle branch reentry. In: Huang SKS, ed. *Radiofrequency catheter ablation of cardiac arrhythmias: basic concepts and clinical applications.* Armonk, NY: Futura Publishing, 1994:479–490.)

prolonged His-Purkinje conduction before ablation, criteria for permanent pacemaker implantation after ablation of the right bundle branch are not well defined. We consider implantation of a permanent pacemaker if the HV interval is 90 msec or longer after ablation. However, in most patients, the HV increase after right bundle branch ablation is small, and permanent pacemaker implantation is unnecessary.

Blanck and colleagues (12) described a cumulative experience from one center in 48 patients with bundle branch reentrant ventricular tachycardia. The clinical presentation was syncope or sudden death in 38 patients and sustained palpitations during wide QRS tachycardia in 5 patients. Structural heart disease was present in 45 of the 48 patients. Idiopathic dilated cardiomyopathy and coronary artery disease were the anatomic substrates in 19 (39%) and 24 (50%) of the patients, respectively. Two patients had severe aortic regurgitation, and three patients had no structural heart disease. All 48 patients had His-Purkinje system disease. Bundle branch reentrant tachycardia had a left bundle branch block contour (46 patients) or right bundle branch block contour (5 patients). Interfascicular bundle branch reentrant tachycardia was initiated in two patients. Ventricular tachycardia of a myocardial origin was also induced in 11 patients. Management of bundle branch reentry included transcatheter bundle branch ablation in 28 patients and antiarrhythmic drug therapy in 16 patients. Four patients had an ICD. After a follow-up period of 15.8 months for 42 patients, there were 13 deaths from congestive heart failure, 4 from sudden cardiac deaths, 3 from nonsudden cardiac deaths, and 3 from noncardiac causes. Congestive heart failure was the most common cause of death in this population.

CONCLUSIONS

Bundle branch reentrant ventricular tachycardia is not uncommon in patients with His-Purkinje conduction delay and structural heart disease. Bundle branch reentrant ventricular tachycardia may be highly malignant, frequently causing syncope or cardiac arrest. Unique ventricular pacing protocols may be necessary to induce bundle branch reentrant ventricular tachycardia in the electrophysiology laboratory. The tachycardia can be eliminated with right bundle branch ablation, but patient survival is limited by the presence of underlying left ventricular dysfunction. In these patients, ICD therapy should be considered instead of or in addition to ablation.

ACKNOWLEDGEMENTS

The authors appreciate the expert secretarial assistance of Kathy Orchin in the preparation of this manuscript.

REFERENCES

1. Morady F, Harvey M, Kalbfleisch SJ, et al. Radiofrequency catheter ablation of ventricular tachycardia in patients with coronary artery disease. *Circulation* 1993;87:363–372.
2. Stevenson WG, Khan H, Sager P, et al. Identification of reentry circuit sites during catheter mapping and radiofrequency ablation of ventricular tachycardia late after myocardial infarction. *Circulation* 1993;88:1647–1670.
3. Kim YH, Sosa-Suarez G, Tranton TG, et al. Treatment of ventricular tachycardia by transcatheter radiofrequency ablation in patients with ischemic heart disease. *Circulation* 1994;89:1094–1102.
4. Wilber DJ, Kopp DE, Glascock DN, et al. Catheter ablation of the mitral isthmus for ventricular tachycardia associated with inferior infarction. *Circulation* 1995;92:348–349.
5. Wellens HJJ, Rodriguez LM, Smeets JL. Ventricular tachycardia in patients with structurally normal hearts. In: Zipes DP, Jalife J, eds. *Cardiac electrophysiology: from cell to bedside*, 3rd ed. Philadelphia: WB Saunders, 2000:640–656.
6. Brooks R, Burgess JH. Idiopathic ventricular tachycardia: a review. *Medicine (Baltimore)* 1988;67:271–272.
7. Belhassen B, Viskin S. Idiopathic ventricular tachycardia and fibrillation. *J Cardiovasc Electrophysiol* 1993;354–356.
8. Mont L, Seixas T, Brugada P, et al. The electrocardiographic, clinical, and electrophysiologic spectrum of idiopathic monomorphic ventricular tachycardia. *Am Heart J* 1992;124:746.
9. Morady F, Kadish AH, DiCarlo L, et al. Long-term results of catheter ablation of idiopathic right ventricular tachycardia. *Circulation* 1990;82:2093–2098.
10. Klein LS, Shih H-T, Hackett FK, et al. Radiofrequency catheter ablation of ventricular tachycardia in patients without structural heart disease. *Circulation* 1992;85:1666–1671.
11. Caceras J, Jazayeri M, McKinnie J, et al. Sustained bundle branch reentry as a mechanism of clinical tachycardia. *Circulation* 1989;79:256.
12. Blanck Z, Dhala A, Deshpande S, et al. Bundle branch reentrant ventricular tachycardia: cumulative experience in 48 patients. *J Cardiovasc Electrophysiol* 1993;4:253–262.
13. Buxton AE, Waxman HL, Marchlinski FE, et al. Right ventricular tachycardia: clinical and electrophysiologic characteristics. *Circulation* 1983;68:917–927.
14. Chiladakis JA, Vassilikos V, Maounis T, et al. Unusual features of right and left idiopathic ventricular tachycardia abolished by radiofrequency catheter ablation. *Pacing Clin Electrophysiol* 1998;21:1831–1834.

15. Mitrani R, Klein LS, Miles WM, et al. Regional cardiac sympathetic denervation in patients with ventricular tachycardia in the absence of coronary artery disease. *J Am Coll Cardiol* 1993;22:1344–1353.
16. Wichler T, Hindricks G, Lerch H, et al. Regional myocardial sympathetic dysinnervation in arrhythmogenic right ventricular cardiomyopathy: an analysis using 123I-meta-iodobenzyguanidine scintigraphy. *Circulation* 1994;89:667–683.
17. Carlson MD, White RD, Trohman RG et al. Right ventricular outflow tract ventricular tachycardia: detection of previously unrecognized anatomic abnormalities using cine magnetic resonance imaging. *J Am Coll Cardiol* 1994;24:720–727.
18. Markowitz SM, Litvak BL, Ramirez de Arellano EA, et al. Adenosine-sensitive ventricular tachycardia: right ventricular abnormalities delineated by magnetic resonance imaging. *Circulation* 1997;96:1192–1200.
19. Globits S, Kreiner G, Frank H, et al. Significance of morphological abnormalities detected by MRI in patients undergoing successful ablation of right ventricular outflow tract tachycardia. *Circulation* 1997;96:2633–2640.
20. Merino JL, Jimanez-Borreguero J, Peinado R, et al. Unipolar mapping and magnetic resonance imaging of "idiopathic" right ventricular outflow tract ectopy. *J Cardiovasc Electrophysiol* 1998;9:84–87.
21. Yamauchi Y, Nogami A, Naito S, et al. Catheter ablation for ventricular tachycardia from a diverticulum at the right ventricular outflow tract. *Pacing Clin Electrophysiol* 1998;21:1835–1836.
22. Mera F, Walter PF, Langberg JJ. Right ventricular outflow tract ventricular tachycardia as a result of blunt chest trauma. *Pacing Clin Electrophysiol* 1998;21:2147–2148.
23. Rahilly GT, Prystowsky EN, Zipes DP, et al. Clinical and electrophysiology findings in patients with repetitive monomorphic ventricular tachycardia and otherwise normal electrocardiogram. *Am J Cardiol* 1982;50:459–468.
24. Lerman BB, Stein K, Engelstein ED, et al. Mechanism of repetitive monomorphic ventricular tachycardia. *Circulation* 1995;92:421–429.
25. Vijgen J, Hill P, Biblo LA, et al. Tachycardia-induced cardiomyopathy secondary to right ventricular outflow tract ventricular tachycardia: improvement of left ventricular systolic function after radiofrequency catheter ablation of the arrhythmia. *J Cardiovasc Electrophysiol* 1997;8:445–450.
26. Lerman BB, Belardinelli L, West GA, et al. Adenosine-sensitive ventricular tachycardia: evidence suggesting cyclic AMP-mediated triggered activity. *Circulation* 1986;74:270–280.
27. Lerman BB, Stein KM, Markowitz SM. Mechanisms of idiopathic left ventricular tachycardia. *J Cardiovasc Electrophysiol* 1997;8:571–583.
28. Belhassen B, Rotmensch HH, Laniado S. Response of recurrent sustained ventricular tachycardia to verapamil. *Br Heart J* 1981;46:679–682.
29. Zipes DP, Foster PR, Troup PJ, et al. Atrial induction of ventricular tachycardia: reentry versus triggered automaticity. *Am J Cardiol* 1979;44:1–8.
30. Lin FC, Finely CD, Rahimtoola SH, et al. Idiopathic paroxysmal ventricular tachycardia with a QRS pattern of right bundle branch block and left axis deviation: a unique clinical entity with specific properties. *Am J Cardiol* 1983;52:95–100.
31. German LD, Packer DL, Bardy GH, et al. Ventricular tachycardia induced by atrial stimulation in patients without symptomatic cardiac disease. *Am J Cardiol* 1983;52:1202–1207.
32. Ward DE, Nathan AW, Camm AJ. Fascicular tachycardia sensitive to calcium antagonists. *Eur Heart J* 1984;5:896–905.
33. Sung RJ, Keung EC, Nguyen NX, et al. Effects of β-adrenergic blockade on verapamil-responsive and verapamil-irresponsive sustained ventricular tachycardias. *J Clin Invest* 1988;81:688–699.
34. Ohe T, Shimomura K, Aihara N, et al. Idiopathic sustained left ventricular tachycardia: clinical and electrophysiological characteristics. *Circulation* 1988;77:560–568.
35. Wen MS, Yeh SJ, Wang CC, et al. Radiofrequency ablation therapy in idiopathic left ventricular tachycardia with no obvious structural heart disease. *Circulation* 1994;89:1690–1696.
36. Bogun F, El-Atassi R, Daoud E, et al. Radiofrequency ablation of idiopathic left anterior fascicular tachycardia. *J Cardiovasc Electrophysiol* 1995;6:1113–1116.
37. Rodriguez LM, Smeets JLRM, Timmermans C, et al. Radiofrequency catheter ablation of idiopathic ventricular tachycardia originating in the anterior fascicle of the left bundle branch. *J Cardiovasc Electrophysiol* 1996;7:1211–1216.
38. Diker E, Tezcan K, Özdemir M, et al. Adenosine sensitive left ventricular tachycardia. *Pacing Clin Electrophysiol* 1998;21:134–136.
39. Damle RS, Landers M, Kelly PA, et al. Radiofrequency catheter ablation of idiopathic left ventricular tachycardia originating in the left anterior fascicle. *Pacing Clin Electrophysiol* 1998;21:1155–1158.
40. Nogami A, Naito S, Tada H, et al. Verapamil-sensitive left anterior fascicular ventricular tachycardia: results of radiofrequency ablation in six patients. *J Cardiovasc Electrophysiol* 1998;9:1269–1278.
41. Okumura K, Matsuyama K, Miyagi H, et al. Entrainment of idiopathic ventricular tachycardia of left ventricular origin with evidence of reentry with an area of slow conduction and effect of verapamil. *Am J Cardiol* 1988;62:727–732.
42. Nakagawa H, Beckman KJ, McClelland JH, et al. Radiofrequency catheter ablation of idiopathic left ventricular tachycardia guided by a Purkinje potential. *Circulation* 1993;88:2607–2617.
43. Wen MS, Yeh SJ, Wang CC, et al. Successful radiofrequency ablation of idiopathic left ventricular tachycardia at a site away from the tachycardia exit. *J Am Coll Cardiol* 1997;30:1024–1031.
44. Lai LP, Lin JL, Hwang JJ, Huang SKS. Entrance site of the slow conduction zone of verapamil-sensitive idiopathic left ventricular tachycardia: evidence supporting macroreentry in the Purkinje system. *J Cardiovasc Electrophysiol* 1998;9:184–190.
45. Pfammatter JP, Paul T. Idiopathic ventricular tachycardia in infancy and childhood. *J Am Coll Cardiol* 1999;33:2067–2072.
46. O'Conner BK, Case CL, Sokoloski MC, et al. Radiofrequency catheter ablation of right ventricular outflow tachycardia in children and adolescents. *J Am Coll Cardiol* 1996;27:869–874.
47. Saul JP, Hulse JE, Papagiannis J, et al. Late enlargement of radiofrequency lesions in infant lambs. Implications for ablation procedures in small children. *Circulation* 1994;90:492–499.
48. Gursoy S, Brugada J, Souza O, et al. Radiofrequency ablation of symptomatic but benign ventricular arrhythmias. *Pacing Clin Electrophysiol* 1992;15:738–741.
49. Zhu DW, Maloney JD, Simmons TW, et al. Radiofrequency catheter ablation for management of symptomatic ventricular ectopic activity. *J Am Coll Cardiol* 1995;26:843–849.
50. Lauck G, Burkhardt D, Manz M. Radiofrequency catheter ablation of symptomatic ventricular ectopic beats originating in the right outflow tract. *Pacing Clin Electrophysiol* 1999;22:5–16.
51. Lauribe P, Shah D, Jaïs P, et al. Radiofrequency catheter ablation of drug refractory symptomatic ventricular ectopy: short- and long-term results. *Pacing Clin Electrophysiol* 1999;22:783–789.

52. Wellens HJJ. Radiofrequency catheter ablation of benign ventricular ectopic beats: a therapy in search of a disease? *J Am Coll Cardiol* 1995;26:850–851.
53. Fontaine G, Tonet J, Frank R. Ventricular tachycardia in arrhythmogenic right ventricular dysplasia. In: Zipes DP, Jalife J, eds. *Cardiac electrophysiology: from cell to bedside*, 3rd ed. Philadelphia: WB Saunders, 2000:546–555.
54. Stark SI, Artur A, Lesh MD. Radiofrequency catheter ablation of ventricular tachycardia in right ventricular cardiomyopathy: use of concealed entrainment to identify the slow conduction isthmus bounded by an aneurysm and the tricuspid annulus. *J Cardiovasc Electrophysiol* 1996;7:967–971.
55. Ellison KE, Friedman PL, Ganz LI, Stevenson WG. Entrainment mapping and radiofrequency catheter ablation of ventricular tachycardia in right ventricular dysplasia. *J Am Coll Cardiol* 1998;32:724–728.
56. Harada T, Aonuma K, Yamauchi Y, et al. Catheter ablation of ventricular tachycardia in patients with right ventricular dysplasia: identification of target sites by entrainment mapping techniques. *Pacing Clin Electrophysiol* 1998;21:2547–2550.
57. Marcus FI. Idiopathic ventricular fibrillation. *J Cardiovasc Electrophysiol* 1997;8:1075–1083.
58. Brugada J, Brugada R, Brugada P. Right bundle-branch block and ST-segment elevation in leads V_1 through V_3. A marker for sudden death in patients without demonstrable structural heart disease. *Circulation* 1998;97:457–460.
59. Gussak I, Antzelevitch C, Bjerregaard F, et al. The Brugada syndrome: clinical, electrophysiologic and genetic aspects. *J Am Coll Cardiol* 1999;33:5–15.
60. Wilber DJ, Baerman J, Okshansky B, et al. Adenosine-sensitive ventricular tachycardia: clinical characteristics and response to catheter ablation. *Circulation* 1993;87:126–129.
61. Coggins DL, Lee RJ, Sweeney J, et al. Radiofrequency catheter ablation as a cure for idiopathic tachycardia of both left and right ventricular origin. *J Am Coll Cardiol* 1994;23:1333–1341.
62. Krebs ME, Krause PC, Engelstein ED, et al. Ventricular tachycardias mimicking those arising from the right ventricular outflow tract. *J Cardiovasc Electrophysiol* 2000;11:45–51.
63. Goyal R, Harvey M, Daoud EG, et al. Effect of coupling interval and pacing cycle length on morphology of paced ventricular complexes: implications for pace mapping. *Circulation* 1996;94:2843–2849.
64. Chinushi M, Aizawa Y, Ohhira K, et al. Repetitive ventricular responses induced by radiofrequency ablation for idiopathic ventricular tachycardia originating from the outflow tract of the right ventricle. *Pacing Clin Electrophysiol* 1998;21:669–678.
65. Peeters HAP, Sippens-Groenewegen A, Schoonderwoerd BA, et al. Body-surface QRST integral mapping. Arrhythmogenic right ventricular dysplasia versus idiopathic right ventricular tachycardia. *Circulation* 1997;95:2668–2676.
66. Peeters HAP, Sippens-Groenewegen A, Wever EFD, et al. Clinical application of an integrated 3-phase mapping technique for localization of the site of origin of idiopathic ventricular tachycardia. *Circulation* 1999;99:1300–1311.
67. Kamakura S, Shimizu W, Matsuo K, et al. Localization of optimal ablation site of idiopathic ventricular tachycardia from right and left ventricular outflow tract by body surface ECG. *Circulation* 1998;98:1525–1533.
68. Gepstein L, Hayam G, Ben-Haim SA. A novel method for nonfluoroscopic catheter-based electroanatomical mapping of the heart. *Circulation* 1997;95:1611–1622.
69. Nademanee K, Kosar EM. A nonfluoroscopic catheter-based mapping technique to ablate focal ventricular tachycardia. *Pacing Clin Electrophysiol* 1998;21:1442–1447.
70. Schilling RJ, Peters NS, Davies DW. Feasibility of a noncontact catheter for endocardial mapping of human ventricular tachycardia. *Circulation* 1999;99:2543–2552.
71. Miles WM, Engelstein ED, Olgin JE, et al. Slow pathway ablation using nonfluoroscopic guidance for His bundle localization during energy delivery [Abstract]. *Circulation* 1997;96:I-452.
72. Wellens HJJ, Smeets JLRM. Idiopathic left ventricular tachycardia: cure by radiofrequency ablation. *Circulation* 1993;88:2978–2979.
73. Rodriguez L-M, Smeets JLRM, Timmermans C, et al. Predictors for successful ablation of right- and left-sided idiopathic ventricular tachycardia. *Am J Cardiol* 1997;79:309–314.
74. Aizawa Y, Chinushi M, Kitazawa H, et al. Spatial orientation of the reentrant circuit of idiopathic left ventricular tachycardia. *Am J Cardiol* 1995;76:316–319.
75. Page RL, Shenasa H, Evans JJ, et al. Radiofrequency catheter ablation of idiopathic recurrent ventricular tachycardia with right bundle branch block, left axis morphology. *Pacing Clin Electrophysiol* 1993;16:327–336.
76. Suwa M, Youeda Y, Nagao H, et al. Surgical correction of idiopathic paroxysmal ventricular tachycardia possibly related to left ventricular false tendon. *Am J Cardiol* 1989;64:1217–1220.
77. Thakur RK, Klein GJ, Sivaram CA, et al. Anatomic substrate for idiopathic left ventricular tachycardia. *Circulation* 1996;93:497–501.
78. Lin F-C, Wen M-S, Wang C-C, et al. Left ventricular fibromuscular band is not a specific substrate for idiopathic left ventricular tachycardia. *Circulation* 1996;93:525–528.
79. Mandrola JM, Klein LS, Miles WM, et al. Radiofrequency catheter ablation of idiopathic ventricular tachycardia in 57 patients: acute success and long term follow-up [Abstract]. *J Am Coll Cardiol* 1995;25:19A.
80. Calkins H, Kalbfleisch SJ, El-Atassi R, et al. Relation between efficacy of radiofrequency catheter ablation and site of origin of idiopathic ventricular tachycardia. *Am J Cardiol* 1993;71:827–833.
81. Arruda M, Chandrasekaran K, Reynolds D, et al. Idiopathic epicardial outflow tract ventricular tachycardia: implications for radiofrequency catheter ablation [Abstract]. *Pacing Clin Electrophysiol* 1996;19:611A.
82. Callans DJ, Menz V, Schwartzman D, et al. Repetitive monomorphic tachycardia from the left ventricular outflow tract: electrocardiographic patterns consistent with a left ventricular site of origin. *J Am Coll Cardiol* 1997;29:1023–1027.
83. Stellbrink C, Diem B, Schauerte P, et al. Transcoronary venous radiofrequency catheter ablation of ventricular tachycardia. *J Cardiovasc Electrophysiol* 1997;8:916–921.
84. Arruda M, Wilber D, Marinchak R, et al. The value of epicardial mapping of ventricular tachycardia from the coronary venous system: a prospective multicenter study [Abstract]. *J Am Coll Cardiol* 1999;816.
85. Sosa E, Scanavacca M, D'Avila A, Pilleggi F. A new technique to perform epicardial mapping in the electrophysiology laboratory. *J Cardiovasc Electrophysiol* 1996;7:531–536.
86. Sosa E, Scanavacca M, D'Avila A, et al. Radiofrequency catheter ablation of ventricular tachycardia guided by nonsurgical epicardial mapping in chronic Chagasic heart disease. *Pacing Clin Electrophysiol* 1999;22:128–130.
87. Yeh SJ, Wen MS, Wang CC, et al. Adenosine-sensitive ventricular tachycardia from the anterobasal left ventricle. *J Am Coll Cardiol* 1997;30:1339–1345.
88. Shimoike E, Ohba Y, Yanagi N, et al. Radiofrequency catheter ablation of left ventricular outflow tract tachycardia: report of two cases. *J Cardiovasc Electrophysiol* 1998;9:196–202.

89. Friedman PL, Stevenson WG, Bittl JA, et al. Left main coronary artery occlusion during radiofrequency catheter ablation of idiopathic outflow tract ventricular tachycardia [Abstract]. *Pacing Clin Electrophysiol* 1997;20:1184A.
90. Hachiya H, Aonuma K, Yamauchi Y, et al. The electrocardiographic characteristics of left ventricular outflow tract tachycardia [Abstract]. *Pacing Clin Electrophysiol* 1999;22:733.
91. Nakagawa H, Yamanashi WS, Pitha JV, et al. Comparison of in vivo tissue temperature profile and lesion geometry for radiofrequency ablation with a saline-irrigated electrode versus temperature control in a canine thigh muscle preparation. *Circulation* 1995;91:2264–2273.
92. Zipes DP, de Joseph RL, Rothbaum DA. Unusual properties of accessory pathways. *Circulation* 1974;49:1200.
93. Akhtar M, Damato AN, Batsford WP, et al. Demonstration of reentry within the His-Purkinje system in man. *Circulation* 1974;50:1150.
94. Akhtar M, Gilbert C, Wolf FG, et al. Reentry within the His-Purkinje system: elucidation of reentrant circuit using right bundle branch and His bundle recordings. *Circulation* 1978;58:295–304.
95. Reddy CP, Slack JD. Recurrent sustained ventricular tachycardia: report of a case with His-bundle branches reentry as the mechanism. *Eur J Cardiol* 1980;11:23–31.
96. Welch WJ, Strasberg B, Coelho A, et al. Sustained macroreentrant ventricular tachycardia. *Am Heart J* 1982;104:166–169.
97. Lloyd EA, Zipes DP, Heger JJ, et al. Sustained ventricular tachycardia due to bundle branch reentry. *Am Heart J* 1982;104:1095–1097.
98. Touboul P, Kirkorian G, Atallah G, et al. Bundle branch reentry: a possible mechanism of ventricular tachycardia. *Circulation* 1983;67:674.
99. Merino JL, Carmona JR, Fernandez-Lozano I, et al. Mechanisms of sustained ventricular tachycardia in myotonic dystrophy. Implications for catheter ablation. *Circulation* 1998;98:541–546.
100. Negri SM, Cowan MD. Becker muscular dystrophy with bundle branch reentry ventricular tachycardia. *J Cardiovasc Electrophysiol* 1998;9:652–654.
101. Narasimhan C, Jazayeri MR, Sra J, et al. Ventricular tachycardia in valvular heart disease: facilitation of sustained bundle-branch reentry by valve surgery. *Circulation* 1997;96:4307–4313.
102. Chien WW, Scheinman MM, Cohen TJ, Lesh MD. Importance of recording the right bundle branch deflection in the diagnosis of His-Purkinje reentrant tachycardia. *Pacing Clin Electrophysiol* 1992;15:1015–1024.
103. Crijns HJGM, Smeets JLRM, Rodriguez LM, et al. Cure of interfascicular reentrant ventricular tachycardia by ablation of the anterior fascicle of the left bundle branch. *J Cardiovasc Electrophysiol* 1995;6:486–492.
104. Blanck Z, Deshpande S, Jazayeri MR, Akhtar M. Catheter ablation of the left bundle branch for the treatment of sustained bundle branch reentrant ventricular tachycardia. *J Cardiovasc Electrophysiol* 1995;6:40–43.
105. Mehdirad AA, Keim S, Rist K, et al. Asymmetry of retrograde conduction and reentry within the His-Purkinje system: a comparative analysis of left and right ventricular stimulation. *J Am Coll Cardiol* 1994;24:177–184.
106. Denker S, Shenasa M, Gilbert C, et al. Effects of abrupt changes in cycle length on refractoriness of the His-Purkinje system in man. *Circulation* 1983;67:60–68.
107. Denker S, Lehman M, Mahmud R, et al. Facilitation of macroreentry within the His-Purkinje system with abrupt changes in cycle length. *Circulation* 1984;69:26–32.
108. Touboul P, Kirkorian G, Atallah G, et al. Bundle branch reentrant tachycardia treated by electrical ablation of the right bundle branch. *J Am Coll Cardiol* 1986;7:1404–1409.
109. Tchou P, Jazayeri M, Denker S, et al. Transcatheter electrical ablation of the right bundle branch: a method of treating macro-reentrant ventricular tachycardia due to bundle branch reentry. *Circulation* 1988;78:246–257.
110. Langberg JJ, Desai J, Dullet N, et al. Treatment of macroreentrant ventricular tachycardia with radiofrequency ablation of the right bundle branch. *Am J Cardiol* 1989;63:1010–1013.
111. Cohen T, Chien W, Luri K, et al. Radiofrequency catheter ablation for treatment of bundle branch reentrant ventricular tachycardia: results and long-term follow-up. *J Am Coll Cardiol* 1991;18:1767–1773.
112. Miles WM. Bundle branch reentrant tachycardia: a chance to cure? *J Cardiovasc Electrophysiol* 1993;4:263–265.
113. Klein LS, Miles WM. Ventricular tachycardia in patients with normal hearts. *Cardiol Rev* 1993;1:336–339.
114. Miles WM, Klein LS. Radiofrequency ablation of idiopathic ventricular tachycardia and bundle branch reentrant tachycardia. In: Singer I, ed. *Interventional cardiology*. Baltimore: Williams & Wilkins, 1996:383–412.
115. Klein LS, Miles WM, Zipes DP. Ablation of idiopathic ventricular tachycardia and bundle branch reentry. In: Zipes DP, ed. *Catheter ablation of arrhythmias*. Armonk, NY: Futura Publishing, 1994:259–276.
116. Klein LS, Miles WM. Ablative therapy for ventricular arrhythmias. *Progr Cardiovasc Dis* 1995;37:225–242.
117. Klein LS, Zipes DP, Miles WM. Ablation of ventricular tachycardia in patients without coronary artery disease and ventricular tachycardia due to bundle branch reentry. In: Huang SKS, ed. *Radiofrequency catheter ablation of cardiac arrhythmias: basic concepts and clinical applications*. Armonk, NY: Futura Publishing, 1994:479–490.

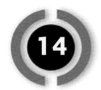

RADIOFREQUENCY CATHETER ABLATION OF VENTRICULAR TACHYCARDIA IN PATIENTS WITH CORONARY ARTERY DISEASE

• • •

ROSS D. FLETCHER, PAMELA KARASIK

One of the earliest tachyarrhythmias to be addressed by catheter ablation was ventricular tachycardia, often occurring in patients with coronary artery disease. The first intracardiac target structure to be ablated using percutaneous catheters was the atrioventricular (AV) node (1,2) to improve rate control during atrial fibrillation. Soon thereafter, catheter ablation was shown to be effective in ablating ventricular tachycardia. Even though the initial series was only three cases, the investigators (3,4) informally postulated that the success in these cases would dramatically change the way we treated ventricular tachycardia. This prediction has not been realized, in part because of the effectiveness of newer antiarrhythmic drugs and of antitachycardia and defibrillation devices. In retrospect, it seems that one of the cases might have been bundle branch reentry, which has proven an easy target for ablation.

During the same period, surgical and electrophysiology teams in Paris (5) and Philadelphia (6) were demonstrating success against ventricular tachycardia using surgical procedures. The success of the endocardial "Philadelphia peel" resection further encouraged those in the field determined to use catheters for mapping and ablation. Several investigators amassed a sizable experience in catheter ablation with direct current (DC) shock, called *fulguration* by Guy Fontaine (7,8).

The success rates for DC shock might have reflected the large lesion size. The use of catheters in the catheterization laboratory eliminated the risks of anesthesia and cross-clamp times in the operating room. This allowed increased time for careful mapping of sustained arrhythmia and the ability to readily return to the catheterization laboratory to ablate a recurrence. In our institution, catheter ablation has always been used to reverse incessant ventricular tachycardia before declaring failure. Incessant tachycardia was the indication that encouraged catheter ablation of ventricular tachycardia before many other arrhythmias were attempted.

◉ INDICATIONS

In patients with coronary disease, incessant ventricular tachycardia that is unresponsive to all other forms of therapy remains one of the primary indications for ablation therapies. In one study, a multivariate analysis showed incessant tachycardia as the only consistent predictor for success. Frequent recurrent ventricular tachycardia is a common additional indication, but the advent of advanced antiarrhythmic pharmacologic agents such as intravenous and oral amiodarone and advanced antitachycardia and defibrillation devices have made ablation therapy for ventricular tachycardia less necessary. However, the use of implantable devices has provided new indications. Recurrent ventricular tachycardia unresponsive to pacing therapy and requiring frequent cardioversions often is a target for ablation therapy. An implanted device cannot specifically detect slow, sustained ventricular tachycardias occurring at rates that overlap the sinus rates. The device cannot be set to detect and treat only the slow ventricular tachycardia without also detecting and treating sinus tachycardia. Antitachycardia and pacing therapies are sometimes uncomfortable and occasionally inappropriate antitachycardia therapy for sinus tachycardia sometimes may induce ventricular tachycardia or ventricular fibrillation. These slow ventricular tachycardia rhythms are therefore best managed as targets for ablation therapy. In some patients, sinus rhythm after shock can rise above the tachycardia rate resulting in inappropriate therapy for delivered on sinus tachycardia. The explanations for post-shock sinus tachycardia include response to pain, fear of further shocks, compensation for a period of hypotension, and possibly, inhibition of endocardial vagal enervation. In a patient with an implantable cardioverter-defibrillator (ICD) and frequent ventricular tachycardia, ablation therapy is recommended in the American College of Cardiology guidelines as a class 1 indication (9).

The success rates of many investigators (10–13) for ablation of individual "target" ventricular tachycardia morphologies are quite high. Although these patients may have ventricular tachycardia recurrences, ventricular tachycardia is often greatly modified. A newer definition for success states that if ventricular tachycardia recurs less frequently and is easily reverted by the device, or the target ventricular tachycardia does not recur, the ablation procedure is considered successful.

Familiarity with the pathophysiology of ventricular tachycardia in coronary disease is important for achieving successful ablations. Most of the cases of ventricular tachycardia in coronary artery disease consist of reentrant circuits within or around scarred myocardium or aneurysms, which is discussed later in this chapter in the section on arrhythmia localization (14,15). Neurohormonal modulation and increased stretch enhance the circuits in the fixed substrate in coronary disease. These factors can facilitate the circuits and produce clinical events that would not be possible without increased sympathetic influence or dilated ventricles resulting from heart failure. The success of ablation may be related to the time of ablation from the index myocardial infarction. In one study, if the ablation was performed less than 2 years after myocardial infarction, the recurrence rate was zero. In the group who underwent ablative therapy more than 2 years after myocardial infarction, the recurrence rate was 62% (16).

● PREPARATION

The success of ablating ventricular tachycardia depends on a careful analysis of all data before the procedure, a well-defined and coordinated plan for executing mapping, and a clear knowledge of the ablating device. Most investigators start with an idea of the probable location of the target ventricular tachycardia. Standard ventriculography and coronary arteriography reveal discrete aneurysms or scars. Thrombus in the left ventricle is detected by imaging techniques and is a relative contraindication to an ablation for several reasons. The risk of thromboembolic events is higher, and the thrombus itself may impair the ability to completely ablate the tachycardia circuit. Echocardiography and ventriculography can reveal the presence of clot but may underestimate the incidence. Altmose and colleagues (17) reported on the incidence of clot in post-myocardial infarction patients undergoing ventriculotomy for ventricular tachycardia surgery (after mapping). Twenty-six percent were found to have unsuspected thrombus. Those with anterior myocardial infarctions and aneurysms had the highest incidence of thrombus, whereas those with inferior myocardial infarction had a 10% incidence. Despite this, the preoperative risk of an embolic event during the preoperative mapping procedures was small, and postoperatively, there was a 2% incidence of central nervous system embolism.

The most important data come from the 12-lead electrocardiogram (ECG) during spontaneous ventricular tachycardia. The morphology allows recognition of the target ventricular tachycardia when it occurs in the electrophysiology laboratory. All

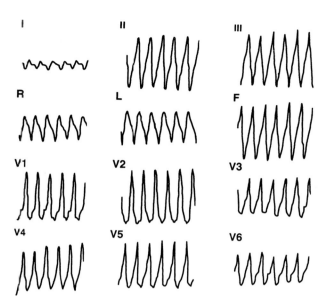
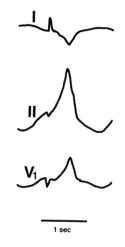

FIGURE 14-1. Ventricular tachycardia (VT) in a patient after repair of tetralogy of Fallot. The VT has an inferior axis and right bundle branch block (RBBB) morphology in V_1. Although this usually represents a left ventricular origin, in this patient, the pace map from the outflow of the right ventricle (right side) reproduced the I, II, and V_1 morphology of the VT. This RBBB morphology of the VT emanates from the repaired outflow of the right ventricle.

monomorphic, sustained ventricular tachycardias induced during the procedure need to be considered possible future clinical problems and may have caused episodes in the past that were not clinically documented. Different morphologies may represent alternative exit sites from the same reentrant circuit.

Common rules that predict location have been defined in the surgical ablation experience. In general, if V_4, V_5, and V_6 are negative, the tachycardia arises from the apical half of the ventricles. If V_4, V_5, and V_6 are positive, the tachycardia arises from the basal half of the ventricles. If V_1 is positive, the tachycardia is from the left ventricle (18,19). We have had exceptions to these rules. A patient with a large right ventricle from repaired tetralogy of Fallot and persistent pulmonary insufficiency offers an example of a ventricular tachycardia with right bundle branch block configuration in V_1 (Fig. 14-1). The V_1 during tachycardia and pace mapping from the right ventricular outflow showed a similar upright QRS in V_1. A negative QRS in V_1, which appears like left bundle branch block, usually indicates origin in the septum, but a right ventricular origin occurred in 36%. A wide (>0.04 msec), small R in V_1 before the deep S may indicate right ventricular free wall origin. Although uncommon, ventricular tachycardia origin from the right ventricle does occur in patients with coronary artery disease and should be considered if all areas in the left ventricle map inappropriately late. Negative QRS in leads II and III and aVF usually indicate a site on the inferior surface of the heart. As the QRS in these leads becomes more positive, the origin is higher in the ventricle.

OVERVIEW OF THE ELECTROPHYSIOLOGY LABORATORY

After the preliminary data have been fully analyzed and suspected sites of altered anatomy are well in mind, the electrophysiology laboratory is prepared for the case. Despite the wide range of equipment available in a modern electrophysiology laboratory, a careful plan for recording and pacing must be established so that mapping proceeds quickly and methodically. Although patience and tenacity are the best qualities for success, systematic and rapid recording and analyzing of sites are essential. Knowledge of the coronary anatomy, the ventricular anatomy, and the ejection fraction are critical for a safe, successful procedure. The target ventricular tachycardia ideally should be hemodynamically tolerated, with the patient free from angina and having a systolic blood pressure greater than 90 mm Hg. Newer mapping systems use a noncontact electrode, which makes possible mapping of a single beat of the ventricular tachycardia.

The indications for ablation may be expanded to patients with unstable rhythms in the future.

Patients are prepared for the ablation in much the same way as for a diagnostic electrophysiology procedure, with some important exceptions. Although antiarrhythmic medications are typically withheld for a diagnostic study, if an otherwise unstable ventricular tachycardia is rendered slower and more suitable for mapping, the drug should be continued. However, if the tachycardia is more difficult to induce, the drug should be discontinued for five half-lives. Patients are brought to the laboratory in the fasting, unsedated state with an indwelling Foley catheter in place. This improves patient comfort during what is often an extended procedure and allows the medical staff to monitor volume status. Conscious sedation is provided using a combination of midazolam, fentanyl, and propofol. In a large series of ablation patients reported by O'Brien and coworkers, doses were 0.5 to 7 mg (total) of midazolam and 25 to 100 mcg of fentanyl, and propofol was administered as a continuous infusion of 20 to 30 mcg/kg/min (20). Sedation can be performed by nurses trained in administration of conscious sedation or by anesthesiology personnel. Approximately 1% of sedated patients require mechanical ventilation.

Venous access is obtained through the right and left femoral veins, and arterial access is obtained through the right femoral artery. Continuous arterial monitoring is performed in every patient through the femoral sheath side arm or a radial arterial line.

Intracardiac recordings are obtained from the His position and the right ventricular apex. Often, a catheter is placed in the high right atrium as well. The right ventricular catheter is critical for recording and providing a site for ventricular tachycardia induction. Although standard quadripolar catheters are suitable for this purpose, we use a monophasic action potential catheter with orthogonal pacing. A separate quadripolar catheter is placed in the inferior vena cava for unipolar recording or pacing when combined with the ablation catheter. If a catheter has been placed initially in the high right atrium, it can be withdrawn or advanced to either vena cava and used as the indifferent electrode. In the past, unipolar electrodes were placed proximally on pacing catheters to achieve convenient unipolar pacing. New catheter designs promise to include proximal electrodes for unipolar pacing or recording. Unipolar pacing most accurately reflects events at the tip of the catheter. Pacing near the threshold value with the ablation tip negative (i.e., cathodal polarity) is rarely inaccurate and produces fewer artifacts on the recording channel (21).

For mapping and ablating, a steerable quadripolar catheter with a 4-mm electrode tip is most commonly used. Early in the development of ablation therapy, 1- and 2-mm tip catheters produced inadequate lesions and quickly developed coagulum associated with high impedance rises (22). Larger electrodes (e.g., 8 mm) have since been used. Ablation catheters come in a variety of curves. A short radius is required for sites in the outflow tract, and a long radius curve may be more valuable in seeking sites on the free wall or under the mitral valve.

The retrograde aortic approach through the right femoral artery is most commonly used to access the left ventricle. Care should always be given to crossing the aortic valve, because the structure can be damaged by aggressive manipulation. Although this is the most common method of mapping the left ventricle, in certain patients, a transseptal approach may be necessary. A variety of transseptal sheaths are available. We use a standard Mullins sheath. Several different mapping and ablation catheters are commercially available. Steerable quadripolar catheters with 4-mm tip electrodes are available in a wide range of curves and lengths. The 8-mm tip electrodes are available as well, but they should be used with caution because they can create larger and deeper lesions and generally require more power than is commonly available on standard radiofrequency generators. Catheters with cooled tips and alternative energy sources are under clinical investigation.

After the left ventricle has been accessed, all patients are anticoagulated with 5,000 units of heparin. We administer 1,000 to 2,000 units of heparin per hour for the duration of the procedure to maintain an activated clotting time of 300 seconds.

After the catheters are properly positioned, attempts are made to induce the clinical ventricular tachycardia. We use standard programmed electrical stimulation protocols, beginning with the least aggressive and increasing aggressiveness as needed. The ability to induce the relevant tachycardia may present the biggest impediment to a successful procedure. If the standard protocol is unsuccessful at inducing the tachycardia, several maneuvers can be attempted. First, if the patient is overly sedated, discontinue sedation. Isoproterenol (Isuprel) and special pacing techniques described later may be necessary for induction. In some laboratories, pace mapping during sinus rhythm is the first maneuver. This technique can identify a target area in which more detailed mapping can be performed (23). Sometimes, tachycardias are induced that do not appear to be the clinical tachycardia. On rare occasions, the dominant ventricular tachycardia does not allow a second, often slower ventricular tachycardia to be expressed. Usually, we do not try to ablate ventricular tachycardia unless it has been documented to have clinical significance. Occasionally, a "new" morphology is easily induced after an initial apparently successful ablation. These may represent a new exit for the original tachycardia. We ablate these new sites, particularly if they are closely related to the original ablation site. We have encountered patients in whom a nonclinical ventricular tachycardia becomes incessant after the primary ventricular tachycardia has been ablated. Those patients require ablation of the second focus. Ortiz and associates presented data on a small group of patients with coronary artery disease who underwent radiofrequency ablation of ventricular tachycardia. Although a nonclinical ventricular tachycardia was induced in many of the patients, only one patient had a recurrence of ventricular tachycardia, and it had not been induced in the laboratory (24).

Radiofrequency generators for ablation may be manually controlled or have thermistor feedback with automatic temperature or wattage control. These devices are helpful in that they automatically power off in the case the impedance rises, thereby minimizing the risk of coagulum formation on the catheter tip. The temperature data is useful in assessing the degree of myocardial contact. If adequate temperature cannot be reached, there is usually poor contact between the myocardium and the ablation catheter. If the output drops to very low wattage, it suggests that the tip of the catheter is too deeply embedded in the myocardium and is not being adequately cooled by the blood pool. In some patients, the impedance remains high despite absence of coagulum formation.

A second, indifferent electrode placed on the thorax may lower the impedance and allow for adequate heating.

Other information can be used to assess catheter contact. The unipolar electrogram recorded between the mapping catheter and a catheter placed in the inferior vena cava with low-frequency settings of 0.05 to 1 Hz can record the ST segment at the point of contact. As pressure on the myocardium increases, the ST segment initially elevates. Elevations greater than 1 to 2 mV may signal perforation of the ventricular wall. If a perforation occurs, the ST segment depresses, and the usually negative QRS becomes positive (Fig 14-2). There are areas in the right ventricular cavity near the base that produce ST depression with initial contact and not elevation (25). These areas should not be interpreted as perforation.

During radiofrequency energy delivery, some patients experience discomfort. Deeper anesthesia to prevent movement leading to displacement of the catheter may be needed. Special consideration should be given to patients with markedly depressed ejection fractions (<20%). Although they may tolerate prolonged procedures, we have found that hemodynamic deterioration occurs after return to the intensive care unit. Even when an anesthesiologist has provided controlled sedation and invasive hemodynamic monitoring with no perturbations during the procedure, some patients become unstable. We advocate prophylactic intraaortic balloon pump insertion and invasive hemodynamic monitoring in the sickest patients in whom a prolonged procedure is anticipated.

We prefer to deliver radiofrequency current during the ventricular tachycardia. If no effect is seen within 30 seconds, energy delivery is terminated, and mapping continues. If the ventricular tachycardia terminates, radiofrequency delivery is continued for 60 to 120 seconds. Attempts at reinduction are done after termination of the tachycardia. If no further ventricular tachycardia is induced, we wait 30 to 60 minutes and repeat the induction protocol. At the conclusion of the procedure, the activated clotting time is measured. When less than 150 seconds, the sheaths are removed, and the patient is transferred to the medical intensive care unit. We no longer measure creatine phosphokinase levels after ablation, because we found that few patients leak enzyme after delivery of radio-

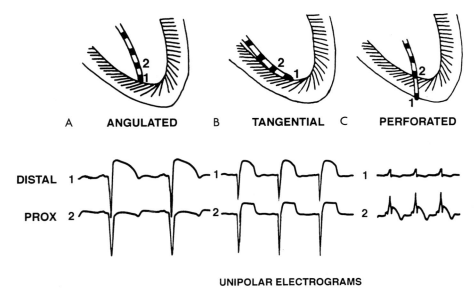

FIGURE 14-2. **A:** The ST segment deviation is higher on the tip than the proximal electrode when the tip is against the ventricular wall. **B:** The ST may be elevated in both leads when they are equally against the ventricular wall. **C:** If the catheter perforates, the ST inverts, and the QRS becomes upright.

frequency energy. Some centers perform an electrophysiology study the next day, but others wait for a clinical event.

● RECORDING, PACING, AND FLUOROSCOPIC TECHNIQUE

The ability to safely manipulate the exploring catheter throughout the left ventricle and achieve consistent contact on left ventricular sites is usually the most difficult part of the procedure and requires persistence. Sometimes, a fresh operator "finds" the spot because more experienced operators have fallen into a routine that prevents access to the correct location.

Recognizing when the catheter is in a good location is much easier than getting it there. The use of electrogram recordings and the classic responses to pacing identify fruitful ablation sites. The commonly used criteria are based on reliable models of reentrant ventricular tachycardia and systematic studies of success rates. The common pathway of a reentrant ventricular tachycardia circuit is identified by these techniques. If it exists on a narrow isthmus, the tachycardia can be eliminated with radiofrequency energy administered through an electrode as small as 4 mm. Before radiofrequency ablation, DC shocks were effective in part because they created a larger lesion (26), and mapping techniques could therefore be less precise. The earliest successful ablation using open-heart surgery excised a sizable patch of endocardium and allowed less precise mapping (27). The techniques used in these early methods for ablation have been adapted and refined for the more precise mapping required for radiofrequency ablation (28, 29). In good hands, the success rates with radiofrequency ablation are as good as with DC ablation.

A systematic exploration requires the ability to place each catheter site on a general map of the left ventricular and right ventricular endocardium. Several maps have been developed for endocardial mapping. These include two apical, five middle, and five basal locations. These are on three septal, five inferior, and posterolateral walls and on four anterior positions (30,31) (Fig. 14-3). Frame-grabbing fluoroscopic images in two planes—left anterior oblique (LAO) and right anterior oblique (RAO) or frontal and lateral—are most helpful when determining the location of the catheter. Ideally, biplane fluoroscopy can be used. Analyzing the catheter locations is especially helpful when dealing with failure or a recurrence. The exact degree of LAO or RAO should be used for each new catheter position so that catheter positions can be superimposed on each other to create a real image map. For example, 30-degree RAO and 60-degree LAO provide convenient orthogonal views. The exact degree of RAO and LAO used is

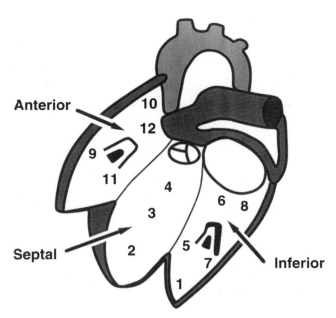

FIGURE 14-3. An example of left ventricular positions for endocardial mapping. (Adapted from Josephson ME, Horowitz LN, Spielman SR, et al. Role of catheter mapping in the preoperative evaluation of ventricular tachycardia. *Am J Cardiol* 1982; 49:207–220, with permission.)

not as important as consistently using the same angle in a given case. Each view needs to be numbered and related to recording sites. Modern electrophysiologic, computerized recorders allow frame grabbing of a digital fluoroscopic image to be automatically placed in the record at the time the electrophysiologic tracings are recorded. When this feature is not available, placing incremental radiopaque numbers in the fluoroscopic or cine path for each site can number sequential cine film recordings. A small area of interest usually contains many mapped sites. Relatively minor changes can obtain a more ideal pace map during sinus rhythm or earlier, more discrete electrograms during ventricular tachycardia, or better pace mapping during ventricular tachycardia. Identifying regions in the heart that are not close to good ablation sites allows the team to focus on more fruitful areas. Systematic mapping allows the physician to determine when no left ventricular site is present and directs attention to the right ventricle. Right ventricular tachycardia accounts for a small but distinct percentage of successful ablation sites in coronary artery disease.

With modern recorders, there is virtually no limi-

tation of leads. Ventricular tachycardia should be recorded with the 12 leads as they have been placed in the electrophysiology laboratory. Arm leads on the shoulders and leg leads on the hips do not reproduce exactly the 12-lead ECG that was recorded in the emergency room or critical care unit (CCU) during the clinical ventricular tachycardia. As often as possible in the electrophysiology laboratory leads should be placed in the standard 12-lead positions. When anterior defibrillation pads are placed low, the V_1 and V_2 are displaced laterally. If special leads were used in the CCU, they can be included as a bipolar lead at standard ECG recording frequencies such as a 0.05-Hz, low-frequency setting. The MCL_1 lead is a bipolar monitoring lead, whose positive electrode is on the V_1 position and whose negative electrode is on the left shoulder. This lead is commonly used in the CCU to simulate V_1 but often is different from a standard recording of V_1. Notice the critical difference in the standard V_1 and MCL_1 in Figure 14-4. A major clinical error was made in this case as the clinicians assumed the rSR' in MCL_1 indicated a supraventricular origin of the tachycardia. The early rise to peak in the true V_1 would favor ventricular tachycardia with 1:1 retrograde conduction to the atrium.

Before pacing, the ventricular capture threshold should be evaluated using a pulse width of 2 msec. The operator sets the output to twice the threshold value and makes certain the ventricle is sensed before pacing to avoid pacing in the vulnerable period. Many programmed stimulators sense in sinus rhythm but pace S_1 at a fixed rate. Custom stimulators made for our laboratory and some commercial units could sense a premature ventricular beat during the S_1 drive and reset the S_1 count to 1 or continue at the next expected number. At the very least, all stimulators should sense the last QRS before pacing and pace at an interval likely to miss the vulnerable period. In ventricular tachycardia patients, recurrent inadvertent inductions with paced R on T can cause the patient to rapidly deteriorate.

Ventricular tachycardia induction for purposes of ablation especially in coronary artery disease, should be done as mildly as possible with longer S_1 drive cycles (600 msec) and as few extrastimuli as possible. The least aggressive protocol induces the slowest ventricular tachycardia and is unlikely to induce nonclini-

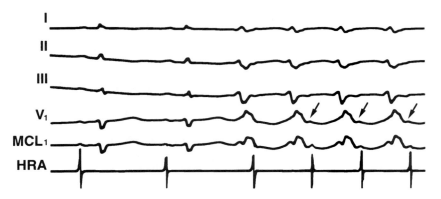

FIGURE 14-4. The MCL_1 showed rSR′, but the V_1 recorded simultaneously in an electrophysiology laboratory showed an early rise to peak, revealing its ventricular origin as confirmed by intracavitary recordings.

cal arrhythmias. The ventricular tachycardia is targeted with whatever technique is required. Sometimes, this means not just S_2, S_3, and S_4, but occasionally an S_5 and commonly the use of isoproterenol. When isoproterenol is required to induce the target ventricular tachycardia, it is given initially as 0.5 mcg/min and increased gradually to a maximum of 3 mcg/min or a change in sinus rate of greater than 20 bpm. Caffeine (125 mg, given intravenously) may be helpful. On occasion, a long setup cycle in the drive train aids tachycardia induction. This is achieved by setting the S_1 intervals to seven cycles at 600 msec. The S_1S_2 is set to a long interval, which is limited by the atrial rate. Ventricular pacing must be pure on the eighth beat. The S_2S_3 becomes the S_1S_2. S_3S_4 is the S_2S_3. This long setup cycle before the premature beats extends refractory periods to allow unidirectional block and reentrant ventricular tachycardia (32). Pacing from the left ventricle may be necessary to induce the clinical ventricular tachycardia.

When the target ventricular tachycardia occurs, it is recorded in the laboratory with 12 leads and used as the reference morphology for all future pacing studies. Copies should be easily seen by those manipulating catheters and those monitoring and recording events. The ablation catheter should be moved to a suspected area. The onset of the earliest QRS on any of the 12 leads is determined. The lead, which shows the clearest and earliest break from baseline, is chosen to measure the onset of QRS in all subsequent interventions. It is important that this QRS onset be easily seen and reproduced. The 12-lead ECG should always be recorded at a high-frequency filter setting of 100 Hz. The ECG technician's temptation to provide "smooth" tracings with 50- or even 25-Hz high-frequency filters should be discouraged. The onset of the electrogram record on the ablation catheter and the time relationship with the earliest QRS onset is measured. If the ventricular tachycardia is hemodynamically tolerated, the catheter is slowly manipulated to obtain an earlier electrogram site. When the ventricular tachycardia is no longer tolerated or the mapping is complete, the ventricular tachycardia is reverted with the pacing technique least likely to produce ventricular fibrillation or polymorphic ventricular tachycardia.

Once ventricular tachycardia can be reliably induced and reverted by pacing, diagnostic pacing during the ventricular tachycardia is started. Typically, pacing at twice threshold requires less than 1 mA. Pacing from the standard 4-mm tip of an ablation catheter usually requires 3 to 5 mA to capture, but in areas of scar, it may require current as high as 12 to 15 mA. Some investigators recommend high outputs, such as 35 to 45 mA, when pace mapping scars. This level is rarely necessary, and it may cause pacing of sites remote to the electrode position.

The S_1 of the stimulator is set 20 to 50 msec shorter than the measured ventricular tachycardia cycle length. Pacing is attempted during ventricular tachycardia, always sensing the first QRS to avoid unduly premature pacing intervals. Short pacing intervals not only run the risk of R on T starting rapid tachycardia, but more likely, short pacing intervals may revert the tachycardia or cause misleading delays between stimulus and QRS. At pacing intervals close to the ventricular tachycardia cycle length, it frequently requires eight S_1s to ensure full capture. Late partial capture with a large component of the ventricular tachycardia morphology can give the erroneous impression that the paced QRS is identical to the ventricular tachycardia. If the QRS morphology changes during pacing, the pacing site is not in the final common pathway.

MAPPING AND PACING RESPONSE

The expected electrograms and response to pacing depend on current models for ventricular tachycardia in coronary artery disease (33). Most frequently, ablatable reentrant circuits require a substrate of scar caused by myocardial infarction. This scar may or may not be an anatomic aneurysm, but the substrate should contain the barriers and the areas of slow conduction necessary for monomorphic reentrant ventricular tachycardia (34,35). The models presented by Stevenson and colleagues are legitimate simplifications of what is often a more complex electrophysiologic source of clinical ventricular tachycardia (36–38). They make the most theoretical sense of the findings during ventricular tachycardia mapping and help localize targets for ablating ventricular tachycardia. The target of ablation therapy is the common pathway, which has an exit and an entrance connected by an inner loop (Fig. 14-5). Other loops with longer paths or slower conduction can also connect the exit of the common pathway with the entrance, but the pathway that leaves the common pathway first and returns to the entrance earliest is the dominant inner loop. If this loop is ablated, the tachycardia could be sustained through a slower outer loop at a longer cycle length. The exit from the common pathway often branches into several exit pathways before the QRS on the external ECG is inscribed. Ablating after the exit from the common pathway but before the QRS does not stop the tachycardia but may change the QRS morphology. However, when the common pathway is ablated, the tachycardia cannot be sustained.

The common pathway is most amenable to ablation therapy when it narrows to a small isthmus and can be bridged by the 4-mm tip of an ablation catheter. The earliest sites may not be in as narrow a region as electrograms in mid-diastole. Some (39) have recommended an electrogram to QRS (EGM-QRS)

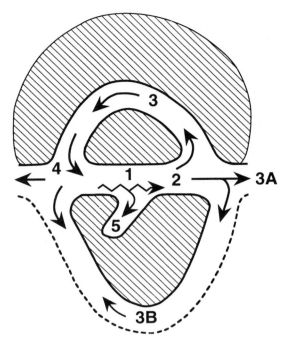

FIGURE 14-5. Ventricular tachycardia reentrant circuit shows the common pathway (1) exiting (2) to an inner loop (3), which reenters at the entrance (4) of the common pathway. The impulse passes from the exit (2) to exit pathway (3A) and simultaneously travels around an outer loop (3B) back to the entrance of the common pathway. (Adapted from Stevenson WG, Khan H, Sager P, et al. Identification of reentry circuit sites during catheter mapping and radiofrequency ablation of ventricular tachycardia late after myocardial infarction. *Circulation* 1993;88:1647–1670, with permission.)

duration no earlier than 70% of the ventricular tachycardia cycle length (1) (Fig. 14-6). However, electrograms that are quite early with an EGM-QRS duration of less than 30% of the ventricular tachycardia cycle length are often recorded from areas emanating from the exit from the common pathway (2) (Fig. 14-6) and include exit pathways and the early portions of the inner and outer loops. Only rarely does ablating a site with these shorter EGM-QRS times revert the ventricular tachycardia and prevent its induction. The exact onset of the electrogram in the common pathway can be misinterpreted if the gain on the amplifier is relatively low. High gain is important for recording the onset of consistent, small electrograms that are often seen in the common pathway. Many feel the onset of the electrogram is more important than whether the electrogram is discrete or continuous,

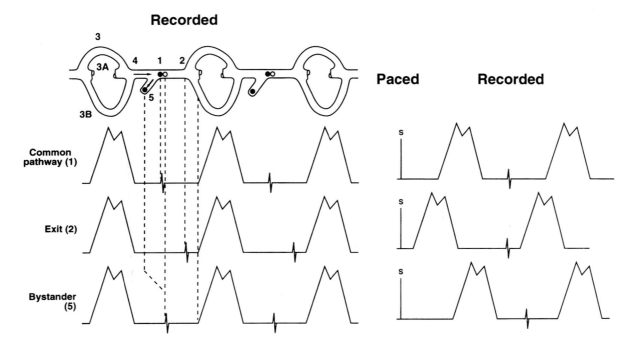

FIGURE 14-6. The loop diagram is made into a continuous horizontal diagram to depict several beats of ventricular tachycardia. Classic recordings from the common pathway (1), exit pathway (2), and a bystander pathway (5) correspond to their respective positions in the continuous loop. The electrogram to QRS (EGM-QRS) duration of the bystander pathway appears earlier than the common pathway but results from the conduction time from the common pathway to the recording spot on the bystander circuit. The paced versus recorded panel *(right)* shows that the stimulus to QRS (S-QRS) duration is equal to the EGM-QRS duration in the common pathway (1) and the exit site (2), but the S-QRS duration is longer than the EGM-QRS duration in the bystander pathway (5).

but isolated diastolic potentials may imply a narrow discrete isthmus amenable to ablation by 4-mm electrode ablating surfaces (40,41).

Pacing during the tachycardia provides better localization. If the paced QRS is identical to the target ventricular tachycardia in all 12 leads, the catheter is in the reentrant circuit or in a bystander circuit. Capture of the common pathway is determined by noting that the stimulus to QRS (S-QRS) time equals the EGM-QRS duration and that these intervals are longer than 30 msec.

Bystander circuits can have intermediate EGM-QRS values that simulate common pathway recordings (5) (Fig.14-6), but stimulation from the exploring catheter during ventricular tachycardia can indicate the origin of the electrogram to be outside the reentrant circuit. In such instances, there is a mismatch between recorded EGM-QRS and S-QRS. Conduction into a bystander pathway makes the recorded electrogram of the bystander pathway appear closer to onset of the QRS. It is closer to the QRS by the amount of time it takes to conduct from the bystander pathway's origin in the common pathway to the recording site in the bystander pathway. When paced, the S-QRS value includes the time it takes to conduct from the site on the bystander pathway to the common pathway. It also includes the time it takes to conduct from this point through the common pathway to its exit. The S-QRS includes the relatively short time it takes to transmit from the exit of the common pathway to the subsequently inscribed QRS. Recording in the common pathway, however, always has an S-QRS equal to the EGM-QRS. When the S-QRS and the EGM-QRS are equal (<20 msec), the catheter is in the reentrant circuit.

Pacing from the recording site during ventricular

tachycardia allows comparison of S-QRS with EGM-QRS and allows assessment of entrainment (42,43). The ventricular tachycardia is entrained when the ventricular tachycardia continues after the pacing is stopped and the last paced QRS has the same morphology as the ventricular tachycardia. Entrainment can often occur when the paced area is in the ventricular tachycardia circuit or when the excitable gap of the ventricular tachycardia circuit is entered from a site outside the reentrant circuit (44,45). More rapid pacing during ventricular tachycardia, by as much as 100 msec less than the ventricular tachycardia cycle length, is often done to confirm no change of the QRS and therefore no progressive fusion. Entrainment with fusion indicates catheter sites at the entrance and exit of the slow zone or pacing has engaged the excitable gap from outside the tachycardia circuit (46). Concealed (47) entrainment is present if, when pacing at 20 to 50 msec less than the ventricular tachycardia cycle length, the ventricular tachycardia morphology is unchanged, and the return beat is advanced (Fig.14-7A).

If the paced QRS is not identical to the ventricular tachycardia, fusion may be occurring. Fusion is more likely to be seen with pacing at faster intervals, such as 100 msec shorter than the ventricular tachycardia cycle. If the QRS is altered more with a more rapid pacing rate, progressive fusion exists (48). When progressive fusion occurs in classic entrainment, it specifically indicates a site in the outer loop or entrance to the common pathway. Even when progressive fusion occurs with entrainment, the last paced QRS is always similar to the tachycardia (Fig. 14-7B), because the fusion occurs between the previous orthodromically conducted beat in the ventricular tachycardia circuit and depolarization of ventricular myocardium conducted antidromically from the stimulation site. The stimulation itself also enters the tachycardia circuit and conducts orthodromically to the next QRS. If pacing is continued, this orthodromically conducted QRS fuses with antidromic conduction from the next stimulus. The last stimulus in the train fuses with the previous QRS and conducts orthodromically to a QRS, which contains no antidromic component, and therefore is identical to the QRS of the native ventricular tachycardia. For all types of entrainment, the last paced QRS is the same as the QRS of the ventricular tachycardia. Progressive fusion with entrainment usually does not indicate a position in the common pathway. It is important to view the next to the last paced QRS to determine if an exact morphologic match has been achieved. If pacing produces a QRS morphology identical to the ventricular tachycardia at the faster pacing rate and there is no change in QRS even at faster paced rates, entrainment is concealed, and the pacing is occurring in the common pathway.

After concealed entrainment without fusion is established, the interval between the last stimulus and

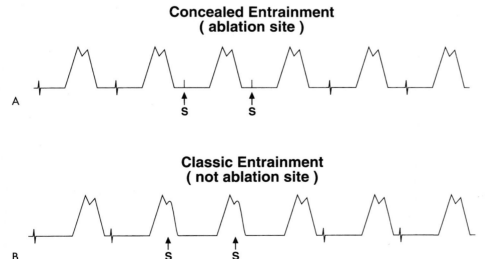

FIGURE 14-7. A: Stimulation during concealed entrainment advances the QRS with no change in QRS morphology and indicates a position of the catheter in the common pathway. The postpacing interval (PPI) is equal to the ventricular tachycardia cycle length (VTCL). B: Stimulation with entrainment and fusion. The first paced beat fuses with the prior VT reentrant beat and advances the next QRS. The last paced beat fuses with the previous QRS but causes a normal VT complex on the last paced beat. A faster pace rate would cause more fusion (i.e., progressive fusion). The PPI is longer than the VTVL. This does not represent a good ablation site.

the local electrogram of the first ventricular tachycardia QRS is measured as the postpacing interval (PPI) and compared to the ventricular tachycardia cycle length. If the catheter is in the circuit, the first postpacing interval will be equal to the ventricular tachycardia cycle length. The circuit includes the common pathway and its exit, along with the inner loop and its entrance. When the pacing site is not in the ventricular tachycardia circuit, the PPI usually is longer than the ventricular tachycardia cycle length. This includes bystander sites, exit pathway, and sites distant from the reentry loop. Although the common pathway, the exit, inner loop, and the entrance sites all have a PPI equal to the ventricular tachycardia cycle length, they are distinguished from each other by the EGM-QRS duration. Often, the current required to capture the ventricle during pace mapping saturates the recording amplifiers and obliterates the signal on the ablation catheter. Soejima and coworkers has reported on the use of the n + 1 interval for entrainment mapping (49). The duration of S-QRS is measured after the last captured beat, S-QRS n + 1. This value is compared with the EGM n + 3 and the QRS n + 4. If the difference is zero, the catheter is in the common pathway.

Although there are many possible recordings and pacing responses to specific areas in and around the ventricular tachycardia circuit, the only response that need be remembered during mapping is the response when in the common pathway. All other responses are not in the common pathway. Recognizing a good position is usually easy if the ventricular tachycardia can be initiated and is hemodynamically stable.

Table 14-1 suggests an orderly assessment of recording and pacing. The first step is to search for an exact 12-lead pace map while pacing in sinus rhythm. When exact or close, the ventricular tachycardia is induced, and a search is made for the earliest electrogram during ventricular tachycardia. The examiner then paces during ventricular tachycardia at 20 to 50 msec less than the ventricular tachycardia cycle length value. When consistent capture is achieved, the paced 12-lead QRS morphology is matched with the target ventricular tachycardia value. When the paced QRS is an exact match in all 12 leads of the external ECG, the EGM-QRS is compared with the S-QRS to see if they are within 20 msec. If ventricular tachycardia is sustained after pacing is stopped, entrainment has probably occurred. The PPI is measured and compared with the next ventricular tachycardia cycle. If they are equal (<30 msec), the catheter is in the reentrant circuit, and therapeutic ablation should proceed. Pacing at a more rapid rate, 100 msec shorter than the ventricular tachycardia cycle length, excludes progressive fusion. The catheter often requires adjustment by small amounts to closely match the ventricu-

TABLE 14-1 • ASSESSMENT OF RECORDING AND PACING

Site	Distant (6)	Common Pathway (1) Ablate	Exit (2)	Inner Loop (3)	Exit Path (3A)	Outer Loop (3B)	Entrance (4)	Bystander Pathway (5)
Sinus rhythm								
(1) Pacemap QRS in 12-lead match	No	Yes/no	Yes/rarely no	Yes/no	No close match	No	Yes/rarely yes	Yes/rarely no
Ventricular tachycardia								
(2) Record earliest EGM <70% VTCL	After QRS	Before QRS—30 to 70% VTCL	Before QRS—30 to 0% VTCL	Before QRS	Before QRS	After QRS	Before QRS	Before QRS shorter than S-QRS
(3) Pace—50 msec shorter than VTCL								
Ablation criteria								
QRS in 12-lead match	No	Yes	Yes	Yes	No (minor)	No	Yes	Yes
S-QRS equals EGM QRS	>>	=	=	= or <	=	>	= or <	>
PPI equals VTCL		=	= or >	=	= or >	=	=	>
(4) Pace—100 msec shorter than VTCL								
QRS in 12-lead match	No	Yes	Yes	Yes	No	Yes/no	No (fusion)	Yes
PPI equals VTCL	>	=	=	> or =	>	=	=	>

VTCL, ventricular cycle length; PPI, postpacing interval.

lar tachycardia in all 12 leads of the external ECG. The first pacing intervention, a pace map in sinus rhythm, can be valuable for general localization. It may not match the ventricular tachycardia morphology in all 12 leads, whereas pacing from the same site during the reentrant ventricular tachycardia does produce an exact match. In sinus rhythm, the paced rhythm may propagate retrogradely or antidromically and anterogradely or orthodromically from the area of slow conduction and may not produce an exact match of all 12 leads even when pacing in the area of slow conduction. In one series, the site of concealed entrainment rarely produced an exact pace map during sinus rhythm (11). However, when pacing well into the common pathway of slow conduction during ventricular tachycardia, the returning waveform of the ventricular tachycardia prevents antidromic conduction. Orthodromic conduction proceeds slowly, but when it exits the common pathway, the QRS is early and exactly matches the clinical tachycardia in all 12 leads. This event is concealed entrainment. No amount of prematurity is likely to create any of the progressive fusion seen in classic entrainment. When entrainment is concealed, a position well within the common pathway is likely, and the site is a good site for ablation.

The negative findings that mandate repositioning include an electrogram that is in or after the QRS onset or is exceedingly short, such as 20 to 30 msec. In this case, the catheter is not on the common pathway. If the paced QRS during ventricular tachycardia does not match exactly, concealed entrainment has not occurred, and the catheter needs to be repositioned. If the S-QRS is greater or less than the EGM-QRS, or the PPI is greater than the ventricular tachycardia cycle length, the catheter is not in the reentrant circuit. When one of these negative findings exists, the catheter should be repositioned to a better location.

All the measurements can be made using a simple four-beat analysis at the termination of pacing during ventricular tachycardia (Fig. 14-8). After the catheter is guided to a probable ventricular tachycardia site by pace mapping, the ventricular tachycardia should be induced. The physician then paces at 20 to 50 msec less than the ventricular tachycardia cycle length and must ensure that pacing captures the QRS. When the QRS stops walking through the stimulation artifact, capture is likely. After termination of pacing, the last two intervals paced and the first two intervals not paced are 'frozen' on the screen. The first two QRS intervals are measured to confirm that the R-R interval is less than the ventricular tachycardia cycle length and equal to the S-S interval. The last two paced beats are compared with the first two postpacing beats of the ventricular tachycardia. The paced QRS in all 12 leads is compared with the adjacent ventricular tachycardia morphology. It is important to note whether the electrogram is isolated or continuous. The S-QRS and the EGM-QRS are then compared. If the paced and ventricular tachycardia QRS values match, and these intervals do not differ by more than 20 msec, the circuit was paced. If the first PPI equals the next interval, which is the ventricular tachycardia cycle length, the circuit was paced. If the PPI does not equal the ventricular tachycardia cycle length, a bystander pathway was paced.

After as many positive attributes as possible have been identified, an attempt to ablate the site is made. In the best of hands, the perfect site may not be recorded and paced. The lack of a perfect site, with all criteria met, does not mean that the rhythm cannot be ablated. The electrophysiologist carefully samples the area where most of the criteria are met. Ablation with radiofrequency current can be successful in these sites and should be attempted. Sometimes, more than one lesion is required at closely related sites. Creating a continuous lesion toward fixed nonconductive structures such as the mitral valve may prove successful where exact criteria cannot be recorded.

Stevenson and associates (37), Fitzgerald and colleagues (50), and Bogun and associates (51) reported systematic studies of ventricular tachycardia ablation. The most reliable positive findings, as documented with the percentage of times the ventricular tachycardia was terminated by ablation, are shown in Table 14-2.

The higher percentage of patients with concealed entrainment and with success after ablation reported by Bogun and associates (51) is probably due to a high percentage of their patients with slow ventricular tachycardia (mean ventricular tachycardia cycle length of 500 msec) and incessant tachycardia (50%). Most were treated with antitachycardia devices (72%)

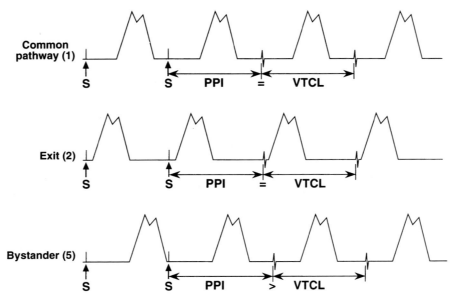

FIGURE 14-8. A simple analysis can be done when pace mapping during ventricular tachycardia (VT) by freezing on screen the last two paced beats and the first two beats of the ventricular tachycardia. This allows comparison of the morphology of paced and VT beats, a comparison of the stimulus to QRS (S-QRS) and electrogram to QRS (EGM-QRS) duration, and comparison of the postpacing interval (PPI) and the VT cycle length (VTCL). Because the last paced beat in entrainment is always the VT morphology, the next to last paced beat or first beat in the four-beat analysis should be compared with the VT morphology to detect fusion forms. The common pathway (1) has identical QRS morphology with intermediate EGM-QRS, S-QRS that is equal to EGM-QRS, and PPI that is longer than VTCL. The exit pathway (2) is the same beat with short EGM-QRS and S-QRS. The bystander pathway (5) has a good pace map, but the S-QRS is longer than the EGM-QRS, and the PPI is longer than the VTCL.

TABLE 14-2 • OUTCOMES FOR VENTRICULAR TACHYCARDIA ABLATION

	Stevenson et al. (37)[a]	Bogun et al. (50)[a]
Pacing during VT at long cycle lengths:		
Reproduces VT morphology in 12 leads and shows concealed entrainment (CE)	17%	54%
S-QRS >60 msec, <70% VTCL and CE	36%	71%
EGM-QRS equal to the S-QRS (<20 msec) and CE	24%	82%
Has PPI = VTCL (<30 msec) and CE	25%	45%
Mid-diastolic isolated potential and CE	45%	67%
Not dissociated from VT	NA	89%

PPI, postpacing interval; VTCL, ventricular cycle length; NA, not available.

and were on antiarrhythmic medications. Their success rates were higher and the rate of success with each criteria was likewise higher, but the relative value of the several criteria was similar. The only criterion that was not proportionately similar was the PPI that was equal to the ventricular tachycardia cycle length. This may result from a variation in technique. Stevenson and associates (37) took care to pace and record unipolar signals, whereas Bogun and associates (51) used a separate bipolar pair to pace and record. Nonetheless, the two studies are largely in agreement about the relative value of the criteria for successful ablation. A series of 15 patients by El-Shalakany (52) and colleagues found that a successful radiofrequency ablation was predicted if the following three criteria were met: (1) an exact 12-lead pace map during entrainment; (2) return cycle length of up to 10 msec of the ventricular tachycardia cycle length; and (3) presystolic potential (<70% of the ventricular tachycardia cycle length) to QRS within 10 msec of the S-QRS interval. Ventricular tachycardia was terminated with one current application in 19 sites that met all three criteria. An alternative method for pacing during ventricular tachycardia is the use of single premature paced beats. A single premature paced beat can fuse with the previous beat of the tachycardia and advance the next beat of the tachycardia when entrainment has occurred. When concealed entrainment occurs, only the advanced beat of the tachycardia is seen. When the premature paced beat has an S-QRS equal to EGM-QRS and has a PPI equal to the ventricular tachycardia cycle length, the catheter is on the common pathway. A particularly close localization is indicated when further prematurity does not capture the ventricle but extinguishes the tachycardia. This is thought to result from concealed conduction in the common pathway and is confirmed by several laboratories to be a sign of a successful ablation site (52–56).

Single-paced premature beats from the right ventricular apex have been used during ventricular tachycardia to reset the tachycardia and their associated isolated diastolic potentials (57). If a premature beat from the right ventricle captures the ventricle and then advances a QRS identical to the ventricular tachycardia, entrainment has occurred. If the ablation catheter records the isolated diastolic potential with an EGM-QRS of the entrained ventricular tachycardia beat, identical to the EGM-QRS of the spontaneous ventricular tachycardia, the isolated diastolic potential is associated with the ventricular tachycardia circuit. Ablation of these sites produces excellent results (72% successful). When the EGM-QRS of the paced QRS is not the same, the electrogram is dissociated, and ablation is unsuccessful. Because the recording catheter is not the pacing catheter, this technique has the advantage of easily seeing the electrogram during pacing. Although this is a recently reported technique and isolated diastolic potentials are not found in all patients, it adds to our armamentarium for identifying ablation sites by pacing during tachycardia.

⊙ ABLATION WITH RADIOFREQUENCY CURRENT

After a site is mapped, radiofrequency current is the therapy of choice. All machines that deliver continuous, unmodulated radiofrequency energy at 500 to 750 kHz and are designed for electrocautery have worked well in the unipolar mode in human arrhythmia ablation. Modern equipment designed for human ablation should allow rapid switching from recording and pacing to ablation. This is important because the catheter position identified may not be stable. An unchanging electrogram often indicates good contact. ST elevation from a unipolar, low-frequency electrogram also indicates good contact. Steady rise in thermistor temperature also indicates good contact. The thermistor temperature of 60°C ensures cell death. Avoiding temperatures above 90°C prevents coagulation and inordinate rises in impedance. An effective standard dose for ventricular tachycardia is 30 W for 1 minute. When possible, ablation should begin with the patient in ventricular tachycardia. When ventricular tachycardia reverts during radiofrequency, the application is commonly successful. Reversion of ventricular tachycardia usually occurs in less than 20 seconds. If ventricular tachycardia has not reverted in 20 to 30 seconds; further energy application rarely causes reversion. A 30- or 60-second application should be used when the ablation energy reverts the ventricular tachycardia.

A common practice is to create a second lesion in the same area. If the site was well chosen and the ventricular tachycardia reverted early (<10 seconds), a second application is unnecessary. Attempts to reinduce the tachycardia in the next few minutes should be made before the catheter is moved, since the catheter pressure on a well-chosen site can itself prevent ventricular tachycardia. A second attempt to reinduce should be made after the catheter has been moved. Some investigators have suggested delivering radiofrequency energy until the site under the catheter can no longer be captured with a pacing stimulus, ensuring complete ablation of the site.

If the impedance rises to more than 100 Ω, the catheter should be removed and the coagulum at the tip cleaned before it is reinserted. Electrical stunning from energy at a site near the common pathway may recover in 60 minutes and allow the ventricular tachycardia to be induced. Edema and transient inability of cells to be excited from the ablation may clear at a later date and allow induction of the ventricular tachycardia that had been noninducible earlier. Recurrence may develop and is available for further mapping and ablation in most cases. If the ventricular tachycardia target is no longer inducible, the ablation procedure is stopped.

Occasionally, other monomorphic tachycardias become inducible, or rarely, a slower, incessant ventricular tachycardia appears. If the tachycardia is incessant, an attempt should be made to locate its origin and ablate it. If a monomorphic ventricular tachycardia is seen that was not recorded clinically, there is a good chance it may become clinically significant. All clinically identified targets should be ablated. A new ventricular tachycardia that is not incessant and is difficult to induce can be ignored until it becomes clinically significant. After ablation, the patient can be returned to his/her monitored bed. Monitoring after the procedure can assess success and allow rapid response to any new or recurrent ventricular tachycardia.

Evaluation of the patient after ablation is difficult. Partial successes are important for individual patients. Absence of the clinical ventricular tachycardia is an obvious success. No recurrence of the target ventricular tachycardia is important if the target was relatively slow and prevented adequate recognition by antitachycardia pacing and defibrillating devices. If ventricular tachycardia with a similar morphology and rate does not recur, the ablation procedure is considered a success. If ventricular tachycardia recurs but can be suppressed with drugs that were not previously effective, ablation is considered a partial success.

CASE STUDIES

An interesting example of the application of the principle of ablation in patients with coronary disease is patient W, who had recurrent ventricular tachycardia for 6 months. The patient had no response to standard antiarrhythmics and only a partial response to amiodarone. The ventricular tachycardia could be induced after amiodarone but at a slower rate. Because of side effects, the dose was reduced to 100 mg every other day. The amiodarone was discontinued 2 weeks before coronary artery bypass surgery. The same monomorphic ventricular tachycardia recurred after coronary artery bypass grafting in the postoperative period.

Amiodarone was restarted. An electrophysiology study 10 days after amiodarone was restarted failed to induce ventricular tachycardia. Amiodarone again was not tolerated and discontinued. One month after discharge, the patient had an episode of clinical ventricular tachycardia. Two distinct morphology types had been seen clinically, both at relatively slow rates. An antitachycardia device could be used, but the rate of the tachycardia would overlap with the patient's sinus rate, making detection and treatment difficult.

An electrophysiology study for ablation initially reproduced two morphologically distinct ventricular tachycardia (VT) events, with VT-1 and VT-2 seen clinically. Pace mapping during sinus rhythm rapidly demonstrated a good morphologic match in all 12 leads for VT-1. The fluoroscopic image of the ablation catheter position in RAO and LAO views placed the site on the inferior septum (Fig. 14-9). Ventricular tachycardia induction showed a relatively early EGM-QRS. During concealed entrainment, the S-QRS was 94 msec (Fig. 14-10), which was equal to the EGM-QRS. Pacing from this site reverted to VT-2 without capturing the ventricle (Fig. 14-11). Radiofrequency energy delivery of 30 W for 60 seconds also reverted to VT-2 (Fig. 14-12). Ventricular tachycardia-1 was no longer inducible. Ventricular tachycardia-2 had a left bundle branch block morphology with a more horizontal axis.

Pace mapping high under the tricuspid valve from the right ventricle produced an exact morphology map but with short EGM-QRS (36 msec) and S-QRS (40 msec) (Fig. 14-13). Ablation at this probable exit site did not prevent induction of ventricular tachycardia. On the left ventricular septal wall opposite the right ventricular exit site, a long S-QRS was seen with a perfect 12-lead match of VT-1 morphology (Fig. 14-14). Pacing from this site extinguished VT-2 without capturing the ventricle and then paced with a VT-1 morphology (Fig. 14-15). The catheter positions for the previous attempt at extinguishing VT-2 from the right ventricle and the new position in the left ventricle are quite close (Fig. 14-9B). The decision to ablate this site, despite the inability to induce VT-1, was based on the fact that VT-2 could be reverted by pacing from this site without capturing the myocardium, and intermediate diastolic potentials at the previous ECG-QRS interval were recorded during pacing (Fig. 14-15). Ventricular tachycardia

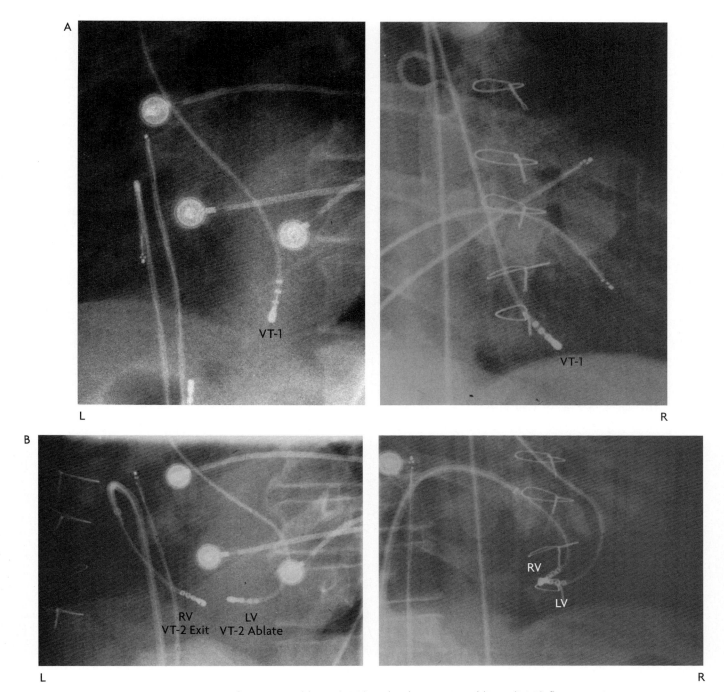

FIGURE 14-9. Left anterior oblique (LAO) and right anterior oblique (RAO) fluoroscopic images of ventricular tachycardia (VT) events. **A:** Ablation catheter on site, which successfully ablated VT-1. **B:** Right ventricular (RV) catheter at an unsuccessful site near the exit of VT-2 with the left ventricular (LV) catheter on the site where VT-2 was ablated from the left ventricle.

390 I. INTERVENTIONAL TECHNIQUES FOR ABLATION OF TACHYCARDIAS

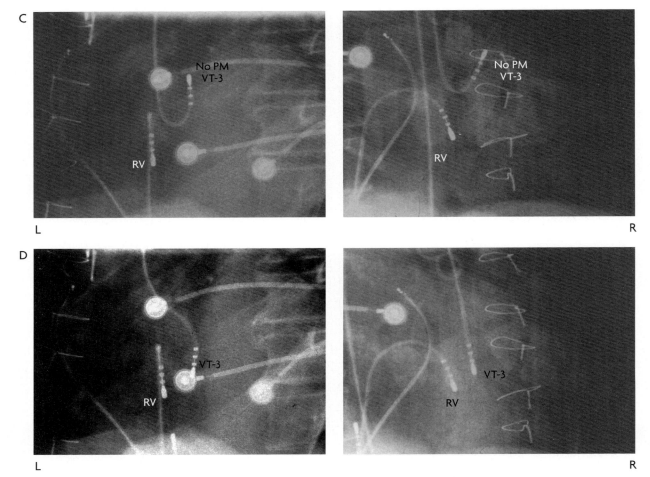

FIGURE 14-9. *(continued)* **C:** The ablation catheter is in the LV outflow with a close but not exact pace map for VT-3. **D:** The ablation catheter is in the medial LV outflow tract, where VT-3 had an exact pace map during VT, had concealed entrainment, and was ablated.

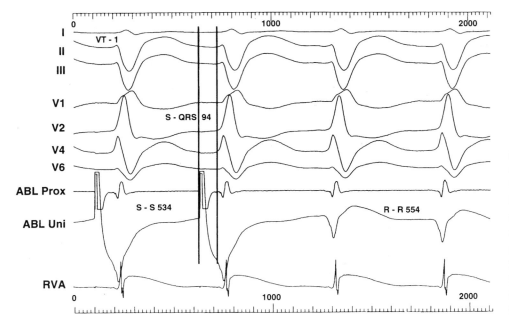

FIGURE 14-10. Pacing during ventricular tachycardia (VT) event VT-1, which was 20 msec less than the VT cycle length (VTCL), showed capture with a perfect match between the paced and spontaneous VT QRS. The stimulus to QRS (S-QRS) duration was an intermediate 94 msec, equal to the electrogram recorded shortly thereafter.

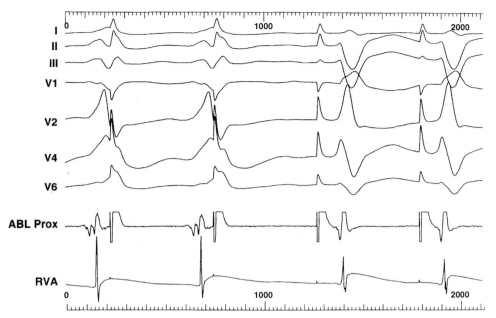

FIGURE 14-11. Ventricular tachycardia (VT) event VT-2 stops after the second stimulus, which failed to capture the ventricle. The third and fourth stimuli exactly reproduce the morphology of VT-1, with a stimulus to QRS (S-QRS) duration of 100 msec.

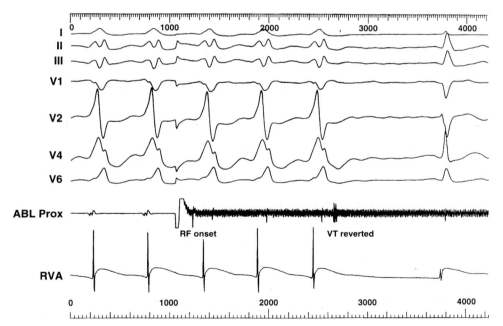

FIGURE 14-12. Ventricular tachycardia (VT) event VT-2 stops after 1.8 seconds of radiofrequency energy applied at the VT-1 site. VT-1 could not be induced after catheter placement. The catheter position is shown in Figure 14-9A.

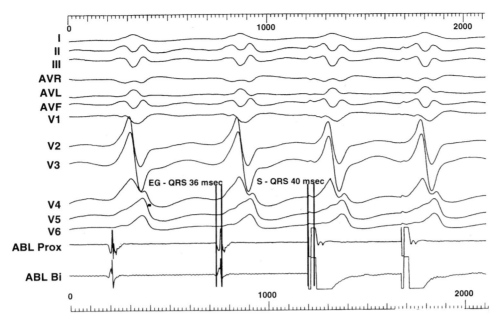

FIGURE 14-13. Ventricular tachycardia (VT) event VT-2 morphology was closely matched by pacing in the right ventricle (RV) under the tricuspid valve, with a short stimulus to QRS (S-QRS) duration (40 msec) that was approximately equal to the electrogram to QRS (EGM-QRS) duration (36 msec). The right ventricular catheter position is shown in Figure 14-9B.

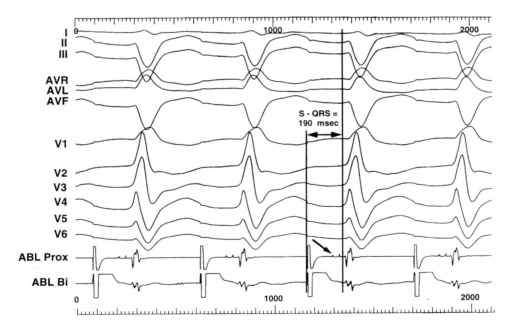

FIGURE 14-14. From the opposite side of the septum, the pace map produced an exact match of ventricular tachycardia (VT) event VT-1, with a stimulus to QRS (S-QRS) duration of 190 msec and clear diastolic potentials *(arrow)*. The left ventricular catheter position is shown in Figure 14-9B.

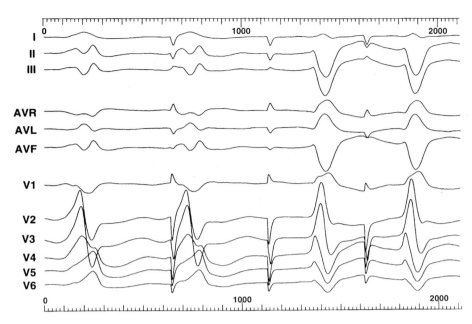

FIGURE 14-15. Pacing stopped the ventricular tachycardia (VT) event VT-2 without capture and then produced an exact match of VT-1 with a long (200-msec) stimulus to QRS (S-QRS) interval. The left ventricular catheter position is shown in Figure 14-9B.

VT-1 became noninducible before radiofrequency energy delivery in the VT-1 position, indicating possible temporary mechanical injury of the reentrant circuit. After radiofrequency energy at the left ventricular site, VT-2 was reverted (Fig. 14-16), and neither VT-1 nor VT-2 could be induced. However, a new, slow, incessant ventricular tachycardia (VT-3) was evident at 95 bpm. An attempt to map VT-3 to lateral outflow did not produce a successful map (Fig. 14-17), and the catheter position is depicted in Figure 14-9C. After a catheter change to one with a shorter radius, VT-3 was mapped to the medial left ventricular outflow (Fig. 14-9D). A perfect pace map was achieved, with EGM-QRS equal to the S-QRS (Figs. 14-18 and 14-

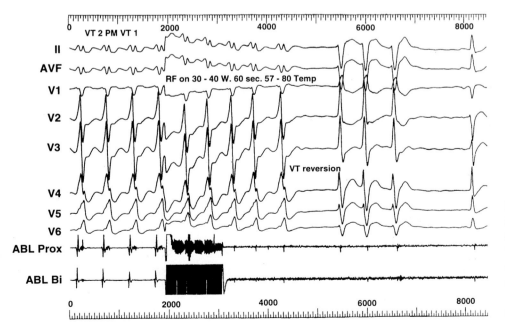

FIGURE 14-16. Radiofrequency application of 30 W for 60 seconds at a temperature of 68°C reverted the ventricular tachycardia (VT) event VT-2, after which it could not be induced. The left ventricular catheter position is shown in Figure 14-9B.

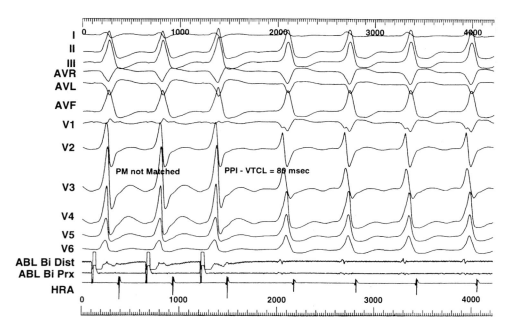

FIGURE 14-17. Pace map during ventricular tachycardia was not matched in V_1 leads I. The postpacing interval (PPI) and VT cycle length (VTCL) difference was of 80 msec. The catheter position is shown in Figure 14-9C.

19). The incessant VT-3 stopped during ablation (Fig. 14-20). After all three ventricular tachycardia sites were ablated, no ventricular tachycardia could be induced with or without isoproterenol.

A good clinical result was achieved despite three separate ventricular tachycardia morphologies. All three probably originated from different levels of the same scar. Ventricular tachycardia-1 and VT-2 were closely linked, with one exiting the left septum and the other exiting the right. The slower VT-3 may have been facilitated through an outer loop after the inner loop was ablated. It is important to recognize and discard catheter-induced tachycardia, which occurred in this case (Fig. 14-21). The rates are often irregular, with large early electrograms and associated ST deviation on the ablation catheter. Although the

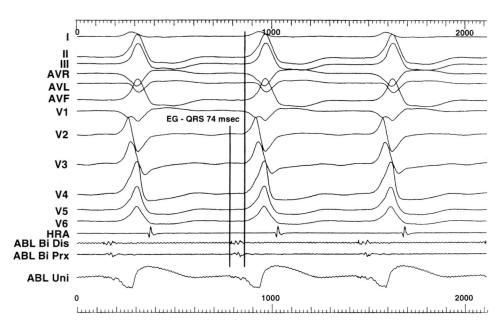

FIGURE 14-18. An earlier electrogram was present at a lower medial site. The electrogram to QRS (EGM-QRS) duration was 74 msec.

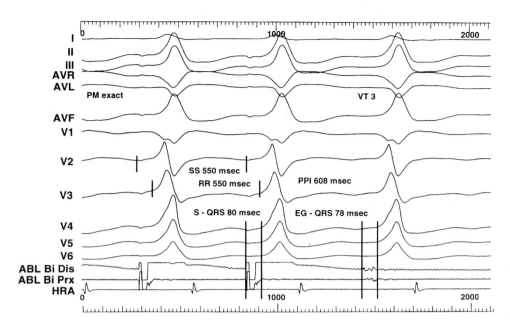

FIGURE 14-19. The stimulus to QRS (S-QRS) duration equaled the electrogram to QRS (EGM-QRS) duration, with a perfect pace map for ventricular tachycardia (VT) event VT-3.

case was not classic, many of the standard principles were used to achieve a good clinical outcome.

Patient M had recurrent ventricular tachycardia reverted by 0.6-J biphasic shocks. Antitachycardia pacing was successful only at rapid rates. The far-field electrogram from his device displayed ventricular tachycardia and then postshock sinus tachycardia (Fig. 14-22), which was also shocked needlessly. Later, this ventricular tachycardia became incessant. This patient had two indications for ablation of this target ventricular tachycardia. The first was the inability to distinguish sinus tachycardia from ventricular tachycardia. The second is that the tachycardia became incessant. Catheters were manipulated until the early EGM-QRS was found (Fig 14-23). Radiofrequency at 30 W for 60 seconds reverted the ventricular tachycardia

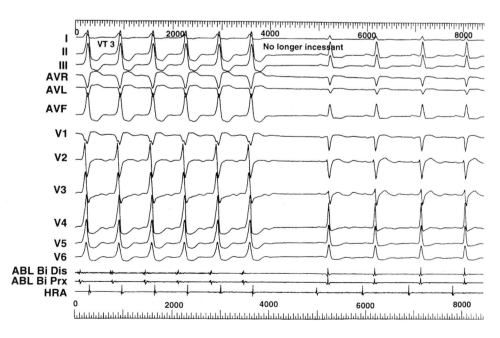

FIGURE 14-20. The incessant ventricular tachycardia (VT) event VT-3 stopped during radiofrequency ablation, after which no VT could be induced. The catheter position is shown in Figure 14-9D.

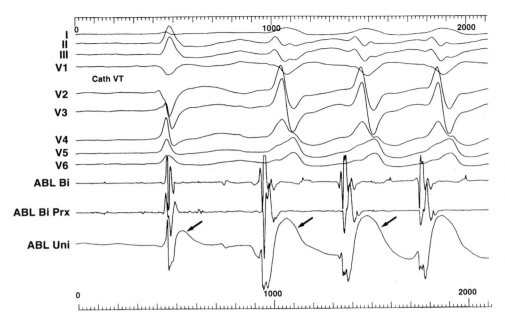

FIGURE 14-21. One of many examples of catheter-induced ventricular tachycardia (VT) during this case has a large early electrogram and associated ST elevation on the unipolar recording from the tip of the catheter. These VTs are frequently irregular and can be more difficult to distinguish when the catheter is close to the VT site.

(Fig. 14-24). The patient never had a ventricular tachycardia recurrence after the successful ablation in 3 years of follow-up.

Patient AG is a 63-year-old man with coronary artery disease who presented with sustained ventricular tachycardia 3 months after a large anterior myocardial infarction. The ejection fraction was 35%. He was initially treated with amiodarone, with a subsequent negative electrophysiologic study. However, he developed mild pulmonary toxicity, and after discontinuing amiodarone, he received a non-thoracotomy defibrillator. Over the next year, he experienced an increasing number of defibrillating shocks. Amiodarone was restarted. He then experienced recurrences of a slow, sustained ventricular tachycardia with rates that overlapped with his sinus mechanism. It was de-

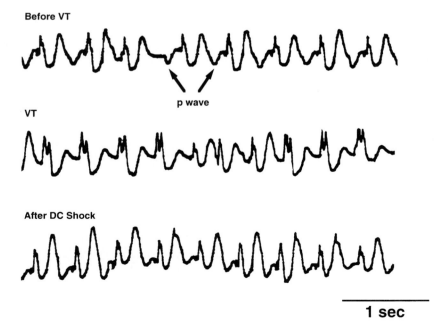

FIGURE 14-22. The patient's implantable defibrillator was capable of recording and storing a far-field electrocardiogram in which P waves could be seen and the conducted QRS morphology defined *(top)*. With the onset of ventricular tachycardia (VT) close to the sinus tachycardiac rate, the defibrillator recognized the event and shocked *(middle)*. Immediately after the shock, the patient's sinus tachycardia accelerated *(bottom)*, causing the defibrillator to shock the patient inappropriately two more times.

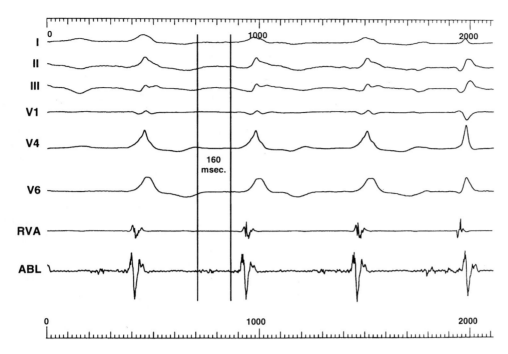

FIGURE 14-23. An early electrogram was recorded during incessant ventricular tachycardia.

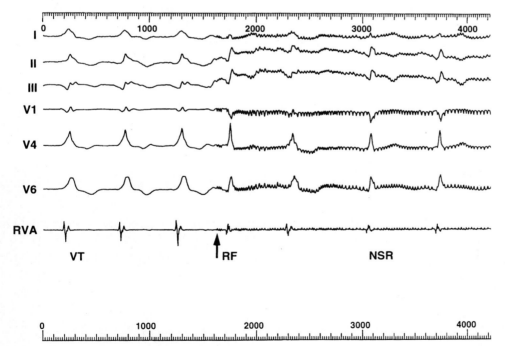

FIGURE 14-24. The incessant ventricular tachycardia (VT) reverted shortly after application of radiofrequency energy. The VT never recurred after this successful ablation.

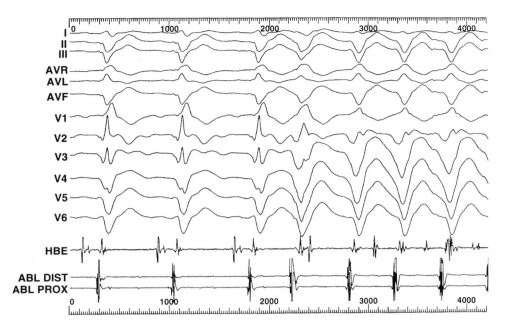

FIGURE 14-25. Clinical ventricular tachycardia (VT) occurred spontaneously when the patient was awake. The true morphology of the VT was consistent with an apical position.

cided to take the patient for ablative therapy to eliminate the dominant clinical ventricular tachycardia. The clinical ventricular tachycardia could only be induced when the patient was awake (Fig. 14-25). The clinical tachycardia had a superior axis and deep negative forces out to lead V_6. The tachycardia was mapped to the left ventricular apex along the septum (Fig. 14-26). Complicating the ablation was the appearance of what seemed to be a second wide complex tachycardia at the same rate as the clinical arrhythmia (Fig. 14-27). Closer scrutiny revealed that the QRS morphology was identical to the normal QRS and that a His bundle recording and then a P wave preceded each beat. This was a sinus tachycardia that overlapped with the ventricular tachycardia. In this case, it was difficult to find an ideal pace map, and the best site still had a PPI less than the ventricular tachycardia cycle length (Fig. 14-28). Despite that fact, the ventricular tachycardia terminated with radiofrequency energy application (Fig. 14-29). The

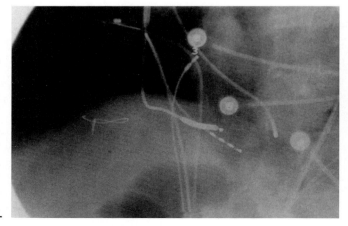
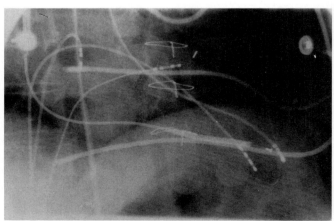

FIGURE 14-26. Left anterior oblique (LAO) and right anterior oblique (RAO) radiographs show the apical and inferior position of the ablation catheter.

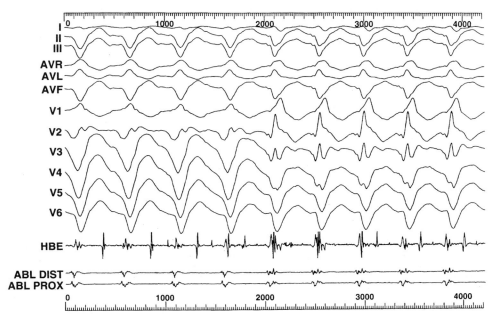

FIGURE 14-27. The left side of the tracing shows the clinical ventricular tachycardia. There is a morphologic change at beat 5. Careful scrutiny of the HBE channel shows an atrial and His bundle deflection preceding each subsequent beat, consistent with a supraventricular tachycardia.

patient has not had a recurrence of sustained ventricular tachycardia in 24 months.

Patient JB was a 45-year-old man with coronary artery disease and with an old inferior wall myocardial infarction. He presented with ventricular tachycardia to another institution and underwent ablation. He did well until 9 months later, when he presented to our hospital with a recurrence of his clinical arrhythmia.

At that time, coronary angiography demonstrated patent arteries and a fixed inferior wall defect. Several sites were mapped to the left ventricle. Initially, a good 12-lead morphologic match was found, but the activation sequence during pacing was not identical to that during the clinical tachycardia (Fig. 14-30). During pace mapping, the QRS onset to proximal coronary sinus time was 37 msec, compared with 15

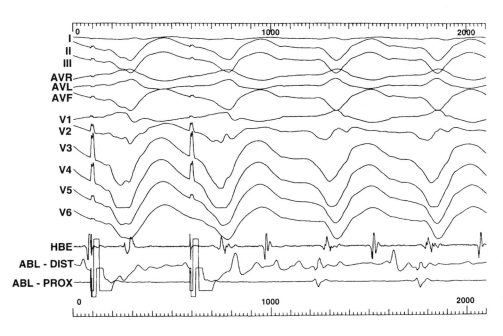

FIGURE 14-28. Pace mapping during ventricular tachycardia. Notice the subtle differences in lead II.

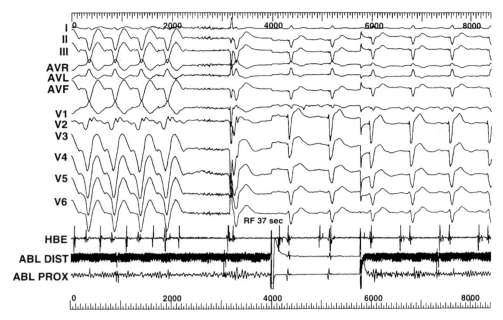

FIGURE 14-29. Termination of ventricular tachycardia with radiofrequency energy.

msec during the tachycardia. Further mapping identified a site where the activation map was identical during pacing and during the spontaneous arrhythmia (Fig. 14-31). Radiofrequency delivery at this site terminated the arrhythmia within 7 seconds (Fig. 14-32). There has not been a recurrence in several years.

Patient JE was a 57-year-old man with a long history of ventricular tachycardia and dilated cardiomyopathy. His case exemplifies some of the difficulties and challenges in managing these patients. In 1987, an epicardial ICD was implanted. At that time, he was treated with amiodarone, tocainide, and inderal. Over the next 10 years, he did well with no device activity until 1997, when he experienced six appropriate ICD shocks over a 6-month period. He was on the same medical regimen and underwent a nonin-

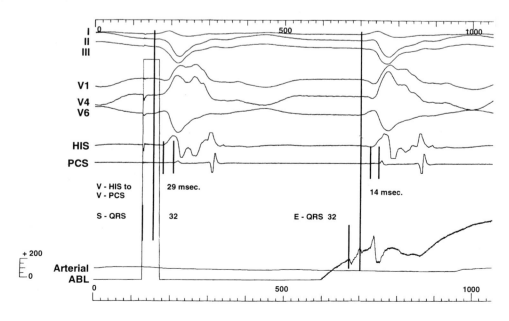

FIGURE 14-30. Pace mapping during ventricular tachycardia showed a good match, but the activation sequence did not. The length of QRS onset to proximal coronary sinus (PCS) was 29 msec during pacing, and the QRS to PCS duration was 14 msec during tachycardia.

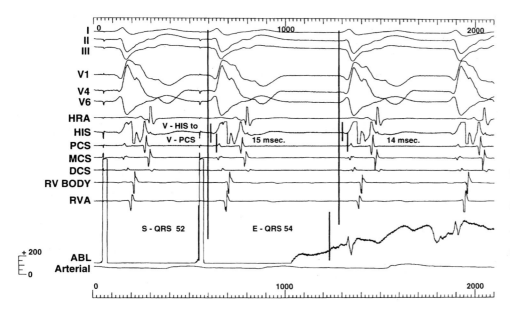

FIGURE 14-31. This site has an identical pace map and activation sequence. The time for V-H to V-PCS is 15 msec during pacing and 14 msec during tachycardia. The stimulus to QRS (S-QRS) duration is 52 msec, and the electrogram to QRS (EGM-QRS) duration is 54 msec.

vasive electrophysiologic study. The ventricular tachycardia cycle length was 430 msec and was terminated with RAMP pacing in 75% of attempts. Low-energy cardioversion restored normal sinus rhythm when the pacing was unsuccessful. He continued to do well with no device activity until September 1999, when he presented in sustained ventricular tachycardia. Despite intravenous administration of high-dose amiodarone and a beta blocker, he remained in ventricular tachycardia. Although he could be returned to sinus rhythm with cardioversion, the ventricular tachycardia returned after the first sinus beat.

The patient was taken to the electrophysiology laboratory for ablation. He had a severely dilated ventricle with multiple wall motion abnormalities and an end-systolic dimension of 91 mm. The left ventricle was extensively mapped. Initial early times and 12/12-lead pace maps were identified on the inferobasal

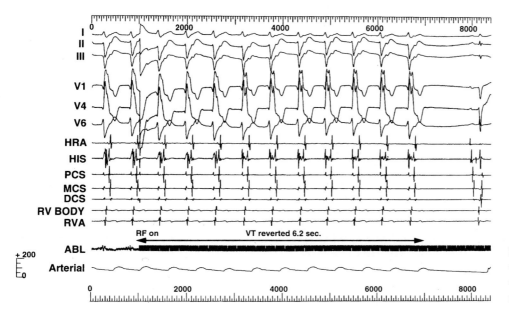

FIGURE 14-32. Termination of ventricular tachycardia occurred within 6.2 seconds of the onset of radiofrequency energy.

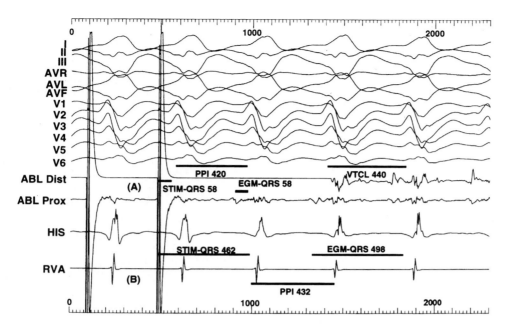

FIGURE 14-33. Entrainment mapping of the clinical ventricular tachycardia (VT). The pace map is a 12/12 match. A: The stimulus to QRS duration (S-QRS) is 58 msec. The postpacing interval (PPI) is 420 msec, and the VT cycle length (VTCL) is 440 msec. The electrogram to QRS (EGM-QRS) duration is 58 msec. Radiofrequency energy delivered at this site did not eliminate the VT. B: Reassessment of this site suggests the measurements found may be more accurate. The S-QRS duration is 462 msec, and the EGM-QRS duration is 498 msec, placing the catheter at a site remote from the common pathway.

segment of the left ventricle. Entrainment mapping was done for the ventricular tachycardia (Fig. 14-33). At first glance, the S-QRS of 58 msec seems to equal the EGM-QRS, and the PPI is within 20 msec of the ventricular tachycardia cycle length. The pace map is identical to the spontaneous ventricular tachycardia, and this appears to be an excellent target for radiofrequency energy delivery. The first ablation resulted in ventricular tachycardia termination. However, ventricular tachycardia remained easily inducible. Slight manipulation of the mapping catheter then demonstrated a markedly prolonged S-QRS of 318 msec and EGM-QRS of 50 msec (Fig. 14-34). Review of the earlier site showed that the S-QRS was 462 msec and that the EGM-QRS was 498 msec, putting our catheter far from the common pathway of the circuit.

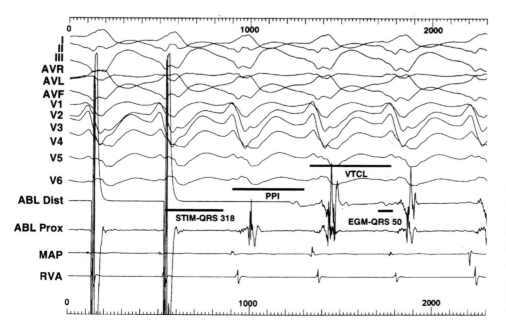

FIGURE 14-34. After slight manipulation of the ablation catheter, pace mapping was a 12/12 match. The stimulus to QRS (S-QRS) duration is 318 msec, the electrogram to QRS (EGM-QRS) duration is 50 msec, and the postpacing interval (PPI) is longer than the ventricular tachycardia cycle length (VTCL).

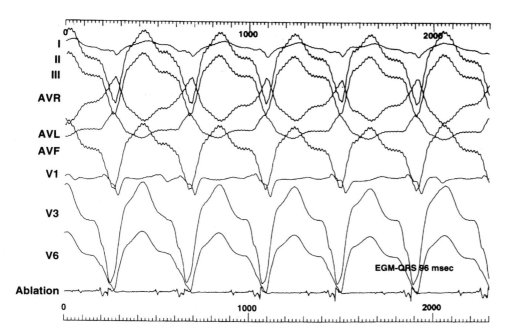

FIGURE 14-35. During ventricular tachycardia mapping, the ablation catheter is placed in a small apical aneurysm. The electrogram to QRS (EGM-QRS) duration is 96 msec.

After extensive mapping, it appeared that the tachycardia circuit was very large, with a long blind loop segment, which yielded good pace maps but did not allow for tachycardia termination. The procedure was aborted after 12 hours, and the patient remained in ventricular tachycardia. He was referred and accepted for heart transplantation but died awaiting a donor.

Patient PK is a 54-year-old man with coronary artery disease. Following a myocardial infarction, he presented with stable monomorphic ventricular tachycardia with right bundle branch block and a superior axis. Ventricular tachycardia was inducible during electrophysiologic study. He underwent implantation of an automatic cardioverter-defibrillator.

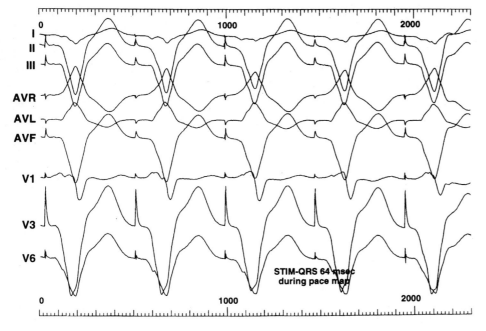

FIGURE 14-36. Pace mapping of the clinical ventricular tachycardia (VT) demonstrates a perfect match, with a stimulus to QRS (S-QRS) duration of 64 msec, which was shorter than the electrogram to QRS (EGM-QRS) duration seen in Figure 14-35. Radiofrequency energy delivered at this site eliminated the VT.

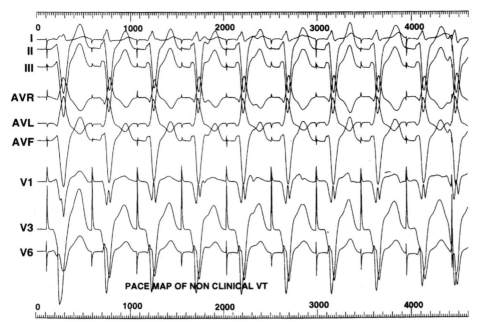

FIGURE 14-37. Pace map of nonclinical ventricular tachycardia (VT). This VT was mapped to the septal aspect of the aneurysm, where the electrogram to QRS (EGM-QRS) duration was 90 msec. The pace map was a perfect match, and the stimulus to QRS (S-QRS) was 100 msec. Radiofrequency energy delivered at this site eliminated this second VT.

The night after implantation, he had more than 100 episodes of ventricular tachycardia that were not suppressed by procainamide. He underwent ablation the next day. The clinical ventricular tachycardia was mapped to a small apical aneurysm (Fig. 14-35). The EGM-QRS was 96 msec. Pace mapping at that site (Fig. 14-36) showed a perfect match but a S-QRS of 64 msec. Radiofrequency energy delivery at this site resulted in termination of ventricular tachycardia. However, a second nonclinical ventricular tachycardia was induced and mapped to the septal aspect of the aneurysm (Fig. 14-37). The EGM-QRS was 90 msec, with a perfect pace map and S-QRS of 100 msec. Ablation terminated the ventricular tachycardia.

◉ LIMITATIONS

As with any procedure, there may be limitations that affect success. Investigators have reported success rates as low as 50% and as high as 80%, and recurrences can be as common (58). A key to success is often careful patient selection. The hemodynamically compromised patient who has difficulty tolerating ventricular tachycardia may not be the ideal candidate. Recognizing that the nature of the disease is one of multiple ventricular tachycardia morphologies with a high recurrence rate is crucial. The intracardiac anatomy is such that identifying the exact position with a small 4-mm-tip catheter can be difficult.

Although the procedure is vastly safer than DC current ablation, there are reports of complications from radiofrequency ablation (59). Procedural complications have been reported with DC and with radiofrequency ablation. Pericardial tamponade from perforation leading to the patient's death has been reported (60,61). Perforation, when it occurs, is as commonly caused by catheter manipulation in an anticoagulated patient as by the ablation energy. Small, asymptomatic pericardial effusions that resolve spontaneously have been reported in as many as 6% of patients. Transient heart block has occurred in patients who receive radiofrequency to the basal septum. There have been reports of the sudden death in patients who have undergone radiofrequency ablation.

◉ CONCLUSIONS

Ablation of ventricular tachycardia in patients with coronary artery disease has been life saving, especially when the ventricular tachycardia is incessant and unresponsive to antiarrhythmic therapy. As a primary therapy, ablation has not been used because of its intermediate success rate (50% to 70%). As mapping techniques are improved, the procedure may be conducted earlier in the course of disease. For example, ventricular tachycardias that use a narrow isthmus of conducting tissue between a scar from myocardial infarction and the mitral valve's fibrous ring are ablated when a line of radiofrequency block can be paced on this isthmus (62). One or two monomorphic ventricular tachycardias in a patient can be ablated, which should be attempted earlier when one of the ventricular tachycardias prevents adequate antitachycardia pacing. New catheter developments may allow fine adjustment and "roll" to difficult locations, have a longer ablation surface, or use energies designed to create larger lesions. Mapping systems are becoming commercially available that use a "locating catheter" and computer programs to identify sites of earliest activation, hoping to limit the need for fluoroscopy. The ablation site can be determined from short runs of ventricular tachycardia. Catheters able to map the venous system of the ventricles may improve our ability to localize tachyarrhythmias. These developments may allow ablation to be the therapy of choice for monomorphic ventricular tachycardia. As with all procedures, the more frequently the ventricular tachycardias are addressed, the more likely the necessary advances will occur.

REFERENCES

1. Scheinman MM, Morady F, Hess DS, Gonzales R. Catheter-induced ablation of the atrioventricular junction to control refractory supraventricular arrhythmias. *JAMA* 1982;248:851–855.
2. Gallagher JJ, Svenson RH, Kasell JH, et al. Catheter technique for closed-chest ablation of the atrioventricular conduction system. *N Engl J Med* 1982;306:194–200.
3. Hartzler GO. Electrode catheter ablation of refractory focal ventricular tachycardia. *J Am Coll Cardiol* 1983;2:1107–1113.
4. Hartzler GO, Giorgi LV. Electrode catheter ablation of refractory focal ventricular tachycardia: continued experience [Abstract]. *J Am Coll Cardiol* 1984;3:512.
5. Guiradon G, Fontaine G, Frank R, et al. Encircling endocardial ventriculotomy: a new surgical treatment for life-threatening ventricular tachycardias resistant to medical treatment following myocardial infarction. *Ann Thorac Surg* 1978;26:438.
6. Josephson ME, Harken AH, Horowitz LN. Long-term results of endocardial resection for sustained ventricular tachycardia in coronary disease patients. *Am Heart J* 1982;104:51–57.
7. Fontaine G, Frank R, Tonet JL, et al. Catheter ablation of ventricular tachycardia [Abstract]. *Eur Heart J* 1984;5[Suppl]:I-127.
8. Fontaine G, Frank R, Tonet J, Grosgogeat Y. Identification of a zone of slow conduction appropriate for ventricular tachycardia ablation: theoretical considerations. *Pacing Clin Electrophysiol* 1989;12:262–267.
9. Lee B, Gottdeiner JS, Fletcher RD, et al. Transcatheter ablation: comparison between laser photoablation and electrode shock ablation. *Circulation* 1985;71(3):579–584.
10. Morady F, Scheinman MM, DiCarlo LA, et al. Catheter ablation of ventricular tachycardia with intracardiac shocks: results in 33 patients. *Circulation* 1987;75:1037–1049.
11. Morady F, Frank R, Kou WH, et al. Identification and catheter ablation of a zone of slow conduction in the reentrant circuit of ventricular tachycardia in humans. *J Am Coll Cardiol* 1988;11:775–782.
12. Morady F, Kadish A, Rosenheck S, et al. Concealed entrainment as a guide for catheter ablation of ventricular tachycardia in patients with prior myocardial infarction. *J Am Coll Cardiol* 1991;17:678–689.
13. Morady F, Harvey M, Kalbfleisch SJ, et al. Radiofrequency catheter ablation of ventricular tachycardia in patients with coronary artery disease. *Circulation* 1993;87:363–372.
14. DeBakker JM, VanCapelle FJ, Janse MJ, et al. Reentry as a cause of ventricular tachycardia in patients with chronic ischemic heart disease: electrophysiologic and anatomic correlation. *Circulation* 1988;77:589–606.
15. Kay GN, Epstein AE, Plumb VJ. Region of slow conduction in sustained ventricular tachycardia: direct endocardial recordings and functional characterization in humans. *J Am Coll Cardiol* 1988;11:109–116.
16. Strobel JS, Plumb VJ, Epstein ED. Interval between myocardial infarction and catheter ablation of ventricular tachycardia: the strongest predictor of the long term results of catheter ablation. *Pacing Clin Electrophysiol* 1999;22(4)[Pt II]:140a.
17. Altmose GT, Jayachandran V, Al-Sheikh T, et al. Left ventricular mural thrombus observed at surgery: implications of catheter mapping and ablation. *Pacing Clin Electrophysiol* 1999;22(4)[Pt II]:138a.
18. Josephson ME, Horowitz LN, Farshidi A, Kastor JA. Recurrent sustained ventricular tachycardia. *Circulation* 1978;57:431–438.
19. Kienzle MG, Miller J, Falcone RA, et al. Intraoperative endocardial mapping during sinus rhythm: relationship to site of origin of ventricular tachycardia. *Circulation* 1984;70:957–965.
20. O'Brien JJ, Fallon SL, Tracy CM. Anesthetic methodology during radiofrequency catheter ablation [Abstract]. *Pacing Clin Electrophysiol* 1996;19(4)[Pt II]:219a.
21. Kadish AH, Childs K, Schmaltz S, Morady F. Differences in QRS configuration during unipolar pacing from adjacent sites: implications for the spatial resolution of pace-mapping. *J Am Coll Cardiol* 1991;17:143–151.
22. Langberg JJ, Calkins H, El-Atassi R, et al. Temperature monitoring during radiofrequency catheter ablation of accessory pathways. *Circulation* 1992;86:1469–1474.
23. Gonska B, Cao K, Schaumann A. Catheter ablation of ventricular tachycardia in 136 patients with coronary artery disease: results and long-term follow-up. *J Am Coll Cardiol* 1995;24:1506–1514.
24. Ortiz M, Almendral J, Villacastin J, et al. Radiofrequency catheter ablation of ventricular tachycardia in patients with coronary artery disease, relation between the inducibility of nonclinical

tachycardias and clinical outcome after a long term follow-up [Abstract]. *Pacing Clin Electrophysiol* 1999;22(4)[Pt II]:394a.
25. Fletcher RD, Swartz JF, Lee B, et al. Advances in catheter ablation: use of unipolar electrograms. *Pacing Clin Electrophysiol* 1989;12(4)[Pt II]:225a.
26. Garan H, Kuchar D, Freeman C, et al. Early assessment of the effect of map-guided transcatheter intracardiac electric shock on sustained ventricular tachycardia secondary to coronary artery disease. *Am J Cardiol* 1988;61(13):1018–1023.
27. El-Sherif N, Mehra R, Gough WB, et al. Reentrant ventricular arrhythmias in the late myocardial infarction period: interruption of reentrant circuits by cryothermal techniques. *Circulation* 1983;68:644–656.
28. Gallagher JD, Del Rossi AJ, Fernandez J, et al. Cryothermal mapping of recurrent ventricular tachycardia in man. *Circulation* 1985;71:733–739.
29. Downar E, Harris L, Mickleborough LL, et al. Endocardial mapping of ventricular tachycardia in the intact human ventricle: evidence of reentrant mechanisms. *J Am Coll Cardiol* 1988;11:783–791.
30. Josephson ME, Horowitz LN, Spielman SR, et al. Role of catheter mapping in the preoperative evaluation of ventricular tachycardia. *Am J Cardiol* 1982;49:207–220.
31. Josephson ME. *Clinical cardiac electrophysiology.* Philadelphia: Lea & Febiger 1993:789.
32. Littmann L, Svenson RH, Gallagher JJ, et al. High grade entrance and exit block in an area of healed myocardial infarction associated with ventricular tachycardia with successful laser photoablation of the anatomic substrate. *Am J Cardiol* 1989;64:122–124.
33. El-Sherif N, Scherlag B, Lazzara R, Hope R. Re-entrant ventricular arrhythmias in the late myocardial infarction period. 1. Conduction characteristics in the infarction zone. *Circulation* 1977;55:686–702.
34. Debakker JM, VanCapelle FJ, Jansen MJ, et al. Reentry as a cause of ventricular tachycardia in patients with chronic ischemic heart disease: electrophysiologic and anatomic correlation. *Circulation* 1988;77:589–606.
35. Downar E, Kimber S, Harris L, et al. Endocardial mapping of ventricular tachycardia in the intact human heart. II. Evidence for multiuse reentry in a function sheet of surviving myocardium. *J Am Coll Cardiol* 1992;20:869–878.
36. Stevenson WG, Weiss JN, Wiener I, Nadamanee K. Slow conduction in the infarct scar: relevance to the occurrence, detection, and ablation of ventricular reentry circuits resulting from myocardial infarction. *Am Heart J* 1989;117:452–464.
37. Stevenson WG, Nademanee K, Weiss JN, et al. Programmed electrical stimulation at potential ventricular reentry circuit sites: a comparison of observations in humans with predictions from computer simulations. *Circulation* 1989;80:793–806.
38. Frazier DW, Stanton MS. Resetting and transient entrainment of ventricular tachycardia. *Pacing Clin Electrophysiol* 1995;18:1919–1946.
39. Stevenson WG, Khan H, Sager P, et al. Identification of reentry circuit sites during catheter mapping and radiofrequency ablation of ventricular tachycardia late after myocardial infarction. *Circulation* 1993;88:1647–1670.
40. Stevenson W, Weiss J, Wiener I, et al. Resetting of ventricular tachycardia: implications for localizing the area of slow conduction. *J Am Coll Cardiol* 1988;11:522–529.
41. Brugada P, Abdollah H, Wellens HJJ. Continuous electrical activity during sustained monomorphic ventricular tachycardia. *Am J Cardiol* 1985;55:402–411.
42. Waldo AL, Henthorn RW. Use of transient entrainment during ventricular tachycardia to localize a critical area in the reentry circuit for ablation. *Pacing Clin Electrophysiol* 1989;12:231–244.
43. MacLean WA, Plumb VJ, Waldo AL. Transient entrainment and interruption of ventricular tachycardia. *Pacing Clin Electrophysiol* 1981;4:358–366.
44. Mann D, Lawrie G, Luck J, et al. Importance of pacing site in entrainment of ventricular tachycardia. *J Am Coll Cardiol* 1985;5:781–787.
45. Anderson KP, Swerdlow CD, Mason JW. Entrainment of ventricular tachycardia. *Am J Cardiol* 1984;53:335–340.
46. El-Sherif A, Gough W, Restivo M. Reentrant ventricular arrhythmias in the late myocardial infarction period: mechanisms of resetting, entrainment, acceleration, or termination of reentrant tachycardia by programmed electrical stimulation. *Pacing Clin Electrophysiol* 1987;10:341–371.
47. Rosenthal ME, Stamato NJ, Almendral JM, et al. Resetting of ventricular tachycardia with electrocardiographic fusion: incidence and significance. *Circulation* 1988;77:581–588.
48. Henthorn RW, Okumura K, Olshansky B, et al. A fourth criterion for transient entrainment: the electrogram equivalent of progressive fusion. *Circulation* 1988;77:1003–1012.
49. Soejima K, Stevenson WG, Delacretaz E, et al. Stimulus-QRS (n + 1): a new measure for entrainment mapping [Abstract]. *Circulation* 1998;98:I-348a.
50. Fitzgerald DM, Friday KJ, Yeung Lai Wah JA, et al. Electrogram patterns predicting successful catheter ablation of ventricular tachycardia. *Circulation* 1988;77:806–814.
51. Bogun F, Bahu M, Knight BP, et al. Comparison of effective and ineffective target sites that demonstrate concealed entrainment in patients with coronary artery disease undergoing radiofrequency ablation of ventricular tachycardia. *Circulation* 1997;94:183–190.
52. El-Shalakany A, Hadjis T, Papageorgiou P, et al. Entrainment/mapping criteria for the prediction of termination of ventricular tachycardia by single radiofrequency lesion in patients with coronary artery disease. *Circulation* 1999;17:2283–2289.
53. Ruffy F, Friday KJ, Southworth WF. Termination of ventricular tachycardia by single extrastimulation during the ventricular effective refractory period. *Circulation* 1983;67:457–459.
54. Shoda M, Kasanuki H, Ohnishi O, et al. Electrophysiologic properties of substrate critical to perpetuation of reentrant ventricular tachycardia: observations based on termination of tachycardia by a non-propagated extrastimulus [Abstract]. *Circulation* 1992;86:I-132.
55. Garan H, Ruskin JN. Reproducible termination of ventricular tachycardia by a single extrastimulus within the reentry circuit during the ventricular effective refractory period. *Am Heart J* 1988;116:546–550.
56. Podczeck A, Borggrefe M, Martinez-Rubio A, Breithardt G. Termination of re-entrant ventricular tachycardia by subthreshold stimulus applied to the zone of slow conduction. *Eur Heart J* 1988;9:1146–1150.
57. Ruffy R. Termination of ventricular tachycardia by nonpropagated local depolarization: further observations on entrainment of ventricular tachycardia from an area of slow conduction. *Pacing Clin Electrophysiol* 1990;13:852–858.
58. O'Callaghan PA, Ruskin J, McGovern BA, et al. Resetting of mid-diastolic potentials localizes successful sites for radiofrequency ablation in patients with ventricular tachycardia due to coronary artery disease. *J Am Coll Cardiol* 1996;27:76a.
59. Morady F, Harvey M, Kalbfleisch SJ, et al. Radiofrequency

catheter ablation of ventricular tachycardia in patients with coronary artery disease. *Circulation* 1993;87:363–372.
60. Kim YH, Sosa-Suarez G, Trouton TG, et al. Treatment of ventricular tachycardia by transcatheter radiofrequency ablation in patients with ischemic heart disease. *Circulation* 1994;89:1094–1102.
61. Borggrefe M, Breithardt G, Podczeck A, et al. Catheter ablation of ventricular tachycardia using defibrillator pulses: electrophysiological findings and long-term results. *Eur Heart J* 1989;10:591–601.
62. Belhassen B, Miller HI, Geller E, Laniado S. Transcatheter electrical shock ablation of ventricular tachycardia. *J Am Coll Cardiol* 1986;1347–1355.
63. Wilber DJ, Kopp DE, Glascock DN, et al. Catheter ablation of the mitral isthmus for ventricular tachycardia associated with inferior infarction. *Circulation* 1995;92:12.

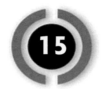

SURGICAL TECHNIQUES FOR ABLATION OF SUPRAVENTRICULAR TACHYCARDIAS
• • •

GERARD M. GUIRAUDON, GEORGE J. KLEIN, RAYMOND YEE

July 2000 was the 10th anniversary of the dramatic advent of catheter ablation for supraventricular tachycardias. This chapter reviews the ebbing of surgery in the treatment of supraventricular tachycardias.

Supraventricular tachycardias are classified according to the site of their working mechanism, which is essentially a reentry mechanism (1). Atrial tachycardias are associated with their electrocardiographic tachycardia patterns: focal atrial tachycardias, atrial flutter, and atrial fibrillation. Atrioventricular (AV) nodal tachycardias are reentrant tachycardias confined to the AV nodal region. Wolff-Parkinson-White syndrome requires the entire heart and an obligatory accessory atrioventricular connection.

The rationale for interventions in supraventricular tachycardias is based on the arrhythmogenic target (i.e., arrhythmogenic anatomic substrate). Identification of the arrhythmogenic anatomic substrate is achieved by electrophysiologic mapping of the cardiac activation sequence. The current rationale is to neutralize the arrhythmogenic anatomic substrate using various physical means: exclusion or ablation using various sources of energy such as cryoablation (2–4), direct current shock (5–7), or radiofrequency electrical energy (8–10). Radiofrequency is the preferred energy because it can be delivered on target by intracardiac catheters and is safe. The ways in which the targeted tissues are approached and the therapy that is delivered define the type of intervention.

Surgery is defined by a transparietal approach (i.e., median sternotomy) that requires general anesthesia with tracheal intubation and is associated with various adjunct maneuvers, such as cardiopulmonary bypass, cardiotomy, and aortic cross-clamping with cardioplegic myocardial preservation, before the ablative therapy can be delivered. Each of the various steps used to approach the arrhythmogenic target is associated with inherent morbidity and mortality (11,12). The surgical risk consequently is essentially associated with the delivery of therapy and not with the therapy itself.

Catheter techniques are much less invasive. After venous or arterial puncture (or both), the catheter follows chartered natural routes to the heart and the arrhythmogenic target. Side effects and complications have become minimal with the dramatic progress in skill (13), techniques, applied anatomy, and technology.

Electrophysiologic interventions using surgical or catheter delivery are the only curative interventions. Other electrophysiologic interventions using drugs or antitachycardia devices are only palliative. His bundle ablation combined with permanent cardiac pacing may be used in selected patients.

When feasible, catheter ablation using radiofrequency electrical energy is the preferred first therapy. This principle implies that patients with Wolff-Parkinson-White syndrome and AV nodal reentrant tachycardias are effectively and safely cured by catheter ablation techniques (14). Patients with atrial flutter also benefit from catheter ablation techniques (15,16). Focal atrial tachycardias may be controlled by using catheter ablation in selected patients (17).

Atrial fibrillation is still approached surgically in a number of patients, while catheter or other ways of delivery are being developed (18–21). In this chapter, we review the historical contribution of surgical approaches to treating Wolff-Parkinson-White syndrome, AV nodal reentrant tachycardia, focal tachycardias, and atrial flutter. The surgical interventions used to control atrial fibrillation are discussed, and their contribution to future catheter delivery is contemplated. Because catheter ablation techniques may fail, patients should not be denied the benefit of a curative intervention, and surgeons should stay current with all methods.

⊙ WOLFF-PARKINSON-WHITE SYNDROME

The first successful surgical ablation of an accessory atrioventricular connection was performed by Sealy and colleagues in 1968 (22). Along with the development of surgical practice came a better understanding of cardiac anatomy and accessory atrioventricular connection, anatomy, and electrophysiology. This knowledge paved the way to advanced surgical techniques with high efficacy and low morbidity and to catheter techniques (13).

The accessory atrioventricular connection in Wolff-Parkinson-White syndrome is distinct from the normal AV nodal–His bundle system and crosses over the atrioventricular attachment. Successful techniques for ablation of the accessory connection requires in-depth knowledge of the complex anatomy of the atrioventricular attachment (23,24) (Figs. 15-1 and 15-2). The atrioventricular attachment joins the atrial myocardium and the ventricular myocardium at the level of their atrioventricular orifices. The complexity of the attachment is determined by the anatomy of the left ventricle, which has a single myocardial opening (i.e., left ventricular ostium) that accommodates the inflow (i.e., mitral valve) and outflow (i.e., aortic valve) orifices. Consequently, the atrioventricular attachment is composed of two segments: the annular and the nonannular. The annular attachment is a simple fibrotic structure, the atrioventricular annulus (or lamina), that joins the adjacent atrial and ventricular rims of the atrioventricular orifices. The annular attachment is close to the coronary sulcus, which encircles the base of the heart around the annular atrioventricular attachment. The coronary sulcus is divided into four regions or segments: the left free wall, posterior septal, right free wall, and anterior septal (right coronary fossa) regions. These regions are arbitrarily defined, and their limits are not materialized by specific anatomic landmarks or partitions. This absence of clear limits is the source of confusion, particularly for the anterior septal and posterior septal regions. The nonannular attachment is composed of the aortic annuli and their appended membranous structures, including the membranous septum, the right fibrous trigone, and the intervalvular trigone (i.e., subaortic curtain). Part of the nonannular attachment is septal: the membranous septum. Another complex segment of the heart septum can be added to the atrioventricular attachment—the triangle of Koch—which comprises two important features, the AV node and the atrioventricular myocardial septum (i.e., posterior superior process of the left ventricle) covered by septal atrial myocardium. The atrioventricular myocardial septum is called the midseptum by catheter interventionists.

The accessory atrioventricular connections are made of strands of working myocardium that bypass the atrioventricular attachment (25,26). The typical accessory atrioventricular connections cross the annular attachment, with most being paraannular (27,28). Atypical accessory atrioventricular connections have been found in all parts of the nonannular attachment: within the atrioventricular myocardial septum (i.e., posterior septal or midseptal pathways), adjacent to the membranous septum (i.e., para-Hisian anterior septal pathways), within the membranous pathway (i.e., membranous pathways with aberrant preexcitation), and over the intervalvular trigone (i.e., atypical posterior septal pathways). Two subvarieties of typical

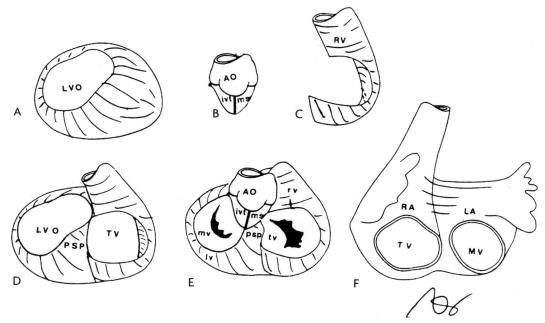

FIGURE 15-1. Construction of the atrioventricular attachment. The ventricles are viewed from behind; the atria are viewed from the front. **A:** Left ventricle with its single orifice: the left ventricular ostium (LVO). **B:** Aortic root with its appended membranous cuff, the aortoventricular membrane. Depicted are the aortic root, the intervalvular trigone (IVT), and the membranous septum (MS). Between the IVT and MS, appended at the nadir of the noncoronary cusp, is the right fibrous trigone, which is a cordlike structure, not a triangular structure. **C:** The right ventricular free wall. **D:** Attachment of the right ventricular free wall to the left ventricle and formation of the tricuspid valve (TV) orifice. The triangular segment of the left ventricular wall between the TV orifice and the LVO is the posterosuperior process (PSP) of the left ventricle. Covered by the right atrial wall, it constitutes the muscular atrioventricular septum in the anterior segment of the triangle of Koch (i.e., midseptum of cardiologic interventionists). **E:** Addition of the aortic annuli and its aortoventricular membrane, which attaches to the LVO and delineates the mitral valve (MV) orifice. **F:** Anterior view of the atria. The two atrioventricular orifices are widely separated, as are the tricuspid and ventricular atrioventricular orifices. The segment between the orifices constitutes the complex atrioventricular septum (i.e., triangle of Koch). AO, aorta; LA, left atrium; RA, right ventricle; RV, right ventricle.

pathways deserve mention: the posterior septal pathway with slow decremental conduction associated with the permanent form of junctional reentrant tachycardia (i.e., Coumel's tachycardias) (29,30) and the right free wall pathway with anterograde decremental conduction (i.e., atriofascicular pathway associated with left bundle branch block pattern tachycardias) (31–34).

Surgical Techniques

The evolution of the surgical techniques for Wolff-Parkinson-White syndrome exemplifies the new surgical philosophy of attaining efficacy with minimal risk of side effects. Surgical risk is associated with every step that is used to approach the accessory atrioventricular connection, including general anesthesia, median sternotomy, cardiopulmonary bypass, aortic cross-clamping, myocardial preservation, and cardiotomy (11,12). Each step uses techniques that are associated with inherent morbidity and mortality. The ablation of the accessory atrioventricular connection is the most benign part of the intervention. On the basis of these premises, which advocate simplified approaches, we developed in 1983 a variant surgical technique, the epicardial approach (35), aimed at de-

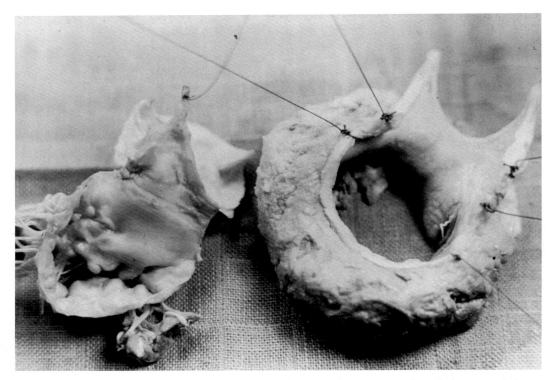

FIGURE 15-2. Dissection of a heart specimen depicting the aortic annuli with the appended aortoventricular membrane **(A)**, including the mitral valve and the left ventricular ostium **(B)**.

creasing risk because the surgical ablation could be carried out without the need for aortic cross-clamping and cardiopulmonary bypass.

Two surgical approaches were described, the endocardial approach and the epicardial approach. The endocardial approach was pioneered and perfected by Sealy (22,36–38), Cox (39), and Gallagher (40). This surgical success constitutes a landmark in the history of cardiac arrhythmias. The epicardial approach combines epicardial exposure and cryoablation of the atrioventricular attachment (35,41,42).

The heart is exposed by a median sternotomy. After extensive examination of cardiac anatomy, epicardial mapping is carried out to confirm the location of the accessory atrioventricular connection established during preoperative electrophysiologic studies. Exploring electrodes are positioned along the atrial and ventricular side of the coronary sulcus at predetermined sites during atrial or ventricular pacing (or both) and atrioventricular reentrant tachycardias. Mapping of the entire ventricles is used in rare, specific cases.

Epicardial mapping is limited by the anatomy of the sulcus and the location of the accessory atrioventricular connection. Because of the depth of the sulcus, the exploring electrode is remote from the atrioventricular annulus and the accessory atrioventricular connection. Epicardial mapping cannot identify the very site of preexcitation, as endocardial mapping does, but identifies a region. Cardiac mapping and electrophysiologic testing using pacing techniques are repeated at each step of surgical ablation to confirm suppression of the conduction of the recognized accessory atrioventricular connection and to potentially identify a second undiagnosed connection.

The Endocardial Approach

The endocardial approach combines an atrial incision along the atrioventricular annulus in the region of interest and an extensive dissection of the entire region of the coronary sulcus. The left free wall connections are approached by using a conventional exposure of the mitral valve similar to the one used for mitral valve surgery. The entire left free wall region is dissected through a semicircular atrial incision along the mitral valve annulus from the right to the left trigone. The coronary sulcus dissection involves the identification of coronary artery and vein and the separation of the atrial and ventricular wall from all attachments to divide all potential pathway insertions. The dissection is carried out under aortic cross-clamping and cardioplegic cardiac arrest.

The posterior septal, right free wall, and anterior septal regions are approached through a right atriotomy. Endocardial mapping and para-Hisian dissection can be carried out on the normothermic beating heart. However, most of the extensive dissection of the region of interest is performed under aortic cross-clamping and cold cardioplegic arrest.

The endocardial approach is associated with excellent efficacy. Surgical morbidity associated with cold cardioplegic cardiac arrest and cardiopulmonary bypass is significant (39,40).

The Epicardial Approach

The epicardial approach combines epicardial dissection of the coronary sulcus and exposure and cryoablation of the atrioventricular attachment (i.e., annulus) (41,42).

The typical accessory atrioventricular connection can be ablated by using this approach on the beating heart without the need for cardiopulmonary bypass. The left free wall dissection is carried out by exposing the left coronary sulcus with the use of a sling (43) (Fig. 15-3). The atrioventricular attachment is exposed by dissection of the fat pad along the left ventricular wall. The obtuse cardiac vein is divided for better exposure, and the coronary arteries are carefully isolated. The posterior region is well exposed by deflecting the heart upward using a rigid, pledgeted suture. The right free wall and anterior septal regions are easily exposed. These typical accessory atrioventricular connections within the coronary sulcus are easily ablated with the high efficacy and minimum morbidity associated with median sternotomy (42).

Atypical accessory atrioventricular connections require endocardial dissection carried out on the normothermic beating heart. Para-Hisian anterior septal connections are ablated by using discrete dissection

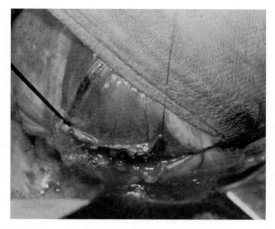

FIGURE 15-3. Surgery for Wolff-Parkinson-White syndrome includes exposure and dissection of the left atrioventricular sulcus on the beating heart (sling exposure).

of the atrial myocardium overlying the atrial membranous septum (44). We have ablated three atypical posterior pathways located over the intervalvular trigone region using discrete cryoablation (45).

Atypical Intramembranous Pathways

We have operated on four patients with aberrant preexcitation and surgically documented intramembranous pathways. The area of aberrant preexcitation was over the right ventricular infundibulum (three patients) or the ventricular septum (one patient) (46). The pathways were ablated by discrete cryoablation of the atrial membranous septum or of the ventricular attachment. These membranous accessory pathways are characteristically located within the membranous septum, with an atrial insertion in the atrial septum and a ventricular insertion at various sites in the septum along the membranous septum attachment to the ventricular septum. The membranous pathway differs from the so-called intermediate pathways (47), which have normal anatomic features and function and are located in the midseptal region.

Other Variant Preexcitation

In 1988, we documented in two patients that the anatomic substrate of the so-called Mahaim fibers associated with left bundle branch block pattern tachycardias was a right ventricular free wall accessory pathway with antegrade decremental conduction and a His bundle–like connection along the right ventricular free wall (i.e., atriofascicular fiber) (31–34). Since then, surgical and catheter ablation techniques have revealed that almost all patients with the electrophysiologically documented Mahaim entity have a right free wall accessory pathway and that the site of preexcitation is close to the atrioventricular groove or at the right ventricular apex (48). In five patients, biopsy specimen findings from the right atrium documented the presence of AV nodal cells at the atrial insertion of the pathway. Our surgical experience comprises 13 patients (49). The surgical technique that is used in this setting is identical to that used for right free wall accessory pathway dissection combined with endocardial cryoablation.

Permanent Form of Junctional Reciprocating Tachycardia

Surgical dissection of the posterior septal region has documented that the permanent form of junctional reciprocating tachycardia (i.e., Coumel's tachycardia) is associated with a posterior septal slow pathway, with decremental retrograde conduction. A conventional posterior septal dissection using the epicardial approach uniformly ablates the pathway (30).

Coronary Sinus Diverticulum

Coronary sinus diverticulum is associated with posterior septal pathways that exhibit maximal preexcitation and a short antegrade refractory period (Fig. 15-4). During surgery, coronary sinus diverticulum is readily visible. Diverticulum is composed of a pouch and a neck that opens into the coronary sinus proximal to the midcardiac vein. The neck diameter is 5 to 10 mm. Intramyocardial cardiac veins open into the coronary sinus diverticulum (50). Accessory pathway conduction is usually interrupted when the neck of the diverticulum is divided, a finding suggesting that the accessory pathway is part of the diverticulum. This anomaly is commonly associated with a very short antegrade refractory period in the pathway. Studies have documented the role of venous anomalies in posterior septal pathways (51).

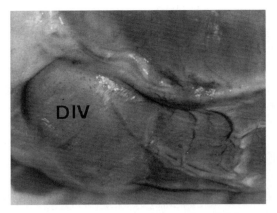

FIGURE 15-4. Coronary sinus diverticulum (DIV).

Multiple Accessory Pathways

Because epicardial mapping is insufficiently discriminating within a region, we defined multiple accessory pathways as widely separated sites of preexcitation in distinct regions (52). Preoperative electrophysiologic studies identify the presence of multiple pathways in about 7% of patients (53). A second pathway can become apparent only after ablation of the dominant accessory pathway. Most unexpected pathways that are detected intraoperatively are posterior septal pathways capable of only retrograde atrioventricular conduction. Multiple accessory pathways are ablated in sequence. If possible, the accessory pathway that does not require cardiopulmonary bypass is ablated first.

Associated Cardiac Lesions

Two congenital cardiac abnormalities are associated with the preexcitation syndrome: Ebstein's anomaly and the coronary sinus diverticulum. Symptomatic Wolff-Parkinson-White syndrome associated with Ebstein's anomaly does not necessarily require anatomic repair, but all such surgical repairs of Ebstein's anomaly should be combined with ablation of the associated preexcitation syndrome.

Our surgical strategy for concomitant cardiac procedures (i.e., coronary artery bypass grafting and valve replacement) is to ablate the accessory pathway first as an independent procedure and then to perform the associated cardiac surgical procedure. Before the chest is closed, four pairs of temporary pacing electrodes are attached to the cardiac chambers for postoperative electrophysiologic testing.

Results and Applications

Before the era of catheter ablation, we reported 502 patients who were operated on before August 1990. In all, 500 patients were cured without any mortality and with low morbidity (mean follow-up, 4 years). These results were similar to those from other reported series (28).

After the introduction of catheter ablation, between August 1990 and August 1993, we operated on 51 patients (35 men and 16 women, ages 9 to 63 years) who were referred for surgical ablation from within our institution and elsewhere (54). During the same period, 375 patients with problematic Wolff-Parkinson-White syndrome underwent catheter ablation procedures at our hospital. Surgical ablation was the initial therapy for 26 patients because of physician preference in 23 and because of the need for concomitant cardiac surgical procedures in 3. Surgical treatment was carried out after attempted catheter ablation in 22 patients, 3 of whom had urgent surgical intervention.

Previous catheter ablation was not associated with added surgical difficulties, and all pathways were ablated intraoperatively on the first attempt using the epicardial approach. Visible epicardial lesions produced by radiofrequency energy were observed in eight patients at the site of the accessory pathway (Fig. 15-5).

Operative therapy gave some insights into the mechanism responsible for the failure of catheter ablation during the learning period: inadequate localization of the accessory pathway was suggested in four patients in whom there were discrepancies between the intraoperative and preoperative localization of the pathway. Inadequate positioning of the catheter off the atrioventricular ring was observed in two patients; the catheter was in the obtuse marginal vein in one and in the left atrial appendage in the other. In most cases, adequate localization of the accessory pathway and the radiofrequency-induced lesions suggested inadequate contact of the catheter with the atrioventric-

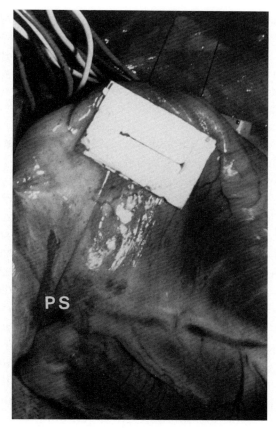

FIGURE 15-5. Operative view of the inferior surface of the heart of a patient after attempted radiofrequency energy ablation. Ecchymosis is seen on the posterior septal region (PS).

ular annulus or with an accessory pathway coursing at a distance from the annulus.

There was a significant preponderance of right free wall pathways after catheter ablation, which suggests that a subepicardial location of the pathways may be a source of failed ablation, as we observed in one patient with a well-defined subepicardial atrioventricular myocardial bundle. Brodman and associates reported similar observations in the setting of intraoperative right free wall bundles (55). Sealy (37) reported that anterior right ventricular free wall pathways could be subepicardial, as shown by findings observed during atrioventricular fat pad dissection using the endocardial approach. We previously reported that inferior right free wall pathways have mostly "deep" paraannular or subendocardial locations, but anterior right ventricular free wall pathways have epicardial locations because accessory pathway conduction usually is interrupted early during epicardial dissection. Rosenberg and colleagues identified a long subepicardial accessory pathway in the right ventricular position in a heart specimen (56). The subepicardial location of right free wall pathways makes them less amenable to catheter ablation. Nonetheless, catheter techniques can be successful by ablating the atrial insertion of the accessory pathway, even if the pathway is distant from the atrioventricular annulus.

Surgical ablation laid the groundwork for catheter ablation by elucidating the anatomic characteristics of the atrioventricular attachments and the surgical anatomy of the accessory atrioventricular connection. With the advent of surgical ablation, nonpharmacologic electrophysiologic interventions became established as the primary choice for patients facing lifelong dependency on drug treatment. Concerns about surgical morbidity encouraged the development of surgical techniques associated with minimal morbidity by suppressing as many ancillary techniques as possible.

Catheter ablation has eclipsed surgical ablation as the primary nonpharmacologic therapy. Nonetheless, surgical ablation continues to have a limited role in the management of patients in whom catheter ablation has failed as the result of anatomic complexities or congenital heart lesions.

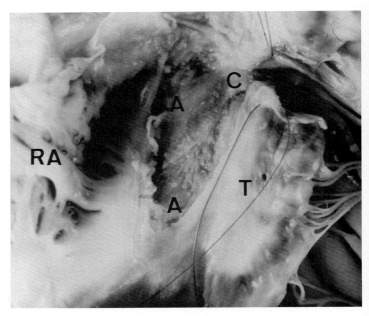

FIGURE 15-6. Dissection of the greater atrioventricular (AV) nodal area. The compact AV node (C) is exposed. A, AV atrial inputs; RA, right atrium; T, tricuspid valve.

⦿ ATRIOVENTRICULAR NODAL REENTRANT TACHYCARDIAS

AV nodal reentrant tachycardia is a common supraventricular tachycardia. It was long accepted that the reentrant mechanism was within the compact AV node (57). Because this concept precluded a direct surgical approach to disable the reentrant mechanism, His bundle ablation was the electrophysiologic intervention used in severe resistant cases. However, an inadvertent cure of a patient with AV nodal reentrant tachycardia after attempted surgical ablation of the AV node suggested that discrete lesions of the AV node could interrupt the tachycardia (58). Marques-Montes and colleagues (59) and Johnson and coworkers (60) were the first to report effective surgical approaches to the AV nodal region to interrupt AV nodal reentrant tachycardias (Fig. 15-6).

The rationale of surgical approaches was consistent with AV nodal physiology as described by basic scientists (61) and with AV nodal anatomy (62). To reconcile data from various disciplines, the concept of a greater AV nodal area that encompasses the AV node and its atrial input was described (63).

The reentrant mechanism, within the greater AV nodal area, uses atrial inputs as limbs or segments of the reentrant circuit. Surgical approaches suggested that modification or ablation of at least one atrial input was associated with disabling of the reentrant mechanism. Johnston and colleagues were the first to report two sites of atrial retrograde activation over the coronary sinus os and at the apex of the triangle of Koch, consistent with the posterior (coronary sinus) atrial inputs and the superficial atrial input (currently labeled anterior, referring to the anterior septal position), respectively. Direct surgical approaches to the AV node for treating AV nodal reentrant tachycardia use sharp dissection of the AV nodal atrial inputs guided by endocardial mapping (60) or not (63), or use cryomodification (i.e., perinodal cryoablation) (64).

Map-Guided Ablation of Atrial Inputs

On the normothermic heart during AV nodal reentrant tachycardia, atrial mapping of the triangle of Koch is carried out. The earliest atrial activation is near the apex (i.e., type A or common type) or near the coronary sinus os (i.e., type B or uncommon type). Most patients have only one type of tachycardia, but some have two.

Cardiac dissection is then carried out on the cold arrested heart. In type A tachycardia, atrial inputs are divided superior (posterior) to the tendon of Todaro. In type B tachycardias, the posterior septal area around the coronary sinus os, inferior (anterior) to the tendon of Todaro, is extensively dissected. Johnson and colleagues (65) reported no mortality for 72 patients. Two patients had permanent complete heart block, and three had early relapses of their tachycardia. During long-term follow-up (6 to 40 months), the clinical cure rate was 93% (90% in sinus rhythm).

Anatomically Guided Dissection of Atrioventricular Nodal Atrial Inputs

In AV nodal skeletonization (66), the dissection is carried out on the normothermic beating heart in two steps while the atrioventricular conduction is continuously monitored. First, using a technique similar to that used for Wolff-Parkinson-White syndrome, the anterior septal and posterior septal regions are dissected by using an epicardial approach. Then cardiopulmonary bypass is instituted using double venous cannulae combined with snaring of the vena cavae. The heart is electrically fibrillated before the right atriotomy is performed along the exposed tricuspid valve annulus in the anterior septal region and the atrioventricular fat pad in the right free wall region. The atrial septum is inspected for defect, and a patent foramen ovale is closed. The heart is then defibrillated.

Skeletonization of the AV node is then carried out. The right atriotomy is extended up to the atrial membranous septum. The tendon of Todaro is identified. The inferior medial (septal) wall of the right atrium is incised along the septal segment of the tricuspid valve annulus below the atrial membranous septum. A plane of dissection is found between the septal right atrial wall and the subjacent intermediate AV node. The septal atrial wall is then opened, and the intermediate AV node is exposed. The AV node is identified by its oblique pale myocardial fibers mixed with yellowish fatty streaks. It is dissected from surrounding tissue to separate posterior (coronary sinus) and superficial (anterior) atrial inputs, but the deep (left) atrial input is spared.

Forty-six patients were described in one series (63). There were 38 females and 8 males between the ages of 9 and 71 years (mean, 36 years). Five patients had associated arrhythmias that were concomitantly surgically ablated; three had Wolff-Parkinson-White syndrome, and two had Mahaim fibers. There were no surgical complications. Three patients had second-degree heart block with adequate ventricular heart rate during treadmill testing. Dual AV nodal pathway physiology was detected in four patients postoperatively, with two having inducible tachycardias. During long-term follow-up, three patients had clinical recurrences of their tachycardias. The three patients underwent a successful repeat dissection. After a mean follow-up of 17 months (range, 1 to 45 months), all patients were free of arrhythmias and off antiarrhythmic drugs.

Perinodal Cryoablation

The surgery is carried out on the normothermic beating heart and exposure of the triangle of Koch (64). Atrioventricular conduction is continuously monitored. Cryoablation uses a cryoprobe that is 3 mm in diameter and cooled at $-60°C$ for 2 minutes or less until transient heart block occurs. Three cryolesions are placed along the tendon of Todaro between the coronary sinus orifice and the apex of the triangle of Koch. Three cryolesions are then placed along the septal segment of the tricuspid annulus. Two more cryolesions are placed at the base of the triangle above the coronary sinus os to connect the previous application and circumscribe the AV nodal area. Twenty patients were reported; all patients were free of tachyarrhythmia in the short and long term.

Results and Applications

Surgical techniques for AV nodal reentrant tachycardias are no longer used. Ablation using catheter delivery is associated with excellent control of the tachycardia and with more discrete electrophysiologic changes (67).

⦿ ATRIAL TACHYCARDIAS

Focal atrial tachycardias are classified into two subgroups. Ectopic atrial tachycardias originate from outside the sinus node area, and sinus node tachycardias originate from within the sinus node area.

Ectopic Atrial Tachycardias

Ectopic atrial tachycardias are rare in the adult population (0.5% to 1%) and most common in children (10% of supraventricular tachycardias) (68). During electrophysiologic studies, they have the characteristics of automatic focus tachycardias. During tachycardia, the P-wave morphology significantly differs from that of sinus node P waves. The site of origin is mostly within the right atrial wall (68%) along the crista terminalis, the left atrial free wall (26%), and the interatrial septum (6%). The tachycardia is frequently incessant. These characteristics explain why tachycardia-induced dilated cardiomyopathy is frequently present (60% of cases).

Ectopic atrial tachycardias are potentially severe arrhythmias and should be controlled by using electrophysiologic intervention. Surgical techniques are considered only after attempted catheter ablation. Because ectopic atrial tachycardias are not inducible, preoperative catheter mapping must be obtained to precisely localize the site of origin.

Surgical techniques use resection, cryoablation, and exclusion, singly or in combination. Resection applies to right atrial free wall and right and left appendage locations. Appendectomies may not require cardiopulmonary bypass. Right atrial excision is repaired by using an autologous pericardial patch. Cryoablation can be combined with resection but is particularly convenient for septal locations. Exclusion is used essentially for the left atrial locations.

Our experience comprises five patients; none of them had incessant tachycardia associated with tachycardia-induced dilated cardiomyopathy (69). Three patients had a right free wall tachycardia localized over the inferior segment of the crista terminalis and underwent extensive right free wall resection combined with autologous pericardial patch reconstruction. One patient had a right atrial appendage tachycardia. The right atrial appendage was resected without using cardiopulmonary bypass. One patient had a left atrial tachycardia. Because the location of the tachycardia was not accurately determined, a left atrial exclusion was carried out.

There were no surgical complications. No patient had recurrence of tachycardia. The patient with left atrial exclusion developed AV nodal conduction disturbances associated with syncopal ventricular pauses during long-term follow-up. A permanent pacemaker was implanted.

Lowe and colleagues (68), in a review of the literature, described 125 patients with ectopic atrial tachycardias. Fifty-two patients were treated with antiarrhythmic drugs; 46 (89%) of them were controlled. Seventy-three patients were treated with surgical techniques; 56 (89%) were cured. Surgical techniques are indicated only after attempted catheter ablation.

Sinus Node Tachycardias

Sinus node tachycardias comprise inappropriate sinus node tachycardias and reentrant sinus node tachycardias. Surgical experience with inappropriate sinus tachycardias documented that surgical ablation was associated with good short-term results (69) but poor long-term results (70) complicated with atrial fibrillation and atrioventricular conduction disturbances. These surgical results suggest that catheter ablation (71) or other ablative techniques (72) are only palliative. Catheter ablation in patients with reentrant sinus node tachycardias (73) attains good results, consistent with those obtained by surgical ablation.

Atrial Flutter

Atrial flutter was first characterized by its electrocardiographic pattern (74) as a rapid, regular atrial tachycardia associated with a typical sawtooth configuration of the atrial electrogram on the surface electrocardiogram. Atrial flutter in humans has been classified as common if negative flutter waves are present in leads II, III, and aVF and as uncommon if flutter waves are positive in these same leads (75). The common flutter was labeled type 1, and the uncommon flutter was labeled type 2 (76).

A large body of experimental (77–80) and clinical (80–87) evidence documents that atrial flutter is associated with a macro-reentry mechanism associated with a large excitable gap in the right atrium and an area of slow conduction in the triangle of Koch. Studies showed that the common and uncommon types share the same mechanism or location (88,89).

The reentry circuit is determined by the functional anatomy of the right atrium. The area of slow conduction at the base of the triangle of Koch in the area of the coronary sinus os occupies a narrow segment (i.e., isthmus) between the inferior vena cava and the tricuspid valve orifices (Fig. 15-7). The reentrant activation exits the area of slow conduction and propagates rapidly by the anterior and middle internodal pathways, which are anterior to the fossa ovalis. The reentrant activation then circulates through the sinus node area, travels caudally within the crista terminalis, and returns to the base of the triangle of Koch, where the slow-conducting isthmus channels and slows the activation before it exits again. The fossa ovale and transversal relatively slow conduction (i.e., anisotropic) helps to create a zone of septal block (90).

Cardiac mapping during electrophysiologic studies and before surgical ablation confirms the functional anatomy of the reentrant circuit (Fig. 15-8). The area of slow conduction within the isthmus at the base of the triangle of Koch is identified as the arrhythmogenic anatomic substrate, although the open circuit circulating along the rapidly conducting bundle may also be obligatory for the perpetuation of the flutter and could be considered as a second arrhythmogenic anatomic substrate.

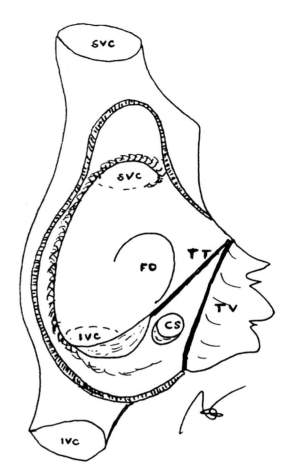

FIGURE 15-7. In this depiction of the right atrium, the right atrial free wall has been excised. The isthmus is described by the inferior vena cava (IVC) orifice, the tendon of Todaro (TT), and the tricuspid valve (TV). The isthmus is divided by the coronary sinus orifice (CS). FO, foramen ovale; SVC, superior vena cava.

orifice and the tricuspid valve annulus at the base of the triangle of Koch, using cryoablation. We used a different rationale in our first case: A right atrial transection was carried out to interrupt the two limbs of the circuit (internodal pathways and crista terminalis).

Intraoperative Cardiac Mapping

We obtained four intraoperative maps at surgery. Epicardial maps in two patients confirmed the slow conduction over the isthmus and circular activation of the right atrium, whereas the left atrium received col-

Surgical Rationale

The current accepted rationale is to ablate the slow conducting isthmus between the inferior vena cava

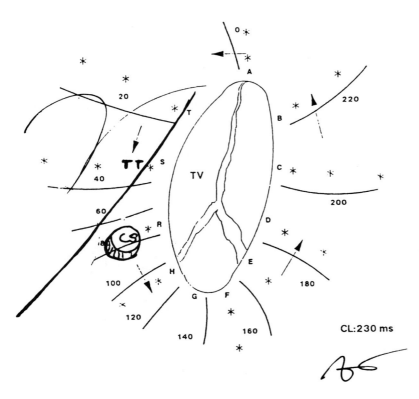

FIGURE 15-8. Intraoperative map of atrial flutter. The activation *(arrows)* circulates around the tricuspid valve (TV) annulus. CS, coronary sinus, TT, tendon of Todaro.

lateral activation from the circuit. Endocardial cardiac mapping in two patients documented circular activation in one patient around the tricuspid annulus and an area of slow conduction in the isthmus, with apparent circular activation within the isthmus, in the other patient.

Surgical technique used epicardial extensive cryoablation of the area bounded by the tricuspid annulus, the coronary sinus os, and the orifice of the inferior vena cava. In four patients, endocardial cryoablation was used with extensive ablation of the base of the triangle of Koch.

Results and Applications

Our experience comprises seven male patients (33 to 63 years old) with problematic symptoms (4 to 20 years' duration). No patient had associated structural heart disease. All patients had the common form. Preoperative electrophysiologic studies confirmed the typical characteristics of the flutter with an area of slow, fragmented conduction in the coronary sinus os region and a large, excitable gap within the right atrium.

Postoperatively, there were no complications. At predischarge electrophysiologic studies, atrial flutter was not inducible. During long-term follow-up, one patient had recurrence of atrial fibrillation and underwent a corridor operation 1 year later. The six other patients were free of arrhythmia without taking antiarrhythmic drugs with follow-up periods of 16, 9, 8, 3, and 2 years, respectively. Successful surgical ablation combined with intraoperative mapping confirmed the mechanism of the atrial flutter.

ATRIAL FIBRILLATION

Atrial fibrillation is the most common supraventricular arrhythmia but has only recently been approached surgically. Atrial fibrillation is a complex arrhythmia without a discrete anatomic substrate. Surgical rationales that are used for other supraventricular tachycardias do not apply; new surgical concepts and rationales had to be developed.

Atrial Functional Anatomy

Atrial fibrillation dramatically alters atrial functional anatomy (91). The atria are two compliant pouches between the venous return and the ventricles. They harbor two critical structures: the sinus node and the AV node. The atria are small (60 mL) and cannot function as a reservoir. The role of atrial contraction is defined by the Frank-Starling law, which applies to the failing heart. The normal ventricle is a sucking pump with active diastole and does not require atrial contraction to enhance its function (92). Chronotropic function is the primary determinant of increased cardiac output during exercise, with increased contractility (i.e., humoral regulation). Atrial contraction is critical to sustain cardiac function of the failing heart (93). However, the respective role of chronotropic function with regular rhythm and atrial contraction has not been elucidated.

Prevention of intracavitary thrombus is a major function of the atria. Alterations of atrial geometry (i.e., dilatation), pathology alteration of the atrial wall (i.e., endothelium), and contraction (i.e., left atrial appendage washout) are the accepted causes of intracavitary thrombus and systemic emboli in atrial fibrillation. The left atrial appendage with its special morphology and physiology is the primary culprit (94).

Atrial Pathology

Atrial fibrillation is commonly associated with primary structural heart disease. Atrial pathology in this setting has been well reported (95,96). Some work has focused on myocardial pathology associated with lone atrial fibrillation, which seems to develop in the absence of clinically detectable structural heart disease (97,98). We have reported atrial myocardial pathology in 12 patients with lone atrial fibrillation who underwent a *corridor operation* (99,100). There was a dramatic decrease in nerve endings and ganglion cells in all heart specimens, a finding that is consistent with the concept of cardioneuropathy or the role of the autonomic nervous system in atrial fibrillation. Myocardial pathology was present in all patients but one. Myocardial hypertrophy was observed in four patients, suggesting a tachycardia-related mechanism.

Atrial myocardiopathy was present in six patients; adiposis, fibrosis, or both were associated with moderate myocardial hypertrophy. Because biopsies were obtained from the high right atrium, sinus node tissue was present in four heart specimens. The sinus node was abnormal in three, with hypocellularity and fatty infiltration. In two, the sinus node artery presented with fibromuscular hyperplasia. None of the patients with sinus node pathology presented with sinus node dysfunction.

Mechanism

Atrial fibrillation is characterized by its electrocardiographic pattern of rapid irregular atrial activation associated with irregular ventricular contractions. Moe speculated, on a computer model, that atrial fibrillation was associated with simultaneous multiple wavelets of activation (101). Allessie and colleagues confirmed similar findings in animal experiments (102) that common atrial fibrillation is of the random reentry type (Fig. 15-9). Four to six wavelets are moving randomly. Their activation front usually is narrow. Wavelets are short lasting, but new wavelets are generated by division of existing wavelets. Atrial vulnera-

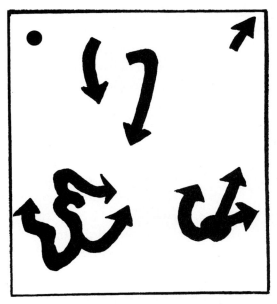

FIGURE 15-9. Schematic depiction of intraatrial random reentry.

bility or atrial propensity to sustain atrial fibrillation is determined by atrial surface area (i.e., size), morphology, anatomic obstacle, and spatial distribution of nonhomogeneous electrophysiologic characteristics (i.e., dispersion) (103). These characteristics may vary over time according to the underlying pathology and duration of the atrial fibrillation, a self-aggravating and perpetuating mechanism. Atrial fibrillation begets atrial fibrillation by modifying electrophysiologic characteristics (i.e., atrial remodeling) (104).

This mechanism may not be the only one that is observed in clinical fibrillation. Atrial flutter with chaotic left atrial activation, multiple atrial foci, or both conditions may be present.

Although established atrial fibrillation is not focal, there are experimental suggestions that the presence of a critical segment of atrial tissue with a very short refractory period may be mandatory for the perpetuation of fibrillation. Morillo and colleagues were able to interrupt and prevent atrial fibrillation by focal cryoablation in an animal model (105). These studies and their potential development may dramatically modify the future of interventional approaches.

Clinical Presentations and Problematic Symptoms

Patients with atrial fibrillation present with three orders of symptoms: those associated with the arrhythmia itself, those related to associated structural heart disease, and those associated with intracavitary thrombosis.

Symptoms associated with atrial fibrillation are well identified in patients with lone atrial fibrillation. Many patients with lone atrial fibrillation are asymptomatic, with a stroke as the initial presentation in 25%. Other patients have palpitations associated with panic syndrome, posttachycardia syndrome, or both. Exercise capacity may be altered during the attacks.

Symptoms related to associated structural heart disease may predominate and may obscure symptoms associated with atrial fibrillation, which is an aggravating factor. Risk of stroke has been well studied, as has its prevention (106).

Surgical Rationales

Surgical rationales are based on the random intraatrial reentry mechanism, although this mechanism may not be present in all patients with atrial fibrillation. Three elementary concepts are used: exclusion, fragmentation, and channeling (Fig. 15-10).

Exclusion is used to isolate the fibrillating atrium (i.e., left atrial exclusion in patients with mitral valve disease) and to protect critical function (i.e., corridor operation, which isolates sinus node and AV node from the rest of fibrillating atria).

Fragmentation uses atriotomies to produce semiexcluded atrial segments. Random reentry cannot be sustained in each semi-isolated segment because of reduced size (i.e., critical surface area), but all segments can contract sequentially in harmony.

Channeling is aimed at modifying the geometry of atrial tissue. A two-dimensional surface area is transformed into a unidimensional surface (i.e., strips of atrial tissue). It is believed that a unidimensional strip of atria cannot sustain reentry.

Several surgical techniques have been described: the left atrial exclusion; the corridor operation, based on an excluded channel that harbors the sinus node and the AV node; the maze operation, which combines subtotal exclusion of the left atrium with channeling and fragmentation; the compartment operation; and the spiral operation, which channels the entire left atrium and fragments the right atrium.

All surgical techniques are associated with resection of the left atrial appendage, which is documented as the main site of intracavitary thrombus. Each technique is aimed at restoring sinus node chronotropic function, whereas the other atrial functions are restored to various degrees. An inherent limitation to all surgical techniques is the potential for sinus node dysfunction, which may require permanent pacing after surgery.

Surgical Techniques

Corridor Operation

A strip or channel of atrial tissue (i.e., a corridor) is isolated to restore sinus node function (107–109)

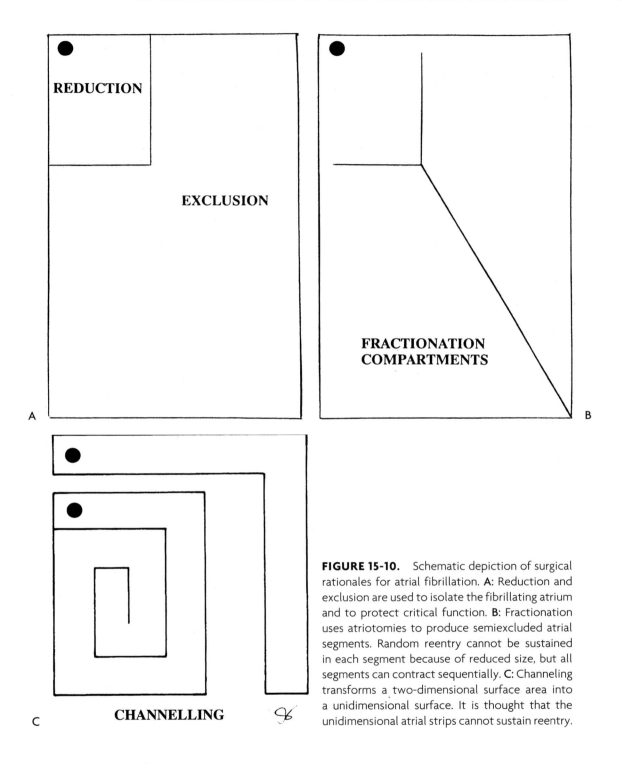

FIGURE 15-10. Schematic depiction of surgical rationales for atrial fibrillation. **A:** Reduction and exclusion are used to isolate the fibrillating atrium and to protect critical function. **B:** Fractionation uses atriotomies to produce semiexcluded atrial segments. Random reentry cannot be sustained in each segment because of reduced size, but all segments can contract sequentially. **C:** Channeling transforms a two-dimensional surface area into a unidimensional surface. It is thought that the unidimensional atrial strips cannot sustain reentry.

(Fig. 15-11). The strip of atrial tissue has a small surface area and should not be able to sustain atrial fibrillation. The corridor operation is performed under cardiopulmonary bypass and cold cardioplegic cardiac arrest (Fig. 15-12). The surgical technique comprised exclusion of the left atrial free wall by using a horseshoe incision along the attachment of the left atrial wall onto the atrial septum. The ends of the left atrial incision attach onto the mitral valve annulus in the anterior and posterior commissure regions. The pos-

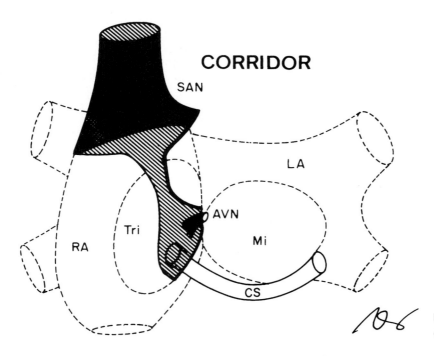

FIGURE 15-11. Schematic depiction of the corridor operation.

terior commissure area (i.e., posterior septal region) must be carefully dissected, including the coronary sinus, to attain uniform exclusion of the left atrium. Cryosurgical ablation at the mitral valve annulus ensures complete exclusion; construction of the corridor uses a horseshoe incision attaching onto the tricuspid annulus and circumscribing the corridor, which includes a cuff of right atrium that harbors the sinus node region, the AV node region, and a strip of atrial septum bridging the two nodes.

We have reported our experience with nine patients with drug-refractory atrial fibrillation who underwent this operation. Four patients had chronic atrial fibrillation, and five had paroxysmal atrial fibrillation; the mean duration of symptoms was 12 ± 8 years. The patients were between the ages of 25 and 68 years (mean, 48 ± 12 years). At the preoperative electrophysiologic study, no patient had evidence of an accessory atrioventricular pathway or AV node reentry. Sinus node recovery time could not be determined in five patients because of recurrent atrial fibrillation during or before programmed stimulation.

At operation, the corridor of atrial tissue connecting the sinus and AV nodes was successfully isolated from the remaining left and right atrial tissue in all patients. There were no perioperative complications. One patient required early reoperation for recurrent atrial fibrillation before hospital discharge. At the predischarge electrophysiologic study, the corridor operation remained isolated in all patients except one who had intermittent conduction between the corridor

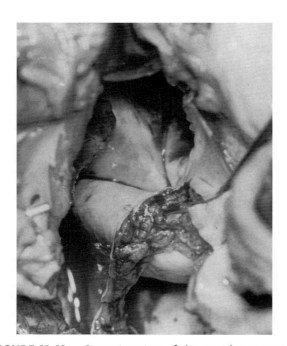

FIGURE 15-12. Operative view of the corridor operation.

and excluded right atrium. One patient had nonsustained atrial fibrillation, and one had atrial tachycardia evidence in the corridor. Atypical AV node reentry of uncertain significance was induced in one other patient.

At exercise testing before discharge, the heart rate in the nine patients increased from a mean of 78 ± 20 to 114 ± 17 bpm, and the maximal heart rate achieved ranged from 41% to 84% (mean, 68 ± 17%) of the predicted maximal heart rate based on age and gender criteria.

The total follow-up time was 191 months (mean, 21 months; range, 3 to 52 months). Seven patients remain free of symptomatic supraventricular tachycardia. Two patients (cases 6 and 7) have had recurrences of atrial fibrillation during follow-up. The arrhythmia in one of these patients has been well controlled with propafenone, with no recurrence in the past 36 months; the other patient has experienced paroxysmal episodes of atrial fibrillation (approximately weekly) while taking quinidine and verapamil.

A permanent ventricular pacemaker was implanted in three patients after surgery. In two patients, a pacemaker was implanted after symptomatic sinus pauses, and a pacemaker was implanted prophylactically when prolonged sinus pauses were demonstrated at the postoperative electrophysiologic study. A patient who had undergone previous cardiac surgery and pacemaker implantation had an atrial pacemaker reimplanted postoperatively because of prolonged sinus pauses associated with bradycardia-dependent atrial arrhythmias.

These initial results demonstrate that the corridor operation can maintain sinus rhythm in patients with atrial fibrillation. Since then, four additional patients have had a corridor operation. Improved selection criteria allowed normal sinus node function after surgery.

Gursoy and colleagues reported five patients with the corridor operation for lone atrial fibrillation. Sinus node chronotropic function was normal postoperatively, with good exercise tolerance (110).

Vigano and colleagues reported 13 patients (nine males and four females) with the corridor operation for paroxysmal lone atrial fibrillation (10 patients) and three atrial flutter (3 patients) (111). The follow-up period ranged from 9 to 47 months. There were no surgical complications. All patients were in sinus rhythm and had adequate exercise capacity. No patients were on antiarrhythmic drugs or had a pacemaker implanted.

Van Hemel and colleagues reported 36 patients with the corridor operation for paroxysmal lone atrial fibrillation (112). The follow-up period was 41 ± 16 months. Thirty-one patients had successful construction of the corridor. Twenty-five patients were arrhythmia free without medication (4-year actuarial freedom, 72 ± 9%). Twenty-six patients had normal sinus node function at rest and during exercise (4-year actuarial freedom of sinus node dysfunction, 81 ± 7%). Five patients had pacemakers implanted.

Overall, the corridor operation gave good control of the arrhythmia and restored sinus rhythm, with good functional capacity. One patient from Utrecht, the Netherlands, ran a marathon.

Maze Operation

Since the first report (113), the maze operation has undergone many modifications and alterations by its designer and others. The master plan comprises a subtotal left atrial exclusion and multiple atriotomies combined with cryoablation. One left atriotomy divides the circular cuff of the left atrium around the mitral valve. Multiple right and septal atriotomies fragment and channel the right atrium and septum (Fig. 15-13).

Cox and colleagues (114–118) reported 87 patients treated with the maze procedure for atrial flutter or fibrillation. The average age of the 64 male and 23 female patients was 54 years. The presenting arrhythmia was paroxysmal atrial flutter in 6 patients, paroxysmal atrial fibrillation in 37 patients, and chronic atrial fibrillation in 44 patients. All patients had failed extensive medical therapy, with an average of five drugs per patient; 36% had failed amiodarone.

Forty-three patients (49%) had paroxysmal atrial flutter or fibrillation, and 44 patients (51%) had chronic atrial fibrillation. The first 33 patients had the standard maze procedure; the remainder had variants that did not differ significantly from the original technique but were aimed at better preservation of sinus node function. Twenty-four patients had concomi-

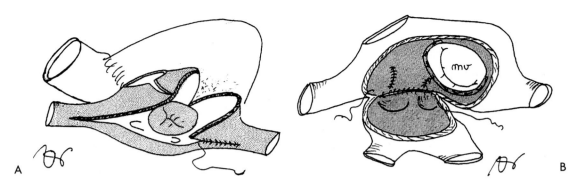

FIGURE 15-13. Maze operation. **A:** Atrial incision. **B:** Left atrial incisions.

tant cardiac repair, and seven had previous cardiac surgery.

Three patients died during surgery. Two patients had postoperative transient ischemic attacks. Early in the series, patients had postoperative fluid retention and pulmonary edema. This was caused by atrial natriuretic factor and was treated by spironolactone, which is now routinely prescribed. In the first three months after surgery, 47% of patients had recurrence of atrial fibrillation or flutter. Of the 78 patients with more than three months of follow-up, 32 required permanent AAIR pacing. Some patients had sinus node dysfunction before surgery. All patients were assessed in terms of exercise tolerance, arrhythmia (i.e., Holter monitoring), and cardiac function (i.e., atrial contraction). Overall, atrial fibrillation or flutter was controlled by surgery alone in 71 of 78 patients, whereas 32 patients (41%) required pacemaker implantation.

Left Atrial Isolation

Graffigna and colleagues reported left atrial isolation in 184 patients with concomitant mitral valve surgery (119). Seventy-one percent of patients returned to sinus rhythm after surgery, whereas 19% of patients with only mitral valve surgery returned to sinus rhythm (not a controlled trial; $p < 0.001$). Patients with restored sinus rhythm had significant improvement of their exercise capacity.

Fragmentation or Compartment Operation

Shyu and colleagues (120) reported their experience with the compartment operation (i.e., open corridor) in 22 patients. All patients had concomitant mitral valve surgery. The compartment operation is best described as an open corridor operation; the atriotomy that normally isolates the left atrium and the corridor itself are left incomplete and allow persistent connections between the three constructed segments of atria.

The compartment operation was not associated with increased surgical morbidity. Fourteen patients (64%) were in sinus rhythm at 6 months of follow-up. Atrial mechanical function, as assessed by echo Doppler studies, was not always present after restoration of sinus rhythm.

Spiral Operation

We designed a surgical technique to control atrial fibrillation based on channeling of the right and left atria, with special concern for patients with mitral valve dysfunction associated with chronic atrial fibrillation. Cardiac physiology and clinical studies emphasize the critical additional benefit of restored sinus rhythm after surgical correction of mitral valve disease. Atrial pathology and its problematic symptoms (e.g., atrial fibrillation) and mitral valve disease are two sides of the same coin and should be addressed routinely in a two-pronged operation.

We wanted to design adjunct atriotomies aimed at disabling atrial fibrillation as a simple extension of the atriotomies that are used to explore the mitral valve. For mitral exposure, we selected the vertical transseptal approach, or *transplant incision* (a term coined by Duran), because it has become the exposure of choice for mitral valve surgery. The spiral combines channeling of the right atria by using the transseptal approach

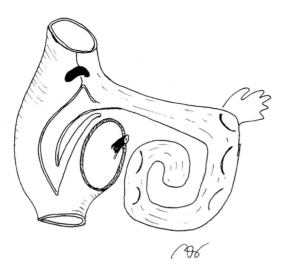

FIGURE 15-14. Spiral operation.

and the left atrium by transforming the left atrium into a circumvoluted (spiral) strip like an orange peel of atrial tissue. We anticipated that the spiral operation would restore sinus rhythm and contraction of the entire left atrium, including the posterior wall, which is recognized as a site of thrombosis along with the left atrial appendage.

The heart is exposed through a median sternotomy. Cardiopulmonary bypass is attached to the patient by using double venous cannulation; the superior vena cava can be directly cannulated according to surgeon's preference or cardiac anatomy. Cardioplegic solution is easily delivered by means of the exposed coronary sinus os. Surgery is performed in three steps: the modified extended transseptal approach, mitral valve surgery (if indicated), and spiraling of the left atrium combined with left atrial appendage exclusion (Fig. 15-14).

Modified Vertical Transseptal Approach

A quasi-circumferential incision (i.e., transplant incision) of the right atrium is performed (121). The right atrial free wall is incised along the right atrioventricular sulcus and is prolonged by the vertical septal incision through the fossa ovale. The incision of the superior wall (roof) of the left atrium extends from the septal incision and curves to reach the mitral valve annulus. The mitral valve is exposed by using stay sutures, and mitral valve surgery is performed. Spiraling of the left atrium is performed by using a left atrial incision that is started at the mitral valve annulus in the left posterior septal region. The incision circumscribes the right pulmonary veins and proceeds transversely to circumscribe the left pulmonary veins, traveling at the inferior pole of the left atrial appendage orifice. At that point, the incision involves the left atrial posterior wall. The extent of the spiraling incision depends on the posterior wall. The spiral incision can be done by using conventional radiofrequency cauterization. The incision is not transmural, with coagulation of the deeper layer by heat energy. The spiral incision is easy and is rapidly repaired by running sutures for safety, as well as other atriotomies.

Our initial experience comprised six patients: three with lone atrial fibrillation and three with mitral valve disease. Early good results need longer follow-up to be reliably assessed.

Results and Applications

Surgical techniques may interrupt atrial fibrillation. The surgical rationales are based on the site of the origin of atrial fibrillation, as in left atrial exclusion, or based on neutralizing the reentrant mechanism of atrial fibrillation (i.e., random reentry). However, surgical successes are not irrefutable evidence that the surgical rationales are true and do not exclude the possibility of other underlying mechanisms.

Surgical failures can be classified in four groups: failure to interrupt atrial fibrillation, failure to reestablish sinus node function with adequate chronotropic response to exercise, failure to restore atrial contraction, and failure to prevent intraatrial thrombus formation and its associated systemic embolic events.

Failure to Interrupt Atrial Fibrillation

The identical atrial fibrillation mechanism could be present postoperatively because the surgical rationale is inappropriate, because the working mechanism is a variant of the one that is currently accepted (focal mechanism?), or because the surgery was not adequately executed. Failure to interrupt atrial fibrillation may be an illusion because a new atrial tachycardia, such as multifocal atrial tachycardia that can mimic the clinical presentation of atrial fibrillation, is present after surgery. Catheter electrophysiologic studies have limited power to distinguish among these various mechanisms. These postoperative arrhythmias may be transitory but are disturbing evidence that our understanding of atrial fibrillation is rudimentary and that there may be more than one working mechanism.

Failure to Restore Sinus Node Function

Sinus node dysfunction may be present before surgery and is part of atrial fibrillation pathophysiology. It can be induced surgically because of the site of atriotomies or associated ischemic changes. Although AAIR pacemaker implantation can restore atrial contraction and chronotropic function, sinus dysfunction is a significant setback.

Atrial Contraction

Loss of atrial contraction can be part of surgical design (i.e., corridor or left atrial exclusion) or may occur because of electromechanical dissociation. Atria may not contract because of irreversible myocardial damage (99,100,120,122).

Myocardial Pathology

Severe cardiac pathology, including the sinus node, was present in all our patients, and some had primary atrial cardiomyopathy. Some patients may have irreversible tachycardia-induced cardiomyopathy. Underlying cardiac pathology has been overlooked in most studies.

Surgical Indication

The surgical indication is for arrhythmia is controversial. Other nonpharmacologic electrophysiologic intervention provides excellent control of arrhythmia with fewer side effects and less risk. Mitral valve disease that requires concomitant mitral valve surgery seems to be the indication of choice.

Direct atrial surgery combined with mitral valve surgery is used extensively by some surgical teams (123–127). Concomitant surgery for atrial fibrillation seems to be a benign adjunct to mitral valve surgery, although it may increase surgical risk in various ways: atriotomies, prolongation of aortic cross-clamping time, and prolongation of cardiopulmonary bypass time. Mitral valve disease associated with atrial fibrillation is a complex entity with multiple components, such as valvular anatomy, left ventricular function, left atrial dimension, duration of symptoms, age, and sex. Studies show that left ventricular function is the main independent prognostic marker. One review (128) of long-term follow-up of patients after mitral valve repair showed no difference between patients with or without atrial fibrillation in terms of survival or morbidity. Despite the large number of patients who have had combined surgery for atrial fibrillation, no comparative, randomized series has been published. Atrial fibrillation may have the same value as ventricular arrhythmia in patients with coronary artery disease. The premier marker of survival is cardiac function.

CONCLUSIONS

If electrophysiologic assessment of atrial fibrillation becomes more precise, new rationales guided by atrial mapping may develop. Some atrial fibrillations may be associated with a focal, perpetuating site that could be ablated.

However, it should be expected that surgery for atrial fibrillation will share the fate of other surgical approaches to supraventricular arrhythmias. Surgical techniques are associated with significant morbidity and should be only temporarily necessary. Surgical approaches offer an opportunity to collect data and assess new rationales and techniques that could be delivered by less invasive approaches.

Catheter ablation techniques have been used to control atrial fibrillation. For example, Haissaguerre and colleagues used catheter ablation techniques for unusual forms of atrial fibrillation (18). Common forms of lone atrial fibrillation have been successfully approached by using catheter techniques (19–21). These developments suggest that catheter ablation of atrial fibrillation may be common practice in the foreseeable future.

REFERENCES

1. Guiraudon GM, Klein GJ, Yee R. Surgery for cardiac tachyarrhythmias. *Highlights* 1990;6:5–10.
2. Guiraudon GM. Cryoablation, a versatile tool in arrhythmia surgery [Editorial]. *Ann Thorac Surg* 1987;43:129–130.
3. Harrison L, Gallagher JJ, Kasell J, et al. Cryosurgical ablation of the AV node–His bundle: a new method for producing AV block. *Circulation* 1977;55:463.
4. Klein GJ, Harrison L, Ideker RF, et al. Reaction of the myocardium to cryosurgery: electrophysiology and arrhythmogenic potential. *Circulation* 1979;59:364–372.
5. Warin JF. Catheter ablation of accessory atrioventricular connections. In: Touboul P, Waldo AL, eds. *Atrial arrhythmias: current concepts and management.* St. Louis: Mosby–Year Book, 1990:476–487.
6. Warin J-F, Haissaguerre M, Lemetayer P, et al. Catheter ablation of accessory pathways with a direct approach: results in 35 patients. *Circulation* 1988;78:800–815.
7. Brugada P, Wellens HJJ. Where to fulgurate in supraventricular tachycardia. In: Fontaine G, Scheinman MM, eds. *Ablation in cardiac arrhythmias.* Mount Kisco, NY: Futura, 1987:141–149.
8. Jackman WM, Wang X, Friday KJ, et al. Catheter ablation of accessory atrioventricular pathways (Wolff-Parkinson-White syndrome) by radiofrequency current. *N Engl J Med* 1991;324:1605–1611.
9. Calkins H, Sousa J, El-Atassi R, et al. Diagnosis and cure of the Wolff-Parkinson-White syndrome or paroxysmal supraventricular tachycardias during a single electrophysiologic test. *N Engl J Med* 1991;324:1612–1662.
10. Leather RA, Leitch JW, Klein GJ, et al. Radiofrequency catheter ablation of accessory pathways: a learning experience. *Am J Cardiol* 1991;68:1651–1655.
11. Kirklin JW. The science of cardiac surgery. *Eur J Cardiothorac Surg* 1990;4:63–71.
12. Buckberg GD. Myocardial protection: an overview. *Semin Thorac Cardiovasc Surg* 1993;5,2:98–106.
13. Scheinman MM. North American Society of Pacing and Electrophysiology (NASPE) survey on radiofrequency catheter ablation: implications for clinicians, third party insurers, and government regulatory agencies. *Pacing Clin Electrophysiol* 1992;15:2228–2231.
14. Scheinman MM. Catheter ablation: present role and projected impact on health care for patients with cardiac arrhythmia. *Circulation* 1991;83:1489–1498.
15. Kirkorian G, Moncada E, Chevalier P, et al. Radiofrequency ablation of atrial flutter: efficacy of an anatomically guided approach. *Circulation* 1994;90:2804–2814.
16. Olshansky B, Okumura K, Henthorn R, et al. Atrial mapping of human atrial flutter demonstrates reentry in the right atrium. *J Am Coll Cardiol* 1988;7:194A.
17. Chen SA, Chiang CE, Yang CJ, et al. Radiofrequency catheter ablation of sustained intra-atrial reentrant tachycardia in adult patients. *Circulation* 1993;88:578–587.
18. Haissaguerre M. Marcus FI, Fischer B, Clementy J. Radiofrequency catheter ablation in unusual mechanisms of atrial fibrillation: report of 3 cases. *J Cardiovasc Electrophysiol* 1994;5:743–751.
19. Haissaguerre M, Gencel L, Fischer B, et al. Successful catheter ablation of atrial fibrillation. *J Cardiovasc Electrophysiol* 1994;5:1045–1052.
20. Elvan A, Pride HP, Eble JN, Zipes DP. Radiofrequency catheter ablation of the atria reduces the inducibility and duration of atrial fibrillation in dogs. *Circulation* 1995;91:2235–2244.
21. Swarz J. Pellersels G, Silvers J, et al. A catheter-based approach to atrial fibrillation in humans [Abstract]. *Circulation* 1994;90[Suppl 4]:I-335.
22. Sealy WC, Hattler BG, Blumennschein SD, et al. Surgical treatment of Wolff-Parkinson-White syndrome. *Ann Thorac Surg* 1969;8:1–11.
23. Guiraudon GM. Anatomy of atrioventricular attachments, connections and junction: in medio stat virtus [Editorial]. *J Am Coll Cardiol* 1994;24:1732–1734.
24. McAlpine WA. *Heart and coronary arteries: an anatomical atlas for clinical diagnosis, radiological investigation, and surgical treatment.* New York: Springer-Verlag, 1975.
25. Wood FC, Wolferth CC, Geckeler GD. Histologic demonstration of accessory muscular connections between auricle and ventricle in a case of short PR interval and prolonged QRS complex. *Am Heart J* 1943;25:454–462.
26. Hackel DB. Anatomic basis for preexcitation syndromes. In: Benditt DG, Benson DW, eds. *Cardiac preexcitation syndromes: origins, evaluation and treatment.* Boston: Martinus Nijhoff, 1986:31–40.
27. Guiraudon G, Klein G, Sharma A, Yee R. Regional subclassification of accessory pathways in the Wolff-Parkinson-White syndrome based on dissection and electrophysiology [Abstract]. *Pacing Clin Electrophysiol* 1989;12[Suppl 1]:653.
28. Guiraudon GM, Klein GJ, Yee R. Surgery for Wolff-Parkinson-White syndrome and supraventricular tachycardias. In: Josephson ME, Wellens HJJ, eds. *Tachycardias: mechanisms and management.* Mount Kisco, NY: Futura Publishing, 1993:479–504.
29. Coumel P, Cabrol C, Fabiato A, et al. Tachycardie permanente par rythme réciproque. 1. Preuves du diagnostic par stimulation auriculaire et ventriculaire. *Arch Mal Coeur* 1967;60:1830.
30. O'Neill BJ, Klein GJ, Guiraudon GM, et al. Results of operative therapy in the permanent form of junctional reciprocating tachycardia. *Am J Cardiol* 1989;63:1074–1079.
31. Klein GJ, Guiraudon GM, Kerr CR, et al. "Nodoventricular" accessory pathway: evidence for a distinct accessory atrioventricular pathway with atrioventricular node-like properties. *J Am Coll Cardiol* 1988;11:1035–1040.
32. Gallagher JJ. Variants of preexcitation: update 1984. In: Zipes DP, Jalife J, eds. *Cardiac electrophysiology and arrhythmias.* Orlando, FL: Grune & Stratton, 419–433.
33. Cappato R, Schluter M, Weib C, et al. Catheter-induced mechanical conduction block of right-sided accessory fibers with Mahaim-type preexcitation to guide radiofrequency ablation. *Circulation* 1994;90:282–290.
34. Grogin HR, Lee RJ, Kwasman M, et al. Radiofrequency catheter ablation of atriofascicular and nodoventricular Mahaim tracts. *Circulation* 1994;90:272–281.
35. Guiraudon GM, Klein GJ, Gulamhusein S, et al. Surgical repair of Wolff-Parkinson-White syndrome: a new closed-heart technique. *Ann Thorac Surg* 1984;37:67–71.
36. Sealy WC. Kent bundles in the anterior septal space. *Ann Thorac Surg* 1983;36:180–186.
37. Sealy WC. The evolution of the surgical methods for interruption of right free wall Kent bundles. *Ann Thorac Surg* 1983;36:29–36.
38. Sealy WC, Gallagher JJ. The surgical approach to the septal area of the heart based on experiences with 45 patients with Kent bundles. *J Thorac Cardiovasc Surg* 1980;79:542–551.
39. Cox JL, Gallagher JJ, Cain ME. Experience with 118 consecutive patients undergoing operation for the Wolff-Parkinson-White syndrome. *J Thorac Cardiovasc Surg* 1985;90:490–501.
40. Gallagher JJ, Sealy WC, Cox JL, et al. Results of surgery for preexcitation in 200 cases [Abstract]. *Circulation* 1981;64[Suppl IV]:146.

41. Guiraudon GM, Klein GJ, Sharma AD, et al. Closed heart technique for Wolff-Parkinson-White syndrome: further experience and potential limitations. *Ann Thorac Surg* 1986;42: 651–657.
42. Guiraudon GM, Klein GJ, Sharma AD, et al. Surgery for the Wolff-Parkinson-White syndrome: the epicardial approach. *Semin Thorac Cardiovasc Surg* 1989;1:21–33.
43. Guiraudon GM, Klein GJ, Yee R, et al. Surgical epicardial ablation of left ventricular pathway using sling exposure. *Ann Thorac Surg* 1990;50:968–971.
44. Guiraudon GM, Klein GJ, Sharma AD, et al. Surgical approach to anterior septal accessory pathways in 20 patients with the Wolff-Parkinson-White syndrome. *Eur J Cardiothorac Surg* 1988;2:201–206.
45. Guiraudon GM, Klein GJ, Sharma AD, et al. "Atypical" posterior septal accessory pathway in the Wolff-Parkinson-White syndrome. *J Am Coll Cardiol* 1988;12:1605–1608.
46. Teo WS, Guiraudon GM, Klein GJ, et al. A unique preexcitation pattern related to an atypical anteroseptal accessory pathway. *Pacing Clin Electrophysiol* 1992;15[Pt 1]:1696–1701.
47. Gallagher JJ, Selle JG, Sealy WC, et al. Intermediate septal accessory pathways (IS-AP): a subset of preexcitation at risk for complete heart block/failure during WPW surgery [Abstract]. *Circulation* 1986;74[Suppl 2]:387.
48. Murdock CJ, Klein GJ, Guiraudon GM, et al. Epicardial mapping in patients with "nodoventricular" accessory pathways. *Am J Cardiol* 1991;68:208–214.
49. Guiraudon CM, Guiraudon GM, Klein GJ. "Nodal ventricular" Mahaim pathway: histologic evidence for an accessory atrioventricular pathway with AV node-like morphology [Abstract]. *Circulation* 1988;78[Suppl II]:II-40.
50. Guiraudon GM, Guiraudon CM, Klein GJ, et al. The coronary sinus diverticulum: a pathological entity associated with the Wolff-Parkinson-White syndrome. *Am J Cardiol* 1988;62: 733–735.
51. Arruda MS, Beckman KJ, McClelland JH, et al. Coronary sinus anatomy and anomalies in patients with posteroseptal accessory pathway requiring ablation within a venous branch of the coronary sinus [Abstract]. *J Am Coll Cardiol* 1994;23:224A.
52. Guiraudon GM, Klein GJ, Sharma AD, et al. Multiple accessory pathways—the elusive posterior septal pathways: experience with 17 patients [Abstract]. *Pacing Clin Electrophysiol* 1988; 11[Suppl]:935.
53. Gallagher JJ, Sealy WC, Kasell J, et al. Multiple accessory pathways in patients with the pre-excitation syndrome. *Circulation* 1976;54:571–590.
54. Guiraudon GM, Guiraudon CM, Klein GJ, et al. Operation for the Wolff-Parkinson-White syndrome in the catheter ablation era. *Ann Thorac Surg* 1994;57:1084–1088.
55. Brodman R, Fisher J, Mitsudo S, et al. Kent pathways visualized in situ and removed at operation. *Am J Cardiol* 1983;51: 1457–1458.
56. Rosenberg HS, Klima T, McNamara DG, Leachman RD. Atrioventricular communication in the Wolff-Parkinson-White syndrome. *Am J Clin Pathol* 1971;56:79–90.
57. Sharma AD, Yee R, Guiraudon GM, Klein GJ. AV nodal reentry: current concepts and surgical treatment. In: Zipes DP, Rowlands DJ, eds. *Progress in cardiology*. Philadelphia: Lea & Febiger, 1988:129–145.
58. Pritchett ELC, Anderson RW, Benditt DG, et al. Reentry within the atrioventricular node: surgical cure with preservation of atrioventricular conduction. *Circulation* 1979;60: 440–446.
59. Marquez-Montes J, Rufilanchas JJ, Esteve JJ, et al. Paroxysmal nodal reentrant tachycardia, surgical cure with preservation of atrioventricular conduction. *Chest* 1983;83:690–694.
60. Ross DL, Johnson DC, Denniss AR, et al. Curative surgery for atrioventricular junctional ("AV nodal") reentrant tachycardia. *J Am Coll Cardiol* 1985;6:1282–1392.
61. Meijler FL, Janse MJ. Morphology and electrophysiology of the mammalian atrioventricular node. *Physiol Rev* 1988;68: 608–647.
62. Anderson RH, Becker AE, Brechenmacher C, et al. The human atrioventricular junctional area: a morphological study of the A-V node and bundle. *Eur J Cardiol* 1975;3:11–25.
63. Guiraudon GM, Klein GJ, van Hemel N, et al. Anatomically guided surgery to the AV node. AV nodal skeletonization: experience in 46 patients with AV nodal reentrant tachycardia. *Eur J Cardiothorac Surg* 1990;49:441–464.
64. Cox JL, Holman WL, Cain ME. Cryosurgical treatment of atrioventricular node reentrant tachycardia. *Circulation* 1987; 76:1329–1336.
65. Johnson DC, Nunn GR, Meldrum-Hanna W. Surgery for atrioventricular node reentry tachycardia: the surgical dissection technique. *Semin Thorac Cardiovasc Surg* 1989;1:53–57.
66. Guiraudon GM, Klein GJ, Sharma AD, et al. Skeletonization of the atrioventricular node surgical alternative for AV nodal reentrant tachycardia: experience with 32 patients. *Ann Thorac Surg* 1990;49:565–572.
67. Natale A, Wathen M, Wolfe K, et al. Comparative atrioventricular node properties after radiofrequency ablation and operative therapy of AV node reentry. *Pacing Clin Electrophysiol* 1993;16[Pt I]:971–977.
68. Lowe JE, Hendry PJ, Packer DL, Tang AS. Surgical management of chronic ectopic atrial tachycardia. *Semin Thorac Cardiovasc Surg* 1989;1:58–66.
69. Guiraudon GM, Klein GJ, Yee R. Supraventricular tachycardias: the role of surgery. *Pacing Clin Electrophysiol* 1993;16[Pt II]:658–670.
70. Sharma AD, Klein GJ, Guiraudon GM, et al. Paroxysmal sinus tachycardia: further experience with subtotal right atrial exclusion suggesting diffuse atrial disease [Abstract]. *J Am Coll Cardiol* 1986;7:128.
71. Morillo CA, Klein GJ, Thakur RK, et al. Mechanism of "inappropriate" sinus tachycardia: role of sympathovagal balance. *Circulation* 1994;90:873–877.
72. Gomes A, Mehta D, Langan MN. Sinus node reentrant tachycardia. *Pacing Clin Electrophysiol* 1995;18[Pt I]:1045–1057.
73. Sanders WE, Sorrentino RA, Greenfield RA, et al. Catheter ablation of sinoatrial node reentrant tachycardia. *J Am Coll Cardiol* 1994;23:926–934.
74. Jolly WA, Ritchie WT. Auricular flutter and fibrillation. *Heart* 1910;2:177.
75. Prinzmetal M. *The auricular arrhythmias*. Springfield, IL: Charles C Thomas, 1952.
76. Wells JL, et al. Characterization of atrial flutter: studies in man after open heart surgery using fixed atrial electrodes. *Circulation* 1979;60:665–673.
77. Lewis T, Freil HS, Stroud WD. Observations upon flutter and fibrillation. II. The nature of auricular flutter. *Heart* 1920;7: 191.
78. Boineau JP, Schuessler RB, Mooney CR, et al. Natural and evoked atrial flutter due to circus movement in dogs. *Am J Cardiol* 1980;45:1167–1181.
79. Allessie MA, Lammers WJ, Bonke IM, et al. Intraatrial reentry as a mechanism for atrial flutter induced by acetylcholine in rapid pacing in the dog. *Circulation* 1984;70:123–135.
80. Page P, Plumb VJ, Okumura K, et al. A new model of atrial flutter. *J Am Coll Cardiol* 1986;8:872–879.

81. Puech P, Latour H, Grolleau R. Le flutter et ses limites. *Arch Mal Coeur* 1970;63:116–144.
82. Klein GJ, Guiraudon GM, Sharma AD, et al. Demonstration of macro-reentry and feasibility of operative therapy in the common type of atrial flutter. *Am J Cardiol* 1986;57:587–591.
83. Disertori M, Inama G, Vergara G, et al. Evidence of a reentry circuit in the common type of atrial flutter in man. *Circulation* 1983;67:434–440.
84. Waldo AL, MacLean WA, Karp RB, et al. Entrainment and interruption of atrial flutter with atrial pacing: studies in man following open heart surgery. *Circulation* 1977;56:737–745.
85. Waldo AL, Carlson MD, Biblo LA, et al. The role of transient entrainment in atrial flutter. In: Touboul P, Waldo AL, eds. *Atrial arrhythmias: current concepts and management*. St. Louis: Mosby–Year Book, 1990:210.
86. Cosio FG. Endocardial mapping of atrial flutter. In: Touboul P, Waldo AL, eds. *Atrial arrhythmias: current concepts and management*. St. Louis: Mosby–Year Book, 1990:229.
87. Chauvin M, Brechenmacher C, Voegltin JR. Applications de la cartographie endocavitaire a l'étude du flutter auriculaire. *Arch Mal Coeur* 1983;76:1020–1030.
88. Cosio FG, Goicolea A, Lopez-Gil M, et al. Atrial endocardial mapping in the rare form of atrial flutter. *Am J Cardiol* 1990;66:715–720.
89. Puech P, Gallay P, Grolleau R. Mechanism of atrial flutter in humans. In: Touboul P, Waldo AL, eds. *Atrial arrhythmias: current concepts and management*. St. Louis: Mosby–Year Book, 1990:190.
90. Allessie MA, Rensma W, Brugada J, et al. Modes of atrial reentry. In: Touboul P, Waldo AL, eds. *Atrial arrhythmias: current concepts and management*. St. Louis: Mosby–Year Book, 1990:112.
91. Guiraudon GM, Guiraudon CM. Atrial functional anatomy. In: Kingma JH, van Hemel NM, Lie KI, eds. *Atrial fibrillation: a treatable disease?* Boston: Kluwer, 1992:23.
92. Robinson TF, Factor SM, Sonnenblick EH. The heart as a suction pump. *Sci Am* 1986;254:84–91.
93. Lamas GA. Physiological consequences of normal atrioventricular conduction: applicability to modern cardiac pacing. *J Card Surg* 1989;4:89–98.
94. Gosselink AT, Crijns HJGM, Lie KI. Risk and prevention of embolism in atrial fibrillation. In: Kingma JH, van Hemel NM, Lie KI, eds. *Atrial fibrillation: a treatable disease?* Boston: Kluwer, 1992:237.
95. James TN. Diversity of histopathologic correlates of atrial fibrillation. In: Kulbertus HE, Olson SB, Schlepper M, eds. *Atrial fibrillation*. Modudal, Sweden: Astra, 1982:13.
96. Bharati S, Lev M. Histology of the normal and diseased atrium. In: Falk RH, Podrid PJ, eds. *Atrial fibrillation: mechanisms and management*. New York: Raven, 1992:15.
97. Frustaci A, Caldarulo M, Buffon A, et al. Cardiac biopsy in patients with "primary" atrial fibrillation: histologic evidence of occult myocardial diseases. *Chest* 1991;100(2):303–306.
98. Sekiguchi M, Hiroe M, Kasanuki H, et al. Experience of 100 atrial endomyocardial biopsies and the concept of atrial cardiomyopathy [Abstract]. *Circulation* 1984;70[Suppl 2]:118.
99. Guiraudon CM, Ernst NM, Guiraudon GM, et al. The pathology of drug resistant lone atrial fibrillation in eleven surgically treated patients. In: Kingma JH, van Hemel NM, Lie KI, eds. *Atrial fibrillation: a treatable disease?* Boston: Kluwer, 1992:41.
100. Guiraudon CM, Ernst NM, Klein GJ, et al. The pathology of intractable "primary" atrial fibrillation [Abstract]. *Circulation* 1992;86[Suppl 1]:4:I-662.
101. Moe GK. On the multiple wavelet hypothesis of atrial fibrillation. *Arch Int Pharmacodyn* 1962;140:183.
102. Allessie MA, Lammers WJEP, Bonke FIM. Experimental evaluation of Moe's multiple wavelet hypothesis of atrial fibrillation. In: Zipes DP, Jalife J, eds. *Cardiac electrophysiology and arrhythmias*. New York: Grune & Stratton, 1985:265.
103. Allessie M, Kirchhof C. Termination of atrial fibrillation by class IC antiarrhythmic drugs, a paradox? In: Kingma JH, van Hemel NM, Lie KI, eds. *Atrial fibrillation: a treatable disease?* Boston: Kluwer, 1992:265.
104. Wijffels M, Kirchhof C, Frederiks J, et al. Atrial fibrillation begets atrial fibrillation [Abstract]. *Circulation* 1993;86[Suppl 1]:I-18.
105. Morillo CA, Klein GJ, Jones DL, et al. Experimental atrial fibrillation: evidence for a focal mechanism [Abstract]. *Am Coll Cardiol* 1993;21:183A.
106. Stroke Prevention in Atrial Fibrillation Study Group Investigators. Preliminary report of the Stroke Prevention in Atrial Fibrillation study. *N Engl J Med* 1990;322:863–868.
107. Guiraudon GM, Campbell CS, Jones DL, et al. Combined sino-atrial node atrio-ventricular isolation: a surgical alternative to His bundle ablation in patients with atrial fibrillation [Abstract]. *Circulation* 1985;72[Suppl 2]:II-220.
108. Leitch JW, Klein G, Yee R, et al. Sinus node–atrioventricular node isolation: long term results with the corridor operation for atrial fibrillation. *J Am Coll Cardiol* 1991;17:970–975.
109. Guiraudon GM, Klein GJ, Guiraudon CM, Yee R. Treatment of atrial fibrillation: preservation of sinoventricular impulse conduction (the corridor operation). In: Olsson SB, Allessie MA, Campbell RWF, eds. *Atrial fibrillation: mechanisms and therapeutic strategies*. Armonk, NY: Futura Publishing, 1994:349.
110. Gursoy S, de Bruyne B, Atie J, et al. Interatrial dissociation following the corridor operation: role of atrial contraction in thrombogenesis [Abstract]. *Eur Heart J* 1991;12[Suppl]:337.
111. Vigano M, Graffigna A, Pagnani F, et al. The surgical treatment for supraventricular arrhythmias. In: D'Alessandro LC, ed. *Heart surgery*. Rome: Casa Editrice Scientifica Internazionale, 1993:403.
112. van Hemel NM, Defaux JJAMT, Kingma JH, et al. Long-term results of the "corridor" operation for atrial fibrillation. *Br Heart J* 1994;71:170–176.
113. Cox JL, Canavan TE, Schuessler RB. The surgical treatment of atrial fibrillation. II. Intra-operative electrophysiologic mapping and description of the electrophysiologic basis of atrial flutter and atrial fibrillation. *J Thorac Cardiovasc Surg* 1991;101:406–426.
114. Cox JL. Evolving applications of the maze procedure for atrial fibrillation. *Ann Thorac Surg* 1993;55:578–580.
115. Cox JL, Boineau JP, Schuessler RB, et al. Successful surgical treatment of atrial fibrillation: review and clinical update. *JAMA* 1991;266:1976–1980.
116. Cox JL, Boineau JP, Schuessler RB, et al. Five-year experience with the maze procedure for atrial fibrillation. *Ann Thorac Surg* 1993;56:814–824.
117. Cox JL, Boineau JP, Schuessler RB, et al. Surgical interruption of atrial reentry as a cure for atrial fibrillation. In: Olsson SB, Allessie MA, Campbell RWF, eds. *Atrial fibrillation: mechanisms and therapeutic strategies*. Armonk, NY: Futura Publishing, 1994:373–404.
118. Cox JL, Schuessler RB, Cain ME, et al. Surgery for atrial fibrillation. *Semin Thorac Cardiovasc Surg* 1989;1:67–73.
119. Graffigna A, Ressia L, Pagnani F, et al. Left atrial isolation for the treatment of atrial fibrillation due to mitral valve disease: hemodynamic evaluation. *New Trends Arrhyth IX* 1993;4:1069.
120. Shyu K-G, Cheng J-J, Chen J-J, et al. Recovery of atrial function after atrial compartment operation for chronic atrial fibril-

lation in mitral valve disease. *J Am Coll Cardiol* 1994;24: 392–398.
121. Guiraudon GM, Ofiesh JG, Kaushik R. Extended vertical trans-septal approach to the mitral valve. *Ann Thorac Surg* 1991; 52:1058–1060.
122. Feinberg MS, Waggoner AD, Kater KM, et al. Restoration of atrial function after the maze procedure for patients with atrial fibrillation: assessment by Doppler echocardiography. *Circulation*, 1994;90[Suppl 2]:II-285.
123. Brodman RF, Frame R, Fisher JD, et al. Combined treatment of mitral stenosis and atrial fibrillation with valvuloplasty and left atrial maze procedure [Letter]. *J Thorac Cardiovasc Surg* 1994;107:622.
124. Hioki M, Ikeshita M, Iedokoro Y, et al. Successful combined operation for mitral stenosis and atrial fibrillation. *Ann Thorac Surg* 1993;55:776–778.
125. Bonchek LI, Burlingame MW, Worley SJ, et al. Cox/maze procedure for atrial septal defect with atrial fibrillation: management strategies. *Ann Thorac Surg* 1993;55:607–610.
126. McCarthy PM, Cosgrove DM, Castle LW, et al. Combined treatment of mitral regurgitation and atrial fibrillation with valvuloplasty and the maze procedure. *Am J Cardiol* 1993;71: 483–486.
127. Kosakai Y, Kawaguchi AT, Isobe F, et al. Cox maze procedure for chronic atrial fibrillation associated with mitral valve disease. *J Thorac Cardiovasc Surg* 1994;108:1049–1055.
128. Chua YL, Schaff HV, Orszulak TA, Morris JJ. Outcome of mitral valve repair in patients with preoperative atrial fibrillation. *J Thorac Cardiovasc Surg* 1994;107:408–415.

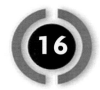

SURGICAL APPROACH TO ATRIAL FLUTTER AND ATRIAL FIBRILLATION

• • •

T. BRUCE FERGUSON, JR., JAMES J. MCKINNIE

The paradigm for ablative therapy of supraventricular and ventricular arrhythmias has continued to be tested during the past 10 years of remarkable advances in cardiac electrophysiology. The three components of this paradigm are elucidation of mechanisms of the arrhythmia, demonstration of the anatomic location of the arrhythmia circuit, and application of effective ablative techniques.

The role that experimental and clinical intraoperative mapping played in the development of procedures for reentrant atrioventricular, AV nodal, and ventricular arrhythmias has been critical in terms of mechanism elucidation and in terms of therapy design and implementation. Initial application of this paradigm in the surgical arena ultimately produced the knowledge base that has resulted in the successful ablation of most supraventricular arrhythmias using interventional electrophysiologic catheter-based techniques. This has been possible with supraventricular and focal ventricular arrhythmias because there is an underlying anatomic substrate that is critical for the initiation and maintenance of each of these arrhythmias.

Atrial fibrillation, however, has presented a different sort of challenge. Despite the fact that it is the most common pathologic rhythm, it remains in many ways the least well understood. Moreover, the clinical spectrum that encompasses atrial fibrillation is extremely broad and complex. This chapter examines surgical approaches to this common arrhythmia.

⦿ EARLY EXPLANATIONS OF ATRIAL FIBRILLATION AND ATRIAL FLUTTER

More than any other type of arrhythmia, elucidation of the mechanism of atrial fibrillation has depended on the development of sophisticated, multichannel, computerized mapping systems for experimental and clinical investigations. The rudimentary information obtained from early single-point intraoperative mapping systems about Wolff-Parkinson-White syndrome, ventricular tachycardia, and even atrial flutter could not be obtained from atrial fibrillation because of its complexity.

On the basis of intuition, observation, and early mapping data, Moe originally described atrial fibrillation as consisting of multiple wavelets occurring simultaneously and transiently throughout the atrial tissue (1). Allessie, in numerous experimental studies over the years, has developed the leading circle concept for atrial fibrillation, in which the reentrant circuit does not depend on an anatomic obstacle or an area of conduction block for maintenance of the arrhythmia (2,3). The only absolute requirement is that the wavelength of the circuit be short enough to be self-sustaining (i.e., to complete the circuit) within the anatomic space that is available to that circuit. In this model, if the wavelength is lengthened, then the circuit can be interrupted by coming into contact with an area of conduction block or with a fixed anatomic obstacle, such as the orifices of the vena cavae or pulmonary veins or the annuli of the mitral and tricuspid valves. However, Boineau demonstrated experimentally that atrial flutter depended on fixed anatomic obstacles or abnormalities in the atrial myocardium and functional factors such as nonuniform repolarization for maintenance of the large macro-reentrant circuits that are seen with induced atrial flutter (4). These early experimental studies suggested what to look for in interpreting the multipoint activation maps and set the stage for the mapping studies that were to come.

⦿ COMPUTERIZED MAPPING STUDIES OF THE ATRIUM

The computerized mapping systems that were developed for experimental and clinical studies were multichannel systems capable of recording a large number of unipolar or bipolar electrograms simultaneously. These recordings were made from custom-designed epicardial or endocardial templates. Later, these templates were designed to be form-fitting so as to capture the maximal amount of simultaneous activation points. Simultaneous limb-lead electrocardiographic recordings were obtained as well, and the digitized data were analyzed with several automated steps using high-resolution graphics capabilities. Output generation included individual electrogram data and activation-time maps. These data were recorded simultaneously and used for the generation of activation-time maps. The 250-channel experimental system and the 160-channel front-end system used in the operating room that was interfaced to the same computer and data storage system have been previously described (5). A second 256-channel experimental system was used for the canine experimental preparations described later for the maze and radial incision approach studies (6).

Two custom-designed sets of epicardial templates were designed to map the atria, one set for animal studies with 250 bipolar electrodes and one set for humans with 156 bipolar points (7,8). The human epicardial set consisted of three templates, one for the right atrial free wall (80 electrode pairs), one for the posterior left atrial tissue beneath the posterior septum and pulmonary veins (44 electrode pairs), and one for the transverse sinus to map the anterior right and left atrial tissue (32 electrode pairs) (Fig. 16-1).

Methods of Experimental and Clinical Mapping Studies

Several animal models were developed and used to map atrial fibrillation. A canine model of mitral insufficiency that avoided manipulation of the atria produced enlarged atria that were easily induced into atrial fibrillation or atrial flutter, although spontaneous atrial fibrillation was uncommon (9). It was determined that large dogs (>35 kg) could be induced into atrial fibrillation or atrial flutter with programmed stimulation, with or without neostigmine, which enhanced vagal tone and shortened atrial refractory periods. A third model that was developed in our laboratory by Yamauchi and colleagues involved anastomosis of the innominate artery with a pulmonary vein (10). This model produced atrial enlargement and significant atrial hypertrophy. This model was particularly useful for studies of atrial flutter.

Intraoperative mapping in humans was performed by using the 160-channel system described earlier. Patients undergoing surgery for Wolff-Parkinson-White syndrome, AV node reentrant tachycardia, or ectopic atrial tachycardias were induced into atrial fibrillation and atrial flutter by programmed stimulation (7,8).

Results of Computerized Mapping Studies for Atrial Fibrillation

Multipoint mapping in animal models demonstrated a wide spectrum of activation patterns during induced tachyarrhythmias (11). Atrial fibrillation also occurred with an activation pattern similar to that proposed by

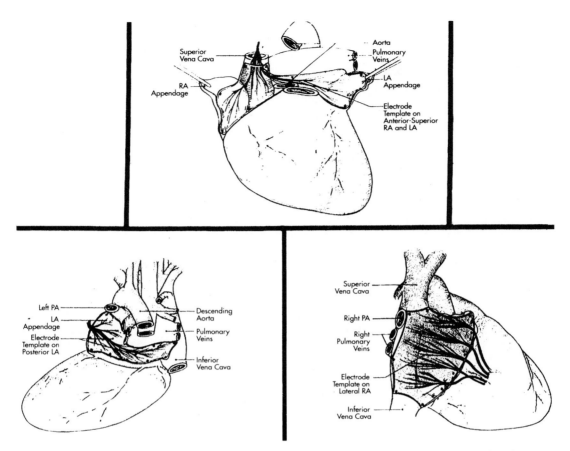

FIGURE 16-1. Positioning of form-fitting atrial epicardial templates containing 156 bipolar electrode pairs. **Lower right panel:** The template on the right side (80 electrodes) covers the lateral right atrium. **Upper panel:** The transverse sinus electrode (32 electrode pairs) covers the anterior right and left atria and the medial portion of the left atrial appendage. **Lower left panel:** The posterior atrial template (44 electrode pairs) covers the posterior left atrium. In addition to these epicardial templates, the lateral right atrial template can be replaced by a right atrial septal template placed through a right atriotomy for use in mapping the right atrial septal tissue. (From Cox JL, Schuessler RB, D'Agostino HJ, et al. The surgical treatment of atrial fibrillation. II. Intraoperative electrophysiologic mapping and description of the electrophysiologic basis of atrial flutter and atrial fibrillation. *J Thorac Cardiovasc Surg* 1991; 101:406–426, with permission.)

Moe (1) in his multiple wavelet hypothesis (Fig. 16-2). In the example in Figure 16-2, the fibrillation is characterized by multiple changing reentrant circuits, with the wavefronts interacting with multiple arcs of conduction block and slow conduction. The average local cycle length was about 90 to 100 msec in the left atrium and 110 to 120 msec in the right atrium. Mapping of the conduction pattern during normal sinus rhythm in this animal demonstrated no abnormal or slow conduction, even though the atria were enlarged.

During induced atrial fibrillation in humans, the spectrum of activation patterns was similar to that seen in the animal models. Most commonly, there were multiple dynamic wavefronts interacting with multiple changing arcs of block and slow conduction. In Figure 16-3, an example of activation maps of three separate 1-second intervals are shown during a run of induced atrial fibrillation in a patient with Wolff-Parkinson-White syndrome. The disparate and transient nature of these wavefronts over time (i.e., the duration of the entire sequence was 3 seconds) is

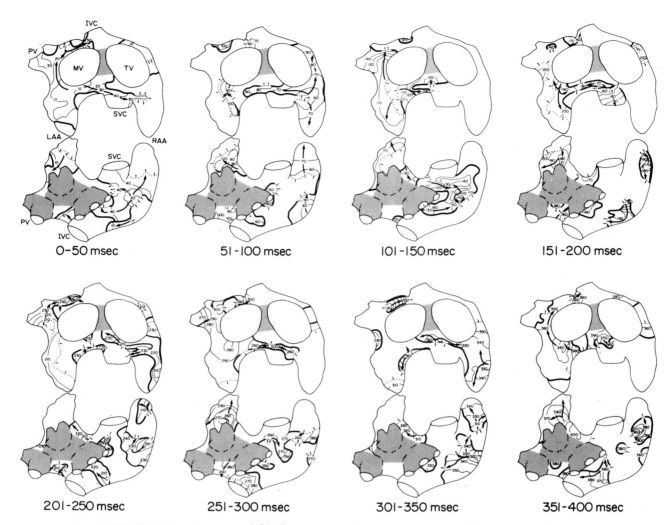

FIGURE 16-2. Canine atrial fibrillation. Activation sequence maps of 400 msec of atrial activation are shown by schematic drawings of the atria of a dog in which atrial enlargement was produced by severing the chordae of the mitral valve through the pulmonary veins. The maps are divided into consecutive 50-msec intervals. The thin dashed line with small arrows demarcates the beginning and end of the 50-msec windows. The thick arrows illustrate the direction of the spreading wavefronts. The arcs of functional block and cycle lengths ranged from 90 to 120 msec. IVC, inferior vena cava; LAA, left atrial appendage; MV, mitral valve annulus; PV, pulmonary veins; RAA, right atrial appendage; SVC, superior vena cava; TV, tricuspid valve annulus. (From Ferguson TB Jr, Schuessler RB, Hand DE, et al. Lessons learned from computerized mapping of the atrium. *J Electrophysiol* 1993;26:210–219, with permission.)

clearly seen. As demonstrated in the animals, normal sinus rhythm and paced activation sequence maps demonstrated no evidence of abnormal conduction in these patients.

Comparison of the canine and human data showed several interesting similarities and differences that are worth noting. Normal sinus rhythm and pacing showed the same activation patterns without areas of conduction block. However, in humans, the total activation time during normal sinus rhythm was about 110 to 120 msec, which was about twice that seen in the dog (50 to 70 msec). During atrial flutter, the activation patterns in humans and dogs suggested that in most cases the reentrant circuit involved an anatomic obstacle. In both groups, a single reentrant circuit resulting in atrial flutter was demonstrated to exist

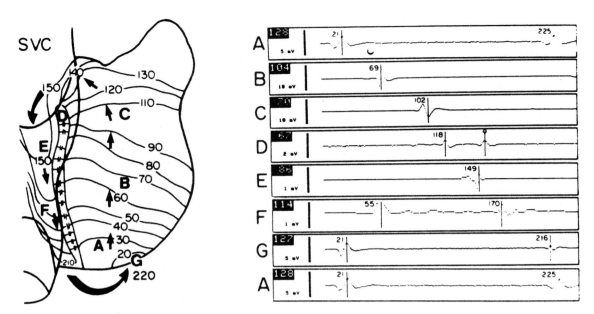

FIGURE 16-3. Human atrial flutter. The A through G labels on the electrograms *(right)* correspond to the letters on the electrophysiologic map denoting the location of seven selected electrodes of the 80 electrodes covering the posterior right atrium. Notice the large reentrant circuit *(arrows)* rotating around an area of functional block (-BB-) along the crista terminalis. The numbers on the map and beside each electrogram represent the isochrones in milliseconds. (From Cox JL, Schuessler RB, D'Agostino HJ, et al. The surgical treatment of atrial fibrillation. II. Intraoperative electrophysiologic mapping and description of the electrophysiologic basis of atrial flutter and atrial fibrillation. *J Thorac Cardiovasc Surg* 1991;101:406–426, with permission.)

without involvement of an anatomic obstacle, but these circuits were almost always transient and unstable. The cycle length during human atrial flutter (200 to 240 msec) was approximately twice that seen in dogs (100 to 130 msec).

During atrial fibrillation, the spectrum of activation patterns in both groups were similar, and the fibrillatory cycle length in humans was approximately twice that observed in the dogs. These findings are consistent with the longer atrial refractory periods that are observed in humans compared with dogs (11).

Results of Computerized Mapping Studies for Atrial Flutter

Experimental mapping demonstrated that at the simplest level there is atrial flutter where a single reentrant circuit activates the remainder of the atria passively and in a one-to-one fashion. These reentrant circuits were located in the left or right atrium but were most common on the right side. Most appeared to rotate around natural anatomic obstacles such as the superior vena cava, inferior vena cava, pulmonary veins, or some combination of these, connected by lines of functional block. Even when only a single anatomic structure was involved, the circuit was enlarged by functional block extending from the anatomic hole, confirming Boineau's earlier work (9).

More complex patterns of atrial flutter were mapped as well, including a single reentrant circuit in the left atrium with fibrillatory conduction into the right atrium. Because of the "clinical" appearance of this arrhythmia on the limb-lead electrocardiogram, it was originally thought to be atrial fibrillation rather than atrial flutter. If the ventricular response was 2:1 and regular, then this supraventricular activation appeared similar to atrial flutter, but in other circumstances in which fibrillatory conduction occurred proximal to the AV node and the ventricular response was irregular, this pattern of supraventricular activation appeared similar to atrial fibrillation.

Analysis of the epicardial human mapping data demonstrated that the activation sequences in humans were similar to those seen in the dog models. During atrial flutter, the data suggested that the reentrant circuits rotated around anatomic obstacles. However, initially, these reentrant circuits appeared to be confined to the right atrium. Arcs of functional block regularly connected the superior vena cava and the inferior vena cava, producing a large circuit that rotated in either a clockwise or a counterclockwise direction. The left atrium was activated passively from this right-sided circuit (Fig. 16-4).

These data suggested that common atrial flutter in humans results from reentry within the right atrium. Left atrial activation may or may not be passive. In typical flutter, there appears to be caudocranial activation along the right atrial septum with craniocaudal activation of the right atrial free wall. Most important, there exists a zone of slow conduction in the low right atrium. The typical flutter morphology may be

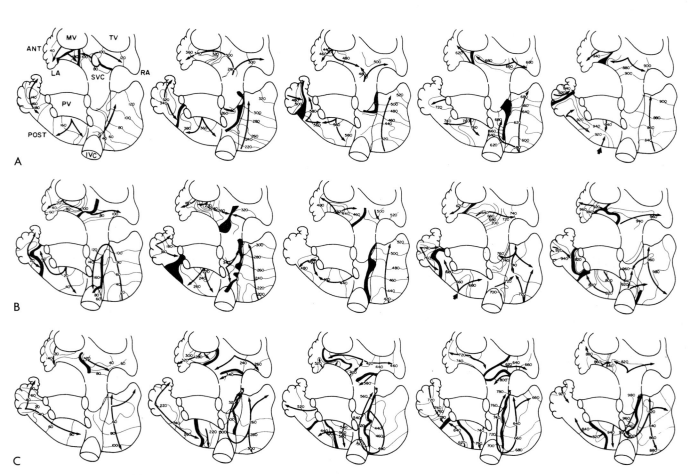

FIGURE 16-4. Human atrial fibrillation. Activation sequence maps of a single run of atrial fibrillation in a patient with Wolff-Parkinson-White syndrome are shown on a schematic drawing of the human atria. Each panel illustrates 1 second of data at different times during the fibrillation. The drawings indicate the arcs of functional block *(thick black lines)*, isochrones *(thin black lines)* every 20 msec, and the direction of the spread of activation *(arrows)*. **A, B and C:** The arrow shows the site of atrial insertion where an accessory pathway is conducting wavefronts from the ventricle. ANT, anterior; IVC, inferior vena cava; LA, left atrium; MV, mitral valve annulus; POST, posterior; PV, pulmonary veins; RA, right atrium; SVC, superior vena cava; TV, tricuspid valve annulus. (From Ferguson TB Jr, Schuessler RB, Hand DE, et al. Lessons learned from computerized mapping of the atrium. *J Electrophysiol* 1993;26:210–219, with permission.)

simulated by rapid pacing from the os of the coronary sinus, now recognized as the exit from the slow zone. The isthmus of slow conduction appears to be in part defined by anatomic landmarks (Figs. 16-5 and 16-6). The posterolateral extent of the slow zone (i.e., the entrance) is formed by the space between the posterolateral inferior vena cava right atrial junction, and the tricuspid annulus. The medial border of the slow zone (i.e., the exit) is between the coronary sinus ostium and the tricuspid annulus. The inferior extent of the isthmus is the fixed barrier that is formed by the tricuspid annulus. What forms the superior and posterior portion of this area, and therefore prevents impulse conduction between the inferior vena cava and the coronary sinus ostium, is uncertain. Data combining intracardiac ultrasound imaging with entrainment techniques suggest that both the crista terminalis in the anterior, lateral, and inferior right atrium and its extension as the eustachian valve, act as lines of bidirectional block (i.e., barriers) during typical atrial flutter in humans.

As demonstrated by catheter ablation studies in patients with atrial flutter, the isthmus of slow conduction in the low right atrium can be ablated as far lateral as the posterolateral inferior vena cava and right atrial junction and as far medial as the space between the coronary sinus os and the tricuspid annulus, suggesting these locations as the entrance and exit, respectively, of the protected isthmus (Fig. 16-6). A remarkably consistent finding in patients with typical atrial flutter is a region of long conduction time from the low posterolateral right atrial free wall to the low posteromedial (posteroseptal) right atrium. This region of 2 to 3 cm accounts for 100 to 150 msec of activation time during the isoelectric portion of the surface flutter wave. This has important implications for surgical ablation during concomitant intracardiac procedures.

More than one type of atypical atrial flutter exists. In some cases, the circuit seems identical to that of typical atrial flutter, with a slow zone in the low right atrium, but the tachycardia circles in a clockwise rather than counterclockwise fashion. This form of atypical flutter can be successfully ablated in the same manner as type I flutter. In other cases, the low right atrium does not seem to be a critical isthmus, and barriers that are responsible for creating a protected slow zone have not been identified. Whether these are true leading circle reentrant tachycardias or have critical zones in the unmapped left atrium is incompletely understood (12).

To overcome the limitations of epicardial mapping, new sets of endocardial animal and human elec-

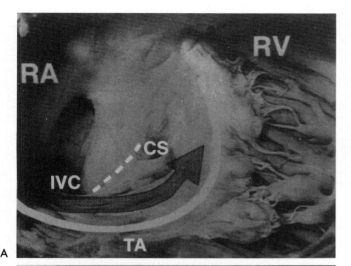
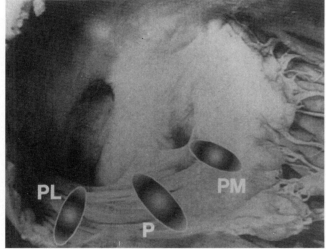

FIGURE 16-5. A: Diagram of the zone of slow conduction in the low right atrium (RA) bounded by the tricuspid annulus (TA), the inferior vena cava (IVC), and the coronary sinus (CS) os. Placement of an ablation lesion such that it completely bridges the slow zone from the tricuspid annulus to the CS, the IVC, or both interrupts the reentrant circuit in common atrial flutter. B: Ablation can be accomplished at the low posterolateral atrium (PL), at the midpoint of the slow zone in the posterior right atrium (P), or near the exit at the low posteromedial right atrium (PM). (From Lesh MD. Radiofrequency catheter ablation of atrial tachycardia and flutter. In: Zipes DP, Jalife J, eds. *Cardiac electrophysiology.* Philadelphia: WB Saunders, 1994:1467, with permission.)

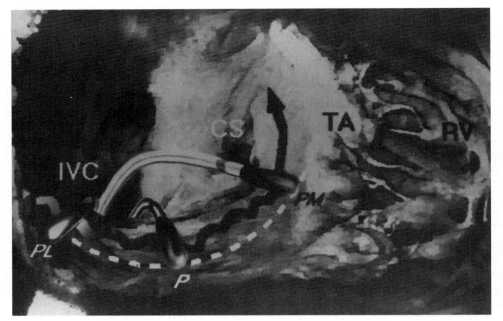

FIGURE 16-6. Catheter positions for ablation of atrial flutter are shown in the right atrium (RA). The reentrant circuit is depicted *(curved arrow)*. Ablation was accomplished in the posteromedial right atrium (PM) in 10 patients, the posterior right atrium (P) in 4 patients, and posterolateral atrium (PL) in 3 patients. CS, coronary sinus; IVC, inferior vena cava; TA, tricuspid annulus. (From Lesh MD, VanHare GF, Epstein LM, et al. Radiofrequency catheter ablation of atrial arrhythmias. *Circulation* 1994; 89:1074–1089, with permission.)

trodes were developed. This permitted simultaneous recording from the endocardial right free wall and septum in conjunction with the left atrial epicardial data (Fig. 16-7). The human epicardial electrodes were reconstructed as three-dimensional epicardial electrodes using the new molding techniques to give better coverage of the epicardial surface (Fig. 16-8).

Using these new templates in patients with atrial fibrillation, atrial flutter, and paroxysmal atrial fibrillation, mapping studies confirmed many of the earlier

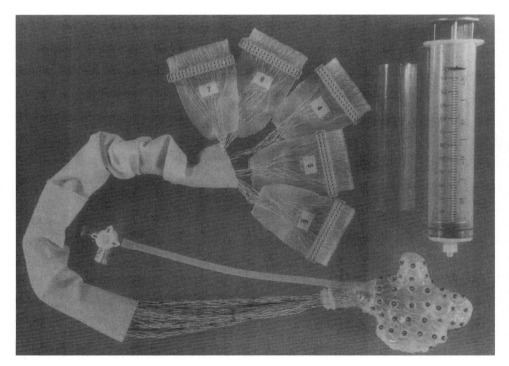

FIGURE 16-7. Inflatable three-dimensional endocardial right atrial electrode array with 80 electrode points. The connectors are labeled (4 through 8). The tube on the right side is wrapped around the collapsed electrode array to facilitate entry into the right atrium. (From Ferguson TB Jr, Schuessler RB, Hand DE, et al. Lessons learned from computerized mapping of the atrium. *J Electrophysiol* 1993;26:210–219, with permission.)

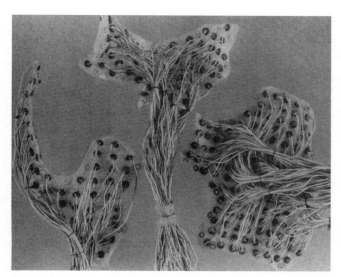

FIGURE 16-8. Molded three-dimensional (form-fitting) atrial epicardial templates for human mapping in conjunction with the inflatable endocardial electrode array. (From Ferguson TB Jr, Schuessler RB, Hand DE, et al. Lessons learned from computerized mapping of the atrium. *J Electrophysiol* 1993;26:210–219, with permission.)

observations and permitted the documentation of complete flutter loops in the right atrium that involved the septum in dogs and humans. The animal studies also demonstrated complete reentrant flutter circuits on the left side involving the pulmonary veins. Another interesting finding in the dog was that the left and right atrial septum could become dissociated during atrial flutter (13). Histologic examination of the septum showed that the two surfaces are separated by a thin layer of connective tissue. This is consistent with the disparate embryologic development of the right and left septal surface (14).

In the human mapping studies, atrial flutter in one patient was observed originating from the left atrium with passive activation of the right atrium. In a second patient with spontaneous atrial flutter, five different reentrant circuits of flutter were mapped, some originating in the right atrium and some in the left. In canine and human studies, the markedly increased complexity of the fibrillatory patterns of atrial fibrillation compared with atrial flutter was demonstrated, including the presence of multiple circuits at one time, the transient nature of the circuits, and the migratory nature of the circuits over the surface of the atria (Fig. 16-9). These data indicated that the para-

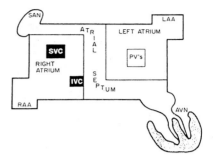
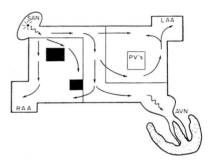
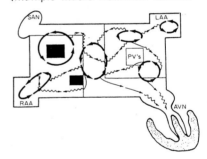

FIGURE 16-9. **A:** Schematic diagram of the right and left atrial anatomy. Electrical activity must propagate around the fixed anatomic obstacles of the superior vena cava (SVC), inferior vena cava (IVC), and pulmonary veins (PV's). **B:** During normal sinus rhythm, the electrical impulse is generated within the sinoatrial node (SAN) and propagates across the right and left atria and the atrial septum to the atrioventricular node (AVN) and then to the ventricles. Under normal circumstances, there is a collision of two portions of the sinus impulse beneath the PV posteriorly (upper portion of left atrium). **C:** Complex atrial fibrillation is characterized by multiple macro-reentrant circuits *(thick arrows)* and variable passive atrial conduction *(thin arrows)*. LAA, left atrial appendage; RAA, right atrial appendage. (From Cox JL, Schuessler RB, D'Agostino HJ, et al. The surgical treatment of atrial fibrillation. II. Intraoperative electrophysiologic mapping and description of the electrophysiologic basis of atrial flutter and atrial fibrillation. *J Thorac Cardiovasc Surg* 1991;101:406–426, with permission.)

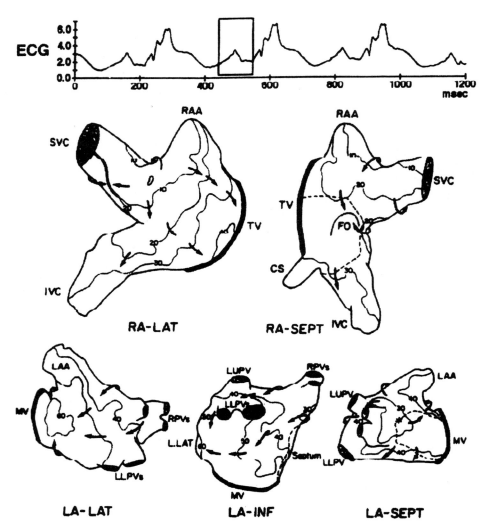

FIGURE 16-10. Atrial endocardial activation maps during sinus rhythm in a normal dog. The boxed area on the electrocardiogram is the data window analyzed to construct the activation maps. The atria were mapped endocardially with 212 unipolar electrodes mounted on sponge forms that were molded to fit the canine atria. The electrode molds were inserted into the atria through biventriculotomies across the atrioventricular valve annuli while the animal was supported by normothermic cardiopulmonary bypass. The wide QRS configuration in the electrocardiogram was the consequence of the ventriculotomies. The two middle maps represent the lateral (LAT) and septal (SEPT) surfaces of the right atrial (RA) endocardium. The three lower maps represent the left lateral (LLAT), inferior (INF), and septal aspects of the left atrium (LA). The sinus node is indicated as an oval on the right atrium at the junction with the superior vena cava (SVC). The border of the interatrial septum *(dashed line)* and the activation sequence *(arrows)* are indicated. The asterisk in the left atrial septum indicates the earliest activation site of the left atrial endocardium. FO, fossa ovalis; IVC, inferior vena cava; LAA, left atrial appendage; LLPVs, left lower pulmonary veins; LUPV, left upper pulmonary vein; MV, mitral valve; RPVs, right pulmonary veins; RAA, right atrial appendage; TV, tricuspid valve. (Adapted from Nitta T, Lee R, Schuessler RB, et al. Radial approach: a new concept in surgical treatment for atrial fibrillation. I. Concept, anatomic and physiologic bases and development of a procedure. *Ann Thorac Surg* 1999;67:27–35, with permission.)

digm that had worked in the past for development of surgical procedures to cure arrhythmias would have to be changed in the case of atrial fibrillation (9).

Nitta and colleagues (15), working in Boineau's laboratory, published the endocardial activation sequence of the left atrium in a normal dog. They demonstrated two paths between the sinus node and the interatrial septum: one clockwise and one counterclockwise around the superior vena cava. These pathways merge and activate the septum in the posterior region of the anterior limbus (Fig 16-10). Left atrial activation begins at the posterior superior septum. The posterior left atrium was activated by a wavefront propagating inferiorly from the superior left atrium through the atrial tissue between the right and left upper pulmonary veins. This activation sequence can be completely interrupted by a pulmonary vein isolation procedure, as occurs in the surgical maze or catheter-maze procedure.

In summary, mapping studies at Washington University between 1983 and 1998 in canine models and in patients undergoing surgical ablation of other supraventricular arrhythmias demonstrated that atrial flutter resulted from a macro-reentrant circuit that was thought to occur only on the right side of the atrium, with passive depolarization of the left atrial tissue (Fig. 16-11A). Atrial fibrillation was initially demonstrated to be considerably more complex, with multiple circuits present. These circuits occurred simultaneously on both the right and left atria. The inability to map the atrial septum and the orifices of the pulmonary veins, however, led to the development of second-generation, form-fitting, experimental endocardial templates for the canine studies and an endocardial right atrial template for the patient studies. These second-generation experimental maps demonstrated that atrial flutter circuits could involve the fixed anatomic obstacles of the right and left atrium and adjacent areas of conduction block and that they frequently involve the septal and pulmonary vein tissue, with passive depolarization of the contralateral atrium (Fig. 16-11B). In contrast to this single-circuit mechanism, atrial fibrillation was confirmed to result from various degrees of multiple reentrant circuits occurring transiently and migrating over the surface of both atria. The "single" clinical arrhythmia of atrial fibrillation could result from a spectrum of endocardially or epicardially mapped arrhythmias, ranging from rapid atrial flutter with variable atrioventricular block (Fig. 16-11C, D) on one end to very fine multicircuit atrial fibrillation on the other end (Fig. 16-11E).

Concepts for Surgical Intervention Based on Mapping Data

Early attempts at surgical interruption of the stable, single reentrant circuits that occur in atrial flutter resulted in atrial fibrillation. Subsequently, this development was also seen in some studies after catheter ablation of atrial flutter (16). These attempts were not specifically designed to interrupt the more recently recognized isthmus of critical slow conduction, which may account for the surgical failure (8).

The problem that atrial fibrillation presented was even more difficult because there were no fixed critical anatomic sites to ablate, the atrial fibrillation was characterized by a dynamic and continuously changing pattern of activation, and the spectrum of clinical atrial fibrillation encompassed an extremely wide range of supraventricular mapping activation patterns. This situation created a dilemma. Extensive computerized intraoperative mapping would be required for patients with atrial fibrillation, with the necessity of almost instantaneous data output, or using intraoperative mapping as a guide to ablative correction of atrial fibrillation would have to be abandoned.

The key to solving this dilemma lay in the work done at Washington University about 80 years earlier by Walter Garrey (17) and by Sir Thomas Lewis (18). They made two important observations. The first was that a minimum mass of tissue was required to support fibrillation in the atria. The second observation, critical for the development of the surgical procedure, was summarized by Garrey: "Any sufficiently narrow bridge of cardiac muscle, whether auricular or ventricular, will suffice to prevent the spread of the fibrillary state, but will allow individual impulses to pass." Subdividing the atria into small parts, which would prevent fibrillation by decreasing the critical mass below that capable of sustaining atrial fibrillation, would not allow impulses originating in the sinus node to control the heart rate or permit sequential

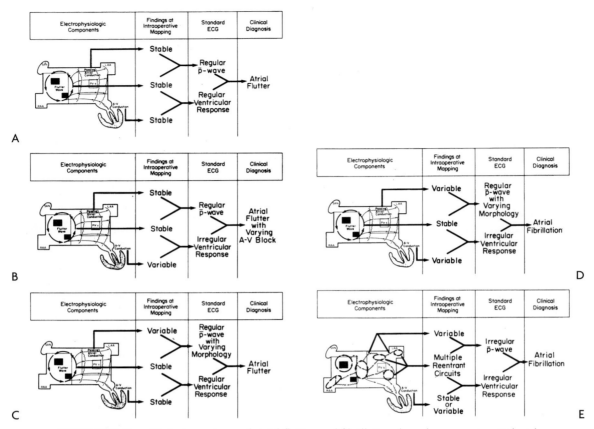

FIGURE 16-11. Clinical spectrum of atrial flutter and fibrillation, based on experimental and clinical mapping data. **A:** Electrophysiologic basis of standard electrocardiographic findings in the simplest type of atrial flutter. **B:** Atrial flutter with varying atrioventricular (AV) block. **C:** Atrial flutter with variable p wave architecture. **D:** "Simple" clinical atrial fibrillation has a single reentrant circuit in which the atrial events are identical to flutter. Variable AV node conduction causes an irregular ventricular response. **E:** Complex atrial fibrillation with multiple reentrant circuits simultaneously present. AVN, atrioventricular node; IVC, inferior vena cava; LAA, left atrial appendage; PV, pulmonary veins; RAA, right atrial appendage; SAN, sinoatrial node; SVC, superior vena cava. (From Cox JL, Schuessler RB, D'Agostino HJ, et al. The surgical treatment of atrial fibrillation. II. Intraoperative electrophysiologic mapping and description of the electrophysiologic basis of atrial flutter and atrial fibrillation. *J Thorac Cardiovasc Surg* 1991;101:406–426, with permission.)

activation and contraction of the entire atrium. However, if an isthmus of tissue was left between the subdivisions, a normal sinus node depolarization could activate the entire atria, preserving a chronotropic response and (theoretically) atrial transport function, while at the same time eliminating the flutter or fibrillation.

On the basis of these observations and the mapping data, it was decided to design a surgical procedure that would eliminate all potential reentrant circuits around anatomic obstacles, subdivide the atrium such that each subdivision was less than the critical mass needed to maintain fibrillation, and preserve the continuity of each division so that an impulse originating in the sinus node would activate the entire atria (19).

SURGICAL THERAPIES FOR ATRIAL FLUTTER AND ATRIAL FIBRILLATION

Surgery for Atrial Flutter

Attempts to interrupt the large macro-reentrant right-sided circuits that are responsible for type I flutter by a right atrial free wall incision experimentally and clinically resulted in the recurrence of a new flutter circuit, often involving the surgical incision as a focus of reentry (8,13) or atrial fibrillation (16). Patients with flutter who had concomitant surgical procedures were subjected to the application of cryolesions to the area of critical slow conduction in the lower right atrium (Figs. 16-5 and 16-6), in the same area where radiofrequency ablation is performed, with excellent success. Because this can often be achieved with less invasive catheter techniques (8,20), surgical intervention is usually reserved for patients who are concomitantly undergoing other types of cardiac surgical procedures.

Correlation of Electrophysiology with Anatomy for Ablation of Atrial Fibrillation

Moe and colleagues (21,22) hypothesized that atrial fibrillation was maintained by multiple independent wavelets activating the atria irregularly, very rapidly, and in a random fashion (23). Allessie and colleagues (24,25) generally confirmed this hypothesis but estimated that an average of only four to six independent wandering wavelets must be present to maintain the fibrillatory process (26). This group (27) demonstrated regional entrainment of atrial fibrillatory wavelets, suggesting that stimulating a short excitable gap in the macro-reentrant circuits could interfere with the fibrillatory process. Conversely, perpetuation of fibrillation may involve one or more additional mechanisms to the multiple wavelet concept. The first is a background "stable circuit" activity that may account for the apparent transitions from fibrillation to flutter (28), and the second is a site of abnormal impulse formation. Such sites have been identified, particularly in the vicinity of the pulmonary vein orifices, and focal ablation of "atrial fibrillation" at these sites has been reported (29). These abnormal sites may be caused by atrial disease or may be the consequence of fibrillation-induced ion-channel remodeling (28). Jalife (30) suggested that atrial fibrillation might not be a random process, but rather one with an underlying organization process. This issue has not been conclusively settled.

The question of whether critical anatomic sites play a role in atrial fibrillation has not been completely answered (31). Documenting the correlation between this electrophysiologic concept and the complex anatomy of the atrium has been more difficult. In an isolated right atrial preparation, Schuessler and colleagues (32) showed that at short refractory periods (<95 msec), atrial reentrant circuits that are unassociated with anatomic obstacles can become stable and dominate activation. These investigators also demonstrated the three-dimensional nature of these electrophysiologic circuits superimposed on the thin, flat atrium (33). Waldo demonstrated in a sterile pericarditis model (34) the conversion of flutter to fibrillation and vice versa. Flutter, in this model, depends on a line of functional block in the right atrium, which on shortening resulted in the development of fibrillation. Other studies (35–37) have suggested that a critical mass of atrial tissue, by definition primarily in a two-dimensional array, is necessary to maintain the fibrillatory process. It is still unclear whether it is the mass or the surface area of tissue that is necessary for sustained fibrillation to occur (38). Further complicating these issues are the effects of intraatrial pressure (39,40) and volume (12,41,42) on the development, maintenance, and ablation of atrial fibrillation.

Several additional important electrophysiologic considerations have been demonstrated (9,43,44). These studies suggested that experimental and clinical atrial flutter and atrial fibrillation can be thought of as a continuum, extending from a single, macro-reentrant circuit of right-sided atrial flutter at one end to multiple, simultaneous macro-reentrant circuits over the entire surface of the right and left atria. These studies also suggested that flutter depended on anatomic obstacles on the right and left sides of the heart (i.e., the superior and inferior caval orifices, the annuli of the atrioventricular valves, and the pulmonary veins) (43). Fibrillation was demonstrated to be independent of any anatomic obstacles for either initiation or maintenance, in contrast to all other types of supraventricular and ventricular arrhythmias previously evaluated. This anatomic independence allowed these circuits to be transient in both time and space on the surface of the atrium, suggesting that considerations such as number of wavelets, surface area of tissue, and perhaps intraatrial size, volume, or pressure are the most important factors to consider in the ablation of atrial fibrillation. At a minimum, these studies from Washington University suggested that any type of map-directed intervention to interrupt these circuits would be difficult (44,45). This fact distinguished atrial fibrillation from all other types of supraventricular and ventricular arrhythmias that had been cured with map-directed surgical therapy before this time.

The Concept of an Ablative Cure of Atrial Fibrillation

The definition of an ablative cure as applied to atrial fibrillation (46) includes elimination of the clinical arrhythmia, maintenance of sinoatrial nodal tissue as the driving impulse for the heart, maintenance of intact atrioventricular conduction, and restoration of atrial transport function. Ideally, if these criteria could be accomplished, the risk of subsequent thromboembolic events related to the presence of atrial fibrillation could be reduced. The appropriateness of any intervention must be judged against these five criteria; to the degree that one or more are not successfully achieved, the catheter-based or surgical therapy may be considered less than optimal.

In general, the greater the risk of morbidity and mortality associated with a procedure, the closer to a complete cure the procedure should come. This conceptualization was used in deriving the five criteria for a successful procedure for curing the arrhythmia of atrial fibrillation. Other investigators have argued that there are limits to this association between surgical risk and surgical cure as they pertain to combined procedures for atrial fibrillation and other associated cardiac diseases. For example, the electroanatomic circumstances in which the fibrillation occurs (i.e., idiopathic, associated with a congenital heart defect such as atrial septal defect, or associated with mitral valvular disease) may also need to be taken into account in examining the criteria for applicability and efficacy of procedures designed to surgically eliminate atrial fibrillation.

Technical Modifications of the Maze Procedure for Atrial Fibrillation

The early experience with the maze procedure (maze I), which has undergone two technical modifications (maze II and III) since the description of the original operation (47), documented that atrial fibrillation could be cured. This surgical experience generated additional considerations regarding the electroanatomic origin of atrial flutter and fibrillation in these patients with primarily idiopathic disease (48):

1. The local effective refractory periods (ERPs) of the left atrium appear to be shorter than those in the right atrium.
2. Because of the longer ERPs and therefore longer reentrant circuits on the right side, atrial flutter is more likely to occur on the basis of reentry in the right atrium.
3. Because of the shorter ERPs and therefore shorter reentrant circuits on the left side, atrial fibrillation is more likely to occur on the basis of reentry in the left atrium.

To eliminate the recurrence of flutter and fibrillation, a procedure that involves both sides of the atrial tissue appears to be necessary in this setting.

The first maze I procedure was performed in September 1987. That patient was followed for 6 months, and then the second procedure was performed. This observation process was repeated until the safety and efficacy of the initial operative approach were documented. As is the case with most new techniques, information obtained during the early experience is used to modify subsequent approaches. Early follow-up examinations of maze procedure patients documented four sequelae of the initial operative approach (19):

1. An inability to achieve maximal heart rates with exercise, called a blunted chronotropic response to exercise
2. An inability to document left atrial transport function in 30% of patients despite the presence of right atrial transport in all patients
3. Requirement for new pacemaker implantation in more than 40% of patients
4. Technical difficulty with performing the procedure in patients who had undergone previous cardiac surgery because of the necessity to alter placement of the suture lines

The inappropriate response to exercise and the pacemaker requirement were initially attributed to possible devascularization of the sinoatrial node by the surgical incisions in this region. Elimination of one incision and movement of the medial superior vena cava incision more posteriorly were the modifications that were made (Figs. 16-12 through 16-14), and these were tested and verified in the experimental laboratory. Subsequent analyses suggested alternative explanations for each of these findings.

The results of the maze I procedure indirectly confirmed the findings of Boineau and colleagues regarding the atrial pacemaker complex (49,50). They had documented in dogs an area of sinoatrial nodal tissue extending along the junction of the superior vena cava and right atrial junction. Pacemaker cells that are capable of firing at a lower rate were located at the caudal end of this complex, while pacemaker cells that are capable of more rapid intrinsic depolarization rates were located more superiorly and anteriorly. Neurocardiogenic influences are thought to play an

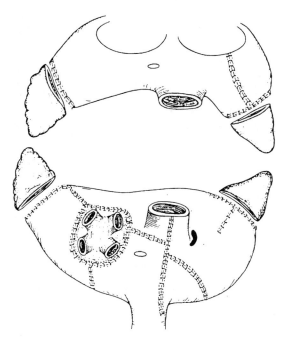

FIGURE 16-13. Schematic depiction of the maze III procedure. The view is the same as in Figure 16-12, but notice the absence of the incision across the top of the atrium. The sinus node is depicted as the black kidney-shaped structure and the atrioventricular node as the open oval circle. The actual sinus node complex encompasses the tissue anterior and lateral (to the right in the lower part) to the superior vena cava, between the suture lines. (Ferguson TB Jr, Cox JL. Arrhythmia surgery. *Coron Artery Dis* 1996;7:36–44, with permission.)

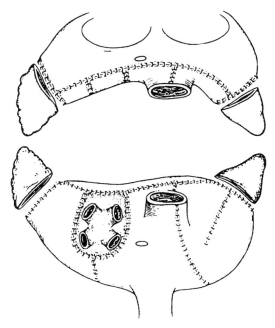

FIGURE 16-12. Schematic depiction the maze I procedure. The top shows the anterior aspect of the atria; the bottom shows the posterior atria. The incision across the top of the atria on both views transected Bachmann's bundle. This incision, along with the anterior incision down to it on the superior vena cava, probably accounted for the blunted sinus node response by interrupting the contiguity of the atrial pacemaker complex. (From Ferguson TB Jr, Cox JL. Arrhythmia surgery. *Coron Artery Dis* 1996;7:36–44, with permission.)

important role in influencing the dominant pacemaker site at any given time (49,51). The maze I operation surgically eliminated conduction from impulses arising in this anteromedial area to the remaining atrial tissue, accounting for the blunted response to exercise.

Pacemaker implantation was initially required in approximately 40% of patients (52). Although DDDR devices were implanted (because the natural history of the conduction abnormality was unknown), all of the patients required only atrial chamber pacing. This was either for a junctional rhythm with a slow or absent sinoatrial response or for a chronotropically incompetent sinoatrial node response at rest, usually below 40 bpm. A few patients had undergone previous implantation of a pacemaker (usually a VVIR following AV node ablation) in conjunction with their paroxysmal or chronic atrial fibril-

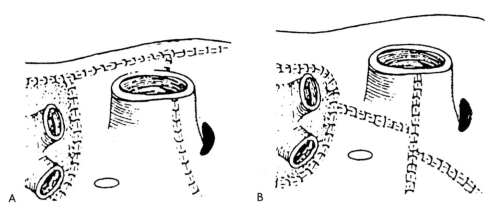

FIGURE 16-14. **A:** Close-up view of the superior vena cava region of the heart, depicting the maze I incisions and their proximity to Bachmann's bundle anteriorly and the sinus node complex anterolaterally. **B:** Same view as in **A** for the maze III procedure. (From Ferguson TB Jr, Cox JL. Arrhythmia surgery. *Coron Artery Dis* 1996;7:36–44, with permission.)

lation, and these patients were upgraded to dual-chamber systems. Careful analysis of the preoperative electrophysiologic data (i.e., Holter or event monitoring, preoperative electrophysiologic study, hospital monitoring) documented that most patients who required a pacemaker for atrial pacing postoperatively had evidence of sick sinus syndrome demonstrable on the preoperative data. This analysis encompassed the first 106 patients in the series, 47 of whom had undergone the maze I or II procedure and 60 of whom had undergone the maze III procedure (Table 16-1).

Atrial transport function impairment on the left side after the maze I and II procedures was thought to be related to impairment of right-to-left atrial conduction. Both of these procedures divided Bachmann's bundle (51), a thick bundle of atrial tissue that runs across the top of the atrial septum posterior to the aorta to rapidly (approximately 40 msec) conduct the sinoatrial impulse to the left side of the atrium. Surgical interruption of the bundle resulted in a 350- to 400-msec conduction time through the "maze" from the right to the left. In some cases, this resulted in left atrial systole occurring when the mitral apparatus was closed during isovolumic contraction or ventricular systole. Eliminating the surgical division of Bachmann's bundle prevented this intraatrial conduction delay, and this modification was incorporated into the maze III procedure.

TABLE 16-1 • RESULTS OF PREOPERATIVE CLINICAL AND ELECTROPHYSIOLOGIC EVALUATION OF SINUS NODE FUNCTION, 9/87–12/93

	Pacemaker		No Pacemaker	
	No.	%	No.	%
Total patients[a]	43		60	
EPS +	13	30.2	2	3.3
Holter +	12	27.9	2	3.3
Clinical assessment +	6	13.9	1	1.6
Evaluation	12	27.9	55	91.7
Prior PM placement	10			
SSS	6			
His ablation	3			
HOCM	1			
New postoperative implant	33			
Sinus bradycardia	20			
Junctional rhythm	11			

EPS, electrophysiologic study; PM, pacemaker; SSS, sick sinus syndrome; +, positive (study).
[a] Total number of maze procedure patients is 106.

Maze III Procedure for Atrial Fibrillation

Experimental and clinical studies addressing various conditions led to the development of the maze III procedure, which rectified some of these considerations to some degree (53–55) (Fig. 16-15).

The following analysis compares the results from the maze I and II procedures with those from the maze III procedure. The maze II procedure was an intermediate modification between I and III that was used in only 15 patients. This was technically more complicated to perform and was further modified into the technically straightforward maze III procedure.

Representative data are presented here (Table 16-2). A total of 139 consecutive patients underwent surgical intervention through January 1995 (56). The mean age was 52 ± 11.5 years. Fifty-five percent of patients had paroxysmal fibrillation or flutter; 45% had chronic atrial fibrillation at the time of surgery. Arrhythmia intolerance was the indication for surgical intervention in 65% of cases, and drug intolerance was present in 11%. A previous thromboembolic event was present as the symptom for surgery in the remaining 24%. Only a small percentage of patients had abnormal ventricular function preoperatively. Thirty-one percent of patients underwent a concomitant cardiac surgical operation at the time of the maze procedure.

There were three perioperative deaths in this series (2.2%), one in the I/II group and two in the III group. There was one late death at 4 years.

Forty-seven patients underwent the I/II procedure, while the remaining 92 had the maze III procedure performed. Except for the difference in patients undergoing reoperation, the patient demographics were similar.

Perioperative complications for the two groups are listed in Table 16-2. The incidence of atrial arrhyth-

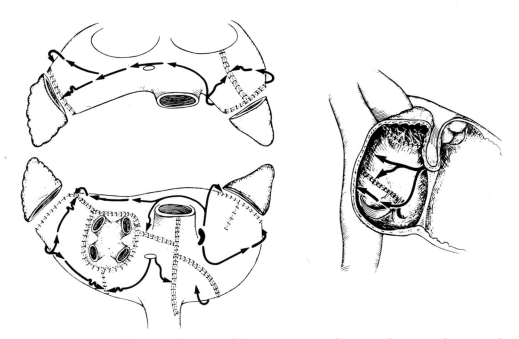

FIGURE 16-15. Schematic depiction of the maze III procedure provides a two-dimensional representation of the pattern of atrial activation postoperatively. On the left, the atria are depicted as if viewed from the posterior direction with the back of both atria in the lower panel; the atria are then divided in a sagittal plane, and the anterior halves of the atria are flipped up in the upper panel. On the right, the surface of the right atrial septum is shown. Appropriately placed atrial incisions direct the sinus impulse from the sinoatrial node to the atrioventricular node along a specified route. The atrial myocardium, except the appendages and pulmonary veins, is electrically activated. (From Cox JL. Evolving applications of the maze procedure for atrial fibrillation. *Ann Thorac Surg* 1993;55:578–580, with permission.)

TABLE 16-2 • COMPARISON OF MAZE I/II AND MAZE III CLINICAL EXPERIENCE

Characteristic	Maze I/II		Maze III	
	n	%	n	%
Demographics				
Patients	47		92	
Mean age (yr)	51 ± 12		54 ± 11	
Males	33	77	64	70
Preop arrhythmia				
Paroxysmal	25	53	53	58
Chronic	22	47	39	42
Prior surgery	13	27	4	4
Concomitant surgery	15	32	39	42
Perioperative complications				
Death	1	2.1	2	2.2
Atrial arrhythmias	19	40.4	38	41.3
Fluid retention	7	14.8	6	6.5
Bleeding	3	6.4	2	2.2
Stroke	1	2.1	0	
Transient ischemic attack	1	2.1	1	1.1
Myocardial infarction	0		1	1.1
Long-term follow-up				
Total patients	47		92	
Procedure survivors	46		90	
Pacemakers				
Total	25	54.3	25	27.8
New	20		17	
Preop sick sinus syndrome	18		15	
Percent of pacemakers		72		60
Preop pacemaker	5		8	
Percent of pacemakers		20		32
Iatrogenic injury	1	4.5	1	1.2
Patients >3 mo follow-up	46		78	
Transient ischemic attack	1	2.2	1	1.3
Blunted sinus response	31	67.4	6	1.7
Arrhythmia recurrence	9	19.6	0	
Atrial flutter	6	13.1	0	
Atrial fibrillation	3	6.5	0	
Atrial transport function				
Patients analyzed	43		53	
Left atrium	30	69.8	48	90.5
Right atrium	43	100	52	98.1

mias was similar. These were thought to be related to shortening of atrial refractoriness as a result of surgical intervention. As the atrium healed, refractoriness returned to normal. The reentrant circuits that were responsible for the perioperative arrhythmias became extinguished against the surgical suture lines and the fixed anatomic obstacles of the left and right atria (48, 55). The incidence of the remaining complications in each group is low and is similar between the two groups and similar to those for other open-heart procedures (57).

Table 16-1 illustrates the follow-up data for these patients. All operative survivors were at risk for requiring pacemaker implantation. This requirement was reduced from 54.3% (25 of 46) in the I/II group to 27.8% (25 of 90) in the maze III group. Most patients requiring pacemaker implantation continued to have evidence of sick sinus syndrome preoperatively or had already undergone implantation of a pacemaker system for conduction system disease. Only two pacemaker patients have sustained an iatrogenic injury: one patient in the I/II group with devascularization of the sinus node and one patient in the maze III group with an anomalous coronary sinus repair and postoperative complete heart block. This patient was the only patient in the entire series requiring ventricular pacing.

Late follow-up (>3 months) was available for all but one patient in the maze I/II group and for 78 of 92 patients in the maze III group. Transient ischemic attacks occurred in 3% of the I/II group and in 1% of the maze III group. The incidence of a blunted response to exercise was reduced from 65% to 8%, most likely for the reasons outlined previously. Nine of 46 patients had a late recurrence of fibrillation ($n = 3$) or flutter ($n = 6$) in the maze I/II group. All were effectively controlled with medication. There were no recurrences during late follow-up after the maze III procedure.

Forty-three of 46 group I and II patients underwent postoperative evaluation for transport function; 53 of 98 group III patients were evaluated. Right atrial transport function was present in all 43 group I/II patients. Of the 53 patients receiving follow-up for transport function in the III group, 52 (98%) had right atrial transport present. In the I/II group, 30 (70%) of 43 patients had left atrial transport, while 48 (90%) of 53 patients in the III group had documented left-sided atrial function present. With the III modification, right-sided transport and left-sided transport occur in 98% and 90% of patients, respectively.

Quantitative analysis of atrial function by other investigators in patients after the maze procedure revealed that the left atrial transport function was significantly less than that in normal control subjects, whereas the right atrial function was comparable (58–61). The two primary reasons hypothesized for this are the large amount of atrial tissue isolated with the pulmonary veins and the discordant activation and contraction of the adjacent atrial tissue, particularly on the left side. Total atrial activation time was prolonged (even with the maze III procedure), creating desynchronized atrioventricular contraction coupling. These data take into account studies that document that it can take up to 6 months for function to return to a stable baseline (15). Lack of left-sided atrial transport remained a problem in late follow-up with the maze III procedure.

Whether long-term freedom from fibrillation would decrease the theoretical risk of thromboembolism compared with a control population was unclear, in part because of the low incidence of events in patients this age with lone fibrillation (62,63). However, the procedure did not increase the incidence of thromboembolism.

⦿ ATRIAL FIBRILLATION AND STRUCTURAL DISEASE OF THE HEART

Are there fundamental differences between fibrillation resulting from valvular disease and fibrillation arising as the idiopathic form of the arrhythmia? Demographic (35,36,41), echocardiographic (39,40), and electrophysiologic (32–34) data are suggestive. If this could be demonstrated, these differences may permit an alteration in the surgical technique that does not significantly compromise the concept or the success rate of the procedure in this setting. For example, alterations in effective refractory periods have been demonstrated to play a fundamental role in the genesis (64) and termination (65) of atrial fibrillation. Isobe and colleagues demonstrated that an acute increase in volume (and pressure) results in an abrupt increase in the disparity of refractory periods of the right and left atrium (66) and that this was correlated with the inducibility of atrial fibrillation; these changes were reversible by decreasing intraatrial volume. These studies were performed by using an autoperfused heart preparation developed for arrhythmia study in our laboratory (67). Using this same model, we demonstrated that acute shortening of the atrial refractory periods precedes the spontaneous development of atrial fibrillation, independent of volume and pressure considerations. Volume overload and hypertrophy are expected to play a role in the setting of valvular disease that may not be as prominent in idiopathic disease.

Overall, the results from these reported surgical experiences and experimental studies suggest that regional isolation of larger segments of the left atrium or the entire left atrium may be feasible in selected, higher-risk patients. However, the interaction between a greater amount of tissue isolated to eliminate atrial fibrillation and greater impairment of postoperative atrial transport is perhaps more important in patients with concomitant organic heart disease and changes in ventricular compliance (68).

Additional data suggest that sinus node automaticity (69) may play a role in the reinitiation of fibrillation in certain circumstances, perhaps in contrast to the clinical association between sick sinus syndrome and atrial fibrillation (70). Approximately 30% to 35% of patients in the Washington University maze group had evidence of sick sinus syndrome preoperatively in primarily idiopathic disease. This may suggest a higher degree of the contribution of right atrial electrophysiology to fibrillation in idiopathic disease patients compared with earlier observations about the left atrial contribution in valvular patients.

After the initial experience with the maze procedure, there was interest in combining it with procedures for other concomitantly addressed cardiac disease processes. Guidelines for patient selection suggested that patients with concomitant disease should ideally be younger than 70 years of age, have normal ventricular function, have had embolic events related to long-standing (>1 year) fibrillation, be medically refractory and severely symptomatic, have a left atrial dimension greater than 60 mm, and have an easily reparable valve lesion (71).

These selection criteria were independently addressed by the Mayo Clinic group in reviewing their experience with mitral valve repair in 323 patients with preoperative atrial fibrillation between 1980 and 1991 (72). In a late follow-up evaluation of this series, atrial fibrillation was present in 5% of patients with preoperative sinus rhythm, 80% of patients with preoperative chronic atrial fibrillation, and 0% of patients with preoperative recent-onset atrial fibrillation. The prevalence of late thromboembolic events was similar for patients with preoperative sinus rhythm and patients with preoperative atrial fibrillation, and the survival rates of the two groups were not different. These findings suggested that a concomitant procedure for atrial fibrillation in this setting should have negligible morbidity and no adverse effect on operative mortality.

Modified Maze Procedure for Rheumatic Mitral Valve Disease

Around the world, where the incidence of rheumatic mitral disease remains high, several investigators have modified the maze procedure in its application to combined procedures (Table 16-3). Most modifications appear to be in the setting of rheumatic mitral disease; presumably, the motivation for the modifications is to simplify the overall operative procedure as a response to concerns similar to those expressed by the Mayo group. Others have suggested, on the basis of preliminary mapping studies of human fibrillation in association with valvular heart disease, that the fibrillatory mechanism in this setting may primarily involve the left side of the atria (73,74), and as a result, surgical procedures that address only the left atrium are all that are required in this setting.

The largest experience with combined antifibrillatory and valve procedures has apparently been accumulated in Japan, where the nationwide response to a survey was reported at the meeting of the International Society of Cardiothoracic Surgeons in Japan. From 30 institutions, a total of 230 patients were reported; 196 patients underwent some form of combined mitral plus (modified) maze procedure. Twenty-one patients had concomitant repair of an atrial septal defect, and only 3 of 230 had idiopathic atrial fibrillation.

The myriad surgical modifications to the maze procedure have been reviewed by Ferguson (75) and Ferguson and McKinnie (76). Kawaguchi and colleagues (77) reported 51 patients undergoing a modified maze procedure plus valvular surgery and compared these results to historical disease- and procedure-matched controls without an antifibrillatory procedure. Morbidity and mortality were similar in both groups; the recurrence rate for fibrillation in the surgical group was 8%, compared with 90% in the non-atrial fibrillation group. In a follow-up study, Isobe and Kawashima (78) examined the efficacy of the surgical maze III in patients with mitral valve disease and chronic atrial fibrillation. In their analysis, patients with a cardiothoracic ratio less than 70% and a left atrial systolic dimension less than 80 mm were predicted to maintain sinus rhythm postoperatively. Izumoto and

TABLE 16-3 • ATRIAL FIBRILLATION SURGICAL EXPERIENCE

Study	Operation[a]	Eliminate RC	Decreases FM	Surgical Technique Side	Technical Difficulty[b]	Late SR	Eliminate AF	Late Atrial Transport Function	Number Of Patients	Pacemaker Implant
Lone AF										
Cox (48)	1	Yes	No	L, R	3+	80%	93%	80%	75	40%
Ferguson (47)	2	Yes	No	L, R	3+	100%	100%	90%	106	28%
McCarthy (71)	1	Yes	No	L, R	3+	100%	Yes	99%	14	NR
Morris (95)	2	Yes	No	L, R	3+	100%	100%	95%	37	0%
Defauw (96)	3	No	Yes	L, R	1+	Yes	No	No	21	50%
Combined valve and AF procedure										
Nitta (93)	4	Yes	No	L, R	3+	92.30%	92.30%	Diminished	13	15.40%
Nitta (93)	5	Yes	No	L, R	2+	90%	90%	100%	10	10%
Nitta (94)	5	Yes	No	L, R	2+	90.60%	90.60%	90.60%	32	6.30%
Kawaguchi (77)	6	Yes (?)	No (?)	L, R	2+	92%	92%	Yes	51	NR
Sueda (86)	7	Yes	No	L	2+	85%	85%	82%	13	NR
Shyu (83)	8	No	Yes	L, R	1+	64%	64%	64%	22	NR
Itoh (88)	4	Yes	No	L, R	3+	100%	Yes	Yes	15	NR
Isobe (78)	9	Yes	No	L, R	3+	90%	85%	Yes	85	NR

AF, atrial fibrillation unable to be controlled medically; FM, ???; L, left; NR, not reported; R, right; RC, reentrant circuits; SR, sinus rhythm.
[a] Operations: 1, maze I or II; 2, maze III; 3, corridor procedure; 4, maze III + valve; 5, radial incision approach + valve; 6, unspecified modification to maze III; 7, pulmonary versus isolation + areas of cryoablation; 8, left and right compartmentalization procedure; 9, modified maze III + valve.
[b] Technical difficulty of the antiarrhythmic portion of the procedure uses a 1 to 4 (most difficult) scale.

coworkers (79) described their experience with 87 patients with mitral disease. Approximately 80% of patients had cure of atrial fibrillation (76,80). By way of comparison, Crijns and associates (81) examined 74 patients with chronic atrial fibrillation after mitral valve surgery presenting for cardioversion. In 7 years of follow-up, 52.7% of patients were in chronic atrial fibrillation; preoperative chronic atrial fibrillation was the most significant risk factor for poorer arrhythmic outcome.

Kamata and colleagues (82) examined the factors that predicted sinus rhythm restoration in this patient population. A preoperative atrial fibrillatory wave (>1.0 mm) and a left atrial diameter (<65 mm) were predictors of sinus rhythm postoperatively in the patients with chronic atrial fibrillation. This group (80) also documented diminished circadian changes in low frequency to high frequency ratio in a subset of postoperative patients with normal sinus rhythm but frequent premature atrial contractions compared with patients with normal sinus rhythm but without premature atrial contractions.

Shyu and colleagues (83) reported 22 patients (16 with rheumatic heart disease) who underwent an atrial compartment procedure in combination with mitral valve surgery. This procedure was either a left atrial isolation procedure or a biatrial isolation procedure. Fourteen of 22 patients were in sinus rhythm at 6-month follow-up; all 14 (most with rheumatic disease) had evidence of left and right atrial mechanical function at this time, although in many patients it took between 2 and 6 months for detectable function to return after surgery. Sueda and colleagues (84) described a modified left-sided maze technique that isolates the pulmonary veins, amputates the left atrial appendage, and uses cryolesions to regionally isolate a large portion of the posterolateral left atrial tissue. They used this technique in 13 patients with mitral valve disease, demonstrating sinus rhythm and atrial transport in 11 of 13 patients at late follow-up. All 11 patients had right atrial contraction by echocardiography, and nine (82%) had left atrial contraction, similar to the experience that has accrued with the standard maze technique. This group (85,86) has described a right atrial separation procedure for the ablation of atrial fibrillation associated with an atrial septal defect. These two groups' efforts support the concept that atrial fibrillation associated with mechanical heart disease may be approached by focusing on that atrial chamber associated with the structural disease (87).

Itoh and colleagues (88) performed a combined maze and valve procedure in 15 patients. Postoperative echocardiographic findings in this group demonstrated that in elderly (>60 years) patients with significant increases in left atrial volume (up to three times normal), effective left atrial systole despite sinus rhythm could not be demonstrated. In younger patients with smaller atria, contractions were readily apparent.

It is unclear whether these or any modifications of the maze technique can be as effective as the maze procedure itself in the setting of concomitant structural disease (53,89). Alternatively, it is unclear whether it is justified to accept a slightly higher fibrillation recurrence rate in order to minimize overall operative mortality and morbidity in this setting of combined procedures for mitral valve disease. Further complicating this dilemma is the fact that many patients with rheumatic mitral disease have impaired ventricular function at the time of surgery. From a functional point of view, it is precisely this group of patients for whom restoration of sinus rhythm and atrial transport would provide the greatest benefit (15, 90,91).

Radial Incision Approach to Atrial Fibrillation

Although the maze procedure has been demonstrated to be effective in the cure of atrial fibrillation with an extremely low incidence of thromboembolic complications after the procedure, the cardiology and cardiac electrophysiology community has been reluctant to send patients for surgical cure. There are three principal reasons for this: the perception that the maze is a technically complicated procedure, the absence of left atrial transport function in up to 10% of patients long-term, and the anticipation of a successful catheter-based intervention (20,29).

Nitta and colleagues, working in Boineau's laboratory at Washington University, addressed the second major problem with the maze procedure: impaired left atrial transport function postoperatively (15,92, 93). Based on careful examination of atrial blood sup-

Maze Procedure

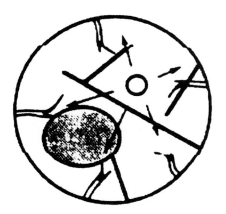

Radial Approach

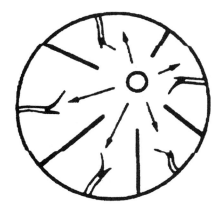

FIGURE 16-16. The maze procedure and the radial approach. The larger outer circle denotes the atria, and its outer limit is bounded by the atrioventricular annular margins. The small circle indicates the sinoatrial node, and the shaded area indicates the isolated portion of the atrium. Arrows indicate the activation wavefront from the sinoatrial node, radiating toward the annular margins. The atrial coronary arteries, arising at the atrioventricular groove, are also schematically drawn. The radial approach *(right)* preserves a more physiologic activation sequence and preserves blood supply to most atrial segments, whereas the atrial incisions of the maze procedure *(left)* desynchronizes the activation sequence, and some of the incisions cross the atrial coronary arteries. (From Nitta T, Lee R, Schuessler RB, et al. Radial approach: A new concept in surgical treatment for atrial fibrillation. I. Concept, anatomic and physiologic bases and development of a procedure. *Ann Thorac Surg* 1999;67:27–35, with permission.)

ply and electrophysiologic activation (Fig. 16-16), they developed a technically simpler procedure that results in a more physiologic electrical activation sequence (Fig. 16-17). This is accomplished by eliminating the pulmonary vein isolation portion of the maze procedure (Fig. 16-18) and therefore eliminating any large area of inert or noncontractile tissue (15, 60) (Fig. 16-19). In the maze procedure, for instance, this pulmonary vein isolation area has been shown in human cadaver hearts to comprise 35% of the endocardial surface and 28% of the weight (61).

Most importantly, this procedure has been demonstrated in extensive experimental studies (15,92) to improve postoperative left atrial transport function compared with the maze procedure. The left atrial contribution to ventricular filling was larger, probably because of a more physiologic atrial activation sequence. The atrial filling fraction, peak velocity of the E wave, peak velocity of the A wave, the E/A ratio, and the left atrial reservoir function (as determined by the peak velocity and the time-velocity interval of the systolic inflow from the pulmonary veins into the left atrium [S wave]) are the measures of atrial function after the procedure. Table 16-4 compares these procedures and provides normal data. Although the radial incision approach improves atrial transport compared with the maze procedure, there still remains a deficit compared with normal atrial function. Both procedures result in decreased atrial reservoir function probably because of impaired compliance of the atrium.

In humans, it requires approximately 6 months for atrial function to return to a stable baseline after the maze III procedure (89). The initial clinical experience with the radial incision approach documented similar findings to the experimental studies when compared with a group of maze patients (94). Two modifications were made from the depicted canine preparation in the patients (93). First, to block the activation propagating from the pulmonary vein orifices, the posterior left atrium around each pulmonary vein was cryoablated circumferentially. Second, the

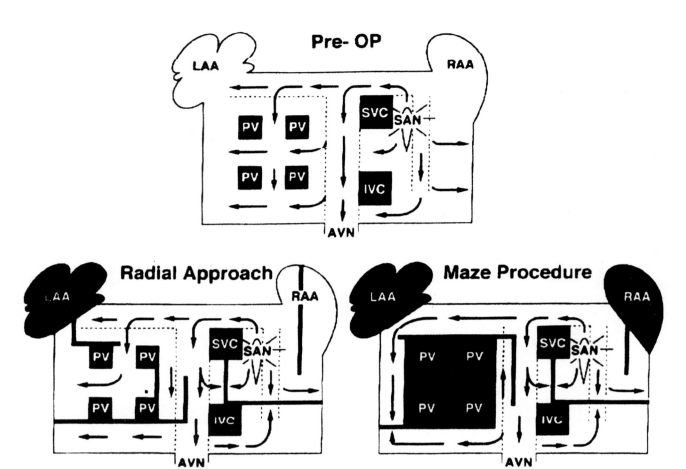

FIGURE 16-17. Anatomic correlation between the atrial incisions and the atrial activation pattern during sinus rhythm in normal atria and in the atria after the maze procedure or the radial approach. The surgical incisions *(thick lines)*; the atrial part that is surgically isolated or excised *(solid area)*; Bachmann's bundle *(dashed lines)* among the atrial appendages, the interatrial septum, and the crista terminalis; and the activation sequence *(arrows)* are identified. AVN, atrioventricular node; FO, fossa ovalis; IVC, inferior vena cava; LAA, left atrial appendage; LLPVs, left lower pulmonary veins; LUPV, left upper pulmonary vein; MV, mitral valve; RPVs, right pulmonary veins; RAA, right atrial appendage; SAN, sinoatrial node; SVC, superior vena cava; TV, tricuspid valve. (From Nitta T, Lee R, Schuessler RB, et al. Radial approach: a new concept in surgical treatment for atrial fibrillation. I. Concept, anatomic and physiologic bases and development of a procedure. *Ann Thorac Surg* 1999;67:27–35, with permission.)

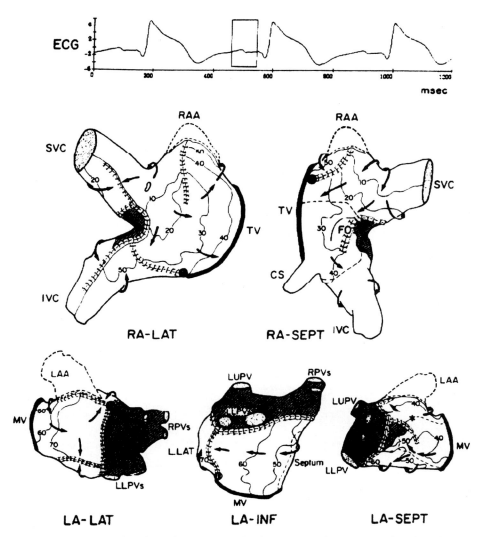

FIGURE 16-18. Atrial endocardial maps made during sinus rhythm 6 weeks after the maze procedure. The shaded area denotes the electrically isolated region. AVN, atrioventricular node; FO, fossa ovalis; IVC, inferior vena cava; LAA, left atrial appendage; LLPVs, left lower pulmonary veins; LUPV, left upper pulmonary vein; MV, mitral valve; RPVs, right pulmonary veins; RAA, right atrial appendage; SAN, sinoatrial node; SVC, superior vena cava; TV, tricuspid valve. (From Nitta T, Lee R, Watanabe H, et al. Radial approach: a new concept in surgical treatment for atrial fibrillation. II. Effects and atrial contribution to ventricular filling. *Ann Thorac Surg* 1999;67:36–50, with permission.)

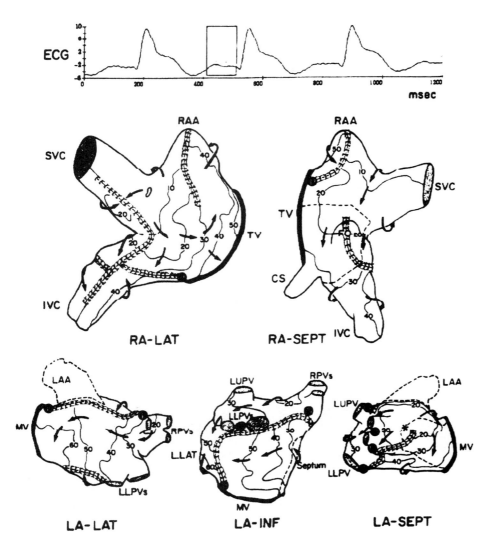

FIGURE 16-19. Atrial endocardial maps made during sinus rhythm 6 weeks after the radial approach. AVN, atrioventricular node; FO, fossa ovalis; IVC, inferior vena cava; LAA, left atrial appendage; LLPVs, left lower pulmonary veins; LUPV, left upper pulmonary vein; MV, mitral valve; RPVs, right pulmonary veins; RAA, right atrial appendage; SAN, sinoatrial node; SVC, superior vena cava; TV, tricuspid valve. (From Nitta T, Lee R, Watanabe H, et al. Radial approach: a new concept in surgical treatment for atrial fibrillation II. Effects and atrial contribution to ventricular filling. *Ann Thorac Surg* 1999;67:36–50, with permission.)

TABLE 16-4 • ECHOCARDIOGRAPHIC DOPPLER DATA FOR MAZE III AND THE RADIAL INCISION APPROACH

Site	Variable	Preoperative	RIA	Maze III
Transmitral	Peak E/A	1.68 ± 0.35^a	1.70 ± 0.40	3.49 ± 1.66^b
	AFF (%)	33.1 ± 6.9	20.0 ± 7.3	14.8 ± 5.0^c
Transtricuspid	Peak E/A	0.64 ± 0.13	1.03 ± 0.32	0.88 ± 0.31
	AFF (%)	58.9 ± 6.3	47.2 ± 13.4	48.0 ± 14.0
Pulmonary venous	Peak S (cm/sec)	23.4 ± 4.7	14.8 ± 6.1	14.9 ± 9.8
	Si (cm)	2.5 ± 1.5	1.5 ± 0.8	1.7 ± 1.2

AFF, atrial filling fraction, an index of atrial contribution to ventricular filling; Peak E/A, ratio of peak E wave to A wave; Peak S, peak velocity of the S wave; RIA, radial incision approach; Si, time-velocity integral of the S wave, an index of left atrial reservoir function.
[a] All values are given as the mean ± standard deviation.
[b] $p < 0.05$, maze versus before operation and RIA.
[c] $p < 0.005$, maze versus before operation.
Adapted from Nitta T, Lee R, Watanabe H, et al. Radial approach: a new concept in surgical treatment for atrial fibrillation. II. Electrophysiologic effects and atrial contribution to ventricular filling. *Ann Thorac Surg* 1999;67:36–50, with permission.

atrial tissue between the upper and lower pulmonary vein orifices was cryoablated in the patients to allow the lateral left atrium to be activated from the posterior left atrium through the left inferior left atrium between the left lower pulmonary vein orifice and the lower left atrial incision (Fig. 16-20). The remainder of the radial incision procedure was performed as described in the canine studies (15,92).

The radial incision approach represents a technically more feasible and perhaps improved surgical approach for the ablation of atrial fibrillation, alone or in combination with organic heart disease. The success of this approach also provides important additional information about the mechanism and effects of ablative components that may lead ultimately to a less invasive but equally effective cure for patients not requiring concomitant surgical intervention.

◉ CONCLUSIONS

The maze III procedure can cure most patients with idiopathic, nonrheumatic atrial fibrillation who are refractory to medical therapy. Combining the maze procedure with mitral valve repair in patients with degenerative disease has demonstrated promising results, provided that ventricular function is normal and that repair can be easily accomplished. Worldwide, in the setting of rheumatic disease, some investigators have modified the maze III procedure as part of a concomitant procedure. The long-term results of these modifications document that morbidity is not increased and that the success rate is almost equal to that of the maze III procedure without treating concomitant disease.

The lack of success in restoring left-sided atrial transport function led to the development of the radial incision approach. The experimental and clinical results with this technique suggest important new principles on which the ultimate ablative procedures for this ubiquitous arrhythmia will ultimately be based.

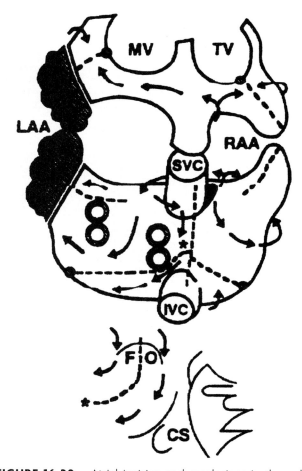

FIGURE 16-20. Atrial incision and cryolesions in the radial incision approach. The upper, middle, and lower panels represent the superior and posterior epicardium and the interatrial septum, respectively. The small, dark region of the right atrium at the junction with the superior vena cava (SVC) represents the sinus node. The activation sequence *(arrows)* after the procedure, the atrial incisions *(broken lines)*, and the excised left atrial appendage *(shaded region)*, and the cryolesions *(shaded circles)* at the atrioventricular valve annuli are identified. All the pulmonary vein orifices are cryoablated circumferentially *(shaded)*. The middle and lower panels show the epicardial and endocardial aspects *(asterisks)* of the identical sites. AVN, atrioventricular node; CS, coronary sinus; FO, fossa ovalis; IVC, inferior vena cava; LAA, left atrial appendage; LLPVs, left lower pulmonary veins; LUPV, left upper pulmonary vein; MV, mitral valve; RPVs, right pulmonary veins; RAA, right atrial appendage; SAN, sinoatrial node; TV, tricuspid valve. (From Nitta T, Ishii Y, Ogasawara O, et al. Initial experience with the radial incision approach for atrial fibrillation. *Ann Thorac Surg* 1999; 68:805–811, with permission.)

REFERENCES

1. Moe GK. On the multiple wavelet hypothesis of atrial fibrillation. *Arch Int Pharmacodyn Ther* 1962;140:183–188.
2. Allessie MA, Bonke FIM, Schopman FJG. Circus movement in rabbit atrial muscle as a mechanism of tachycardia. III. The

"leading circle" concept: a new mode of circus movement in cardiac tissue without the involvement of an anatomical obstacle. *Circ Res* 1977;41:9–18.
3. Allessie MA, Lammers WJEP, Bonke FIM, et al. Experimental evaluation of Moe's multiple wavelet hypothesis of atrial fibrillation. In: Zipes DP, Jalife J, eds. *Cardiac electrophysiology and arrhythmias*. New York: Grune & Stratton, 1985:265–276.
4. Boineau JP, Schuessler RB, Mooney CR, et al. Natural and evoked atrial flutter due to circus movements in dogs. *Am J Cardiol* 1980;45:1167–1181.
5. Peirick J, Pogwizd SM, Watchmaker GP, et al. The evolution of intraoperative electrophysiologic mapping procedures to guide cardiac arrhythmia surgery. In: Cox JL, ed. *Cardiac arrhythmia surgery: state of the art reviews*. Philadelphia: Hanley & Belfus, 1990:93–121.
6. Branham BH, Bi X, Cox JL. A system for accurate interactive 3-D display of cardiac electrical activity.
7. Canavan TE, Schuessler RB, Boineau JP, et al. Computerized global electrophysiological mapping of the atrium in patients with the Wolff-Parkinson-White Syndrome. *Ann Thorac Surg* 1989;46:223–231.
8. Canavan TE, Schuessler RB, Cain ME, et al. Computerized global electrophysiological mapping of the atrium in a patient with multiple supraventricular tachyarrhythmias. *Ann Thorac Surg* 1988;46:232–235.
9. Cox JL, Schuessler RB, D'Agostino HJ, et al. The surgical treatment of atrial fibrillation. II. Intraoperative electrophysiologic mapping and description of the electrophysiologic basis of atrial flutter and atrial fibrillation. *J Thorac Cardiovasc Surg* 1991;101:406–426.
10. Yamauchi S, Shuman TS, Kawamoto T, et al. Extent of surgery necessary to ablate atrial flutter [Abstract]. *Circulation* 1990;82[Suppl III]:III-144.
11. Ferguson TB Jr, Schuessler RB, Hand DE, et al. Lessons learned from computerized mapping of the atrium. *J Electrophysiol* 1993;26:210–219.
12. Allessie MA, Rensma PL, Brugada J, et al. Pathophysiology of atrial fibrillation. In: Zipes DP, Jalife J, eds. *Cardiac electrophysiology*. Philadelphia: WB Saunders, 1990:548–558.
13. Rodefeld MD, Bromberg BI, Huddleston CB, et al. Ablation of atrial flutter in a canine model of the modified Fontan operation [Abstract]. *Circulation* 1995;92:[Suppl I]:I-766.
14. Stone CM, Chang BC, Schuessler RB, et al. Independent activation of the right and left side of the atrial septum [Abstract]. *Circulation* 1989;80[Suppl II]:95.
15. Nitta T, Lee R, Schuessler RB, et al. Radial approach: a new concept in surgical treatment for atrial fibrillation. I. Concept, anatomic and physiologic bases and development of a procedure. *Ann Thorac Surg* 1999;67:27–35.
16. Saoudi N, Atallah G, Kirkorian G, Touboul P. Catheter ablation of the atrial myocardium in human type I atrial flutter. *Circulation* 1990;81:762–771.
17. Garrey WE. Auricular fibrillation. *Physiol Rev* 1924;4:215–250.
18. Lewis T, Drury AN, Iliescu CC. A demonstration of circus movement in clinical flutter of the auricles. *Heart* 1921;8:341–359.
19. Cox JL, Boineau JP, Schuessler RB, et al. A review of surgery for atrial fibrillation. *J Cardiovasc Electrophysiol* 1991;2:541–561.
20. Lesh MD, VanHare GF, Epstein LM, et al. Radiofrequency catheter ablation of atrial arrhythmias. *Circulation* 1994;89:1074–1089.
21. Moe GK, Abildskov JA. Atrial fibrillation as a self-sustaining arrhythmia independent of focal discharge. *Am Heart J* 1959;58:59–70.
22. Moe GK, Rheinboldt WC, Abildskov JA. A computer model of atrial fibrillation. *Am Heart J* 1964;67:200–220.
23. Hoffman BF, Rosen MR. Cellular mechanisms for cardiac arrhythmias. *Circ Res* 1981;49:1–15.
24. Allessie MA, Lammers WJEP, Bonke FIM, Hollen J. Experimental evaluation of Moe's multiple wavelet hypothesis of atrial fibrillation. In: Zipes DP, Jalife J. eds. *Cardiac electrophysiology and arrhythmias*. Orlando, FL: Grune & Stratton, 1985:265–275.
25. Allessie MA, Brugada J, Boersma L, et al. Mapping of atrial fibrillation in man. *New Trends Arrhyth* 1990;6:787–790.
26. Konings KTS, Kirchhof CJHJ, Allessie MA. Different degrees of complexity of excitation patterns during atrial fibrillation in man studied by high-resolution mapping [Abstract]. *Eur Heart J* 1992;13:80.
27. Kirchhof CJHJ, Chorro F, Scheffer GJ, et al. Regional entrainment of atrial fibrillation studied by high-resolution mapping in open-chested dogs. *Circulation* 1993;88:736–749.
28. Allessie MA, Chorro EJ, Wijffels MCEF, et al. What are the electrophysiological mechanisms of perpetuation of atrial fibrillation. In: Raviele A, ed. *Cardiac arrhythmias*. Berlin: Springer-Verlag, 1997:3–11.
29. Haissaguerre M, Jais P, Shah D, et al. Spontaneous initiation of atrial fibrillation by ectopic beats originating in the pulmonary veins. *N Engl J Med* 1998;339:659–666.
30. Jalife J, Berenfeld O, Skanes A, Mandapati R. Mechanisms of atrial fibrillation: mother rotors or multiple daughter wavelets, or both. *J Cardiovasc Electrophysiol* 1998;9:S2–S12.
31. Benditt DG, Samniah N, Fahy GJ, et al. Atrial fibrillation: defining potential curative ablation targets. *J Interv Card Electrophysiol* 2000;4:141–147.
32. Schuessler RB, Grayson TM, Bromberg BI, et al. Cholinergically mediated tachyarrhythmias induced by a single extrastimulus in the isolated canine right atrium. *Circ Res* 1992;71:1254–1267.
33. Schuessler RB, Kawamoto T, Hand DE, et al. Simultaneous epicardial and endocardial activation sequence mapping in the isolated canine right atrium. *Circulation* 1993;88:250–263.
34. Ortiz J, Niwano S, Abe H, et al. Mapping the conversion of atrial flutter to atrial fibrillation and atrial fibrillation to atrial flutter. *Circ Res* 1994;74:882–894.
35. Petersen P, Kastrup J, Brinch K, et al. Relation between left atrial diameters and duration of atrial fibrillation. *Am J Cardiol* 1987;60:382–384.
36. Sanfilippo AJ, Abascal VM, Sheenan M, et al. Atrial enlargement as a consequence of atrial fibrillation. *Circulation* 1990;82:792–797.
37. York TC, Landa JF. Minimal mass required for induction of a sustained arrhythmia in isolated atrial segments. *Am J Physiol* 1962;202:232–236.
38. Wijffels MCEF, Kirchof CJHJ, Dorland R, Allessie MA. Atrial fibrillation begets atrial fibrillation: a study in awake chronically instrumented goats. *Circulation* 1995;92:1954–1968.
39. Barbier P, Alioto G, Buazzi MD. Left atrial and ventricular filling in hypertensive patients with paroxysmal atrial fibrillation. *J Am Coll Cardiol* 1994;24:165–170.
40. Vulliemin P, Bufalo AD, Schlaepfer J, et al. Relation between cycle length, volume and pressure in type I atrial flutter. *Pacing Clin Electrophysiol* 1994;17:1391–1398.
41. Gosselink ATM, Crijns HJGM, Hamer HPM, et al. Changes in left and right atrial size after cardioversion of atrial fibrillation: role of mitral valve disease. *J Am Coll Cardiol* 1993;22:1666–1672.
42. Vaziri SM, Larson MG, Benjamin EJ, Levy D. Echocardiographic predictors of nonrheumatic atrial fibrillation. *Circulation* 1994;89:724–730.

43. Boineau JP, Schuessler RB, Mooney CR. Natural and evoked atrial flutter due to circus movement in dogs: role of abnormal atrial pathways, slow conduction, nonuniform refractory period distribution and premature beats. *Am J Cardiol* 1980;45:1167–1181.
44. Cox JL, Schuessler RB, D'Agostino JH, et al. The surgical treatment of atrial fibrillation. III. Development of a definitive surgical procedure. *J Thorac Cardiovasc Surg* 1991;101:569–583.
45. Cox JL, Boineau JP, Schuessler RB, et al. Electrophysiologic basis, surgical development and clinical results of the maze procedure for atrial flutter and fibrillation. In: Karp RB, Wechsler AS, eds. *Advances in cardiac surgery 1995.* Vol 6. St. Louis: Mosby–Year Book, 1995:1–67.
46. Ferguson TB Jr. Surgery for atrial fibrillation. *Coron Artery Dis* 1995;6:121–128.
47. Cox JL. The surgical treatment of atrial fibrillation. IV. Surgical technique. *J Thorac Cardiovasc Surg* 1991;101:584–592.
48. Cox JL, Boineau JP, Schuessler RB, et al. Five year experience with the maze procedure for atrial fibrillation. *Ann Thorac Surg* 1993;56:814–824.
49. Boineau JP, Schuessler RB, Mooney CR, et al. Multicentric origin of the atrial depolarization wave: the pacemaker complex. *Circulation* 1978;58:1036–1048.
50. Boineau JP, Schuessler RB. Reflections on the establishment of the electrophysiologic basis for cardiac arrhythmia surgery. In: Cox JL, ed. *Cardiac arrhythmia surgery: state of the art reviews.* Philadelphia: Hanley & Belfus, 1990:1–17.
51. Randall WC, Ardell JL. Nervous control of the heart: anatomy and pathophysiology. In: Zipes DP, Jalife J. eds. *Cardiac electrophysiology: from cell to bedside.* Philadelphia: WB Saunders, 1990:291–299.
52. Ferguson TB Jr, Kater KM, Boineau JP, Cox J. The requirement for permanent pacemaker therapy following the maze procedure for atrial fibrillation: incidence and therapeutic indications [Abstract]. *Pacing Clin Electrophysiol* 1994;17:862.
53. Cox JL, Boineau JP, Schuessler RB, et al. Modification of the maze procedure for atrial flutter and atrial fibrillation. I. Rationale and surgical results. *J Thorac Cardiovasc Surg* 1995;110:473–484.
54. Ferguson TB Jr. Surgical approach to atrial flutter and atrial fibrillation. In: Singer I, ed. *Interventional electrophysiology.* Baltimore: Williams & Wilkins, 1997:595–640.
55. Cox JL. The maze III procedure for treatment of atrial fibrillation. In Sabiston DC, ed. *Atlas of cardiothoracic surgery.* Philadelphia: WB Saunders, 1995:460–475.
56. Ferguson TB Jr. Surgery for atrial fibrillation. In: Zipes DP, ed. *Coronary artery disease: review in depth.* Vol (2):1995;121–128.
57. Ferguson TB Jr, Cox JL. Complications related to the surgical treatment of supraventricular and ventricular cardiac arrhythmias. In: Waldhausen JA, Orringer MB, eds. *Complications in cardiothoracic surgery.* St. Louis: Mosby–Year Book, 1990:303–315.
58. Feinberg MS, Waggoner AD, Kater DM, et al. Restoration of atrial function after the maze procedure for patients with atrial fibrillation: assessment by Doppler echocardiography. *Circulation* 1994;90[Suppl II]:II-285–II-292.
59. Itoh T, Okamoto H, Nimi T, et al. Left atrial function after Cox's maze operation concomitant with mitral valve operation. *Ann Thorac Surg* 1995;60:354–359.
60. Yashima N, Nasu M, Kawazoe K, Jiramori K. Serial evaluation of atrial function by Doppler echocardiography after the maze procedure for chronic atrial fibrillation. *Eur Heart J* 1997;18:496–502.
61. Tsui SS, Grace AA, Ludman PF, et al. Maze 3 for atrial fibrillation: two cuts too few? *Pacing Clin Electrophysiol* 1994;17:2163–2166.
62. Atrial Fibrillation Investigators. Risk factors for stroke and efficacy of antithrombotic therapy in atrial fibrillation: analysis of pooled data from five randomized controlled trials. *Arch Intern Med* 1994;154:1449–1457.
63. Kopecky SL, Gersh BJ, McCoon MD, et al. The natural history of lone atrial fibrillation: a population-based study over three decades. *N Engl J Med* 1987;317:669–674.
64. Rensma PL, Allessie MA, Lammers WJEP. Length of excitation wave and susceptibility to reentrant atrial arrhythmias in normal conscious dogs. *Circ Res* 1988;62:395–410.
65. Asano Y, Saito J, Matsumoto K, et al. On the mechanism of termination and perpetuation of atrial fibrillation. *Am J Cardiol* 1992;69:1033–1038.
66. Isobe FM. Personal communication.
67. Glick DB, Cronin CS, Jaquiss RDB, Ferguson TB Jr. The extended use of the autoperfusing heart-lung preparation for electrophysiologic studies. *Surg Forum* 1993;44:309–311.
68. Manning WJ, Silverman DI, Katz SE, et al. Impaired left atrial mechanical function after cardioversion: relation to the duration of atrial fibrillation. *J Am Coll Cardiol* 1994;23:1535–1540.
69. Kirchhof CJHJ, Allessie MA. Sinus node automaticity during atrial fibrillation in isolated rabbit hearts. *Circulation* 1992;86:263–271.
70. Page PL. Sinus node during atrial fibrillation. *Circulation* 1992;86:334–336.
71. McCarthy PM, Cosgrove DM, Castle LW, et al. Combined treatment of mitral regurgitation and atrial fibrillation with valvuloplasty and the maze procedure. *Am J Cardiol* 1992;71:483–486.
72. Chua YL, Schaff HV, Orszulak TA, Morris JJ. Outcome of mitral valve repair in patients with preoperative atrial fibrillation: should the maze procedure be combined with mitral valvuloplasty? *J Thorac Cardiovasc Surg* 1994;107:408–415.
73. Harada A, Sasaki K, Fukushima T, et al. Atrial activation during chronic atrial fibrillation in patients with isolated mitral valve disease. *Ann Thorac Surg* 1996;61:104–112.
74. Hioki M, Ikeshita M, Iedokoro Y, et al. Successful combined operation for mitral stenosis and atrial fibrillation. *Ann Thorac Surg* 1993;55:776–778.
75. Ferguson TB Jr. Modifications to the maze procedure for surgical ablation of atrial fibrillation. In: Singer I, Barold SS, Camm AJ, eds. *Nonpharmacological therapy of arrhythmias in the 21st century: the state of the art.* Armonk, NY: Futura Publishing, 1998:655–667.
76. Ferguson TB Jr, McKinnie JJ. Operative approach to atrial fibrillation. *Cardiac Electrophysiol Rev* 1999;3:103–105.
77. Kawaguchi AT, Kosaki Y, Isobe F, et al. Risk and benefit of combined maze procedure for atrial fibrillation associated with valvular heart diseases [Abstract]. *J Am Coll Cardiol* 1994;23(2):459–469.
78. Isobe F, Kawashima Y. The outcome and indications of the Cox maze III procedure for chronic atrial fibrillation with mitral valve disease. *J Thorac Cardiovasc Surg* 1998;116:220–227.
79. Izumoto H, Kawazoe K, Kitahara H, Kamata J. Operative results after the Cox/maze procedure combined with a mitral valve operation. *Ann Thorac Surg* 1998;66:800–804.
80. Kamata J, Kawazoe, Izumoto H, et al. Predictors of sinus rhythm restoration after the Cox maze procedure concomitant with other cardiac operations. *Ann Thorac Surg* 1997;64:394–398.
81. Crijns HJGM, Van Gelder IC, Brugemann J. Atrial fibrillation after valve replacement: concomitant preventive surgery or postoperative cardioversion? *Cardiol Rev* 1998;15:18–21.
82. Kamata J, Nakai K, Chiba N, et al. Electrocardiographic nature

83. Shyu K, Cheng J, Chen J, et al. Recovery of atrial function after atrial compartment operation for chronic atrial fibrillation in mitral valve disease. *J Am Coll Cardiol* 1994;24:392–398.
84. Sueda T, Okada K, Hirai S, et al. Right atrial separation for chronic atrial fibrillation with atrial septal defects. *Ann Thorac Surg* 1997;64:541–542.
85. Sueda T, Imai K, Okada K, et al. Right atrial separation for chronic atrial fibrillation with atrial septal defect and aortic valvular regurgitation in an elderly patient. *Ann Thorac Cardiovasc Surg* 1998;4:44–46.
86. Sueda T, Imai K, Orihashi K, et al. Efficacy of a left atrial procedure for treatment of chronic atrial fibrillation in elderly patients. *Ann Thorac Cardiovasc Surg* 1998;4:201–204.
87. Ferguson TB Jr. The future of arrhythmia surgery. *J Cardiovasc Electrophysiol* 1994;5:621–634.
88. Itoh T, Okamoto H, Ogawa Y. Left atrial function after the Cox/maze operation in mitral valvular disease patients [Abstract]. *Jpn Heart J* 1994:35.
89. Kosakai Y, Kawaguchi AT, Isobe F, et al. Modified maze procedure for patients with atrial fibrillation undergoing simultaneous open heart surgery. *Circulation* 1995;92[Suppl II]:II-359–II-364.
90. Cox JL. Evolving applications of the maze procedure for atrial fibrillation. *Ann Thorac Surg* 1993;55:578–580.
91. Kono T, Sabbah HN, Rosman H, et al. Left atrial contribution to ventricular filling during the course of evolving heart failure. *Circulation* 1992;86:1317–1322.
92. Nitta T, Lee R, Watanabe H, et al. Radial approach: a new concept in surgical treatment for atrial fibrillation. II. Electrophysiologic effects and atrial contribution to ventricular filling. *Ann Thorac Surg* 1999;67:36–50.
93. Nitta T, Ishii Y, Ogasawara O, et al. Initial experience with the radial incision approach for atrial fibrillation. *Ann Thorac Surg* 1999;68:805–811.
94. Ishii Y, Nitta T, Fujii M, et al. Serial change in the atrial transport function after the radial incision approach. *Ann Thorac Surg* 1999;63(3):805–810.

ROLE OF INTRAOPERATIVE MAPPING IN VENTRICULAR ARRHYTHMIA SURGERY

• • •

JOHN M. MILLER, GREGORY T. ALTEMOSE, MARK A. COPPESS, YOUSUF MAHOMED

Surgery was the first form of therapy that offered a potential cure for life-threatening ventricular arrhythmias. A variety of surgical techniques were developed in the 1970s and 1980s in an attempt to improve the antiarrhythmic effect of surgery and decrease operative risk (1–3). These innovations, as well as other improvements in surgical techniques such as myocardial preservation, have resulted in excellent survival and success rates for ventricular arrhythmia surgery. However, these procedures are rarely performed today, having been largely supplanted by the implantable cardioverter-defibrillator (ICD).

Implantable cardioverter defibrillator offers rescue rather than cure from the arrhythmia; episodes still occur, but their worst consequence—death—is almost completely averted. The device is relatively easy to implant, and patient recovery is much quicker than with the open-heart surgical procedures needed for curative surgery. Nonetheless, there is still a place in the electrophysiologist's arsenal for surgical therapy of ventricular arrhythmias. Occasionally, a patient presents with frequent recurrences of drug-refractory, sustained, hemodynamically unstable ventricular arrhythmias. Having not responded to drug therapy, such a patient would likely suffer frequent implantable cardioverter defibrillator discharges, and catheter ablation probably would be unsatisfactory because of poor hemodynamics. In this scenario as well as in others, surgery would be a good option. Most surgical centers employ some form of intraoperative electrophysiologic mapping during the arrhythmia to guide the surgical procedure. The purpose of this chapter is to review the role of intraoperative mapping in the surgical treatment of ventricular arrhythmias in man. The discussion in this chapter focuses on sustained, uniform-morphology ventricular tachycardia and less so on ventricular fibrillation.

◉ SUBSTRATES OF VENTRICULAR ARRHYTHMIAS AMENABLE TO DIRECT SURGICAL THERAPY

Surgical therapy has been applied to a number of different clinical circumstances, including different arrhythmia substrates or pathophysiologic settings in which ventricular arrhythmias arise (Table 17-1). Understanding of the pathophysiologic substrate is useful in planning what type of mapping procedure, criteria, and surgical approach to use. Most of these substrates consist of some form of structural heart disease that provides the setting for sustained, uniform-morphology ventricular tachycardia, although the clinical presentation (i.e., first recorded rhythm) may be ventric-

TABLE 17-1 • SUBSTRATES FOR SURGICALLY TREATABLE VENTRICULAR ARRHYTHMIAS

Substrate	Arrhythmia	Pathophysiology	Surgical Intervention
Structural heart disease present			
Postmyocardial infarction	VT	Reentry involving surviving subendocardial myocytes insulated from others by scar tissue	Resection or cryoablation of myocytes in circuit
Repaired congenital heart disease	VT	Reentry around ventricular incision or septal defect repair, bounded by nonconductive barrier (valve annulus, other incision)	Extend incision to nonconductive barrier
Arrhythmogenic right ventricular dysplasia	VT	Reentry involving surviving myocytes insulated from others by scar or fat tissue	Incision of circuit; right ventricular disarticulation
Chagasic cardiomyopathy	VT	Reentry involving surviving myocytes insulated from others by scar tissue	Resection or cryoablation of myocytes in circuit
Sarcoid cardiomyopathy	VT	Reentry; exact pathoanatomy unclear	Resection or cryoablation of myocytes in circuit
Idiopathic dilated cardiomyopathy	VT	Reentry; exact pathoanatomy unclear	Resection or cryoablation of myocytes in circuit
Structural heart disease minimal or absent			
Right ventricular outflow tract VT	VT	Triggered or automatic focus in right ventricular outflow tract, usually septal aspect	Resection or cryoablation of arrhythmogenic myocytes
Left septal (verapamil-sensitive) VT	VT	Reentry involving distal Purkinje network; possible role of left ventricular false tendon	Cryoablation of myocytes in circuit; division of false tendon (?)
Severe ischemia	VF	Subtotal occlusion of proximal coronary artery	Revascularization

VT, ventricular tachycardia; VF, ventricular fibrillation.

ular fibrillation because of deterioration of a very rapid rhythm after ischemia develops. In some cases, there is no discernible myocardial disease; rather, severe ischemia, neural input, or drug or electrolyte abnormalities have caused the arrhythmia. The initial rhythm in most of these settings is ventricular fibrillation, for which intraoperative mapping techniques are not yet available. Because intraoperative mapping currently has no meaningful role in these settings, they are not discussed further in this chapter.

The preponderance of experience in ventricular arrhythmia surgery exists in patients with the post–myocardial infarction substrate. Coronary artery occlusion causes death of most myocytes within the infarct zone. Surviving myocytes are separated by collagenous scar that replaces the dead myocytes (4). When these surviving cells are connected to others and to more normal myocardium at the periphery of the infarct zone, a potential circuit exists. These surviving cells are generally near the endocardial surface (perhaps prevented from dying by proximity to oxygen and nutrients from left ventricular cavitary blood). Other substrates of ventricular tachycardia to which surgical therapy has been applied include ventricular tachycardia after repair of congenital heart disease (5), arrhythmogenic right ventricular dysplasia (6), myocardial tumors (7), Chagas' disease, and some cases of ventricular tachycardia arising in the absence of overt structural heart disease. Included in the latter group are patients with idiopathic ventricular tachycardia arising from the right ventricular outflow tract (8) and the so-called Purkinje-based, verapamil-sensitive ventricular tachycardia arising in the left ventricular septum (9). Surgical therapy has occasionally been applied to sarcoid cardiomyopathy or nonischemic idiopathic dilated cardiomyopathy. Relatively little information is available concerning the exact pathophysiologic substrates in these disorders.

Surgical procedures that are not designed primarily to be antiarrhythmic but that are performed on patients with potential arrhythmia substrates include septal myomectomy for hypertrophic obstructive cardiomyopathy (10), free wall myomectomy (i.e., Batista procedure) for dilated cardiomyopathy (11), and laser transmyocardial revascularization (12). Whether these procedures ameliorate or aggravate ventricular arrhythmias is not yet clear.

● MAPPING EQUIPMENT

The tools used for acquiring electrophysiologic mapping information from the heart have changed significantly over the years, although the fundamental characteristics are the same. Recordings of cardiac electrical activity are obtained by contact with an electrode. The signal is amplified, filtered, recorded, and displayed for analysis of morphology and timing. Unipolar and bipolar signals have been used, as well as a wide range of filter settings. For the first decade of intraoperative cardiac mapping, most centers acquired mapping information using a single electrode that was moved from site to site in the heart. As technology improved, multipolar mapping electrodes became available for obtaining more information simultaneously from a larger area. Eventually, computer algorithms were developed to assist in the analysis of complex recordings. Most centers at which surgical therapy of ventricular arrhythmias is performed now employ sophisticated computerized mapping systems capable of acquiring data from more than 250 sites simultaneously with online analysis capability. This information is typically displayed as isochronal lines showing regions having equal timing of activation (13) (Fig. 17-1). With the capability of simultaneously recording from nearly the entire heart has come the possibility of analyzing activation differently, using isopotential mapping (i.e., displaying lines of equivalent voltage) (14,15) or vector mapping (i.e., displaying direction of wave front propagation at each point). Each method (i.e., unipolar or bipolar recording; iso-

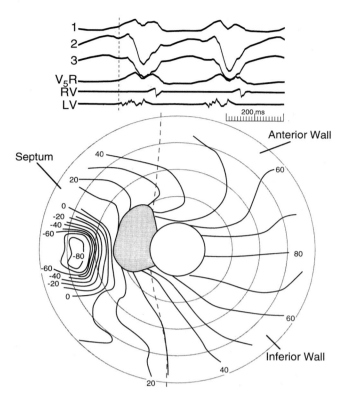

FIGURE 17-1. Isochronal map of ventricular tachycardia in a patient with a prior anterior myocardial infarction. At the top are four surface ECG leads and right and left ventricular reference electrograms during ventricular tachycardia (VT); at the bottom is a bull's-eye (polar) display of ventricular activation during VT. The apex is at the center and base at the outer ring (rings spaced 1 cm apart). The septum is indicated on the left. During this VT, activation spread centrifugally from an area of about 1 cm^2 to the rest of the endocardium, as shown by isochrones (lines of equivalent timing; numbers are milliseconds before QRS onset). More closely spaced isochrones indicate slowed conduction.

chronal, isopotential, and vector mapping) has its advantages and disadvantages, but a more detailed discussion of these features is beyond the scope of this chapter.

● MAPPING TECHNIQUES

The purpose of electrophysiologic mapping is to determine the location of tissues that must be ablated to cure the patient of the arrhythmia while leaving nonarrhythmogenic myocardium unaffected. Mapping data can be obtained during ventricular tachycardia, during sinus rhythm, atrial fibrillation and other fundamental rhythms, or during ventricular pacing. The best characterized of these techniques is *activation mapping during ventricular tachycardia,* in which the timing of activation during uniform-morphology ventricular tachycardia at any site is compared with that of a reference—usually the onset of the surface QRS complex. In the original mapping studies, sites from which activations were recorded in the latter half of diastole were considered to be close to the "site of origin" of ventricular tachycardia, a term with little meaning when discussing a circuit. The concept behind this was that, although ventricular tachycardia was known to consist of continuous propagation of current within a circuit, sites activated during the surface electrocardiogram (ECG) diastole must contain relatively few myocytes (i.e., such that they generated no discernible ECG deflection) and have abnormally slow intercellular conduction (i.e., prolonged, often fractionated electrograms). These data were obtained by moving a single electrode from site to site, with the sites separated by approximately 1 cm. This technique lacked the resolution to record isolated mid-diastolic potentials that have subsequently been determined to be the most favorable sites for ablation (16–18) (Fig. 17-2). Nonetheless, this technique was validated by ablating or removing ventricular tachycardia sites of origin and thereby rendering ventricular tachycardia noninducible at postoperative electrophysiologic study.

The concept of searching for diastolic electrograms has since been refined to seeking isolated mid-diastolic potentials that are almost always associated with but separate from a systolic potential (Fig. 17-2). Mapping studies have shown that, in at least some cases, these recordings are made from myocytes that are within a relatively narrow corridor between lines of functional or anatomic block. These types of potentials can be recorded in up to 80% of patients with careful mapping (19–21).

When activation mapping during ventricular tachycardia cannot be performed, *sinus rhythm mapping* is a reasonable alternative. The principle behind this technique is that the electrophysiologic abnormalities that are necessary for reentrant ventricular tachycardia to occur (especially slow conduction) are manifested as abnormal electrograms during sinus rhythm. These abnormalities have been characterized as fractionated (i.e., multicomponent, high fre-

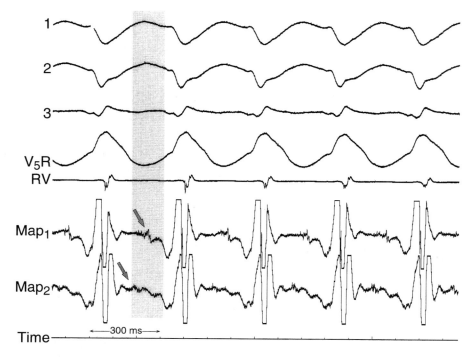

FIGURE 17-2. Mid-diastolic potential in ventricular tachycardia (VT). Four surface ECG leads are shown with reference electrograms from the right ventricle (RV) and two bipolar recordings from the mapping electrode (Map$_1$ and Map$_2$). Arrows denote potentials occurring in mid-diastole.

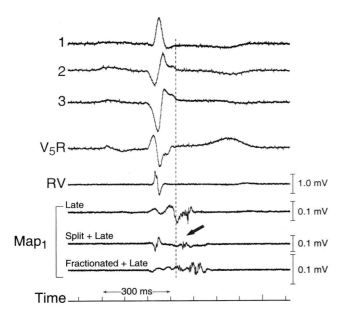

FIGURE 17-3. Electrogram types during sinus rhythm. Recordings are similar to those in Figure 17-2. Amplitude calibration marks (in millivolts [mV]) are shown at right. The right ventricular (RV) electrogram is a normal recording; Map_1 recordings are all abnormal and were obtained at different times from various sites and then time aligned.

quency, and prolonged), split (i.e., having at least two discrete components separated by 30-msec isoelectric interval), late (i.e., with some portion of the electrogram outlasting the end of the surface QRS complex), or simply abnormally prolonged or low amplitude potentials (22,23) (Fig. 17-3). Sinus rhythm mapping has been shown to have poor specificity (i.e., large areas of abnormal electrograms exist although ventricular tachycardia circuits incorporate small portions of these) and sensitivity (i.e., areas critical for reentry may have relatively normal electrograms in sinus rhythm). It is not a preferred method of mapping (22–25). If uniform-morphology ventricular tachycardia cannot be initiated, mapping in sinus rhythm to identify and ablate regions from which fragmented electrograms can be recorded has been used successfully to prevent arrhythmia recurrences (26,27).

Ventricular pace mapping has been used to determine target areas for ablation. Using this technique, the heart is paced at various sites, and the resulting 12-lead ECG is compared with that of the ventricular tachycardia (28) (Fig. 17-4). A 'match' indicates that pacing and the ventricular tachycardia are arising from the same area. This technique has the obvious limitation of ECG lead positioning because of the open chest and an open heart without cavitary blood. Like sinus rhythm mapping, pace mapping is neither sensitive nor specific enough to be useful as a sole tool to guide surgical ablation.

During the surgical procedure, time is critical. Decisions must be made relatively quickly about what areas of the heart must be ablated or removed and what method is best suited to this purpose without incurring unnecessary damage to nonarrhythmogenic myocardium. A close working relationship between the surgeon, who obtains mapping data and performs the ablative procedure, and the electrophysiologist, who interprets mapping information and directs the surgeon's attention to areas requiring ablation, is essential. What follows is a description of a typical intraoperative mapping session in a patient with post-infarct ventricular tachycardia. Although the details vary for other substrates, the basic principles remain the same.

The heart is exposed through median sternotomy, and a pericardial cradle is constructed. Arterial and venous cannulas are placed for cardiopulmonary bypass. Pacing and reference electrodes are attached to the heart and tested. Mapping electrodes (single or multipolar arrays) are likewise tested. Epicardial mapping of sinus rhythm or ventricular tachycardia may be performed at this time, while the heart is still closed, filled with blood, and under relatively normal loading conditions. Some groups employ an electrode-studded balloon for endocardial mapping of the closed heart (29). This device is introduced through a purse-string left atriotomy. Because of the space the balloon occupies in the left ventricle, the patient must be on cardiopulmonary bypass for these studies. In most cases of post-infarct ventricular tachycardia, areas that require ablation for cure of ventricular tachycardia are on the endocardial surface, and most groups therefore do not routinely perform epicardial mapping but proceed directly to endocardial mapping. Mapping is typically performed after instituting cardiopulmonary bypass and entering the left ventricular cavity through a wide incision in the infarct or aneurysm. The surgeon then makes a visual inspection of the endocardial surface for the presence of

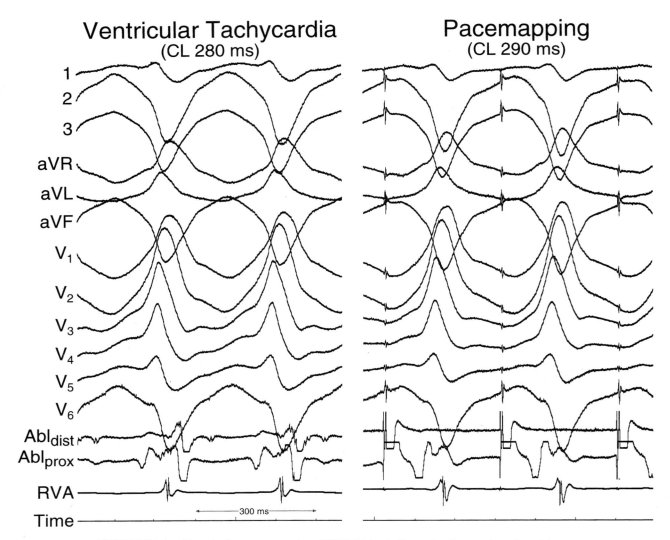

FIGURE 17-4. Ventricular pace mapping. All 12 ECG leads (from the electrophysiology laboratory) and intracardiac recordings from the distal (dist) and proximal (prox) ablation (Abl) catheter electrode and right ventricular apex (RVA) are shown during ventricular tachycardia (VT) *(left)*, and pacing from the ablation site is recorded. The paced QRS complexes are identical to those during VT, indicating that ventricular activation proceeds in the same manner in both circumstances. Pacing is at a rate slightly slower than VT to ensure that entrainment of VT is not occurring.

friable thrombus, which is removed at this time to prevent subsequent dislodgement and possible embolization. The perfusionist must maintain the blood perfusate temperature at 37.5°C to 38°C during the mapping process to counteract myocardial cooling caused by radiant heat loss from the heart's surface that may preclude initiation or maintenance of sustained arrhythmias.

Endocardial mapping can be performed during sinus rhythm or ventricular tachycardia using various electrode arrays or hand-held probes. Ventricular tachycardia is initiated using programmed stimulation or burst pacing. The mode of ventricular tachycardia initiation required in the operating room usually is similar to that encountered in the clinical electrophysiology laboratory (i.e., if single or double extrastimuli usually initiated ventricular tachycardia in the laboratory, a similar stimulation protocol elicits ventricular tachycardia during surgery). In approximately 5% of cases, ventricular tachycardia cannot be initiated during surgery despite reliable initiation preoperatively. After ventricular tachycardia has been initiated, mapping of the entire endocardial surface or within a smaller region is dictated by the morphologic appearance of the induced ventricular tachycardia. If the ventricular tachycardia appears similar to a morphology that was mapped in the electrophysiology laboratory preoperatively, mapping should begin in the region suggested by the prior data (30,31). Alternatively, features of the ECG during ventricular tachycardia can often help in directing attention toward certain areas (32–34). Sites with isolated, low-amplitude, mid- or late diastolic potentials are sought. If possible, attempts should be made to corroborate the mapping information by observing the behavior of the potential during spontaneous changes in ventricular tachycardia cycle length (Fig. 17-5) or by using pacing maneuvers (i.e., entrainment or single-beat resetting) or physical maneuvers such as focal pressure or cooling to slow or terminate the ventricular tachycardia (Fig. 17-6). It is not always feasible to perform these techniques, but they can be useful tools in differentiating tissues that participate in reentry from those that are passively activated (35).

After a ventricular tachycardia morphology has been satisfactorily mapped, an attempt is made to initiate other ventricular tachycardia morphologies. Multiple ventricular tachycardia morphologies are the rule in post-infarct ventricular tachycardia and may simply be different ECG manifestations of the same circuit (i.e., different directions of rotation within the same circuit or different "exit points" from the same circuit) or represent completely different circuits (36, 37). When no additional ventricular tachycardias can be initiated, a quick review of the data should be conducted to ensure that all ventricular tachycardias have been adequately mapped before concluding this portion of the procedure.

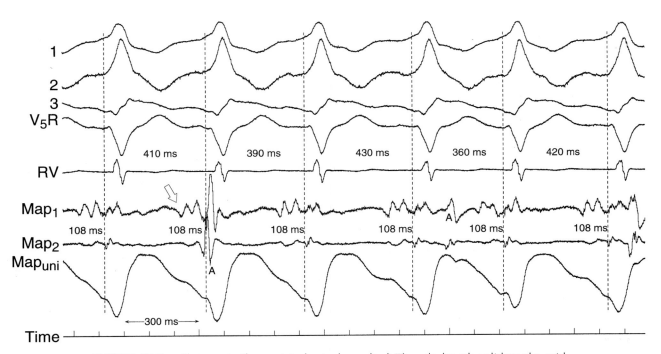

FIGURE 17-5. Changes in the ventricular tachycardia (VT) cycle length validate the mid-diastolic potential. Recordings are similar to those in Figure 17-2. Ventricular tachycardia is shown with marked variability in the RR intervals; this affords an opportunity to observe the behavior of a diastolic potential (arrow). The diastolic potential maintains a constant relationship to the onset of the next QRS complex (dashed lines). A, atrial electrogram (near mitral annulus); uni, unipolar.

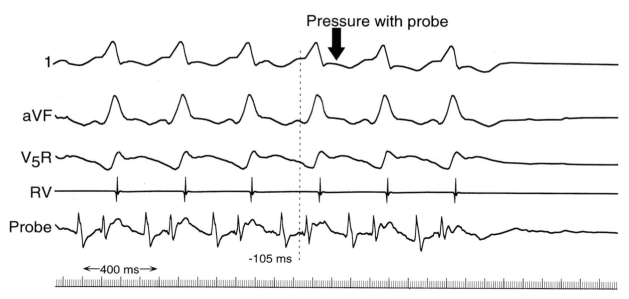

FIGURE 17-6. Pressure termination of ventricular tachycardia (VT). Recordings are similar to those in Figure 17-2. During VT, the probe electrogram shows a low-amplitude mid-diastolic recording. Pressure with the mapping probe results in termination of VT after the inscription of the mid-diastolic potential.

After mapping has been completed, the ablation portion of the procedure can begin. The most commonly used methods of surgical ablation are subendocardial resection (38), in which the superficial 2 to 3 mm of endocardium and subjacent tissue of the area implicated by mapping are removed as a sheet by sharp dissection and encircling endocardial ventriculotomy (1), involving an endocardial incision about halfway through the myocardial wall thickness and circumscribing the arrhythmogenic areas indicated by mapping. The original intent of the encircling endocardial ventriculotomy was to "wall off" the arrhythmia, such that it might continue but not spread to the rest of the heart (much like right ventricular disarticulation for arrhythmogenic right ventricular dysplasia), but it probably works more by incising critical circuit components.

Ablation can also be achieved by applying a cryoprobe to freeze tissue (to −70°C or colder for 2 to 3 minutes) focally, regionally, or as an encircling procedure (39). Using this method, ablation of large areas can take up to 30 minutes, and many centers therefore use cryoablation as an adjunct to treat areas that are not readily amenable to resection or incision, such as papillary muscles and deep septal sites.

Myocardial ablation can be performed while the heart is still beating. This affords the opportunity for immediate assessment of the efficacy of ablation by attempting to reinitiate ventricular tachycardia with programmed stimulation (40). If ventricular tachycardia can be reinitiated, mapping is repeated. This usually points to a deeper septal or epicardial site that can be ablated with the cryoprobe. Repeated cycles of stimulation, mapping, and ablation are performed until ventricular tachycardia is no longer inducible. This process can be concluded more rapidly when working on a normothermic, beating heart than when the heart must be cooled for ablation and rewarmed for repeat stimulation.

Early mapping and surgical studies demonstrated that almost all cases of post-infarct ventricular tachycardia required endocardial ablation for cure, and routine epicardial mapping was abandoned. The role of the epicardium and deeper myocardial layers has recently been reexamined (41–44). This is because of the availability of more sophisticated mapping equipment (particularly intramyocardial multipolar plunge electrodes and biventricular mapping arrays) and techniques, such as restimulation after myocardial ablation or resection. Some studies have shown regions of reentry outside the endocardium and even some cases in which ventricular tachycardia could be terminated by epicardial or right ventricular septal cryoablation. This finding confirms participation of these regions in reentry, but does not necessarily indicate that the endocardium is passively activated. There have, however, been cases in which epicardial laser photoablation has been the sole means of ventricular tachycardia termination after ablation attempts at multiple endocardial sites had failed (45). It is not clear why a higher proportion of ventricular tachycardias in more recent series appear to have critical sites of reentry in areas other than the endocardium. One possible explanation is a change in the nature of the substrate because of innovations in therapy of acute myocardial infarction (e.g., limitation of infarct size by early reperfusion, changes in ventricular remodeling due to beta blocker and angiotensin-converting enzyme inhibition). Inferior infarct-related ventricular tachycardia appears to have a disproportionately high likelihood of requiring epicardial ablation in recent series. This is in the face of the nearly uniform success achieved with a modified endocardial approach to ventricular tachycardia surgical ablation (46).

After mapping and ablation have been accomplished, the ventriculotomy is repaired, and other surgical procedures, such as bypass grafting, valve repair or replacement, are performed if needed. Some authorities have advocated performing coronary artery bypass grafting at the beginning of the procedure before the mapping portion to improve myocardial perfusion during induced ventricular tachycardia. It is not clear whether this confers the intended benefit, since myocardial oxygen demands are relatively low because the heart is unloaded from most mechanical work during the mapping portion of the surgery (i.e., left ventricle is open). Residual effects of myocardial cooling and high potassium concentrations in cardioplegic solutions used during bypass grafting may prevent arrhythmia initiation if it is attempted afterward. For these reasons, most groups perform mapping and arrhythmia ablation before administering cardioplegia solution for bypass grafting or valve surgery.

PREOPERATIVE MAPPING STUDIES

Because intraoperative mapping time is relatively limited, it stands to reason that the physician should have as much information as possible available prior to entering the operating room. In theory, this includes catheter mapping data. However, this information may be of limited value in that, if catheter mapping had correctly identified the optimal site for ablation, the arrhythmia related to that site would likely have been successfully ablated and would not need surgical attention. If catheter mapping data suggested a particular site but radiofrequency energy delivery there had no effect on the ventricular tachycardia, the reliability of the catheter mapping data might be questioned. As a practical matter, extensive catheter mapping data is rarely available before surgery except in cases of failed catheter ablation attempts. Features of the 12-lead ECG during ventricular tachycardia can still be used to help guide mapping efforts to particular regions of the heart (32,33). Having ECG recordings of as many ventricular tachycardia morphologies as possible can be useful in this regard, as well as providing a checklist of ventricular tachycardia morphologies for which attempts at initiation and mapping should be made.

IS MAPPING NECESSARY?

The sophistication and capabilities of currently available intraoperative mapping equipment are impressive. Paradoxically, many investigators are advocating arrhythmia surgery without performing mapping studies. In this approach, the ablation procedure is directed against visibly abnormal, scarred endocardium, including papillary muscles (necessitating mitral valve replacement) (47–49). This sentiment is based on nearly equivalent antiarrhythmic results of surgery regardless of whether mapping was used, the perception that the time spent during mapping increases the operative risk, and the expense and complexity of available mapping systems. Although the first two contentions are difficult to prove, the third contention is valid. Mapping systems are costly and complicated to use and are used relatively infrequently, providing a relatively poor return on a considerable financial investment.

Comparing results of current series to those conducted earlier in the experience with surgical management of ventricular tachycardia (i.e., historical controls) is not entirely valid, since there have been substantial improvements in surgical management unrelated to the arrhythmia portion of the procedure. These include better myocardial preservation, better conduits for bypass grafting, mechanically more advantageous ventricular closure techniques, and more potent inotropic agents for postoperative care. Improved patient selection for surgical therapy probably has led to improved survival (50–52). In the largest series, one from the University of Pennsylvania, practically no patient selection was applied (53–55). Only on rare occasions were patients turned down for surgery, probably leading to a higher overall operative mortality.

Balanced against the view that mapping is unnecessary in ventricular tachycardia surgery are arguments that suggest it has a definite beneficial role:

1. There is a relationship between the completeness of mapping as judged at the time of surgery and antiarrhythmic outcome. In a consecutive series of 100 patients who underwent surgical therapy for post-infarct ventricular tachycardia, 88% of those in whom all ventricular tachycardias were adequately mapped were cured of ventricular tachycardia (i.e., no inducible ventricular tachycardia at postoperative electrophysiologic study and no arrhythmias during follow-up), whereas 69% of those in whom 51% to 99% of ventricular tachycardias were mapped and 53% of those in whom less than 50% of ventricular tachycardias were mapped were cured of ventricular tachycardia (56).

2. Visually guided surgery cannot be applied in patients who have ventricular tachycardia early after myocardial infarction, before scar has developed (<2 to 3 months). In this small but important subset of patients with ventricular tachycardia, the only way to identify regions responsible for the arrhythmia is using mapping (27,57,58).
3. In patients in whom critical components of the ventricular tachycardia circuit lie outside the region of visible scar—such as deep septal, right ventricular wall, epicardial, or endocardial sites outside the scarred territory—mapping is the only method to discover these areas (41,43). Visually directed surgery eliminates only ventricular tachycardias related to visible scar but in none of these types of cases.

◉ PROBLEMS WITH INTRAOPERATIVE MAPPING

A variety of problems can interfere with successful gathering of critical data during intraoperative mapping. Since many of these are unpredictable and there is little time to spare during the procedure, the electrophysiologist must be prepared for any eventuality and have alternate plans.

In some cases, no mappable arrhythmia can be initiated, which may result from a lack of inducibility of any arrhythmia, initiation of only nonsustained ventricular tachycardia, or initiation of only ventricular fibrillation. Causes of the first situation include excessive myocardial cooling, inadvertent damage to critical circuit components during ventriculotomy or removal of adherent endocardial thrombus, or absence of mechanical loading conditions necessary for ventricular tachycardia initiation. If only nonsustained ventricular tachycardia is induced, administration of procainamide into the perfusate often facilitates initiation of sustained ventricular tachycardia. When ventricular fibrillation is repeatedly initiated, especially when this was not the case before surgery, the presence of myocardial hypothermia or ischemia must be suspected. If the latter exists, further attempts to initiate ventricular tachycardia should be halted and the heart allowed to rest, or the mapping portion of the procedure should end. In patients with inferior infarction, elevation of the cardiac apex to access the inferior wall may result in kinking of the left anterior descending artery and resultant anterior wall ischemia. If no arrhythmia can be initiated, it is still possible to perform sinus rhythm mapping. The limitations of this procedure have been discussed.

There may be uncertainty about the reference for timing of the recordings. Since the ideal target sites for ablation are those from which middle to late diastolic electrograms are recorded, it follows that the physician must be able to accurately determine the beginning and the end of diastole. In some cases, particularly rapid ventricular tachycardias, this can be problematic (Fig. 17-7). When faced with this problem, a burst of overdrive pacing during ventricular tachycardia can produce a short pause after cessation of pacing (Fig. 17-8). When the same ventricular tachycardia resumes after this, one can more easily tell where the QRS starts. If this maneuver is not helpful, it is often best to terminate the arrhythmia and attempt to reinitiate one that is more amenable to mapping. Alternatively, procainamide administration can often slow the ventricular tachycardia rate enough that QRS complexes are more discrete, making the onset more definitive.

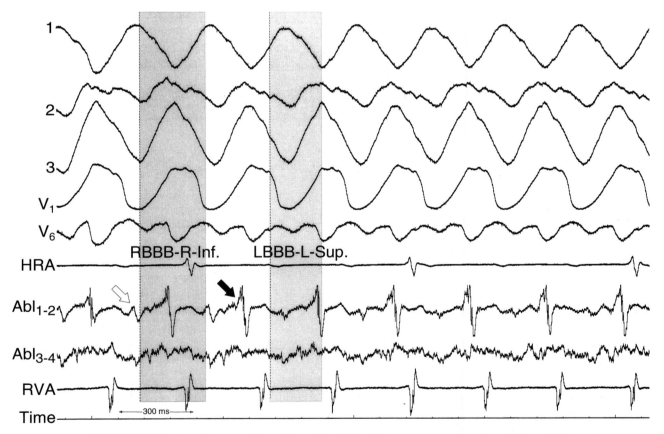

FIGURE 17-7. Rapid ventricular tachycardia (VT) with some uncertainty about where QRS begins. In this example from the electrophysiology laboratory, it is not clear where the QRS complex begins and ends in the rapid VT. Two plausible options are shown, indicated by dashed lines at QRS onset and shading for its duration. If the right bundle branch block, right inferior axis (RBBB-R-Inf) choice is correct, a diastolic potential in Abl$_{1-2}$ *(white arrow)* is minimally presystolic and unlikely to be involved in the reentrant circuit. If the VT is a left bundle branch block, left superior axis morphology (LBBB-L-Sup), the diastolic potential *(black arrow)* is large and within mid-diastole and may be involved in reentry.

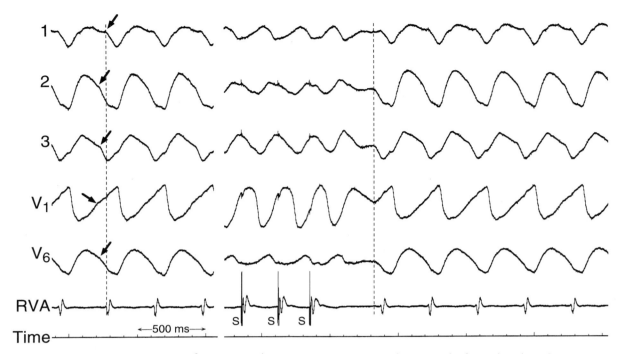

FIGURE 17-8. Use of pacing to determine QRS onset. In this example from the clinical electrophysiology laboratory, the rapid ventricular tachycardia (VT) has unclear QRS morphology; in the left panel, possible QRS onsets *(arrows)* are designated in each surface lead. The most obvious inflection point is in lead 1 *(dashed line)*. In the right panel, the last three paced complexes of a pacing train delivered during VT are followed by a short pause, after which VT resumes. This pause provides the opportunity to see where the QRS starts *(dashed line)*. This occurs slightly earlier than the event in the left panel.

There may be uncertainty about the timing of local activations. The multicomponent, complex electrograms recorded in diseased myocardium can make reliable determination of the exact timing of local activation problematic (in immediate contact with the electrode). A variety of criteria have been proposed for the most accurate definition of local activation (Fig. 17-9), including onset of any electrical activity, the earliest high-frequency signal, the most rapid crossing of the baseline, and others. Most evidence points to the deflection with the highest dV/dt in the unipolar recording, or the peak voltage in a bipolar signal, as the best indicators of local activation (59–61) (Fig. 17-10). When moved from site to site, recordings from a unipolar electrode may be difficult to interpret because of baseline drift and amplifier saturation. However, newer mapping systems with larger multipolar electrode arrays may be positioned once and remain in stable contact thereby obviating this limitation.

Intermittent potentials may be observed during ventricular tachycardia. During ventricular tachycardia mapping in scarred endocardium, it is possible to record low-amplitude diastolic potentials that are not present on every beat. This phenomenon, referred to as *local conduction failure* or *exit block*, is not caused by far-field atrial potentials or poor electrode contact but does indicate intermittent activation of cells under the recording electrode (Fig. 17-11). This has been observed in 64% of individual ventricular tachycardias during intraoperative mapping and during at least one ventricular tachycardia in 86% of patients (35). The pattern of block is typically 2 : 1, although Wenckebach and more complex patterns may be observed. Although the cells from which these potentials are recorded are clearly not integral in the ventricular

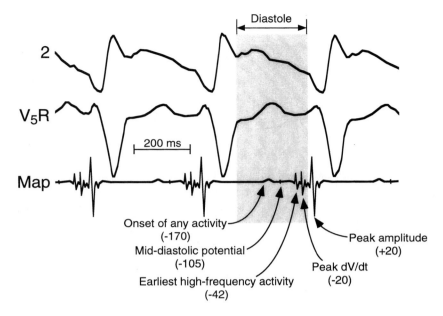

FIGURE 17-9. A complex intracardiac electrogram with several possible interpretations about the timing of local activation. Two surface ECG leads and an intracardiac recording (Map) during ventricular tachycardia (VT) are shown, and diastole is the shaded area. Arrows indicate points within the electrogram at which local activation may be designated. The low-amplitude bump at −170 msec is probably a local T wave from the prior beat. Using low-amplitude mid-diastolic potentials, the earliest high-frequency activity or peak dV/dt (slow rate) leads to an interpretation of the site as near or within the VT circuit, whereas taking the peak amplitude as local activation leads to the site's being interpreted as outside the circuit.

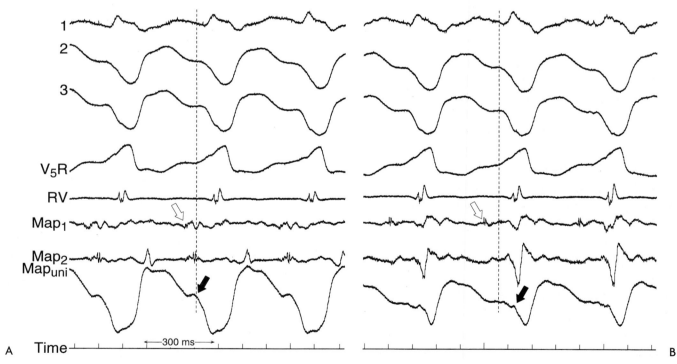

FIGURE 17-10. Comparison of unipolar and bipolar signals. Recordings from two sites during the same ventricular tachycardia (VT) are shown. In each, a diastolic potential is present in Map$_1$ (i.e., bipolar); the white arrow points to its peak voltage as the timing of local activation. A unipolar recording from one Map$_1$ electrode is shown with its corresponding point of activation (maximum dV/dt) *(black arrow)*. Dashed lines indicate QRS onset. Notice the closer similarity of timing of bipolar and unipolar activations in **A** and a sharper bipolar potential in **B**, indicating that each contains useful information.

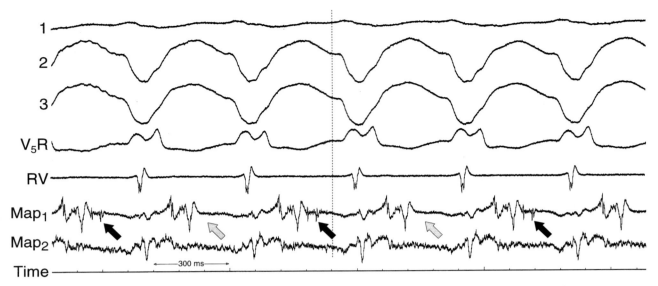

FIGURE 17-11. Intermittent appearance of a potential during ventricular tachycardia (VT). QRS onset *(dashed line)* is indicated, and two discrete potentials in diastole *(black arrows)* are absent on alternate beats *(gray arrows)*. The timing of these potentials is such that they could be designated within the reentrant circuit if not for the fact that the tachycardia continues without them.

tachycardia circuit, the potentials often occur in mid-diastole (Fig. 17-11) and can mislead the electrophysiologist into thinking that he or she is recording from part of the actual ventricular tachycardia circuit. This pitfall can be avoided by observing more than one or two ventricular tachycardia cycles.

Spurious (nonphysiologic) recordings may be obtained. Recordings from an electrode with poor contact or broken electrical continuity can yield spurious data. These recordings may be interpreted by automated computer systems as valid signals and analyzed, resulting in misleading isochronal mapping plots. Vigilant surveillance of the quality of the signals coming into the system is important. The electrophysiologist should not allow the computer to function autonomously without adequately screening and editing its input (Fig. 17-12).

It is also possible for general equipment failure to occur during intraoperative mapping. If a computerized system suddenly becomes inoperative, recovery is more difficult than with older systems because of the complexity and relative lack of user-serviceable components or bypasses.

CONCLUSIONS

The heyday of surgical therapy for ventricular tachycardia has passed and with it the need for widespread expertise in intraoperative mapping of arrhythmias. Ironically, this has occurred at a time when powerful mapping and analysis tools have become available to facilitate surgical therapy of ventricular tachycardia. There will probably always be at least a limited role for surgical therapy of ventricular tachycardia, but is there a need for mapping, with evidence that similar antiarrhythmic results can be obtained without it? In up to 25% of patients, critical elements of ventricular tachycardia circuits exist outside the boundary of visible scar tissue that would ordinarily be removed or otherwise ablated. In some cases, these critical circuit components are epicardial or intramural, and because mapping provides the only way to determine which ventricular tachycardias have critical circuit components in such unusual areas, the surgical team should be prepared to do some mapping, even if only a visually directed procedure is planned. A good working relationship between electrophysiologist and surgeon

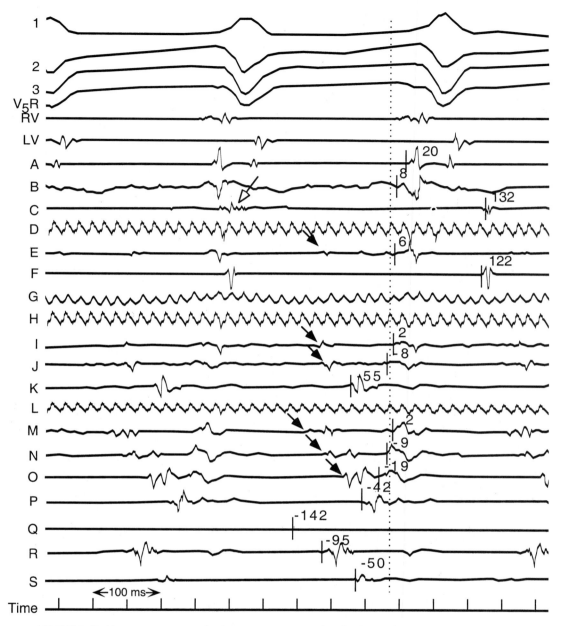

FIGURE 17-12. Spurious signals during computerized multielectrode mapping. Four surface ECG leads are shown with right (RV) and left (LV) ventricular reference electrograms and 19/20 electrode recordings from a multipolar electrode array during ventricular tachycardia (VT). QRS onset *(dotted line)* is indicated, and computer-derived activations *(vertical lines)* are shown on the electrograms with corresponding timing relative to QRS onset. At electrode C, an activation *(white arrow)* was marked despite an unstable recording. Low-amplitude, mid-diastolic potentials *(dark arrows)* may have been important during VT, but they were ignored by the computer algorithm. Electrodes D, G, H, and L show a 60-Hz artifact; computer-derived activations have been edited out. In Q, the computer mistook a bit-error signal for a local activation. This example shows why interaction with computerized systems is important for accuracy.

is critical for obtaining the optimal outcome from these demanding procedures.

REFERENCES

1. Guiraudon G, Fontaine G, Frank R, et al. Encircling endocardial ventriculotomy: a new surgical treatment for life-threatening ventricular tachycardias resistant to medical treatment following myocardial infarction. *Ann Thorac Surg* 1978;26:438–444.
2. Gallagher JJ, Anderson RW, Kasell J, et al. Cryoablation of drug-resistant ventricular tachycardia in a patient with a variant of scleroderma. *Circulation* 1978;57:190–197.
3. Josephson ME, Harken AH, Horowitz LN. Endocardial excision: a new surgical technique for the treatment of recurrent ventricular tachycardia. *Circulation* 1979;60:1430–1439.
4. Fenoglio JJ, Pham TD, Harken AH, et al. Recurrent sustained ventricular tachycardia: structure and ultrastructure of subendocardial regions in which tachycardia originates. *Circulation* 1983;68:518–533.
5. Harken AH, Horowitz LN, Josephson ME. Surgical correction of recurrent sustained ventricular tachycardia following complete repair of tetralogy of Fallot. *J Thorac Cardiovasc Surg* 1980;80:779–781.
6. Guiraudon GM, Klein GJ, Gulamhusein SS, et al. Total disconnection of the right ventricular free wall: surgical treatment of right ventricular tachycardia associated with right ventricular dysplasia. *Circulation* 1983;67:463–470.
7. Guiraudon G, Fontaine G, Frank R, et al. Surgical treatment of ventricular tachycardia guided by ventricular mapping in 23 patients without coronary artery disease. *Ann Thorac Surg* 1981;32:439–450.
8. Fontaine G, Guiraudon G, Frank R, et al. Surgical management of ventricular tachycardia unrelated to myocardial ischemia or infarction. *Am J Cardiol* 1982;49:397–410.
9. Suwa M, Yoneda Y, Nagao H, et al. Surgical correction of idiopathic paroxysmal ventricular tachycardia possibly related to left ventricular false tendon. *Am J Cardiol* 1989;64:1217–1220.
10. Fighali S, Krajcer Z, Leachman RD. Septal myomectomy and mitral valve replacement for idiopathic hypertrophic subaortic stenosis: short- and long-term follow-up. *J Am Coll Cardiol* 1984;3:1127–1134.
11. Suma H, Isomura T, Horii T, et al. Two-year experience of the Batista operation for non-ischemic cardiomyopathy. *J Cardiol* 1998;32:269–276.
12. Gassler N, Stubbe HM. Clinical data and histological features of transmyocardial revascularization with CO_2 laser. *Eur J Cardiothorac Surg* 1997;12:25–30.
13. Miller JM, Harken AH, Hargrove WC, Josephson ME. Pattern of endocardial activation during sustained ventricular tachycardia. *J Am Coll Cardiol* 1985;6:1280–1287.
14. Harada A, D'Agostini HJ, Schuessler RB, et al. Potential distribution mapping: new method for precise localization of intramural septal origin of ventricular tachycardia. *Circulation* 1988;78:
15. Harada A, Tweddell JS, Schuessler RB, et al. Computerized potential distribution mapping: a new intraoperative mapping technique for ventricular tachycardia surgery. *Ann Thorac Surg* 1990;49:649–655.
16. Stevenson WG, Khan H, Sager P, et al. Identification of reentry circuit sites during catheter mapping and radiofrequency ablation of ventricular tachycardia late after myocardial infarction. *Circulation* 1993;88:1647–1670.
17. Bogun F, Bahu M, Knight BP, et al. Comparison of effective and ineffective target sites that demonstrate concealed entrainment in patients with coronary artery disease undergoing radiofrequency ablation of ventricular tachycardia. *Circulation* 1997;95:183–190.
18. El-Shalakany A, Hadjis T, Papageorgiou P, et al. Entrainment/mapping criteria for the prediction of termination of ventricular tachycardia by single radiofrequency lesion in patients with coronary artery disease. *Circulation* 1999;99:2283–2289.
19. de Bakker JM, Janse MJ, Van Capelle FJ, Durrer D. Endocardial mapping by simultaneous recording of endocardial electrograms during cardiac surgery for ventricular aneurysm. *J Am Coll Cardiol* 1983;2:947–953.
20. Harris L, Downar E, Mickleborough L, et al. Activation sequence of ventricular tachycardia: endocardial and epicardial mapping studies in the human ventricle. *J Am Coll Cardiol* 1987;10:1040–1047.
21. Downar E, Saito J, Doig JC, et al. Endocardial mapping of ventricular tachycardia in the intact human ventricle. III. Evidence of multiuse reentry with spontaneous and induced block in portions of reentrant path complex. *J Am Coll Cardiol* 1995;25:1591–600.
22. Cassidy DM, Vassallo JA, Buxton AE, et al. The value of catheter mapping during sinus rhythm to localize site of origin of ventricular tachycardia. *Circulation* 1984;69:1103–1110.
23. Cassidy DM, Vassallo JA, Buxton AE, et al. Catheter mapping during sinus rhythm: relation of local electrogram duration to ventricular tachycardia cycle length. *Am J Cardiol* 1985;55:713–716.
24. Cassidy DM, Vassallo JA, Miller JM, et al. Endocardial catheter mapping in patients in sinus rhythm: relationship to underlying heart disease and ventricular arrhythmias. *Circulation* 1986;73:645–652.
25. Kienzle MG, Miller JM, Falcone RA, et al. Intraoperative endocardial mapping during sinus rhythm: relationship to site of origin of ventricular tachycardia. *Circulation* 1984;70:957–965.
26. Bourke JP, Campbell RWF, Renzulli A, et al. Surgery for ventricular tachyarrhythmias based on fragmentation mapping in sinus rhythm alone. *Eur J Cardiothorac Surg* 1989;3:401–406.
27. Bourke JP, Hilton CJ, McComb JM, et al. Surgery for control of recurrent life-threatening ventricular tachyarrhythmias within 2 months of myocardial infarction. *J Am Coll Cardiol* 1990;16:42–48.
28. O'Keefe DB, Curry PVL, Prior AL, et al. Surgery for ventricular tachycardia using operative pace-mapping. *Proc Br Coll Surg* 1980;43:116–121.
29. Mickleborough LL, Harris L, Downar E, et al. A new intraoperative approach for endocardial mapping of ventricular tachycardia. *J Thorac Cardiovasc Surg* 1988;95:271–280.
30. Josephson ME, Horowitz LN, Spielman SR, et al. Comparison of endocardial catheter mapping with intraoperative mapping of ventricular tachycardia. *Circulation* 1980;61:395–404.
31. Hauer RN, de Zwart MT, de Bakker JM, et al. Endocardial catheter mapping: wire skeleton technique for representation of computed arrhythmogenic sites compared with intraoperative mapping. *Circulation* 1986;74:1346–54.
32. Miller JM, Marchlinski FE, Buxton AE, Josephson ME. Relationship between the 12-lead electrocardiogram during ventricular tachycardia and endocardial site of origin in patients with coronary artery disease. *Circulation* 1988;77:759–766.
33. Kuchar DL, Ruskin JN, Garan H. Electrocardiographic localization of the site of origin of ventricular tachycardia in patients with prior myocardial infarction. *J Am Coll Cardiol* 1989;13:893–900.
34. Davis LM, Byth K, Uther JB, Ross DL. Localisation of ventricu-

lar tachycardia substrates by analysis of the surface QRS recorded during ventricular tachycardia. *Int J Cardiol* 1995;50:131–142.
35. Miller JM, Vassallo JA, Hargrove WC, Josephson ME. Intermittent failure of local conduction during ventricular tachycardia. *Circulation* 1985;72:1286–1292.
36. Miller JM, Kienzle MG, Harken AH, Josephson ME. Morphologically distinct sustained ventricular tachycardias in coronary artery disease: significance and surgical results. *J Am Coll Cardiol* 1984;4:1073–1079.
37. Waspe LE, Brodman R, Kim SG, et al. Activation mapping in patients with coronary artery disease with multiple ventricular tachycardia configurations: occurrence and therapeutic implications of widely separate apparent sites of origin. *J Am Coll Cardiol* 1985;5:1075–1086.
38. Horowitz LN, Harken AH, Kastor JA, Josephson ME. Ventricular resection guided by epicardial and endocardial mapping for treatment of recurrent ventricular tachycardia. *N Engl J Med* 1980;302:589–593.
39. Guiraudon GM, Thakur RK, Klein GJ, et al. Encircling endocardial cryoablation for ventricular tachycardia after myocardial infarction experience with thirty-three patients. *Am Heart J* 1994;128:982–989.
40. Haines DE, Lerman BB, Kron IL, DiMarco JP. Surgical ablation of ventricular tachycardia with sequential map-guided subendocardial resection: electrophysiologic assessment and long-term follow-up. *Circulation* 1988;77:131–141.
41. Kaltenbrunner W, Cardinal R, Dubuc M, et al. Epicardial and endocardial mapping of ventricular tachycardia in patients with myocardial infarction. Is the origin of the tachycardia always subendocardially localized? *Circulation* 1991;84:1058–1071.
42. Littmann L, Svenson RH, Chuang CH, et al. Neodymium:YAG contact laser photocoagulation of the in vivo canine epicardium: dosimetry, effects of various lasing modes, and histology. *Lasers Surg Med* 1993;13:158–167.
43. Page PL. Surgical treatment of ventricular tachycardia. Indications and results. *Arch Mal Coeur Vaiss* 1996;89:115–121.
44. Pfeiffer D, Moosdorf R, Svenson RH, et al. Epicardial neodymium:YAG laser photocoagulation of ventricular tachycardia without ventriculotomy in patients after myocardial infarction. *Circulation* 1996;94:3221–3225.
45. Selle JG, Svenson RH, Gallagher JJ, et al. Surgical treatment of ventricular tachycardia with Nd:YAG laser photocoagulation. *Pacing Clin Electrophysiol* 1992;15:1357–1361.
46. Hargrove WC, Miller JM, Vassallo JA, Josephson ME. Improved results in the operative management of ventricular tachycardia related to inferior wall infarction: importance of the annular isthmus. *J Thorac Cardiovasc Surg* 1986;92:726–732.
47. Moran JM, Kehoe RF, Loeb JM, et al. Extended endocardial resection for the treatment of ventricular tachycardia and ventricular fibrillation. *Ann Thorac Surg* 1982;34:538–552.
48. Moran JM, Kehoe RF, Loeb JM, et al. The role of papillary muscle resection and mitral valve replacement in the control of refractory ventricular arrhythmia. *Circulation* 1983;68:154–160.
49. Landymore RW, Kinley CE, Gardner M. Encircling endocardial resection with complete removal of endocardial scar without intraoperative mapping for the ablation of drug-resistant ventricular tachycardia. *J Thorac Cardiovasc Surg* 1985;89:18–24.
50. Van Hemel NM, Kingma JH, Defauw JAM, et al. Left ventricular segmental wall motion score as a criterion for selecting patients for direct surgery in the treatment of postinfarction ventricular tachycardia. *Eur Heart J* 1989;10:304–315.
51. Nath S, Haines DE, Kron IL, et al. Regional wall motion analysis predicts survival and functional outcome after subendocardial resection in patients with prior anterior myocardial infarction. *Circulation* 1993;88:70–76.
52. Bourke JP, Gray J, Hilton CJ, et al. Identifying patients at low risk of death from cardiac failure after operation for postinfarct ventricular tachycardia. *Ann Thorac Surg* 1999;67:404–410.
53. Miller JM, Kienzle MG, Harken AH, Josephson ME. Subendocardial resection for ventricular tachycardia: predictors of surgical success. *Circulation* 1984;70:624–631.
54. Miller JM, Gottlieb CD, Hargrove WC, Josephson ME. Factors influencing operative mortality in surgery for ventricular tachycardias [Abstract]. *Circulation* 1988;78:44.
55. Hargrove WC, Josephson ME, Harken AH, Miller JM. Endocardial resection for ventricular tachycardia in 353 patients. (Abstract) *J Am Coll Cardiol* 1994;23:480A.
56. Miller JM, Gottlieb CD, Marchlinski FE, et al. Does ventricular tachycardia mapping influence the success of antiarrhythmic surgery? (Abstract) *J Am Coll Cardiol* 1988;11:112A.
57. DiMarco JP, Lerman BB, Kron IL, Sellers TD. Sustained ventricular tachyarrhythmias within 2 months of acute myocardial infarction: results of medical and surgical therapy in patients resuscitated from the initial episode. *J Am Coll Cardiol* 1985;6:759–768.
58. Miller JM, Marchlinski FE, Harken AH, et al. Subendocardial resection for sustained ventricular tachycardia in the early period after acute myocardial infarction. *Am J Cardiol* 1985;55:980–984.
59. Damiano RJ, Blanchard SM, Asano T, et al. The effects of distant potentials on unipolar electrograms in an animal model utilizing the right ventricular isolation procedure. *J Am Coll Cardiol* 1988;11:1100–1109.
60. Biermann M, Shenasa M, Borggrefe M, et al. The interpretation of cardiac electrograms. In: Biermann M, Shenasa M, Borggrefe M, et al, eds. *Cardiac mapping.* Mount Kisco, NY: Futura Publishing, 1991:11–34.
61. Anderson KP, Walker R, Fuller M, et al. Criteria for local electrical activation: effects of electrogram characteristics. *IEEE Trans Biomed Eng* 1993;40:169–181.

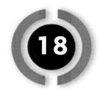

VENTRICULAR TACHYCARDIA SURGICAL TECHNIQUES
• • •

GERARD M. GUIRAUDON, GEORGE J. KLEIN, COLETTE M. GUIRAUDON

Surgical approaches to ventricular tachycardias first addressed manifest pathology (1) without comprehensive understanding of the underlying mechanism. Based on pathophysiology and guided by intraoperative mapping, direct approaches were attempted in the mid-1970s (2,3). Unfortunately, interventions on left-sided ventricular tachycardias were associated with severe side effects, which hampered the development and acceptance of the surgical techniques. The current surgical techniques are limited to a few selected patients. In this chapter, we review the history and contributions of surgical approaches to less invasive techniques, particularly catheter ablation (4). The chapter is organized around a series of theses that address specific experiences gained from surgical approaches to ventricular arrhythmias.

Ventricular tachycardia can be interrupted using interventions based on preoperative electrophysiologic testing and intraoperative cardiac mapping (5, 6). The initial experience was based on three patients operated on in 1973. One patient had an idiopathic dilated cardiomyopathy, and two had arrhythmogenic right ventricular dysplasia. An incision (i.e., ventriculotomy) performed at the earliest epicardial activation site during ventricular tachycardia interrupted the ventricular tachycardia in each of the three patients. The surgical rationale was similar to the one used in ablation of the atrioventricular accessory pathway in the Wolff-Parkinson-White syndrome (7). Although at that time our depth of knowledge was rather shallow, good fortune brought us success and the opportunity to advance.

◉ THE CONCEPT OF ARRHYTHMOGENIC SUBSTRATE

The area of myocardium located around the early activation during ventricular tachycardia and the area where slow conduction or delayed or fragmented activation (i.e., fractionation) were recorded were identified as the part of myocardium where the reentrant mechanism was located. These areas were defined as arrhythmogenic (8).

Cardiac mapping was a critical guide to identifying the arrhythmogenic substrate. Cardiac mapping could be carried out epicardially or endocardially. Unfortunately, technology and intraoperative conditions for mapping severely limited the quality of information obtained. It was exceptionally possible to pinpoint the reentrant loop with its necessary slow conduction segment. Mapping essentially identified an area around the earliest activation during the tachycardia or an area where abnormal activation was recorded.

Mapping, despite its limitations, was definitely established as a critical guide (9,10).

A better definition of the arrhythmogenic substrate was achieved. It was defined as the segment of ventricular myocardium necessary but not sufficient for the tachycardia to be initiated and sustained. The necessary segment of the reentrant loop is rarely anatomically delineated (e.g., a conducting bundle), but it is usually functionally defined. The link may have complex morphology, with ramifications associated with dead-end pathways or multiple vicarious pathways. These so-called necessary links associated with slow conduction are found mostly in pathologic myocardium that exhibits a nonhomogeneous structure with an excess of fibrosis or other connective tissue and a disarray of myocardial cells or bundles. The anatomy of the substrate can be viewed at the microscopic and macroscopic levels. At the microscopic level, the anatomic substrate appears complex and small. Analysis at the macroscopic level shows that the slow conduction pathway appears unique and has the form of a simple channel (figure-of-eight model [11]) and that the greater the mass of pathologic tissue, the greater is the arrhythmogenicity (12). This is particularly true for the infarct scar and for arrhythmogenic right ventricular dysplasia.

Arrhythmogenicity varies over time. The pathology can be progressive and can be modified by other factors. The other factors, which are included with nonnecessary and nonsufficient factors, may involve the rest of the ventricles, the autonomic nervous system, the blood supply (i.e., coronary artery disease), and various other factors. These factors can be major determinants in setting the condition for arrhythmias to initiate or sustain. Arrhythmogenicity is not confined to the substrate as defined earlier (13). Identification and localization of the substrate can be achieved by using electrophysiologic testing, anatomic landmarks, or both.

⊙ THERAPEUTIC TRIAD: THE TARGET, THE BULLET, AND THE GUN

Our experience with surgery for arrhythmias helped us to understand the anatomy of every therapeutic intervention, which reconciles three elements: the target, the bullet, and the gun (14–16).

The target is the arrhythmogenic substrate and based on the documented pathophysiology of disease or symptoms to be addressed. For ventricular tachycardias, the target is not discrete and nonprogressive, as in the atrioventricular accessory connection of the Wolff-Parkinson-White syndrome. The target is elusive and multiple, with vicarious targets at different sites. The target is difficult to localize with certainty using the current technologies.

The bullet is the physical agent aimed at neutralizing the target. Because of the pathophysiology and the absence of a discrete target, large "bullets" were used to neutralize as large a target as possible. Two rationales for interventions were described:

1. Ablation aims at neutralizing a certain mass of myocardium and uses incision, excision, or modification of targeted tissue by various energies, such as cryoablation, radiofrequency current, microwave energy, and laser energy (2,3).
2. Exclusion aims at confirming the arrhythmia mechanism within a large substrate when the substrate is too large to be resected or ablated without severe compromise of cardiac function (2,17).

The gun is the way to deliver the bullet on target. There are many methods of delivery. Cardiac interventions consist of surgery and catheter ablation.

The surgical route for ventricular arrhythmia, especially the ones associated with coronary artery disease, requires a number of steps: general anesthesia with tracheal intubation, median sternotomy, cardiac mapping used to delineate the substrate, cardiopulmonary bypass, aortic cross-clamping with concomitant myocardial preservation, and left ventriculotomy. At that point, the management of the substrate (i.e., bullet) can be delivered according to rationale and surgical technique. Each step, including the management of substrate, is associated with inherent risks (18,19). The overall risk is the summation of each element of risk.

Surgical risk was less for patients with arrhythmogenic right ventricular dysplasia, because aortic cross-clamping was not used, and essentially, the left ventricle was left intact. Side effects are consequences that do not affect the target. This definition showed us that most of the surgical delivery meets the definition of side effect and is associated with major mortality and morbidity. A poorly defined target is associated with the risk of undue collateral damage to the myocardium, postoperative left ventricular dysfunction, and death. Unfortunately, less invasive techniques could not be delineated for the Wolff-Parkinson-White syndrome, for example.

ARRHYTHMOGENIC RIGHT VENTRICULAR DYSPLASIA

Although surgery for control of ventricular tachycardia associated with arrhythmogenic right ventricular dysplasia was limited to very few patients, the surgical experience with arrhythmogenic right ventricular dysplasia has made dramatic contributions to the understanding of ventricular tachycardia mechanism and the associated substrate. The rationales for surgical "ablation" and exclusion were initially developed for and applied to patients with arrhythmogenic right ventricular dysplasia (2,17).

Arrhythmogenic right ventricular dysplasia is a recently identified clinical entity (20). The lesions involve the right ventricular free wall and, to a lesser extent, the left ventricle. The right ventricular free wall is dilated, and the patient presents with large, dome-shaped bulges over the infundibulum, apex, and basal portion of the inferior right ventricular wall. These bulging areas are akinetic or dyskinetic. Right ventricular trabeculations are increased in size and number. The subepicardial fat is abundant, and the myocardium is infiltrated or replaced by fat. This fatty infiltration gives the myocardium its characteristic appearance. Microscopic examination shows fatty infiltration and hypertrophy or degeneration of myocardial cells. Patchy subendocardial fibrosis may be observed.

Well-recognized clinical characteristics make identification of the disease easy. Surgery for arrhythmogenic right ventricular dysplasia has evolved over time. From 1973 through 1981, we operated on 12 patients with problematic, drug-resistant tachycardias (3). Discrete ventriculotomy and resection at the site of epicardial breakthrough (i.e., origin) of ventricular activation during ventricular tachycardia, at the site of late diastolic activation during sinus rhythm (i.e., arrhythmogenic area), or at both sites were performed. There were no intraoperative complications. All patients were discharged free of tachycardia. During long-term follow-up (mean, 36 months), five patients had recurrences. In two patients, tachycardias were not problematic and were not treated. Longterm recurrence of tachycardia probably was associated with the large amount of abnormal right ventricular wall left intact. Consequently, the entire right ventricular wall was isolated after 1981 (17). Since then, we have carried out a right ventricular free wall disconnection in 10 patients (21). Surgery was indicated for patients failing nonsurgical electrophysiologic interventions. One patient died perioperatively of malignant hyperthermia. One patient had early recurrence of left ventricular tachycardia. During long-term follow-up, three patients with a low left ventricular ejection fraction preoperatively (0.44, 0.35, 0.30) died of congestive heart failure 5 months, 3 years, and 11 years postoperatively. The six other patients with good left ventricular function had excellent control of arrhythmia with preserved cardiac function.

Right ventricular free wall disconnection for arrhythmogenic right ventricular dysplasia is feasible and associated with long-term good results in selected patients (22,23), as corroborated by others' experience. Our experience suggests that patient selection is essentially based on left ventricular function. A normal left ventricular ejection fraction implies that the left ventricle is not involved in the pathologic process and that good cardiac function and arrhythmia control can be anticipated postoperatively. Right ventricular free wall disconnection is confined to a small number of patients with preserved left ventricular function after well-documented failure of nonsurgical electrophysiologic interventions.

VENTRICULAR TACHYCARDIAS AFTER ACUTE MYOCARDIAL INFARCTION: THE ELUSIVE TARGET

In the 1970s, attempted surgical approaches to ventricular tachycardia after acute myocardial infarction were based on a rationale similar to the one used successfully for arrhythmogenic right ventricular dysplasia. It was anticipated that cardiac mapping would be an effective guide for surgery and that interrupting ventricular tachycardia would prolong life. These assumptions were made without a correct appreciation of the magnitude of myocardial pathology, complexity of substrate, and associated left ventricular dysfunction.

Epicardial mapping failed to provide reliable guidance, but at least indicated that the arrhythmogenic substrate was endocardial, and that the endocardium should be mapped (8). Unfortunately, failure to interrupt the tachycardia after epicardial mapping was blamed on mapping instead of the mapper (i.e., blame the messenger), and the pursuit of experience using endocardial mapping was stalled.

Surgical pathology documented that the lesions were mostly endocardial and that the endocardial fibrosis was a discrete landmark for subendocardial lesions (24,25). This series of attempted map-guided interventions was productive and allowed us to describe the first direct surgical approach to ventricular tachycardias after acute myocardial infarction based on exclusion of the entire potentially arrhythmogenic myocardium—the border zone identified by the endocardial fibrosis. The encircling endocardial ventriculotomy was based on, but did require, mapping guidance at the time of surgery (24). Shortly thereafter, Josephson and his colleagues in Philadelphia described a more limited endocardial approach based on intraoperative mapping (26). In the following decades, the acceptance of surgery as a safe and effective therapeutic system was hampered by the complexity of the substrate and inherent mismatch between target and bullet and by the severe side effects associated with surgical techniques on left ventricular function.

The dilemma was compounded by the fact that the patients with resistant, life-threatening ventricular arrhythmias usually presented with associated severe left ventricular dysfunction. The less invasive interventions used to control ventricular arrhythmias, such as transvenous implantable cardioverter-defibrillators (ICDs), confirmed the initial hypothesis that surgical approaches failed to document: control of ventricular arrhythmias in patients with significant left ventricular dysfunction prolongs life, as shown in the Multicenter Automatic Defibrillator Implantation Trial (MADIT) and Antiarrhythmics Versus Implantable Defibrillators (AVID) trials (27,28). In cardiac physiology, pacing and pumping are two sides of the same coin, with potentially equal value. Pacing (rhythm) cannot be restored at the expense of pumping.

Status of Surgery for Ventricular Tachycardia after Acute Myocardial Infarction

Surgery for ventricular arrhythmia has declined dramatically in the recent years. Two surgical papers were eulogies in praise of direct surgery for ventricular tachycardias associated with coronary artery disease (29,30), mourning the disappearance of referrals. Surgery for ventricular tachycardia never really developed. The number of patients operated on was negligible compared with the patient population. The most active centers rarely performed more than 10 operations per year.

The advent of nonsurgical interventions is the accepted reason for the decline. Better, less invasive, more effective interventions (i.e., ICD, catheter ablation, and antiarrhythmic drugs) were designed to control arrhythmia. Better prevention of arrhythmia was associated with aggressive management of acute coronary artery thrombosis to avoid myocardial necrosis. The patient population characteristics changed, and therefore the management approach changed. Surgical indications for ventricular tachycardia are governed by an imperative *no-no rule*: no mortality; no failure to control the arrhythmia.

Patient Selection

Appropriate patient selection designed to avoid surgical mortality has been exemplified by van Hemel and colleagues (31,32). Using the left ventricular score system of the Coronary Artery Surgery Study (CASS), they were able to operate on more than a hundred patients without a mortality. Arrhythmia surgery can be safely carried out if three or more of the nine segments identified on the left and right anterior oblique views are contracting normally. Other investigators have successfully selected patients using similar methods such as excess ejection fraction (33) or center-line chord motion analysis (34). This patient population with preserved left ventricular function has a low surgical risk but also good long-term survival, whatever the therapy (35).

Amiodarone has been suggested as a risk factor. In one retrospective study, Mickleborough reported that amiodarone was the only cause of death (36). Although consistent with other experience, these results remained questionable because large surgical series using amiodarone preoperatively in large doses did not report any excessive morbidity or mortality (37).

Criteria for successful surgical ablation of arrhythmias are not well defined and vary from one series to another. Monomorphic sustained ventricular tachycardia of one of two morphologies associated with a discrete arrhythmogenic scar (e.g., aneurysm) are ideal indicators. The site of origin of the tachycardia and the location of the infarct scar are associated with inconsistent results. A septal origin is reported to be difficult (33) or easy (38) to ablate. The inferior wall location is reported as a risk for failure (33) or not (38).

Surgical techniques deal with two issues: value of intraoperative mapping and best ablative techniques associated with minimal damages to contracting myocardium and left ventricular function. Intraoperative mapping functions as a guide for surgical ablation and as a research tool to retrospectively analyze surgical failures or explore pathophysiology of the scar. As a research tool, comprehensive intraoperative mapping has dramatically contributed to basic and applied science, such as identification of epicardial breakthrough in inferior scars (38) or the understanding of activation of deep septal origin of the tachycardias (37) or subendocardial arrhythmogenic pathways (39). As an intraoperative guide, cardiac mapping has significant limitations. Cardiac mapping is not feasible in all patients and, when feasible, is frequently incomplete. Promoters of intraoperative mapping explain surgical failure to control the arrhythmia by incomplete or misleading mapping (40). Some investigators did not observe any improvement in arrhythmia control after starting to use a more sophisticated mapping system. Rokkas reported a new way to map ventricular tachycardia using multiplexed electrodes, epicardial sock, and an endocardial balloon, using potential distribution mapping that can be available to the surgical team almost on line (41). In simple terms, better results are associated with extensive, comprehensive mapping when multiple tachycardia morphologies associated with multiple sites of origin are identified, and extensive ablation of arrhythmogenic scar is performed accordingly (42): the more ablation, the better. All potentially arrhythmogenic tissues should be ablated as long as it can be done without damaging normal myocardium with or without supporting mapping data. This concept has been successful at our institution (43,44) and many others (45,46). This approach is used successfully when mapping is not feasible or deemed incomplete (32,33,34,38,43).

The ablative technique did not seem critical. Excision, incision, cryoablation, and laser photocoagulation seem to accomplish similar goals and could be used selectively or in combination. Moosdorf documented that laser photocoagulation can be applied successfully epicardially on the closed, beating heart (47). If confirmed, these results can encourage epicardial laser ablation of ventricular tachycardias using minimally invasive techniques (e.g., VATS).

Does refinement in patient selection allow surgical ablation to fare better? All surgical series are cohort descriptive studies. However, the 5-year survival and freedom from arrhythmia rates do not seem dramatically better than with other interventions. Van Hemel and colleagues published a randomized study comparing antiarrhythmic drug and surgical therapy (40). They could not document any advantage to the surgical technique that was associated with a higher risk of total cardiac death. Despite inherent limitations, this remarkable study by a well-experienced center shows that surgical ablation, even in very selected patient population with preserved left ventricular function, is not a first choice, but just an option.

Current Approach

Patients with ventricular arrhythmia associated with coronary artery disease must have complete assessment in terms of cardiac functional anatomy and electrophysiology. When indicated, myocardial revascularization must be performed. This has been documented to decrease arrhythmic death (48), especially in patients with ischemia induced arrhythmia (49). In a small group of patients, concomitant ablation of ventricular arrhythmia can be carried out if it is associated with no additional risk and deemed highly effective. After successful revascularization, patients are reassessed, and the appropriate electrophysiologic intervention is selected. Surgical ablation of arrhythmia in patients who do not require coronary artery bypass grafting may be indicated in very few selected patients.

CONCLUSIONS

Future surgical approaches can be anticipated. At the minimalist level, video-assisted thoracic surgery combined with sophisticated robotic technologies may allow a safe delivery of ablative energy on target with minimal side effects (50,51). At the maximalist level, mechanical cardiac assist, including permanently implanted left ventricular assist devices (52–55), may describe a fundamentally different rationale. Prolonged mechanical assist can be associated with myocardial remodeling, reversal of myocardial lesions, and restoration of left ventricular contractility. Concomitant remodeling of substrate can disable current arrhythmogenic substrate, or arrhythmogenic substrate can be ablated safely under mechanical assist using less invasive approaches such as catheter ablation.

REFERENCES

1. Couch OA. Cardiac aneurysm with ventricular tachycardia and subsequent excision of aneurysm. *Circulation* 1959;20:251–253.
2. Guiraudon G, Frank R, Fontaine G. Interet des cartographies dans le traitement chirurgical des tachycardies ventriculaires rebelles recidivantes. *Nouv Presse Med* 1974;3:321.
3. Guiraudon G, Fontaine G, Frank R, et al. Surgical treatment of ventricular tachycardia guided by ventricular mapping in 23 patients without coronary artery disease. *Ann Thorac Surg* 1981; 32:439–450.
4. Morady F, Frank R, Kou WH, et al. Identification and catheter ablation of a zone of slow conduction in the reentrant circuit of ventricular tachycardia in humans. *J Am Coll Cardiol* 1988; 11:775–782.
5. Boineau JP, Cox JL. Slow ventricular activation in acute myocardial infarction: a source of reentrant premature ventricular contractions. *Circulation* 1973;48:702.
6. Fontaine G, Guiraudon G, Frank R, et al. Epicardial mapping and surgical treatment in 6 cases of resistant ventricular tachycardia not related to coronary artery disease. In: Wellens HJJ, Lie KL, Janse MJ, eds. *The conduction system of the heart.* Leiden: HE Stenfert Korese, 1976:545.
7. Guiraudon GM. Surgical treatment of Wolff-Parkinson-White syndrome—a retrospectroscopic view. *Ann Thorac Surg* 1994; 58:1254–1261.
8. Fontaine G, Guiraudon G, Frank R, et al. Stimulation studies and epicardial mapping in ventricular tachycardia: study of mechanisms and selection for surgery. In: Kulbertus HE, ed. *Reeintrant arrhythmias.* Lancaster, UK: MTP Press, 1977: 334–350.
9. Klein GJ, Ideker RE, Smith WM, et al. Epicardial mapping of the onset of ventricular tachycardia initiated by programmed stimulation in the canine heart with chronic infarction. *Circulation* 1979;60:1375–1384.
10. de Bakker JMT, Janse MJ, Van Capele FJL, Durrer D. Endocardial mapping by simultaneous recording of endocardial electrograms during cardiac surgery for ventricular aneurysm. *J Am Coll Cardiol* 1983;2:947–953.
11. El Sherif N, Mehra R, Gough WB, Zeiler RH. Ventricular activation pattern of spontaneous and induced ventricular rhythms in canine one-day-old myocardial infarction: evidence of focal and reentrant mechanisms. *Circ Res* 1982;51:152–166.
12. Blanchard SM, Walcott GP, Wharton JM, Ideker RE. Why is catheter ablation less successful than surgery for treating ventricular tachycardia that results from coronary artery disease? *Pacing Clin Electrophysiol* 1994;17[Pt I]:2315–2335.
13. Coumel P. Cardiac arrhythmias and the autonomic nervous system. *J Cardiovasc Electrophysiol* 1993;4:338.
14. Guiraudon GM, Klein GJ, van Hemel N, et al. Atrial flutter: lessons from surgical interventions (musing on atrial flutter mechanism). *Pacing Clin Electrophysiol* 1996;19[Pt II]: 1933–1938.
15. Guiraudon GM. Surgery without interventions? *Pacing Clin Electrophysiol* 1998;21[Pt II]:2160–2165.
16. Guiraudon GM. Musing while cutting. *J Card Surg* 1998;13: 156–162.
17. Guiraudon GM, Klein GJ, Gulamhusein S, et al. Total disconnection of right ventricular free wall: surgical treatment of right ventricular tachycardia associated with right ventricular dysplasia. *Circulation* 1983;67:463–470.
18. Kirklin JW. The science of cardiac surgery. *Eur J Cardiothorac Surg* 1990;4:63–71.
19. Buckberg GD. Myocardial protection: an overview. *Semin Thorac Cardiovasc Surg* 1993;5:98–106.
20. Marcus FI, Fontaine GH, Guiraudon G, et al. Right ventricular dysplasia: a report of 24 cases. *Circulation* 1982;65:384.
21. Guiraudon GM, Klein GJ, Guiraudon C, et al. Long term prognosis of patients with right ventricular free wall disconnection for arrhythmogenic right ventricular dysplasia: left ventricular ejection fractions as a marker of outcome. *Pacing Clin Electrophysiol* 1996;19[Pt II]:628.
22. Misaki T, Watanabe G, Iwa T, et al. Surgical treatment of arrhythmogenic right ventricular dysplasia: long-term outcome. *Ann Thorac Surg* 1994;58:1380–1385.
23. Doig C, Nimkhedkar K, Bourke JP, et al. Acute and chronic hemodynamic impact of total right ventricular disarticulation. *Pacing Clin Electrophysiol* 1991;14[Pt II]:1971–1975.
24. Guiraudon G, Fontaine G, Frank R, et al. Encircling endocardial ventriculotomy: a new surgical treatment for life-threatening ventricular tachycardias resistant to medical treatment following myocardial infarction. *Ann Thorac Surg* 1978;26: 438–444.
25. Mallory CK, White PD, Salgedo-Salgar J. The speed of healing of myocardial infarction. *Am Heart J* 1931;18:647.
26. Josephson ME, Harden AH, Horowitz LN. Endocardial excision: a new surgical technique for the treatment of recurrent ventricular tachycardia. *Circulation* 1979;60:1430–1439.
27. Moss AJ, Hall WJ, Cannon DS, et al, for the Multicenter Auto-

matic Defibrillator Implantation Trial investigators. Improved survival with an implanted defibrillator in patient with coronary disease at high risk for ventricular arrhythmia. *N Engl J Med* 1996;335:1933–1940.
28. The Antiarrhythmics Versus Implantable Defibrillators (AVID) investigators. A comparison of antiarrhythmic-drug therapy with implantable defibrillators in patients resuscitated from near-fatal ventricular arrhythmias. *N Engl J Med* 1997;337:1576–1583.
29. Page PL. Surgical treatment of ventricular tachycardia. *Arch Mal Coeur* 1996;89:115–121.
30. Selle JG. Reflections on definitive surgical treatment of postinfarction ventricular tachycardia. *Ann Thorac Surg* 1994;58:1287–1290.
31. Hemel NM van, Kingma JH, Defauw JAM, et al. Left ventricular segmental wall motion score as a criterion for selecting patients for direct surgery in the treatment of post-infarction ventricular tachycardia. *Eur Heart J* 1989;10:304–315.
32. Hemel NM van, Defauw JAM, Kingma JH, et al. Risk factors of map-guided surgery for postinfarction ventricular tachycardia. A 12-year experience [Abstract]. *Eur Heart J* 1992;13:1662.
33. Lee R, Mitchell JD, Garan H, et al. Operation for recurrent ventricular tachycardia. *J Thorac Cardiovasc Surg* 1994;107:732–742.
34. Nath S, Haines DE, Kron IL, et al. Regional wall motion analysis predicts survival and functional outcome after subendocardial resection in patients with prior anterior myocardial infarction. *Circulation* 1993;88:70–76.
35. Willems AR, Tijssen JGP, Van Capelle FJl, et al. Determinants of prognosis in symptomatic ventricular tachycardia or ventricular fibrillation late after myocardial infarction. *J Am Coll Cardiol* 1990;16:521–530.
36. Mickleborough LL, Maruyama H, Mohamed S, et al. Are patients receiving amiodarone at increased risk for cardiac operations? *Ann Thorac Surg* 1994;58:622–629.
37. Kawamura Y, Page PL, Cardinal R, et al. Mapping of septal ventricular tachycardia: clinical and experimental correlations. *J Thorac Cardiovasc Surg* 1996;112:914–925.
38. Selle JG, Svenson RH, Gallagher JJ, et al. Surgical treatment of ventricular tachycardia with Nd:YAG laser photocoagulation. *Pacing Clin Electrophysiol* 1992;15:1357–1361.
39. de Bakker JMT, van Capelle FJL, Jansen MJ, et al. Macroreentry in the infarcted human heart: the mechanism of ventricular tachycardia with a "focal" activation pattern. *J Am Coll Cardiol* 1991;18:1005–1014.
40. Hemel NM van, Kingma JH, Defauw JJAM, et al. Continuation of antiarrhythmic drugs or arrhythmia surgery after multiple drug failures: a randomized trial in the treatment of postinfarction ventricular tachycardia. *Eur Heart J* 1996;17:564–573.
41. Rokkas CK, Nitta T, Schuessler RB, et al. Human ventricular tachycardia: precise intraoperative localization with potential distribution mapping. *Ann Thorac Surg* 1994;57:1628–1635.
42. Miller JM, Kienzle MG, Harken AH, Josephson ME. Morphologically distinct sustained ventricular tachycardias in coronary artery disease: significance and surgical results. *J Am Coll Cardiol* 1984;4:1073–1079.
43. Guiraudon GM, Thakur RK, Klein GJ, et al. Encircling endocardial cryoablation for ventricular tachycardia after myocardial infarction: experience with 33 patients. *Am Heart J* 1994;128:982–989.
44. Thakur RK, Guiraudon GM, Klein GJ, et al. Intraoperative mapping is not necessary for ventricular tachycardia surgery. *Pacing Clin Electrophysiol* 1994;17[Pt II]:2156–2162.
45. Ostermeyer J, Gorggrefe M, Breithardt G, Bircks W. Direct, electrophysiology guided operations for malignant ischemic ventricular tachycardia. *Pacing Clin Electrophysiol* 1994;17[Pt II]:550–551.
46. Niebauer MJ, Kirsh M, Kadish A, et al. Outcome of endocardial resection in 33 patients with coronary artery disease: correlation with ventricular tachycardia morphology. *Am Heart J* 1992;124:1500–1506.
47. Moosdorf R, Pfeiffer D, Schneider C. Jung W. Intraoperative laser photocoagulation of ventricular tachycardia. *Am Heart J* 1994;127:1133–1138.
48. Kelly P, Ruskin JN, Vlahakes GJ, et al. Surgical coronary revascularization in survivors of prehospital cardiac arrest: its effects on inducible ventricular arrhythmias and long-term survival. *J Am Coll Cardiol* 1990;15:267–273.
49. Berntsen RF, Gunnes P, Liet M. Rasmussen K. Surgical revascularization in the treatment of ventricular tachycardia and fibrillation exposed by exercise-induced ischaemia. *Eur Heart J* 1993;14:1297–1303.
50. Benetti FJ. Cirurgia coronaria directa con bypass de vena safena sin circulation extracorporea o parada cardaca: communicacion previs. *Arg Cardiol* 1980;8:3.
51. Buffolo E, Andrade JC, Suzzi J, et al. Direct myocardial revascularization without cardiopulmonary bypass. *Thorac Cardiovasc Surg* 1985;33:26–29.
52. Bergsland J, Hasnan J, Lewin N, et al. Coronary artery bypass grafting without cardiopulmonary bypass—an attractive alternative in high risk patients. *Eur J Cardiothorac Surg* 1997;2:876–880.
53. Mancini Donna M, Beniaminovitz A, Levin Howard, et al. Low incidence of myocardial recovery after left ventricular assist device implantation in patients with chronic heart failure. *Circulation* 1998;98:2382–2389.
54. Rose EA, Moskowitz AJ, Packer M, et al. The REMATCH trial: rationale, design and end points. *Ann Thorac Surg* 1999;67:723–730.
55. Mussivand TM, Masters RG, Hendry PJ, Keon WJ. Totally implantable intrathoracic ventricular assist device. *Ann Thorac Surg* 1996;61:444–447.

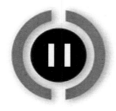

ADVANCES IN IMPLANTABLE CARDIOVERTER-DEFIBRILLATORS AND PACEMAKER THERAPY

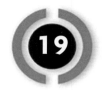

IMPLANTATION OF CARDIOVERTER-DEFIBRILLATORS IN THE ELECTROPHYSIOLOGY LABORATORY

• • •

ADAM ZIVIN, GUST H. BARDY

As the spectrum of indications for implantable cardioverter-difibrillator (ICD) implantation continues to widen to include primary prevention, techniques and devices that minimize the morbidity of implantation are increasingly critical in satisfying the goals of this therapy. ICDs implanted in the 1980s required a sternotomy or thoracotomy for placement of epicardial defibrillation patch electrodes and, because of size, abdominal placement of the generator. With the advent of transvenous defibrillation leads in the early 1990s, thoracotomy was no longer necessary, but device size still necessitated abdominal placement and subcutaneous tunneling of the lead from the subclavian region down to the generator. Because of the requirement for tunneling, adequate pain control with local anesthesia remained difficult, and most ICDs continued to be implanted in the operating room under general anesthesia.

Similar to the evolution of pacemaker therapy, the technology for defibrillators has progressed rapidly, and size has been reduced dramatically. Early pacemakers weighed 250 g, occupied 110 cc, and required abdominal placement by surgeons in the operating room, but the newest pacing devices are smaller than 30 g and 15 cc (1–3). In adults, nearly all current-generation devices are placed in the pectoral region by nonsurgeons. Advances in ICD pulse generator technology have reduced the pulse generator volume to 39 to 60 cc and weights to 75 to 115 g, depending on features and manufacturer (4,5). These features allow prepectoral implantation in most patients. The implantation techniques differ little from those of pacemaker implantation, making implantation in the electrophysiology laboratory or cardiac catheterization laboratory practical and safe. In this chapter, we describe the equipment, personnel, and techniques required for safe and effective implantation in the electrophysiology laboratory.

◉ BENEFITS OF THE ELECTROPHYSIOLOGY LABORATORY ENVIRONMENT FOR IMPLANTABLE CARDIOVERTER-DIFIBRILLATOR IMPLANTATION

Numerous published reports have demonstrated the safety of ICD implantation by nonsurgeons in the electrophysiology laboratory for abdominal and pectoral implants and under general anesthesia or local anesthesia with sedation (6–16). Implantation success rates and rates of acute and late complications are comparable to the published experience in the operating room (17,18).

The electrophysiology-catheterization laboratory offers several potential benefits compared with the standard operating room. First, all of the necessary equipment to implant an ICD is already present, including high-quality rhythm-monitoring equipment, external defibrillators, and hemodynamic monitoring systems. The fluoroscopic equipment is likely to be far superior to the portable C-arm usually found in an operating room. This is particularly helpful for thinner leads and positioning within the coronary sinus, when required. The nursing and ancillary support staff in the electrophysiology laboratory are familiar and comfortable with the techniques and equipment involved and with the management of patients with arrhythmias and congestive heart failure. It has been our experience that cardiologists' access to the operating rooms is often hampered by previously scheduled operative procedures that run over the allotted schedule, add-on surgical cases that take priority over elective cardiac device implantation, and a number of other logistic factors that result in frequent delays, patient and physician frustration, and increased hospitalization costs. These factors should not be taken lightly, given that each day a patient spends in the hospital on a telemetry-monitored ward increases hospital costs and the risk of nosocomial infections, medication errors, and other problems. For a procedure such as ICD implantation, which is relatively minor from a surgical standpoint, the electrophysiology laboratory with dedicated equipment and personnel is far more efficient, and the cost advantage of this approach has been demonstrated (9,15). The potential for cost containment may be one of the strongest arguments for ICD implantation in the electrophysiology laboratory.

Drawbacks to the electrophysiology laboratory are few. Laminar air flow, which is present in most operating rooms and absent in the typical electrophysiology-catheterization laboratory, can be adequately addressed and in a cost-effective fashion by directing air-conditioning flow across the surgical field. Visualization issues have also been raised as a possible drawback. However, very good portable surgical lights are available and, given the rather limited surgical dissection field necessary for the pectoral ICD implant, can be more than adequate.

SELECTION OF IMPLANTABLE DEVICES

ICD devices have been significantly reduced in size to the current 40- to 60-cc "can" size, which allows subcutaneous pectoral implantation in most patients (19,20). Pectoral ICDs have a number of advantages over abdominal ICD devices. The surgical procedure is less extensive, reducing risk and allowing implantation without general anesthesia, often as an outpatient procedure. Single-chamber unipolar devices can be used in combination with a single lead in the right ventricle (single or dual coil), simplifying implantation and minimizing hardware and the risk of subsequent lead failure. Given that ICD can size will continue to decrease over time, the techniques described here are limited to pectoral implantation using a subcutaneous or, in select circumstances, a subpectoral approach.

ELECTROPHYSIOLOGY LABORATORY NEEDS

Equipment

The basic equipment required in the electrophysiology laboratory is listed in Table 19-1. Cardiac monitoring systems capable of displaying multiple surface

TABLE 19-1 • BASIC EQUIPMENT REQUIRED FOR CARDIOVERTER-DEFIBRILLATOR IMPLANTATION IN THE ELECTROPHYSIOLOGY LABORATORY

Continuous electrocardiographic monitoring equipment
Two external defibrillators
Multipositional fluoroscopic unit
Noninvasive blood pressure monitoring equipment
Oxygenation saturation monitor
Suction apparatus
Laminar air flow or directional air conditioning unit
Surgical overhead lighting (portable)
Pericardiocentesis tray
Intubation tray
Portable oxygenation canisters
Electrocautery unit
Surgical instrument tray
Crash cart

electrocardiographic (ECG) leads are sufficient. A fluoroscopic system capable of multiple-angle views is advisable. Confirmation of lead placement is often enhanced with right anterior oblique, left anterior oblique, and anteroposterior projections. A ceiling-mounted or portable surgical lighting system is especially important. For cephalic dissection and for subpectoral implantation, it may be preferable to have at least two portable operative overhead lights, although this is not absolutely necessary. A backup external defibrillation system is critical for safe implantation of ICDs, and two external defibrillators should be in the room for connection to the patient before the procedure. A peripheral pulse oximeter is usually adequate for monitoring oxygen saturation, and we advocate end-tidal carbon dioxide (CO_2) monitoring with face-mask oxygenation for heavy, conscious sedation. For procedures performed under general anesthesia in the electrophysiology laboratory, a standard operating room ventilator cart is used. A complete "crash cart," including intubation tray and supplies for emergent pericardiocentesis and chest tube placement, also should be in the room. For most cases, noninvasive blood-pressure monitoring is adequate, although the capability for continuous invasive monitoring of arterial pressure and right heart pressures may be appropriate in rare cases.

The surgical equipment is standard, including sterile suctioning apparatus and electrocautery. A standard surgical tray usually has all the required surgical instruments. The minimal surgical tools are listed in Table 19-2.

TABLE 19-2 • BASIC SURGICAL INSTRUMENTS FOR USE IN CARDIOVERTER-DEFIBRILLATOR IMPLANTATION

Instrument	Use
Scalpels	
Number 10 blade	Skin incision
Number 11 blade	Cephalic venotomy
Forceps	
Adson	Skin closure
DeBakey	General use
Dietrich	Holding cephalic vein during venotomy
Retractors	
Weitlaner (small, medium)	General use
Richardson	Retracting skin for pocket formation
Army-Navy	General use
Rake (small, medium)	Skin retraction
Vein retractor	Cephalic dissection
Scissors	
Tenotomy scissors	Cephalic venotomy
Metzenbaum	General use, blunt dissection
Mayo	General use, suture
Clamps	
Mosquito	General use
Right angle	Placement of ties around cephalic vein
Towel clips	General use
Needle holders (short, medium)	Suturing
Suture	
Nonabsorbable braided suture	Anchoring leads and pulse generator
2-0 and 3-0 absorbable monofilament or braided suture	Pocket closure
Skin stapler, Steri-Strips	Skin closure

Personnel

The individuals involved in ICD implantation should be thoroughly familiar with all equipment and with the general laboratory environment. Besides the implanting electrophysiologist, support staff should include a circulating nurse and a dedicated nurse trained in analgesia whose sole responsibility is to monitor the patient's airway, oxygenation, and level of sedation. The circulating nurse is generally responsible for running the external defibrillator for rescue as directed by the implanting physician and for ensuring that the needed supplies and instruments are available. An additional scrub nurse can be helpful to assist with retraction and cephalic vein cutdown in difficult cases and can be one of the primary individuals responsible for maintenance of sterile procedure.

⊙ PREOPERATIVE PREPARATION OF THE PATIENT

Part of the preoperative assessment for pectoral implantation is evaluation of the patient's body habitus.

Attention should be directed at subcutaneous space, any pectoral or chest wall deformities that may present problems for placement and positioning of the device, and an estimation of the length of leads necessary. The problem of too much lead redundancy should not be overlooked, because the excess could affect pocket size and device fit, as well as increase the likelihood of lead fractures in subsequent years if kinks develop in the redundant lead. With recent-generation ICDs in the 40-cc range, subcutaneous placement is appropriate and desirable in most patients. In those with minimal subcutaneous tissue or significant cosmetic concerns, subpectoral generator placement is appropriate. Either approach can be performed safely without general anesthesia (21,22). We do not advocate subpectoral placement as standard practice because of the additional technical challenges subpectoral location presents at implantation and at the time of generator replacement.

Patients who are anticoagulated with warfarin should have three to four doses held before surgery to allow the INR to fall to 1.5 (23). For atrial fibrillation, prosthetic valves, or other conditions such as severely reduced left ventricular function without a history of thromboembolism, preoperative admission for heparin is not necessary (24). If not anticoagulated, the annual risk of thromboembolism in these patients is approximately 5% to 12%. Four to 7 days off anticoagulation subjects the patient to minimal incremental risk. These patients can have warfarin restarted the evening after the procedure, and heparinization, if used, should be held for 6 to 12 hours after implantation and restarted without a bolus to reduce the risk of pocket hematoma formation. In patients with recent peripheral thromboembolism due to atrial fibrillation, the estimated rate of recurrence is 0.5% per day in the first month if not anticoagulated, and these patients should receive periprocedural heparin (25,26). Similarly, the risk of recurrent venous thrombosis in the first month in non-anticoagulated patients is estimated at 40%, and at least postprocedural heparin is appropriate (24). In patients without recent thromboembolism, the value of postoperative heparinization has not been demonstrated, and it increases the risk of bleeding and large pocket hematomas, with their attendant risks for wound infection and incision dehiscence. The decision to heparinize should be made on a case-by-case basis, especially for chronically anticoagulated patients with prosthetic valves in the mitral position, history of stroke or peripheral embolism, or recurrent venous thrombosis. Particularly for patients with coronary disease, we do not routinely ask them to stop aspirin therapy in preparation for device implantation.

Before the patient arrives in the electrophysiology laboratory, the room should be regarded like any surgical room in terms of sterile procedure. All personnel entering the laboratory are masked with appropriate foot and head covers. If laminar air flow is not available, the air conditioning unit is activated to circulate air across the operative table. If necessary, the patient's chest should be shaved at the time the chest is prepped, preferably using clippers. Two pairs of adhesive defibrillation pads should be placed. One set is positioned anteroposteriorally, with the anterior patch placed over the sternum in the vicinity of V_4 and the posterior patch left of midline below the scapula. For pectoral implantation, this placement keeps the patches out the operating field and allows palpation of important anatomic landmarks. A second set of defibrillation patches is placed conventionally, with the anterior patch below and slightly lateral to the cardiac apex and the posterior patch over the right scapula. Two systems are required, not only for the uncommon event of technical failure, but for management of rare cases of ventricular fibrillation that are refractory to standard external defibrillation but may respond to combination or rapid, sequential external shocks (27). Except in the case of uncompensated heart failure with severe left ventricular dysfunction, we try to avoid invasive right heart monitoring because it can interfere with electrode positioning and carries risk.

The surgical site is then sterilely prepped, covered with iodophor, and draped with sterile towels and a sterile drape. Both sides of the chest should be prepped in the event of an inability to achieve venous access on the left side. The prepped area should be extended enough to allow quick access to the whole chest should emergent pericardiocentesis or thoracentesis be required.

All patients should receive prophylactic intravenous antibiotics. The value of preoperative prophylactic antibiotics has been demonstrated conclusively (28–31). The principle is to select an antibiotic with as narrow a spectrum of coverage as possible that covers the appropriate organisms. For pacemaker or defibrillator implantation, a single dose of intravenous antibiotic appropriate for gram-positive infections should be administered ideally 30 minutes to 1 hour, but not more than 2 hours, before the procedure (32, 33). This allows time for tissue concentration to reach a therapeutic level. Current recommendations call for a first-generation cephalosporin or, for patients with a history of an immediate hypersensitivity reaction β-lactam antibiotics, clindamycin or vancomycin. Cefazolin, with a half-life of 1.8 hours, can provide adequate coverage for the duration of a typical ICD implantation, and its efficacy for surgical prophylaxis has been demonstrated (34). If the procedure is complicated and extends beyond 3 hours, an additional dose of antibiotic should be given. With the emergence of vancomycin-resistant bacterial strains of *Enterococcus, Staphylococcus aureus,* and *Staphylococcus epidermidis,* the use of vancomycin should be reserved for patients who have significant allergy to other antibiotics, for those who have been recently treated as inpatients with penicillin-like drugs, or for hospitalized patients with a high incidence of methicillin-resistant *S. aureus* (MRSA) (32,35,36). Although commonly given, additional postoperative antibiotic administration is not of proven benefit and increases the likelihood of colonization with resistant organisms and infection with *Clostridium difficile* if continued for more than 24 to 48 hours (34,37). If postoperative antibiotics are given, a single dose 4 to 6 hours after completion is more than adequate.

⦿ ANESTHESIA

Conscious Sedation Versus General Anesthesia

Most patients who are stable enough to undergo ICD implantation can undergo the procedure safely with local anesthesia and sedation (8,14,38–41). Patients who are difficult to sedate adequately or who have obstructive sleep apnea or severe obstructive lung disease (COPD) may be easier to manage if mechanically ventilated, although the risks and complications of mechanical ventilation need to be considered. Local anesthesia for pocket formation and conscious to heavy sedation for ventricular fibrillation testing is usually adequate and safe; however, close attention by a dedicated nurse to airway management and to the level of sedation is imperative.

Although defibrillator implantation has traditionally been done under general anesthesia in the operating room or electrophysiology laboratory, numerous studies have demonstrated the feasibility of implantation with local anesthesia and light sedation, with heavier sedation used only for brief periods during defibrillation testing (8,13,15,16,38–42). This is not surprising given the similarity between implantation of defibrillators and implantation of pacemakers, which is rarely done under general anesthesia. Patient tolerance of the procedure is excellent, especially with the use of agents having an amnestic effect. Implantation time is not increased by the need for intermittent dosing of sedation, and total case time is reduced compared with cases done under general anesthesia because of elimination of ventilator setup, intubation, extubation, and frequently invasive hemodynamic monitoring required by the anesthesiologist (14). Although the safety of sedation by trained nurses has been demonstrated, no study has ever confirmed a safety benefit to anesthesia administered by an anesthesiologist (40,42). It has been our experience that complications related to fluid overload and the administration of vasopressors are more common when an anesthesiologist or nurse anesthetist is involved because of standard anesthesiology procedures and lack of familiarity with managing patients with severely impaired left ventricular function, arrhythmias, and chronic hypotension (43). This has been especially true for cases done under local anesthesia and sedation when the margin for error in fluid management is less. On the other hand, airway management and anesthetic administration is performed with greater ease and facility by a trained anesthesiologist. In the final analysis, it should be the implanting physician's preference that prevails in the choice between conscious sedation and general anesthesia.

For standard ICD implantation, we advocate conscious sedation similar to what is used for electrophysiologic studies or pacemaker implantation. This may include midazolam (Versed) and fentanyl, with local 1% lidocaine at the incision site. Typical starting doses for conscious sedation are 2 to 3 mg of midazolam given intravenously and 50 mcg of fentanyl. Dosing must be adjusted based on patient age, lean body weight, liver and pulmonary function, and clinical status. Additional doses of 1 to 2 mg of midazolam and 50 mcg of fentanyl, respectively, can be administered throughout the procedure as needed. Cumulative doses of 10 mg of midazolam and 250 mcg of fentanyl are rarely required. If fentanyl or other opioids are used, postprocedural nausea can be a problem, but premedication with intravenous administration of an antiemetic such as 0.5 to 0.625 mg of droperidol (Inapsine), 5 to 10 mg of prochlorperazine (Compazine), or 5 to 10 mg of metoclopramide (Reglan) is effective and contributes to a mild sedating effect (44–47).

In all but the most fragile patients, step-down defibrillation threshold testing (DFT) can be performed safely without general anesthesia, despite potential effects on cardiac hemodynamics (14,40). Immediately before ventricular fibrillation induction, methohexital (Brevital), propofol (Diprivan), or additional midazolam can be given if needed for deeper sedation. Methohexital, an ultrashort-acting barbiturate, is ideal for sedation before ventricular fibrillation induction but dosing is highly variable, and great care must be taken in its administration. An initial dose of 0.5 to 1.0 mg/kg body weight is recommended, with lower starting doses especially important in patients with poor left ventricular systolic function or who have received prior respiratory depressants such as midazolam. Duration of action is 5 to 7 minutes, and additional doses can be given if needed. Propofol, by virtue of its short duration of action, is also ideal for this purpose, and starting doses are similar. Etomidate has been used because of its lesser effect on blood pressure, but it causes involuntary muscle movements in 8% to 10% of patients, which may create confusing artifacts on the ECG monitor (41). Local hospital regulations may affect the choice of agent used; for example, propofol is often restricted to use by anesthesiologists or nurse anesthetists. The optimal level of sedation is one that leaves the patient with no recollection of the testing procedure but does not impair intrinsic respiration. Meticulous attention to patient respiration, blood pressure, and level of consciousness is essential throughout implantation and testing, and continuous monitoring of oxygen saturation and expiratory CO_2 is advocated. An Ambu bag should be immediately accessible in the event of apnea, and personnel trained in general endotracheal intubation and the appropriate equipment should be available at all times when employing deep sedation.

Our standard intraoperative testing protocol is to perform a limited step-down DFT determination with one induction at 10 J, and a second at 5 J, if the initial 10-J test is successful, and at 20 J if not. In most patients, this process can define a DFT of 10 J or less, allowing first-shock programming at 10 to 20 J and minimizing the number of inductions required. The lower the first energy, the faster the charge time and the lower the likelihood that the patient will lose consciousness before being shocked, an important issue for ICD patients who drive.

Anesthesia and Defibrillation Threshold Testing

Whether mode of anesthesia affects defibrillation thresholds is of concern for ensuring the reliability of backup external defibrillation and predicting the validity of DFTs determined at the time of implantation. Fortunately, clinical studies comparing general anesthesia with sedation concluded that the type of anesthesia has no significant effect on defibrillation threshold. When used for general anesthesia, acute and chronic (1 month) defibrillation thresholds did not differ between inhalational isoflurane and intravenous propofol (48). Similarly, when comparing general anesthesia with local anesthesia and sedation, no significant difference in implant DFT was found (14). Animal studies comparing the effect of pentobarbital, methohexital, and halothane on the DFT in 18 mongrel dogs found no significant effect of anesthetic agent on DFT (49). If lidocaine is used for local anesthesia, the issue of systemic absorption of lidocaine and its potential effect on the DFT needs to be addressed. Previous studies in patients undergoing electrophysiologic studies who had 1% lidocaine used as a local anesthetic found that significant systemic absorption occurs (50). Data for animals have shown that lidocaine in therapeutic to toxic levels may increase the defibrillation threshold, but this occurred only with pentobarbital anesthesia, not with halothane or chloralose, suggesting an interaction between barbiturates and lidocaine possibly related to alpha-adrenergic blockade (51,52). There are limited data, however, to suggest that lidocaine has a significant effect on DFT in humans, with the systemic levels resulting from local anesthesia usually insignificant, and consequently unlikely to be of clinical importance (53).

⊙ IMPLANTATION TECHNIQUE FOR THE PECTORAL IMPLANTABLE CARDIOVERTER-DEFIBRILLATOR

Although we advocate placement of the ICD generator in the subcutaneous region if possible, the subpectoral approach also is described for the few patients for whom this approach may be necessary. Whether a single-chamber (single-lead) or dual-chamber defibrillator is to be implanted, the approach is similar. The left side of the chest is preferable for unipolar "active can" systems because it provides a better shocking vector. However, right-sided implantation has been tested and usually results in adequate defibrillation thresholds (54).

The initial incision is made approximately 3 cm below the clavicle, extending from the midclavicular region to just above the deltopectoral groove (Fig. 19-1). Alternatively, the incision can be made over

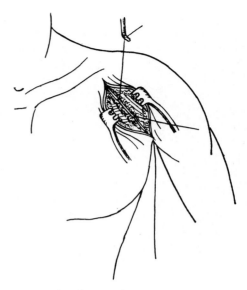

FIGURE 19-2. The alternate location for the incision overlies the deltopectoral groove. This facilitates exposure of the cephalic vein while allowing subclavian vein puncture if needed. The pocket should be made medial to the incision to keep the generator out of the shoulder joint.

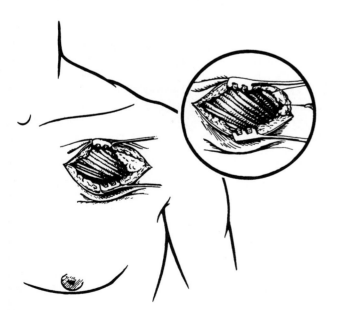

FIGURE 19-1. The initial incision for placement of a pectoral defibrillator can is made approximately 3 cm below the clavicle, extending from the midclavicle to the deltopectoral groove.

the deltopectoral groove to facilitate visualization and isolation of the cephalic vein if desired (Fig. 19-2). Use of the cephalic vein is recommended as a means to avoid crush injury to the lead from a medial subclavian entry site that brings the lead through the costoclavicular ligament (55). The incision is carried down to the prepectoralis fascia, and the cephalic vein is identified using blunt dissection along the fat pad that overlies the deltopectoral groove (Fig. 19-2). Care must be taken in the dissection as the cephalic vein may lie superficially within the groove and can be associated with a small venous and an arterial plexus. After the vein is isolated, loose ties are applied distally and proximally around the vein. If a subclavian puncture is to be used instead of or in addition to cephalic access, it is performed at this point using a modified Seldinger approach, staying in the lateral one third of the subclavian vein. If subcutaneous generator placement is planned, the pocket can be made at this point. We prefer to make the pocket using electrocautery just above the prepectoralis fascia, because this approach minimizes bleeding and helps avoid subcutaneous hematoma formation.

After access is obtained, leads are placed. With light tension applied to the proximal tie of the cephalic

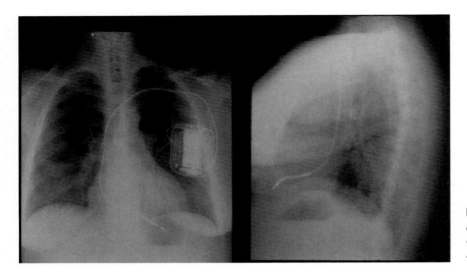

FIGURE 19-3. Posteroanterior and lateral chest radiographs of a unipolar defibrillator with the defibrillation lead in the right ventricular apex.

vein, a small incision (approximately one third of the width of the vein) is made in the vein with tenotomy scissors or a number 11 scalpel blade, and a lead is advanced and positioned in the right ventricular apex (Fig. 19-3). If difficulty is encountered advancing the lead directly into the vein, a guide wire can be placed first and an introducer sheath advanced over the guide wire in standard fashion. Lead sensing and capture are verified at this point.

The leads should be anchored in a position that minimizes the risk of lead fracture and interference with the field current when using the active can. Figure 19-4 shows the leads exiting the cephalic vein and entering the header block. The leads should be anchored to the prepectoralis fascia in such a way that a gentle curve exists at the exit site of the subclavian or cephalic vein. For the unipolar system, the leads should ideally be positioned clockwise along the edge of the can and enter the medially directed header block to minimize the length of lead coiled between the active can and chest wall.

After the leads are connected to the ICD header block, the generator can be positioned in the pocket. Care must be given to the lateral margin of the can, which should be at least 2 cm from the deltopectoral groove to avoid mechanical irritation of the shoulder region, which could produce long-term impairment in arm motion, especially abduction and internal rotation. A loose anchoring tie attached to the underlying muscle and device header is then used to avoid excessive movement of the can after the pocket is closed.

SINGLE LEAD ENTERING CEPHALIC VEIN

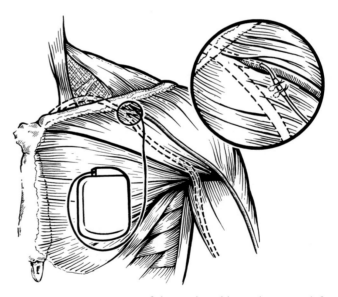

FIGURE 19-4. Position of the implantable cardioverter-defibrillator within the subcutaneous pocket with the lead entering the cephalic vein. The cephalic vein should be used whenever possible to minimize the risk of crush injury to the right ventricular lead in the first rib–clavicular space or by entrapment in the costoclavicular ligament. The lead should be anchored to the underlying muscle with two or three nonabsorbable 1-0 sutures around the Silastic anchoring collar. The device should be positioned with the header block oriented medially to avoid unnecessary lead contortion. (From Bardy GH, Raitt MH, Jones GK. Unipolar defibrillation systems. In: Singer I, ed. *Implantable cardioverter defibrillators.* Armonk, NY: Futura Publishing, 1994, with permission.)

If the subcutaneous space is insufficient, subpectoral placement of the generator can avoid undue tension along the incision that could lead to mechanical breakdown of the pocket. For the subpectoral approach, dissection is required down to the pectoralis fascia, where the fibrous band separating the inferior (sternal) portion of the pectoralis major muscle from the clavicular head can be identified (Fig. 19-5A). The two portions of the pectoralis major can then be separated using blunt dissection. In separating the two heads, gentle separation of a small portion can be done with blunt dissection followed by insertion of a finger between the two muscle heads and gentle separation along the fibrous sheath. Care should be taken to avoid tearing the fascia and exposing underlying muscle fibers, because this can lead to bleeding and formation of a pocket hematoma. The other important structure to identify is the thoracoacromial neurovascular bundle, which descends vertically on the underbelly of the pectoralis major muscle (Fig. 19-5B). Attempts should be made to avoid unnecessary damage to this structure when dissection is performed. After the muscle is separated, the submuscular space is accessible (Fig. 19-5C). Often, the neurovascular bundle can be dissected free to allow medial or lateral displacement, allowing entrance into the submuscular space without damage to the bundle. Exposed at this point are the intercostal muscles, the pectoralis minor muscle, the thoracoacromial neurovascular bundle, and ribs, whose periosteal tissues can serve as an anchoring site for the ICD (Fig. 19-5D). Figure 19-5E shows the ICD positioned beneath the pectoralis major muscle and connected to the right ventricular lead as it exits the cephalic vein. The pulse generator is oriented somewhat differently than with a subcutaneous insertion to better accommodate the lead as it descends through the pectoralis muscle between the clavicular and sternal muscle bundles. Ultimately, the direction of the connector block is best guided by the amount of redundant lead remaining and the natural curve of the lead.

Dual-Chamber and Biventricular Pacing Implantable Cardioverter-Defibrillators

Dual-chamber ICDs fall into two major categories: those capable of defibrillation in the ventricle and pacing and sensing in the atrium and those with atrial defibrillation as well. For the former, placement of the atrial lead is fundamentally no different from placement of an atrial pacemaker lead, and for this reason, the specific techniques are not discussed here (see Chapter 30). It is worth mentioning, however, that placement of the atrial lead is somewhat more critical to minimize the chance of sensing problems that may compromise the efficacy of dual-chamber algorithms designed to enhance tachycardia detection specificity and sensitivity. It is always preferable to place the atrial lead in the right atrial appendage if possible. If stable placement of the atrial lead in the appendage is not possible, careful attention should be paid to potential far-field R-wave sensing, particularly if the atrial lead is placed on the septum. This should be done before closing the generator pocket in the event that lead repositioning is necessary. Figure 19-6 shows posteroanterior and lateral chest radiographs for a recent-generation, dual-chamber ICD.

Biventricular Implantable Cardioverter-Defibrillators

Biventricular pacing represents the most recent attempt at achieving hemodynamic improvement in patients with severe congestive heart failure. Multicenter, randomized trials are underway to examine the value of biventricular pacing, which is sometimes referred to as *cardiac resynchronization*. Limited early data suggest that this therapy may be beneficial in patients with medically refractory congestive heart failure and intraventricular conduction delays, typically manifested as left bundle branch block (56,57). ICDs with biventricular pacing capability integrate this pacing modality into a dual-chamber ICD. Depending on the outcome of biventricular pacing trials and the outcome of ongoing primary prevention trials of ICD therapy, biventricular pacing ICDs may become increasingly common in patients with congestive heart failure and primary or secondary indications for ICD therapy.

Venous access for these devices is achieved in a standard fashion. Because biventricular ICDs require the placement of three leads—an atrial lead, a right ventricular defibrillation lead, and a coronary sinus

START OF SEPARATION OF CLAVICULAR HEAD OF PECTORALIS MAJOR FROM STERNAL PORTION OF PECTORALIS MAJOR

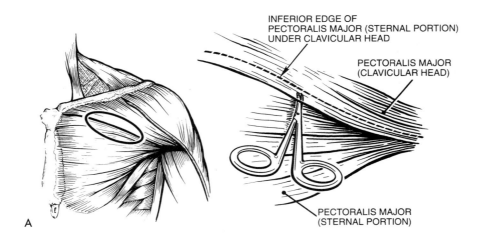

A

LOCATION OF SUBMUSCULAR POCKET

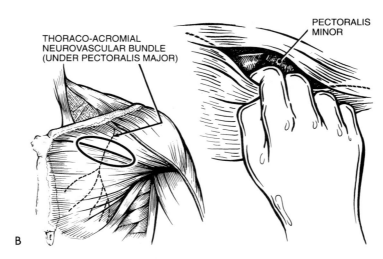

B

CROSS-SECTION OF SEPARATIONS OF PECTORALIS MAJOR

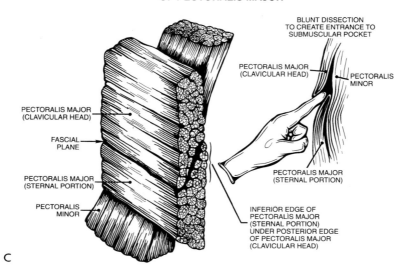

C

SUBMUSCULAR ANATOMY

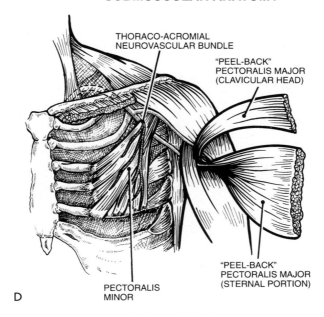

SUBMUSCULAR DEVICE PLACEMENT

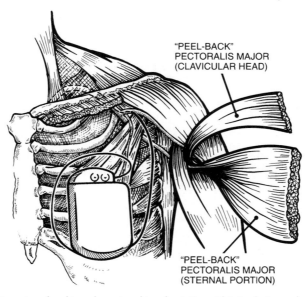

FIGURE 19-5. Steps involved in subpectoral implantation. This technique should be reserved for patients with inadequate subcutaneous tissue. **A:** After dissection down to the superficial pectoralis fascia, the fibrous band *(circled)* separating the sternal from the clavicular head of the pectoralis major can be identified. **B:** The course of the thoracoacromial neurovascular bundle *(dotted line)* lies under the pectoralis major. Attention must be paid to avoid damage to this structure during dissection. Damage to this nerve bundle can result in weakening and atrophy of the pectoralis major, with loss of forward power in the left upper arm. Blunt dissection using Metzenbaum scissors allows a finger to be inserted to create an opening between the heads of the pectoralis major for pocket formation. **C:** Overlap between the heads of the pectoralis major and its relationship to the pectoralis minor. The clavicular head overlaps the sternal head by 1 to 2 cm. Blunt dissection using the fingers should therefore be directed upward initially before creating the pocket deep to the sternal head of the muscle. **D:** The two heads of the pectoralis major have been reflected to show the underlying structures, including the pectoralis minor, neurovascular bundle, and ribs. **E:** The implantable cardioverter-defibrillator generator can be anchored to the periosteum of the ribs to prevent device migration. (From Bardy GH, Ralti MH, Jones GK. Unipolar defibrillation systems. In: Singer I, ed. *Implantable cardioverter defibrillators.* Armonk, NY: Futura Publishing, 1994, with permission.)

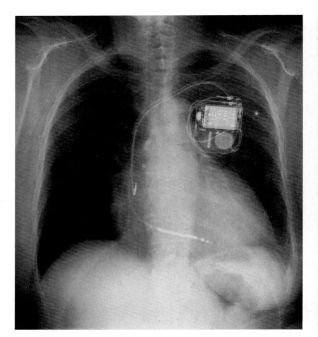 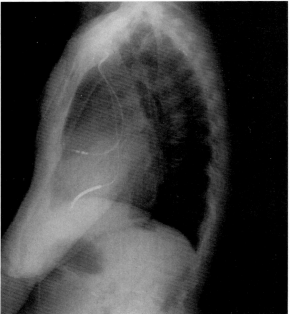

FIGURE 19-6. Posteroanterior and lateral chest radiographs of a dual-chamber implantable cardioverter-defibrillator. In the lateral view, the atrial lead is placed anterior in the atrial appendage, and the right ventricular (RV) lead is anterior in the RV apex.

pacing lead—it is worthwhile attempting cephalic and subclavian access in these cases. The right ventricular defibrillation lead should be placed by means of a cephalic approach if possible to minimize the potential for subclavian crush of the larger lead. The subclavian vein can then be used for introduction of the atrial and coronary sinus leads.

These devices add the additional complexity of left ventricular lead placement by means of the coronary sinus to the standard atrial and ventricular lead implantation process. For optimal resynchronization, the left ventricular lead needs to be placed as far laterally as feasible in one of the lateral or posterolateral branches of the coronary sinus. Coronary sinus angiography greatly facilitates identification of a suitable branch vessel. Guiding sheaths and balloon catheters specifically designed for this purpose are available in Canada and Europe and are undergoing clinical trials in the United States. After introduction of a guide wire through a subclavian or cephalic approach, a slitable guiding sheath is advanced to engage the coronary sinus ostium. Through the guiding sheath, a balloon-tipped catheter with a central lumen is advanced into the proximal coronary sinus for angiography.

The balloon is then gently inflated to occlude the ostium and a small amount of contrast medium injected to opacify the vessel. Coronary sinus angiograms, preferably using right anterior oblique and left anterior oblique projections, should be recorded for reference during lead positioning. The balloon is then deflated and the catheter withdrawn. The coronary sinus lead is advanced through the sheath and guided into one of the lateral branches using the angiogram as a road map. If no purpose-specific introducer sheath is available, it may be helpful to use a guiding sheath designed for coronary interventions or diagnostic coronary angiography to inject contrast into the coronary sinus. A Judkins right coronary catheter, an Amplats left coronary catheter, or a multipurpose coronary catheter usually suffices, depending on the implantation site (i.e., right or left shoulder) and the patient's cardiac anatomy. This angiographic catheter can then be exchanged over a wire for a peel-away introducer sheath. A longer peel-away sheath is recommended if available to provide additional lead support. The lead is guided into the coronary sinus with a stylet.

The exact technique for placement of these left ventricular pacing leads varies somewhat by manufac-

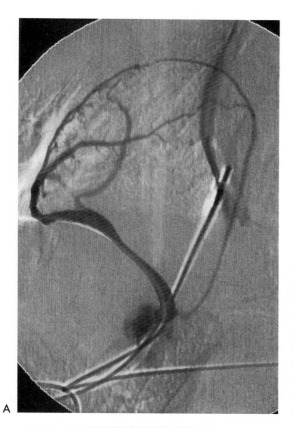
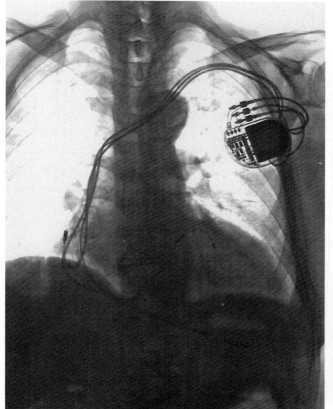
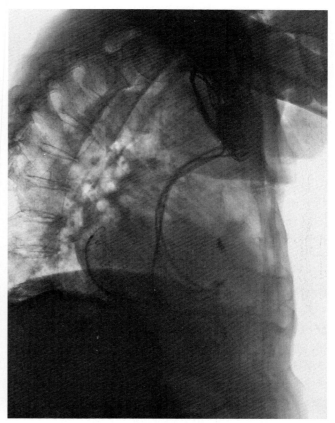

FIGURE 19-7. A: Coronary sinus angiogram is used to guide coronary sinus lead placement. The lateral or posterolateral branches allow for maximum separation between right ventricular (RV) and left ventricular (LV) leads. B: Posteroanterior and lateral chest radiographs of a biventricular pacemaker in place. The atrial lead is positioned anterior in the right atrial appendage, the RV lead in the RV apex (anterior in the lateral view), and the LV lead in a posterolateral branch of the coronary sinus, directed posteriorly in the lateral projection. In case of an ICD, a ventricular defibrillation and pacing lead is positioned in the right ventricle instead of an RV pacing and sensing electrode. (Courtesy of Dr. Daniel Gras.)

turer and lead design. Most have a preformed bend or curve at the distal end, which can be straightened with the stylet to facilitate "steering" the lead into proper position. When advancing the lead into one of the smaller branches, the stylet should be withdrawn slightly to soften the tip of the lead and reduce the chance of perforation. After the distal electrode is fully advanced within the branch vessel, the stylet is withdrawn further, allowing the lead to return to its natural bent position and flex against the vessel wall, gently anchoring the lead. Most pacing leads intended for use in the coronary sinus do not have a conventional helix or tined fixation mechanism. This is done to minimize lead diameter and reduce the chance for trauma to one of these small branches. The lack of a positive fixation mechanism makes removal of the stylet and introducer-guiding sheath a more delicate process, because lead dislodgement is comparatively easy. With one hand stabilizing the lead position at the venous insertion site at the patient's shoulder, the sheath is slit and withdrawn or peeled back slowly under continuous fluoroscopic visualization to ensure that the lead does not pull back out of the vessel during the process. The stylet is then gently withdrawn completely and the lead fixed to the underlying muscle using the anchoring sleeves. The atrial and right ventricular leads are placed in a standard fashion. Posteroanterior and lateral chest radiographs of a biventricular pacemaker are shown in Figure 19-7.

DFT testing of dual-chamber and biventricular pacing ICDs is done as described for single-chamber devices. The primary additional issues relate to sensing, especially crosstalk. This should be evaluated before defibrillation testing to identify potential problems that may result in arrhythmia underdetection or overdetection.

Defibrillation Threshold Testing

DFT testing should be performed before the pocket is closed. Device-based ventricular fibrillation induction is done using low-energy T-wave shock or a synthesized 50-Hz signal. A 10-J shock is used for initial defibrillation because this is effective in more than two thirds to three fourths of cases. We usually deliver the first rescue shock if needed from the ICD and subsequent shocks from the external backup defibrillators. A second induction successfully defibrillated with 5 J may allow programming of a lower-strength first shock (58,59). At this point, the pocket is flushed with antibiotic solution and closed in two or three layers according to physician preference.

OUTPATIENT IMPLANTATION

The safety and feasibility of outpatient implantation of pacemakers has been well documented (23,60–62). Given the relative ease of implantation with current-generation ICDs and the climate of cost containment, consideration of outpatient implantation should be made for patients with adequate personal assistance at home and if the indication for implantation permits.

Patients should be informed not to eat after midnight the night before the procedure and to take their usual medications (except warfarin) with sips of water. Patients should also be reminded that they will not be permitted to drive home and to arrange for transportation. Preoperative laboratories can be drawn and an intravenous line placed in the outpatient surgery or short-stay unit. After the procedure, most patients, in our experience, can be discharged home after 6 to 8 hours of postoperative observation.

The major issues of postoperative care are wound care and control of pain and nausea. Patient compliance is especially important for outpatient care, and detailed instructions need to be given regarding dressing, wound care, and signs of infection or hematoma formation, about which the implanting team should be notified. Preoperative antiemetics are helpful for control of nausea. Rare patients may require a small supply of oral or rectal antiemetics for use at home. We have found oral narcotics for 24 and 48 hours to be sufficient for pain control in most cases. Instructions to the patient to use the prescribed analgesic before maximal discomfort is reached is important for reasonably constant pain control. Within 48 hours, acetaminophen alone is usually adequate.

CONCLUSIONS

The rapid development of ICD technology in the past decade has made the devices similar to pacemakers in terms of implantation. All the equipment required for implantation is available in a well-equipped electrophysiology laboratory, the personnel are familiar with the management of patients with severe cardiac disease, and the safety of ICD placement under local anesthesia with sedation by electrophysiologists and trained nursing personnel has been well documented. The electrophysiology laboratory should be regarded as the first choice for ICD implantation, and many patients undergoing implantation for prophylactic indications can probably have the procedure performed on an outpatient basis without compromising safety or results.

REFERENCES

1. *Pacesetter affinity pacing system: device specifications*. Sylmar, CA: St Jude Medical, 1999.
2. *Kappa technical manual: device specifications*. Minneapolis, MN: Medtronic, 1999.
3. Parsonnet V, Manhardt M. Permanent pacing of the heart: 1952 to 1976. *Am J Cardiol* 1977;39:250–256.
4. *Ventak Mini IV technical manual: device specifications*. Minneapolis, MN: Guidant, 1999.
5. *Gem II: device specifications*. Minneapolis, MN: Medtronic, 1999.
6. Fitzpatrick AP, Lesh MD, Epstein LM, et al. Electrophysiological laboratory, electrophysiologist-implanted, nonthoracotomy-implantable cardioverter/defibrillators [See comments]. *Circulation* 1994;89:2503–2508.
7. Manolis AS, Vassilikos V, Maounis T, et al. Transvenous defibrillator systems implanted by electrophysiologists in the catheterization laboratory. *Clin Cardiol* 1997;20:117–124.
8. Schmitt C, Alt E, Plewan A, Schomig A. Initial experience with implantation of internal cardioverter/defibrillators under local anaesthesia by electrophysiologists. *Eur Heart J* 1996;17:1710–1716.
9. Stamato NJ, O'Toole MF, Enger EL. Permanent pacemaker implantation in the cardiac catheterization laboratory versus the operating room: an analysis of hospital charges and complications. *Pacing Clin Electrophysiol* 1992;15:2236–2239.
10. Strickberger SA, Hummel JD, Daoud E, et al. Implantation by electrophysiologists of 100 consecutive cardioverter defibrillators with nonthoracotomy lead systems. *Circulation* 1994;90:868–872.
11. Strickberger S, Niebauer M, Man K, et al. Comparison of implantation of nonthoracotomy defibrillators in the operating room versus the electrophysiology laboratory. *Am Heart J* 1995;75:255–257.
12. Trappe HJ, Pfitzner P, Heintze J, et al. Cardioverter-defibrillator implantation in the catheterization laboratory: initial experiences in 48 patients. *Am Heart J* 1995;129:259–264.
13. Stix G, Anvari A, Grabenwoger M, et al. Implantation of a unipolar cardioverter/defibrillator system under local anaesthesia. *Eur Heart J* 1996;17:764–768.
14. Stix G, Anvari A, Podesser B, et al. Local anaesthesia versus general anaesthesia for cardioverter-defibrillator implantation. *Wien Klin Wochenschr* 1999;111:406–409.
15. Tung RT, Bajaj AK. Safety of implantation of a cardioverter-defibrillator without general anesthesia in an electrophysiology laboratory. *Am J Cardiol* 1995;75:908–912.
16. van Rugge FP, Savalle LH, Schalij MJ. Subcutaneous single-incision implantation of cardioverter-defibrillators under local anesthesia by electrophysiologists in the electrophysiology laboratory. *Am J Cardiol* 1998;81:302–305.
17. Bardy G, Yee R, Jung W, Investigators for the active can. Multicenter experience with a pectoral unipolar implantable cardioverter-defibrillator. *J Am Coll Cardiol* 1996;28:400–410.
18. Frame R, Brodman R, Gross J, et al. Initial experience with transvenous implantable cardioverter defibrillator lead systems: operative morbidity and mortality. *Pacing Clin Electrophysiol* 1993;16:149–152.
19. Bardy GH, Hofer B, Johnson G, et al. Implantable transvenous cardioverter-defibrillators. *Circulation* 1993;87:1152–1168.
20. Bardy G, Johnson G, Poole J, et al. A simplified, single lead unipolar transvenous cardioversion-defibrillation system. *Circulation* 1993;88:543–547.
21. Jones G, Bardy G. Implantation of ICDs in the electrophysiology laboratory. In: Singer I, editor. *Interventional electrophysiology*, 1st ed. Baltimore: Williams & Wilkins, 1997:725–740.
22. Manolis AS, Chiladakis J, Vassilikos V, et al. Pectoral cardioverter defibrillators: comparison of prepectoral and submuscular implantation techniques. *Pacing Clin Electrophysiol* 1999;22:469–478.
23. Goldstein DJ, Losquadro W, Spotnitz HM. Outpatient pacemaker procedures in orally anticoagulated patients. *Pacing Clin Electrophysiol* 1998;21:1730–1734.
24. Kearon C, Hirsh J. Management of anticoagulation before and after elective surgery [See comments]. *N Engl J Med* 1997;336:1506–1511.
25. Kinch JW, Davidoff R. Prevention of embolic events after cardioversion of atrial fibrillation: current and evolving strategies. *Arch Intern Med* 1995;155:1353–1360.
26. Wolf PA, Kannel WB, McGee DL, et al. Duration of atrial fibrillation and imminence of stroke: the Framingham study. *Stroke* 1983;14:664–647.
27. Cohen T. Innovative emergency defibrillation methods for refractory ventricular fibrillation in a variety of hospital settings. *Am Heart J* 1993;126:962–968.
28. Bluhm G, Jacobson B, Ransjo U. Antibiotic prophylaxis in pacemaker surgery: a prospective trial with local or systemic administration of antibiotics at generator replacements. *Pacing Clin Electrophysiol* 1985;8:661–670.
29. Bluhm GL. Pacemaker infections: a 2-year follow-up of antibiotic prophylaxis. *Scand J Thorac Cardiovasc Surg* 1985;19:231–235.
30. Da Costa A, Kirkorian G, Cucherat M, et al. Antibiotic prophylaxis for permanent pacemaker implantation: a meta-analysis. *Circulation* 1998;97:1796–1801.
31. Mounsey JP, Griffith MJ, Tynan M, et al. Antibiotic prophylaxis in permanent pacemaker implantation: a prospective randomised trial. *Br Heart J* 1994;72:339–343.
32. Gyssens IC. Preventing postoperative infections: current treatment recommendations. *Drugs* 1999;57:175–185.
33. Page CP, Bohnen JM, Fletcher JR, et al. Antimicrobial prophylaxis for surgical wounds: guidelines for clinical care. *Arch Surg* 1993;128:79–88.
34. McDonald M, Grabsch E, Marshall C, Forbes A. Single-versus multiple-dose antimicrobial prophylaxis for major surgery: a systematic review. *Aust N Z J Surg* 1998;68:388–396.
35. Flores PA, Gordon SM. Vancomycin-resistant *Staphylococcus aureus*: an emerging public health threat. *Cleve Clin J Med* 1997;64:527–532.
36. Dellinger EP, Gross PA, Barrett TL, et al. Quality standard

37. Scher KS. Studies on the duration of antibiotic administration for surgical prophylaxis. *Am Surg* 1997;63:59–62.
38. Craney JM, Gorman LN. Conscious sedation and implantable devices: safe and effective sedation during pacemaker and implantable cardioverter defibrillator placement. *Crit Care Nurs Clin North Am* 1997;9:325–334.
39. Lipscomb KJ, Linker NJ, Fitzpatrick AP. Subpectoral implantation of a cardioverter defibrillator under local anaesthesia [See comments]. *Heart* 1998;79:253–255.
40. Natale A, Kearney MM, Brandon MJ, Safety of nurse-administered deep sedation for defibrillator implantation in the electrophysiology laboratory. *J Cardiovasc Electrophysiol* 1996;7: 301–306.
41. Pacifico A, Cedillo-Salazar FR, Nasir N Jr, et al. Conscious sedation with combined hypnotic agents for implantation of implantable cardioverter-defibrillators. *J Am Coll Cardiol* 1997; 30:769–773.
42. Geiger MJ, Wase A, Kearney MM, et al. Evaluation of the safety and efficacy of deep sedation for electrophysiology procedures administered in the absence of an anesthetist. *Pacing Clin Electrophysiol* 1997;20:1808–1814.
43. Tisdale JE, Patel RV, Webb CR, et al. Proarrhythmic effects of intravenous vasopressors. *Ann Pharmacother* 1995;29:269–281.
44. Carroll NV, Miederhoff P, Cox FM, Hirsch JD. Postoperative nausea and vomiting after discharge from outpatient surgery centers. *Anesth Analg* 1995;80:903–909.
45. Chestnut DH, Owen CL, Geiger M, et al. Metoclopramide versus droperidol for prevention of nausea and vomiting during epidural anesthesia for cesarean section. *South Med J* 1989;82: 1224–1247.
46. Trapp LD. An evaluation of droperidol for preventing nausea and vomiting after deep intravenous sedation for ambulatory dental surgery. *Anesth Prog* 1989;36:9–12.
47. Tripple GE, Holland MS, Hassanein K. Comparison of droperidol 0.01 mg/kg and 0.005 mg/kg as a premedication in the prevention of nausea and vomiting in the outpatient for laparoscopy. *Aana J* 1989;57:413–416.
48. Moerman A, Herregods L, Tavernier R, et al. Influence of anaesthesia on defibrillation threshold. *Anaesthesia* 1998;53: 1156–1159.
49. Gill R, Sweeney R, Reid P. The defibrillation threshold: a comparison of anesthetics and measurement methods. *Pacing Clin Electrophysiol* 1993;16:708–714.
50. Broudy D, Kron J, Li C, et al. Lidocaine as local anesthesia for electrophysiologic studies: blood levels and potential effects. *Circulation* 1983;68[Suppl. III]:274.
51. Natale A, Jones DL, Kim YH, Klein GJ. Effects of lidocaine on defibrillation threshold in the pig: evidence of anesthesia related increase. *Pacing Clin Electrophysiol* 1991;14:1239–1244.
52. Kerber RE, Pandian NG, Jensen SR, et al. Effect of lidocaine and bretylium on energy requirements for transthoracic defibrillation: experimental studies. *J Am Coll Cardiol* 1986;7:397–405.
53. Jones D, Klein G, Guiraudon G, et al. Effects of lidocaine and verapamil on defibrillation in humans. *J Electrocardiol* 1991;24: 299–305.
54. Flaker G, Tummala T, Wilson J, for the Worldwide Jewel Investigators. Comparison of right- and left-sided pectoral implantation parameters with the Jewel active can cardiodefibrillator. *Pacing Clin Electrophysiol* 1998;21:447–451.
55. Roelke M, O'Nunain SS, Osswald S, et al. Subclavian crush syndrome complicating transvenous cardioverter defibrillator systems. *Pacing Clin Electrophysiol* 1995;18:973–979.
56. Auricchio A, Klein H, Tockman B, et al. Transvenous biventricular pacing for heart failure: can the obstacles be overcome? *Am J Cardiol* 1999;83:136D–142D.
57. Kerwin WF, Botvinick EH, O'Connell JW, et al. Ventricular contraction abnormalities in dilated cardiomyopathy: effect of biventricular pacing to correct interventricular dyssynchrony. *J Am Coll Cardiol* 2000;35:1221–1227.
58. Strickberger SA, Daoud EG, Davidson T, et al. Probability of successful defibrillation at multiples of the defibrillation energy requirement in patients with an implantable defibrillator. *Circulation* 1997;96:1217–1223.
59. Strickberger SA, Man KC, Souza J, et al. A prospective evaluation of two defibrillation safety margin techniques in patients with low defibrillation energy requirements. *J Cardiovasc Electrophysiol* 1998;9:41–46.
60. Irwin ME, Gulamhusein SS, Senaratne MP, St Clair WR. Outcomes of an ambulatory cardiac pacing program: indications, risks, benefits, and outcomes. *Pacing Clin Electrophysiol* 1994;17: 2027–2031.
61. Huffman M. Pacemaker battery change: an outpatient procedure. *AORN J* 1988;48:733–739.
62. Belott PH. Outpatient pacemaker procedures. *Int J Cardiol* 1987; 17:169–176.

DEFIBRILLATION WAVEFORMS

JIAN HUANG, RAYMOND E. IDEKER

Since defibrillation was first performed, multiple waveforms have been studied for clinical application. Concerned mainly with the reduction of dysfunction, the external defibrillation waveforms evolved from alternating current (AC), monophasic, untruncated capacitor discharge, to Edmark and Lown (Fig. 20-1), to the currently used biphasic truncated capacitor discharge (Fig. 20-2). Because of size and weight restriction, the only feasible waveform for the implantable cardiovertor-defibrillator (ICD) has been a truncated capacitor discharge. Originally, the internal defibrillation waveform was monophasic, but it is now biphasic (Fig. 20-2) because the latter markedly reduces the defibrillation threshold, enabling the implantation of a totally transvenous lead system. Because the mechanisms underlying defibrillation are still being learned, selection of an optimal waveform for defibrillation has been empirical.

MORPHOLOGY OF WAVEFORMS

An electrical shock is thought to defibrillate by causing current to flow through the heart. The current is delivered by a defibrillation shock with a specific waveform. Because defibrillation requires voltages that are much greater than the voltage of the ICD battery, capacitors are used. The defibrillation waveforms can be characterized by tilt, duration, truncation, and number of phases. These characteristics are determined by the waveform generator and resistance of the electrodes and the body, with a variation from 20 to 80 Ω (1). The change of the values of any of these characteristics may have a marked effect on defibrillation efficacy.

Tilt and Duration of Waveforms

A waveform is generated when a capacitor is charged and then allowed to discharge through the resistance of the leads and the body of the patient. The waveform then decays exponentially until it is truncated. The tilt of a waveform is the percent decline of the voltage during the pulse.

$$\text{Tilt} = 1 - \frac{\text{trailing-edge voltage}}{\text{leading-edge voltage}}$$

The trailing-edge voltage (V) delivered is a function of the leading-edge voltage (V_0), the duration (d) of discharge, the resistance (R) of the defibrillation pathway, and the capacitance (C) of the defibrillation capacitor:

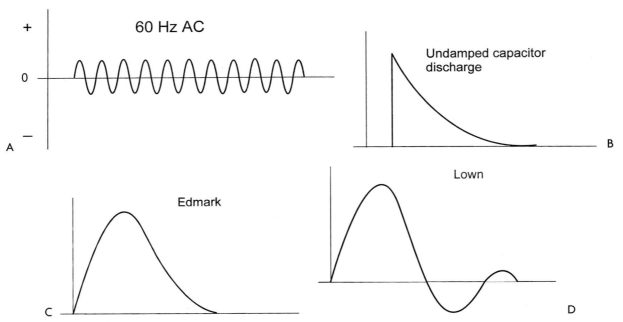

FIGURE 20-1. Transthoracic defibrillation waveforms. **A:** A 60-Hz alternating current (AC) waveform. **B:** Undamped capacitor discharge (exponential decay) waveform. **C:** Critically damped capacitor discharge (Edmark) waveform. **D:** Underdamped capacitor discharge (Lown) waveform.

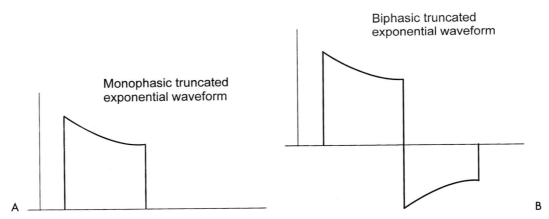

FIGURE 20-2. **A:** Monophasic, truncated, exponential waveform. **B:** Biphasic, truncated, exponential waveform.

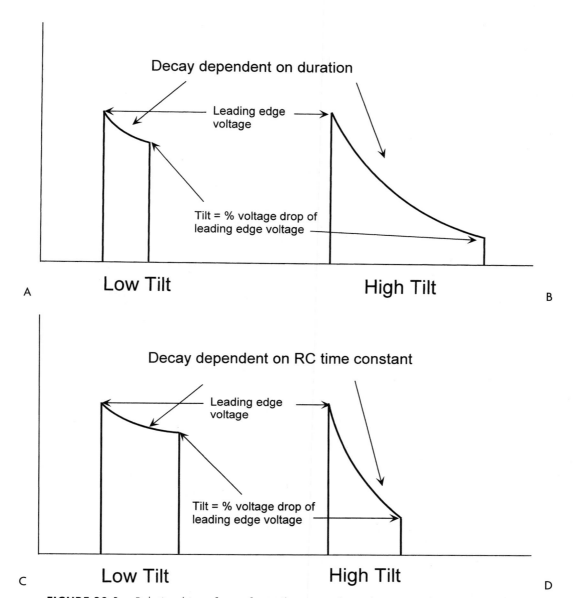

FIGURE 20-3. Relationships of waveform tilt to waveform duration and time constant.

$$V = V_0 \times e^{(-d/RC)}$$

A low defibrillation pathway impedance or a low capacitance leads to a steep decay of the waveform. If the waveform is not truncated, the voltage decays toward zero asymptotically. The waveform can be truncated after a predetermined pulse duration (i.e., fixed duration) or after the voltage has dropped by a predetermined percentage (i.e., fixed tilt). Tilt (T) and duration d of a pulse have the following relationship:

$$T = [1 - e^{(-d/RC)}] \times 100\%$$

The waveform time constant is a measure of how quickly the waveform drops from its initial voltage to 37% of its starting value and is equal to the capacitor size in the defibrillator multiplied by the resistance of the electrode-subject circuit.

Optimal waveform duration and optimal tilt are directly related to the defibrillation pathway resistance for a given individual. Waveform tilt can be altered by changing the duration of waveforms with the same time constant (Fig. 20-3A, B) or by changing the time constant without altering the waveform duration (Fig. 20-3C, D). Tilt can also be altered by changing the

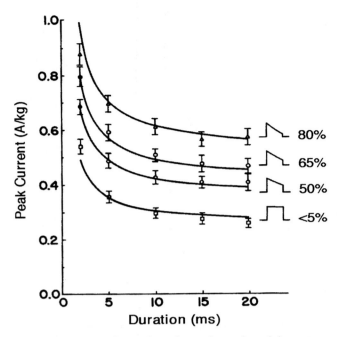

FIGURE 20-4. Relationship of waveform tilt and duration to the internal defibrillation threshold in dogs. The threshold peak current per unit of body weight (amps/kg) is compared with the waveform duration (msec). The percent tilt is given on the right side. The mean ± the standard error is given for each combination of tilt and duration (n = 30). (From Wessale JL, Boulard JD, Tacker WA Jr, Geddes LA. Bipolar catheter defibrillation in dogs using trapezoidal waveforms of various tilts. *J Electrocardiol* 1980;13:359–366, with permission.)

time constant and the waveform duration. Similarly, the waveform time constant and duration can simultaneously be altered in such a way that the waveform tilt remains constant (Fig. 20-4). The data in Figure 20-4 show that, for a constant tilt, the defibrillation threshold decreases as the waveform duration increases, and for a constant duration, the defibrillation threshold (DFT) decreases as the tilt decreases (2).

It is commonly thought that the long, low tail of the exponential waveform shown in Figure 20-1B refibrillates the heart (3). However, this result was for waveforms lasting 16 msec or longer and may not apply to the lower time constant waveform used in ICDs. The results from clinical studies show that the defibrillation threshold does not change significantly for monophasic waveforms with tilts ranging from 50% to 80% (4), but biphasic waveforms with 50% tilt required less energy for defibrillation than 40%, 65%, and 80% tilts (5). One study showed low DFTs resulted from biphasic waveforms using two separate and fully discharging capacitors (6).

Capacitors of the Defibrillator

Current ICDs contain capacitors of 90 to 150 μF. Theoretical models suggest that the stored-energy DFT is minimized when the time constant of the defibrillating waveform is close to the biologic time constant of the heart (7–9). The predicted optimal capacitance is as low as 30 to 50 μF. Smaller capacitance values lower stored energy and require higher leading-edge voltages than do larger capacitors to deliver the same energy (10). The effect of capacitance on DFT has varied in previous reports. Animal studies have shown that, over a wide range of capacitances (90 to 450 μF), stored energies needed at DFT did not differ significantly for low and medium defibrillation pathway resistances (11,12). Human crossover studies comparing this standard capacitance to smaller and larger capacitances have shown that, for lead systems with low defibrillation pathway resistances, current standard capacitances are close to the optimal capacitance with respect to energy. Smaller capacitances are possible for medium pathway resistances and better for high defibrillation pathway resistances (13–16). Larger capacitances had little influence on defibrillation threshold (17).

Biphasic Waveforms

Biphasic waveforms are created by switching the waveform polarity part way through the pulse so that the first part of the waveform is delivered with one polarity and the second part of the waveform is delivered with the opposite polarity. During the past two decades, biphasic waveform defibrillation has attracted clinical and commercial attention in a variety of research models and settings (18–21). Schuder and colleagues reported that, in calves, certain symmetric biphasic waveforms could defibrillate at lower energies and currents than monophasic waveforms of similar durations (18). Dixon and coworkers, using large epicardial patches in dogs, compared multiple bipha-

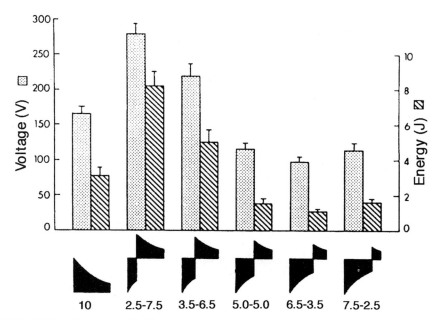

FIGURE 20-5. Internal defibrillation threshold voltage and energy values in dogs for six waveforms of the same total duration (10 msec), demonstrating that the defibrillation threshold is lowest for biphasic waveforms in which the second phase is smaller than the first phase. The mean values and standard deviations are shown. Diagrams of the waveforms are shown below the bar graphs. The biphasic waveform with a second-phase duration equal to the first phase (5/5 msec for first-phase duration/second-phase duration) or shorter than the first phase (6.5/3.5 and 7.5/2.5 msec) had significantly lower leading-edge voltage and energy requirements than other waveforms tested. The biphasic waveforms with shorter first phases than second phases (2.5/7.5 and 3.5/6.5 msec) had significantly higher voltage and energy requirements than the other waveforms tested, including the 10-msec monophasic waveform. The 2.5/7.5 biphasic waveform had significantly higher defibrillation voltage and energy requirements than the 3.5/6.5 msec biphasic waveform. (Adapted from Dixon EG, Tang ASL, Wolf PD, et al. Improved defibrillation thresholds with large contoured epicardial electrodes and biphasic waveforms. *Circulation* 1987;76:1176–1184, with permission.)

sic waveforms with similar monophasic waveforms (20). They demonstrated that biphasic waveforms in which the second phase was shorter or equal to the first phase in duration were more effective than monophasic waveforms of equal duration (Fig. 20-5). Kavanagh and associates used cathodal first-phase catheter electrodes in the right ventricular apex and outflow tract and an anodal electrode over the left side of the chest in dogs that had not undergone a thoracotomy to demonstrate that single-capacitor biphasic waveforms, delivered from a 150-μF capacitor, required less energy and lower leading-edge voltages to defibrillate than did monophasic or double-capacitor biphasic waveforms. Single-capacitor biphasic waveforms have the leading-edge voltage of the second phase equal to the trailing-edge voltage of the first phase. Two capacitors are required to produce a waveform with the leading-edge voltage of the second phase equal to the leading-edge voltage of the first phase. However, not all biphasic waveforms are superior to all monophasic waveforms. Biphasic waveforms that deliver more charge in the second phase require a higher voltage and more energy for defibrillation than do monophasic waveforms of the same total duration (22) (Fig. 20-6). The human clinical studies using biphasic waveforms support the experimental findings that biphasic waveforms with a shorter second phase appear to be more effective (23, 24).

Additional work has also been done to determine

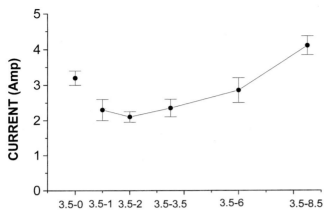

FIGURE 20-6. Scatterplot of internal defibrillation threshold current versus phase-two duration in dogs. Values are given as the mean ± standard deviation. As long as the first phase (3.5 msec) was longer than the second phase, the current threshold decreased as the second phase-two duration increased. As the second-phase duration became longer than the first-phase duration, the defibrillation threshold increased. The waveform labeled 3.5/0 was monophasic. (Adapted from Feeser SA, Tang ASL, Kavanagh KM, et al. Strength-duration and probability of success curves for defibrillation with biphasic waveforms. *Circulation* 1990;82:2128–2141, with permission.)

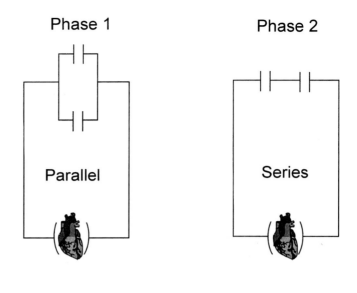

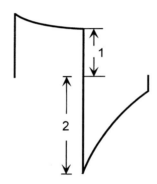

FIGURE 20-7. Parallel and series biphasic waveforms. In phase 1 of the biphasic waveform, the two capacitors are wired in parallel. The equivalent capacitance is twice the value of each of the capacitors. In phase 2, the capacitors are wired in series. The equivalent capacitance is one half of the value of each of the capacitors. Phase 2 leading-edge voltage is twice the phase 1 trailing-edge voltage. (Adapted from Winkle RA, Mead RH, Ruder MA, et al. Improved low energy defibrillation efficacy in man with the use of a biphasic truncated exponential waveform. *Am Heart J* 1989;117:122–127, with permission.)

whether it is beneficial to increase the fraction of the charge stored in the capacitor. The parallel/series configuration of the capacitors allows the possibility of a second phase shorter than or equal to the first phase of the biphasic waveform and makes the total amount of charge delivered equal in the two phases (Fig. 20-7). This configuration defibrillates at a lower leading-edge voltage and total delivered energy (25, 26).

Shock Polarity

Most studies have reported that shock polarity significantly influences the effectiveness of monophasic waveforms for internal defibrillation (27–30), but the results have been inconsistent regarding the influence of polarity on the defibrillation threshold of the biphasic waveform (31–36). Figure 20-8 illustrates the results from one study. Defibrillation thresholds were determined for a 6-msec, truncated, exponential monophasic waveform and a 6- to 4-msec, truncated, exponential biphasic waveform in six pigs (35). Consistent with previous reports, the defibrillation threshold for the monophasic waveform was significantly lower when the right ventricular catheter electrode was an anode than when it was a cathodal catheter electrode (Fig. 20-8). However, for the biphasic waveform, this study did not show a significant effect of polarity on the defibrillation threshold.

The studies that have shown an influence of polarity on the defibrillation efficacy of biphasic waveforms have found that the defibrillation threshold was lowered when the first-phase polarity anodal to the right

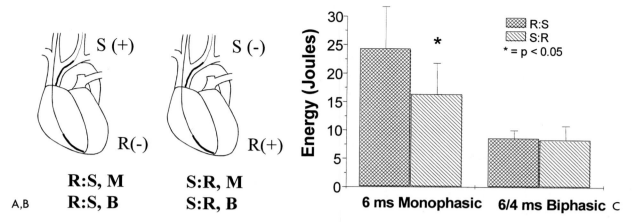

FIGURE 20-8. Effect of shock polarity on defibrillation threshold. Defibrillation catheters were placed in the right ventricular apex (R) and at the junction of the superior vena cava and right atrium (S) of six pigs. Four configurations were tested: R cathode (−) to S anode (+); monophasic waveform (R:S, M) **(A)**; S(−) to R(+), monophasic waveform (R:S, M) **(B)**; R first phase (−) to S first phase (+), biphasic waveform (R:S, B) **(A)**; S first phase (−), biphasic waveform (S:R, B) **(B)**. Means ± standard deviations are given for defibrillation threshold energies **(C)**. For monophasic shocks, the polarity reversal of the right ventricular (RV) electrode from cathode to anode caused a significant decrease in voltage. For biphasic shocks, the threshold energy was significantly lower than for monophasic shocks. However, polarity reversal of the RV electrode from the first-phase cathode to the first-phase anode did not significantly affect defibrillation efficacy. (Adapted from Usui M, Walcott GP, Strickberger SA, et al. Effects of polarity for monophasic and biphasic shocks on defibrillation efficacy with an endocardial system. *Pacing Clin Electrophysiol* 1996;19:65–71, with permission.)

ventricular electrode and the second phase was equal to or shorter than the first phase (31,32). Other studies found no significant difference in defibrillation threshold with reversal of polarity for biphasic waveforms with the second-phase duration shorter than the first-phase duration (37,38). These studies reported that the second-phase duration (37) or total-phase duration (38) affects the defibrillation efficacy of polarity reversal for biphasic waveform. No evidence has been reported in the literature to indicate that a cathodal right ventricular electrode for a biphasic waveform is superior to an anodal right ventricular polarity. Because some of the studies report that polarity makes no difference but other studies report that an anodal first phase is superior, the prudent choice is to use an anodal first-phase polarity to the right ventricular electrode for biphasic shocks as long as there is no detrimental effect on the patient. Because one of the two polarities must be used at the right ventricular electrode, the polarity used may as well be the one that some studies report as better, even if both polarities actually prove to be equally efficacious.

PROPOSED MECHANISMS OF IMPROVED EFFICACY OF BIPHASIC WAVEFORMS

Several theories have been developed to explain the improved defibrillation efficacy of biphasic waveforms. A potential gradient field created by the defibrillation shock extends from the shock electrode through the extracellular space of the heart. Because of this extracellular gradient, current enters the myocardial cells and alters their transmembrane potential. This alteration in transmembrane potential is thought to be responsible for defibrillation. For most defibrillation electrode configurations used with ICDs, the potential gradient field is highly uneven with very high potential gradients adjacent to the defibrillation electrodes and low potential gradients in areas of the heart distant from the electrodes (39) (Fig. 20-9). To successfully defibrillate, a minimum value of potential gradient should be achieved. The minimum potential gradients throughout the myocardium are 6 V/cm for a typical monophasic waveform and 4 V/cm for

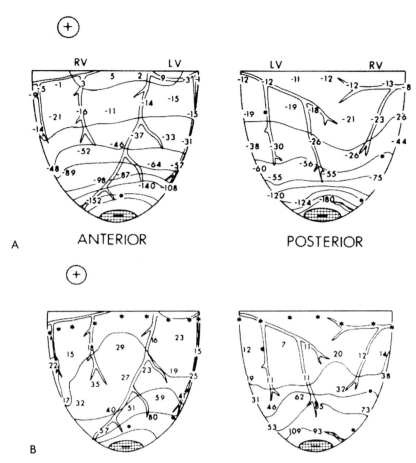

FIGURE 20-9. Epicardial potential (**A**) and potential gradient (**B**) distribution during a very-low-voltage shock in a dog. The maps are displayed as two complementary projections of the ventricles with the anterior left ventricular (LV) and right ventricular (RV) epicardium shown in the left diagram and the posterior left and right ventricular epicardium in the right diagram. The location of a cathodal defibrillation electrode at the apex is indicated by a minus sign within a crosshatched circle. The plus sign within a circle indicates that the location of an anodal defibrillation electrode was on the right atrium. Numbers represent the locations of electrodes with satisfactory recordings and give the potential (mV in **A**) or potential gradient (mV/cm in **B**) for those locations. Closed circles indicate electrode sites where adequate recordings were not obtained. Asterisks indicate electrode sites for which no gradient was calculated because there were neighboring electrodes on only one site. The isopotential lines are 25 mV apart; the isogradient lines are 25 mV/cm apart. The isopotential map (**A**) displays results of a 1-V shock given in electrical diastole during atrial paced rhythm. The voltage drop across the ventricle was 189 mV. The isopotential lines were closer together at the apex than at the base of the heart, indicating a higher gradient at the apex as quantified in **B**, which shows the isogradient map of the same shock. The higher potential gradient area was near the apex, and the lower gradient area was near the base. There was a 102-mV/cm difference between the maximal and minimal gradients on the surface of the heart. (From Chen P-S, Wolf PD, Claydon FJ III, et al. The potential gradient field created by epicardial defibrillation electrodes in dogs. *Circulation* 1986;74:626–636, with permission.)

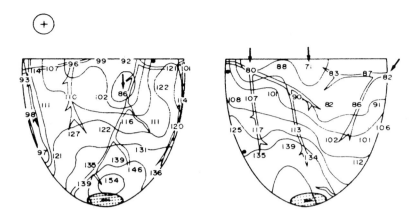

FIGURE 20-10. The isochronal map of the first postshock activation after a 4.9-J, unsuccessful defibrillation shock given during electrically induced fibrillation for the electrode configuration shown in Figure 20-9. The early sites of activation *(arrows)* appeared 71 to 86 msec after the shock and were located at the base of the ventricles where the potential gradient was low, as shown in Figure 20-9. Activation spread away from the base so that the apex was the last region to be depolarized. Isochronal lines are spaced 10 msec apart. (From Chen P-S, Wolf PD, Claydon FJ III, et al. The potential gradient field created by epicardial defibrillation electrodes in dogs. *Circulation* 1986;74:626–636, with permission.)

a biphasic waveform (40,41). Low potential gradients and high potential gradients can cause a defibrillation shock to fail. After a shock that is slightly weaker than that needed to defibrillate, the earliest postshock activation appears where the potential gradient is the lowest (42–44) (Fig. 20-10). For a shock that creates too high a potential gradient, conduction block and tachyarrhythmia foci can occur in the tissue exposed to the high potential gradient (43) (Fig. 20-11).

One possible explanation for why biphasic waveforms are generally more effective than monophasics is that the minimum potential gradient required for defibrillation is about one-third lower for the biphasic than for the monophasic waveform. The higher tolerance that cardiac tissue has for biphasic shocks may also explain the increased defibrillation efficacy, because a biphasic waveform is less likely to cause block and reentry in the high potential gradient area around the shocking electrode than is a monophasic waveform with the same voltage (40). The ratio of the potential gradient, above which detrimental effects occurred, to the minimum potential gradient needed for defibrillation (i.e., the safety factor) (45) is approximately 10:1 (64:6 V/cm) for monophasic waveforms and 17:1 (74:4 V/cm) for biphasic waveforms.

A highly nonuniform epicardial polarization pattern created by a defibrillation shock has been shown by optical mapping technique (46–48). In response to a shock, large regions of the epicardium are depolarized and adjacent large regions are hyperpolarized. Where a large gradient of transmembrane potentials

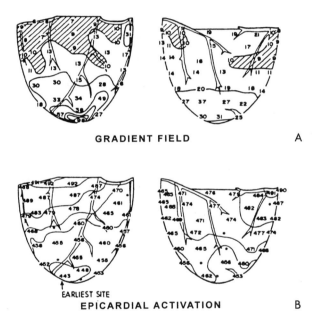

FIGURE 20-11. Example of an arrhythmia arising from the tissue adjacent to a defibrillation electrode. **A:** The potential gradient field is shown for a 284-V shock by means of a cathode on the left ventricle apex and dual anodes on the right atrium and left ventricle base in a dog. Anterior *(left)* and posterior *(right)* views are shown. The crosshatched area indicates a region where the potential gradient was less than 10 V/cm. Isopotential lines are 10 V/cm apart. **B:** The isochronal map illustrates the second beat of ventricular tachycardia that arose immediately after the successful defibrillation shock shown in **A**. The origin of the tachycardia was adjacent to the apical shock electrode. The isochronal lines are spaced 10 msec apart. Time zero is the onset of the shock. (From Wharton JM, Wolf PD, Smith WM, et al. Cardiac potential and potential gradient fields generated by single, combined, and sequential shocks during ventricular defibrillation. *Circulation* 1992;85:1510–1523, with permission.)

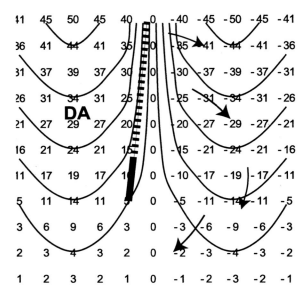

FIGURE 20-12. An idealized diagram is shown of a critical point caused by adjacent regions of depolarized and hyperpolarized transmembrane potential changes caused by a shock. The numbers represent transmembrane changes, with isolines spaced every 10 mV beginning at 45 mV. The directly activated region occurs to the left of the frame line, where depolarized transmembrane potential changes are suprathreshold. Where the transmembrane potential gradient is high, as indicated by closely spaced isolines *(top center)*, conduction can occur into the hyperpolarized region. Below, where the gradient in transmembrane potential is smaller, propagation cannot occur. A critical point is formed at the intersection of the frame and block lines, where one end of the propagating activation front terminates. (Data from Efimov IR, Cheng YN, Biermann M, et al. Transmembrane voltage changes produced by real and virtual electrodes during monophasic defibrillation shocks delivered by an implantable electrode. *J Cardiovasc Electrophysiol* 1997; 8:1031–1045 and from Gillis AM, Fast VG, Rohr S, Kléber AG. Spatial changes in transmembrane potential during extracellular electrical shocks in cultured monolayers of neonatal rat ventricular myocytes. *Circ Res* 1996;79:676–690.)

excites just after the shock at the boundary between depolarized and hyperpolarized regions, an activation front can propagate from the depolarized region into the hyperpolarized region (Fig. 20-12). In the area where the transmembrane potential gradient is smaller, propagation does not occur. A critical point is formed where the propagating activation front terminates (Fig. 20-12). Efimov and colleagues proposed that shocks can initiate a postshock reentrant arrhythmia by this mechanism (46). The second phase of a biphasic waveform may remove much of the transmembrane polarization caused by the first phase so that a critical point is no longer present just after the shock (46). This may partially explain why the biphasic waveform defibrillates more effectively than the monophasic waveform.

A mathematical model based on a resistor and a capacitor in a parallel configuration (Fig. 20-13) can be used to predict if a particular monophasic or biphasic waveform has a low defibrillation threshold (8, 49). According to the model's assumptions, a certain minimum potential difference across the resistor-capacitor network must be achieved by monophasic waveforms and the first phase of biphasic waveforms for successful defibrillation (49). For biphasic waveforms, the magnitude of this minimum potential difference for the first phase is decreased as the second phase decreases the potential difference across the resistor-capacitor network present at the end of the first phase. The optimal second phase of a biphasic waveform should bring the potential difference across the resistor-capacitor circuit quickly back to or slightly past its starting value at the beginning of the first phase (8,49).

Figure 20-14 shows the input waveforms and model response to a series of biphasic waveforms. The input waveform has a time constant equal to 7 msec; phase 1 duration is always 6 msec. Phase 2 duration varies from 1 to 8 msec. The input waveform is always a single capacitor waveform with the leading-edge voltage of the second phase equal to the trailing edge of the first phase. A second phase of 2 msec brings the potential back to its starting level, and a second phase of 3 msec brings the voltage slightly below the starting level. Walcott and colleagues demonstrated in dogs that the biphasic waveforms with this same time constant, 4/2- and 4/3-msec waveforms, defibrillate better than the 4/0-, 4/1-, 4/4-, or 4/8-msec waveforms (49).

Shorter-duration (<12 msec) biphasic waveforms are generally less able to excite myocardium than monophasic waveforms of the same duration, even though such short biphasic waveforms are usually better able to defibrillate (50). The effective refractory period was longer, and the strength interval curve was shifted to the right for a 3.5/2-msec biphasic waveform compared with a 5.5-msec monophasic waveforms when epicardial defibrillation electrodes were used in dogs (51).

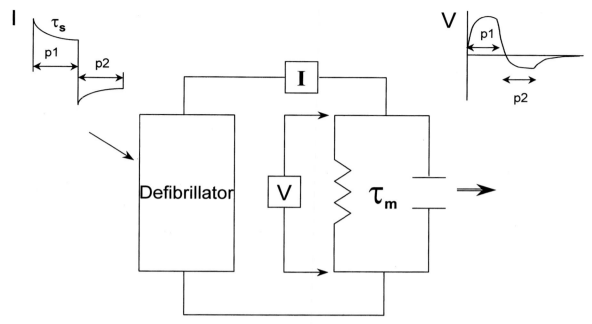

FIGURE 20-13. Diagram shows a parallel resistor-capacitor (RC) circuit model used to predict defibrillation efficacy of different monophasic and biphasic waveforms. The RC circuit has a time constant (τ_m) of 2.8 msec. An input biphasic waveform has a phase 1 duration (p1) and phase 2 duration (p2), and τ_s represents the time constant for the shock waveform. Model response (V) to the input waveform (I).

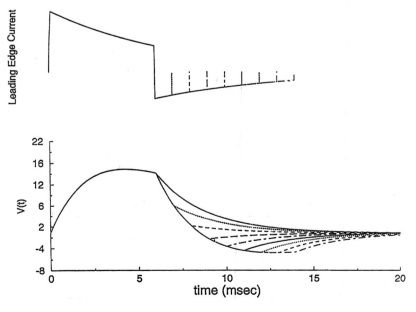

FIGURE 20-14. The resistor-capacitor (RC) model response to a biphasic truncated exponential waveform with a time constant of 7 msec. Leading-edge current of the input waveform was 10 A. **Top:** Shapes of the input waveforms. Phase 1 was truncated at 6 msec. Phase 2 was truncated after 0, 1, 2, 3, 4, 5, 6, 7, and 8 msec. **Bottom:** The model response ($V_{(t)}$) is shown. The model response does not change polarity until the duration of phase 2 is longer than 2 msec. (From Walcott GP, Walker RG, Cates AW, et al. Choosing the optimal monophasic and biphasic waveforms for ventricular defibrillation. *J Cardiovasc Electrophysiol* 1995; 6:737–750, with permission.)

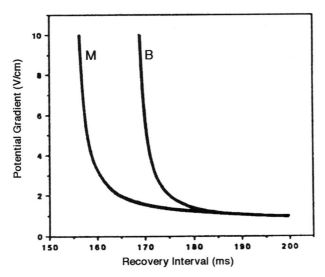

FIGURE 20-15. Monophasic and biphasic strength-interval curves for cardiac stimulation in a dog. The biphasic curve (B) is to the right of the monophasic (M), indicating the biphasic waveform is less able to directly excite relatively refractory myocardium. The absolute refractory period is the asymptote of the strength-interval curve parallel to the y axis, and the diastolic threshold is the asymptote parallel to the x axis. The absolute refractory period was 155 msec for the monophasic curve and 168 msec for the biphasic curve. The monophasic diastolic threshold was 0.7 V/cm, and the biphasic diastolic threshold was 0.6 V/cm. (From Daubert JP, Frazier DW, Wolf PD, et al. Response of relatively refractory canine myocardium to monophasic and biphasic shocks. *Circulation* 1991;84: 2522–2538, with permission.)

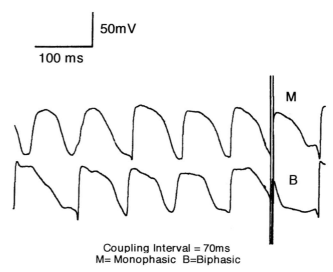

FIGURE 20-16. Examples of action potentials recorded before and after test shocks during ventricular fibrillation. The voltage and time scales are shown in the top left corner. The response to the monophasic shock is greater than that to the same strength of biphasic shock. The monophasic shock induces a new action potential, but the biphasic shock merely causes prolongation of the action potential. (Adapted from Zhou X, Wolf PD, Rollins DL, et al. Effects of monophasic and biphasic shocks on action potentials during ventricular fibrillation in dogs. *Circ Res* 1993;73:325–334, with permission.)

The 2/1-msec biphasic curve was also located to the right of the 3-msec monophasic curve when field stimulation techniques were used to determine the strength duration curves, even though the biphasic waveform has a significantly lower defibrillation threshold (52) (Fig. 20-15). This indicates that the biphasic waveform was less able to excite refractory myocardium. When 5-msec monophasic and 2.5/2.5-msec biphasic shocks were used to create a potential gradient of 5 V/cm at an *in vivo* site in which a microelectrode had been inserted, the monophasic waveform had a larger effect on the action potential than did the biphasic waveform during premature stimulation (53) (Fig. 20-16). The monophasic waveform caused more prolongation of the action potential and was better able to initiate a new action potential. The same results were found when biphasic and monophasic shocks were given during ventricular fibrillation (41).

The efficacy of a defibrillation shock is thought to be related to its ability to prolong the action potential and extend the refractory period without causing a new action potential, allowing resynchronization of the myocardium (53–55). An example of such a response is shown in Figure 20-17. However, recordings made in 10 dogs with floating microelectrodes during shocks delivered after 10 seconds of ventricular fibrillation showed that at five different coupling intervals, with a shock field strength of 5 V/cm, a 2.5/2.5-msec biphasic waveform was less successful than the 5-msec monophasic waveform in prolonging the action potential (Fig. 20-18). Some biphasic waveforms are less able to stimulate a new action potential or cause action potential prolongation than monophasic waveforms, but other biphasic waveforms have

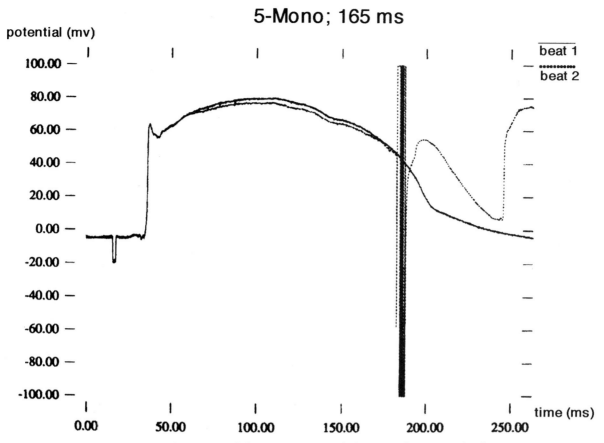

FIGURE 20-17. Prolongation of the action potential duration after an S2 shock. At a 165-msec S1-S2 interval for a 5 msec monophasic shock, action potential prolongation is observed. Two S1-stimulated action potentials are shown. No S2 shock was given during the action potential *(solid line)*. An S2 shock was given during the action potential *(dotted line)*. S1, S1 stimulus artifact; S2, S2 shock artifact. (Adapted from Zhou X, Knisley SB, Wolf PD, et al. Prolongation of repolarization time by electric field stimulation with monophasic and biphasic shocks in open chest dogs. *Circ Res* 1991;68:1761–1767, with permission.)

a markedly lower defibrillation threshold than their corresponding monophasic waveforms.

⊙ ATRIAL AND TRANSTHORACIC DEFIBRILLATION

The superiority of biphasic waveforms has also been shown for atrial defibrillation (56–58). In six patients a 3/3-msec biphasic waveform had a lower atrial defibrillation threshold in terms of energy and voltage than did the corresponding 6-msec monophasic waveform (Fig. 20-19). Results also indicate that a truncated, exponential, biphasic waveform is superior to an Edmark monophasic waveform for external ventricular defibrillation (59). For internal as well as external defibrillation and for ventricular as well as atrial defibrillation, the biphasic waveform is the most effective waveform.

⊙ TRIPHASIC WAVEFORMS

The search continues for a waveform that defibrillates better than the currently available biphasic waveform.

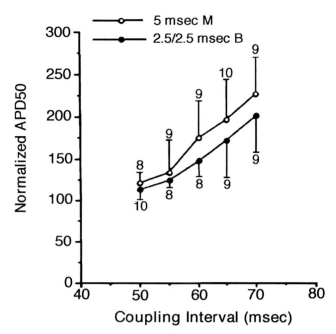

FIGURE 20-18. Relation between the normalized time from the onset of the S1-stimulated action potential to the time for the action potential to return to 50% of its maximum value after the S2 shock (APD$_{50}$) and the S1-S2 coupling interval. On the y axis is the APD$_{50}$ (mean ± standard deviation) expressed as a percent of the APD$_{50}$ if no S2 shock is given. The APD$_{50}$ for the 5-msec monophasic waveform was significantly longer than for the 2.5/2.5-msec biphasic waveform. (From Zhou X, Wolf PD, Rollins DL, et al. Effects of monophasic and biphasic shocks on action potentials during ventricular fibrillation in dogs. *Circ Res* 1993;73:325–334, with permission.)

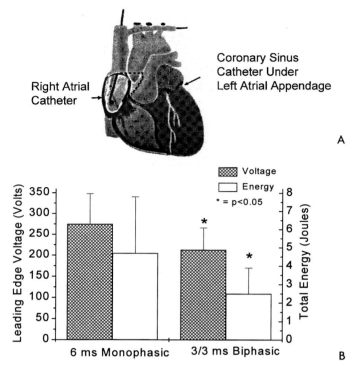

FIGURE 20-19. **A:** Defibrillation catheters were placed in the right atrium and coronary sinus in six patients. **B:** For a 3/3-msec biphasic shock, which was equal in total duration to a 6-msec monophasic shock, the atrial defibrillation threshold voltage and energy were significantly lower than for the monophasic shock. Mean ± standard deviation values are shown. (Adapted from Johnson EE, Yarger MD, Wharton JM. Monophasic and biphasic waveforms for low energy internal cardioversion of atrial fibrillation in humans. *Circulation* 1993;(4)88:I-592, with permission.)

Triphasic waveforms, although initially reported to be less effective than the biphasic waveform (20,60–62), have shown some potential to slightly lower the DFT compared with some biphasic waveforms. A study reported that one type of triphasic waveform was able to lower the defibrillation threshold compared with the performance of a similar biphasic waveform (63,64).

ACKNOWLEDGEMENTS

The authors wish to thank Ms. Kate M. Sreenan for her assistance in the preparation of the manuscript. This work was supported in part by National Institutes of Health research grant HL-42760.

REFERENCES

1. Lawrence JH, Brin KP, Halperin HR, et al. The characterization of human transmyocardial impedance during implantation of the automatic internal cardioverter defibrillator. *Pacing Clin Electrophysiol* 1986;9:745–755.
2. Wessale JL, Boulard JD, Tacker WA Jr, Geddes LA. Bipolar catheter defibrillation in dogs using trapezoidal waveforms of various tilts. *J Electrocardiol* 1980;13:359–366.
3. Schuder JC, Rahmoeller GA, Stoeckle H. Transthoracic ventricular defibrillation with triangular and trapezoidal waveforms. *Circ Res* 1966;19:689–694.
4. Shorofsky SR, Foster AH, Gold MR. Effect of waveform tilt on defibrillation thresholds in humans. *J Cardiovasc Electrophysiol* 1997;8:496–501.
5. Natale A, Sra J, Krum D, et al. Relative efficacy of different tilts with biphasic defibrillation in humans. *Pacing Clin Electrophysiol* 1996;19:197–206.
6. Yamanouchi Y, Brewer JE, Olson KF, et al. Fully discharging phases: a new approach to biphasic waveforms for external defibrillation. *Circulation* 1999;100:826–831.

7. Kroll MW. A minimal model of the monophasic defibrillation pulse. *Pacing Clin Electrophysiol* 1993;16:769–777.
8. Kroll MW. A minimal model of the single capacitor biphasic defibrillation waveform. *Pacing Clin Electrophysiol* 1994;17:1782–1792.
9. Irnich W. The optimum tilt for defibrillation. In: Aubert A, Ector H, Stroobandt R, eds. *Cardiac pacing and electrophysiology.* Dordrecht, The Netherlands: Kluwer Academic Publishers, 1994:381–385.
10. Rist K, Tchou PJ, Mowrey K, et al. Smaller capacitors improve the biphasic waveform. *J Cardiovasc Electrophysiol* 1994;5:771–776.
11. Hahn SJ, Heil JE, Lang DJ. Large capacitor defibrillation waveform reduces peak voltages without increasing energies. *Pacing Clin Electrophysiol* 1995;18:203–207.
12. Hahn AJ, Heil JE, Lin Y, et al. Improved defibrillation with small capacitance and optimized biphasic waveform. *Circulation* 1994;[Suppl. 90](4,Pt. 2):I-175.
13. Swerdlow CD, Kass RM, Chen P-S, et al. Effect of capacitor size and pathway resistance on defibrillation threshold for implantable defibrillators. *Circulation* 1994;90:1840–1846.
14. Swerdlow CD, Kass RM, Davie S, et al. Short biphasic pulses from 90 microfarad capacitors lower defibrillation threshold. *Pacing Clin Electrophysiol* 1996;19:1053–1060.
15. Bahu M, Knight BP, Weiss R, et al. Randomized comparison of a 90 µF capacitor three-electrode defibrillation system with a 125 µF two-electrode defibrillation system. *J Interv Card Electrophysiol* 1998;2:41–45.
16. Block M, Hammel D, Böcker D, et al. Internal defibrillation with smaller capacitors: a prospective randomized cross-over comparison of defibrillation efficacy obtained with 90-µF and 125-µF capacitors in humans. *J Cardiovasc Electrophysiol* 1995;6:333–342.
17. Block M, Hammel D, Böcker D, et al. ICD device size can be reduced by large output capacitance. *Eur Heart J* 1994;15:79.
18. Schuder JC, McDaniel WC, Stoeckle H. Defibrillation of 100-kg calves with asymmetrical, bidirectional, rectangular pulses. *Cardiovasc Res* 1984;18:419–426.
19. Flaker GC, Schuder JC, McDaniel WC, et al. Superiority of biphasic shocks in the defibrillation of dogs by epicardial patches and catheter electrodes. *Am Heart J* 1989;118:288–291.
20. Dixon EG, Tang ASL, Wolf PD, et al. Improved defibrillation thresholds with large contoured epicardial electrodes and biphasic waveforms. *Circulation* 1987;76:1176–1184.
21. Chapman PD, Vetter JW, Souza JJ, et al. Comparative efficacy of monophasic and biphasic truncated exponential shocks for nonthoracotomy internal defibrillation in dogs. *J Am Coll Cardiol* 1988;12:739–745.
22. Feeser SA, Tang ASL, Kavanagh KM, et al. Strength-duration and probability of success curves for defibrillation with biphasic waveforms. *Circulation* 1990;82:2128–2141.
23. Bardy GH, Ivey TD, Allen MD, et al. A prospective randomized evaluation of biphasic versus monophasic waveform pulses on defibrillation efficacy in humans. *J Am Coll Cardiol* 1989;14:728–733.
24. Winkle RA, Mead RH, Ruder MA, et al. Improved low energy defibrillation efficacy in man with the use of a biphasic truncated exponential waveform. *Am Heart J* 1989;117:122–127.
25. Walcott GP, Rollins DL, Smith WM, Ideker RE. Effect of changing capacitors between phases of a biphasic defibrillation shock. *Pacing Clin Electrophysiol* 1996;19:945–954.
26. Yamanouchi Y, Mowrey KA, Nadzam GR, et al. Large change in voltage at phase reversal improves biphasic defibrillation thresholds: parallel-series mode switching. *Circulation* 1996;94:1768–1773.
27. Schuder JC, Stoeckle H, McDaniel WC, Dbeis M. Is the effectiveness of cardiac ventricular defibrillation dependent upon polarity? *Med Instrum* 1987;21:262–265.
28. Strickberger SA, Hummel JD, Horwood LE, et al. Effect of shock polarity on ventricular defibrillation threshold using a transvenous lead system. *J Am Coll Cardiol* 1994;24:1069–1072.
29. Bardy GH, Ivey TD, Allen MD, et al. Evaluation of electrode polarity on defibrillation efficacy. *Am J Cardiol* 1989;63:433–437.
30. O'Neill PG, Boahene KA, Lawrie GM, et al. The automatic implantable cardioverter-defibrillator: effect of patch polarity on defibrillation threshold. *J Am Coll Cardiol* 1991;17:707–711.
31. Natale A, Sra J, Dhala A, et al. Effects of initial polarity on defibrillation threshold with biphasic pulses. *Pacing Clin Electrophysiol* 1995;18:1889–1893.
32. Thakur R, Souza J, Chapman P, et al. Electrode polarity is an important determinant of defibrillation efficacy using a nonthoracotomy system. *Pacing Clin Electrophysiol* 1994;17:919–923.
33. Strickberger SA, Man KC, Daoud E, et al. Effect of first-phase polarity of biphasic shocks on defibrillation threshold with a single transvenous lead system. *J Am Coll Cardiol* 1995;25:1605–1608.
34. Block M, Hammel D, Böcker D, et al. Transvenous-subcutaneous defibrillation leads: effect of transvenous electrode polarity on defibrillation threshold. *J Cardiovasc Electrophysiol* 1994;5:912–918.
35. Usui M, Walcott GP, Strickberger SA, et al. Effects of polarity for monophasic and biphasic shocks on defibrillation efficacy with an endocardial system. *Pacing Clin Electrophysiol* 1996;19:65–71.
36. Huang J, KenKnight BH, Walcott GP, et al. Effect of electrode polarity on internal defibrillation with monophasic and biphasic waveforms using an endocardial lead system. *J Cardiovasc Electrophysiol* 1997;8:161–171.
37. Huang J, KenKnight BH, Walcott GP, et al. Effects of transvenous electrode polarity and waveform duration on the relationship between defibrillation threshold and upper limit of vulnerability. *Circulation* 1997;96:1351–1359.
38. Schauerte P, Schondube FA, Grossmann M, et al. Optimized pulse durations minimize the effect of polarity reversal on defibrillation efficacy with biphasic shocks. *Pacing Clin Electrophysiol* 1999;22:790–797.
39. Chen P-S, Wolf PD, Claydon FJ III, et al. The potential gradient field created by epicardial defibrillation electrodes in dogs. *Circulation* 1986;74:626–636.
40. Yabe S, Smith WM, Daubert JP, et al. Conduction disturbances caused by high current density electric fields. *Circ Res* 1990;66:1190–1203.
41. Zhou X, Wolf PD, Rollins DL, et al. Effects of monophasic and biphasic shocks on action potentials during ventricular fibrillation in dogs. *Circ Res* 1993;73:325–334.
42. Witkowski FX, Penkoske PA, Plonsey R. Mechanism of cardiac defibrillation in open-chest dogs with unipolar DC-coupled simultaneous activation and shock potential recordings. *Circulation* 1990;82:244–260.
43. Wharton JM, Wolf PD, Smith WM, et al. Cardiac potential and potential gradient fields generated by single, combined, and sequential shocks during ventricular defibrillation. *Circulation* 1992;85:1510–1523.
44. Zhou X, Daubert JP, Wolf PD, et al. Epicardial mapping of ventricular defibrillation with monophasic and biphasic shocks in dogs. *Circ Res* 1993;72:145–160.
45. Jones JL, Jones RE. Determination of safety factor for defibrillator waveforms in cultured heart cells. *Am J Physiol* 1982;242:H662–H670.

46. Efimov IR, Cheng Y, Van Wagoner DR, et al. Virtual electrode-induced phase singularity: a basic mechanism of defibrillation failure. *Circ Res* 1998;82:918–925.
47. Efimov IR, Cheng YN, Biermann M, et al. Transmembrane voltage changes produced by real and virtual electrodes during monophasic defibrillation shocks delivered by an implantable electrode. *J Cardiovasc Electrophysiol* 1997;8:1031–1045.
48. Gillis AM, Fast VG, Rohr S, Kléber AG. Spatial changes in transmembrane potential during extracellular electrical shocks in cultured monolayers of neonatal rat ventricular myocytes. *Circ Res* 1996;79:676–690.
49. Walcott GP, Walker RG, Cates AW, et al. Choosing the optimal monophasic and biphasic waveforms for ventricular defibrillation. *J Cardiovasc Electrophysiol* 1995;6:737–750.
50. Knisley SB, Smith WM, Ideker RE. Effect of intrastimulus polarity reversal on electric field stimulation thresholds in frog and rabbit myocardium. *J Cardiovasc Electrophysiol* 1992;3:239–254.
51. Wharton JM, Richard VJ, Murry CE Jr, et al. Electrophysiological effects of monophasic and biphasic stimuli in normal and infarcted dogs. *Pacing Clin Electrophysiol* 1990;13:1158–1172.
52. Daubert JP, Frazier DW, Wolf PD, et al. Response of relatively refractory canine myocardium to monophasic and biphasic shocks. *Circulation* 1991;84:2522–2538.
53. Zhou X, Knisley SB, Wolf PD, et al. Prolongation of repolarization time by electric field stimulation with monophasic and biphasic shocks in open chest dogs. *Circ Res* 1991;68:1761–1767.
54. Dillon SM. Synchronized repolarization after defibrillation shocks: a possible component of the defibrillation process demonstrated by optical recordings in rabbit heart. *Circulation* 1992;85:1865–1878.
55. Kwaku KF, Dillon SM. Shock-induced depolarization of refractory myocardium prevents wave-front propagation in defibrillation. *Circ Res* 1996;79:957–973.
56. Cooper RAS, Alferness CA, Smith WM, Ideker RE. Internal cardioversion of atrial fibrillation in sheep. *Circulation* 1993;87:1673–1686.
57. Keane D, Boyd E, Anderson D, et al. Comparison of biphasic and monophasic waveforms in epicardial atrial defibrillation. *J Am Coll Cardiol* 1994;24:171–176.
58. Johnson EE, Yarger MD, Wharton JM. Monophasic and biphasic waveforms for low energy internal cardioversion of atrial fibrillation in humans. *Circulation* 1993;(4)88:I-592A.
59. Walcott GP, Hagler JA, Walker RG, et al. Comparison of monophasic, biphasic, and the Edmark waveform for external defibrillation. *Pacing Clin Electrophysiol* 1992;15:563A.
60. Manz M, Jung W, Wolpert C, et al. Can triphasic shock waveforms improve ICD therapy in man? *Circulation* 1993;(4)88:I-593.
61. Jung W, Manz M, Moosdorf R, et al. Comparative defibrillation efficacy of biphasic and triphasic waveforms. *New Trends Arrhyth* 1993;9:765–769.
62. Chapman PD, Wetherbee JN, Vetter JW, Troup PJ. Comparison of monophasic, biphasic, and triphasic truncated pulses for non-thoracotomy internal defibrillation. *J Am Coll Cardiol* 1988;11:57A.
63. Huang J, KenKnight BH, Rollins DL, et al. Defibrillation with triphasic waveforms. *Pacing Clin Electrophysiol* 1997;20:1056A.
64. Huang J, KenKnight BH, Smith WM, Ideker RE. Ventricular defibrillation with triphasic waveforms. *Circulation* 2000;101:1324–1328.

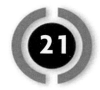

DUAL-CHAMBER SENSING AND DETECTION FOR IMPLANTABLE CARDIOVERTER-DEFIBRILLATORS
• • •

JEFFREY M. GILLBERG, WALTER H. OLSON

Single-chamber implantable cardioverter-defibrillators (ICDs) are highly sensitive for detection of true ventricular tachyarrhythmias. However, inappropriate detection of supraventricular tachycardia (SVT) by ventricular rate–only algorithms during clinical ICD studies has ranged from 20% to 41% (1). The inappropriate ICD therapy (i.e., antitachycardia pacing or shocks) that results can be proarrhythmic (2–6). Painful, inappropriate shocks are frequently repetitive and may cause adverse psychologic consequences (7). In addition to ventricular rate–only algorithms, single-chamber ICDs have optional criteria to discriminate rapidly conducted SVTs from ventricular tachycardia. Sudden-onset and ventricular-interval stability criteria identify rhythms to be supraventricular in origin if the ventricular RR intervals have a gradual onset (e.g., sinus tachycardia) or are irregular (e.g., atrial fibrillation). Electrogram morphology criteria can also identify rhythms to be SVTs if the ventricular electrogram waveform characteristics during high-rate rhythms are similar to beats with known atrial origin. Although these criteria can be configured to improve discrimination of ventricular tachycardia and SVT, loss in sensitivity for ventricular tachyarrhythmias can result without careful programming (8–10). It is intuitive to cardiac electrophysiologists that at least some of the performance issues of these single-chamber detection enhancements can be attributed to a lack of information about atrial activity.

The availability of atrial and ventricular electrograms for dual-chamber ICDs provides the opportunity for new algorithms that may improve specificity of tachyarrhythmia detection compared with methods that use only ventricular electrogram information. The use of atrial rate and atrioventricular (AV) relationships may help in discriminating rapidly conducted atrial flutter, atrial fibrillation, or sinus tachycardia from ventricular tachyarrhythmias.

The tachyarrhythmia detection algorithms used in dual-chamber ICDs from ELA Medical (Montrouge, France), Guidant (St. Paul, MN), (see Chapter 22) and Medtronic (Minneapolis, MN) have been described (11,12). Clinical performance of these algorithms has been reported, although not with the same set of tachyarrhythmias or performance metrics (13–19). In this chapter, we use widely accepted electrophysiologic principles to define generally applicable building blocks for the design of any dual-chamber tachyarrhythmia detection algorithm. We also describe specific building blocks and their selective use by the PR Logic dual-chamber detection algorithm available in Medtronic dual-chamber ICDs (i.e., Gem DR, Gem II DR, Gem III DR and Jewel AF). Examples of spontaneous tachycardias retrieved from Gem

DR device memory are presented to show correct and incorrect rhythm diagnosis. It is hoped that the examples and descriptions presented will enable clinicians to better understand the benefits and shortcomings of the PR Logic detection algorithm. Future directions in dual-chamber detection algorithm design are also discussed.

◉ DUAL-CHAMBER SENSING CONSIDERATIONS

Sensing of intrinsic atrial and ventricular depolarizations is the first step in dual-chamber tachyarrhythmia detection. Reliable sensing is important for proper detection of tachyarrhythmias and for inhibition of pacemaker stimuli (20). Sensing in dual-chamber ICDs is accomplished by designs that integrate two single-chamber sensing systems. Each single-chamber sensing system uses amplifiers, bandpass filters, signal rectifiers, and comparators to identify atrial or ventricular depolarizations (20).

As in single-chamber ICDs, the ventricular sensing channel in dual-chamber ICDs uses bipolar-only electrograms with amplifiers that are about 10 times more sensitive than typical pacemaker sense amplifiers to allow reliable sensing during ventricular fibrillation (VF) with small electrogram amplitudes. High sensitivities are achieved without inappropriate oversensing (e.g., T-wave oversensing, double counting of R waves) through the use of auto-adjusting sensitivity or autogain control (20). The bandpass filters are designed to accept ventricular depolarizations for all rhythms and to reject lower frequency signals such as T waves and higher-frequency signals such as myopotentials and electromagnetic interference. Filters typically reject signals with frequencies lower than about 10 Hz and greater than about 60 Hz.

Reliable sensing of atrial electrograms in dual-chamber ICDs is important to avoid inappropriate detection of supraventricular tachyarrhythmias. The frequency spectra of unipolar and bipolar atrial electrograms has most of the energy in the range of 10 to 50 Hz (21,22). Atrial sense amplifiers can be designed with auto-adjusting sensitivity or autogain control similar to those used for ventricular sensing. In the Gem DR ICD, atrial sensing uses an auto-adjusting sensitivity design with a shorter decay time constant and slightly different bandpass filter characteristics than the ventricular sensing channel. These parameters were selected to optimize sensing of atrial fibrillation and minimize sensing of far-field R waves (FFRWs). Atrial electrograms during atrial fibrillation may be more difficult to sense than ventricular electrograms during ventricular fibrillation because atrial electrograms are generally smaller than ventricular electrograms. For bipolar atrial electrograms from the right atrial appendage, Kerr (23) found in 11 patients that mean peak-to-peak electrogram amplitude in sinus rhythm was 2.6 ± 1.0 mV and not significantly less during paroxysmal atrial fibrillation (2.3 ± 1.3 mV). Mean minimum values were 2.0 ± 0.8 mV in sinus rhythm and 1.4 ± 1.1 mV during atrial fibrillation. The smallest value for atrial fibrillation was 0.7 mV.

Sensing and detection of atrial fibrillation from bipolar atrial electrograms was studied in 80 patients implanted with the Jewel AF dual-chamber ICD. The Jewel AF uses the same auto-adjusting sensitivity design as in the Gem DR. For 31 patients with programmed sensitivity of 0.35 ± 0.14 mV, 295 (91.6%) of 322 device detections were appropriate and only 1 of the 295 episodes was not detected continuously because of atrial undersensing. Atrial sensitivity was programmed to 0.9 mV during this one episode to avoid oversensing of FFRWs. Inappropriate atrial fibrillation or atrial flutter detections (27 of 322) occurred in five patients because of misclassification of FFRWs that were sensed on the atrial channel. Device memory recorded 90 episodes longer than 1 hour for a total of 2,697 hours of continuous atrial fibrillation detection (24).

Dual-chamber pacemakers and ICDs use blanking periods after paced and sensed events to avoid oversensing and double counting of cardiac activity. Blanking periods and pacemaker refractory periods are also used to prevent undesirable behavior such as pacemaker-mediated tachycardia caused by retrograde P waves. The Gem dual-chamber ICDs have zero cross blanking in the atrium after ventricular-sensed events and only 30 msec after ventricular-paced events to allow reliable sensing and detection of atrial tachyarrhythmias. All sensed, refractory sensed, and paced events from the atrium and the ventricle are used by the PR Logic dual-chamber detection algorithm. However, the Gem dual-chamber ICDs use postventricular atrial blanking and refractory periods to exclude some of these events from pacemaker timing calculations. Atrial events sensed during postventricular blanking and refractory periods are shown on the marker channel and are labeled as atrial refractory (AR). The blanking periods in Gem dual-chamber ICDs are indicated by the dark rectangles on the marker channel portion of Figure 21-1, which also shows the surface electrocardiogram (ECG), atrial bipolar electrogram, and right ventricular coil-can electrogram. The marker channel represents atrial-sensed and -paced events as vertical lines above the horizontal line and ventricular-sensed and -paced events as vertical lines below the horizontal line. Blanking periods for each chamber are indicated by rectangles above the horizontal line for atrial amplifier blanking or below the horizontal line for ventricular blanking. The blanking periods in the atrium after atrial-sensed and -paced events (AS, AP) and the blanking periods in the ventricle after ventricular-sensed and -paced events (VS, VP) are called same-chamber blanking. Same-chamber blanking periods are artificial absolute refractory periods used to ensure each depolarization is sensed only once. Same-chamber blanking in Gem dual-chamber ICDs is 100 msec in the atrium and 120 msec in the ventricle. After paced events, the blanking period is longer (nominally, 200 to 240 msec) to prevent oversensing of the pacing artifact and the evoked response. The blanking periods in the ventricle after atrial-sensed or -paced events and in the atrium after ventricular-sensed or -paced events are called cross-chamber blanking. In Gem dual-chamber ICDs, cross-chamber blanking

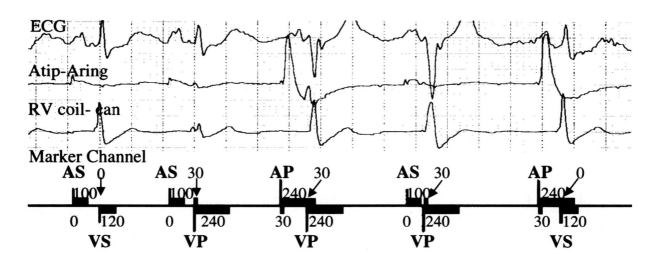

Same-chamber blanking:
240 ms after A or V pace (nominal)
120 ms after V sense
100 ms after A sense

Cross-chamber blanking:
30 ms after opposite chamber pace
0 ms after opposite chamber sense

FIGURE 21-1. Blanking periods in the Gem DR dual-chamber defibrillator. A real-time strip with the surface electrocardiogram, atrial electrogram (AEGM), ventricular electrogram (VEGM), and marker channel shows the same-chamber and cross-chamber blanking periods used by the Gem DR during sensed and paced events. The blanking periods are illustrated with dark rectangles on the dual-chamber marker channel. There is zero atrial blanking after ventricular-sensed (VS) events and only 30-msec atrial blanking after ventricular-paced (VP) events to achieve reliable atrial sensing during rapid ventricular rhythms. AS, atrial-sensed event; AP, atrial-paced events.

after paced events is very short (30 msec), and there is no cross-chamber blanking after atrial or ventricular sensed events. The primary purpose of cross-chamber blanking is to prevent oversensing of the pacing artifact after a paced event in the opposite chamber. Cross-chamber blanking can also be used after sensed events to avoid oversensing a depolarization in the opposite chamber. Cross-chamber blanking in the atrium after a ventricular-sensed event must be minimized in a tachyarrhythmia device to avoid undersensing the atrial rhythm particularly during fast ventricular rates. Long atrial cross-blanking periods preclude reliable sensing of most atrial rhythms, especially atrial tachycardias. However, short atrial cross-blanking periods may result in inappropriate atrial sensing of far-field ventricular depolarizations (i.e., FFRWs).

Figure 21-2 presents stored Gem DR strips illustrating reliable atrial sensing during rapidly conducted atrial fibrillation (left panel) and atrial oversensing of FFRWs during sinus tachycardia (right panel). The top tracing is the A_{tip} to A_{ring} electrogram from a closely spaced atrial bipole, and the middle tracing is the ventricular electrogram. The dual-chamber marker channel shows numeric values for the PP and RR intervals (in milliseconds), with atrial events marked above and ventricular events marked below the horizontal line. During atrial fibrillation, reliable sensing of all atrial events (i.e., atrial sense [AS] for

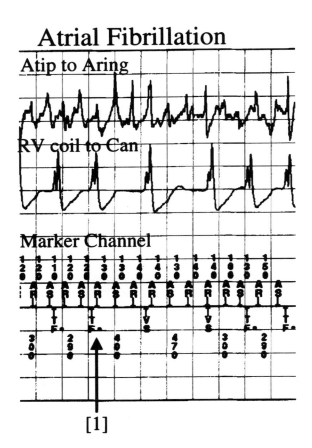
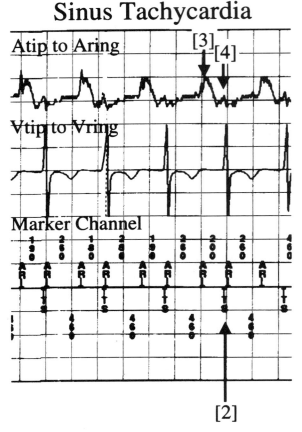

FIGURE 21-2. Benefit and consequence of minimal cross-chamber blanking on atrial sensing. Stored strips from the Gem DR implantable cardioverter-defibrillator (with 0-msec cross-chamber blanking after sensed events) during atrial fibrillation with rapid conduction *(left)* and sinus tachycardia with far-field R waves *(right)*. Minimal cross-chamber blanking allows reliable sensing of atrial fibrillation [1] but may also allow oversensing of far-field R waves on the atrial amplifier [2].

atrial events outside of pacemaker refractory periods, and atrial refractory [AR] for atrial events within pacemaker refractory periods) can be seen even for atrial events that occur soon after ventricular events (Fig. 21-2 [1]) because there is no cross-chamber blanking after sensed events. However, atrial oversensing of FFRWs may occur, as shown by [2]. FFRW oversensing generally occurs when the P wave [3] amplitude is not much larger than the FFRW [4] amplitude on the atrial electrogram. As demonstrated in an acute study, as bipolar electrode spacing decreases, the size of the FFRW relative to the local P waves decreases (25). To minimize the oversensing of FFRWs, use of an active fixation atrial lead placed on the high lateral wall (26) and bipolar electrode spacing of 10 mm or less is recommended (standard atrial bipole spacing is 15 to 17 mm).

⊙ DUAL-CHAMBER TACHYARRHYTHMIA DETECTION: THE BUILDING BLOCK MODEL

Dual-chamber ICDs perform tachyarrhythmia detection using a microprocessor and digital electronics to analyze and combine information derived from intracardiac atrial and ventricular electrograms. Detection processes are driven by timing information derived from sensed intrinsic atrial and ventricular depolarizations, as well as the pacemaker stimuli generated by the ICD.

Dual-chamber tachyarrhythmia detection is generally performed in a stepwise process using a series of "building blocks" of physiologically relevant information extracted from two simultaneous electrograms. Table 21-1 presents a list of general tachyarrhythmia detection building blocks for dual-chamber ICDs, along with the potentially relevant information provided by each and its possible weaknesses. Some of these building blocks have not yet been incorporated into any commercially available dual-chamber ICD, and different algorithm designers have selected different combinations of the available information. The design of a complete dual-chamber detection algorithm must consider the clinical significance and weaknesses of each building block and must consider how combinations of building blocks can be used to form the detection decision.

Dual-Chamber Detection Building Blocks

The first five building blocks in Table 21-1 are applicable to single-chamber ICDs, because these blocks are derived using only ventricular information. The *RR interval* analysis building block classifies ventricular intervals into zones by programmable cycle length (or rate) thresholds, and various counting schemes and logic are used to detect and classify tachyarrhythmias (20). All single and dual-chamber ICDs use this building block as the most basic method of detection. When used alone, RR interval analysis provides the highest sensitivity for detection of true ventricular tachyarrhythmias but may result in inappropriate detection of SVT for ventricular cycle lengths that overlap with cycle lengths during ventricular tachycardia or ventricular fibrillation. The *RR regularity* building block is used in single and dual-chamber ICDs to discriminate between regular ventricular intervals due to monomorphic ventricular tachycardia and irregular ventricular intervals due to rapidly conducted atrial fibrillation. This method of ventricular tachycardia/atrial fibrillation discrimination may lose effectiveness as ventricular rates during atrial fibrillation increase (27) and may be ineffective for rhythms with regular ventricular response such as 2:1 atrial flutter. RR regularity criteria may withhold detection inappropriately for polymorphic ventricular tachycardia with variable cycle lengths. The *RR onset* building block is used to discriminate sudden onset ventricular tachycardia from gradual onset SVT rhythms such as sinus tachycardia. However, if ventricular tachycardia arises during sinus tachycardia, this method may cause true ventricular tachycardia to not be detected (9,10), and SVT with sudden onset (e.g., atrial tachycardia) may be treated inappropriately. The *ventricular electrogram morphology* (VEGM) building block can identify rhythms to be SVT if the ventricular electrogram waveform characteristics during high rate rhythms are similar to beats with known atrial origin. This method may be confounded by conduction aberrancy during SVTs or by changes in the normal electrogram mor-

TABLE 21-1 • GENERAL DUAL-CHAMBER DETECTION BUILDING BLOCKS

Dual-Chamber Detection-Building Blocks[a]	Purpose or Information	Potential Weaknesses
Ventricle Only		
RR intervals	Identifies high ventricular rates	SVT with high ventricular rates that overlap with VT/VF rates
RR regularity	Discrimination of monomorphic VT (regular cycle lengths) from rapid AF (irregular cycle lengths)	May lose effectiveness as ventricular rates during AF increase; 2:1 atrial flutter has regular RR intervals. May cause underdetection of VT with irregular RR intervals
RR onset	Identifies sudden ventricular rate changes	Not specific for atrial or ventricular tachyarrhythmias; may miss VT arising during sinus tachycardia
VEGM morphology	Abnormal ventricular electrogram morphology may indicate ventricular tachyarrhythmias.	Confounded by conduction aberrancy or changes in "normal" VEGM morphology
Ventricular extrastimuli	Intervals after entrainment of VT by burst pacing are less variable than intervals after burst pacing during SVT.	Sensitive to single interval measurement, potential detection time delay, and potential proarrhythmia
Atrium Only		
PP intervals	Identifies high atrial rates	High atrial rates may be present during true VT/VF
PP regularity	Regular atrial rates may indicate organized atrial activity.	Little benefit for ventricular tachyarrhythmia characterization
PP onset	Identifies sudden atrial rates changes	Not specific for atrial or ventricular tachyarrhythmias (e.g., VT with 1:1 retrograde association)
AEGM morphology	Identifies atrial tachyarrhythmias and/or retrograde conduction	Confounded by far-field R waves and changes in "normal" AEGM morphology
Atrium and Ventricle		
PR patterns/relationships	Consistent PR patterns or relationships usually indicate SVT.	AV reentrant tachycardia and VT with 1:1 retrograde conduction
PR dissociation	PR dissociation may indicate VT.	Rapidly conducted atrial fibrillation may be associated
Chamber of Origin	Identifies if atrium leads ventricle or ventricle leads atrium at tachycardia onset	Can be fooled by single oversensed or undersensed event
Atrial extrastimuli	Discrimination of 1:1 rhythms using ventricular response to atrial extrastimuli	Primarily aids diagnosis for 1:1 rhythms, concerns for VT detection delay and proarrhythmia

AEGM, atrial electrogram; AF, atrial fibrillation; AV, atrioventricular; SVT, supraventricular tachycardia; VEGM, ventricular electrogram; VF, ventricular fibrillation; VT, ventricular tachycardia.
[a] Physiologically relevant information from general building blocks such as these may be combined to form a dual-chamber detection algorithm.

phology. The use of *ventricular extrastimuli* has been proposed as a method for discriminating between SVT and ventricular tachycardia. The first postpacing interval after the entrainment of ventricular tachycardia by two sets of pacing bursts was shown to be less variable than the same intervals measured during bursts delivered during SVT (28). This method has not been incorporated into ICDs because of concerns for delays in ventricular tachycardia detection (i.e., at least two sequences of burst pacing are required) and potential risk, although possibly quite small, of ventricular tachycardia induction by the burst pacing trains.

Table 21-1 also describes four dual-chamber detection building blocks that can be derived from the atrial electrogram alone. The building blocks—*PP interval* (i.e., atrial cycle length), *PP regularity, PP onset,* and *atrial electrogram morphology* (AEGM)—can help identify the presence of atrial tachyarrhythmias but must be used in conjunction with other criteria to be useful for ventricular tachyarrhythmia detection. The morphology of the atrial electrogram may be useful for classifying atrial tachyarrhythmias and discriminating between antegrade and retrograde conduction (29), but it may be confounded by FFRWs and changes in normal atrial electrogram morphology.

The final four building blocks described in Table 21-1 are based on combinations of atrial and ventricular information. The *PR patterns/relationships* building block can help to identify consistent AV patterns that are likely present during some SVTs. However, tachyarrhythmias such as ventricular tachycardia with 1 : 1 retrograde conduction and AV reentrant tachycardia may also have repeating patterns. Similarly, *PR dissociation* may help to indicate the presence of ventricular tachycardia during SVT but may be confounded by ventricular tachyarrhythmias that conduct retrograde to the atrium. The *chamber of origin* can be used to help discriminate between ventricular tachycardia and SVT rhythms with 1 : 1 association by identifying whether the atrium precedes the ventricle or vice versa at the time of tachycardia onset. At the start of spontaneous ventricular tachycardia, an intrinsic atrial event usually does not occur between the last sinus ventricular event and the first ectopic ventricular event. Conversely, at the start of an SVT, there is an atrial event before every ventricular event. Decisions made by this building block depend heavily on the critical timing of onset patterns and may be fooled by a single oversensed or undersensed event. The use of *atrial extrastimuli* has been proposed as a means of discriminating between SVT and ventricular tachycardia with 1 : 1 association. One method is to use a single atrial extrastimulus and examine the timing of the next ventricular event (30,31); if the rhythm is SVT, the atrial extrastimuli should shorten the following RR interval. For SVTs, this extrastimulus method may fail if the antegrade premature conduction is too early and blocks at the AV node. It may also fail for slow ventricular tachycardia if ventricular capture occurs. Such atrial extrastimuli may be proarrhythmic for the atrium or the ventricle.

No dual-chamber detection algorithm makes use of all the building blocks listed in Table 21-1. Each ICD manufacturer has designed different methods of computing the building blocks and different methods of combining a subset of the available information. The simplest dual-chamber detection algorithms have used PP intervals (atrial rate) in combination with RR intervals, RR regularity, and RR onset. More sophisticated algorithms have integrated the PP intervals, PR patterns, and PR dissociation with ventricular rate detection algorithms. The specific building blocks used and the order and methods used to combine them can serve as a high-level description of the detection algorithm. However, assessment of algorithm performance on a specific tachycardia may require more detailed descriptions of the specific computational methods used.

BASIC PR LOGIC DESCRIPTION

The dual-chamber detection algorithm, PR Logic, in Medtronic ICDs uses several basic design principles. High sensitivity for true ventricular tachyarrhythmias is maintained by the underlying ventricular rate–only detection algorithm. PR Logic withholds detection and therapies for rhythms in the ventricular rate detection zones *only* if dual-chamber data positively identify a particular type of SVT. This design principle is critical to improving specificity of detection without compromising detection sensitivity for life-threatening ventricular tachyarrhythmias. The algorithm must ensure prompt detection of ventricular tachycardia or ventricular fibrillation during ongoing SVT such as atrial fibrillation that may cause the atrial rate to remain above the ventricular rate even after the onset of ventricular tachycardia or ventricular fibrillation. The algorithm uses several beats of the rhythm to make decisions to minimize the effects of undersensing or oversensing in the atrial or the ventricular channel and to avoid uncertainty if there are changes in the characteristics of the rhythm being analyzed.

In addition to the standard single-chamber rate detection parameters, PR Logic has four physician-programmable parameters, three ON/OFF switches, and one RR interval–based parameter, the SVT limit.

The three independently programmable ON/OFF switches allow the user to enable or disable SVT rejection for rapidly conducted atrial fibrillation/flutter (AFib/AFlutter), sinus tachycardia (Sinus Tach), and SVTs with nearly simultaneous atrial and ventricular activations such as junctional tachycardia (Other 1 : 1 SVTs). The RR interval–based parameter, SVT limit, defines the shortest ventricular cycle length (or fastest ventricular rate) for which PR Logic withholds therapies for SVTs. The SVT limit parameter is nominally set at the fibrillation detection interval (FDI = 320 msec), but can be adjusted to longer or shorter cycle length values independent of the rate detection zone programming. There are no other numeric parameters to select in programming PR Logic.

The PR Logic SVT rejection criteria apply only during initial detection of tachyarrhythmia episodes. During redetection of tachyarrhythmia episodes, the ventricular rate–only detection criteria are used. PR Logic is designed to perform rhythm classifications within the programmed number of intervals for detection (NID) selected by the user for ventricular rate–only detection. Because PR Logic uses several beats to make decisions, a rolling buffer of recent dual-chamber information is maintained so that rhythm classifications can be made without delay. The recent information maintained by PR Logic is typically no greater than 24 RR intervals. PR Logic uses 6 of the 13 general dual-chamber detection building blocks in Table 21-1.

PR Logic Building Blocks

The six dual-chamber detection building blocks used by PR Logic are described in Table 21-2. The PR Logic building blocks consider all atrial-sensed atrial-refractory sensed, and -paced events as P events and all ventricular-sensed and -paced events as R events. The *RR interval* building block consists of the RR interval counting methods used in the Jewel family of single-chamber ICDs: "N of M" counting for detection of rhythms in the ventricular fibrillation zone and consecutive counting for detection of rhythms in the ventricular tachycardia zone. The median RR interval is calculated and compared with the programmable RR interval threshold, the SVT limit. The SVT limit defines the fastest ventricular rate for which the PR Logic criteria apply. PR Logic can only withhold detection when the median RR interval is greater than or equal to the SVT limit and an SVT has been positively identified. *PP intervals* and *PR patterns* are used to help identify the presence of an SVT, and the *RR regularity* and *PR dissociation* and are used to identify ventricular tachycardia when atrial fibrillation/flutter is present. Because the sensing circuitry has no cross-chamber blanking after sensed events and only 30 msec of cross-chamber blanking after paced events, there is a greater possibility for FFRW oversensing than with a standard dual-chamber pacemaker. *PP intervals, PR patterns*, and *PP regularity* are

TABLE 21-2 • PR LOGIC BUILDING BLOCKS

Building Blocks[a]	PR Logic Approach
RR intervals	"N of M" RR interval counting: identifies rhythms in VF zone Consecutive RR interval counting: identifies rhythms in VT zone Median RR interval: detection is never withheld for rhythms with median RR interval ≤SVT limit
PP intervals	Median PP interval: one of several criteria to recognize atrial fib/flutter if median PP ≤94% of median RR
PR patterns	Pattern syntax: used to identify sinus tachycardia, atrial fib/flutter, junctional tachycardia AF evidence counter: one of several criteria to identify atrial fib/flutter with a nonspecific pattern FFRW patterns: help identify FFRW oversensing during 2:1 rhythms
RR regularity	One of several criteria used to identify VT during atrial fib/flutter
PR dissociation	One of several criteria that helps identify VT or VF during atrial fibrillation
PP regularity	Identifies short-long PP intervals during 2:1 rhythm to help identify FFRW oversensing

AF, atrial fibrillation; FFRW, far-field R waves; SVT, supraventricular tachycardia; VF, ventricular fibrillation; VT, ventricular tachycardia.
[a] PR Logic uses several of the general dual-chamber detection building blocks listed in Table 21-1.

used to help identify the presence of consistent FFRW oversensing during 2:1 rhythms.

The RR-onset building block has not been incorporated into PR Logic because of concern about underdetection of spontaneous ventricular tachycardia during sinus tachycardia. Atrial and ventricular electrogram morphology building blocks have not yet been incorporated into PR Logic, primarily because of computational limitations. The chamber of origin building block has not been used in PR Logic because it can be heavily influenced by a single event that may be oversensed, undersensed, or blanked. Atrial and ventricular extrastimuli have not yet been included, but if proven safe (i.e., not proarrhythmic) and effective with clinically insignificant detection delays, these methods may provide yet another method of arrhythmia discrimination in the future.

PR Logic: Clinical Inductive Model

Classification of tachyarrhythmias by humans is generally approached with an inductive reasoning methodology, in which the final rhythm diagnosis is made using several layers of information incorporated with the process of elimination. Simple, unambiguous episodes may be classified with the most basic level of information, but challenging episodes require more information to ensure accuracy of the classification. The rhythm classification process used by PR Logic

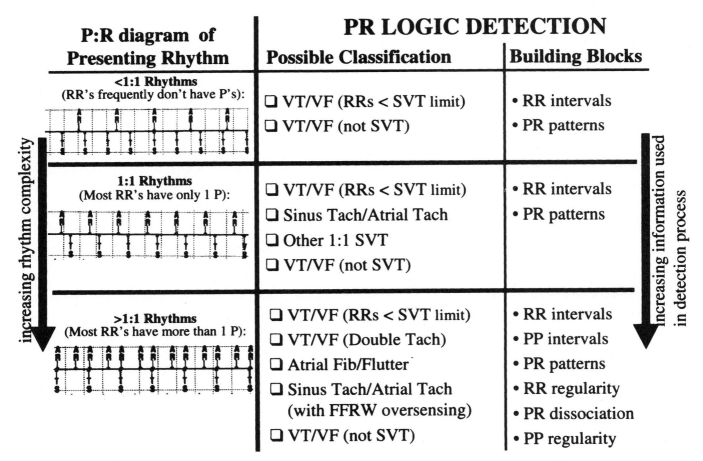

FIGURE 21-3. Clinical decision process for PR Logic. The rhythm types are represented using PR marker diagram examples *(left)* from the least complex *(top)* to the most complex *(bottom)*. A list of possible PR Logic decisions *(middle)* and the building blocks *(right)* used are shown for each of the rhythm types.

can be described in a manner that emulates this human diagnostic process.

As shown in Figure 21-3, the clinical decision process for PR Logic can be divided into three sections, with each corresponding to a different level of complexity of the rhythm being classified. Rhythm types are represented using PR marker diagrams on the left of Figure 21-3, and the rhythm complexity increases with the number of atrial events (Ps) between ventricular events (Rs). The least complex rhythm (Fig. 21-3, upper left) has a <1 : 1 pattern; RR intervals frequently do not have Ps. PR patterns for rhythms in this class have no more than 3 RRs of every 5 with 1 P event. The PR pattern cannot recognize SVT for this class of rhythms, and the detection decision is based exclusively on the RR interval analysis. The next level of complexity (Fig. 21-3, second row) consists of rhythms with a 1 : 1 pattern. PR patterns are considered 1 : 1 when most RR intervals have 1 P event and no more than 1 RR of every 5 has 0 or 2 Ps. Separate PR patterns incorporating PR relationships are used to describe "associated" 1 : 1 SVT rhythms (sinus/atrial tachycardia and junctional tachycardia) and to discriminate these 1 : 1 SVTs from ventricular tachycardia with 1 : 1 retrograde conduction. Rhythms at the third level of complexity are >1 : 1; most RR intervals have more than 1 P event. As shown in Figure 21-3 (bottom row), all six of the PR Logic building blocks are used to classify >1 : 1 rhythms. PR patterns, PP intervals, and PP regularity are used to define and discriminate sinus tachycardia with atrial oversensing of FFRW from atrial fibrillation/flutter. Direct measures of PR dissociation and RR interval regularity, as well as PR patterns, are used to identify the presence of double tachycardia (i.e., VT/VF during atrial fibrillation/atrial flutter) to maintain high sensitivity for true ventricular tachyarrhythmias. At each level of the detection process, when PR Logic cannot recognize SVT or when the ventricular rate gets too fast (RR intervals get shorter than the programmable SVT limit), the detection decision defaults to the RR interval–based criterion.

PR Logic Rhythm Classification

Figure 21-4 presents a decision tree diagram summarizing the possible PR Logic rhythm classifications and decision flow at each of the three levels of rhythm complexity (increasing complexity from left to right). Although the actual computational flow of PR Logic (described later) is different from that portrayed by Figure 21-4, this decision tree provides a clinically meaningful description of the PR Logic decision process. The combinations of dual-chamber detection building blocks used in the decision process are shown in each of the rectangles. Rhythm decisions are shown by the solid-line ovals for ventricular tachycardia, fast ventricular tachycardia (FVT), and ventricular fibrillation (VT/FVT/VF) and double tachycardia decisions (i.e., therapy delivered) and by the dotted-line ovals for the SVT decisions (i.e., therapy withheld). This summary assumes that all three of the PR Logic SVT rejection criteria are turned ON. This diagram can be used for selective programming of the SVT rejection criteria by assuming a NO result for decisions involving an SVT criterion that is OFF. The double tachycardia criteria are always enabled if one or more of the SVT rejection criteria are ON. Starting from the top, the entire decision tree is evaluated on every ventricular event until VT/FVT/VF or double tachycardia is detected (at which point therapy is initiated). The PR Logic decision tree is not evaluated during redetection, because PR Logic only applies during initial detection of tachyarrhythmia episodes. The decision process starts by determining if the ventricular rate is too fast to apply PR Logic (Fig. 21-4, top). If the median RR interval is less than the SVT limit, PR Logic defaults to the RR interval–based detection of VT/FVT/VF. If not, then one of the three "branches" of the tree is traversed, depending on the presenting PR diagram. The <1 : 1 rhythm branch is shown on the far left of Figure 21-4. For this class of rhythms, there are not enough P events to consider the rhythm to be any type of SVT, and the rhythm decision is VT/FVT/VF according to the RR interval–based detection.

The center branch of Figure 21-4 is for 1 : 1 rhythms (i.e., rhythms that are primarily 1 : 1 with no more than 1 atrial undersense or oversense every 5 RR intervals). As shown in Figure 21-4, 1 : 1 rhythms may be classified as sinus tachycardia, junctional tachycardia, or ventricular tachycardia. The sinus tachycardia classification is evaluated first, and if the pattern criterion is met (which requires

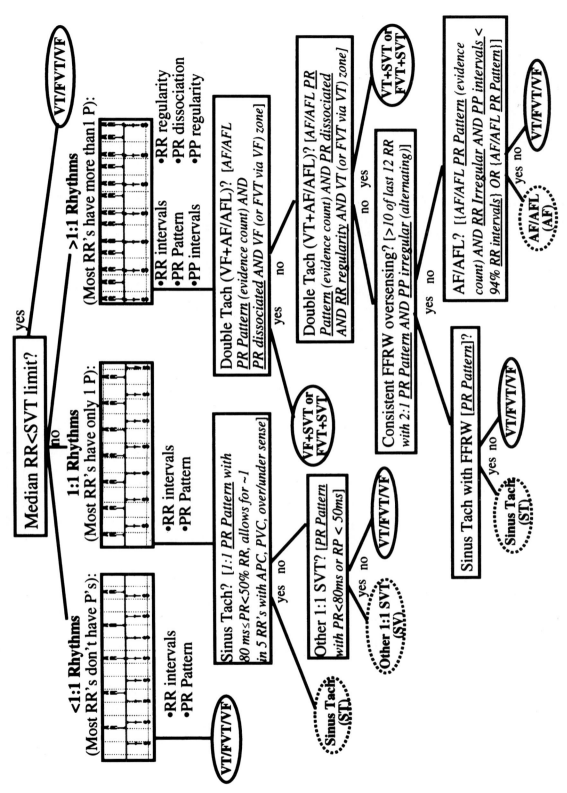

FIGURE 21-4. PR Logic clinical decision tree diagram for Gem DR and Gem II DR. The entire rhythm classification process is tested on each ventricular event. The decision tree diagram assumes that all three of the PR Logic supraventricular tachycardia (SVT) rejection criteria are programmed ON. The ovals show the rhythm classifications, with the dotted line ovals denoting classification as an SVT. For each of the three main branches of the tree diagram, detection is withheld only if PR Logic positively identifies the rhythm as an SVT. The actual computational flow of PR Logic is slightly different, as shown in Figure 21-14.

80 msec ≤ PR < 50% RR), the rhythm is classified as sinus tachycardia (ST). If the rhythm is not ST, the Other 1 : 1 SVT criterion is evaluated. If the pattern for junctional rhythm is met (requiring PR < 80 msec or RP < 50 msec), the rhythm is classified as SV (Other 1 : 1 SVT). Rhythms with repeating 1 : 1 patterns with PR ≥50% of the RR interval and RP ≥50 msec are classified as VT/FVT/VF by RR interval–based criterion. This classification assumes that the pattern may result from retrograde conduction, and for safety, the rhythm must be classified as a ventricular tachyarrhythmia. If the rhythm is dissociated, no consistent 1 : 1 pattern can be identified, and the rhythm classification defaults to VT/FVT/VF by RR interval–based detection.

The far right branch of Figure 21-4 is for >1 : 1 rhythms, which are rhythms with more than 1 P event for most RR intervals. PR Logic first checks for the presence of double tachycardia (i.e., ventricular tachycardia or ventricular fibrillation arising during atrial fibrillation/atrial flutter). When double tachycardia is detected, the rhythm is treated with the zone-appropriate programmed VT/FVT/VF therapy. Rhythms conducting into the ventricular fibrillation zone that have PR dissociation are classified as VF + SVT (i.e., ventricular fibrillation during atrial fibrillation/atrial flutter). Rhythms in the ventricular tachycardia zone that are PR dissociated and have regular RR intervals are classified as VT + SVT (i.e., ventricular tachycardia during atrial fibrillation/atrial flutter). If a rhythm is not detected as double tachycardia, PR Logic combines the PP intervals, PR pattern, RR regularity, and PP regularity to determine whether the rhythm is either atrial fibrillation/flutter or sinus tachycardia with consistent FFRW oversensing, in which case VT/FVT/VF detection is withheld. If the rhythm is not identifiable as SVT, VT/FVT/VF detection occurs.

◉ DETAILED PR LOGIC BUILDING BLOCKS AND GEM DR EXAMPLES

The overview of PR Logic previously presented describes how PR Logic works at the most basic level of understanding. The following discussion reinforces these concepts through examples of PR Logic detection at each of the three levels of rhythm complexity: <1 : 1, 1 : 1, and >1 : 1 rhythms. The examples presented are spontaneous tachycardias that were recorded by and retrieved from patients with Gem DR devices. A deeper level of understanding can be achieved by study of the PR Logic building blocks and how they were combined to form the rhythm classifications. The building blocks are described in more detail in the boxed text as they are used in the examples.

The <1:1 Rhythms

To be considered a <1 : 1 rhythm, RR intervals must frequently have 0 P events, with no more than 3 RRs of every 5 having 1 P event. PR pattern analysis cannot recognize SVT for these rhythms, and the detection decision is based exclusively on the RR interval analysis.

Building Block 1: RR Intervals. RR intervals are used to estimate the ventricular cycle length and for the counting algorithms of ventricular rate–only tachyarrhythmia detection. Ventricular cycle length is estimated by the median of the last 12 RR intervals, updated on each ventricular event. The median statistic is used because it is not as sensitive to occasional undersensing or oversensing as the mean value or other statistics. The ventricular cycle length counting algorithms used by PR Logic are identical to the methods used in the Jewel family of single-chamber ICDs and consists of two counters (one for ventricular fibrillation and another for ventricular tachycardia) and three rate detection zones that use these two counters. The ventricular fibrillation rhythm counter nominally requires that 18 of the last 24 RR intervals be less than the fibrillation detection interval (FDI). This counter is very sensitive to ensure rapid detection of ventricular fibrillation even if some undersensing occurs. The ventricular tachycardia counter nominally requires 16 consecutive RR intervals be less than the tachycardia detection interval (TDI) but greater than or equal to the FDI; the TDI is required to be longer than the FDI. This counter is much more specific because sensing of ventricular tachycardia is rarely a problem and rejection of variable atrial fibrillatory rhythms is important
Continued, p. 535

(32). There is also a combined count criterion that accelerates detection of rhythms that straddle the ventricular tachycardia and ventricular fibrillation detection zones. Combined count is applicable for episodes when the ventricular fibrillation counter is at least 6 and allows detection to occur when the sum of the ventricular tachycardia and ventricular fibrillation counters reaches 7/6 of the programmed number of intervals to detect ventricular fibrillation.

The RR interval building block also allows ventricular rate–only detection to occur in a third rate zone, the FVT zone. The purpose of the FVT zone is to allow a third set of programmable antitachycardia therapies that are generally more aggressive than standard ventricular tachycardia therapies for faster tachycardias that may not require defibrillation. RR intervals are defined to be in the FVT zone if they have cycle lengths between the FDI and the fast tachycardia interval (FTI). The intervals in the FVT zone are always counted as a part of the ventricular tachycardia or the ventricular fibrillation counter, depending on how FTI is programmed. When the FTI is less than the FDI, the FVT zone is a subset of the ventricular fibrillation zone, and all RR intervals less than the FDI are counted on the ventricular fibrillation counter (FVT via VF). When the FTI is greater than the FDI, the FVT intervals are counted on the ventricular tachycardia counter (FVT via VT). The decision to deliver FVT, VT, or VF therapy is made with the last eight RR intervals before the ventricular tachycardia or ventricular fibrillation counter is satisfied. For FVT via VF, FVT therapy is delivered if all of the last eight intervals are in the FVT zone. For FVT via VT, FVT therapy is delivered if any of the last eight beats are in the VF or FVT zone.

Figure 21-5 presents an example of spontaneous ventricular tachycardia that was detected when the ventricular tachycardia counter reached 12, the programmed number of intervals for detection (NID). The strip shows atrial and ventricular electrograms, dual-chamber marker channel with numeric values for the PP and RR intervals, and a rhythm annotation showing the detection result. The rhythm annotation indicates when VT/FVT/VF detection and therapy occurred and includes beat-by-beat rhythm classification (AF for atrial fibrillation/flutter, ST for sinus tachycardia, SV for Other 1 : 1 SVT) when PR Logic withholds VT/FVT/VF detection. The interval versus time plot in Figure 21-5 shows patterns of the atrial intervals (squares) and ventricular intervals (circles) versus time for a longer period before and after detection of the tachyarrhythmia. The lower right part of Figure 21-5 is an enlarged portion of the PR marker diagram with a summary of the PR Logic rhythm classification. All rhythm example figures in this chapter have a strip, interval plot, and enlarged portion of the marker diagram with a similar format. The rhythm annotation shows when ventricular tachycardia detection occurred (Fig. 21-5, VT at [2], also shown on the marker channel as TD). The ventricular events with cycle length in the ventricular tachycardia zone are labeled Tachy Sense (TS). Atrial and ventricular intervals are shown versus time for approximately 15 seconds before detection of ventricular tachycardia and for approximately 25 seconds after the first antitachycardia pacing (ATP) therapy started.

The atrial and ventricular intervals are nearly identical to each other (left side of the interval plot). At the onset of the ventricular tachycardia, the strip and interval plot show the sudden shortening of ventricular intervals to a cycle length that was clearly shorter than the atrial intervals [1]. There was no change in atrial intervals after the onset of ventricular tachycardia. FFRWs can be seen on the atrial electrogram channel. However, there was no oversensing of FFRWs on the atrial amplifier, as shown by the marker channel. After the ventricular tachycardia began [1], there were not enough P events between R events for the PR Logic pattern analysis to positively identify an SVT, and the rhythm therefore was detected when the ventricular tachycardia counter reached 12.

The 1 : 1 Rhythms

Rhythms are considered to be 1 : 1 when most RR intervals have only 1 P event, and no more than 1 RR of every 5 has 0 or 2 Ps. Separate PR patterns incorporating PR relationships describe associated 1 : 1 SVT rhythms (i.e., sinus/atrial tachycardia and junctional tachycardia) and discriminate these 1 : 1 SVTs from ventricular tachycardia with 1 : 1 retrograde conduction.

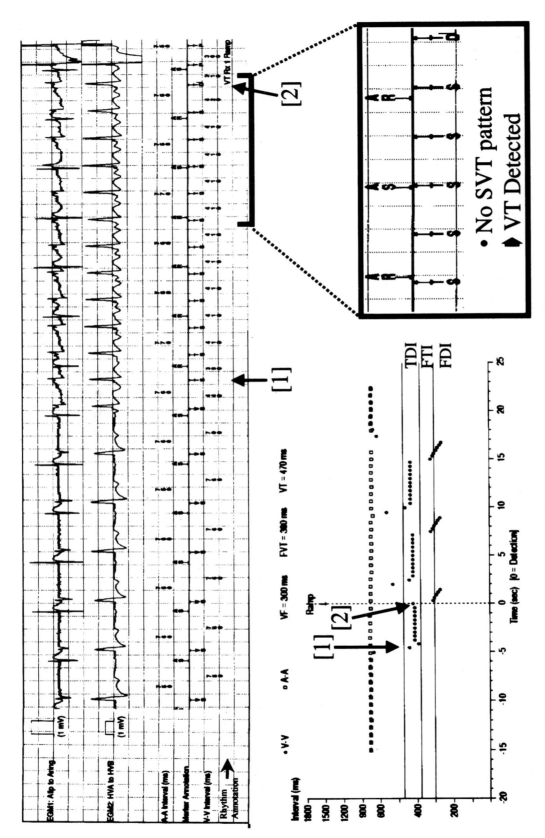

FIGURE 21-5. Detection of spontaneous ventricular tachycardia (VT). The stored Gem DR implantable cardioverter-defibrillator strip shows detection of VT [2] and start of antitachycardia pacing (ATP) therapy when the VT counter reached the number of intervals for detection (NID = 12). The strip shows the bipolar atrial electrogram (EGM), the right ventricular coil-to-can EGM, the dual-chamber marker channel, and the rhythm annotation. The interval versus time plot shows that the RR intervals suddenly shortened at the onset of VT [1]. The ventricular EGM morphology also changed after the onset of VT. The interval plot shows that VT was terminated after the third sequence of ramp ATP.

Building Block 2: PR Pattern. The PR pattern building block is illustrated in Figure 21-6. As shown at the top of Figure 21-6A, pattern analysis is performed for each ventricular event using the two previous RR intervals. The first stage of the pattern analysis is to form couple codes represented as letters of the alphabet (i.e., letters A through Q, Y, and Z) based on the number of atrial events and their timing relative to the ventricular events. Zero, one, two, or more atrial events for each RR interval are classified according to their proximity to the R events. Each RR interval is divided into three regions for the purpose of classifying the P events as shown in Figure 21-6A. If a P event is less than 80 msec before a ventricular event or less than 50 msec after a ventricular event, that P event is considered "junctional"; these fixed 50- and 80-msec boundaries exclude antegrade or retrograde conduction and were determined by consensus of electrophysiologists as the shortest antegrade and retrograde conduction time that could be expected in typical ICD patients. For defining the boundary between antegrade and retrograde conduction, an RR interval adaptive threshold (50% of the current RR interval) is used. If a P event occurs such that the PR interval is less than 50% of the current RR interval and greater than or equal to 80 msec, the P event is considered antegrade. If the P event occurs such that the PR interval is greater than or equal to 50% of the current RR interval and the RP interval is greater than or equal to 50 msec, it is considered retrograde. The antegrade-retrograde boundary was selected to maximize sensitivity for detecting ventricular tachycardia with 1 : 1 retrograde conduction using PR timing derived from human intracardiac electrogram recordings of ventricular tachycardia with 1 : 1 retrograde conduction. The antegrade-retrograde boundary is fixed at 50% of the RR interval in the Gem DR and Gem II DR ICDs; a programmable parameter, the "1 : 1 VT-ST Boundary," has been added to PR Logic in the Gem III DR ICD to allow changing this boundary to values from 35% to 85% of the RR interval.

The next stage of the pattern analysis is to form strings of couple codes from successive pairs of RR intervals after every R event in the cardiac rhythm being analyzed. Each RR interval and its P event(s) are used twice, first as the most recent RR interval for one couple code and then the same RR interval

Continued

and its P event(s) are used as the second most recent RR interval for the next couple code. This process of computing couple codes forms a string of letters that is compared with sequences of letters known to occur during one of the specific SVTs recognized (i.e., the SVT syntax). For example, in sinus tachycardia, sequences such as AAA, ABCEA, ADEA, ABZAA, or ALMAA are allowed. The pattern ABCEA is typical for a premature ventricular contraction (PVC) in sinus tachycardia as shown for the sinus tachycardia rhythm in Figure 21-6A. The pattern matching is continuous and analogous to a word-processing spelling checker. The sinus tachycardia syntax patterns are like words in a spelling checker dictionary. The unknown rhythm being classified is like the stream of new text being evaluated by the spelling checker. Sinus tachycardia is no longer recognized if the string of letters no longer matches the sinus tachycardia patterns and is analogous to the spelling checker stopping for an unknown word. Each of the SVT patterns is recognized through the use of separate counters that count up by 1 when a letter matches one of the predefined strings and that reset to 0 or count down exponentially when a letter does not match the predefined strings. A particular SVT pattern is recognized when its counter reaches the value of 6 and is unrecognized when its counter has decremented to a value below 6. The sinus tachycardia pattern counter has a maximum value of 13 and has two stages in which different decrement properties are used. When the counter has not yet reached its recognition threshold of 6, it is reset to 0 when a couple code does not match the predefined syntax. After the counter reaches 6, it decrements by 4, 8, 16, and so on (i.e., exponential countdown) to a minimum value of 0 for each ventricular event for which no match is seen. The exponential decay (i.e., decrement value) is reset to 4 when the counter reaches 6 for the first time after counting up from 0 and when it reaches the maximum value of 13. The exponential decrement property and the counter maximum of 13 (with recognition threshold at 6) allow the sinus tachycardia pattern to remain recognized for occasional occurrences of couple codes that are not in the predefined syntax. The Other 1 : 1 SVT counter has a maximum value of 6 and resets to 0 when a couple code does not match the predefined strings. The Other 1 : 1 SVT pattern counter does not have the exponential decrement property.

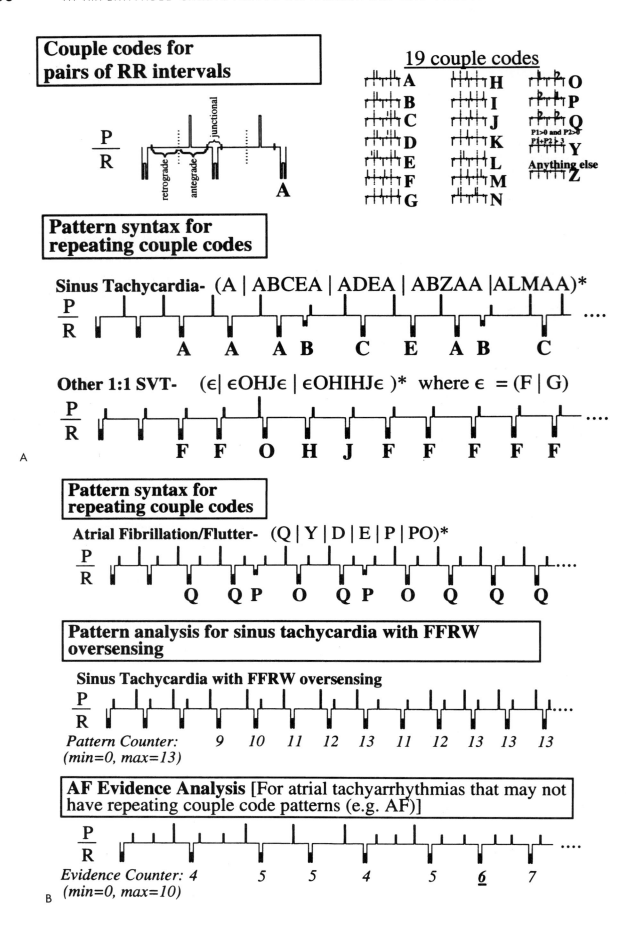

For 1 : 1 rhythms, the PR relationship (i.e., PR interval) plays an important role in PR Logic rhythm classification. Only 1 : 1 patterns with PR intervals primarily in the antegrade or junctional regions of the RR interval can be classified as SVT. Figure 21-7 shows an example of sinus tachycardia in the ventricular tachycardia zone that would have resulted in inappropriate therapy by single-chamber, rate-only detection. The ST rhythm annotations starting on the left side of the strip [1] indicate that ventricular rate–only detection was being withheld by PR Logic. The ventricular events labeled TS (Tachy Sense) and FS (Fibrillation Sense) had cycle lengths in the ventricular tachycardia zone and ventricular fibrillation zone, respectively. Ventricular tachycardia would have been detected when the ventricular tachycardia counter reached the programmed NID of 16. However, the annotation shows ST to indicate that the sinus tachycardia SVT rejection criteria was withholding detection. The PR pattern for this rhythm was 1 : 1, with PR intervals in the antegrade region of the RR interval. The couple codes for this rhythm were mainly A's, and the sinus tachycardia pattern criterion was satisfied, so ventricular tachycardia detection was withheld. The ST annotations continued until PR Logic was no longer withholding detection because one long RR interval after a PVC reset the ventricular tachycardia counter to 0 [2]. The ST annotations resumed when the ventricular tachycardia counter reached 16 again [3]. The ST annotations stopped again when the sinus tachycardia slowed, and the RR intervals increased to values above the TDI [4]. The interval plot shows a 1 : 1 tachycardia in the ventricular tachycardia zone that was neither detected nor treated.

Figure 21-8 shows an example of junctional tachycardia in the ventricular tachycardia zone that would have resulted in inappropriate therapy by single-chamber, rate-only detection. The SV rhythm annotation on this strip indicates that ventricular tachycardia detection was being withheld by the Other 1 : 1 SVT criterion. The PR pattern for this rhythm was 1 : 1, with PR intervals in the junctional region of the RR interval. The couple codes for this rhythm were primarily F, and the pattern syntax for Other 1 : 1 SVT was satisfied, allowing ventricular tachycardia detection to be withheld. The PR pattern changed for a single RR interval [1] because of a premature atrial event, after which the prior PR pattern resumed. This slight disturbance did not cause the SV rhythm classification to change because the resulting couple code sequence was allowed by the predefined Other 1 : 1 SVT pattern syntax. Spontaneous termination of the junctional tachycardia occurred as shown on the interval plot by a sudden slowing of atrial and ventricular rates to cycle lengths outside of the ventricular tachycardia detection zones.

Figure 21-9 shows an example of spontaneous ven-

FIGURE 21-6. **A:** PR Logic pattern analysis for 1:1 rhythms. On every ventricular event, the preceding two RR intervals and intervening P events are analyzed. The number and timing of the P events are used to classify the current ventricular event as one of the 19 couple codes (represented by letters of the alphabet). There are two types of 1:1 supraventricular tachycardias (SVTs) represented by pattern syntax. Each SVT has a pattern syntax that allows some deviation from the "pure" rhythm, such as premature ventricular contraction (PVC) or premature atrial contraction (PAC). For example, pure sinus tachycardia is AAA–, but sinus tachycardia is still recognized when the string ABCEA occurs because of a PVC as shown. **B:** PR Logic pattern analysis for >1:1 rhythms. The AFib/AFlutter is recognized using a pattern syntax for atrial fibrillation/flutter with regular atrioventricular (AV) conduction *(top)* or atrial fibrillation evidence analysis *(bottom)* that can identify atrial fibrillation when PR relationships are highly variable. The AFib/AFlutter pattern syntax allows for some deviation of a pure 2:1 or 3:1 rhythm as shown. Atrial fibrillation evidence analysis determines if the atrial fibrillation evidence counter is incremented by 1, decremented by 1, or remains at the same value using the number of P events in each RR interval. The pattern analysis for sinus tachycardia with far-field R waves (FFRWs) *(center)* does not use couple codes, but rather uses the number and relative position of P events within a single RR interval to determine patterns. PR Logic combines the sinus tachycardia with an FFRW pattern counter with the PP regularity building block to classify rhythms as sinus tachycardia with FFRW oversensing.

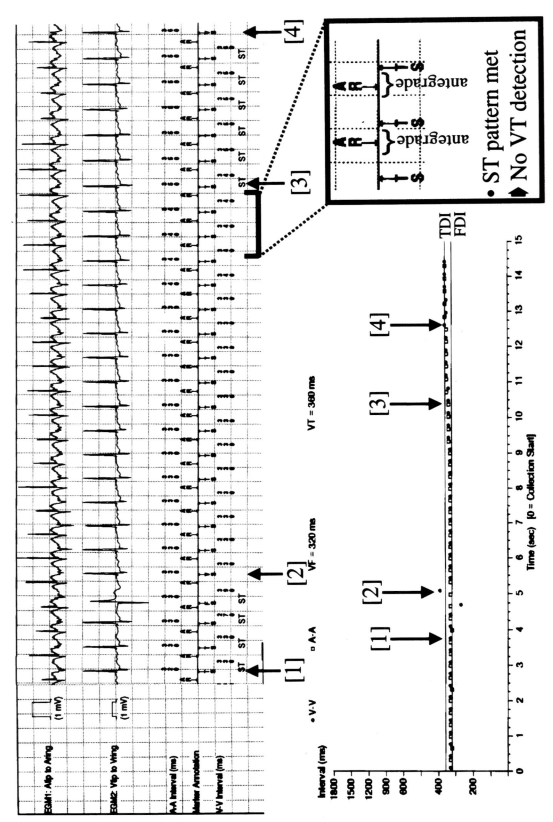

FIGURE 21-7. Ventricular tachycardia (VT) detection appropriately withheld during sinus tachycardia. This example is a stored supraventricular tachycardia (SVT) episode showing sinus tachycardia that was not detected as VT because of the sinus tachycardia criterion (ST) of PR Logic. The ST annotations [1] indicated that the rhythm was classified as sinus tachycardia at the left of the strip. These annotations continued until the VT counter was reset to 0 by one long RR interval after a premature ventricular contraction (PVC) [2]. The ST annotations resumed [3] when the VT counter reached the programmed number of intervals for detection (NID = 16) again. The ST annotations stopped on the far right side of the strip because the RR intervals increased to values greater than the tachycardia detection interval (TDI = 360 msec) [4]. The interval plot shows a 1:1 tachycardia in the VT zone that was neither detected nor treated.

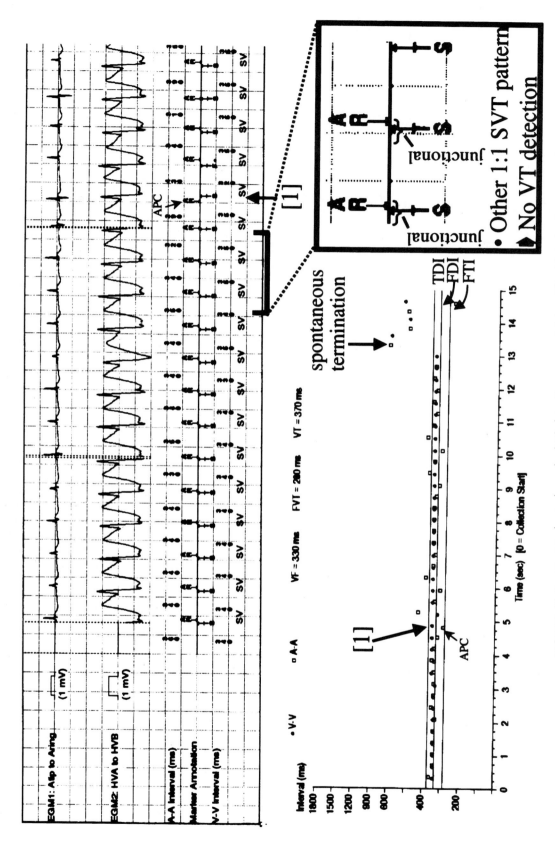

FIGURE 21-8. Ventricular tachycardia (VT) detection appropriately withheld during junctional tachycardia. This example is a stored supraventricular tachycardia (SVT) episode showing a junctional tachycardia that was not detected as VT because of the Other 1:1 SVT criterion (SV) of PR Logic. The RR intervals were in the VT zone (tachycardia detection interval [TDI] = 370 msec), and the number of intervals to detect VT (NID = 12) had been satisfied. Although the PR pattern changed for a single RR interval because of a premature atrial event [1], the SV rhythm classification did not change. The interval plot shows spontaneous termination of the SVT with a sudden slowing of atrial and ventricular rates to cycle lengths outside of the VT zone.

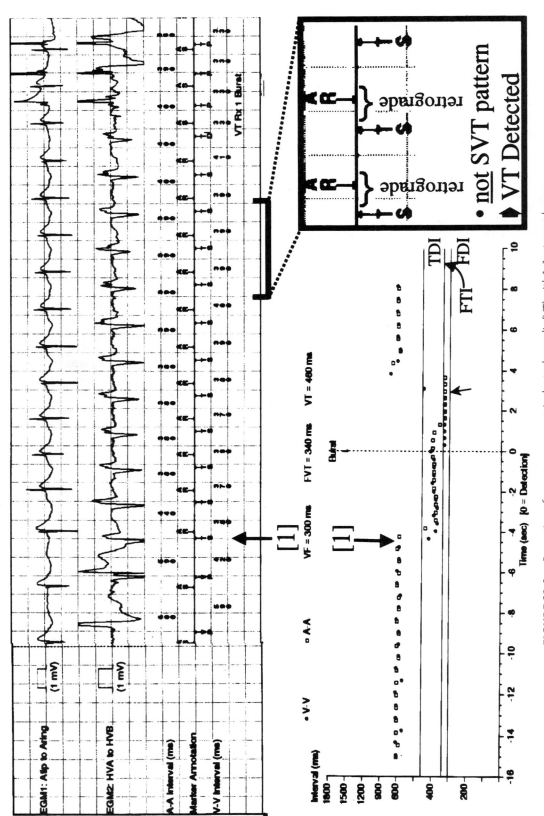

FIGURE 21-9. Detection of spontaneous ventricular tachycardia (VT) with 1:1 retrograde conduction. The interval plot and strip from this stored VT episode shows that first event of the tachycardia was an R event [1], not an atrial event. The ventricular rate accelerates suddenly into the VT zone (tachycardia detection interval [TDI] = 460 msec), followed by atrial rate acceleration due to retrograde conduction of the R events. After these first 2 beats, the rhythm remained 1:1 until the VT counter reached the programmed number of intervals for detection (NID = 16). Although this rhythm had a 1:1 pattern, the PR relationship did not match those expected for sinus tachycardia or Other 1:1 SVT. VT detection occurred because no SVT was identified. As seen on the right side of the interval plot, burst ATP was delivered after VT detection occurred, terminating the VT. Burst pacing seems to have conducted retrograde and accelerated the atrial rhythm (*arrow*); the last of the three short PP intervals was an atrial pace.

tricular tachycardia with 1 : 1 retrograde conduction. The interval plot and strip show the first event of the tachycardia was an R event [1]. Retrograde conduction occurred on the next R event, where there was a sudden shortening of the PP intervals. The rhythm remained 1 : 1 after these first two beats until the ventricular tachycardia counter reached the programmed number of intervals for detection (NID = 12) (VT). Although this rhythm had a 1 : 1 pattern, the PR relationship did not match those expected for sinus tachycardia or Other 1 : 1 SVT, because the P event was consistently occurring in the retrograde region of the RR interval. The couple code (N) generated by this rhythm is not part of the predefined pattern syntax for sinus tachycardia or Other 1 : 1 SVT, and PR Logic did not withhold detection for this 1 : 1 rhythm. Ventricular tachycardia detection occurred when the ventricular tachycardia counter reached 16 because PR Logic had not identified this rhythm to be SVT.

PR Logic defaults to the RR interval–based criterion when the ventricular rate gets too fast. When the median RR interval is less than the SVT limit, the RR interval–based criteria decide the detection outcome. The example in Figure 21-10 was probably a spontaneous atrial tachycardia with aberrant conduction and had median RR intervals less than the SVT limit. It appears that this fast rhythm was being driven by the atrium, as evidenced by the sudden PP interval shortening that preceded the RR interval shortening [1]. The patient's physician confirmed the diagnosis of atrial tachycardia. This 1 : 1 rhythm had PR intervals in the antegrade conduction zone, and the couple code string for this episode consisted of A's. Even though the sinus tachycardia pattern syntax was satisfied, ventricular fibrillation was detected (FD) when the ventricular fibrillation counter criterion was satisfied (12th FS event). Ventricular fibrillation detection occurred because the median RR interval (290 msec) was less than the programmed SVT limit (300 msec), and PR Logic defaulted to the basic RR interval–based rhythm classification.

The >1 : 1 Rhythms

Because of the complexity of >1 : 1 rhythms (most RRs have more than 1 P event), PR patterns and PR relationships may not be enough to make an accurate rhythm diagnosis. For example, the PR patterns previously defined cannot determine if the rhythm is rapidly conducted atrial fibrillation or ventricular tachycardia during atrial fibrillation. PR Logic integrates all six of its building blocks to make rhythm decisions at this level. In addition to PR Patterns, direct measures of PR dissociation and RR interval regularity are used to identify the presence of ventricular tachycardia or ventricular fibrillation during atrial fibrillation/atrial flutter (i.e., double tachycardia) to maintain high detection sensitivity. PR patterns, PR relationships, and PP regularity are used to define and discriminate sinus tachycardia with FFRW oversensing on the atrial lead from atrial tachyarrhythmias with rapid ventricular responses. If the combination of the PR Logic building blocks cannot recognize SVT, VT/FVT/VF is detected when the RR interval criterion is satisfied. When the ventricular rate becomes too fast (i.e., median RR intervals become shorter than the programmable SVT limit), the detection decision defaults to the RR interval only criterion.

Building Block 2: PR Pattern (continued). As shown in Figure 21-6B, there are predefined patterns for recognition of >1 : 1 rhythms such as atrial fibrillation/flutter with regular ventricular response (e.g., 2 : 1 or 3 : 1 atrial flutter) and sinus tachycardia with FFRW oversensing. The atrial fibrillation/flutter pattern is recognized using a pattern counter that increments by 1 when a letter (i.e., couple code) matches the predefined syntax and resets to 0 when a letter does not match the predefined string. The AFib/AFlutter pattern is recognized when the counter reaches its maximum value of 6.

The sinus tachycardia with FFRW pattern counter does not use couple codes, but rather uses the number and relative position of P events within a *single* RR interval to determine patterns. The pattern derived from a single RR interval is used because the couple code description results in ambiguities that make the pattern recognition less specific for sinus tachycardia with FFRW oversensing. As shown in Figure 21-6B, the sinus tachycardia with FFRW pattern counter is incremented by 1 when there are 1 or 2 P events within an RR interval with one of the P events in the antegrade region of the RR interval. *Continued,* p. 545

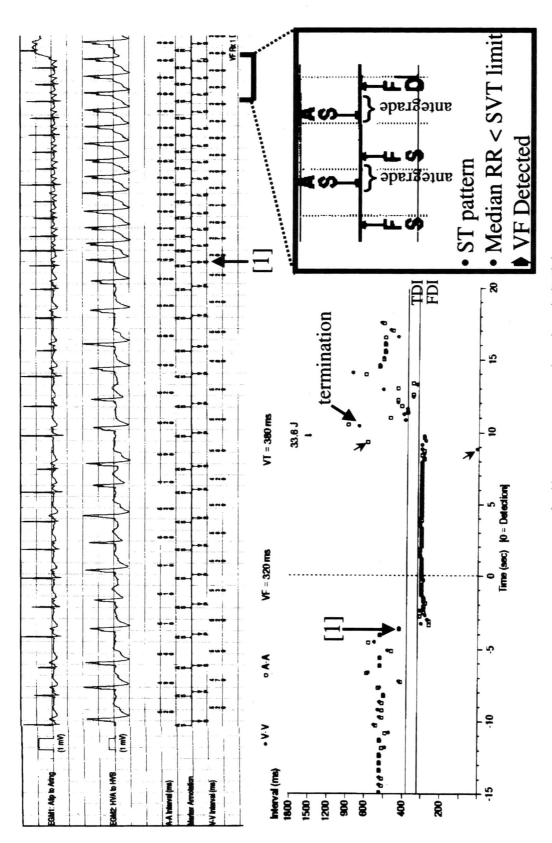

FIGURE 21-10. Detection of sudden-onset supraventricular tachycardia (SVT) due to a median RR interval less than the SVT limit. This spontaneous atrial tachycardia with aberrancy had median RR intervals of 290 msec, which was less than the SVT limit of 300 msec. The PP interval shortening preceded the RR interval shortening at the arrhythmia onset [1]. Although the PR pattern satisfied the sinus tachycardia pattern, ventricular fibrillation (VF) detection occurred when the VF counter was satisfied because the median RR interval was less than the SVT limit, and PR Logic was not applied. The interval plot shows that a shock was delivered and terminated the rapidly conducted atrial tachycardia. The short RR interval and long PP interval before termination *(small arrows)* occurred at the end of the capacitor charging period. The interval from the previous ventricular event to the charge end is reported as an RR interval of less than 100 msec *(small arrow)*. A blanking period on the atrial and ventricular sense amplifiers is started after charge end to avoid oversensing and resulted in a long PP interval *(small arrow)*.

Building Block 2: PR Pattern (continued). There is a predefined set of patterns based on single RR intervals that allow the counter to also be incremented for isolated premature atrial contractions and PVCs. The sinus tachycardia with FFRW oversensing pattern is recognized when the counter reaches 6. The counter has a maximum value of 13 and has two stages with different decrement properties. When the counter has not yet reached the recognition threshold of 6, it is reset to 0 for patterns not in the predefined set. After the counter reaches 6, it decrements by 2, 4, 8, and so on (i.e., exponential countdown) to a minimum value of 0 for each ventricular event that does not match. The exponential decay (i.e., decrement value) is reset to 2 when the counter reaches 6 for the first time after counting up from 0 and when it reaches the maximum value of 13. The exponential decrement property and the counter maximum of 13 (with a recognition threshold at 6) allows the sinus tachycardia with a FFRW pattern to remain recognized for occasional occurrences of patterns that are not in the predefined syntax. PR Logic combines the sinus tachycardia and FFRW pattern counter with the PP regularity building block to classify rhythms as sinus tachycardia with FFRW oversensing.

To recognize atrial tachyarrhythmias with no repeating couple code patterns, PR Logic uses an up-down atrial fibrillation evidence counter that has a maximum value of 10 and a minimum value of 0 (Fig. 21-6B, bottom). Atrial fibrillation evidence is recognized when the counter reaches 6 and stays recognized until the counter falls below 5. The atrial fibrillation evidence counter increments for a given RR interval if there are 2 or more intervening P events, unless 1 P event is identified as a FFRW oversense, in which case the evidence counter is unchanged. The atrial fibrillation evidence counter decrements when there are 0 or 1 intervening P events, unless there is 1 P event with a significantly different PR interval than the previous PR interval, in which case the evidence counter is unchanged. This counter is used to help identify atrial fibrillation when PR relationships during atrial fibrillation are highly variable.

Building Block 3: RR interval Regularity. RR interval regularity is determined by a measurement called *modesum*. The last 18 RR intervals are analyzed *Continued*

Building Block 3: RR interval Regularity (continued). by generating a histogram with 10-msec bins and by comparing the sum of the number of intervals in the two largest bins to the total number of intervals. The higher this ratio, the more regular is the rhythm (e.g., ventricular tachycardia or atrial flutter with 2 : 1 conduction has a high modesum ratio). For an irregular rhythm, such as the ventricular response to atrial fibrillation or ventricular fibrillation, the modesum ratio is low. This measure can tolerate moderate undersensing or oversensing.

Building Block 4: PR Dissociation. PR dissociation is computed from a recent series of PR intervals. On every ventricular event, the mean of the most recent 8 PR intervals is computed. An individual ventricular event is judged dissociated if the absolute difference between the current PR interval and the average is greater than 40 msec or if there are no P events in the current RR interval. A rhythm is considered dissociated if at least four of the last eight ventricular events are dissociated.

Building Block 5: PP Intervals. The median PP interval is computed to estimate the atrial cycle length. The median PP interval is updated on every ventricular event based on the previous 12 PP intervals. The median statistic is used because it is not as sensitive to limited undersensing or oversensing as the mean value or other statistics.

PR Logic identifies the presence of double tachycardia by combining several of the PR Logic building blocks. PR Logic detects double tachycardia in the ventricular tachycardia detection zone (VT + SVT) when the following criteria are simultaneously satisfied:

- Ventricular tachycardia counter satisfied (or VT detection by combined count)
- Evidence of atrial fibrillation or flutter (i.e., AF evidence)
- PR dissociation
- Regular RR intervals (modesum ≥14/18)

These criteria are derived from the expectation that ventricular tachycardia during atrial fibrillation should have regular RR intervals but is dissociated from atrial activations. PR Logic also detects double tachycardias in the ventricular fibrillation detection zone (VF + SVT) when the following criteria are simultaneously satisfied:

- Ventricular fibrillation counter satisfied (or VF detection by combined count)
- Evidence of atrial fibrillation or flutter (i.e., AF evidence)
- PR dissociation

The RR regularity criterion is not included for the detection of VF + SVT, because ventricular fibrillation or rapid polymorphic ventricular tachycardia may have irregular RR intervals. Figure 21-11 is an example of appropriate detection of double tachycardia (i.e., spontaneous ventricular tachycardia during atrial fibrillation) that was promptly detected and terminated with burst ATP therapy. The strip shows atrial fibrillation on the atrial electrogram that was appropriately sensed. Sudden onset of a regular ventricular rate occurred [1], and the rhythm was detected as VT + SVT (i.e., double tachycardia) by PR Logic near the end of the strip (VT). At the time of detection, the ventricular tachycardia counter was satisfied (NID = 16), and atrial fibrillation evidence, PR dissociation, and RR regularity (modesum ≥14/18) were all satisfied. These are the building block criteria that must be simultaneously satisfied for PR Logic to classify rhythms as VT + SVT.

Figure 21-12 shows a similar strip and interval plot where rejection of atrial fibrillation/flutter prevented inappropriate ventricular tachycardia detection. The atrial tachyarrhythmia at the start of the strip had a 2 : 1 ventricular response that was in the ventricular tachycardia zone (TS markers), and the atrial fibrillation annotations show that the PR Logic AFib/AFlutter rejection criterion was withholding ventricular tachycardia detection and therapy [1]. The ventricular rate remained in the ventricular tachycardia zone, and detection continued to be withheld for many beats. The atrial cycle lengths lengthened slightly after the ventricular event labeled [2], and conduction to the ventricles slowed to be outside of the ventricular tachycardia zone. The atrial fibrillation annotations stopped at the first RR interval greater than the TDI [2] because the ventricular tachycardia counter was reset to 0. In this example of atrial fibrillation/atrial flutter with regular RR intervals, the atrial fibrillation/flutter pattern syntax was satisfied because the rhythm was 2 : 1 (the couple codes were Q), and ventricular tachycardia detection was withheld. Three of the four criteria for double tachycardia were satisfied by this example. The ventricular tachycardia counter was satisfied, there was evidence of atrial fibrillation, and the RR intervals were regular. However, PR dissociation was not satisfied, which ruled out the double tachycardia classification. Because the AFib/AFlutter rejection criterion was satisfied and double tachycardia had not been detected, ventricular tachycardia detection was withheld.

Atrial fibrillation with irregular ventricular response cannot be reliably defined by a predetermined pattern syntax. PR Logic uses a different combination of building blocks within the AFib/AFlutter criterion that withholds detection for atrial fibrillation/atrial flutter with irregular RR intervals. Detection is withheld for atrial fibrillation/atrial flutter with irregular RR intervals when RR regularity ≤9/18 if the atrial fibrillation evidence counter is satisfied and the median PP interval is less than the median RR interval.

Oversensing of FFRWs as P waves on the atrial amplifier is more likely for dual-chamber defibrillators than for dual-chamber pacemakers because of differences in blanking periods. PR Logic uses the PP regularity building block in conjunction with PR pattern criterion to discriminate between 2 : 1 atrial tachyarrhythmias and sinus tachycardia or atrial tachycardia with consistent FFRW oversensing.

Building Block 6: PP Regularity. An algorithm for identifying FFRW oversensing during sinus tachycardia uses PP regularity and PR patterns for 2 : 1 rhythms. FFRWs are identified when there are exactly 2 Ps for each RR interval, consistent alternation of PP intervals (>30 msec), low RP interval variability (<50 msec), and consistent RP intervals or PR intervals (<20 msec from the average RP or PR). Consistent alternation of PP intervals is needed to avoid misclassifying the rhythm as 2 : 1 atrial flutter. One of the P events must be close to the R event (PR < 60 msec or RP < 160 msec). In the Gem DR and Gem II DR, these criteria must be met for
Continued, p. 550

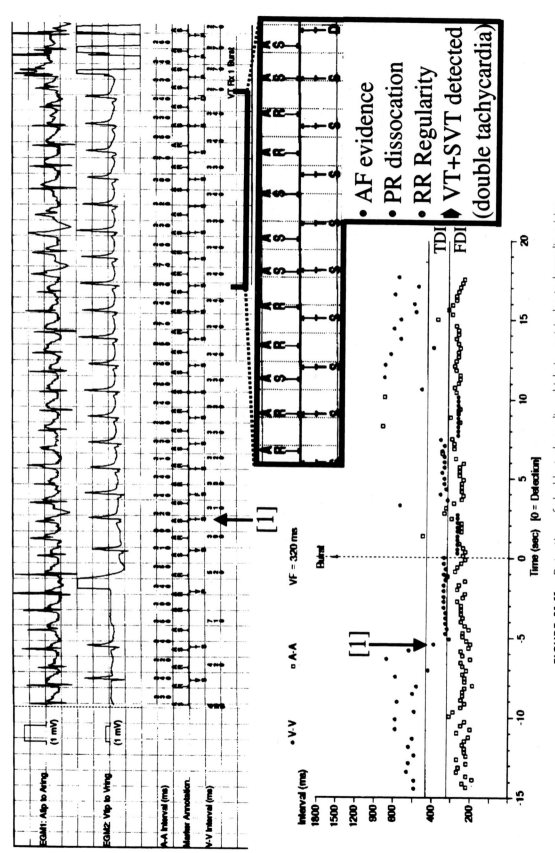

FIGURE 21-11. Detection of double tachycardia, which is ventricular tachycardia arising during atrial fibrillation (AF). The strip shows AF that was appropriately sensed and sudden onset of VT with regular ventricular cycle lengths in the VT zone (tachycardia detection interval [TDI] = 430 msec) [1]. The PR Logic building block criteria for AF evidence, PR dissociation, and RR regularity were satisfied simultaneously when the VT counter reached the number of intervals for detection (NID = 16), and the rhythm was detected as VT + SVT (double tachycardia). On the far right side of the interval plot, the rhythm remained in atrial fibrillation after VT was terminated by two sequences of burst pacing.

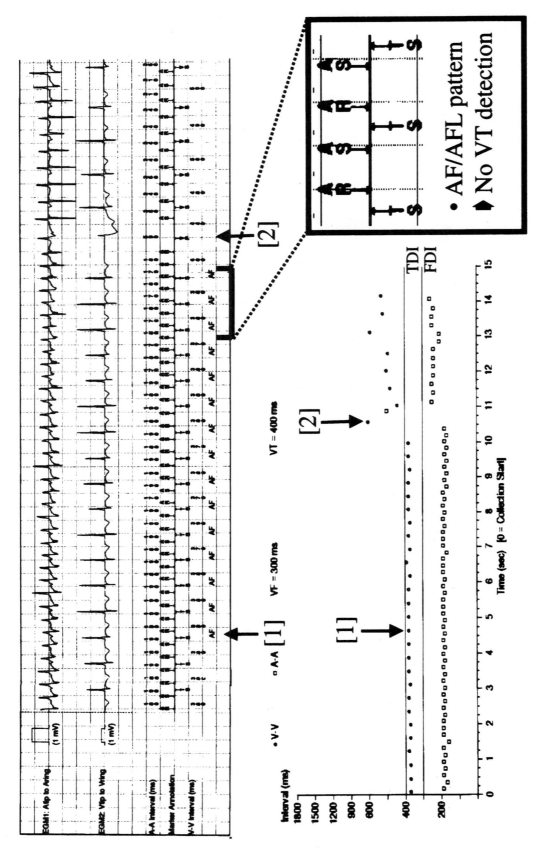

FIGURE 21-12. Detection appropriately withheld for rapidly conducted atrial fibrillation or atrial flutter (AF/AFL). This stored supraventricular tachycardia (SVT) episode shows AF/AFL with ventricular rates in the ventricular tachycardia (VT) zone (tachycardia detection interval [TDI] = 400 msec) that was not detected because of the AFib/AFlutter criterion in PR Logic. On the left side of the strip, the rhythm had a 2:1 ventricular response in the VT zone (TS markers) and was annotated as AF because the PR Logic classified the rhythm as AF/AFL [1]. The atrial tachyarrhythmia changed slightly at [2], causing the ventricular cycle lengths to be outside of the VT zone and more irregular, as shown on the right side of the interval plot.

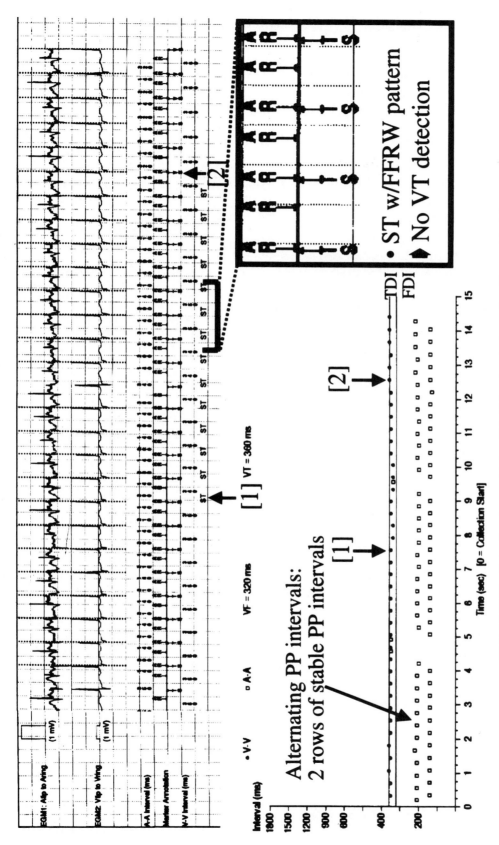

FIGURE 21-13. Detection appropriately withheld for sinus tachycardia with consistent far-field R-wave (FFRW) oversensing. This stored supraventricular tachycardia (SVT) episode shows sinus tachycardia that had consistent FFRW oversensing. The RR intervals were in the VT zone (tachycardia detection interval [TDI] = 360 msec) and the rhythm annotation was ST when the VT counter reached the programmed number of intervals for detection (NID = 16) [1] because the PR pattern for sinus tachycardia with FFRW oversensing was recognized, and FFRWs were identified in 10 of the last 12 RR intervals. The alternating PP interval characteristic used by PR Logic to identify FFRW oversensing can be seen on the interval versus time plot. The rhythm annotations stopped after the first RR interval outside the VT zone [2] reset the VT counter to 0.

> **Building Block 6: PP Regularity (continued).**
> 10 of the last 12 RR intervals to reject P events as FFRWs in the Sinus Tach and AFib/AFlutter SVT criteria. PR Logic in the Gem III DR has been modified to relax this criterion to 4 of the last 12 RR intervals in the Sinus Tach criterion only.

Figure 21-13 demonstrates sinus tachycardia that had consistent FFRW oversensing. In this example, the rhythm annotation was ST [1] because the PR pattern for sinus tachycardia with FFRW oversensing was recognized, and FFRWs were identified in 10 of the last 12 RR intervals. The alternating PP interval characteristic used by PR Logic to identify FFRW oversensing can be seen on the interval versus time plot as two rows of stable PP intervals. Although there were some events for which FFRW oversensing is not apparent (i.e., "breaks" in the rows of PP intervals), this rhythm consistently had FFRW oversensing in at least 10 of the last 12 RR intervals. The rhythm annotations stopped after the first RR interval outside the ventricular tachycardia zone reset the ventricular tachycardia counter to 0 [2]. This rhythm also satisfied the atrial fibrillation/flutter pattern criterion previously described. However, PR Logic did not classify the rhythm as atrial fibrillation because FFRW oversensing was consistently identified as the source of a 2:1 PR rhythm pattern. If there had been fewer than 10 of the last 12 RR intervals with a 2:1 pattern due to FFRW oversensing, PR Logic could have classified the rhythm as atrial fibrillation if the AFib/AFlutter criterion remained satisfied (Fig. 21-4, lower portion of the right branch of the PR Logic decision tree).

● ADVANCED PR LOGIC DESCRIPTION AND EXAMPLES

The examples that have been presented were selected to illustrate the basic operation of dual-chamber detection decisions with PR Logic. This section presents and explains more complex and challenging examples of dual-chamber detection and provides more detailed descriptions of PR Logic.

PR Logic Computational Flow

The computational flow of PR Logic is shown in Figure 21-14. This diagram applies only during initial detection and not during redetection of VT/FVT/

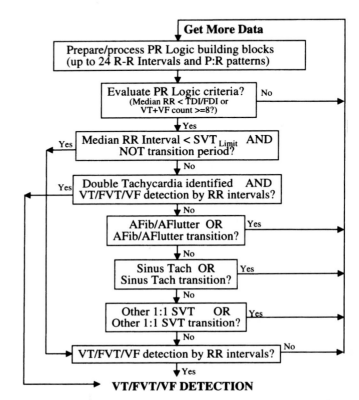

FIGURE 21-14. PR Logic computational flow diagram. The entire process is repeated on each new ventricular event starting with the preparation of new PR, RP, PP, and RR patterns and timing information for the PR Logic building blocks. The next block starts the evaluation of the PR Logic criteria when the ventricular rate gets fast (i.e., median RR interval less than the tachycardia detection interval [TDI] or sum of VT and VF counters is 8 or more) to reduce the computational burden at slow ventricular rate, thereby increasing the implantable cardioverter-defibrillator longevity. When evaluation of PR Logic is required, rhythms with a median RR interval less than the SVT limit are detected by the single-chamber detection criteria without considering the PR Logic algorithm. If the median RR interval is greater than or equal to the SVT limit and double tachycardia (VT/FVT/VF + SVT) is not detected, the three PR Logic criteria for identifying SVTs are tested in the order shown. If any one of the PR Logic SVT criteria is satisfied, inappropriate detection is avoided. If an SVT is not positively identified, VT/FVT/VF is detected when the RR interval–based criterion is satisfied. VT/FVT/VF, ventricular tachycardia, fast ventricular tachycardia, and ventricular fibrillation.

VF episodes. PR Logic is reenabled after termination of a VT/FVT/VF episode when there are 8 consecutive RR intervals longer than the RR interval detection zones. At the top of Figure 21-14, dual-chamber timing information necessary for computing the PR Logic building blocks is collected and prepared on every ventricular event. Each of the PR Logic building blocks is updated to ensure the output of all building blocks is available on every ventricular event. The PR Logic criteria are evaluated only when the ventricular rate becomes fast, as when the median RR interval is less than TDI (or FDI if no ventricular tachycardia zone is programmed) or when the sum of the ventricular tachycardia and ventricular fibrillation counters is 8 or higher. This condition for evaluating the PR Logic criteria helps to reduce the computational burden at slow rates and thereby increases ICD longevity. The PR Logic criteria continue to be evaluated until the median RR interval is greater than or equal to the TDI (or FDI if there is no ventricular tachycardia zone programmed) and the sum of the ventricular tachycardia and ventricular fibrillation counters is less than 8. When the median RR interval is less than the SVT limit, the PR Logic criteria are skipped, and rhythm classification defaults to RR interval–based detection. When the median RR interval is greater than or equal to the SVT limit, the double tachycardia criteria are evaluated first to maintain high sensitivity for ventricular tachyarrhythmias that arise during atrial fibrillation/atrial flutter. When double tachycardia is recognized, zone-appropriate VT/FVT/VF therapies are delivered. If double tachycardia is not recognized, the SVT rejection criteria are evaluated in the order shown: Atrial Fibrillation/Flutter, Sinus Tach, and Other 1 : 1 SVT. If SVT is recognized, the RR interval–based detection criteria are "bypassed" (right arrows). If SVT is not recognized, VT/FVT/VF detection may occur by means of the RR interval–based criterion.

As shown in Figure 21-14, the evaluation of the PR Logic criteria is arranged in a hierarchic manner, with the double tachycardia criteria evaluated first, then SVT criteria, and finally the RR interval–based criterion. Table 21-3 lists the combinations of dual-chamber detection building blocks used for each of the PR Logic criteria. For a particular PR Logic criterion to be satisfied, the corresponding set of elements must be satisfied. Detection of double tachycardia in the ventricular fibrillation zone (or FVT via VF zone) or the ventricular tachycardia zone (or FVT via VT zone) requires atrial fibrillation evidence and PR dissociation to be recognized. Detection of double tachycardia in the ventricular tachycardia zone also requires regular RR intervals (modesum $\geq 14/18$), but RR intervals do not need to be regular for detection of double tachycardia in the ventricular fibrillation zone (i.e., VF or rapid polymorphic ventricular tachycardia may have irregular RR intervals). There are two different ways for the *AFib/AFlutter* criterion and *Sinus Tach* criterion to be satisfied as shown in Table 21-3 by the OR condition in their description. The *AFib/AFlutter* criterion can be satisfied when the *AFib/AFlutter* pattern syntax (if AV conduction is regular) is satisfied (but not because of FFRW oversensing) or when the atrial fibrillation evidence counter is satisfied (but not because of FFRW oversensing), the RR intervals are irregular (modesum $\leq 9/18$), and the median PP interval is less than 0.94 of the median RR interval. The *Sinus Tach* criterion can be satisfied when the sinus tachycardia pattern is recognized or when the sinus tachycardia with FFRW pattern is recognized and there is consistent FFRW oversensing.

Each of the three criteria for identifying SVT (i.e., *AFib/AFlutter*, *Sinus Tach*, and *Other 1 : 1 SVT*) has a "transition" property that continues to withhold detection for several ventricular events after the criterion is no longer satisfied. During the transition period, PR Logic attempts to reestablish the same SVT or recognize a different SVT. The transition property helps to avoid inappropriate detection of VT/FVT/VF when there are transitions between different types of SVT. As shown in Figure 21-14, detection is withheld if an SVT criterion is satisfied or PR Logic is in a transition period. In the Jewel AF, Gem DR, and Gem II DR, the duration of the transition period is six ventricular events. The transition period is 10 ventricular events in the Gem III DR. During the transition period, all PR Logic criteria that are at the same level or higher in the computational hierarchy than the most recently satisfied SVT criterion are evaluated, but criteria that are lower in the hierarchy are not evaluated. Because the RR interval criterion is lowest in the hierarchy, VT/FVT/VF detection is

TABLE 21-3 • PR LOGIC CRITERIA AND COMBINATIONS OF DUAL-CHAMBER DETECTION BUILDING BLOCKS

PR Logic Criteria	Description		
Ventricular rate too fast to apply PR logic	Median RR interval <SVT limit		
Double tachycardia-VF (or FVT via VF) zone	Median RR interval ≥SVT limit VF (or FVT via VF) by RR intervals AF evidence PR dissociation		
Double Tachycardia-VT (or FVT via VT) zone	Median RR interval ≥SVT limit VT (or FVT via VT) by RR intervals AF evidence PR dissociation Regular RR intervals (modesum ≥ 14/18)		

AFib/AFlutter	AFib/AFlutter with pattern
	  Median RR interval ≥SVT limit
	  <10/12 FFRWs
	  AF or AFL pattern
		OR	AFib/AFlutter with AF evidence
			  Median RR interval ≥SVT limit
			  <10/12 FFRWs
			  Median PP interval <0.94 median RR interval
			  AF evidence
			  Irregular RR intervals (modesum ≤9/18)

Sinus Tach	Sinus tachycardia
	  Median RR interval ≥SVT limit
	  Sinus Tach pattern
		OR	Sinus tachycardia with FFRWs
			  Median RR interval ≥SVT limit
			  ≥10/12 FFRWs (≥4/12 FFRWs in Gem III DR)
			  Sinus Tach with FFRW pattern

Other 1:1 SVTs	Median RR interval ≥SVT limit Other 1:1 SVT pattern		

AF, atrial fibrillation; AFL, atrial flutter; FFRW, far-field R waves; FVT, fast ventricular tachycardia; SVT, supraventricular tachycardia; tach, tachycardia; VF, ventricular fibrillation; VT, ventricular tachycardia.

withheld during the transition period unless double tachycardia is recognized. The double tachycardia criteria and SVT criteria at the same level or higher in the hierarchy can be satisfied at any time during the transition period, thereby ending the transition period. However, SVT criteria lower in the hierarchy may only be satisfied after the transition period expires. If SVT cannot be reestablished or if a different SVT cannot be recognized after the transition period expires, VT/FVT/VF is detected. As indicated in Figure 21-14, if the median RR interval becomes less than the SVT limit, the PR Logic SVT criteria are overridden, but only after an existing transition period has expired.

Advanced and Challenging Examples

Figure 21-15 illustrates the effect of the transition period on VT/FVT/VF detection. In this example, sinus tachycardia was appropriately recognized and annotated as ST [1]. Ventricular tachycardia spontaneously occurred during sinus tachycardia with no change in RR cycle length [2] but with a change in ventricular electrogram morphology and gradual PR dissociation. The gradual PR dissociation can also be seen on the interval versus time plot by the slightly increased atrial cycle lengths relative to the ventricular cycle lengths and the variable timing between the atrial and ventricular events. Because the atrial and ventricular events are no longer associated after ventricular tachycardia initiated, the sinus tachycardia pattern counter decreased exponentially after a few beats of ventricular tachycardia because of the gradual PR dissociation. The sinus tachycardia pattern counter decreased to below the threshold of 6; the sinus tachycardia criterion was no longer satisfied, and the transition period started [3]. The rhythm annotation remained ST during the transition period even

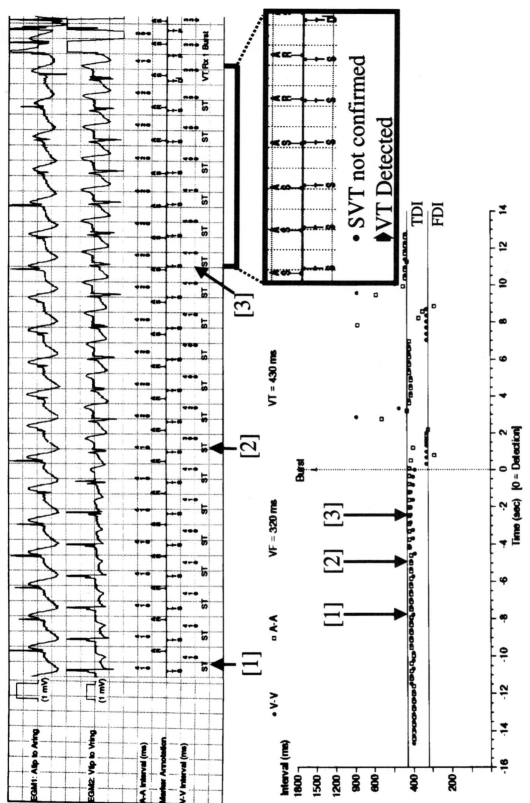

FIGURE 21-15. Detection of spontaneous ventricular tachycardia (VT) during sinus tachycardia. On the left side of the strip, the rhythm was sinus tachycardia with RR intervals in the VT zone (tachycardia detection interval [TDI] = 430 msec) and the Sinus Tach criterion was withholding VT detection [1]. VT occurred spontaneously [2] with the same RR cycle length as the sinus tachycardia. After a few beats of VT, the Sinus Tach criterion was no longer satisfied, and the transition period (during which PR Logic tries to reestablish supraventricular tachycardia [SVT]) started [3]. The rhythm annotation remains ST during the transition period even though the PR Logic sinus tachycardia criterion was no longer satisfied. SVT was not reestablished, and VT detection occurred when the transition period expired. Burst ATP therapy was delivered, and the VT was terminated. As shown on the interval plot, sinus tachycardia remained in the VT zone and a second sequence of burst ATP was delivered because the PR Logic criteria do not apply during redetection.

though the PR Logic *Sinus Tach* criterion was no longer satisfied. The rhythm annotation indicated that PR Logic was still withholding therapy but did not explicitly indicate that the decision process had entered the transition period of 6 ventricular events when PR Logic tried to reestablish the presence of SVT. Because none of the SVT criteria was satisfied, ventricular tachycardia detection occurred when the transition period expired.

Tip: When VT/FVT/VF detection occurs after a transition period expires, the point at which SVT was no longer recognized by PR Logic (i.e., start of the transition period) can be determined by counting backward *n* ventricular events from the point of detection, for which *n* is the number of beats in the transition period ($n = 6$ beats for the Jewel AF, Gem DR, and Gem II DR and $n = 10$ beats for the Gem III DR).

Figure 21-16 is an example of ventricular tachycardia with 1 : 1 retrograde conduction that blocked, showing the effect of the transition period on detection of ventricular tachycardia. Spontaneous onset of ventricular tachycardia can be seen on the interval plot [1], with sudden RR interval shortening preceding the PP interval shortening. The electrograms at onset are not seen on the strip. As shown on the interval plot, 1 : 1 retrograde conduction to the atrium was established after two beats of ventricular tachycardia. The retrograde conduction time (or RP interval) was unusually long, and the PR interval fell into the antegrade region of the RR interval. The PR Logic pattern analysis inappropriately classified the rhythm as sinus tachycardia temporarily [2]. As shown by [3], there was intermittent retrograde conduction block after a few seconds of consistent retrograde conduction. This block resulted from what appears to be retrograde Wenckebach conduction and caused the sinus tachycardia pattern counter to decrease. The sinus tachycardia pattern counter dropped below 6, and the sinus tachycardia criterion was no longer satisfied at [4]. This also marks the start of the transition period of six ventricular events during which ventricular tachycardia detection continued to be withheld (rhythm annotation continued to be ST). PR Logic had not identified the presence of an SVT, so ventricular tachycardia was detected when the transition period expired (i.e., right side of strip [VT]).

Ventricular tachycardia with sustained 1 : 1 retrograde conduction is rare, and it is even more unusual to observe retrograde conduction with RP conduction times that result in P waves falling in the antegrade region of the RR interval. In an analysis of 667 spontaneous VT/VF episodes, 642 were monomorphic ventricular tachycardia, and only 17 (2.6%) of 642 had 1 : 1 retrograde conduction. Nine (1.4%) of 642 had long RP conduction times falling into the antegrade region. All of these episodes were spontaneously terminated within 30 ventricular events, or developed retrograde block and were detected as ventricular tachycardia in a manner similar to the example in Figure 21-16.

Figure 21-17 presents a rare example of a nonsustained ventricular tachycardia with 1 : 1 retrograde conduction lasting approximately 22 beats that was classified as sinus tachycardia by PR Logic. At [1] in Figure 21-17, the onset of the ventricular tachycardia was indicated by the ventricular electrogram morphology change and the sudden increase in ventricular rate. There was a warm-up period of a few beats until retrograde conduction was consistent. Retrograde conduction times were long, such that the P waves fell into the antegrade region of the RR interval, resulting in the misclassification of rhythm as ST [2] when the ventricular tachycardia counter reached 16. At [3], the ventricular tachycardia terminated spontaneously, and the ST annotations stopped because the ventricular intervals were longer than the ventricular tachycardia detection interval and the ventricular tachycardia counter was reset to 0.

Figure 21-18 presents an example of ventricular tachycardia during atrial fibrillation/atrial flutter that was detected as VT + SVT (i.e., double tachycardia) by the PR Logic detection algorithm. The rhythm was atrial fibrillation/atrial flutter when the ventricular tachycardia started spontaneously [1]. The *AFib/AFlutter* criterion was satisfied when the ventricular tachycardia counter reached 16, shown by the atrial fibrillation rhythm annotations [2]. As summarized in Table 21-3, double tachycardia detection in the ventricular tachycardia zone requires four PR Logic building blocks to be satisfied simultaneously: RR interval criterion, atrial fibrillation evidence, PR dissociation, and RR regularity (modesum $\geq 14/18$). In this episode, the ventricular tachycardia counter, atrial

21. DUAL-CHAMBER ICD SENSING AND DETECTION   555

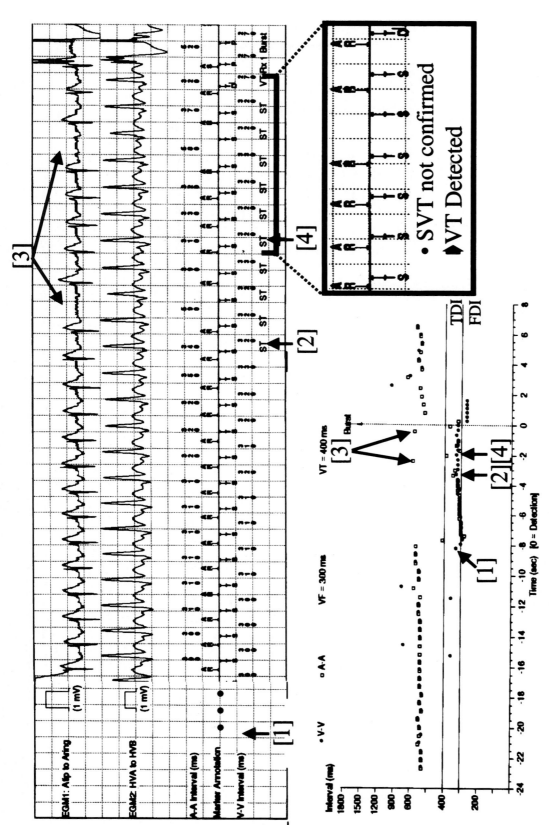

FIGURE 21-16. Detection of ventricular tachycardia (VT) with 1:1 retrograde conduction. Spontaneous onset of VT can be seen on the interval plot [1] with sudden shortening of the RR interval into the VT zone (tachycardia detection interval [TDI] = 400 msec) preceding shortening of the PP interval. PR Logic temporarily classifies the rhythm as sinus tachycardia (ST) [2] because the retrograde conduction (i.e., RP interval) was unusually long, resulting in a P event in the antegrade portion of the RR interval. Retrograde block occurred at [3], causing the sinus tachycardia pattern counter to decrease. At [4], the sinus tachycardia criterion was no longer satisfied, and the transition period began. VT detection occurred when the transition period expired (on the right of the strip [VT]) because PR Logic had not reestablished supraventricular tachycardia (SVT). As shown on the interval plot, VT was terminated by a single burst of antitachycardia pacing therapy.

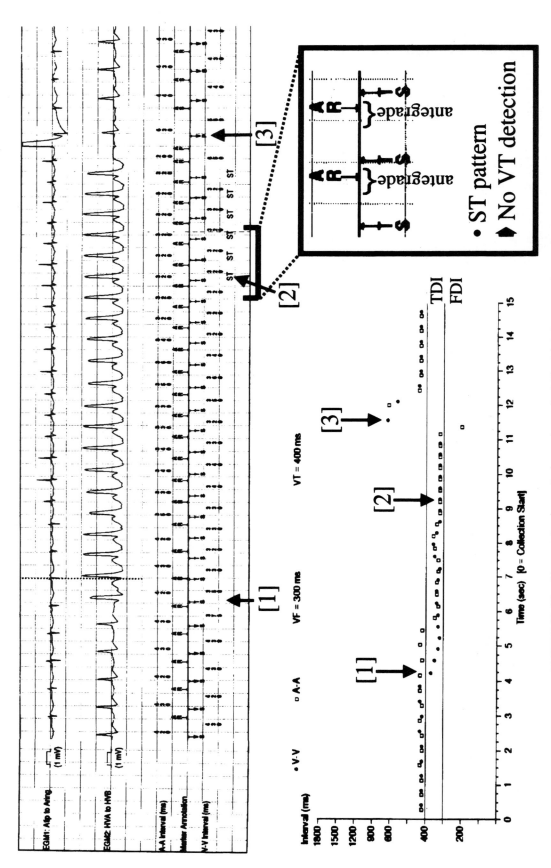

FIGURE 21-17. Nonsustained ventricular tachycardia (VT) with 1:1 retrograde conduction. This is a rare example of nonsustained VT that was classified as sinus tachycardia (ST) by PR Logic because of the long 1:1 retrograde conduction, sometimes causing P events to occur in the antegrade region of the RR interval. There was a sudden shortening of ventricular cycle length in the VT zone (tachycardia detection interval [TDI] = 400) and sudden change in ventricular electrogram morphology at the onset of VT [1]. When the VT counter reached the programmed number of intervals for detection (NID = 16), the ST annotations begin because the sinus tachycardia criterion was satisfied [2]. VT spontaneously terminated, and ST annotations stopped because of RR intervals outside of the VT zone [3].

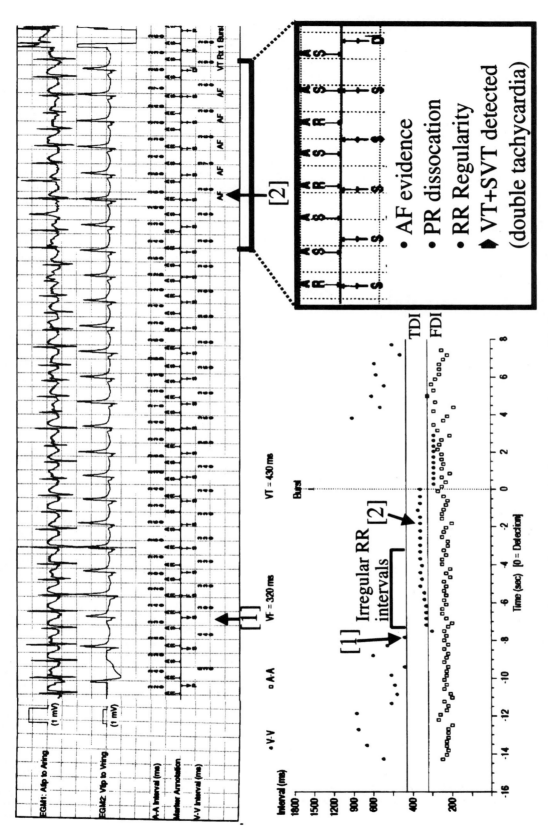

FIGURE 21-18. This is an example of appropriate detection of double tachycardia, or ventricular tachycardia during atrial fibrillation (VT + SVT), although after the rhythm was initially classified as atrial fibrillation (AF) for 5 beats. VT started spontaneously with a sudden shortening of RR intervals into the VT zone (tachycardia detection interval [TDI] = 430 msec) [1]. When the VT counter was initially satisfied by reaching the programmed number of intervals for detection (NID = 16), the rhythm classification was AF [2]. The rhythm was not immediately classified as double tachycardia because the RR intervals were initially irregular, as shown on the interval plot. After five ventricular events of rhythm classified as AF, RR regularity became 14/18, and VT + SVT was detected. The right side of the interval plot shows termination of VT after a single burst of antitachycardia pacing, followed by continuing AF.

fibrillation evidence, and PR dissociation were all satisfied, but RR regularity was <14/18 until the ventricular event where VT + SVT detection occurred. As shown in Figure 21-14, rhythm classification as double tachycardia requires no transition period, and detection occurs immediately (and overrules the *AFib/AFlutter* rhythm classification) when all four of the required building blocks are satisfied simultaneously. Recall that the RR regularity criterion uses the *modesum,* defined as the sum of the number of intervals in the two largest bins of the RR interval histogram based on the last 18 RR intervals. For the RR regularity criterion to be satisfied, the two largest bins must sum to at least 14 (ratio of ≥14/18). In this episode, the RR modesum was 12/18 at the point labeled [2] in Figure 21-18. Although the rhythm was quite regular at cycle length 360 msec at [2], the previous 18 intervals showed some variability of ventricular cycle lengths from 330 to 360 msec. The RR modesum remained at 12/18 or 13/18 until the VT + SVT was detected (VT), when modesum reached 14/18. The slightly irregular RR intervals at the onset of this spontaneous ventricular tachycardia episode (as shown on the interval plot) delayed VT + SVT detection for 5 RR intervals after the ventricular tachycardia counter was satisfied. It is somewhat common for spontaneous ventricular tachycardias to exhibit some irregularity at the onset. When the number of intervals to detect ventricular tachycardia is 16 and ventricular tachycardia occurs spontaneously during atrial fibrillation, there may be episodes for which ventricular tachycardia detection is delayed slightly. This delay is not expected for episodes in the ventricular fibrillation zone, because the RR regularity criterion is not used to identify VF + SVT double tachycardias.

Tip: The rhythm annotations on the Gem DR and Gem II stored strips do not show double tachycardia rhythm classifications. This information can be found in the text portion of the episode record.

Based on an unpublished review of 667 spontaneous VT/VF episodes from 50 patients enrolled in the Gem DR clinical trial, delays in VT/VF detection were seen in 20 episodes from six patients. Detection delays were only seen for episodes of double tachycardia (similar to Fig. 21-18) and for episodes of ventricular tachycardia with 1 : 1 retrograde conduction with long retrograde conduction times (similar to Fig. 21-16). Detection delays were seen for 11 of 60 episodes of double tachycardia. The median delay seen in these 11 episodes was 2 ventricular events, with a range of 1 to 5 ventricular events. Detection delays were seen for 9 of 17 episodes of ventricular tachycardia with 1 : 1 VA conduction. The median delay seen for these 9 episodes was 8 ventricular events, with a range of 1 to 40 ventricular events.

Figure 21-19 presents an example of ventricular tachycardia during atrial fibrillation/atrial flutter that was detected as ventricular tachycardia (but not as double tachycardia) by PR Logic. The classification was ventricular tachycardia, not VT + SVT, in this episode because the *AFib/AFlutter* criterion that was initially withholding detection became unsatisfied before the double tachycardia detection criterion was satisfied. The rhythm was atrial fibrillation/atrial flutter with an irregular ventricular response before the spontaneous onset of ventricular tachycardia [1]. There was no stored electrogram for this portion of the episode. The ventricular tachycardia initially had irregular ventricular cycle lengths with some RR intervals falling in the ventricular fibrillation zone (FS) and some in the ventricular tachycardia zone (TS). After the RR interval detection criterion was satisfied [3], the rhythm was annotated as atrial fibrillation because the double tachycardia criterion was not yet satisfied and the *AFib/AFlutter* criterion was satisfied. The double tachycardia criterion was not satisfied before detection because of the irregular RR intervals at the onset of the ventricular tachycardia. The RR modesum was 11/18 at [3] and was 13/18 at detection (VT). The RR intervals were irregular enough at the onset of the ventricular tachycardia to cause the RR modesum to be ≤9/18 initially, which allowed the "AFib/AFlutter with atrial fibrillation evidence" criterion to be satisfied (Table 21-3). The atrial fibrillation/flutter pattern criterion was not satisfied because of several pairs of RR intervals with two consecutive 1 : 1 beats. None of the couple codes in the atrial fibrillation/flutter pattern syntax allow two consecutive 1 : 1 beats. After the RR interval modesum reached 10/18, the *AFib/AFlutter* criterion was no longer satisfied, and the transition period of six ventricular events started [2]. SVT was not reestablished, and ventricular tachycardia was detected (VT) when the transition period expired.

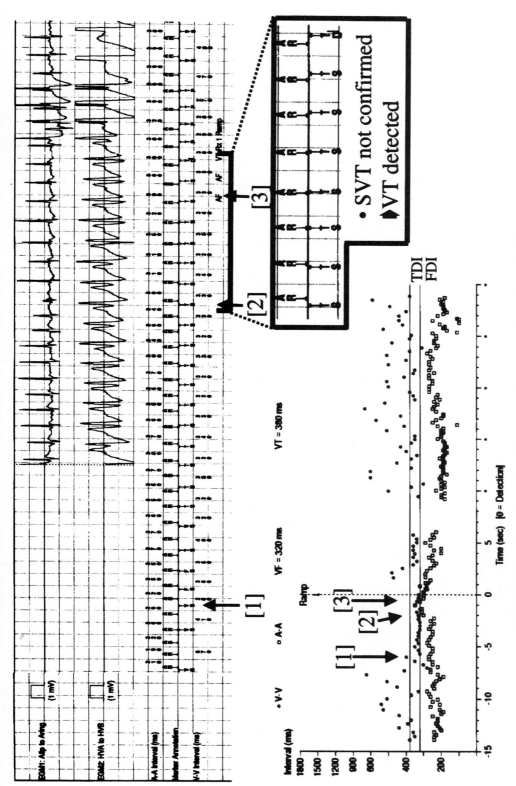

FIGURE 21-19. Detection of double tachycardia as ventricular tachycardia (VT), not as ventricular tachycardia during atrial fibrillation (VT + SVT). The classification was VT, not VT + SVT, in this episode because the AFib/AFlutter criterion was initially withholding detection and became "unsatisfied" before the double tachycardia detection criterion was satisfied. The rhythm was atrial fibrillation (AF) with an irregular ventricular response before the spontaneous onset of VT [1]. The AFib/AFlutter criterion was initially satisfied but then was no longer satisfied at [2]. The RR interval detection criterion was satisfied at [3], and the rhythm annotation was AF even though the transition period had started at [2]. The RR regularity portion of the double tachycardia criterion was not satisfied during or after the transition period, and VT detection occurred (VT) after the transition period expired because supraventricular tachycardia could not be reestablished. The interval plot shows the RR interval irregularity near the onset of the VT. The missing section of the interval plot (at about 6 seconds) resulted from conservation of implantable cardioverter-defibrillator memory during a period in which no therapies were delivered. This missing section was also annotated on the electrogram strip (not shown).

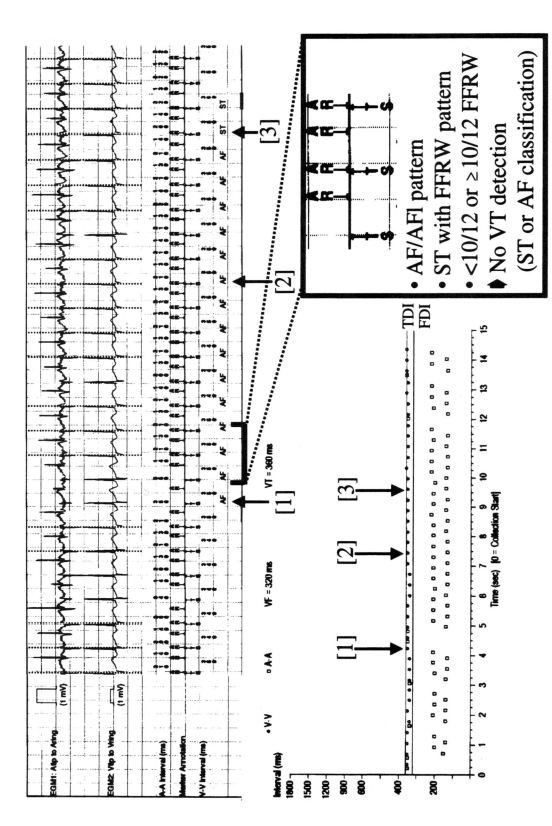

FIGURE 21-20. Sinus tachycardia with far-field R-wave (FFRW) oversensing classified as atrial fibrillation (AF) and then as sinus tachycardia (ST). The rhythm was in the ventricular tachycardia (VT) detection zone (tachycardia detection interval [TDI] = 360 msec) and was classified as AF when the VT counter was satisfied by reaching the programmed number of intervals for detection (NID = 16) [1]. The AF classification occurred initially because there were fewer than 10 of the last 12 RR intervals with FFRW oversensing. As the rhythm progressed, FFRW oversensing was more consistent and caused the AFib/AFlutter criterion to become "unsatisfied," and a transition period started [2]. The sinus tachycardia criterion was not evaluated during the transition period because it is lower in the computational hierarchy than the AFib/AFlutter criterion, as addressed in Figure 21-14. When the transition period expired, the sinus tachycardia criterion was satisfied, and the rhythm classification changed to ST [3]. The ST rhythm annotations stopped on the right side of the strip after the first RR interval longer than the TDI reset the VT counter to 0.

Tip: PR Logic SVT criterion may be satisfied before rhythm annotations are displayed, because rhythm annotations are only displayed when the RR interval–based criterion is satisfied (i.e., ventricular tachycardia, ventricular fibrillation, or combined count reaches NID).

The example in Figure 21-20 shows how the transition counter can interact with the rhythm classification and hierarchy. This is an example of sinus tachycardia with FFRW oversensing that was in the ventricular tachycardia zone, but ventricular tachycardia detection was withheld because of rhythm classification as atrial fibrillation and as ST. At the point labeled [1] in Figure 21-20, the rhythm was initially classified as atrial fibrillation. Classification as ST was not possible initially because PR Logic in the Gem DR requires that FFRW oversensing be identified in at least 10 of the last 12 RR intervals. As seen from the interval plot, before [1], the FFRW oversensing was intermittent, and there were fewer than 10 FFRWs in the last 12 RR intervals. The number of RR intervals with FFRW oversensing increased, and at [2], there were exactly 10 RR intervals of the last 12 with FFRW oversensing. At this point, the *AFib/AFlutter* criterion was no longer satisfied because there were at least 10 of 12 FFRWs (Table 21-3), and a transition period of 6 RR intervals started. The atrial fibrillation annotations continued, and the *Sinus Tach* criterion was not evaluated during the transition period because it is lower in the computational hierarchy than the *AFib/AFlutter* criterion (Fig. 21-14). When the transition period expired, the *Sinus Tach* criterion was evaluated and was satisfied, and the rhythm classification changed to ST [3] (i.e., PR Logic criteria higher in the hierarchy were not satisfied).

◉ CLINICAL PERFORMANCE OF DUAL-CHAMBER SENSING AND DETECTION

The performance of the PR Logic detection algorithm was studied as part of the Gem DR clinical study. Three hundred patients (238 male) with an average age of 64 years (standard deviation, 13 years) were studied with a mean follow-up time of 1.7 months and a cumulative follow-up time of 495 months (33).

Arrhythmic episodes were documented by stored electrograms and marker data. All spontaneous episodes that occurred when at least one of the three PR Logic SVT criteria was programmed "ON" were included. No episodes were excluded for any reason, including sensing problems and median RR intervals less than the SVT limit. There were a total of 1,092 episodes from 96 patients. The stored episodes were classified as ventricular tachycardia or ventricular fibrillation or as SVT without a coexistent ventricular tachyarrhythmia. Calculations were made from the perspective of the ability of the ICD to accurately detect ventricular tachycardia or ventricular fibrillation (true positive); accurately detect SVT (i.e., withhold therapies for ventricular tachycardia or ventricular fibrillation) without coexistent ventricular tachycardia or ventricular fibrillation (true negative); falsely detect SVT as ventricular tachycardia or ventricular fibrillation (false positive); and falsely detect ventricular tachycardia or ventricular fibrillation as SVT (false negative). The definition for false negative and true negative is constrained to include only rhythms that meet the ventricular rate–only detection criterion without ventricular rate detection enhancements such as stability or sudden onset. Tachycardias with a ventricular rate slower than the slowest VT/FVT/VF detection zone did not contribute to the false-negative or true-negative numbers because the ICD diagnostics were designed specifically for rhythms within programmed VT/FVT/VF detection zones.

The PR Logic detection results for the 1,092 tachycardia episodes are presented in Figure 21-21, where the episodes were categorized as true positives, false positives, true negatives, and false negatives. There were a total of 795 spontaneous VT/FVT/VF episodes, all of which were detected appropriately using PR Logic (100% sensitivity). Of these 795 spontaneous VT/FVT/VF episodes, 80% (638 of 795) had a median ventricular cycle length greater than or equal to the programmed SVT limit, which means that PR Logic was applied to these episodes, and all were appropriately classified as VT, FVT, or VF. There were a total of 296 episodes of true SVT in 42 patients. The single-chamber, RR interval–based detection algorithm would have detected all 296 of these SVTs inappropriately. PR Logic positively identified 214

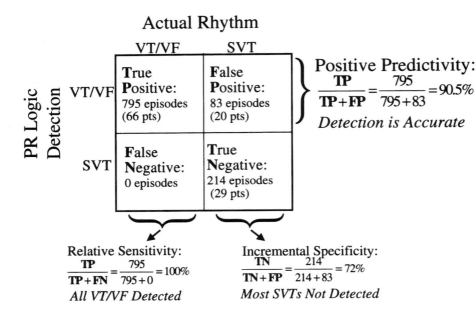

FIGURE 21-21. Gem DR PR Logic tachyarrhythmia detection results: 1,092 spontaneous sustained tachycardias from 96 patients. No episodes were excluded for any reason.

of these 296 episodes as SVT and withheld VT/FVT/VF detection. PR Logic classified 181 (85%) of 214 episodes as *Sinus Tach* in 20 patients, 31 (14%) of 214 episodes as atrial fibrillation or flutter in 8 patients, and 2 (1%) of 214 episodes as *Other 1 : 1 SVT* in 2 patients. Despite the dual-chamber PR Logic detection algorithm, 83 of these episodes from 20 patients were detected inappropriately as VT/FVT/VF. Incremental specificity or reduction of inappropriately detected episodes compared with the single-chamber, rate-only detection was 72%. Adjusting for multiple episodes in each patient using the generalized estimating equations (GEE) model, the specificity improvement over RR interval–only detection was 63% (95% CI: 49%–75%). The positive predictive value, defined as the correct classification of VT/VF by the PR Logic algorithm, was 90.5% (795 of 878), or 78.7% as adjusted using the GEE model (95% CI: 69.1%–86.0%).

Discussion and Examples of Supraventricular Tachycardia Episodes Classified as VT/FVT/VF

In the Gem DR study, PR Logic positively identified 214 of 296 SVT episodes as SVT and withheld VT/FVT/VF detection. However, there were 83 SVTs in 20 patients with RR intervals in the VT, FVT, or VF zone that were inappropriately classified and detected as VT/FVT/VF or as double tachycardia. Twenty-eight SVT episodes classified as VT/FVT/VF in three patients did not receive therapy because ventricular tachycardia therapies were programmed OFF. Eighty-eight percent (73 of 83) of all inappropriate ventricular tachycardia or ventricular fibrillation detections resulted from one of the following three rhythm categories:

- Sinus tachycardia or atrial tachycardia with intermittent atrial oversensing of FFRWs: two patients, 39 (47%) of 83 episodes
- Sinus tachycardia or atrial tachycardia with long PR intervals: 8 patients, 24 (29%) of 83 episodes
- Atrial fibrillation with rapid conduction into the ventricular fibrillation zone: 3 patients, 10 (12%) of 83 episodes

Other reasons for inappropriate detection of SVT as VT/FVT/VF were two episodes from two patients with median RR intervals less than the SVT limit (which effectively disabled PR Logic). Six episodes from three patients that were 1 : 1 SVTs with short and variable PR intervals. One episode of atrial fibrillation with AV dissociation and regular ventricular intervals that was mistaken for ventricular tachycardia during atrial fibrillation. Atrial sensing was in general very good, with only one episode of inappropriate detection caused by atrial undersensing during atrial fibrillation.

The following examples illustrate inappropriate detection of SVTs as VT/FVT/VF and point out enhancements that have been made to PR Logic in the Gem III DR that will help reduce inappropriate detections. Figure 21-22 presents an example in which PR Logic did not withhold therapy for sinus tachycardia with intermittent FFRW oversensing. Gradual acceleration of the ventricular rate into the ventricular tachycardia zone can be seen on the left side of the interval plot. The first of 16 consecutive RR intervals in the ventricular tachycardia zone is marked by [1]. Notice the alternating pairs of PP intervals on the interval plot, indicating possible FFRW oversensing. Examination of the atrial electrogram and marker channel reveals FFRWs that were sensed intermittently. Unlike the examples shown in Figures 21-13 and 21-20, there were not enough oversensed FFRWs for PR Logic to reliably classify this rhythm as SVT, and inappropriate ventricular tachycardia detection occurred when the ventricular tachycardia counter reached the programmed number of intervals for detection (NID = 16). In the Gem DR and Gem II DR, FFRW oversensing must be identified in at least 10 of the last 12 RR intervals for classification as sinus tachycardia with FFRW oversensing. To help avoid this type of inappropriate detection, PR Logic in the Gem III DR has been modified to require identification of FFRW oversensing in at least 4 of the last 12 RR intervals for rhythm classification as sinus tachycardia with FFRW oversensing.

Inappropriate detection due to SVT in the VT/VF zones with intermittent FFRW oversensing on the atrial lead may be avoided through careful placement of an atrial lead with close tip-ring spacing (10 mm), or careful programming of atrial sensitivity. Retrospective analysis of the Gem DR clinical data indicated that atrial lead placement on the lateral wall significantly reduced the amount of FFRW oversensing without causing significant atrial undersensing (26). Attention to atrial lead positioning during implantation to maximize the P-wave to R-wave ratio while maintaining adequate P-wave amplitude and atrial pacing thresholds may help prevent FFRW oversensing. Changing atrial sensitivity from the nominal value of 0.3 mV to larger values may eliminate FFRW oversensing, but atrial undersensing during normal sinus rhythm or atrial fibrillation may occur. As a last resort, increasing atrial sensitivity to smaller values (e.g., 0.15 mV) may make FFRW oversensing more consistent and allow PR Logic to appropriately withhold detection for SVTs. However, it is recommended that the performance of PR Logic be assessed with the patient's clinical tachyarrhythmias, because there is a remote chance that consistent FFRW during VT or VF may cause PR Logic to classify the rhythm as *Other 1 : 1 SVT*. This could happen when very low atrial rates occur during ventricular tachycardia, and consistent FFRW oversensing causes the PR pattern to appear as a junctional rhythm. The *Other 1 : 1 SVT* criterion should be programmed OFF for the first month after implantation to avoid inappropriate withholding of detection and therapy in case the atrial lead dislodges into the ventricle.

Figure 21-23 presents a Gem DR example of when PR Logic did not withhold therapy for sinus tachycardia or atrial tachycardia with long PR intervals (i.e., PR ≥50% of RR). The gradual acceleration of ventricular rate into the ventricular tachycardia zone can be seen on the interval plot. The first of 16 consecutive intervals in the ventricular tachycardia zone is shown at [1]. Notice that the pattern was 1 : 1, with PR intervals that were consistently ≥50% of the RR interval and in the retrograde region as defined in Figure 21-6A. Because the PR intervals occurred in the retrograde region, the *Sinus Tach* criterion was not satisfied, and ventricular tachycardia was detected when the ventricular tachycardia counter reached 16. Inappropriate detection of ventricular tachycardia occurred because the PR interval was on the wrong side of the antegrade-retrograde conduction boundary and caused this sinus tachycardia to be mistaken for ventricular tachycardia with 1 : 1 VA conduction. The clinical incidence of 1 : 1 SVT with long PR intervals is low (approximately 3% of patients in this study, and in the single center experience reported by Wolpert (34). However, patients with 1 : 1 SVT (i.e., atrial tachycardia or sinus tachycardia) with rates that overlap with the ventricular tachycardia detection zone and long PR intervals (PR ≥50% of the

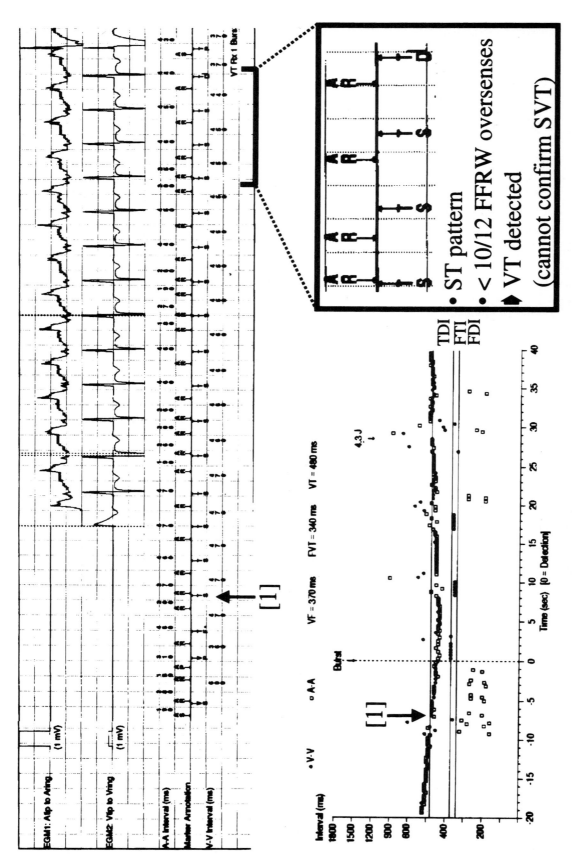

FIGURE 21-22. PR Logic in the Gem DR was unable to withhold detection for this sinus tachycardia (ST) with intermittent far-field R-wave (FFRW) oversensing. The first RR interval in the ventricular tachycardia (VT) zone (tachycardia detection interval [TDI] = 480 msec) occurred at [1]. VT detection occurred as shown on the right of the strip when the VT counter was satisfied by reaching the programmed number of intervals for detection (NID = 16). FFRW oversensing was too frequent for the sinus tachycardia pattern syntax to be satisfied and not frequent enough for the ST with FFRW oversensing criteria to be satisfied.

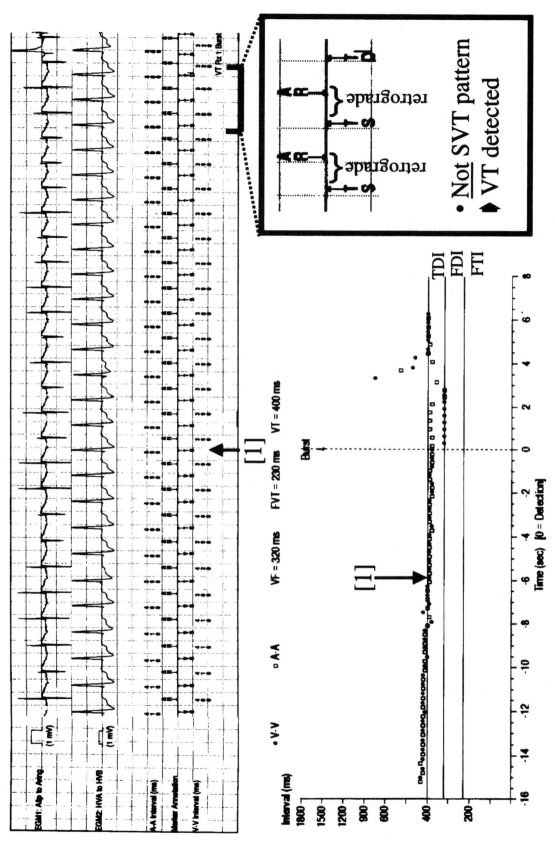

FIGURE 21-23. PR Logic in the Gem DR was unable to withhold detection for this supraventricular tachycardia (SVT) with long PR intervals. The rhythm was sinus tachycardia with long PR intervals and RR intervals in the ventricular tachycardia (VT) detection zone (tachycardia detection interval [TDI] = 400 msec). The long PR intervals (i.e., PR ≥50% RR) caused the P events to occur in the retrograde region of the RR interval, and rhythm classification therefore could not be SVT. The first of 16 consecutive intervals in the VT zone is shown at [1]. Because the PR intervals occurred in the retrograde region, the sinus tachycardia criterion was not satisfied, and VT was detected when the VT counter reached the programmed number of intervals for detection (NID = 16).

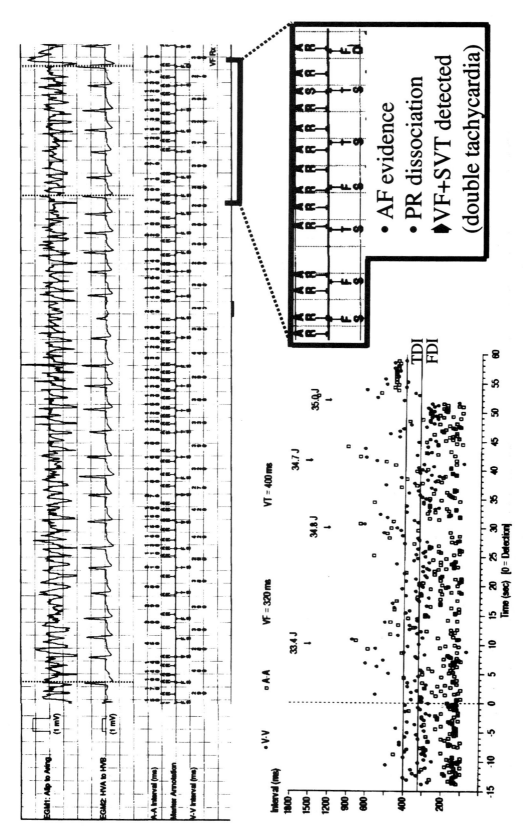

FIGURE 21-24. PR Logic was unable to withhold detection for this episode of atrial fibrillation (AF) with rapid conduction into the ventricular fibrillation (VF) detection zone. The rhythm was AF with some RR intervals in the VF zone (fibrillation detection interval [FDI] = 320 msec), and the median RR interval was greater than the SVT limit (300 msec). The rhythm was classified as VF + SVT when the RR interval VF detection criterion was satisfied (FD), because there was evidence of AF and PR dissociation occurring simultaneously. The VF + SVT criterion does not require RR intervals to be regular because VF or rapid polymorphic VT may have irregular intervals.

RR interval) may receive inappropriate therapies despite the *Sinus Tach* rejection criterion. A programmable parameter, the "1 : 1 VT-ST Boundary," has been added to PR Logic in the Gem III DR to allow customizing the antegrade-retrograde boundary. This PR Logic enhancement can help eliminate inappropriate therapy in patients with PR ≥50% RR interval during 1 : 1 SVT.

Figure 21-24 presents an example of atrial fibrillation with rapid conduction into the ventricular fibrillation zone that was inappropriately classified as double tachycardia (VF + SVT). The onset of the rapid conduction cannot be seen in this episode. Ventricular fibrillation detection was programmed to detect when 12 of the last 16 intervals are in the ventricular fibrillation zone (FS). The ventricular fibrillation counter was only at 9 at the point of detection; ventricular fibrillation detection occurred because the combined count (sum of the VF and VT counters) reached 14. The rhythm was classified as VF + SVT, because there was evidence of atrial fibrillation and PR dissociation present simultaneously when the combined count criterion was satisfied. Recall that RR regularity is not part of the double tachycardia criterion for rhythms in the ventricular fibrillation zone, because true ventricular fibrillation during atrial fibrillation may have irregular RR intervals. By design, PR Logic has less power to withhold detection and therapy for atrial fibrillation in the ventricular fibrillation zone (and FVT via VF), even when the median RR interval is greater than or equal to the SVT limit. However, the discrimination capability of PR Logic is the same in the VT and VF zone for atrial tachyarrhythmias that have AV association such as 2 : 1 atrial fibrillation or flutter, sinus tachycardia, and Other 1 : 1 SVT, assuming the median RR interval is greater than or equal to the SVT limit. When inappropriate detection of atrial fibrillation in the ventricular fibrillation zone occurs clinically, one solution may be to reprogram the detection zones such that the ventricular rates during atrial fibrillation are in the ventricular tachycardia detection zone (or FVT via VT). Programming the number of intervals to detect ventricular fibrillation to the nominal value of 18 of 24 or possibly even higher may reduce the chances of inappropriate detection. However, care must be taken in making these changes so that true ventricular fibrillation is not underdetected.

CONCLUSIONS

Dual-chamber tachyarrhythmia detection algorithms can be thought of as combinations of building blocks derived from ventricular-only, atrial-only, and combined atrial and ventricular information. The PR Logic dual-chamber detection algorithm combines 6 dual-chamber building blocks to perform rhythm classification: PP intervals, RR intervals, PR patterns, RR regularity, PR dissociation, and PP regularity. PR Logic has three independently programmable "ON/OFF" switches for rejection of three specific types of SVT (i.e., atrial fibrillation/atrial flutter, sinus tachycardia, and junctional tachycardia) and a single SVT limit cycle length parameter to define the shortest ventricular cycle length for which detection can be withheld. PR Logic has been shown to reduce the number of inappropriate detections of SVT as VT or VF compared with single-chamber, ventricular rate–only detection. However, some SVTs that conduct rapidly into the VT, FVT, or VF detection zones may still be detected inappropriately as VT/FVT/VF.

As shown by the examples presented in this chapter, the behavior of dual-chamber tachyarrhythmia detection algorithms can be as straightforward as single-chamber algorithms or can be more complex. Episode strips with atrial and ventricular intracardiac electrograms, marker channel, and rhythm annotations can be used to diagnose arrhythmias and explain dual-chamber detection results. The details of the PR Logic dual-chamber detection algorithm have been described at different levels of detail by the clinical decision process diagram (Fig. 21-3), the detailed decision tree diagram (Fig. 21-4), the list of PR Logic criteria (Table 21-3), and the computational flow diagram (Fig. 21-14). These figures and table may be used to explain why PR Logic classified a rhythm in a particular way. SVT rhythm classifications are annotated only when RR interval–based detection was already satisfied, and annotations continue to be displayed during transition periods, even when the SVT rejection criteria are no longer satisfied. Determining whether the rhythm classification was double tachycardia (e.g., VT + SVT, FVT + SVT, VF + SVT) or "plain" VT/FVT/VF can help to determine whether detection occurred because one of the double tachycardia criteria was satisfied or an SVT was not recognized (or became "unrecognized").

Direct comparisons of the performance of the available dual-chamber detection algorithms is difficult because published studies vary significantly in the number and type of tachyarrhythmia episodes, the evaluation criteria, the number of patients studied, and methods for excluding certain types of episodes. Equally difficult is the comparison of dual-chamber tachyarrhythmia detection with single-chamber tachyarrhythmia detection using enhancements such as sudden onset, stability, and ventricular electrogram morphology (35).

None of the dual-chamber ICDs available uses all the information available from atrial and ventricular electrograms for rhythm classification. As advances are made in the microelectronics available for ICDs, more sophisticated detection algorithms that more fully integrate the available information will be developed. Future concepts for improving dual-chamber detection in ICDs may include the use of atrial and ventricular electrogram morphology and possibly even atrial and ventricular extrastimuli to improve classification of challenging tachycardias.

ACKNOWLEDGEMENTS

The authors gratefully acknowledge helpful reviews from Robert Stadler, Mark Brown, and Jim Willenbring and are grateful to Jean Hayman for figure and bibliography preparation and administrative support.

REFERENCES

1. Jenkins JM, Caswell SA. Detection algorithms in implantable cardioverter-defibrillators. *Proc IEEE* 1996;84:428–445.
2. Johnson NJ, Marchlinski FE. Arrhythmias induced by device tachycardia therapy due to diagnostic nonspecificity. *J Am Coll Cardiol* 1991;18:1418–1425.
3. Reiter MJ, Mann DE. Sensing and tachyarrhythmia detection problems in implantable cardioverter-defibrillators. *J Cardiovasc Electrophysiol* 1996;7:542–558.
4. Swerdlow CD, Chen PS, Kass RM, et al. Discrimination of ventricular tachycardia from sinus tachycardia and atrial fibrillation in a tiered-therapy cardioverter-defibrillator. *J Am Coll Cardiol* 1994,23:1342–1355.
5. Schaumann A, von zur Mühlen F, Gonska B-D, Kreuzer H. Enhanced detection criteria in implantable cardioverter-defibrillators to avoid inappropriate therapy. *Am J Cardiol* 1996;78[Suppl 5A]:42–50.
6. Pinski SL, Fahy GJ. The proarrhythmic potential of implantable cardioverter-defibrillators. *Circulation* 1995;92:1651–1664.
7. Dougherty CM. Psychological reactions and family adjustment in shock versus no shock groups after implantation of internal cardioverter defibrillator. *Heart Lung* 1995;24:281–291.
8. Duru F, Schönbeck M, Lüscher TF, Candinas R. The potential for inappropriate ventricular tachycardia confirmation using the intracardiac electrogram (EGM) width criterion. *Pacing Clin Electrophysiol* 1999;22:1039–1046.
9. Swerdlow CD, Ahern T, Chen PS. Underdetection of ventricular tachycardia by algorithms to enhance specificity in a tiered-therapy cardioverter-defibrillator. *J Am Coll Cardiol* 1994;24:416–424.
10. Brugada J, Mont L, Figueiredo M. Enhanced detection criteria in implantable defibrillators. *Cardiovasc Electrophysiol* 1998;9:261–268.
11. Bhandari AK. Arrhythmia detection algorithms in dual chamber ICDs. *Cardiac Electrophysiol Rev* 1998;2:305–307.
12. Olson WH. Dual chamber sensing and detection for implantable cardioverter-defibrillators. In: Singer I, Barold SS, Camm AJ, eds. *Nonpharmacological arrhythmias for the 21st century: the state of the art.* Armonk, NY: Futura Publishing, 1998:385–421.
13. Sadoul N, Henry C, on behalf of Defender Investigator Group. Long term performance of a dual chamber detection algorithm, the PARAD algorithm, programmed with nominal settings in patients with implantable cardioverter-defibrillators [Abstract]. *Pacing Clin Electrophysiol* 1999;22[Pt II]:A125.
14. Kuck KH, Cappato R, Aliot E, et al, on behalf of IDEF05 Study Group. First clinical results with a new dual chamber implantable cardioverter defibrillator capable of treating slow VTs [Abstract]. *Pacing Clin Electrophysiol* 1999;22[Pt II]:A74.
15. Kouakam C, Klug D, Jarwé M, et al. Analysis of dual-chamber implantable cardioverter defibrillators electrograms for discrimination of ventricular from supraventricular tachycardia: implication for ICD specificity and programming [Abstract]. *Pacing Clin Electrophysiol* 1999;22[Pt II]:A125.
16. Kühlkamp V, Dörnberger V, Mewis C, et al. Clinical experience with the new detection algorithms for atrial fibrillation of a defibrillator with dual chamber sensing and pacing. *J Cardiovasc Electrophysiol* 1999;10:905–915.
17. Wilkoff BL, Kühlkamp V, Gillberg JM, et al, for the Gem DR 7271 Worldwide Investigators. Performance of a dual chamber detection algorithm (PR Logic) based on the worldwide Gem DR clinical results [Abstract]. *Pacing Clin Electrophysiol* 1999;22[Pt II]:720.
18. Swerdlow CD, Gunderson BD, Gillberg JM, et al. Discrimination of concurrent atrial and ventricular tachyarrhythmias from rapidly conducted atrial arrhythmias by a dual-chamber ICD [Abstract]. *Pacing Clin Electrophysiol* 1999;22[Pt II]:775.
19. Kühlkamp V, Dörnberger V, Suchalla R, et al. Specificity and sensitivity of a detection algorithm using patterns, AV association and rate analysis for the differentiation of supraventricular tachyarrhythmias and ventricular tachyarrhythmias [Abstract]. *Pacing Clin Electrophysiol* 1999;22[Pt II]:823.
20. Olson WH. Tachyarrhythmia sensing and detection. In: Singer I, ed. Implantable cardioverter-defibrillator. Armonk, NY: Futura Publishing, 1994:71–107.
21. Kleinert M, Elmquist H, Strandberg H. Spectral properties of atrial and ventricular endocardial signals. *Pacing Clin Electrophysiol* 1979;2:11–18.

22. Goldreyer BN, Almquist CK, Beck RC, Olson WH. Waveform and frequency analysis of unipolar, bipolar, and orthogonal atrial electrograms. *Pacing Clin Electrophysiol* 1986;9(2):283A.
23. Kerr CR, Mason MA. Amplitude of atrial electrical activity during sinus rhythm and during atrial flutter–fibrillation. *Pacing Clin Electrophysiol* 1985;8[Pt I]:348–355.
24. Swerdlow CD, Schols W, Dijkman B, et al. Detection of atrial fibrillation and flutter by a dual-chamber implantable cardioverter-defibrillator. *Circulation* 2000;101(8):878–885.
25. Adler SW, Brown ML, Nelson LK, Mehra R. Interelectrode spacing and right atrial location, both influence far-field ventricular electrogram amplitude [Abstract]. *Pacing Clin Electrophysiol* 1999;22[Pt II]:877.
26. Gunderson BD, Gillberg JM, Pearson AM, et al for Gem DR Clinical Worldwide Investigators. Atrial sensing during detection of spontaneous tachyarrhythmias in a dual-chamber implantable cardioverter-defibrillator [Abstract]. *Pacing Clin Electrophysiol* 1999;22[Pt II]:803.
27. Kühlkamp V, Mewis C, Suchalla R, et al. Rate dependence of R-R stability during atrial fibrillation and ventricular tachyarrhythmias. *Circulation* 1998;98(17):I-713A.
28. Arenal A, Almendral J, Villacastin J, et al. First postpacing interval variability during right ventricular stimulation: a single algorithm for the differential diagnosis of regular tachycardias. *Circulation* 1998;98:671–677.
29. Jung J, Strauss D, Sinnwell T, et al. A new method for discrimination of antegrade from retrograde atrial activation. *Pacing Clin Electrophysiol* 1998;21(4):918A.
30. Munkenbeck FC, Bump TE, Arzbaecher RC. Differentiation of sinus tachycardia from paroxysmal 1:1 tachycardias using single late diastolic atrial extrastimuli. *Pacing Clin Electrophysiol* 1986;9[Pt I]:53–64.
31. Jenkins J, Noh KH, Bump T, et al. A single atrial extrastimulus can distinguish sinus tachycardia from 1:1 paroxysmal tachycardia. *Pacing Clin Electrophysiol* 1986;9[Pt II]:1063–1068.
32. Anderson MH, Murgatroyd FD, Hnatkova K, et al. Performance of basic ventricular tachycardia detection algorithms in implantable cardioverter defibrillators. *Pacing Clin Electrophysiol* 1997;20[Pt I]:2975–2983.
33. Wilkoff BL, Gillberg JM, Hillman S, Larsen JS. Clinical experience with detection of spontaneous ventricular arrhythmias by a new dual chamber defibrillator in a multicenter study. *Circulation* 1998;17:I-289A.
34. Wolpert C, Jung W, Spehl S, et al. Potential pitfalls of a new dual-chamber detection algorithm: implications for patient selection and device programming. *Eur Heart J* 1999;20[Suppl]:110A.
35. Wilkoff B, Kühlkamp V, Vdosin K, et al. Critical analysis of dual-chamber implantable cardioverter-defibrillator arrhythmia detection: results and technical considerations. *Circulation* 2001;103:381–386.

ATRIAL DEFIBRILLATION WITH IMPLANTABLE CARDIOVERTER-DEFIBRILLATORS
• • •

STEVEN D. GIROUARD, MILTON M. MORRIS, HENDRIK LAMBERT, ULRICH MICHEL,
MICHAEL E. BENSER, BRUCE H. KENKNIGHT, DOUGLAS J. LANG

The normal, resting heartbeat is usually imperceptible, but when heart rate deviates from the normal, narrow range, symptoms emerge. The symptoms associated with irregular heart rhythms are highly varied. The severity of arrhythmia symptoms is typically associated with concomitant changes in cardiac output. During an arrhythmia, cardiac output depression is determined primarily by the heart chamber that the arrhythmia involves (i.e., atria or ventricles) and the type of arrhythmia present (i.e., bradyarrhythmia or tachyarrhythmia). For supraventricular tachyarrhythmias such as atrial fibrillation, symptoms may be mild, moderate or severe.

The treatment of symptoms and thromboembolic complications associated with atrial fibrillation constitutes a major health care problem in monetary terms (1) and in terms of reduced quality of life (2). Medical therapies remain palliative and commonly produce unwanted side effects themselves. Surgical therapy may be effective but is highly invasive and carries its own risk profile (3). New therapeutic strategies for atrial fibrillation treatment are needed, and several new strategies for the management of symptoms caused by atrial fibrillation have been proposed (4). These multifaceted strategies ultimately will be based on etiologic factors and will likely involve cardioactive medicines, ablation, and implanted devices for termination of atrial fibrillation and maintenance of normal rhythm (5–7).

This chapter describes implantable defibrillator technology for the treatment of atrial fibrillation. First, we discuss the challenges faced by clinicians treating patients with atrial fibrillation and briefly summarize existing and emerging clinical management strategies. Next, general concepts and mechanisms underlying external and internal electrical cardioversion are described, with attention given to patient issues associated with these therapies. Most of the chapter focuses on the role of implanted devices in atrial fibrillation treatment strategies and highlights issues encountered by developers of implanted devices intended for safe and effective treatment of atrial fibrillation.

ATRIAL FIBRILLATION: A CHALLENGING RHYTHM DISTURBANCE

The social and economic impact of atrial fibrillation is enormous. Although atrial fibrillation remains the most common arrhythmia requiring hospitalization (8), its seemingly benign nature does not attract immediate attention unless it is highly symptomatic. Untreated atrial fibrillation begins to alter the heart muscle as the atria and ventricles experience chronic, elevated rates of activation. These changes are electrophysiologic (i.e., action potential shortening and altered rate adaptation), ultrastructural, and macrostructural (9–11). All of these changes promote the reinitiation or maintenance of atrial fibrillation.

Clinical treatment of atrial fibrillation is a challenge because of several factors. First, the number of patients presenting with atrial fibrillation is astounding compared with the numbers for other cardiac arrhythmias. Estimates suggest that at least 2.2 million Americans experience chronic atrial fibrillation (12). Inclusion of individuals with paroxysmal or persistent atrial fibrillation, who are often untreated, surely makes the number of patients suffering from atrial fibrillation significantly higher. Second, atrial fibrillation can be caused by several mechanisms that act alone or in concert to permit the onset and maintenance of the arrhythmia. The mechanisms underlying the initiation of atrial fibrillation can be acute and reversible or chronic and irreversible. One subset of atrial fibrillation has been linked to the autonomic nervous system (13). The onset of atrial fibrillation can be by adrenergically mediated (14) or cholinergically mediated (15). It is thought that structural changes act to support the reentrant nature of chronic atrial fibrillation. Increased left atrial size from mitral regurgitation may lead to fibrosis and slow conduction (16–18). Third, atrial fibrillation imposes a profound reduction on quality of life by imposing troubling symptoms (i.e., chronic fatigue, chest pain, and reduced exercise capacity) and their attendant psychologic burden (19). Fourth, atrial fibrillation is associated with an ominous increased risk of stroke (20). Although the risk of stroke can be mitigated by appropriate anticoagulation (21–23), the side effects of chronic anticoagulation in the presence and absence of other drugs that have been shown to potentiate their effects produce additional concerns that must be weighed against the benefits.

Atrial fibrillation is a challenging rhythm disturbance because its treatment and long-term management requires substantial health care expenditure (1). Frequent hospitalization for cardioversion and treatment of associated symptoms and comorbid conditions exacerbated by atrial fibrillation divert health care resources away from primary prevention. A rapidly aging population and an incomplete understanding of the mechanisms of atrial fibrillation motivate the exploration of more economical forms of atrial fibrillation management.

HEALTH CARE BURDEN

The absolute extent of the problem, the multitude of therapies, high recurrence rates, and comorbidities associated with atrial fibrillation combine to make the treatment of atrial fibrillation a major public health cost burden. It is estimated that 225,000 patients are admitted to U.S. hospitals each year with a primary diagnosis of atrial fibrillation (24). The typical admission for treatment of atrial fibrillation and its related symptoms and sequelae lasts approximately 4 days and costs more than $6,000 (1). Conventional medical therapy has been unsuccessful at curing atrial fibrillation in most patients. Atrial fibrillation has a prevalence that increases with age (25), and the U.S. population is aging, underscoring the intense search for safe, effective, and less-expensive atrial fibrillation therapies.

The range of contemporary treatment options spans traditional drug therapy, pacing therapy, surgical or ablative compartmentalization of the atria, atrioventricular (AV) nodal ablation and pacemaker implantation, and hybrid combinations. Current state-of-the-art treatment is summarized in Table 22-1.

Atrial fibrillation is often associated with numerous other medical conditions such as mitral valve disease (48), coronary artery disease (12), sick sinus syndrome (49), hypertension (50), cardiomyopathies (51,52), and heart failure (53–55). These concomitant abnormalities increase the complexity of clinical management. Stratification of patients to specific treatment options is guided by the physician's ability to understand the mechanisms of atrial fibrillation initiation and maintenance. It is clear that no one solution is curative or universally palliative in the atrial fibrillation population.

The medical management of patients with atrial fibrillation will continue to evolve. The last two decades have seen tremendous advances in the treatment of atrial fibrillation. Combined with a greater under-

TABLE 22-1 • TREATMENTS FOR ATRIAL FIBRILLATION

Treatment Option	Target	Established Or Emerging Status (references)
Pharmacology	RC/SR	Established (26,27)
Anticoagulation	AC	Established (22,23,28)
AV ablation + pacemaker	RC	Established (29,30)
Internal or external cardioversion	SR	Established (31,32,76,88)
Ablation or surgery	SR	Emerging (33–38,66)
Implantable cardioverter	SR	Emerging (4,39)
Atrial pacing	SR	Emerging (40–44)
Hybrid therapies	SR/RC	Emerging (45–47)

AC, anticoagulation; AV, atrioventricular; RC, rhythm control; SR, sinus rhythm.

standing of basic mechanisms, novel therapies are being developed that will assist in the management of patients in the 21st century. As the population ages, it is expected that the socioeconomic impact of atrial fibrillation will increase proportionately. Identifying specific patients and their likelihood to respond to a particular therapy option will be essential for efficient management of patients and associated health care costs.

● CLINICAL MANAGEMENT STRATEGIES FOR ATRIAL FIBRILLATION

Atrial fibrillation patients typically seek medical attention when the onset or persistence of atrial fibrillation causes symptoms that affect their quality of life. The symptoms associated with atrial fibrillation and their severity are, in general, related to the elevated and irregular ventricular rate, compromised ventricular function, and the extent of underlying heart disease. The most common symptoms are palpitations, fatigue, and lightheadedness. However, more extreme symptoms may occur such as heart failure, angina, and syncope. In the absence of a cure for atrial fibrillation, the physician is forced to manage the symptoms of atrial fibrillation and minimize the risks of stroke and systemic emboli. The standard of care has three main therapeutic objectives: maintenance of sinus rhythm, control of ventricular rate and regularity, and reduction of the risk of systemic emboli and stroke (56).

Maintenance of Sinus Rhythm

It is generally believed that paroxysms of atrial fibrillation "beget" additional paroxysms of atrial fibrillation through a process of electrical (57) and structural (58) alterations of the atria. Over time, paroxysmal atrial fibrillation probably becomes persistent and eventually permanent. Maintaining sinus rhythm minimizes symptomatic time and may help prevent the cascade whereby atrial fibrillation leads to electrophysiologic and structural changes that further facilitate the initiation and maintenance of atrial fibrillation. The strategies employed to maintain sinus rhythm include pharmacologic intervention with antiarrhythmic drugs (59,60), external and internal cardioversion, atrial pacing (61,62), surgical (63) and ablative (64–66) maze procedures, and the implantable atrial defibrillator (IAD) (4). The IAD allows patients or physicians the opportunity to terminate paroxysms of atrial fibrillation early after their onset. Rapid electrical conversion to sinus rhythm using pacing and defibrillation may ultimately prove to alter the natural progression of atrial fibrillation.

Ventricular Rate Control and Rate Regularity

The control of ventricular rate as a therapeutic aim serves two fundamental purposes. First, acutely elevated or irregular ventricular rates lead to patient symptoms of palpitations, dizziness, and fatigue. Second, reducing the ventricular rate lowers the risk of developing tachycardia-induced cardiomyopathies (67). Pharmacologic agents such as calcium channel blockers, beta blockers, and digoxin are typically used to modify AV nodal conduction properties. Ventricular rate control may be obtained through an irreversible procedure of AV nodal ablation and permanent pacemaker implantation (29,30). Alternatively, modern defibrillators with advanced dual-chamber pacing capabilities may provide features to help prevent atrial fibrillation (42,68) or alleviate the symptoms of irregular ventricular rates (69). Features such as rate smoothing have shown promise at reducing symptoms associated with irregular ventricular responses (70).

Reducing the Risk of Systemic Emboli and Stroke

The most serious morbidity risk associated with atrial fibrillation is thrombus formation and stroke. Atrial dyskenesis increases the likelihood of thrombus formation. Patients with atrial fibrillation demonstrate a fivefold increased risk of stroke (71). A review of 32 studies reported that 98% of thromboembolic complications occurred within 10 days after cardioversion (72). Moreover, high-risk patients with prior stroke, hypertension, diabetes, heart failure, and advanced age may have a 5% to 7% yearly risk of stroke or thromboembolism (73). The use of anticoagulation can help to lower the risk of stroke. However, this therapy comes with its own set of risks and comorbidity. No consensus exists on a standard use of anticoagulation therapy in atrial fibrillation patients (74).

● ELECTRICAL CARDIOVERSION: MAINTENANCE OF SINUS RHYTHM

Lown and colleagues presented the first description of high-energy, direct current (DC) cardioversion for the termination of atrial fibrillation in 1962 (75). Since that time, transthoracic cardioversion has been widely used as a means for transiently terminating atrial fibrillation in patients with persistent arrhythmia refractory to medical therapies (76).

Regardless of the method of shock application (i.e., internal or external), it is thought that the mechanism for electrical cardioversion is similar to that suggested by Ideker and colleagues for ventricular defibrillation (77). Defibrillation is successful when a critical mass of fibrillating atrial myocardium experiences a voltage gradient greater than some critical threshold (about 5 V/cm). Optical mapping of atrial transmembrane potential during defibrillation has shown that the applied shock field interacts with atrial myocardium by altering the transmembrane potential at the time of the shock and after the shock. At the cellular level, the membrane potential change of atrial cells is related to the shock timing with respect to the local action potential and the intensity of the local electric field. Membrane potential may depolarize or hyperpolarize during a shock, depending on the relative timing and polarity of the applied field. Gray and colleagues demonstrated that shock repolarization time was 19% longer after successful shocks compared with shocks that failed to defibrillate (78). These investigators described four possible defibrillation attempt outcomes: 1) immediate termination of atrial fibrillation, 2) single postshock activation with return to sinus rhythm, 3) organization of tachycardia for less than 2 seconds, followed by termination, and 4) organization of tachycardia with degeneration to atrial fibrillation. These modes of defibrillation success and failure are consistent with clinical observations.

Transthoracic Cardioversion

In their 1962 publication, Zoll and Linenthal described the first transthoracic termination of atrial fibrillation (79). Under general anesthesia, patients were defibrillated with a 650-V, 60-Hz pulse lasting for 150 msec. In the same year, Lown and colleagues reported the first high-energy DC cardioversion of atrial fibrillation in patients (75). Using the Lown waveform (i.e., critically damped resistor-inductor-capacitor network) with energies up to 400 J, patients were defibrillated under general anesthesia. Today, external cardioversion is common, using monophasic and biphasic waveforms with energies between 100 and 360 J. External cardioversion is effective in about 80% of patients, independent of patch locations and energy level (80). Recurrence of atrial fibrillation is common, resulting in frequent hospital visits for repeat cardioversion.

Internal Cardioversion

In some patients, atrial fibrillation is resistant to cardioversion by high-voltage transthoracic shocks. In an attempt to increase the efficacy of treatment in these patients, Lévy and coworkers reported the first experience with catheter-based internal cardioversion (81). Using a defibrillation vector directed between a catheter in the right atrium and an external skin patch, they were successful in terminating atrial fibrillation previously refractory to external cardioversion. However, shock energies up to 200 J were necessary to terminate atrial fibrillation. Subsequently, numerous experimental and clinical studies showed that atrial defibrillation is feasible at considerably lower energies by using completely transvenous electrode systems (82,83).

Internal cardioversion has several clear advantages over external cardioversion. Most notably, internal cardioversion has a greater success rate (84–86). Internal cardioversion offers reduced risk of skin injury and the requirement for only minimal sedation (87). The primary indication for internal cardioversion is persistent atrial fibrillation that is refractory to external cardioversion (87–90). No data directly compare the incidence of ventricular proarrhythmia by transthoracic and internal cardioversion. However, it has been suggested that use of the more local intracardiac ventricular electrograms, for R-wave synchronization may result in less ventricular proarrhythmia than standard surface electrocardiograms used during transthoracic cardioversion (91,92–97).

Transvenous cardioversion with the right atrial appendage → coronary sinus *(RAA → CS)* vector has been used often with energies typically less than 5 J (93). Even in chronic atrial fibrillation patients previously resistant to external cardioversion, internal cardioversion has been successful at energies less than 10J.

Internal cardioversion has not been shown to improve long-term atrial fibrillation outcomes (i.e., incidence of atrial fibrillation recurrence). In a study in which patients were randomly assigned to either external or internal cardioversion, Levy showed that the higher success rate with internal cardioversion did not correlate with the long-term probability of recurrence of atrial fibrillation for both treatments (84).

Risks of Electrical Cardioversion

The most dangerous complication associated with electrical cardioversion is ventricular proarrhythmia caused by poor shock synchronization to ventricular activation. However, cardioversion is safe if R-wave synchronization is achieved and if the RR intervals preceding shock delivery meet certain cycle length criteria (94–97). First, the preceding cycle must be sufficiently long to prevent a shock on the previous T wave. Second, the shocked interval should not be part of a long-short interval sequence. In the two cases of ventricular proarrhythmia reported (94,98), one or both of these safety criteria were not fulfilled.

The risk of stroke after electrical cardioversion is relatively high because increased blood velocity and improved mechanical performance returns in the hours and days after cardioversion. Dislodgement of thrombi, formed during episodes of atrial fibrillation or in the dyskinetic atria after successful defibrillation, can lead to pulmonary emboli or stroke. To minimize the potential for thrombus formation, anticoagulation is urged, but no clear guidelines exist (99,100). The use of transesophageal echocardiography can mitigate the risk of stroke after cardioversion (101,102).

The additional risks attendant to internal cardioversion not present with transthoracic cardioversion are those associated with venous punctures, endocardial catheter manipulation and insertion of catheters in the coronary sinus. Additional risks include myocardial damage, heart wall perforation, arrhythmia induction, and coronary sinus wall perforation.

⊙ IMPLANTABLE ATRIAL DEFIBRILLATORS

Atrial defibrillation with an implantable device may be accomplished by a stand-alone IAD, such as the Guidant Metrix (Fig. 22-1), or an implantable cardioverter-defibrillator (ICD) that is also capable of ventricular defibrillation, such as the Medtronic, Jewel AF model 7250. The principal components for implantable devices that treat atrial arrhythmias are similar to those necessary for treating ventricular arrhythmias. First, a pulse generator capable of shock-stimulus generation and delivery is needed. Second, two or more electrodes are needed for energy delivery. Third, atrial and ventricular sensing and detection systems are necessary to recognize atrial fibrillation and ensure that atrial shocks are delivered consistently and reliably without inducing ventricular fibrillation. In addition to these device-specific aspects of treating

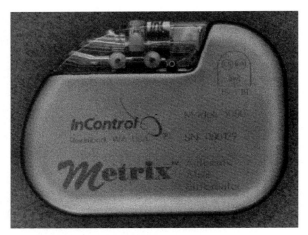

FIGURE 22-1. Metrix stand-alone implantable atrial defibrillator.

atrial arrhythmias, several patient-specific issues must also be considered, such as shock-induced discomfort, patient tolerance, and clinical implications of early recurrence of atrial fibrillation (ERAF) after cardioversion. We first address these factors in the proof of feasibility of atrial therapy with the stand-alone IAD and then consider the integration of atrial therapy into the ICD platform.

Figure 22-1 shows the first commercial IAD, the Metrix (Guidant Corp., St. Paul, MN). This device is implanted in the subcutaneous or submuscular space in the thoracic or abdominal cavity. The 82-g device has a displacement volume of 53 cc. The system requires three leads: a right ventricular bipolar pace/sense lead, a screw-in 6-cm shock coil in the right atrium (Perimeter, model 7205) and a passive-fixation coronary sinus lead with a 6-cm shock coil (Perimeter CS, model 7109). The system was designed to detect atrial fibrillation and deliver R-wave synchronized defibrillation shocks to restore sinus rhythm. In case of shock-induced bradycardia, the Metrix can also pace the right ventricle. The initial model 3000 defibrillator, implanted until September 1996, had an 80-μF capacitor and delivered a 3/3-msec biphasic waveform (maximum energy 3J). Model 3020 has a 160-μF capacitor and delivers a 6/6-msec biphasic waveform (maximum energy, 6 J).

Metrix stores intracardiac electrograms from the prior six successfully terminated atrial fibrillation episodes. The programmer allows visualization of three simultaneous intracardiac electrograms by means of real-time telemetry. The device can be activated directly through the programmer, or it can be programmed for ambulatory use in two different modes:

- Automatic mode: The device is automatically activated at preprogrammed wakeup intervals. An atrial fibrillation detection test is performed and if positive a defibrillation shock is delivered.
- Patient-activated mode: atrial fibrillation detection and defibrillation are initiated by placing a magnet over the IAD (4).

As a first-generation device, the Metrix IAD proved the feasibility of a stand-alone IAD.

Implantable Atrial Defibrillator Thresholds

Critical considerations in the development of atrial defibrillation devices are the shocking vectors that can be used to deliver defibrillation energy and the energy required to terminate chronic atrial fibrillation. Figure 22-2 depicts a number of defibrillation vectors realizable with a standard ICD lead set (Fig. 22-2A) and with a coronary sinus lead added to a standard ICD lead set (Fig. 22-2B). The remainder of this section refers to clinical and experimental studies using vectors depicted in Figure 22-2.

Many atrial defibrillation threshold (A-DFT) studies have been performed in patients with electrically induced atrial fibrillation without a prior history of atrial fibrillation. Using a right atrium–coronary sinus electrode system, Lévy and coworkers assessed A-DFT as a function of atrial fibrillation duration in 141 patients (94). Patients were divided into four groups: no history of atrial fibrillation ($n = 20$), paroxysmal atrial fibrillation (<7 days, $n = 50$), intermediate atrial fibrillation (>7 but <30 days, $n = 18$), and chronic atrial fibrillation (>30 days, $n = 53$). The A-DFT increased as a function of atrial fibrillation duration. Groups with no atrial fibrillation, paroxysmal atrial fibrillation, intermediate atrial fibrillation, and chronic atrial fibrillation had mean A-DFTs of 1.8 ± 1.3, 2.0 ± 1.0, 2.8 ± 1.0, and 3.6 ± 1.4 J, respectively. A related study by Heisel and associates compared A-DFTs in patients with electrically in-

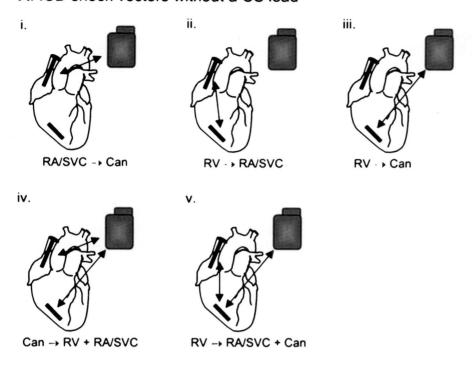
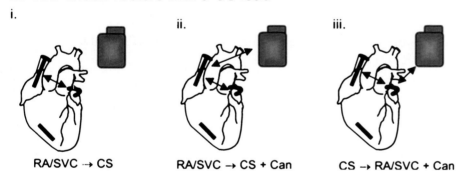

FIGURE 22-2. Numerous defibrillation vectors for implantable cardioverter-defibrillators without (A) and with (B) the use of a coronary sinus catheter.

duced atrial fibrillation to A-DFTs in patients with persistent atrial fibrillation (mean atrial fibrillation duration of 6.6 months). The investigators found a mean A-DFT of 2.0 ± 1.4 J in the induced group, whereas the mean A-DFT for the chronic atrial fibrillation group was 9.2 ± 5.9 J. Similarly, Lau and Lok compared the A-DFTs in patients with acute atrial fibrillation (<1 month) with those with chronic atrial fibrillation (>1 month) and found that patients with chronic atrial fibrillation experienced higher A-DFTs (1.5 ± 1.0 versus 3.6 ± 1.5 J) (103). Over shorter periods of atrial fibrillation, changes in A-DFTs are not clearly observable (104). The data from these studies indicate that there is a relationship between atrial fibrillation duration and the shock strength required to terminate it.

A-DFT increases observed with increased duration of atrial fibrillation are likely caused by a combination of factors. Atrial refractoriness decreases with the duration of atrial fibrillation (105), shortening atrial wavelength and making the atria more vulnerable to atrial fibrillation. Structural changes such as increased left atrial size and atrial fibrosis are associated with atrial fibrillation (16,106). Larger atria are predictive of higher A-DFTs (107). Modeling suggests that increased size may correlate with higher DFTs (108). In contrast, in a sheep model of atrial fibrillation, Power and coworkers did not find a significant change in A-DFT after pacing-induced atrial dilatation (109). In humans, it is difficult to attribute A-DFT increases solely to increases in atrial size.

Antiarrhythmic drugs may alter A-DFT by prolonging refractoriness and wavelength, slowing propagation velocity, or preventing postshock activation. In general, class III agents tend to decrease the A-DFT. For example, Lau and Lok found sotalol significantly reduced the A-DFT in patients with acute atrial fibrillation (<1 month) by 40% (0.9 ± 0.5 versus 1.5 ± 1.0 J). However, this significant effect was lost in patients with chronic atrial fibrillation (>1 month, 3.2 ± 1.2 versus 3.6 ± 1.5 J) (103). The investigators speculated that the low-dose sotalol used in this study may have resulted in an insignificant A-DFT reduction for chronic atrial fibrillation patients. In an acute canine vagal-stimulation model of atrial fibrillation, Baker and coworkers found only a slight and insignificant reduction in A-DFT by sotalol (111). Additional benefits of sotalol have been reported, including ventricular rate control and suppression of the early recurrence of atrial fibrillation after cardioversion (112,113).

Boriani investigated the effect of intravenous flecainide on A-DFT and the success rate for cardioversion of paroxysmal and persistent atrial fibrillation patients (114). Intravenous flecainide increased conversion success of persistent atrial fibrillation and decreased the A-DFT from 4.42 ± 1.37 J to 3.50 ± 1.51 J for the persistent group and from 1.68 ± 0.29 J to 0.84 ± 0.26 J for the paroxysmal atrial fibrillation group. In 14 patients not requiring sedation, the effect of flecainide on A-DFT resulted in significant reduction in shock-induced discomfort score. In addition to lowering A-DFT, intravenous flecainide has been shown to be effective in the treatment of early recurrence of atrial fibrillation (115).

Another antiarrhythmic drug approved for the termination of recent-onset atrial fibrillation or atrial flutter is ibutilide. In a canine model of vagally mediated atrial fibrillation, Khoury and coworkers demonstrated that ibutilide decreased atrial fibrillation cycle length and concomitantly decreased the A-DFT energy by 36% (116). Intravenous ibutilide has also been shown to reduce A-DFTs for transthoracic cardioversion (117,118).

Few data exist regarding the effect of amiodarone on the A-DFT, and the existing data are conflicting. Baker and coworkers studied a vagally mediated canine model of atrial fibrillation and found intravenous amiodarone slightly reduced A-DFT (111). In a prospective, paired human study, Natale and coworkers measured A-DFT first without amiodarone and then began daily administration of the drug (119). In patients in whom cardioversion was required at least 1 month after administration of amiodarone commenced, A-DFTs were significantly increased compared with pretreatment values (15 ± 4 versus 12 ± 4 J). A larger investigation reported by Santini and associates compared the A-DFT of patients pretreated with amiodarone to that of patients without and found that patients pretreated with amiodarone had significantly lower A-DFTs (6.4 ± 1.8 versus 9.2 ± 3.7 J) (120).

Atrial Defibrillation Threshold Optimization

During the development of the Metrix device, various aspects of the IAD system were optimized, including electrodes, shock vectors, and waveforms, to obtain A-DFTs consistent with the output of the system. In a series of reports, Cooper and colleagues compared the efficacy of numerous atrial defibrillation vectors and waveform characteristics in a sheep model (121,122) and human (123,124) atrial fibrillation. Vectors included right-sided only and both left- and right-sided approaches. The studies revealed that energy requirements for single atrial defibrillation shocks were minimized if current was delivered between electrodes in the right atrial appendage and coronary sinus. Further studies showed the lowest A-DFTs result from a distal coronary sinus electrode and an electrode in the right atrial appendage (125,126).

The spatial location of defibrillation electrodes determines the current distribution and resulting voltage gradient during a shock. To minimize A-DFTs, studies demonstrate that right atrial electrodes should be positioned as laterally as possible to maximize the volume of right atrial tissue encompassed by the shock field. Min and coworkers compared the A-DFTs of the $RAA \rightarrow CS$ and $RA/SVC \rightarrow CS$ vectors in a human thorax finite element model and found that the A-DFTs were 1.5 and 4.6 J, respectively (127). Clinical results of Lok and colleagues in patients with chronic atrial fibrillation are consistent with these modeling results. They found high right atrial appendage position yielded the lowest A-DFT (3.9 ± 1.8 J), followed by anterolateral right atrial (4.6 ± 1.8 J) and inferomedial right atrial (6.0 ± 1.7 J) positions (126). These data have been verified in an analogous experimental setup using an acute model of atrial fibrillation in sheep (128). The location of the left-sided shock electrode also has profound effects on the A-DFT. Alt and coworkers found the A-DFT in humans with chronic atrial fibrillation to be greater with a right atrial to left pulmonary artery $(RA \rightarrow LPA)$ configuration (7.2 ± 3.1 J) compared with $RA \rightarrow CS$ (4.1 ± 2.3 J) (129).

Efforts to reduce the A-DFT have also been directed at altering the waveform tilt and phase durations (123,130,131). Lower-tilt, longer waveforms deliver greater energy at lower peak voltages. Such waveforms offer the possibility of cardioversion with less sedation and greater patient tolerance.

Electrode-length also plays a role in determining A-DFT. For the right atrium–coronary sinus defibrillation lead system, Ortiz and coworkers found that atrial defibrillation requirements in the canine model of atrial fibrillation could be minimized using an electrode length of 6 cm for both electrodes (132). Timmermans and colleagues investigated whether longer defibrillation electrodes would lower A-DFTs in humans (133). They evaluated the $RA \rightarrow CS$ vector with different electrode lengths in 15 patients with chronic atrial fibrillation. The length of the right atrium or coronary sinus catheter electrode was increased from 6 to 11 cm, compared with a system with two 6-cm electrodes. No difference was found in A-DFT between the various electrode configurations, but longer electrode lengths yielded significantly lower impedance.

In an attempt to reduce the number of electrodes necessary for atrial defibrillation, investigators have assessed the use of a single-pass, dual-electrode lead (134–137). The distal defibrillation electrode resides in the coronary sinus, and the proximal coil is situated along the lateral right atrium. Clinical data show that such a lead is straightforward to position (134,137). These two studies reported relatively low A-DFTs for chronic atrial fibrillation patients (9.2 ± 5.9 and 5.5 ± 2.7 J).

Detection Algorithms for Implantable Atrial Defibrillators

Detection algorithms are a crucial design aspect for implantable defibrillators. Algorithms are necessary for rhythm discrimination and to guide the safe and effective delivery of therapy to the patient (138–140). These requirements are true for each of three different implantable systems available today: an IAD with stand-alone atrial therapy, an ICD with ventricular tachyarrhythmia therapy (V-ICD), and a combined ICD system with atrial and ventricular therapies (AV-ICD). Each configuration, whether based on single or dual-chamber sensing and detection, could draw on numerous resources for detection: rate or shock channel electrograms, atrial and/or ventricular rates, rate stability, AV interval characteristics, signal morphology, and physiologic sensor signals.

Therapy decision accuracy has traditionally been described using two performance metrics: sensitivity and specificity. In the V-ICD system, *sensitivity* refers to the probability that a ventricular tachyarrhythmia (i.e., ventricular tachycardia or ventricular fibrillation) is appropriately diagnosed, and *specificity* refers to the probability that a supraventricular tachyarrhythmia (i.e., sinus tachycardia, atrial flutter, and atrial fibrillation) is appropriately diagnosed. Ideal operation of an algorithm used to classify rhythms provides 100% sensitivity and 100% specificity. However, in most practical applications, a tradeoff exists whereby an increase in sensitivity comes at the expense of specificity. Because of the life-threatening nature of ventricular arrhythmias, V-ICD systems are optimized for very high sensitivity (>99%), incorporating detection enhancement algorithms to improve specificity without compromising sensitivity.

Performance metrics change for the stand-alone IAD, which must make therapy decisions for sinus rhythm/sinus tachycardia versus atrial fibrillation. IAD sensitivity refers to the probability that atrial fibrillation is properly diagnosed, and IAD specificity refers to the probability that sinus rhythm/sinus tachycardia is properly diagnosed. Because atrial arrhythmias are not immediately life threatening, IAD algorithms are optimized for very high specificity to ensure that atrial therapy is delivered only during an atrial arrhythmia.

The detection architecture in the Metrix IAD follows this paradigm, discriminating non-atrial fibrillation rhythms from atrial fibrillation. Atrial fibrillation detection occurs in three stages. These stages are activated at programmable wakeup intervals. In the first stage, signal collection and qualification occurs. In the second stage, an analysis of the percentage of time the electrogram is proximal to baseline (quiet time) is used to distinguish sinus tachycardia from non-sinus tachycardia. In the third stage, an analysis of baseline crossings is used to distinguish atrial fibrillation from other non-sinus tachycardias.

In the first stage of atrial fibrillation detection, *Signal Collection*, 8 seconds of electrogram information from the $RA \rightarrow CS$ bipole and the right ventricular bipole is analyzed. Signal amplitude, ventricular heart rate, and noise amplitude are confirmed. If unacceptable, an additional 8 seconds of electrogram data are analyzed. This process can be repeated up to six times before the device returns to sleep until the next programmed wakeup interval. However, if the signal is deemed acceptable, the device advances to the second stage.

In the second stage, *Quiet Interval Analysis*, the device analyzes the $RA \rightarrow CS$ electrogram for the percent of time that the electrogram amplitude remains within a positive and a negative sensitivity threshold (Fig. 22-3). A large percentage of quiet time is indicative of sinus rhythm or sinus tachycardia. In contrast, atrial fibrillation typically produces a small percentage of quiet time with electrograms that spend more time away from the baseline. If the percentage of quiet time is greater than the programmed threshold, the device classifies the cardiac rhythm as sinus rhythm and returns to sleep until the end of the next programmed wakeup interval. Conversely, if the percentage of quiet time is below the programmed threshold, the device classifies the cardiac rhythm as *Not sinus rhythm* and progresses to the third stage.

In the third stage, *Baseline Crossing*, after the rhythm has been classified as *Not sinus rhythm*, the same 8-second electrogram is analyzed to determine if the cardiac rhythm is atrial fibrillation. A baseline crossing algorithm tracks the number of times the signal crosses the baseline within a series of detection windows (Fig. 22-4). If the average baseline crossing count within each window is less than a programmable threshold, the device goes back to sleep until the end of the next wakeup interval. If the average baseline crossing count within each window is greater than the programmable threshold, the cardiac rhythm is classified as atrial fibrillation, and the device prepares to give a therapeutic shock.

The Metrix algorithm uses these three stages to balance performance toward specificity (i.e., not treating sinus rhythm or sinus tachycardia), establishing an atrial therapy paradigm for stand-alone IAD and combination AV-ICD devices. The Metrix system was demonstrated through clinical experience to provide mean specificity and sensitivity of 100% and 92.3%, respectively (141). Combination therapy devices should strive to preserve this balance of high sensitivity and specificity. In this way, inappropriate therapy will be minimized.

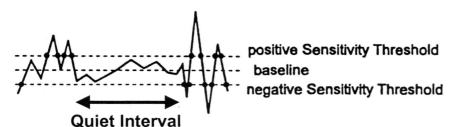

FIGURE 22-3. Schematic of the Metrix AF detection algorithm for quiet interval analysis.

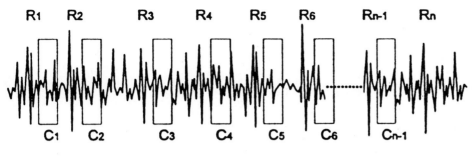

FIGURE 22-4. Schematic of the Metrix AF detection algorithm for baseline crossing analysis.

Atrial Shock Synchronization by Implantable Atrial Defibrillators

Atrial defibrillation shocks are typically delivered synchronized to an R wave to avoid the ventricular vulnerable period and thereby minimize the likelihood of proarrhythmia. Because RR intervals are irregular during atrial fibrillation, the delivery of a properly timed shock depends on accurate sensing of R waves. Ayers and associates investigated the incidence of proarrhythmia during R-wave synchronized atrial shocks $(CS \rightarrow RA)$ in an acute sheep model of atrial fibrillation (96). The incidence of shock-induced proarrhythmia was less than 1%. Two episodes of ventricular fibrillation were induced by shocks delivered on short RR intervals of 198 and 240 msec. Others have studied proarrhythmia by delivering shocks falling within the ventricular vulnerable period. Keelan and colleagues found in canines that atrial shocks delivered more than 380 msec after the preceding R wave were never proarrhythmic (97). Sokoloski and coworkers showed that proarrhythmia was avoided when atrial shocks were delivered after QT + 60 msec (absolute interval of >320 msec) in a canine model (95). Clinically, several groups have delivered shocks on or near the T wave in an effort to establish the zone most vulnerable to ventricular fibrillation induction (142–145). In combination, these groups found that shocks delivered on the rising phase of the T wave were more likely to induce ventricular fibrillation than shocks delivered on the falling phase. None of these studies observed proarrhythmia as a result of shocks delivered on the latter third of the T wave.

To ensure safe delivery of atrial shocks, devices must sense R waves properly and avoid shocking on short RR interval sequences.

Shock Synchronization Algorithm: Metrix Defibrillation System

The Metrix IAD system uses a real-time R-wave synchronization algorithm to time the delivery of defibrillation therapy. The Metrix algorithm senses electrical activity or events from two electrogram channels selected for their complementary sensing characteristics $(RV_{tip} \rightarrow RV_{ring}$ and $RV_{tip} \rightarrow CS_{coil})$. These vectors contain near-field and far-field electrical information, respectively. Both channels are analyzed in four areas: RR interval timing, event activity and timing, R-wave morphology, and signal quality. The overriding intent of the algorithm is to avoid ventricular proarrhythmia by delivering each shock synchronously with a qualified R wave that occurs at the end of a qualified interval. Sixteen individual criteria within the four specific areas must be met to deliver therapy. The minimum RR interval criterion and the long-short criterion are two of the 16 criteria (95–97). The minimum RR interval criterion is designed to avoid shocking during the vulnerable period. The long-short criterion avoids shocking after a RR interval that is preceded by a sufficiently longer interval. Shock synchronization aborts after 90 seconds if no R waves meet all synchronization criteria.

Figure 22-5 shows a Poincaré plane that characterizes an R wave as a point according to its current RR

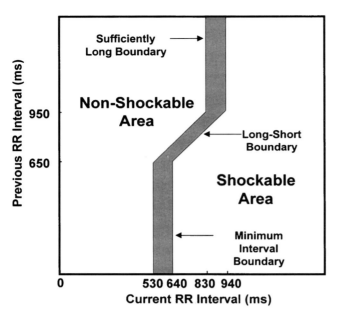

FIGURE 22-5. Depiction of the Metrix R-wave synchronization scheme on the Poincaré plane. The vertical axis represents the previous RR interval, and the horizontal axis represents the current RR interval. Minimum interval, long-short interval, and sufficiently long interval criteria are graphically represented.

interval (horizontal axis) and its previous RR interval (vertical axis). A boundary is used to depict the behavior of the Metrix synchronization algorithm with respect to any RR interval sequence. The Metrix synchronization algorithm uses an SQ interval measurement in the minimum interval criterion, allowing the Metrix device to be sensitive to variations in QS duration. A long QS duration can result in a shift of the T wave toward the next candidate R wave. To characterize the minimum interval and long-short criteria on a Poincaré plane, the minimum (SQ) interval criterion must be translated by adding a QS duration. The location of the boundary is based on the programming of the minimum SQ interval. The figure illustrates a 500-msec minimum SQ interval. The width of the boundary reflects the potential variability of the minimum RR interval due to variations in QS durations. QS durations between 30 and 140 msec are illustrated in Figure 22-5.

The vertical portion of the boundary extending from the horizontal axis represents the minimum interval criterion. No RR interval less than 500 msec + QS duration (i.e., 530 msec, assuming 30-msec QS duration) is identified as shockable. When the boundary reaches a vertical height (i.e., previous RR interval) of 650 msec, it rotates 45-degrees and progresses to a vertical height of 950 msec. This portion of the boundary characterizes the behavior of the long-short criterion. RR intervals between 500 msec + QS duration and 800 msec + QS duration with previous RR intervals no more than 140 msec longer satisfy the minimum interval and long-short criteria. The boundary rotates left to become a vertical line again at 950 msec. RR intervals greater than 800 msec + QS duration are sufficiently long to satisfy the minimum interval and long-short criteria.

Implantable Atrial Defibrillator Clinical Experience: Metrix Phase I

The first implantation of the Metrix device was performed in October 1995 (146). In April 1996, the phase I Metrix multicenter trial was started. The study objectives were safety evaluation and atrial fibrillation detection and treatment efficacy (4). By May 1997, a total of 51 Metrix systems had been implanted in 19 centers.

The patients (40 men, 11 women) were relatively young, suffering from recurrent atrial fibrillation and were at low risk for ventricular arrhythmias. Patients were between 31 and 78 years of age, with a left ventricular ejection fraction of 58 ± 11% and a left atrial size of 4.4 ± 0.8 cm; 36 were classified in New York Heart Association (NYHA) class I, and 15 were in NYHA class II. Before enrollment, all patients were treated with an average of 3.9 class I and III antiarrhythmic drugs. Antiarrhythmic drugs were poorly tolerated or ineffective in controlling atrial fibrillation recurrences.

Because the Metrix IAD has no ventricular defibrillation capability, the long-term efficacy of atrial fibrillation detection and R-wave synchronization are critical safety requirements (141). A total of 2,240 atrial fibrillation detection tests were performed under medical observation: 1,062 during sinus rhythm and 1,178 during atrial fibrillation (141). Each of the tests during sinus rhythm yielded a correct rhythm detection, achieving the design goal of 100% specificity to sinus rhythm. During atrial fibrillation, 109 episodes resulted in a false-negative detection (i.e., determination of sinus rhythm when the patient was in atrial fibrillation), yielding a 92.3% sensitivity for atrial fibrillation detection. However, all of these false-negative episodes were transient, with a correct atrial fibrillation detection in the next cycle of rhythm analysis or after reprogramming.

A total of 242,435 R waves were analyzed during sinus rhythm (71,665) and atrial fibrillation (170,770) (146). During atrial fibrillation, 36% of the R waves analyzed were considered appropriate for shock delivery. The main reason for rejecting R waves for shock was violation of the minimum RR interval criterion. The most important finding was that 100% synchronization accuracy was obtained, with all shock markers being coincident with R waves and none coincident with T waves.

During the phase I trial, 3,719 shocks were delivered with the Metrix system, increasing to more than 10,000 at the end of 1998. Importantly, all shocks were accurately synchronized, and no ventricular proarrhythmia was observed.

All spontaneous episodes were treated under a physician's observation. A total of 231 episodes were treated in 41 patients, with an average of three shocks per episode (4). The device terminated 96% of the episodes. However, often atrial fibrillation recurred within 1 minute after treatment (i.e., early recurrence of atrial fibrillation). Device therapy was repeated, sometimes combined with drug treatment. Taking early recurrence of atrial fibrillation into account, the overall clinical efficacy of the device was 86.3%.

In addition to these treated episodes, 971 nontreated episodes occurred (147). The mean duration of the nontreated episodes was significantly shorter than that of the treated episodes (38 versus 10 hours). Seventy-two percent of the nontreated episodes were shorter than 8 hours, indicating that paroxysmal-atrial fibrillation patients are unlikely to be good candidates for an atrial defibrillator (148).

After July 1997, the Metrix IAD devices were programmed in patient-activated or automatic mode for out-of-hospital atrial fibrillation treatment (149). Most patients (21 of 23) had devices that were programmed in the patient-activated mode. The overall clinical efficacy in treating atrial fibrillation episodes was 87%. However, efficacy rose to 95% when patients returned to the hospital or clinic after failed ambulatory treatment (150).

Later, patients with underlying cardiac disease were implanted with the atrial defibrillator. Daoud described the clinical experience from 91 Metrix patients with different kinds of underlying cardiac disease, including hypertension, valvular disease, ischemic heart disease, and symptoms of heart failure (151). In these patients, 4,005 shocks were delivered, and 33 patients had at least one episode treated in an out-of-hospital setting, with an efficacy ranging from 77% to 95%. No complications or proarrhythmic events were observed during this study.

Preliminary findings from the phase I clinical study suggest that maintenance of sinus rhythm with an IAD prolongs the interval between symptomatic episodes of atrial fibrillation (152,153). Timmermans and colleagues showed that the mean time between atrial fibrillation episodes increased from 1 week at implantation to about 1 month after 90 days. In 16 patients evaluated by Tse and coworkers, the number of hours each patient spent in atrial fibrillation was significantly lower in months 4 through 6 after implantation than in months 1 through 3; moreover, left atrial size decreased. This is consistent with the hypothesis of reverse remodeling of the atrium in the absence of fibrillation (154). However, one report challenges the reverse-remodeling hypothesis. Four Metrix patients who had been arrhythmia free for more than 1,000 hours were submitted to electrophysiologic testing to determine the change in atrial electrical parameters (155). In three of these patients, atrial fibrillation was induced with a single extrastimulus, and in the remaining patient, electrical parameters were unchanged compared with the preimplantation values. The investigators concluded that, despite prolonged periods of sinus rhythm after Metrix implantation, reverse remodeling did not occur in patients with a long history of atrial fibrillation.

Therapy Issues: Pain Perception and Discomfort During Cardioversion

Shock tolerability and patient discomfort remain open issues with atrial cardioversion therapy. For widespread acceptance, patients with an IAD should be able to initiate therapy without sedation or medical assistance. Shock-induced discomfort is a complex problem that may be related to multiple factors, including skeletal muscle contraction, direct nerve stimulation, and psychologic factors (104) such as fear of pain (156) and heightened perception because of preceding shocks (157). The level of discomfort felt by the patient during a defibrillation shock depends on a variety of factors, including shock strength (104, 127,156,158), waveform (158–161), the number of shocks, and shock outcome (127,157,162). Shock vector and patient posture also may play a role in patient perception.

Early reports on patient discomfort focused on shock energy. Data from these studies are inconsistent (162), with severe discomfort reported at energy levels as low as 0.1 (163), 0.4 (164), or 0.5 J (165), whereas in other cases, patients tolerated up to 10 J with only light sedation (166). Two similar studies suggest that the number of shocks rather than energy level is more closely related to pain perception (104, 127). Nonsedated patients were subjected to step-up defibrillation protocols starting at 20 V (104) or 180 V (127). In both studies, most patients received three or four shocks before requesting sedation. Additional investigations have corroborated these findings (157, 164). Jung et al. gave nonsedated patients two consecutive shocks of 1 or 2 J in random order within 3 minutes. All patients reported greater discomfort after the second shock than the first. No patient defined the first shock as intolerable, whereas 40% described the second shock as intolerable. Steinhaus and colleagues, delivered shocks of 0.4 or 2.0 J in random order and found that patient tolerance declined with the number of shocks. No relationship was found between shock strength and discomfort.

If peak voltage is related to pain perception, waveform rounding and other wave shapes may hold promise for reducing shock-related discomfort (158, 159,162,167). Heisel and coworkers investigated pain perception during internal atrial fibrillation cardioversion by using waveforms from two different capacitors: 500 and 60 μF (160). The mean A-DFT for the waveforms tested was comparable (1.6 $\pm$ 1.1 versus 2.0 $\pm$ 0.9 J), but peak voltage was significantly lower for shocks delivered with the 500-μF capacitor (96 $\pm$ 34 versus 245 $\pm$ 64 V). Discomfort was comparable for the two waveforms. Further investigation of the relation between peak voltage and shock discomfort is required.

To clinically manage pain during cardioversion, Timmermans and associates investigated the effect of intranasally administered butorphanol on shock-related discomfort in a double-blind, placebo-controlled study (168). In addition to the standard visual analog scale for evaluation of pain and fear, the pain rating index (PRI) was obtained using the McGill Pain Questionnaire. The study showed that the PRI evaluated pain more accurately than the more commonly used visual analog scale. Intranasal butorphanol decreased or stabilized the value of several pain variables but did not affect fear. The investigators concluded that the favorable effect of butorphanol, the ease of use, and the absence of side effects would make the drug suitable for ambulatory use. They also speculated that anxiety substantially contributes to patient discomfort. These components require further evaluation.

Early Recurrence of Atrial Fibrillation

Early recurrence of atrial fibrillation within the first seconds or minutes after a successful cardioversion to sinus rhythm has been observed clinically after external (169,170) and internal cardioversion (115, 171–173). The mechanisms by which early recurrence of atrial fibrillation occurs are not well understood. Early recurrence of atrial fibrillation has been reported to occur after premature atrial depolarizations (115,172,174). In a retrospective multivariate analysis, Tieleman and coworkers found that the use of intracellular calcium-lowering drugs during atrial fibrillation was the only significant variable related to maintenance of sinus rhythm after cardioversion (175).

Though technical success (i.e., conversion to sinus rhythm) rates of internal cardioversion are high, early recurrence of atrial fibrillation results in a lower clinical success (i.e., conversion to sinus rhythm without early recurrence of atrial fibrillation) rate. Prevalence of early recurrence of atrial fibrillation after internal cardioversion ranges from 13% to 31%

(115,171,172). The occurrence seems to be higher in paroxysmal patients, reaching values as high as 50% (171). A retrospective evaluation of 96 patients implanted with a Metrix atrial defibrillator revealed that 44% of patients experienced at least one occurrence of early recurrence of atrial fibrillation (173,176). However, only 15% of patients frequently experienced early recurrence of atrial fibrillation (>50% of their spontaneous atrial fibrillation episodes). Because early recurrence of atrial fibrillation increases the number of shocks required to produce sinus rhythm, there is a link between early recurrence of atrial fibrillation and therapy tolerance.

IMPLANTABLE DEVICES FOR ATRIAL DEFIBRILLATION: ICDS

The introduction of dual-chamber ICD systems significantly improved the therapy capabilities available to patients with complex bradyarrhythmias and tachyarrhythmias. These systems represent a further development of the fundamental principles of detection, detection enhancements, and therapy, providing increased sophistication in arrhythmia detection and rhythm management for both heart chambers. The ICD system safety and efficacy stems from years of design and clinical evaluation, aimed at providing maximal protection against life-threatening ventricular arrhythmias.

Current V-ICDs with ventricular tachyarrhythmia therapies possess the technologies required for atrial defibrillation. These devices are implanted in the subcutaneous or submuscular thoracic region, use a transvenous catheter situated in the right ventricle, which may be used for R-wave synchronization, and already have defibrillation electrodes, which may be used for atrial defibrillation. The first commercial AV-ICD that provides for ventricular and atrial defibrillation (Medtronic Jewel AF model 7250) uses an atrial pace/sense lead and the same electrodes available for ventricular defibrillation. The device allows for an optional defibrillation lead to be positioned in the coronary sinus. The shock vector for atrial defibrillation may be programmed from the available electrodes. Before addressing the clinical performance of this dual-therapy AVICD device, we first discuss the issues involved in the integration of atrial therapies into an ICD platform.

ICD Atrial Defibrillation Thresholds

Modern ICDs are equipped with a transvenous lead that situates a coil defibrillation electrode in the right ventricle (RV) and often contains a second proximal electrode in the superior vena cava (SVC) or right atrium (RA). Most ICDs use the conductive housing (Can) of the pulse generator as an electrode. For termination of ventricular fibrillation or atrial fibrillation, shock vectors include $RV \rightarrow SVC$, $RV \rightarrow Can$, and $RV \rightarrow SVC + Can$ (Fig. 22-2A). With the addition of a coronary sinus lead, several additional electrode configurations may be used for atrial defibrillation, including the standard $RA \rightarrow CS$ vector used in the IAD (Fig. 22-2B).

Studies have shown that atrial cardioversion is feasible with standard V-ICD lead configurations. For example, consistently low A-DFTs were obtained with the three-electrode $RV \rightarrow SVC + Can$ system, with mean thresholds between 2 and 7 J (177–182). Low (<10 J) A-DFTs have also been obtained with other ICD lead combinations: $RV \rightarrow SVC$ (179), $RV \rightarrow Can$ (180,183), and $RA/SVC \rightarrow Can$ (177). Not all ICD lead combinations, however, yield consistently low A-DFTs (178). In contrast, altering the right atrial electrode position can have a profound effect on ADFT (180).

Further optimization of atrial cardioversion thresholds can be achieved through the use of a coronary sinus lead with an ICD lead system. In patients with no prior history of atrial fibrillation, Desai and coworkers reported A-DFTs for the $RA \rightarrow CS$ system (1.8 J) to be lower than for either of the two ICD configurations tested: $RA \rightarrow Can$ (5.4 J) and $RV \rightarrow SVC$ (4.3 J) (184). Similar results were reported by Saksena in patients with paroxysmal or chronic atrial fibrillation with A-DFTs near 9 ± 9 J for the $RA \rightarrow CS$ vector compared with other more standard ICD configurations, with thresholds ranging from 13 to 20 J (185). These results were reinforced by Min and coworkers using a finite element model of the human thorax (186).

Atrial defibrillation thresholds can be reduced even

further by combining electrodes with the $RA \rightarrow CS$ configuration. Geiger and associates reduced A-DFTs in humans by adding a SVC electrode ($RA + SVC \rightarrow CS$) or a pectoral electrode ($RA \rightarrow CS + cutaneous\ patch$) (187). Min and colleagues found similar threshold results for this second configuration using their finite element model; the $RA \rightarrow CS + Can$ system required 29% lower A-DFT energy than the standard two-electrode configuration (188).

ICD Detection Algorithms for V-ICDs

The detection architecture in a standard V-ICD is designed to classify supraventricular tachycardia (SVT) and ventricular tachycardia or fibrillation (ventricular tachycardia/ventricular fibrillation). The current paradigm in standard V-ICDs is to balance therapy decisions toward maximal sensitivity at a modest cost of specificity. This balance is designed to deliver ventricular therapy for all episodes of ventricular tachycardia/ventricular fibrillation at a cost of treating some SVTs.

The V-ICD systems use ventricular rate and rate duration to start the detection process. Therapy is chosen based on the ventricular rate zone that a rhythm occupies (Fig. 22-6). In certain zones (e.g., sinus rhythm zone), no tachycardia therapy is delivered, and no further detection algorithms are needed. In other zones (e.g., ventricular fibrillation zone) that deliver immediate therapy, the V-ICD has straightforward detection schemes that do not require further enhancements. To optimize specificity in zones that could encounter benign SVTs, detection enhancements are invoked to direct appropriate therapy.

V-ICD Detection: VENTAK AV ICD Family with Atrial View

The VENTAK AV family of ICDs (Guidant Corp.) use A-A and V-V intervals throughout the detection process. After an initial detection by 8 of 10 fast V-V intervals ($>VT\ threshold$), at least 6 of 10 intervals must remain fast during a duration time to avoid resetting detection. After the duration is met, each therapy enhancement that is programmed "ON" is used to classify the cardiac rhythm. The *Onset* algorithm searches backward in time to a pivot defining the onset of the episode. A comparison of the intervals on both sides of this pivot is made to assess whether the onset was sudden or gradual. The *Stability* algorithm calculates a weighted sum of current and previous V-V interval differences. This weighted sum is compared with a programmed threshold to assess whether the rhythm is stable or unstable. The *AF Threshold* criterion is met if 6 of 10 (4 of 10 thereafter) PP intervals are greater than a programmable threshold. The $V_{rate} > A_{rate}$ detection enhancement uses an average of the 10 most recent RR and PP intervals to determine which chamber has a greater rate. If the V_{rate} exceeds the A_{rate} by 10 bpm, the $V_{rate} > A_{rate}$ criterion is met.

When programmed 'ON,' *Onset, Stability, AF Threshold,* and $V_{rate} > A_{rate}$ are collectively used to classify the cardiac rhythm as SVT or ventricular tachycardia after duration is met. If a cardiac rhythm is determined to be an SVT, *Sustained Rate Duration* may be used to override inhibitors.

A convenient way to characterize rhythms according to their atrial and ventricular (AV) rates is the two-dimensional atrial-ventricular rate plane shown in Figure 22-7. Here, the atrial-ventricular rate plane is used to illustrate the VENTAK AV detection architecture with all enhancements turned ON. Detection

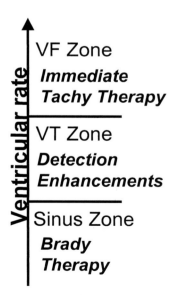

FIGURE 22-6. Depiction of VR device rate zones: sinus zone, ventricular tachycardia (VT) zone, and ventricular fibrillation (VF) zone.

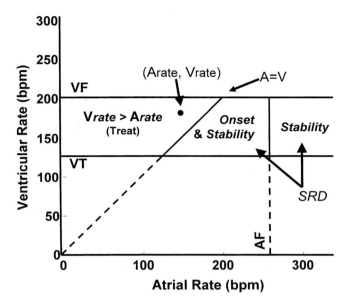

FIGURE 22-7. Depiction of the atrial-ventricular (AV) rate plane for the VENTAK AV family of dual-chamber defibrillators. The ventricular rate is plotted on the vertical axis, and the atrial rate is plotted on the horizontal axis. Rhythms fall on the plane at various points (A_{rate}, V_{rate}). The AV plane is depicted for the VENTAK AV family of devices with all specificity enhancements programmed ON. The plane is shown divided into a single ventricular tachycardia (VT) zone for $125 < V_{rate} < 200$ bpm. A line of identity depicts the $A_{rate} = V_{rate}$. Onset, Stability, and A > AF criteria are used.

enhancements are reserved for cardiac rhythms with ventricular rates in the ventricular tachycardia zone as shown in Figure 22-7. However, the addition of Atrial View allows additional compartmentalization of enhancements by adding atrial rate information. As depicted in Figure 22-7, the stability algorithm is used on rhythms within the ventricular tachycardia zone that have atrial rates greater than the *AF threshold*. If the cardiac rhythm has a stable ventricular response, it is classified as a ventricular tachycardia. Otherwise, the rhythm is classified as atrial fibrillation. The stability and onset algorithms are used on rhythms within the ventricular tachycardia zone that have atrial rates exceeding the ventricular rate but less than the *AF threshold*. If the cardiac rhythm has a sudden onset and a stable ventricular response, it is classified as a ventricular tachycardia. Otherwise, it is classified as an SVT. If the cardiac rhythm has a ventricular rate that is greater than the atrial rate by 10 bpm, it is classified as a ventricular tachycardia.

AF Threshold and A > V allows for use of *onset* and *stability* to classify SVT and atrial fibrillation from 1:1 retrograde ventricular tachycardia and dual tachycardia (e.g., atrial fibrillation with concomitant ventricular tachycardia) that may occupy the ventricular tachycardia zone in the SVT or atrial fibrillation zones.

V-ICD Detection: Gem DR Family of ICDs with PR Logic

The Gem DR family of ICDs (Medtronic, Minneapolis, MN) use PR Logic atrial and ventricular event pattern and rate analysis to discriminate between SVT and ventricular tachycardia rhythms. This algorithm was designed to preserve the V-ICD paradigm of high sensitivity and reserves the use of enhanced detection for cardiac rhythms with median ventricular rates that are slower than a programmable maximum SVT rate. The PR Logic algorithm withholds ventricular therapy if an SVT is positively identified.

The PR Logic algorithm uses several electrogram timing features to help classify cardiac rhythms. The *modesum* algorithm creates a histogram of the last 18 RR intervals and calculates the percentage of intervals in the largest two bins. A large percentage reflects a cardiac rhythm with regular ventricular intervals. The median atrial and ventricular cycle lengths are computed after every ventricular event using the last 12 PP and RR intervals. *PR-dissociation* metric is calculated by measuring the absolute difference between the current PR interval and the mean of the most recent 8 PR intervals. For differences greater than 40 msec, the current PR is considered dissociated. The rhythm is considered dissociated if at least 4 of the last 8 PR intervals are dissociated. *Pattern analysis* parses a cardiac rhythm into a series of coupled RR intervals. Each coupling contains an RR interval and the previous RR interval. These couplings are parsed into zones (i.e., antegrade, retrograde, and junctional) in which atrial events usually occur. A letter is assigned to each coupling by matching the location of naturally occurring P waves within the zones of each coupling to a database of 19 couple codes. Collecting a time sequence of couple codes generates a syntax. Cardiac rhythms such as sinus tachycardia, atrial fibrillation/

atrial flutter, and other SVTs have their own naturally occurring syntax.

Counters for ventricular tachycardia, ventricular fibrillation, and atrial fibrillation are also used in the detection process. The *fibrillation detection interval* (FDI) and *tachycardia detection interval* define the ventricular fibrillation and ventricular tachycardia detection zones. An "X of Y" counter registers intervals for detection in the ventricular fibrillation zone, and a consecutive counter registers intervals for detection in the ventricular tachycardia zone. An atrial fibrillation evidence counter tallies atrial tachyarrhythmias that cannot be described using pattern syntax, it is used to help identify atrial fibrillation when PR relationships during atrial fibrillation are highly variable. On each ventricular event, the atrial fibrillation evidence counter increments by 1, decrements by 1, or remains at the same value depending on the number and pattern of atrial events since the previous ventricular event. PR Logic also uses an algorithm to detect far-field R waves during sinus tachycardia. P events are rejected as far-field R wave if the device senses consistent alternation of PP and RP intervals and low RP interval variability; for every RR interval, two atrial events occur, with one of those two atrial events occurring very close in time to one of the R waves, and the previous two cases occur for 10 of the last 12 RR intervals.

Parameters are programmed with nominal values and the sinus tachycardia, atrial fibrillation, and other 1 : 1 SVT detection criteria are programmed ON. The algorithm collects up to 24 RR intervals and PR patterns. If no high ventricular rates are sensed, no detection occurs, and the device collects additional data. After a high ventricular rate is sensed, the median RR interval is compared with the programmable minimum SVT RR interval. If the median RR interval is smaller than the minimum SVT RR interval, ventricular tachycardia and ventricular fibrillation detection are met. Otherwise, the device checks for dual tachycardia (i.e., ventricular tachycardia or ventricular fibrillation during atrial fibrillation/atrial flutter) by determining the PR relationship. If the PR relationship is greater than 1 : 1 (i.e., atrial fibrillation evidence), the rhythm is *dissociated*, and the RR intervals are regular (i.e., modesum). RR interval regularity is not required if the RR interval are in the ventricular fibrillation zone. If these criteria are met, dual tachycardia is recognized, and zone-appropriate ventricular tachycardia/ventricular fibrillation therapies are delivered. If dual tachycardia is not recognized, syntactic PR patterns, atrial fibrillation evidence counter, modesum, dissociation, and far field R-wave (FFRW) criteria are assessed to positively identify an atrial fibrillation, atrial flutter, SVT, or sinus tachycardia. If none of these rhythms is positively identified, the algorithm detects ventricular tachycardia/ventricular fibrillation by default. A complete description of PR Logic is contained in Chapter 21.

Detection Architecture for a Standard Ventricular ICD

Current devices maintain the V-ICD paradigm by balancing detection toward safety. The VENTAK AV and Gem families of V-ICD devices have provided very high levels of specificity (91% to 100%) in selected patient groups (190–192). Specificity values may be more modest when tested against broader patient groups (193,194).

The AV-ICDs that deliver atrial and ventricular therapies must preserve the sensitivity requirement of the V-ICD. In this way, lethal arrhythmias such as ventricular tachycardia and ventricular fibrillation always receive therapy.

Detection Algorithms for Atrioventricular Implantable Cardioverter-Defibrillators

A method for appropriate integration of detection algorithms should be considered when merging atrial and ventricular therapy in a single device. Designing the method for integration is somewhat trivial when considering "well-behaved" arrhythmia such as ventricular tachycardia with concomitant normal sinus rhythm. However, a device that provides atrial and ventricular therapy must be robust to the most confounding arrhythmia scenarios, such as SVT with a rapid ventricular response. The design challenges reside in the parsing of prevalent and potentially confounding arrhythmias to ensure accurate and safe therapy decisions.

Integration of Atrial and Ventricular Defibrillation Devices: the A-machine and the V-machine

Integration of the IAD and V-ICD detection architectures can be accomplished by assigning priority to the V-ICD. This can be achieved by analyzing the combination device as a V-machine (i.e., V-ICD detection algorithms optimized for high ventricular tachycardia sensitivity) coupled with an A-machine (i.e., IAD detection algorithms optimized for high atrial fibrillation specificity). The performance paradigms of the V-machine and A-machine detection architectures are identical to those of the V-ICD and IAD, respectively. However, the V-machine maintains priority over the A-machine when both are invoked (i.e., elevated atrial and ventricular rates). The V-machine operates whenever ventricular rates are elevated above a minimum ventricular tachycardia rate threshold (Fig. 22-8). The A-machine operates whenever the atrial rate is above a minimum atrial rate threshold *(AT Threshold)* and greater than the ventricular rate. The V-machine controls therapy decisions when ventricular rates are very high, or when the ventricular rate exceeds the *VT Threshold*. When ventricular rates are below the *VT threshold* and atrial rates exceed the *AT threshold*, the A-machine controls atrial therapy decisions, similar to an IAD device.

When ventricular and atrial rates exceed their respective minimum rate thresholds, detection algorithms from the V-machine and A-machine work in tandem, with priority given to the ventricular detection process. If the V-machine determines a ventricular tachycardia/ventricular fibrillation is present, it maintains control of therapy decisions. If the programmed detection enhancements used by the V-machine indicate a SVT rhythm and inhibit ventricular therapy (according to its V-specificity), therapy control is passed to the A-machine, which directs atrial therapy decisions. The A-machine maintains control unless the V-machine changes its rhythm classification to ventricular tachycardia/ventricular fibrillation.

The ventricular tachycardia sensitivity of this combined AV-ICD detection architecture in the zones in which the A- and V-machines overlap is equal to the sensitivity of the V-machine. The sinus tachycardia-specificity of this AV-ICD system is equal to the product of the two specificity values: one from the V-machine and the other from the A-machine. For example, if the V-machine has a 85% specificity to SVT and the A-machine has a 99% specificity to sinus tachycardia, the overall specificity of the AV-ICD to sinus tachycardia would be 84% because of the characteristics of the V-machine. It is clear that for combined AV-ICD systems, improvements in V- and A-detection algorithms are necessary.

Figure 22-9 depicts a population of spontaneous episodes, recorded by VENTAK AV devices, plotted on the two-dimensional AV rate plane. For typical rate threshold settings, a nontrivial number of SVTs are evaluated by the V-machine. Proper device programming of enhancements used to inhibit ventricular therapy when SVTs are detected will be required for these SVTs to receive appropriate atrial therapy from the A-machine. Overlap in rate occurs between atrial fibrillation and other SVT (e.g., atrial flutter and sinus tachycardia). This fact along with the desire to provide tiered atrial therapy, establishes a need for atrial detection enhancements that do not rely solely on rate to further subclassify SVT.

Integration of atrial tachyarrhythmia therapy with a device that provides ventricular tachyarrhythmia therapy needs to preserve the same performance para-

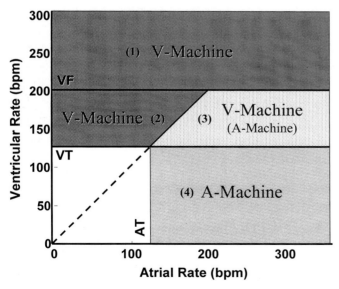

FIGURE 22-8. A breakdown of the atrial-ventricular (AV) rate plane depicting which device (V-machine or A-machine) takes precedence in each rate zone. Zonal performance is optimized to give maximum sensitivity to ventricular tachycardia (VT/VF) while preserving specificity for atrial fibrillation (AF).

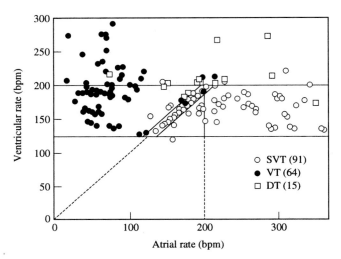

FIGURE 22-9. The atrial-ventricular (AV) rate plane populated by patient data from the VENTAK AV family of devices. Ventricular tachycardia (VT), supraventricular tachycardia (SVT), and dual tachycardia (DT) are depicted on the rate plane. This figure illustrates the need for specificity enhancement and accurate discrimination of atrial and ventricular arrhythmias. Notice the overlap between different arrhythmias and the prevalence of rhythms near the $A_{rate} = V_{rate}$ line of identity.

digms as those in the stand-alone atrial defibrillator and standard ventricular ICD. This can be accomplished through strategic allocation of therapy control to a V-machine and an A-machine and prioritizing this control to the V-machine. This places a strong emphasis on ventricular detection algorithms that are optimized for high sensitivity to ventricular tachycardia but also operate with very high specificity, allowing appropriate hand-off of control to the atrial detection algorithms.

Clinical Experience with Atrioventricular Implantable Cardioverter-Defibrillators: Jewel AF

The first dual-chamber defibrillator is the model 7250 Jewel AF arrhythmia management device (Medtronic Inc., Minneapolis, MN). The Jewel AF is a dual-chamber pacemaker and dual-chamber cardioverter-defibrillator. The device provides for programmable energy delivery including an optional $RA \rightarrow CS$ vector. Multiple programmable atrial therapies are available, including antitachycardia pacing, 50-Hz burst pacing, and automatic or patient-activated R-wave synchronous defibrillation shocks. Ventricular backup therapies include antitachycardia pacing and defibrillation. The Jewel AF incorporates the PR Logic dual-chamber detection algorithm described previously (195,196).

In a multicenter investigation (197) in patients with symptomatic atrial tachycardia (AT), atrial fibrillation, or both, 80 patients were studied, with a mean follow-up of 6 ± 2 months. Fifty-eight patients were Holter monitored to validate detection of AT or atrial fibrillation and to determine sensitivity to detection of AT or atrial fibrillation. Detection was appropriate in 98% of 132 atrial fibrillation episodes and 88% of 190 AT episodes. Intermittent sensing of far-field R waves caused inappropriate detection of 27 AT or atrial fibrillation episodes.

The multiple therapies delivered by the Jewel AF were effective in terminating many atrial arrhythmias. Swerdlow and coworkers reported a 45% termination rate for AT with antitachycardia pacing alone. In a related publication, Swerdlow and colleagues reported the defibrillation success for first shocks programmed to DFT^+, $1.5 \times DFT^+$, $2 \times DFT^+$, and $>2 \times DFT^+$; the corresponding first-shock success rates were 40%, 78%, 73%, and 68%, respectively (198). Overall defibrillation efficacy was 91%. However, in this study, early recurrence of atrial fibrillation was reported as a significant clinical problem (14 of 52 patients) that limited shock success. early recurrence of atrial fibrillation occurred frequently and was independent of shock energy. The researchers suggested, despite the high defibrillation success, an important clinical implication was that early recurrence of atrial fibrillation might limit the clinical efficacy of atrial defibrillation.

CONCLUSIONS

The challenge of managing patients with atrial fibrillation has long been a burden on the medical community. Given the prevalence of atrial fibrillation in the elderly population and the growth of this demographic group the treatment of atrial fibrillation is a burgeoning problem. Until recently, atrial fibrillation management was confined to medical therapy, surgical, ablative, and in-hospital procedures. It has since been shown that internal atrial defibrillation delivered from an implantable device is feasible and effective for the termination of atrial fibrillation. Stand-alone atrial defibrillators and dual-chamber defibrillators that provide electrical therapies for atrial fibrillation are gaining acceptance in the medical community. However, it remains to be demonstrated that device-based control of atrial fibrillation through repeated electrical cardioversion can result in a lower atrial fibrillation burden or reversal of the disease process in humans. The medical-economic outcomes for this new therapeutic approach require time to adequately assess.

The initial experiences with the Metrix and Jewel AF devices demonstrate the safety and efficacy of atrial tachyarrhythmia detection and treatment with implantable devices. Overall defibrillation success can be quite high. More benign pacing therapies appear to be useful in terminating a significant fraction of atrial arrhythmias. However, these data also highlight areas for future improvement. Appropriate detection, early recurrence of atrial fibrillation, and first-shock success remain important problems to solve to ensure widespread patient and physician acceptance of this therapy.

The previous decade of experimental and clinical research has provided tremendous advances in the treatment of atrial fibrillation. It is expected that the medical management of patients with atrial fibrillation will continue to evolve through an industry and medical-community partnership seeking a greater understanding of basic mechanisms of atrial fibrillation, pain, and early recurrence of atrial fibrillation. The delivery atrial defibrillation therapy from an implanted device is emerging as an important weapon in the arsenal for atrial fibrillation treatment in the 21st century.

REFERENCES

1. Dell'Orfano JT, Patel H, Wolbrette DL, et al. Acute treatment of atrial fibrillation: spontaneous conversion rates and cost of care. *Am J Cardiol* 1999;83:788–790.
2. Dorian P, Paquett M, Newman D. Evaluation of quality of life in atrial fibrillation. In: Murgatroyd FD, Camm AJ, eds. *Nonpharmacological management of atrial fibrillation*. Armonk, NY: Futura Publishing, 1997:23–35.
3. Cox JL, Boineau JP, Schuessier RB, et al. Five-year experience with the maze procedure for atrial fibrillation. *Ann Thorac Surg* 1993;56:814–824.
4. Wellens HJ, Lau CP, Luderitz B, et al. Atrioverter: an implantable device for the treatment of atrial fibrillation. *Circulation* 1998;98:1651–1656.
5. Bigger JT Jr. Epidemiological and mechanistic studies of atrial fibrillation as a basis for treatment strategies. *Circulation* 1998;98:943–945.
6. Levy S, Breithardt G, Campbell RW, et al. Atrial fibrillation: current knowledge and recommendations for management, Working Group on Arrhythmias of the European Society of Cardiology. *Eur Heart J* 1998;19:1294–1320.
7. Reuter D, Ayers GM. Future directions of electrotherapy for atrial fibrillation. *J Cardiovasc Electrophysiol* 1998;9[Suppl]:S202–S210.
8. Bialy D, Lehmann MH, Schumacher DN, et al. Hospitalization for arrhythmias in the United States: importance of atrial fibrillation [Abstract]. *J Am Coll Cardiol* 1992;19:41A.
9. Duytschaever M, Danse P, Eijsbouts S, Allesie M. The presence of a supervulnerable period immediately after conversion of atrial fibrillation [Abstract]. *Pacing Clin Electrophysiol* 1999;22[Pt II]:707.
10. Sanfilippo AJ, Abascal VM, Sheehan M, et al. Atrial enlargement as a consequence of atrial fibrillation: a prospective echocardiographic study. *Circulation* 1990;82:792–797.
11. Lau CP, Tse HF. Electrical remodelling of chronic atrial fibrillation. *Clin Exp Pharmacol Physiol* 1997;24:982–983.
12. Kannel WB, Abbott RD, Savage DD, McNamara PM. Epidemiologic features of chronic atrial fibrillation: the Framingham study. *N Engl J Med* 1982;306:1018–1022.
13. Coumel P. Autonomic influences in atrial tachyarrhythmias. *J Cardiovasc Electrophysiol* 1998;7:32–34.
14. Chen PS, Wu TJ, Ikeda T, et al. Focal source hypothesis of atrial fibrillation. *J Electrocardiol* 1998;31[Suppl]:32–34.
15. Coumel P. Neurogenic and humoral influences of the autonomic nervous system in the determination of paroxysmal atrial fibrillation. In: Atteul P, Coumel P, Janse ML, eds. *The atrium in health and disease*. Mount Kisco, NY: Futura Publishing, 1989:213–232.
16. Thamilarasan M, Klein AL. Factors relating to left atrial enlargement in atrial fibrillation: "chicken or the egg" hypothesis. *Am Heart J* 1999;137:381–383.
17. Andersen JS, Egeblad H, Abildgaard U, et al. Atrial fibrillation and left atrial enlargement: cause or effect? *J Intern Med* 1991;229:253–256.
18. Qin Y, Kaibara M, Hirata T, et al. Atrial conduction curves in patients with and without atrial fibrillation. *Jpn Circ J* 1998;62:289–293.
19. Jung W, Lüderitz B. Quality of life in patients with atrial fibrillation. *J Cardiovasc Electrophysiol* 1998;9[Suppl]:S177–S186.
20. The National Heart, Lung and Blood Institute Working Group on Atrial Fibrillation. Risk factors for stroke and efficacy of antithrombotic therapy in atrial fibrillation: current understandings and research imperatives. *J Am Coll Cardiol* 1993;22(7):1830–1834.
21. Akhtar W, Reeves WC, Movahed A. Indications for anticoagulation for atrial fibrillation. *Am Fam Physician* 1998;58:130–136.
22. Albers GW. Choice of antithrombotic therapy for stroke prevention in atrial fibrillation: warfarin, aspirin, or both? *Arch Intern Med* 1998;158:1487–1491.

23. Koefoed BG, Petersen P. Oral anticoagulation in nonvalvular atrial fibrillation. *J Intern Med* 1999;245:375–381.
24. Cairns JA, Connolly SJ. Nonrheumatic atrial fibrillation. Risk of stroke and role of antithrombotic therapy. *Circulation* 1991; 84:469–481.
25. Furberg CD, Psaty BM, Manolio TA, et al. Prevalence of atrial fibrillation in elderly subjects (the cardiovascular health study). *Am J Cardiol* 1994;74:236–241.
26. Olgin JE, Viskin S. Management of intermittent atrial fibrillation: drugs to maintain sinus rhythm. *J Cardiovasc Electrophysiol* 1999;10:433–441.
27. Dell'Orfano JT, Luck JC, Wolbrette DL, et al. Drugs for conversion of atrial fibrillation. *Am Fam Physician* 1998;58:471–480.
28. Gersh BJ. Antithrombotic therapy in nonrheumatic/nonvalvular atrial fibrillation. *J Cardiovasc Electrophysiol* 1999;10:461–471.
29. Touboul P. Atrioventricular nodal ablation and pacemaker implantation in patients with atrial fibrillation. *Am J Cardiol* 1999; 83[Suppl 5B]:241D–245D.
30. Narasimhan C, Blanck Z, Akhtar M. Atrioventricular nodal modification and atrioventricular junctional ablation for control of ventricular rate in atrial fibrillation. *J Cardiovasc Electrophysiol* 1998;9[Suppl 8]:S146–S150.
31. Knight BP, Morady F. Optimal management of the patient with an episode of atrial fibrillation in and out of the hospital: acute cardioversion or not? *J Cardiovasc Electrophysiol* 1999;10:425–432.
32. Miller JM, Jayachandran JV, Coppess MA, Olgin JE. Optimal management of the patient with chronic atrial fibrillation: whom to cardiovert? *J Cardiovasc Electrophysiol* 1999;10:442–449.
33. McComb JM. Surgery for atrial fibrillation. *J Thromb Thrombolysis* 1999;7:39–44.
34. Lesh MD. Progress toward a catheter ablative cure of atrial fibrillation. *J Electrocardiol* 1998;31[Suppl]:71–79.
35. Schwartzman D, Kuck KH. Anatomy-guided linear atrial lesions for radiofrequency catheter ablation of atrial fibrillation. *Pacing Clin Electrophysiol* 1998;21:1959–1978.
36. Wellens HJ, Sie HT, Smeets JL, et al. Surgical treatment of atrial fibrillation. *J Cardiovasc Electrophysiol* 1998;9[Suppl 8]:S151–154.
37. Keane D, Zhou L, Ruskin J. Catheter ablation for atrial fibrillation. *Semin Interv Cardiol* 1997;2:251–265.
38. Sundt TM 3rd, Camillo CJ, Cox JL. The maze procedure for cure of atrial fibrillation. *Cardiol Clin* 1997;15:739–748.
39. Ayers GM, Griffin JC. The future role of defibrillators in the management of atrial fibrillation. *Curr Opin Cardiol* 1997;12:12–17.
40. Levy T, Walker S, Rochelle J, Paul V. Evaluation of biatrial pacing, right atrial pacing, and no pacing in patients with drug refractory atrial fibrillation. *Am J Cardiol* 1999;84:426–429.
41. Ramdat Misier A, Beukema WP, Oude Luttikhuis HA. Multisite or alternate site pacing for the prevention of atrial fibrillation. *Am J Cardiol* 1999;83[Suppl 5B]:237D–240D.
42. Saksena S, Delfaut P, Prakash A, et al. Multisite electrode pacing for prevention of atrial fibrillation. *J Cardiovasc Electrophysiol* 1998;9[Suppl 8]:S155–S162.
43. Papageorgiou P, Monahan K, Anselme F, et al. Electrophysiology of atrial fibrillation and its prevention by coronary sinus pacing. *Semin Interv Cardiol* 1997;2:227–232.
44. Fahy GJ, Wilkoff BL. Pacing strategies to prevent atrial fibrillation. *Cardiol Clin* 1996;14:591–596.
45. Lesh MD, Kalman JM, Roithinger FX, Karch MR. Potential role of "hybrid therapy" for atrial fibrillation. *Semin Interv Cardiol* 1997;2:267–271.
46. Huang DT, Monahan KM, Zimetbaum P, et al. Hybrid pharmacologic and ablative therapy: a novel and effective approach for the management of atrial fibrillation. *J Cardiovasc Electrophysiol* 1998;9:462–469.
47. Artzberger R, Buscemi P. Pharmacological atrial defibrillator: initial experimental studies with rapid intra-atrial infusion of procainamide [Abstract]. *Pacing Clin Electrophysiol* 1997;20[Pt II]:1093.
48. Levy S. Factors predisposing to the development of atrial fibrillation. *Pacing Clin Electrophysiol* 1997;20[Pt II]:2670–2674.
49. De Sisti A, Leclercq JF, Fiorello P, et al. Sick sinus syndrome with and without atrial fibrillation: atrial refractoriness and conduction characteristics. *Cardiologia* 1999;44:361–367.
50. Kowey PR, Marinchak RA, Rials SJ, Filart RA. Management of atrial fibrillation in patients with hypertension. *J Hum Hypertens* 1997;11:699–707.
51. Gallagher MM, Obel OA, Camm JA. Tachycardia-induced atrial myopathy: an important mechanism in the pathophysiology of atrial fibrillation? *J Cardiovasc Electrophysiol* 1997;8:1065–1074.
52. Saxon LA. Atrial fibrillation and dilated cardiomyopathy: therapeutic strategies when sinus rhythm cannot be maintained. *Pacing Clin Electrophysiol* 1997;20[Pt 1]:720–725.
53. Crijns HJ, Van den Berg MP, Van Gelder IC, Van Veldhuisen DJ. Management of atrial fibrillation in the setting of heart failure. *Eur Heart J* 1997;18[Suppl C]:C45–C49.
54. Van den Berg MP, Tuinenburg AE, Crijns HJ, et al. Heart failure and atrial fibrillation: current concepts and controversies. *Heart* 1997;77:309–313.
55. Middlekauf HR, Stevenson WG, Stevenson LW. Prognostic significance of atrial fibrillation in advanced heart failure. *Circulation* 1994;89:724–730.
56. Prystowski EN. Perspectives and controversies in atrial fibrillation. *Am J Cardiol* 1998;82[Suppl 4A]:3I–6I.
57. Wijffels MC, Kirchhof CJ, Dorland R, et al. Electrical remodeling due to atrial fibrillation in chronically instrumented conscious goats: roles of neurohumoral changes, ischemia, atrial stretch, and high rate of electrical activation. *Circulation* 1997;96:3710–3720.
58. Ausma J, Wijffels M, Thone F, et al. Structural changes of atrial myocardium due to sustained atrial fibrillation in the goat. *Circulation* 1997;96:3157–3163.
59. Aliot E. New drugs for atrial arrhythmias. In: Saksena S, Luderitz B, eds. *Interventional electrophysiology: a textbook,* 2nd ed. Armonk, NY: Futura Publishing, 1996:479–492.
60. Wijfells MC, Dorland R, Allessie MA. Pharmacologic cardioversion of chronic atrial fibrillation in the goat by class IA, IC, and III drugs: a comparison between hydroquinidine, cibenzoline, flecainide, and D-sotalol. *J Cardiovasc Electrophysiol* 1999;10:178–193.
61. Saksena S, Prakash A, Mongeon L, et al. Clinical efficacy and safety of atrial defibrillation using biphasic shocks and current nonthoracotomy endocardial lead configurations. *Am J Cardiol* 1995;76:913–921.
62. Daubert C, Gras D, LeClercq C, et al. Biatrial synchronous pacing: a new therapeutic approach to prevent refractory atrial tachyarrhythmias [Abstract]. *J Am Coll Cardiol* 1995;23:230A.
63. Sundt TM III, Camillo CJ, Cox JL. The maze procedure for cure of atrial fibrillation. *Cardiol Clin* 1997;15:739–748.
64. Swartz JF, Perrersels G, Silvers J, et al. A catheter based curative approach for atrial fibrillation in humans [Abstract]. *Circulation* 1994;90[Suppl I]:I-335.
65. Haissaguerre M, Jais P, Shah DC, et al. Right and left atrial

radiofrequency catheter therapy of paroxysmal atrial fibrillation. *J Cardiovasc Electrophysiol* 1996;7:1132–1144.
66. Calkins H, Hall J, Ellenbogen K, et al. A new system for catheter ablation of atrial fibrillation. *Am J Cardiol* 1999;83(5B): 227D–236D.
67. Shinbane JS, Wood MA, Jensen DN, et al. Tachycardia-induced cardiomyopathy: a review of animal models and clinical studies. *J Am Coll Cardiol* 1997;29:709–715.
68. Saksena S, Prakash A, Krol R, Delfaut P. Time dependence and pattern of atrial fibrillation recurrences after single and dual site right atrial pacing [Abstract]. *J Am Coll Cardiol* 1999; 33[Suppl A]:140A.
69. Lau CP, Jiang ZY, Tang MO. Efficacy of ventricular rate stabilization by right ventricular pacing during atrial fibrillation. *Pacing Clin Electrophysiol* 1998;21:542–548.
70. Wittkampf FH, de Jongste MJ, Lie HI, Meijler FL. Effect of right ventricular pacing on ventricular rhythm during atrial fibrillation. *J Am Coll Cardiol* 1988;11:539–545.
71. Wolf PA, Abbott RD, Kannel WB. Atrial fibrillation as an independent risk factor for stroke: the Framingham study. *Stroke* 1991;22:983–988.
72. Berger M, Schweitzer P. Timing of thromboembolic events after electrical cardioversion of atrial fibrillation or flutter: a retrospective analysis. *Am J Cardiol* 1998;82(12):1545–1547, A8.
73. Risk factors for stroke and efficacy from antithrombotic therapy in atrial fibrillation: analysis of pooled data from five randomized controlled trials. *Arch Intern Med* 1994;154: 1449–1457.
74. Mayet J, More RS, Sutton GC. Anticoagulation for cardioversion of atrial arrhythmias. *Eur Heart J* 1998;19:548–552.
75. Lown B, Amarasingham R, Neuman J. New method for terminating cardiac arrhythmias: use of synchronized capacitor discharge. *N Engl J Med* 1962;182:548–555.
76. Van Gelder IC, Crijns HJ. Cardioversion of atrial fibrillation and subsequent maintenance of sinus rhythm. *Pacing Clin Electrophysiol* 1997;20[Pt 2]:2675–2683.
77. Ideker RE, Chen PS, Zhou XH. Basic mechanisms of defibrillation. *J Electrocardiol* 1990;[Suppl 23]:36–38.
78. Gray RA, Ayers G, Jalife J. Video imaging of atrial defibrillation in the sheep heart. *Circulation* 1997;95:1038–1047.
79. Zoll PM, Linenthal AJ. Termination of refractory tachycardia by external countershock. *Circulation* 1962;25:596–602.
80. Mathew TP, Moore A, McIntyre M, et al. Randomized comparison of electrode positions for cardioversion of atrial fibrillation. *Heart* 1999;81:576–579.
81. Levy S, Lacombe P, Cointe R, Bru P. High energy transcatheter cardioversion of chronic atrial fibrillation. *J Am Coll Cardiol* 1988;12:514–518.
82. Keane D, Zou L, Ruskin J. Nonpharmacologic therapies for atrial fibrillation. *Am J Cardiol* 1998;81[Suppl 5A]:41C–45C.
83. Heisel A Jung J. The atrial defibrillator: a stand-alone device or part of a combined dual-chamber system? *Am J Cardiol* 1999; 83(5B):218D–226D.
84. Lévy S, Lauribe P, Dolla E, et al. A randomized comparison of external and internal cardioversion of chronic atrial fibrillation. *Circulation* 1992;86:1415–1420.
85. Paravolidakis KE, Kolettis TM, Theodorakis GN, et al. Prospective randomized trial of external versus internal transcatheter cardioversion in patients with chronic atrial fibrillation. *J Interv Card Electrophysiol* 1998;2:249–253.
86. Alt E, Ammer R, Schmitt C, et al. A comparison of treatment of atrial fibrillation with low-energy intracardiac cardioversion and conventional external cardioversion. *Eur Heart J* 1997;18: 1796–1804.
87. Schmitt C, Alt E, Plewan A, et al. Low energy intracardiac cardioversion after failed conventional external cardioversion of atrial fibrillation. *J Am Coll Cardiol* 1996;28:994–999.
88. Santini M, Pandozi C, Gentilucci G, et al. Intra-atrial defibrillation of human atrial fibrillation. *J Cardiovasc Electrophysiol* 1998; 9[Suppl 8]:S170–176.
89. Cooper RA, Johnson EE, Kanter RJ, et al. Internal cardioversion in two patients with atrial fibrillation refractory to external cardioversion. *Pacing Clin Electrophysiol* 1996;19:872–875.
90. Sopher SM, Murgatroyd FD, Slade AK, et al. Low energy internal cardioversion of atrial fibrillation resistant to transthoracic shocks. *Heart* 1996;75:635–638.
91. Powell AC, Garan H, McGovern BA, et al. Low energy conversion of atrial fibrillation in the sheep. *J Am Coll Cardiol* 1992;20:707–711.
92. Simons GR, Newby KH, Kearney MM, et al. Safety of transvenous low energy cardioversion of atrial fibrillation in patients with a history of ventricular tachycardia: effects of rate and repolarization time on proarrhythmic risk. *Pacing Clin Electrophysiol* 1998;21:430–437.
93. Alt E, Schmitt C, Ammer R, et al. Initial experience with intracardiac atrial defibrillation in patients with chronic atrial fibrillation. *Pacing Clin Electrophysiol* 1994;17[Pt 2]:1067–1078.
94. Levy S, Ricard P, Lau CP, et al. Multicenter low energy transvenous atrial defibrillation (XAD) trial results in different subsets of atrial fibrillation. *J Am Coll Cardiol* 1997;29:750–755.
95. Sokoloski MC, Ayers GM, Kumagai K, et al. Safety of transvenous atrial defibrillation: studies in the canine sterile pericarditis model. *Circulation* 1997;96:1343–1350.
96. Ayers GM, Alferness CA, Ilina M, et al. Ventricular proarrhythmic effects of ventricular cycle length and shock strength in a sheep model of transvenous atrial defibrillation. *Circulation* 1994;89:413–422.
97. Keelan ET, Krum D, Hare J, et al. Safety of atrial defibrillation shocks synchronized to narrow and wide QRS complexes during atrial pacing protocols simulating atrial fibrillation in dogs. *Circulation* 1997;96:2022–2030.
98. Barold HS, Wharton JM. Ventricular fibrillation resulting from synchronized internal atrial defibrillation in a patient with ventricular preexcitation. *J Cardiovasc Electrophysiol* 1997;8: 436–440.
99. Gersh BJ. Antithrombotic therapy in nonrheumatic/nonvalvular atrial fibrillation. *J Cardiovasc Electrophysiol* 1999;10: 461–471.
100. Gallagher MM, Hart CM, Shannon MS, et al. Safety of direct current cardioversion of atrial arrhythmias [Abstract]. *J Am Coll Cardiol* 1998;31[Suppl A]:38A.
101. Main ML, Klein AL. Cardioversion in atrial fibrillation: indications, thromboembolic prophylaxis, and role of transesophageal echocardiography. *J Thromb Thrombolysis* 1999;7:53–60.
102. Blackshear JL, Zabalgoitia M, Pennock G, et al, Stroke Prevention and Atrial Fibrillation and Transesophageal Echocardiography (SPAF-TEE) Investigators. Warfarin safety and efficacy in patients with thoracic aortic plaque and atrial fibrillation. *Am J Cardiol* 1999;83(3):453–455, A9.
103. Lau CP, Lok NS. A comparison of transvenous atrial defibrillation of acute and chronic atrial fibrillation and the effect of intravenous sotalol on human atrial defibrillation threshold. *Pacing Clin Electrophysiol* 1997;20[Pt 1]:2442–2452.
104. Murgatroyd FD, Slade AK, Sopher SM, et al. Efficacy and tolerability of transvenous low energy cardioversion of paroxysmal atrial fibrillation in humans. *J Am Coll Cardiol* 1995;25: 1347–1353.
105. Tieleman RG, Van Gelder IC, Tuinenburg AE, et al. Intraoperative atrial refractory periods in patients with chronic and

paroxysmal atrial fibrillation as compared with sinus rhythm [Abstract]. *Pacing Clin Electrophysiol* 1999;22[Pt II]:816.
106. Andersen JS, Egeblad H, Abildgaard U, et al. Atrial fibrillation and left atrial enlargement: cause or effect? *J Intern Med* 1991; 229:253–256.
107. Carlsson J, Tebbe U, Rox J, et al. Cardioversion of atrial fibrillation in the elderly. *Am J Cardiol* 1996;78:1380–1384.
108. Min X, Mehra R. Relationship between anatomy and ventricular defibrillation thresholds in two human torso models [Abstract]. *Pacing Clin Electrophysiol* 1999;22[Pt II]:823.
109. Power JM, Beacom GA, Alferness CA, et al. Effects of left atrial dilatation on the endocardial atrial defibrillation threshold: a study in an ovine model of pacing induced dilated cardiomyopathy. *Pacing Clin Electrophysiol* 1998;21:1595–1600.
110. Wang J, Liu L, Feng J, Nattel S. Regional and functional factors determining induction and maintenance of atrial fibrillation in dogs. *Am J Physiol* 1996;271[Pt 2]:H148–158.
111. Baker BM, Botteron GW, Ambos D, et al. The effects of amiodarone, sotalol, and procainamide on internal atrial defibrillation threshold [Abstract]. *Circulation* 1995;92:I-473.
112. Juul-Moller S, Edvardsson N, Rehnqvist-Ahlberg N. Sotalol versus quinidine for the maintenance of sinus rhythm after direct current conversion of atrial fibrillation. *Circulation* 1990; 82:1932–1939.
113. Reimold SC. Clinical challenge. I: Control of recurrent symptomatic atrial fibrillation. *Eur Heart J* 1996;17[Suppl C]:35–40.
114. Boriani G, Biffi M, Capucci A, et al. Favorable effects of flecainide in transvenous internal cardioversion of atrial fibrillation. *J Am Coll Cardiol* 1999;33:333–341.
115. Timmermans C, Rodriguez LM, Smeets JL, Wellens HJ. Immediate reinitiation of atrial fibrillation following internal atrial defibrillation. *J Cardiovasc Electrophysiol* 1998;9:122–128.
116. Khoury DS, Assar MD, Sun H. Pharmacologic enhancement of atrial electrical defibrillation efficacy: role of ibutilide. *J Interv Card Electrophysiol* 1997;1:291–298.
117. Stambler BS, Wood MA, Ellenbogen KA. Antiarrhythmic actions of intravenous ibutilide compared with procainamide during human atrial flutter and fibrillation: electrophysiological determinants of enhanced conversion efficacy. *Circulation* 1997; 96:4298–4306.
118. Oral H, Souza JJ, Michaud GF, et al. Facilitating transthoracic cardioversion of atrial fibrillation with ibutilide pretreatment. *N Engl J Med* 1999;340:1849–1854.
119. Natale A, Tomassoni G, Beheiry S, et al. Effect of chronic administration of amiodarone on internal atrial defibrillation [Abstract]. *Circulation* 1998;98[Suppl I]:I-711.
120. Santini M, Pandozi C, Toscano S, et al. Low energy cardioversion of persistent atrial fibrillation. *Pacing Clin Electrophysiol* 1998;21:2641–2650.
121. Cooper RA, Alferness CA, Smith WM, Ideker RE. Internal cardioversion of atrial fibrillation in sheep. *Circulation* 1993;87: 1673–1686.
122. Cooper RA, Smith WM, Ideker RE. Internal cardioversion of atrial fibrillation: marked reduction in defibrillation threshold with dual current pathways. *Circulation* 1997;96: 2693–2700.
123. Cooper RA, Johnson EE, Wharton JM. Internal atrial defibrillation in humans: improved efficacy of biphasic waveforms and the importance of phase duration. *Circulation* 1997;95: 1487–1496.
124. Cooper RA, Plumb VJ, Epstein AE, et al. Marked reduction in internal atrial defibrillation thresholds with dual-current pathways and sequential shocks in humans. *Circulation* 1998; 97:2527–2535.
125. Ayers GM, Ilina M, Wagner D, et al. Cardiac vein electrodes for transvenous atrial defibrillation [Abstract]. *J Am Coll Cardiol* 1993;21:306A.
126. Lok NS, Lau CP, Tse HF, Ayers GM. Clinical shock tolerability and effect of different right atrial electrode locations on efficacy of low energy human transvenous atrial defibrillation using an implantable lead system. *J Am Coll Cardiol* 1997;30: 1324–1330.
127. Min X, Mongeon LR, Mehra R. Low threshold non-CS electrode systems for atrial defibrillation and compared with CS-RA by finite element human thorax model [Abstract]. *Circulation* 1997;96:I-529.
128. Ayers GM, Ilina MB, Wagner DO, et al. Right atrial electrode location for transvenous atrial defibrillation [Abstract]. *J Am Coll Cardiol* 1994;23:125A.
129. Alt E, Schmitt C, Ammer R, et al. Effect of electrode position on outcome of low-energy intracardiac cardioversion of atrial fibrillation. *Am J Cardiol* 1997;79:621–625.
130. Tomassoni G, Newby KH, Kearney MM, et al. Testing different biphasic waveforms and capacitances: effect on atrial defibrillation threshold and pain perception. *J Am Coll Cardiol* 1996;28:695–699.
131. Sra J, Bremner S, Krum D, et al. The effect of biphasic waveform tilt in transvenous atrial defibrillation. *Pacing Clin Electrophysiol* 1997;20:1613–1618.
132. Ortiz J, Niwano S, Abe H, et al. Transvenous atrial defibrillation in two canine models of atrial fibrillation [Abstract]. *J Am Coll Cardiol* 1994;23:125A.
133. Timmermans C, Rodriguez LM, Ayers GM, et al. Effect of electrode length on atrial defibrillation thresholds. *J Cardiovasc Electrophysiol* 1998;9:582–587.
134. Alferness CA, Ilina MI, Wagner DO, et al. Comparison of a dual to a single lead system for transvenous atrial defibrillation [Abstract]. *Pacing Clin Electrophysiol* 1993;16:854.
135. Ayers GM, Tacker WA, Gonzalez X, et al. Experience with a single pass atrial defibrillation lead system [Abstract]. *Circulation* 1995;92:I-472.
136. Heisel A, Jung J, Neuzner J, et al. Low-energy transvenous cardioversion of atrial fibrillation using a single atrial lead system. *J Cardiovasc Electrophysiol* 1997;8:607–614.
137. Tse HF, Lau CP, Yomtov BM, Ayers GM. Implantable atrial defibrillator with a single-pass dual-electrode lead. *J Am Coll Cardiol* 1999;33:1974–1980.
138. Morris MM, KenKnight BH, Warren JA, Lang DJ. A preview of implantable cardioverter defibrillator systems in the next millennium: an integrative cardiac rhythm management approach. *Am J Cardiol* 1999;83(5B):48D–54D.
139. Jenkins JM, Caswell SA. Detection algorithms in implantable cardioverter defibrillators. *Proc IEEE* 1996;84:428–445.
140. Chiang CM, Jenkins JM, DiCarlo LA. Digital signal processing chip implementation for detection and analysis of intracardiac electrograms. *Pacing Clin Electrophysiol* 1994;17:1373–1379.
141. Tse HF, Lau CP, Sra JS, et al. Atrial fibrillation detection and R-wave synchronization by Metrix implantable atrial defibrillator: implications for long-term efficacy and safety. *Circulation* 1999;99:1446–1451.
142. Hauer B, Seidl K, Senges J. The T-wave shock: a new reliable method for induction of ventricular fibrillation in ICD testing. *Z Kardiol* 1995;84:284–288.
143. Hou CJ, Chang-Sing P, Flynn E, et al. Determination of ventricular vulnerable period and ventricular fibrillation threshold by use of T-wave shocks in patients undergoing implantation of cardioverter/defibrillators. *Circulation* 1995;92:2558–2564.
144. Swerdlow CD, Martin DJ, Kass RM, et al. The zone of vulnerability to T-wave shocks in humans [Abstract]. *Pacing Clin Electrophysiol* 1996;19:623.

145. Bhandari AK, Isber N, Estioko M, et al. Efficacy of low-energy T wave shocks for induction of ventricular fibrillation in patients with implantable cardioverter defibrillators. *J Electrocardiol* 1998;31:31–37.
146. Lau CP, Tse HF, Lok NS, et al. Initial clinical experience with an implantable human atrial defibrillator. *Pacing Clin Electrophysiol* 1997;20[Pt 2]:220–225.
147. Lévy S, Rodriguez LM, Camm AJ, et al. Number, duration and frequency of non-treated atrial fibrillation episodes observed during the Metrix automatic atrial defibrillator trial [Abstract]. *Pacing Clin Electrophysiol* 1998;21[Pt II]:811.
148. Josephson ME. New approaches to the management of atrial fibrillation: the role of the atrial defibrillator. *Circulation* 1998;98:1594–1596.
149. Timmermans C, Levy S, Tavernier R, et al. Ambulatory use of the Metrix automatic implantable atrial defibrillator to treat episodes of atrial fibrillation [Abstract]. *Pacing Clin Electrophysiol* 1998;21[Pt II]:811.
150. Timmermans C, Fellows C, Lévy S, et al. Ambulatory use of the Metrix automatic implantable atrial defibrillator to treat episodes of atrial fibrillation [Abstract]. *Eur Heart J* 1998;19:76.
151. Daoud EG, Ayers, G, Fellows C, et al, for the Metrix Investigators. Effect of underlying cardiac disease on the ambulatory use of the Metrix implantable atrial defibrillator [Abstract]. *Pacing Clin Electrophysiol* 1999;22[Pt II]:890.
152. Timmermans C, Wellens HJJ. Effect of device-mediated therapy on symptomatic episodes of atrial fibrillation [Abstract]. *J Am Coll Cardiol* 1998;31[Suppl A]:331A.
153. Tse HF, Lau CP, Yu CM, et al. Effect of the implantable atrial defibrillator on the natural history of atrial fibrillation. *J Cardiovasc Electrophysiol* 1999;10:1200–1209.
154. Wijffels MC, Kirchhof CJ, Dorland R, Allessie MA. Atrial fibrillation begets atrial fibrillation: a study in awake chronically instrumented goats. *Circulation* 1995;92:1954–1968.
155. Rodriguez LM, Timmermans C, Wellens HJ. Are electrophysiological changes induced by longer lasting atrial fibrillation reversible? Observations using the atrial defibrillator. *Circulation* 1999;100:113–116.
156. Lévy S, Ricard P, Gueunoun M, et al. Low-energy cardioversion of spontaneous atrial fibrillation: immediate and long-term results, *Circulation* 1997;96:253–259.
157. Jung J, Heisel A, Fries R, Kollner V. Tolerability of internal low-energy shock strengths currently needed for endocardial atrial cardioversion. *Am J Cardiol* 1997;80:1489–1490.
158. Ammer R, Alt E, Ayers G, et al. Pain threshold for low energy intracardiac cardioversion of atrial fibrillation with low or no sedation. *Pacing Clin Electrophysiol* 1997;20[Pt 2]:230–236.
159. Harbinson MT, Imam Z, McEneaney DJ, et al. Patient discomfort after transvenous catheter cardioversion of atrial tachyarrhythmias with rounded waveforms—initial results [Abstract]. *Circulation* 1996;94:I-67.
160. Heisel A, Jung J, Schubert BD, Michel U. Evaluation of two new biphasic waveforms for internal cardioversion of atrial fibrillation [Abstract]. *Circulation* 1997;96:I-207.
161. Boriani G, Biffi M, Zannoli R, et al. Transvenous internal cardioversion for atrial fibrillation: a randomized study on defibrillation threshold and tolerability of asymmetrical compared with symmetrical biphasic shocks. *Int J Cardiol* 1999;71:63–69.
162. Ayers GM. How can atrial defibrillation be made more tolerable? In: Murgatroyd FD, Camm AJ, eds. *Nonpharmacological management of atrial fibrillation*. Armonk, NY: Futura Publishing, 1997:475–487.
163. Nathan AW, Bexton RS, Spurrell RA, Camm AJ. Internal transvenous low energy cardioversion for the treatment of cardiac arrhythmias. *Br Heart J* 1984;52:377–384.
164. Steinhaus DM, Cardinal D, Mongeon L, et al. Atrial defibrillation: are low energy shocks acceptable to patients? [Abstract]. *Pacing Clin Electrophysiol* 1996;19[Pt 2]:625.
165. Zipes DP, Jackman WM, Heger JJ, et al. Clinical transvenous cardioversion of recurrent life-threatening ventricular tachyarrhythmias: low energy synchronized cardioversion of ventricular tachycardia and termination of ventricular fibrillation in patients using a catheter electrode. *Am Heart J* 1982;103:789–794.
166. Baker BM, Botteron GW, Smith JM. Low-energy internal cardioversion for atrial fibrillation resistant to external cardioversion. *J Cardiovasc Electrophysiol* 1995;6:44–47.
167. Harbinson MT, Allen JD, Imam Z, et al. Rounded biphasic waveform reduces energy requirements for transvenous catheter cardioversion of atrial fibrillation and flutter. *Pacing Clin Electrophysiol* 1997;20[Pt 2]:226–229.
168. Timmermans C, Rodriguez LM, Ayers GM, et al. Effect of butorphanol tartrate on shock-induced discomfort during internal atrial defibrillation. *Circulation* 1999;99:1837–1842.
169. Bianconi L, Mennuni M, Lukic V, et al. Effects of oral propafenone administration before electrical cardioversion of chronic atrial fibrillation: a placebo-controlled study. *J Am Coll Cardiol* 1996;28:700–706.
170. Van Gelder IC, Crijns HJ, Van Gilst WH, et al. Prediction of uneventful cardioversion and maintenance of sinus rhythm from direct-current electrical cardioversion of chronic atrial fibrillation and flutter. *Am J Cardiol* 1991;68:41–46.
171. Lau CP, Tse HF, Ayers GM. Defibrillation-guided radiofrequency ablation of atrial fibrillation secondary to an atrial focus. *J Am Coll Cardiol* 1999;33:1217–1226.
172. Sra J, Biehl M, Blanck Z, et al. Spontaneous reinitiation of atrial fibrillation following transvenous atrial defibrillation. *Pacing Clin Electrophysiol* 1998;21:1105–1110.
173. Reuter DG, Kriplen MM, Hoyt RH, et al. Early recurrence of atrial fibrillation with an implantable atrial defibrillator: incidence, clinical predictors, and time course [Abstract]. *Circulation* 1998;98[Suppl I]:I-191.
174. Tse HF, Lau CP, Ayers GM. Incidence and modes of modes of onset of early reinitiation of atrial fibrillation after successful internal cardioversion, and its prevention by sotalol. *Heart* 1999;82:319–324.
175. Tieleman RG, Van Gelder IC, Crijns HJ, et al. Early recurrences of atrial fibrillation after electrical cardioversion: a result of fibrillation-induced electrical remodeling of the atria? *J Am Coll Cardiol* 1998;31:167–173.
176. Reuter D, Kriplen M, Ayers GM. Mechanisms of atrial fibrillation early recurrences and potential electrophysiological modifications. In: Santini M, ed. *Progress in clinical pacing*. Armonk, NY: Futura, 1998:25–36.
177. Cooklin M, Olsovsky MR, Brockman RG, et al. Atrial defibrillation with a transvenous lead: a randomized comparison of active can shocking pathways. *J Am Coll Cardiol* 1999;34:358–362.
178. Gallik DM, O'Connor ME, Warman E, Swerdlow CD. Optimal defibrillation pathway for an implantable atrial defibrillator without a coronary sinus lead [Abstract]. *Pacing Clin Electrophysiol* 1999;22[Pt II]:826.
179. Heisel A, Jung J, Nikoloudakis N, et al. Transvenous atrial cardioversion of atrial cardioversion threshold in patients with implantable cardioverter defibrillator: influence of active pectoral can. *Pacing Clin Electrophysiol* 1999;22:253–257.
180. Leiberman RA, for the Jewel AF Investigators. Insights into lead configuration and initial atrial defibrillation thresholds in

a dual chamber active can defibrillator [Abstract]. *Pacing Clin Electrophysiol* 1998;21[Pt II]:806.
181. Neri R, Palermo P, Cesario AS, et al. Effect of electrode configuration and capacitor size on internal atrial defibrillation threshold using leads currently used for ventricular defibrillation. *J Interv Card Electrophysiol* 1999;3:149–153.
182. Revishvili AS, Merkely B, Schaldach M. Transvenous ICD leads for single and dual chamber ICDs: actual and future developments. In: Antonioli GE, ed. *Pacemaker leads*. Bologna: Monduzzi Editore, 1997:527–534.
183. Poole JE, Kudenchuk PJ, Dolack GL, et al. Atrial defibrillation using a unipolar, single lead right ventricular to pectoral can system [Abstract]. *J Am Coll Cardiol* 1995;25:110A.
184. Desai PK, Mongeon L, Conlon S, et al. Is energy for transvenous defibrillation of atrial fibrillation (AF) with active pectoral cans feasible? [Abstract]. *Circulation* 1994;90:I-376.
185. Saksena S, Prakash A, Mongeon L, et al. Clinical efficacy and safety of atrial defibrillation using biphasic shocks and current nonthoracotomy endocardial lead configurations. *Am J Cardiol* 1995;76:913–921.
186. Min X, Mongeon L, Mehra R. Analysis of CS-RA, Can-RA, Can-RV and SVC-RV systems for atrial defibrillation by using finite element human thorax model and comparisons with the clinical studies [Abstract]. *Pacing Clin Electrophysiol* 1996;19[Pt 2]:696.
187. Geiger MJ, Mongeon L, Kearney MM, et al. Effects of an additional electrode on atrial defibrillation in patients [Abstract]. *Pacing Clin Electrophysiol* 1996;19[Pt 2]:624.
188. Min X, Mongeon L, Mehra R. An electrode system Can + CS-RA with low atrial defibrillation threshold by finite element human thorax model and comparisons with the clinical data [Abstract]. *Circulation* 1996;94:I-67.
189. Ammer R, Lehmann G, Plewan A, et al. Marked reduction in atrial defibrillation thresholds with repeated internal cardioversion. *J Am Coll Cardiol* 1999;34:1569–1576.
190. Ruppel R, Langes K, Kalkowski H, et al. Initial experience with implantable cardioverter defibrillator providing dual chamber pacing and sensing [Abstract]. *Pacing Clin Electrophysiol* 1997;20:1078.
191. Schuchert A, Kuhl M, Meinertz T. Evaluation of an algorithm designed to differentiate atrial and ventricular arrhythmias [Abstract]. *Pacing Clin Electrophysiol* 1998;21:872.
192. Swerdlow CD, Gunderson BD, Gillberg JM, et al. Discrimination of concurrent atrial and ventricular tachyarrhythmias from rapidly conducted atrial arrhythmias by a dual-chamber ICD [Abstract]. *Pacing Clin Electrophysiol* 1999;22:775.
193. Wilkoff BL, Kuhlkamp V, Gillberg JM, et al. Performance of a dual chamber detection algorithm (PR Logic) based on the worldwide Gem DR clinical results [Abstract]. *Pacing Clin Electrophysiol* 1999;22:720.
194. Morris MM, Marcovecchio AF, KenKnight BH, Lang DJ. Retrospective evaluation of detection enhancements in a dual-chamber implantable cardioverter defibrillator: implications for device programming [Abstract]. *Pacing Clin Electrophysiol* 1999; 22:849.
195. Kaemmerer WF, Olson WH. Dual chamber tachyarrhythmia detection using syntactic pattern recognition and contextual timing rules for rhythm classification [Abstract]. *Pacing Clin Electrophysiol* 1998;18:872.
196. Stanton MS, Hammill SC, Gillberg JM, et al. Clinical testing of a dual chamber combined atrial and ventricular defibrillator [Abstract]. *J Am Coll Cardiol* 1997;29:473.
197. Swerdlow CD, Schols W, Dijkman B, et al. Detection of atrial fibrillation and flutter by a dual-chamber implantable cardioverter-defibrillator. *Circulation* 2000;101:878–885.
198. Swerdlow CD, Bailin SJ, Warman EN, for the Worldwide Model 7250 AF-only Investigators. [Abstract]. *J Am Coll Cardiol* 2000;35:151A.

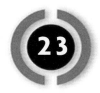

23

TIERED THERAPY FOR IMPLANTABLE CARDIOVERTER-DEFIBRILLATORS:
UNDERLYING PRINCIPLES AND CLINICAL IMPLICATIONS
• • •

MILTON M. MORRIS, STEPHEN J. HAHN, STEPHEN P. MCQUILLAN, BRUCE H. KENKNIGHT,
LYNN S. ELLIOTT, JAMES O. GILKERSON, LORENZO A. DICARLO

Understanding the mechanisms of cardiac tachyarrhythmia and their diverse clinical outcomes enable effective treatment by implantable cardioverter-defibrillator (ICD) device interventions. Tachyarrhythmias are not uniform in their initiation, propagation, or termination. Because of this, programming device intervention using tiered therapy is optimized when there is an understanding of the underlying mechanisms of tachyarrhythmias and use of this information to tailor the specific approach needed.

Because tachyarrhythmias are unique to patients, device interventions must be delivered appropriately to derive clinical benefit. This requires proper device programming to accurately discriminate cardiac rhythms and to deliver the appropriate intervention. Appropriate therapy may include therapy inhibition, antitachycardia pacing (ATP) therapy, low-energy cardioversion (LEC) therapy, or high-energy defibrillation therapy.

This chapter details the rationale for tiered therapy by discussing the linkages between tachyarrhythmia mechanisms and keys to successful therapeutic interventions. The chapter concludes with a description of device programming to achieve tiered therapy.

◉ RATIONALE FOR A TIERED-THERAPY IMPLANTABLE CARDIOVERTER-DEFIBRILLATOR: INTERPLAY OF ARRHYTHMIA MECHANISMS AND THERAPEUTIC INTERVENTIONS

Ectopic Automaticity

Ectopic automaticity is associated with tissue ectopic to the sinoatrial and atrioventricular (AV) nodes (1). This tissue is capable of depolarizing and activating surrounding myocardium at rates faster than sinus rhythm rates. When this occurs, the ectopic tissue becomes the dominant driver of myocardial activation.

Ectopic automaticity is thought to result from slow currents that are different from the slow currents of the sinus node's normal pacemaker activity. Ectopic tissue capable of automaticity may be located in any cardiac chamber. In some cases, it may be present in a portion of the myocardial tissue that is normally exvaginated from the left atrium into the distal pulmonary veins (2). Hallmarks of automaticity include the inability to initiate or to suppress automatic activity with programmed stimulation. Ectopic automatic activity may persist after attempted cardioversion. Examples of clinical tachyarrhythmias caused by ectopic automaticity include some atrial tachycardias and focal initiation of atrial fibrillation (3).

Triggered Rhythms Caused by Early Afterdepolarization

Early afterdepolarizations is believed to be the cause of tachyarrhythmias such as torsades des pointes (4). Early afterdepolarizations are associated with prolonged action potential duration and occur typically during cellular repolarization. The occurrence of a "long-short" sequence of myocardial activation is common but not required before the onset of recurrent, sustained early afterdepolarizations (5). When it does occur, a long-short sequence of myocardial activation is usually generated by ectopic premature activity, most commonly single premature ventricular depolarization. It is the abrupt prolongation of action potential that follows the long-short activation sequence that provides the critical electrophysiologic milieu for early afterdepolarizations to occur. Alternatively, abrupt prolongation of cell recovery may be provoked by an acute neurologic event (e.g., fright) (6) or chronically at patient-specific heart rates known to be critical to the occurrence of afterdepolarizations (7).

The electrophysiologic cellular environment causing early afterdepolarizations can develop genetically (i.e., long QT syndromes) (8) or be acquired as a result of tissue changes caused by ischemia, electrolyte deficiency, or the unwanted effects of Vaughn-Williams class Ia and III drugs known to affect cellular repolarization (9).

Because of its electrophysiologic underpinnings, torsades des pointes cannot be terminated by programmed electrical stimulation. Torsades des pointes has a variable incidence of recurrence after attempted cardioversion. Whenever feasible, a first priority in patient management is reversal of any causes believed to be associated with the occurrence of torsades des pointes. Because heart rate–dependent changes in chronic action potential duration may be critical to the occurrence of torsades des pointes in some patients, chronic overdrive pacing may help to prevent recurrent early afterdepolarizations in patient-specific cases (9). Investigations are under consideration to determine whether rate smoothing may mitigate the prolongation of action potential duration associated with long-short sequences.

Triggered Rhythms Caused by Delayed Afterdepolarization

In contrast to early afterdepolarizations that occur in phase 3 of the action potential (during cell recovery), delayed afterdepolarizations occur in phase 4 (after cell recovery) (10). Although early afterdepolarizations underlie polymorphic tachyarrhythmias such as torsades des pointes, delayed afterdepolarizations underlie monomorphic tachyarrhythmias such as idiopathic ventricular tachycardia originating in the right ventricular outflow tract (11) and some atrial tachycardias (12). Unlike early depolarizations, delayed afterdepolarizations have no known reversible causes.

Delayed afterdepolarizations are attributed to abnormally high intracellular calcium concentrations during phase 4 of action potential (13). It is during this phase of the action potential that affected cells have the potential of reaching their threshold potential for activation repeatedly.

The preceding rate of cell activations appears to be critical to the occurrence of delayed afterdepolarization. Delayed afterdepolarization has been observed to occur at critical activation rates, but not at slower or faster rates. Delayed afterdepolarizations can be induced and terminated using programmed electrical stimulation including burst pacing (14). Because of the critical dependence of delayed afterdepolarizations on preceding heart rate, the incidence of recurrence of tachyarrhythmias manifested by delayed afterdepolarizations is variable after attempted cardioversion.

Reentry

Circulating wavefronts of activation were studied early in the 20th century in isolated preparations from animal models by Mayer, who used rings of excitable tissue from jellyfish, and Mines, who studied rings of excitable tissue excised from tortoise (15,16). These models of healthy tissue demonstrated circulating wavefronts and bidirectional block of electrical activity.

The capability of electrical activation to continue to propagate in a circulating or reentrant manner came to be understood as a phenomenon that depends on suitable cardiac substrate, unidirectional block for initiation, circulation of electrical activation around a central area of block, and across an excitable gap for continuation. In the human heart, suitable cardiac substrate includes the electrophysiologic properties of the AV node and a congenitally acquired accessory bypass tract, in addition to atrial and ventricular tissue, for supraventricular tachycardia (SVT) caused by orthodromic reciprocation (17). In contrast, suitable anatomically or electrically isolated atrial tissue alone provides the milieu for an atrial tachycardia caused by intraatrial reentry (18). Isolated areas of diseased tissue, with inhomogeneous cell-to-cell conduction and disparity of cellular repolarizations beyond normal, could result in monomorphic ventricular tachycardia using a micropathway of intraventricular reentry (19) or a macropathway of His-Purkinje reentry (20).

Entrainment of reentrant pathways in animals and humans can be used to differentiate reentry from other underlying mechanisms of tachyarrhythmias. Entrainment can be demonstrated by the presence of constant fusion, progressive fusion dependent on pacing rate, localized conduction block, and a change of conduction (21,22).

As with delayed afterdepolarization, reentry may be initiated or terminated by programmed electrical stimulation including overdrive pacing. Initiation of reentry occurs by causing unidirectional block and slow conduction retrograde through the site of block by the circulating wavefront (23). Termination of reentry occurs by causing bidirectional wavefront collision orthodromic and antidromic to the direction of the electrical wavefront that otherwise circulates during reentry (24). Bidirectional wavefront collision resulting in termination of reentry can also be accomplished with cardioversion (25).

The conditions that cause reentry to occur or recur spontaneously in humans are multifactorial and poorly understood.

Fibrillation

Whether atrial or ventricular, fibrillation occurs in the setting of diffuse anisotropic conduction and refractoriness. A critical mass of tissues using multiple micro-reentrant wavelets or large macro-reentrant waves has been postulated as necessary for initiation, propagation and continuation of fibrillation (26,27).

One of the factors contributing to the milieu for atrial fibrillation is atrial remodeling, occurring as a result of chronic tachycardia (i.e., tachycardia-induced atrial myopathy) or as a consequence of disease (28,29). Abrupt and rapid firing of focal right atrial, left atrial, or pulmonary intravenous atrial tissue is also recognized as a critical contributor to some occurrences of atrial fibrillation (30). Generally, atrial remodeling is more commonly considered as the primary contributing factor for patients who have clinically evident structural heart disease and persistent or permanent atrial fibrillation (28), whereas focal activity is more commonly associated with patients who appear to have normal hearts and paroxysmal atrial fibrillation. With regard to the ventricle, tissue ischemia and electrolyte disorders appear to be the common final pathways for most ventricular fibrillation (29).

Fibrillation may be induced with aggressive programmed stimulation, including rapid and sustained burst pacing (31), or by depolarization of sufficient tissue (i.e., critical mass) during myocardial recovery from activation (32). Termination is not considered likely without depolarization of sufficient mass (i.e., "critical mass") to cause collision of all propagating wavefronts in addition to any caused by the depolarization itself. Recurrence after attempted defibrillation is variable. In the case of ventricular fibrillation, reversal of ischemia is crucial to minimizing the risk of recurrence.

Overview of Tachyarrhythmias

Tachyarrhythmias are not uniform in their initiation, propagation, or termination. Monomorphic atrial and ventricular tachyarrhythmias, such as atrial tachycardia and ventricular tachycardia, may have more than one potential underlying mechanism. Not all polymorphic ventricular tachyarrhythmias represent primary ventricular fibrillation. The use of electrophysiologic understanding and clinical parameters may be helpful in determining underlying mechanisms and in optimizing the programming and the ultimate success of device interventions.

Arrhythmia initiation or termination by electrical programmed stimulation may suggest reentry or delayed afterdepolarization as an underlying mechanism. Demonstration of entrainment during a tachyarrhythmia is compatible with reentry, in contrast with other arrhythmia mechanisms.

Device shock therapy may be initially successful for arrhythmias having mechanisms other than reentry or fibrillation. Early arrhythmia recurrence after cardioversion is more likely with automaticity than other arrhythmia mechanisms. Reversal of identifiable and treatable causes of arrhythmias is crucial to minimizing the risk of any arrhythmia recurrence after intervention.

The ICD may be confronted with tachyarrhythmias with each form of initiation and propagation. Consequently, ICDs may be programmed to administer tiered therapy whereby tachyarrhythmias with different mechanisms receive different therapy.

⦿ CLINICAL CONSIDERATIONS FOR PROGRAMMABLE DEVICE DESIGN

The key motivating factor for a tiered-therapy device is the recognition that different treatment options are required and delivered based on the type and severity of the arrhythmia. Slow, stable ventricular tachycardias may be well tolerated and are often amenable to fast, simple, and painless pace termination methods. Fast ventricular tachycardias or ventricular fibrillation with their more dire outcomes require more aggressive shock therapy. An ideal device would automatically identify different rhythms and automatically deliver a therapy commensurate with the severity of the arrhythmia. ICDs have made great strides in the discrimination of cardiac rhythms and provide a multitude of flexible therapy options. However, they are not totally automatic devices. Individual patients may present with unique circumstances that require special considerations when selecting therapeutic options.

Current-generation ICDs are designed with a multitude of programmable options that allow the clinician to tailor how the device detects, discriminates between, and treats a variety of different arrhythmias. In addition to understanding the mechanisms of tachycardia, understanding the clinical outcomes afforded by various ICD treatment options is key to developing a logical strategy for programming ICDs. Before entering into a discussion of specific ICD programming, an overview of clinical data supporting the selection and use of various programming options is presented.

Detection

To fulfill its purpose, the ICD must have a process through which cardiac rhythms are placed into appropriate therapy tiers. This process is designed so that lethal tachyarrhythmias such as ventricular fibrillation are rapidly treated with aggressive defibrillation therapy and slow and stable ventricular tachycardia can be initially treated with ATP pacing schemes that are well tolerated by patients. If these pacing schemes fail, the ICD graduates to more aggressive low-energy cardioversion or high-energy defibrillation.

The process by which therapy is tiered involves cardiac rhythm discrimination and is performed by detection algorithms. These detection algorithms are designed to use patient electrogram information collected from sensing electrodes placed within the heart chambers. The detection algorithms use ventricular and atrial heart rate zones to tier cardiac rhythms into different therapy regimens. For example, ventricular fibrillation presents with a very rapid ventricular rate and, with proper programming, is immediately placed into a rate zone where rhythms receive aggressive defibrillation therapy.

ICDs can be programmed with up to three rate zones. These rate zones are created by physician programmable rate thresholds. Rate zones provide a highly sensitive means for detecting potentially lethal arrhythmia. This high sensitivity can come at the expense of specificity whereby nonlethal cardiac rhythms, such as sinus tachycardia and other SVTs, elicit ICD therapy. Consequently, electrogram features such as atrial and ventricular cycle length variability, atrial and ventricular activation patterns, and ventricular electrogram morphology are used to enhance the specificity of detection algorithms used in ICDs. The enhancement in specificity minimizes the likelihood of inappropriate therapy.

Similar to rate zones, most detection enhancements have physician-programmable parameters, whereas others have been designed for ease of use to be ON/OFF or to be automatically programmed based on physician provided patient history regarding frequent occurrence of sinus tachycardia or other SVTs with high ventricular rates. The programming of these parameters have been studied at length (33–42). A single common theme underlying the use of these enhancements is that they all result in an incremental improvement to specificity relative to using rate zones only (33,41,42).

Stability and Onset

In many cases, ventricular tachycardias have a sudden onset (i.e., nonphysiologic and abrupt decrease in RR cycle length from the last normally conducted R wave to the first abnormal R wave) and cause a very regular, or stable, RR cycle length. Conversely, SVTs such as sinus tachycardia more often have gradual onsets and greater variability in RR cycle lengths. Algorithms designed to measure RR cycle length, *Stability* and *Onset,* have been used to distinguish between potentially lethal ventricular tachycardia and nonlethal SVT. *Stability* has been demonstrated in 124 patients to be effective in preventing unnecessary shocks by Shaumann and colleagues (34). With a mean follow-up period of 20 ± 9.4 months, *Stability* measurements for 92% of the ventricular tachycardias were less than 21 msec. Higgins and coworkers studied 22 rhythms from 19 patients and were able to correctly identify 100% of atrial fibrillation episodes (35). *Onset* has also been demonstrated in 27 patients to be effective in preventing unnecessary shocks (36). All sinus tachycardia episodes studied had measured *Onset* values of nearly 0%. Additionally, 68% of atrial arrhythmia SVTs had measured *Onset* values between 0% and 18%, and 84% of true ventricular tachycardias had measured values greater than 18.5%. Shaumann and associates also studied *Onset* in the 124 patients (34). They found that 84% of spontaneous ventricular tachycardia episodes had measured *Onset* values of greater than 20%.

Dual-Chamber Algorithms

Dual-chamber ICDs incorporate electrogram information sensed from the atria into their detection algorithms. *Atrial View* (VENTAK PRIZM DR, Guidant Corp., St. Paul, MN) is an algorithm that uses atrial rate information in concert with ventricular rate information to further enhance detection. The $V_{rate} > A_{rate}$ enhancement calls for therapy when the ventricular rate exceeds the atrial rate, because this is a clear indication of the presence of a potentially lethal arrhythmia. When high atrial rates exceed high ventricular rates (or $A_{rate} > V_{rate}$), *AFib Threshold* allows for therapy inhibition if the atrial rate is greater than a physician programmed threshold. *AFib Threshold* is designed to prevent unnecessary shocks because of atrial fibrillation, the primary cause of inappropriate therapy (36,37). Clinical testing of the AFib Threshold algorithm on induced tachycardia ($n = 52$ patients) at predischarge showed correct classification of atrial fibrillation was between 89% to 100% while preserving 100% correct classification of ventricular tachycardias (38,39).

A Canadian randomized, multicenter trial evaluating atrial sensing to reduce inappropriate defibrillation (ASTRID trial) compared standard ventricular rate–only features (control population) with *Atrial View* features (study population). The objective of the trial was to demonstrate a 1-year reduction in the occurrence and rate of inappropriate therapy and for arrhythmias other than ventricular tachycardia/ventricular fibrillation. One hundred forty-nine patients (79 study and 70 control) were enrolled in the trial meeting standard indications for an ICD. Successful randomization was confirmed by equivalent baseline characteristics for age, gender, arrhythmia history, and medication treatment. The results from this study confirmed the study objectives. With an average follow-up of more than 12 months, 36% of patients in the control group received inappropriate therapy compared with 18% of patients in the study (*Atrial View*) group ($p < 0.01$). Time to first inappropriate therapy was significantly delayed in the study group (147 ± 134 days) compared with the control group (110 ± 108 days, $p < 0.009$, log rank). The primary arrhythmia treated for inappropriate therapy was atrial fibrillation or flutter. There was no significant difference between the two cohorts with respected to inappropriate therapy for ATP or high-energy shocks (129).

Atrial and ventricular event timing methods have also been used for discrimination of SVT and ventricular tachycardia. By analyzing the relationship between atrial and ventricular events, these algorithms are capable of determining which chambers (atria or ventricles) are controlling the ventricular rhythm. The Defender (ELA Medical, Le Plessis-Robinson, France) employs the PARAD algorithm, which uses the variability in PR intervals and the association of atrial and ventricular events to distinguish SVT and ventricular tachycardia. In this algorithm, the presence of stable PR intervals and associated atrial and ventricular events is supporting (not conclusive) evidence of an atrial flutter or sinus tachycardia. Additional parameters may be considered by the ICD when making a final rhythm classification.

Early clinical findings during a follow-up period of $7.1 ± 4.5$ months showed that 176 episodes were stored using the Holter function on the Defender device. The PARAD algorithm recorded a specificity of 96% (49 of 51 SVTs) and a sensitivity of 100% (122 of 122 ventricular tachycardias) (40). Additional clinical results showed a sensitivity of 100% (147 of 147) with oversensing of 13 episodes of atrial fibrillation. The total number of atrial fibrillation episodes was not available.

The PR Logic algorithm (Gem DR, Medtronic, Inc., Minneapolis, MN) uses the basic rate as the underlying detection principle and uses syntactic pattern recognition of P- and R-wave timing and sequence to classify each rhythm. The timing and sequence of P and R events are used to create a "word" through the use of a syntactic code that links such sequences to 19 letters from the alphabet. The word is then compared with words previously defined to represent specific types of SVT (i.e., sinus tachycardia, atrial flutter/atrial fibrillation, or other 1:1 SVT). If the word matches one of the previously defined SVT words, ventricular therapy is withheld.

The PR Logic algorithm has been demonstrated to provide 99.9% sensitivity and 70.2% specificity on a broad data set ($n = 2,457$ spontaneous rhythms) and 100% sensitivity (sustained dual tachycardia) and 94% specificity on a subset of patients with concurrent SVT and ventricular tachycardia (i.e., dual tachycardia) (41,42).

Morphology

Intracardiac electrogram morphology has been proposed for use in reduction of unnecessary therapy provoked by SVT (43–45). Supraventricular tachycardias are similar to normal sinus rhythm in that they use the AV node and His-Purkinje system to facilitate conduction to the ventricles. This results in a consistent pattern of wavefront propagation and consequently a consistent ventricular electrogram morphology. Conversely, ventricular tachycardia episodes originate in the ventricles and though their sites of origin and underlying mechanisms may differ, they typically result in patterns of wavefront propagation and consequently, ventricular morphologies that are distinguishable from SVT.

One morphology algorithm (Contour MD, Angstrom MD, and Profile MD, St. Jude Medical, Inc., St. Paul, MN) measures a percent match between stored normal electrogram beats and eight consecutive beats under analysis (46). The percent match is compared with a programmable threshold. If the percent match is greater than the threshold, the eight consecutive beats would be classified as supraventricular in origin (i.e., SVT). If the percent match is below the programmed threshold, the eight consecutive beats would be classified as ventricular in origin (i.e., ventricular tachycardia).

Antitachycardia Pacing Therapy Delivery

Most patients treated with an ICD have a history of ischemic heart disease. Although several mechanisms exist that are responsible for triggering spontaneous ventricular tachycardia in this population with occlusive coronary artery disease, the dominant mechanism underlying the maintenance of tachyarrhythmia is reentry. Reentry is a pattern of conduction characterized by reciprocating action potential propagation over a fixed or dynamically changing path within ventricular myocardium adjacent to an infarct. It has been suggested that ventricular tachycardia propagating over a fixed path tend to be monomorphic on the surface electrocardiogram (ECG) and that ventricular tachycardia propagating over a dynamically changing path may be polymorphic. In this discussion, we restrict our comments to monomorphic (i.e., uniform) ventricular tachycardia sustained by reentry. Antitachycardia pacing (ATP) therapy is preferred over shock therapy for termination of hemodynamically tolerable ventricular tachycardia, because ATP therapy is most often imperceptible to the patient receiving the therapy.

Although the concept of reentry was first presented and discussed at the beginning of the 20th century, the intricate details surrounding the cellular mechanisms by which reentry is sustained have only recently been described (47–49). During reentry, the action potential propagates in a wave of excitation, that blocks along one path (functional or anatomic) and conducts slowly along a second path. The slow conduction must permit recovery of excitability at the location of block so that the head of the activation wave propagates through this area of block and thereby begins the reciprocating pattern of activation. Because the physical length of the conduction path is typically somewhat longer than the minimum required to sustain reentry, a temporal window exists during which an exogenous wave of activation is able to influence the circulating wave associated with the ventricular tachycardia. This "excitable gap" permits wavefronts produced during ATP therapy to propagate into the excitable gap of the ventricular tachycardia and interrupt the reentrant conduction pattern, resulting in sudden termination of the ventricular tachycardia.

Systematic research (50) conducted over several decades has revealed that exogenous pacing during ventricular tachycardia has several observable effects on reentrant ventricular tachycardia. Activation waves produced by ATP may have no effect, may reset or entrain the ventricular tachycardia, or may terminate the ventricular tachycardia. Several factors may influence the interaction among activation waves responsible for the ventricular tachycardia and those produced by ATP: ventricular tachycardia cycle length, refractory periods at the stimulation site and near the organizing center of the ventricular tachycardia, conduction time from the stimulation site to the organizing center of the ventricular tachycardia, and the duration of the excitable gap. For the ATP therapy to result in termination of the ventricular tachycardia, an ATP activation wave must penetrate the excitable gap and preexcite this area so that conduction of the ventricular tachycardia activation wave fails. When the ventricular tachycardia activation wave fails to propagate, the reentrant ventricular tachycardia terminates.

Critical conditions must coexist in time and space for reentry to be sustained (51). It should not be surprising that several factors can influence whether a particular ATP scheme results in termination of ventricular tachycardia: spontaneous versus induced, coupling interval and cycle length of stimuli relative to ventricular tachycardia cycle length, number and temporal relationship among ATP stimuli, spatial proximity of the stimulation site relative to the ventricular tachycardia circuit, and functional and structural characteristics of the ventricular tachycardia circuit (50).

Spontaneous and Induced Ventricular Tachycardia

Clinical utility of ATP was first demonstrated in the setting of acute electrophysiology study (52,53). Early ATP methods evolved into more systematic schema that were ultimately adapted for automatic therapies delivered by the ICD (54,55). Although many similarities exist among inducible monomorphic ventricular tachycardias and spontaneous ventricular tachycardias treated with device-based ATP, evidence is mounting to suggest that spontaneous ventricular tachycardias may be more amenable to termination by ATP than ventricular tachycardias induced in the electrophysiology laboratory (56). This apparent difference in "terminability" of ventricular tachycardias is most likely caused by subtle differences in the electrophysiologic properties of the myocardial substrate forming the reentrant circuit. Reports suggest that the cycle length of activation for ventricular tachycardias and ventricular fibrillation are shorter when induced in the laboratory compared with those occurring spontaneously (57). Other factors contributing to increased terminability of spontaneous ventricular tachycardia may be involved. For example, autonomic tone and the subsequent reflexive cholinergic and adrenergic responses may importantly influence the spatial distribution of local refractory period and conduction velocity.

Coupling Interval and Stimulation Cycle Length

Coupling interval is a term used to denote the temporal relationship between the local activation time at the stimulation site and time at which the first ATP stimulus is delivered. To increase the probability that the first stimulus results in production and propagation of an action potential, the coupling interval must be shorter than the intrinsic cycle length of the ventricular tachycardia being treated with ATP. This strategy ensures that the first stimulus will fall within a local excitable gap and permit the ATP activation wave to partially or completely penetrate the ventricular tachycardia circuit. The stimulation cycle length determines the frequency at which the ventricular tachycardia circuit is invaded by the wavefronts emanating from the ATP stimulation site. If the ATP cycle length is nearly the same as the ventricular tachycardia cycle length, the ventricular tachycardia may be continuously reset (i.e., entrained) but not terminated. In contrast, if the ATP cycle length is too short compared with the ventricular tachycardia cycle length, the circuit may not be penetrated by wavefronts emanating from the ATP site owing to functional conduction block between the stimulation site and the ventricular tachycardia organizing center. Heuristic testing has revealed that ATP coupling intervals of 81% to 91% are effective and that stimulation cycle lengths corresponding to 81% to 91% produce acceptable clinical results. Because multiple ventricular tachycardia may occur spontaneously in a patient, the ATP algorithm must adapt to the underlying ventricular tachycardia that is being treated.

Stimulation Site

For ATP to be effective, the stimulus must produce a wavefront that propagates to the ventricular tachycardia circuit. Theoretically, stimulation sites near the ventricular tachycardia circuit would be expected to produce more favorable results. However, there are other factors that modulate the importance of stimulation site. For example, if the stimulation site is very near the ventricular tachycardia circuit, but the local refractory period at the stimulation site is too long, the ATP may be less effective than ATP from a site on the opposite side of the heart where the refractory period is shorter. The importance of stimulation site has been appreciated since ATP was first discovered. For implanted devices that deliver ATP, the site of stimulation is constrained to the right ventricle, typically the right ventricular apex. ATP from this site has been shown to be effective.

Antitachyardia Pacing Schema

Many combinations of cycle lengths, number of stimuli, and temporal relationships among stimuli can be programmed. The two most commonly employed ATP schema are *fixed burst* and *autodecremental,* often referred to as *ramp*. Details of these ATP schema are presented in the Therapy Parameters section later in this chapter. The efficacy (i.e., percentage termination) and safety (i.e., percentage acceleration) of these forms of ATP have been compared for induced (58–60) and spontaneous ventricular tachycardias (61, 62).

Antitachyardia Pacing for Spontaneous Ventricular Tachycardia

At least two factors motivate the use of empirical ATP for patients with ICDs. First, although high-voltage shocks are almost uniformly effective in termination of ventricular tachycardia, the psychologic and emotional impact of the shock must be considered. Second, the effectiveness of ATP for spontaneous ventricular tachycardia appears to be much higher than originally anticipated. In a prospective study including 200 patients implanted with ICDs, Schaumann and coworkers (63) studied the safety of empirical ATP in patients who did not undergo demonstration of ATP effectiveness at the time of ICD implantation and hospital discharge. The ATP schema programmed in Schaumann's study was the same for both groups: autodecremental ramp, coupling interval of 81%, and stimulation cycle length of 81% of ventricular tachycardia cycle length. They reported that the overall success of ATP for the prompt termination of spontaneous ventricular tachycardia occurred in 4,845 (94%) of 5,165 trials in 123 of the 200 patients enrolled in the study. Moreover, they showed that the ATP success in the patient group with empirical ATP programming ($n = 146$) was 90% (1,205 of 1,346), whereas the ATP success in the patient group with predischarge ATP testing ($n = 54$) was 95% (3,640 of 3,819). They also reported impressive statistics concerning the success of ATP for spontaneous ventricular tachycardia with rates ≥ 200 bpm (about 80% successful). This important study suggests that physicians should consider programming ATP in all patients, regardless of whether their conditions were such that ventricular tachycardia could be induced at predischarge testing. Because ventricular tachycardia often precedes ventricular fibrillation, ATP should reduce exposure to the emotionally disruptive consequences of high-voltage shocks, thereby improving the quality of life.

Low-Energy Cardioversion

Low-energy cardioversion (LEC) and ATP have been used as the first-tier attempt to treat ventricular tachycardia. Available ICDs allow for programming multiple combinations of ATP, LEC, and high-energy shocks, depending on the appropriate therapy rate zones.

When incorporated into tiered-therapy ICDs, ATP techniques have proven to be effective in terminating sustained monomorphic ventricular tachycardias with the advantages of rapid delivery, acceptable discomfort, and improved device longevity. Low energy conversion has been reported to be as effective as ATP for ventricular tachycardia, but the disadvantages of LEC are patient discomfort, atrial proarrhythmia, and decreased device longevity compared with ATP therapy (64).

The utility of LEC as first-line treatment is controversial. There are generally two schools of thought among physicians about programming tiered shock schemes: those who use LEC in combination with maximum device output and those who program the ICDs to maximum output only. Fotuhi and colleagues maintain the three most important considerations in selecting defibrillation energies are that the shock should be strong enough to defibrillate at least 98% of the time on the first shock, weak enough not to cause severe postshock arrhythmias or reinitiation of fibrillation, but strong enough to compensate for changes of defibrillation requirements over time (65). Selecting the optimal therapy option among these considerations has been the topic of several studies.

The likelihood of using LEC as a therapy option with today's ICD patients depends on an adequate available safety margin (i.e., maximum device output and minimum defibrillation energy) for the patient. A candidate for LEC should have a low (≤ 15 J) defibrillation energy requirement in combination with an optimal lead system configuration using a biphasic shock pulse generator (66).

Defibrillation

When the device detects very fast ventricular tachycardia or ventricular fibrillation or has expended its programmed ATP or LEC attempts, high-energy shocks are the final option. There are three key areas to consider in the delivery of high-energy shock therapy. First, a lead system suitable for the patient must be chosen. The lead system chosen affects the types of shock vectors that can be delivered. Second, the type of shock waveform must be considered, and in some devices this must be selected and programmed. Third, an energy level must be selected. The choice of programmed energy levels is usually made based on the results of defibrillation tests performed with the implanted lead system and device. A basic understanding of defibrillation testing is also required.

Lead Systems and Shock Vectors

The standard for modern ICD systems is a single transvenous lead implanted into the right ventricular apex and used in conjunction with an electrically active ICD pulse generator, the so-called 'hot can.' All major manufacturers offer a single-lead ICD system, and all provide acceptable pacing, sensing, and defibrillation performance. However, different lead models allow choices between single and dual shocking coil leads and between active and passive fixation leads. Studies have demonstrated that the lowest defibrillation thresholds are achieved with the so-called 'TRIAD system,' which uses a dual shocking coil lead, with shocking electrodes placed in the right ventricle and the superior vena cava and a hot can ICD (67). Shocks are delivered from the right ventricular (RV) electrode to the superior vena cava (SVC) and hot can (Can) *(RV → SVC + Can)*. Alternatively, a single shocking coil lead (right ventricular electrode only) and hot can device can be employed in the so-called unipolar configuration *(RV → Can)*. Studies have shown the unipolar system provides acceptable defibrillation performance, and some have suggested it may be preferable for cases where lead extraction is a concern (68,69). Other leads are available that allow shocking electrodes to be placed in a variety of other locations that may be useful for patients with exceptionally high energy requirements. Subcutaneous patches and arrays are most often chosen for such patients. Numerous studies have demonstrated that subcutaneous electrodes lower the defibrillation energy requirements (66,70–73). However, use of these leads is usually limited because they complicate the system, increase procedure times, and have the potential to contribute additional complications such as hematoma, seroma, and skin erosion. Addition of a coronary sinus lead can also be used to reduce defibrillation energy requirements (74,75), but they tend to complicate the system, are more difficult to implant, and increase complications, particularly lead dislodgement.

Shock Waveforms

All ICDs deliver shock therapy by discharging energy from a capacitor. The capacitor discharge creates a waveform with an exponentially decaying voltage and current. Numerous studies have shown that reversing the polarity during the shock to create a "biphasic" waveform reduces defibrillation energy requirements by 30% to 50% (76–79). Most ICDs still offer a selection of monophasic or biphasic waveforms. There are anecdotal reports that monophasic waveforms may be superior in individual patients (80). Because defibrillation is a probabilistic phenomenon, it is difficult to confirm. Still, biphasic waveforms are the standard.

Numerous studies have also shown that halting or truncating the shock improves defibrillation efficacy, a feature found in all ICDs (81–84). Some devices allow programmable selection of the truncation point by selecting the waveform's duration (in milliseconds) or by selecting a tilt (percent drop from initial amplitude). Fixed-tilt waveforms are convenient because they have the added advantage that the total energy delivered remains fixed. The optimal truncation point (as tilt or duration), particularly for biphasic waveforms, is disputed (85–87). Defibrillation does follow a strength-duration relationship similar to pacing, but biphasic waveforms appear to be much less sensitive to duration than monophasic waveforms (88–90). No compelling data show that the available programming options can allow the user to improve defibrillation efficacy compared with the manufacturer's standard settings. However, studies do suggest that the biphasic waveforms available in some devices are superior to those in other devices (91,92).

Most devices allow the selection of the overall polarity of the waveform. The leading edge of the shock is usually delivered such that the right ventricular electrode is negative, also referred to as cathodic or standard polarity. Some studies have shown that defibrillation efficacy is improved (particularly with monophasic waveforms) by reversing this polarity to make the right ventricular electrode positive (anodic) (93–96). Although the data on reversed polarity with biphasic waveforms are not conclusive, it is common practice to try reverse polarity in cases where the standard polarity did not produce an acceptable defibrillation energy.

Appropriate Shock Energies for Ventricular Defibrillation

All ICDs allow the ability to program the energy of the first or second shock before reverting to maximum energy for the remaining shocks, but exactly how to program shock energies remains controversial. Intentionally programming a lower energy may have several benefits, including a shorter time to therapy that decreases the incidence or duration of syncope (97) and increases battery longevity. Conversely, many clinicians prefer to keep all shocks at maximum energy in the belief that this ensures the maximum first-shock success rate. However, some data suggest that delivering the maximum may be unnecessary and even undesirable. High-energy shocks cause temporary bradycardia (AV block) and increased postshock ectopy (98,99), prolong postshock hemodynamic recovery (100), and possibly even fail to defibrillate (101). Most manufacturers recommend that the implanting physician demonstrate two successful defibrillations without a failure at an energy level 10 J below the maximum energy of the device. With these minimal tests and the 10-J "safety margin," significant clinical data indicate that patients are protected against tachyarrhythmic death.

The exact origin of the 10-J safety margin is unclear, but several studies support its safety and efficacy (102). Epstein and associates (103) showed that patients with high intraoperative defibrillation energy requirements (≥ 25 J) and only 0-5 J of safety margin had a lower total mortality than patients without defibrillators, but arrhythmic mortality was higher than in other ICD studies. However, this study did not suggest what the correct safety margin might be.

Block and colleagues (104) showed that mortality was not different between patients with 21-J versus lower intraoperative energy requirements, but patients with the 21-J intraoperative energy requirement tended to have a slightly lower first-shock success rate. However, a low intraoperative energy requirement did not ensure 100% first-shock conversion, and all patients in this study had a minimum 10-J safety margin.

To consider programming a defibrillation energy other than maximum, additional information is needed from implantation defibrillation testing. One such test is the defibrillation threshold (DFT). Defibrillation thresholds are typically measured by repeated fibrillation episodes tested with successively lower energies until the point at which failure to defibrillate occurs. However, defibrillation is known to be a probabilistic phenomenon, with an S-curve transition from energies that nearly always defibrillate to energies that nearly always fail (Figs. 23-1 and 23-2.) The DFT measured in a given patient, using the relatively large differences between energies in an

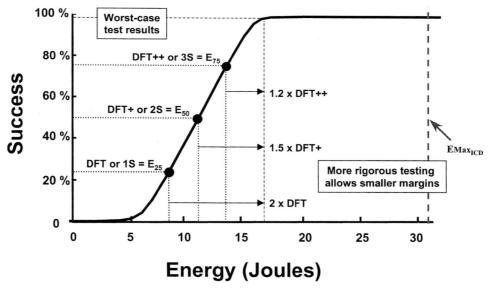

FIGURE 23-1. A typical defibrillation energy versus probability of success curve. When performing defibrillation testing, such as a step-down defibrillation threshold (DFT) protocol, the result may be located at almost any energy along the sloping part of the curve. The predicted worst-case (lowest) percent success levels for three types of energy test protocols (DFT, DFT +, and DFT + +) are shown. Analysis predicts that programming energy to twice the DFT (2 × DFT) can ensure high defibrillation success. Because the more rigorous DFT + and DFT + + methods identify energies higher on the defibrillation success curve, smaller energy margins may be programmed that still achieve consistently high success.

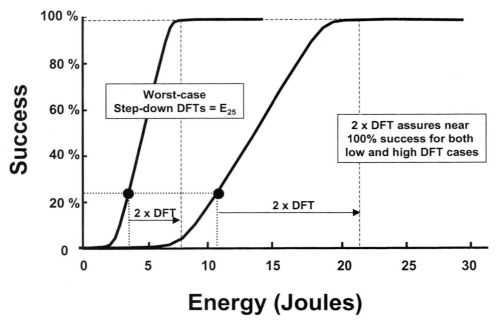

FIGURE 23-2. Defibrillation probability of success curves for patients with high and low energy requirements. Because the probability of success must go to zero at zero energy, the width of the curve must be narrower for patients with lower energy requirements. Analysis predicts the width of the curves are proportional to the overall energy requirement. An energy margin based on a percentage of the measured defibrillation threshold, such as 2 × DFT, may ensure an energy with high success is programmed for each type of patient.

ICD, could occur at almost any energy along the defibrillation probability curve. Knowledge of a reasonably low DFT may be adequate if all shocks are programmed with a very large safety margin (or to maximum energy), but to properly program lower shock energies, it is desirable to know what energy yields a relatively high probability of success (>95%). However, accurate measurement of a point high on the probability of success curve would require many more fibrillation trials than clinically feasible.

Fortunately, alternatives exist. Singer (105) and Lang and coworkers (106) used intraoperative DFT data and mathematical models showing that in the worst case a step-down DFT could result in a defibrillation probability as low as 25% (Fig. 23-1). Estimates of the width of the defibrillation probability of success curve suggested that doubling this worst-case DFT would ensure a better than 95% success rate. ICD patient data demonstrated that the width of the defibrillation probability of success curve is proportional to the overall energy requirements (107) (Fig. 23-2). Safety margins based on a percentage or multiple of the DFT may make better physiologic sense than an absolute margin such as 10 J. The analysis by Singer and by Lang and associates also predicts that use of "enhanced" DFT procedures increase the likelihood of high defibrillation success and allow the use of smaller safety margins. Specifically, a simple reconfirmation of the DFT (two successes without a failure [DFT+]) would require only 1.5 times the DFT+ to ensure a high conversion success rate. Following a similar analysis, a second reconfirmation (three successes without a failure [DFT++]) would require only 1.2 × DFT++ (Fig. 23-1). These latter predictions for DFT+ (two success) and DFT++ (three success) are important because they suggest a systematic method of programming energies for patients with lower energy requirements. These predictions also suggest patients with high energy requirements may be safely programmed to margins less than 10 J if multiple successes can be demonstrated at implantation. A prospective study to test these predicted safety margins is being conducted, and data from several other studies already exist to support this percent safety margin concept.

Strickberger and colleagues used induced ventricular fibrillation episodes to determine the probability of success for a population of patients programmed to different values above DFT (108). Subanalysis suggested 1.7 times the DFT resulted in near 100% success for patients with DFT of more than 6 J, but patients with low DFTs (<6 J) may behave differently, and a 10-J margin may be better in such cases. In a prospective study of patients followed for 1 year,

Neuzner and coworkers (109,110) showed first-shock conversion success was not different between patients programmed to 2 × DFT+ and that for patients programmed to maximum energy. Additional data showed patients programmed to 2 × DFT+ received shock therapy sooner and reduced syncopal episodes (97). Another multicenter trial found no difference in follow-up defibrillation success with first-shock energies programmed to 5 or 10 J above ED_{80} (111). This study used a novel method to estimate the 80% probability of defibrillation success at ICD implantation (ED_{80}). The data support predictions that smaller safety margins can be used if more rigorous implant testing is performed.

PROGRAMMING TIERED-THERAPY IMPLANTABLE CARDIOVERTER-DEFRIBILLATORS: RELEVANT PARAMETERS AND THEIR PURPOSE

Detection Parameters

Rate Zones

Ventricular rate is at the foundation of current and past detection algorithms. Without a high ventricular rate, it is assumed that no ventricular tachycardia or ventricular fibrillation is present. With this is mind, an ICD uses rate thresholds as the first step in detection of ventricular tachycardia or ventricular fibrillation. Most devices are programmable with up to three rate thresholds. The lowest ventricular rate threshold should always be programmed below the slowest ventricular tachycardia that is to receive therapy; 10 bpm is commonly suggested. This ensures that the device can identify the ventricular tachycardia and go through the detection process.

Rate zones also enable detection enhancements to be programmed ON where ventricular rates for SVT overlap with ventricular rates of slower ventricular tachycardias. In this way, detection enhancements do not analyze faster tachycardias such as ventricular fibrillation that are largely distinguishable from SVT by rate only.

Rate zones also allow different (tiered) therapy for tachycardia with different ventricular rates. The physician has the option of programming progressively more aggressive therapy in the higher rate zones. Less aggressive therapies such as ATP and LEC could be reserved for the slow or middle ventricular tachycardia zones.

Detection Durations

Some devices allow physicians to program a duration to therapy delivery after a tachycardia is positively identified. These durations are specific to a rate zone and span from approximately 1 to 60 seconds, with higher rate zones having shorter maximum programmable durations. Durations allow for rhythms to spontaneously convert, which may result in greater patient therapy tolerance and greater device longevity.

Some ICDs allow duration to be programmed for each therapy mode (i.e., ATP or shock) as well. This feature is particularly useful in devices that provide atrial cardioversion therapy because atrial fibrillation episodes typically are not immediately life threatening. Atrial fibrillation therapies are typically given to conscious patients. Atrial fibrillation episodes can spontaneously convert after a short duration, and the frequency of atrial fibrillation episodes can be high; additional time before defibrillation therapy may allow for spontaneous cardioversions and avoid frequent atrial fibrillation defibrillation shocks.

The *Atrial View* allows programming of a *Sustained Rate Duration* (SRD) that is used with detection enhancements. The SRD timer tracks the length of time therapy has been inhibited by a detection enhancement. If an episode persists until the SRD timer expires, the detection enhancement responsible for inhibiting ventricular therapy is overruled, and ventricular therapy is given.

Ventricular RR Interval Regularity

Ventricular RR interval regularity tracks the variability of successive RR intervals. In general, ventricular tachycardias present with regular (or stable) RR intervals, although torsades des pointes is an exception to this rule. When algorithms such as *Stability* (Atrial View) or *modesum* (PR Logic) are programmed ON, "unstable" RR intervals are used as supporting (not conclusive) evidence that a tachycardia is an SVT; additional parameters may be considered by the ICD when making a final rhythm classification. For patients with a history of torsades des pointes, *Stability* may alternatively be used as an accelerator to more aggressive defibrillation therapy. The *modesum* algorithm does not require physician programming. A *Stability* threshold may be programmed by the physician. In general, higher threshold values may make the device less specific (i.e., SVTs have a smaller chance of being correctly identified) and more sensitive (i.e., ventricular tachycardias have a greater chance of being correctly classified).

Ventricular Tachycardia Onset

Certain ICDs use algorithms that measure the suddenness or acceleration with which a ventricular tachycardia occurs. Such algorithms are particularly useful in distinguish 1:1 ventricular tachycardias from sinus tachycardia. *Onset* (Atrial View) can be programmed to measure the suddenness with which a rhythm transitions from a slower rate to a tachycardia. A nonsudden (or gradual) transition is supportive (not conclusive) evidence that a tachycardia is atrial fibrillation, atrial flutter or an ectopic atrial tachycardia. An *Onset* threshold is programmed by the physician as well. In general, lower threshold values may make the device less specific (i.e., SVTs have a smaller chance of being correctly identified) and more sensitive (i.e., ventricular tachycardias have a greater chance of being correctly classified). The PARAD + (ELA Medical, Le Plessis-Robinson, France) employs an acceleration metric for the atrial PP intervals and for ventricular RR intervals (111). The atrial and ventricular *Onset* information is used to determine whether no acceleration, atrial acceleration, or ventricular acceleration occurred. No acceleration is supportive (not conclusive) evidence that a tachycardia is sinus tachycardia. Atrial acceleration is supportive (not conclusive) evidence that a tachycardia is an SVT, and ventricular acceleration is supportive (not conclusive) evidence that a tachycardia is a ventricular tachycardia. Additional parameters may be considered by an ICD when making the final rhythm classification.

Atrial Rate Zones

The Atrial View algorithm uses *AFib Threshold* to inhibit unnecessary ventricular therapy when atrial rates enter an atrial zone defined as atrial rates greater than the *AFib threshold*. *Stability* may be programmed to operate within the atrial zone defined by the *AFib threshold*, thereby steering or guiding the use of *Stability*. The *AF Threshold* allows a physician to program an atrial rate threshold. A tachycardia with an atrial rate above the *AF Threshold* is supportive (not conclusive) evidence that the tachycardia is an SVT (atrial fibrillation in particular). Additional parameters may be considered by the ICD when making a final rhythm classification. In general, higher threshold values for AFib Threshold may make the device less specific (i.e., SVTs have a smaller chance of being correctly identified) and more sensitive (i.e., ventricular tachycardias have a greater chance of being correctly classified).

Atrial and Ventricular Event Relationship

ICDs also track the relationship between atrial and ventricular events to enhance cardiac rhythm discrimination. The PR Logic algorithm acquires information on P and R event patterns and *AV Dissociation* in classifying cardiac rhythms. This algorithm is designed to enhance rate only detection of cardiac rhythms through programming of *SVT Criteria*. The SVT Criteria may be programmed to inhibit therapy for atrial fibrillation or atrial flutter, sinus tachycardia, and/or other 1:1 SVTs individually or in combination. When programmed ON, the Atrial View algorithm uses V > A to compare atrial and ventricular rates with or override other therapy inhibitors such as *Stability* and *Onset*. The PARAD algorithm can also track atrial and ventricular event association or *AV Association*. These algorithms operate on a set of rules that do not require parameter adjustments.

Morphology

Morphology algorithms typically compare a template electrogram representing a normal ventricular cycle to a cycle under analysis during the detection process. The Contour MD, Angstrom MD, and Profile MD devices (St. Jude Medical, Minneapolis, MN) employ the MD algorithm for discrimination of SVT and ventricular tachycardia/ventricular fibrillation using morphology (113). A threshold on *Percent Match* between the template and cycle under analysis can be programmed by the physician. In general, higher threshold values for Percent Match may make the device less specific (i.e., SVTs have a smaller chance of being correctly identified) and more sensitive (i.e., ventricular tachycardias have a greater chance of being correctly classified). Physician interaction may be needed for programming of the MD template.

Therapy Parameters

Various programmable options are available for treating ventricular arrhythmias. In the following sections, we discuss therapies that are useful for ventricular tachycardia and therapies for ventricular fibrillation, such as ATP, LEC, and high-energy shocks.

Antitachycardia Pacing

The first parameter to consider in programming ATP is the time from the last sensed beat to the first pacing stimulus. This is referred to as a delay, R-S1 interval, or coupling interval. This can be programmed as a fixed value in milliseconds or as a percentage of the tachycardia cycle length (typically, 81% to 91%). If multiple attempts of the ATP scheme is desired, this value can be programmed to stay as programmed for the first attempt or to decrement by a fixed value in milliseconds or as a percentage. The sequence of pacing stimuli are typically broken into three main categories: bursts, ramps, and scans.

Figure 23-3 illustrates a burst ATP, which is a sequence of pacing stimuli that are equally spaced in time and remain equally spaced in time over a number of attempts. This time is programmed in milliseconds or as a percentage of the tachycardia cycle length (typically, 81% to 91%), which is referred to as an adaptive burst cycle length. The number of stimuli can be changed incrementally with each new attempt, but the spacing remains constant unless an adaptive burst cycle length is used.

Figure 23-4 illustrates a ramp ATP, which is sequences of pacing stimuli that sequentially decrement in time with respect to each other. The first stimulus is programmed in milliseconds or as a percentage of the tachycardia cycle length. The second and each subsequent stimuli are shortened with respect to its previous stimuli by a programmed amount (in milliseconds). The number of stimuli can be changed incrementally with each new attempt, but the first stimulus timing remains constant (unless an adaptive burst cycle length is used), and the decrement between stimuli remains constant.

Figure 23-5 illustrates a scan ATP, which is a sequence of pacing stimuli that are equally spaced in time (like burst ATP) but decrement by a programmed amount in milliseconds for each new attempt. The time between stimuli is programmed in milliseconds or as a percentage of the tachycardia cycle length. The number of stimuli can be incremented with each new attempt.

There are many variations on these basic schemes, and they can be combined in various ways to create sophisticated ATP schemes. Physicians should refer to the manufacturer's documentation for a complete description of the specific capabilities of a given device.

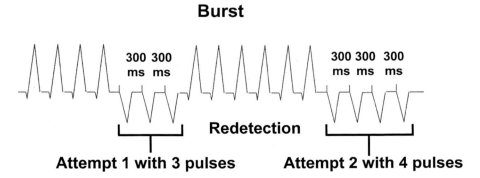

FIGURE 23-3. Burst antitachycardia pacing (ATP) is a sequence of pacing stimuli that are equally spaced in time and remain equally spaced in time over a number of attempts.

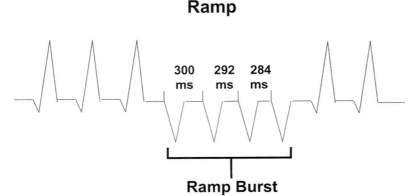

FIGURE 23-4. Ramp antitachycardia pacing (ATP) is a sequence of pacing stimuli that sequentially decrement in time with respect to each other.

High-Energy Shocks

High-energy shocks are useful in terminating ventricular fibrillation. All implanted devices use high-energy capacitors to store the energy. It takes the device some time to charge these capacitors, typically 6 to 12 seconds in a new device and 18 to 30 seconds by the time the device reaches elective battery replacement time (ERI).

By using capacitors to deliver therapy, all ICDs use an exponentially decaying voltage defibrillation waveforms. These waveforms are available in two basic configurations: monophasic and biphasic. Biphasic shocks (Fig. 23-6) switch polarity at some point in the delivery sequence, whereas monophasic shocks maintain polarity throughout the delivery of the shock.

These shocks are generally programmed using the peak voltage, or the energy (measured in Joules). The energy can be specified in terms of the amount of energy *stored* on the capacitors or the amount of energy *delivered* to the heart, depending on the manufacturer. The waveform itself is controlled by the peak voltage to which the capacitors are charged and by the truncation of the delivered waveform. This truncation is referred to as the *tilt* of the waveform and is measured as a percentage of peak voltage to the termination voltage (i.e., an 80% tilt waveform that started with a peak voltage of 100 V would terminate at 20 V). For a biphasic waveform, the two phases can be specified in time, voltage, or percent decay. The waveforms that are specified in terms of time are referred to as *fixed-duration shocks* and those that are

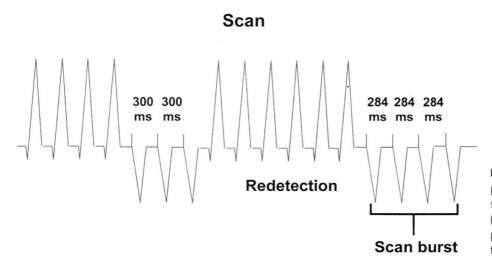

FIGURE 23-5. Scan antitachycardia pacing (ATP) is a sequence of pacing stimuli that are equally spaced in time (like burst ATP), but decrement by a programmed amount in milliseconds for each new attempt.

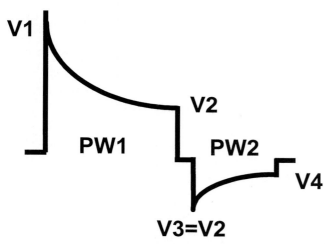

FIGURE 23-6. Biphasic defibrillation waveform. Current devices use capacitors to deliver therapy. Consequently, defibrillation waveforms are exponentially decaying with a time constant related to the system impedance and the capacitance (C) of the capacitors. After a certain duration of time (PW1 + short delay), the device switches polarity and continues discharging its capacitor where it left off. PW1, pulse width of phase 1; PW2, pulse width of phase 2; V1, leading-edge voltage of waveform; V2/V3, falling-edge voltage of phase 1 and leading edge of phase 2, respectively; V4, falling-edge voltage of phase 2.

specified in terms of voltage or percentage and called *adaptive-duration shocks* (or the waveform adapts to the load impedance and has a variable time to ensure the programmed energy is delivered).

The polarity of the leading edge voltage of the delivered shock is also programmable. This can be useful during DFT testing. Changing the initial polarity may improve the effectiveness of the shock in some cases. Implantable cardioverter defibrillators can also be programmed to always deliver a shock after the charging cycle has been initiated or to reconfirm the existence of the arrhythmia after charging has completed, but before delivering the shock.

Low-Energy Cardioversion

Low-energy cardioversion is similar to a high-energy shock, and all of the previously discussed terminology and behavior applies. The main difference is the amount of energy delivered and the arrhythmia being treated. Typically, LEC is programmed from 0.1 J (40 V) to 6 J (300 V) and is typically limited to less than or equivalent to 15 J. This therapy is useful in treating ventricular tachycardias that are resistant to ATP.

Programming to Achieve Optimal Outcomes

The primary discriminator in all marketed ICDs is heart rate. This information is determined by evaluating the intracardiac signal that is presented to a lead typically placed in the right ventricle. Since the infancy of this therapeutic method, rate has been used to initiate tachyarrhythmia decision making. When the heart rate is determined to exceed a programmed threshold and the tachyarrhythmia persists for a programmable duration of time, the device delivers programmed therapy. Consequently, differences in the rates of various ventricular tachyarrhythmias (ventricular tachycardia and ventricular fibrillation in particular) have been used to differentiate tachyarrhythmia that require less aggressive therapy from those that require more aggressive therapy. An example of this strategy is to deliver high-energy shocks for ventricular fibrillation in a fast or high rate zone and ATP for a pace terminable ventricular tachycardia in a slower or lower rate zone.

It is imperative that rate thresholds for these devices be programmed appropriately. This must include a safety margin to allow for variability in tachycardia rates from one arrhythmic episode to the next and for incomplete sensing of all intrinsic complexes. For monomorphic ventricular tachycardias, this margin has traditionally been 10 bpm, and for polymorphic arrhythmias, it is as much as 30% of the native rate.

Unfortunately, all tachyarrhythmias cannot be differentiated by rate alone, and it becomes necessary to use the secondary characteristics of rhythms to enhance the performance of cardiac rhythm discrimination. The rhythm characteristics that are used vary across devices but include RR interval variability, atrial and ventricular event timing and rate comparisons, and morphology of the ventricular electrogram.

Programming of these detection enhancements differs between manufacturers and between models. The clinician must be aware of the specific enhancement that is being programmed, because performance may vary depending on the specific combination of tachyarrhythmias a patient may exhibit.

Common, Population-Based Programming Schemes

It is possible to use standardized programming safely in the ICD general population. This was demonstrated in the ASTRID trial for Atrial View. This prospective study randomized 149 patients with VENTAK AV family of devices to a rate-only arm or to a detection-enhancement arm that employed detection algorithms programmed to a standard set of values. The study showed that the use of the specific settings studied could reduce the time to inappropriate therapy while maintaining the ability to effectively treat malignant arrhythmias. The study also showed the number of patients receiving inappropriate therapies could be reduced by one half (129).

The PR Logic algorithm is designed with population-based programming in mind. By programming a ventricular rate limit, the *SVT Limit*, below which the algorithm operates and selecting what SVT rhythms the device should detect (SVT Criteria), PR Logic employs population based algorithms to guide therapy delivery and inhibition. Clinical experience with 47 patients and 56 episodes of ventricular tachycardia or ventricular fibrillation and 294 episodes of SVT demonstrated that sinus tachycardia, atrial fibrillation, 1 : 1 SVT, and other SVT could be appropriately detected in 91%, 78%, 100%, and 90%, respectively, of cases while maintaining 100% sensitivity using the PR Logic algorithm (114). In a larger study encompassing 2,457 spontaneous episodes, the rate of appropriate detection of SVT was 70.2% (45).

● MILESTONES IN THE DEVELOPMENT OF IMPLANTABLE CARDIOVERTER-DEFIBRILLATORS

The original implantable ventricular defibrillator developed by Michel Mirowski and Morton Mower used a nonprogrammable detection rate and a nonprogrammable discharge to detect and to treat ventricular fibrillation (115). However, the coexistence of other arrhythmias provided the impetus for rapid development of the refinements now included in implantable devices. These refinements allowed concomitant recognition and selective treatment of fast and slow ventricular tachycardias, as well as bradyarrhythmias and SVTs.

Incorporation of therapies complementary to current automated antiarrhythmic treatment is highly desirable if comprehensive therapy is to be provided by implantable devices. As with ventricular tachyarrhythmias, the use of algorithms to detect and to discriminate SVT is proving to be feasible and effective (116). Properly detected, atrial arrhythmias can be terminated by ATP and defibrillation (117,118).

A potential prophylactic role for pacing may also prevent recurrences of atrial fibrillation, but much remains to be clarified. Most studies have evaluated patients with tachycardia-bradycardia syndrome. Whether pacing has a certain role in the prevention of atrial fibrillation in nonbradycardic patients remains to be determined. Methodology must become more uniform to make disparate study results comparable. Studies have been largely single-center trials that used different inclusion criteria, one or more different pacing sites, different pacing modes, and different end points to determine effectiveness. Concurrent administration of antiarrhythmic drugs has confounded the interpretation of some study results. Although arrhythmia frequency has appeared to decrease in some studies (119), it does not appear to have changed in others (120,121), although the duration of recurrences may be decreased (122). Fewer patients with intermittent atrial fibrillation appear to progress to chronic atrial fibrillation (123).

Developers of future devices recognize the desirability of continuing to refine cardiac rhythm discrimination and treatment while incorporating additional therapy modalities. Most immediate among these goals is the use of cardiac resynchronization therapy for chronic heart failure. Studies have demonstrated that appropriately timed cardiac stimulation resynchronizes cardiac contraction by affecting the timing of atrioventricular, interventricular, and intraventricular contractions (122). Cardiac resynchronization results in improved pump function and cardiac energetics (123,125). Early experience with chronic pacing has demonstrated improvements in functional capacity and quality of life (126,127). There also may be a role for cardiac stimulation in the prevention of ventricular tachyarrhythmias in patients with heart failure (128).

CONCLUSIONS

The rapid evolution of ICD systems in concert with carefully designed clinical investigations has led to safe and effective treatment of ventricular tachyarrhythmia in many thousands of patients throughout the world. Whereas the earliest ICD systems delivered high-voltage therapy based on a fixed ventricular activation rate criterion, later versions of the ICD employ programming schemes that allows tiers of therapy to be delivered when the ventricular rate exceeds two or three programmable zone boundaries. Tiered therapy has many advantages; possibly the most significant advantage is the acceptance and long-term tolerability of this lifesaving therapy by patients.

REFERENCES

1. Josephson ME, Spear JF, Harken AH, et al. Surgical excision of automatic atrial tachycardia: anatomic and electrophysiologic correlates. *Am Heart J* 1982;104:1076–1085.
2. Neil CA. Development of the pulmonary veins. *Pediatrics* 1956;18:880–887.
3. Haissaguerre M, Jais P, Shah CD, et al. Spontaneous initiation of atrial fibrillation by ectopic beats originating in the pulmonary veins. *N Engl J Med* 1998;339:659–666.
4. Antzelvitch C, Sicouri S. Clinical relevance of cardiac arrhythmias generated by afterdepolarizations: role of M cells in the generation of U waves, triggered activity and torsade de pointes. *J Am Coll Cardiol* 1994;23:259–277.
5. Kay GN, Plumb VJ, Arciniegas JG, et al. Torsade de pointes: the long-short initiating sequence and other clinical features: observations in 32 patients. *J Am Coll Cardiol* 1983;2:806–817.
6. Bhandari AK, Scheinman M. The long Q-T syndrome. *Mod Concepts Cardiovasc Dis* 1985;54:45–50.
7. Leenhardt L, Glaser E, Burguera M, et al. Short-coupled variant of torsade de pointes: a new electrocardiographic entity in the spectrum of idiopathic ventricular tachyarrhythmias. *Circulation* 1994;89:206–215.
8. Schwartz PG, Priori SG, Locati EH, et al. Long Q-T syndrome patients with mutations of the SCN5A and HERG genes have differential responses to Na^+-channel blockade and to increases in heart rate: implications for gene-specific therapy. *Circulation* 1995;92:3381–3386.
9. Stratmann HG, Kennedy HL. Torsades de pointes associated with drugs and toxins: recognition and management. *Am Heart J* 1987;113:1470–1482.
10. Cranefield PF, Aronson RS. *Cardiac arrhythmias: the role of trigger activity and other mechanisms.* Mt Kisco, NY: Futura Publishing, 1998.
11. Rahilly GT, Prystowsky EN, Zipes DP, et al. Clinical and electrophysiologic findings in patients with otherwise normal electrocardiograms. *Am J Cardiol* 1982;50:459–468.
12. Kimura T, Imanishi S, Atria M, et al. Two differential mechanisms of automaticity in diseased human atrial fibers. *Jpn J Physiol* 1988;8:851–867.
13. Kass RS, Lederer WJ, Tsien RW, et al. Role of calcium in transient inward currents and after contractions induced by stronphanthidin in Purkinje fibers. *J Physiol* 1978;281:187–208.
14. Sung RJ, Shapiro WA, Shen EN, et al. Effects of verapamil on ventricular tachycardias possibly caused by re-entry, automaticity, and triggered activity. *J Clin Invest* 1983;72:350–360.
15. Mayer AG. *Rhythmical pulsation in scyphomedusae.* Publication no. 47. Washington, DC: Carnegie Institution of Washington, 1906:1–62.
16. Mines GR. On dynamic equilibrium in the heart. *J Physiol (Lond)* 1913;46:349–383.
17. Wellens HJJ. Wolff-Parkinson-White syndrome: I. Diagnosis, arrhythmias and identification of the risk patient. *Mod Concepts Cardiovasc Dis* 1983:52:53–56.
18. Coumel P, Flammang D, Attuel P, et al. Sustained intra-atrial reentrant tachycardia: electrophysiologic study of 20 cases. *Clin Cardiol* 1979;2:167–178.
19. Josephson ME, Marchlinski FE, Buxton AE, et al. Electrophysiologic basis for sustained ventricular tachycardia—role of reentry. In: Josephson ME, Wellens HJJ, eds. *Tachycardias: mechanisms, diagnosis, treatment.* Philadelphia: Lea & Febiger, 1984:305–323.
20. Caceres J, Jazayeri M, McKinnie J, et al. Sustained bundle branch reentry mechanism of clinical tachycardia. *Circulation* 1989;79:256–270.
21. Waldo AL, MacLean WAH, Karp RB, et al. Entrainment and interruption of atrial flutter with atrial pacing: studies in man following open heart surgery. *Circulation* 1977;56:737–744.
22. MacLean WAH, Plumb VJ, Waldo AL. Transient entrainment and interruption of ventricular tachycardia. *Pacing Clin Electrophysiol* 1981;4:358–366.
23. Waldo AL. Cardiac pacing: role in diagnosis and treatment of disorders of cardiac rhythm and conduction. In: Rosen MRR, Hoffman BF, eds. *Cardiac therapy.* Boston: Martinus Nijhoff, 1983:299–336.
24. El-Sherif N, Gough WB, Restivo M. Reentrant ventricular arrhythmias in the late myocardial infarction period: 14. Mechanisms of resetting, entrainment, acceleration, or termination of reentrant tachycardia by programmed electrical stimulation. *Pacing Clin Electrophysiol* 1987;10:341–371.
25. Lawn B, DeSilva RA. External cardioversion and defibrillation. In: Alexander RW, Schlant RC, Fuster V, et al, eds. *Hurst's the heart arteries and veins,* vol I, 9th ed. New York: McGraw-Hill, 1998:1003–1006.
26. Winfree AT. Electrical instability in cardiac muscle: phase singularities and rotors. *J Theor Biol* 1989;138:353–405.
27. Jalife J, Davidenko J, Michaels DC. A new perspective on the mechanisms of arrhythmias and sudden cardiac death: spiral waves of excitation in heart muscle. *J Cardiovasc Electrophysiol* 1991;2[Suppl 3]:S133–S152.
28. Takahashi, N, Seki A, Imataka, K, et al. Clinical features of paroxysmal atrial fibrillation: an observation of 94 patients. *Jpn Heart J* 1981;22:143–149.
29. Myerburg RJ, Kessler KM. Management of patients who survive cardiac arrest. *Mod Concepts Cardiovasc Dis* 1986;55:61–66.
30. Chen SA, Tai CT, Yu WC, et al. Right atrial focal atrial fibrillation: electrophysiologic characteristics and radiofrequency catheter ablation. *J Cardiovasc Electrophysiol* 1999;10:328–335.
31. Brugada P, Wellens HJ. Programmed electrical stimulation of the human heart: general principles. In: Josephson ME, Wellens HJJ, eds. *Tachycardias: mechanisms, diagnosis, treatment.* Philadelphia: Lea & Febiger, 1984:61–89.
32. Shibata N, Chen P-S, Dixon EG, et al. Influence of shock

strength and timing on induction of ventricular arrhythmias in dogs. *Am J Physiol* 1988;255(4 PT 2):H891–H901.
33. Brugada J, Mont L, Figueiredo, et al. Enhanced detection criteria in implantable defibrillators. *J Cardiovasc Electrophysiol* 1998; 9:261–268.
34. Schaumann A, von zur Muhlen F, Gonska B, et al. Enhanced detection criteria in implantable cardioverter defibrillators to avoid inappropriate therapy. *Am J Cardiol* 1996;78[Suppl 5A]: 42–50.
35. Higgins SL, Lee RS, Farmer CE, et al. Stability: an ICD detection criteria useful in discriminating atrial fibrillation from ventricular tachycardia. *J Am Coll Cardiol* 1994;23:126A.
36. Neuzner J, Pitschner H, Schlepper M. Programmable ventricular tachycardia detection enhancements in implantable cardioverter defibrillator therapy. *Pacing Clin Electrophysiol* 1995; 18[Suppl II]:539–547.
37. Swerdlow C, Ahern T, Chen P, et al. Underdetection of ventricular tachycardia by algorithms to enhance specificity in a tiered-therapy cardioverter-defibrillator. *J Am Coll Cardiol* 1994;24:416–424.
38. Ruppel R, Langes K, Kalkowski H, et al. Initial experience with implantable cardioverter defibrillator providing dual chamber pacing and sensing. *Pacing Clin Electrophysiol* 1997;20: 1078.
39. Schuchert A, Kuhl M, Meinertz T, et al. Evaluation of an algorithm designed to differentiate atrial and ventricular arrhythmias. *Pacing Clin Electrophysiol* 1998;21:872.
40. Aliot EM, Limousin M, Nitzsche R, et al. Dual chamber implantable cardioverter-defibrillator: a preliminary experience. In: Singer I, Barold SS, Camm AJ, eds. *Nonpharmacological therapy of arrhythmias for the 21st century: the state of the art.* Armonk, NY: Futura Publishing, 1998:423–436.
41. Wilkoff BL, Kuhlkamp V, Gillberg JM, et al. Performance of a dual chamber detection algorithm (PR Logic) based on the worldwide Gem DR clinical results. *Pacing Clin Electrophysiol* 1999;22:720.
42. Swerdlow CD, Gunderson BD, Gillberg JM, et al. Discrimination of concurrent atrial and ventricular tachyarrhythmias by a dual-chamber ICD. *Pacing Clin Electrophysiol* 1999;22:775.
43. Ropella KM, Baerman JM, Sahakian AV, et al. Differentiation of ventricular tachyarrhythmias. *Circulation* 1990;82: 2035–2043.
44. Chiang CM, Jenkins JM, DiCarlo LA. Digital signal processing chip implementation for detection and analysis of intracardiac electrograms. *Pacing Clin Electrophysiol* 1994;17:1373–1379.
45. Baumann LS, Lang DJ. Automatic classification of ventricular and supraventricular tachycardia from a unipolar right ventricular electrogram for implantable cardioverter defibrillators. *Pacing Clin Electrophysiol* 1996;19:583.
46. Schulte B, Sperzel J, Schwarz T, et al. Temporal and exercise-related stability of a new, "morphology-based" arrhythmia detection parameter in implantable defibrillators. *Pacing Clin Electrophysiol* 1999;22:823.
47. Fenoglio JJ, Pham TD, Harken AH, et al. Recurrent sustained ventricular tachycardia: structure and ultrastructure of subendocardial regions in which tachycardia originates. *Circulation* 1983;68:518–533.
48. Wit AL, Dillon S, Ursell PC. Influences of anisotropic tissue structure of ventricular tachycardia. In: Brugada P, Wellens HJJ, eds. *Cardiac arrhythmias: where to go from here?* Mount Kisco, NY: Futura Publishing, 1987:27.
49. El-Sherif N. Reentry revisited. *Pacing Clin Electrophysiol* 1988; 11:1358–1368.
50. Josephson ME. Recurrent ventricular tachycardia. *Clinical Cardiac Electrophysiology: techniques and interpretations* 1993: 417–615.
51. Frame LH, Simson MB. Oscillations of conduction, action potential duration and refractoriness: a mechanism for spontaneous termination of reentrant tachycardias. *Circulation* 1988; 78:1277–1287.
52. Wellens HJJ, Lie KI, Durrer D. Further observations on ventricular tachycardia as studied by electrical stimulation of the heart. *Circulation* 1974;49:647–653.
53. Wellens HJ, Duren DR, Lie KI. Observations on mechanisms of ventricular tachycardia in man. *Circulation* 1976;54: 237–244.
54. Fischer JD, Johnston DR, Kim SG, et al. Implantable pacers for tachycardia termination: stimulation techniques and long-term efficacy. *Pacing Clin Electrophysiol* 1986;9:1325–1333.
55. Charos GS, Haffajee GI, Gold RL, et al. A theoretically and practically more effective method for interruption of ventricular tachycardia: self-adapting autodecremental overdrive pacing. *Circulation* 1986;73:309–315.
56. Gillis AM, Leitch JW, Sheldon RS, et al. A prospective randomized comparison of autodecremental pacing to burst pacing in device therapy for chronic ventricular tachycardia secondary to coronary artery disease. *Am J Cardiol* 1993;72: 1146–1151.
57. Bollman A, Langberg JJ. The relationship between induced and spontaneous ventricular fibrillation. [abstract] *Circulation* 1997;96;I-529.
58. Newman D, Dorian P, Hardy J. Randomized controlled comparison of antitachycardia pacing algorithms for termination of ventricular tachycardia. *J Am Coll Cardiol* 1993;21:1413–1418.
59. Kantoch MJ, Green MS, Tang ASL. Randomized cross-over evaluation of two adaptive pacing algorithms for termination of ventricular tachycardia. *Pacing Clin Electrophysiol* 1993;16: 1664–1672.
60. Calkins H, El-Atassi R, Kalbfleisch S, et al. Comparison of fixed burst versus decremental burst pacing for termination of ventricular tachycardia. *Pacing Clin Electrophysiol* 1993;16: 26–32.
61. Hammill SC, Packer DL, Stanton MS, et al. Termination and acceleration of ventricular tachycardia with autodecremental pacing, burst pacing and cardioversion in patients with an implantable cardioverter defibrillator. *Pacing Clin Electrophysiol* 1995;18:3–10.
62. Peinado F, Almerndral J, Rius T, et al. Randomized, prospective comparison of four burst pacing algorithms for spontaneous ventricular tachycardia. *Am J Cardiol* 1998;82: 1422–1425.
63. Schaumann A, von zur Muhlen F, Herse B, et al. Empirical versus tested antitachycardia pacing in implantable cardioverter defibrillators: a prospective study including 200 patients. *Circulation* 1998;97:66–74.
64. Estes M, Haugh CJ, Wang PJ. Antitachycardia pacing and low-energy cardioversion for ventricular tachycardia termination: a clinical perspective. *Am Heart J* 1997;127:1038–1046.
65. Fotuhi P, Epstein E, Ideker R. Energy levels for defibrillation: what is of real clinical importance? *Am J Cardiol* 1999:83: 24D–33D.
66. Munsif A, Saksena S, DeGroot P, et al. Low-energy endocardial defibrillation using dual, triple, and quadruple electrode systems. *Am J Cardiol* 1997;79:1632–1639.
67. Gold M, Foster A, Shorofsky S. Lead system optimization for transvenous defibrillation. *Am J Cardiol* 1997;80:1163–1167.
68. Bardy G, Johnson G, Poole J, et al. A simplified, single-lead unipolar transvenous cardioversion-defibrillation system. *Circulation* 1993;88:543–547.

69. Haffajee C, Martin D, Bhandari A, et al, for the Jewel Active Can Investigators. A multicenter, randomized trial comparing an active can implantable defibrillator with a passive can system. *Pacing Clin Electrophysiol* 1997;20:215–219.
70. Jordaens L, Trouerbach JW, Vertongen P, et al. Experience of cardioverter-defibrillators inserted without thoracotomy: evaluation of transvenously inserted intracardiac leads alone or with a subcutaneous axillary patch. *Br Heart J* 1993;69:14–19.
71. Saksena S, Tullo N, Krol R, et al. Initial clinical experience with endocardial defibrillation using an implantable cardioverter/defibrillator with a triple-electrode system. *Arch Intern Med* 1989;149:2333–2339.
72. Higgins S, Alexander D, Kuypers C, et al. The subcutaneous array: a new lead adjunct for the transvenous ICD to lower defibrillation thresholds. *Pacing Clin Electrophysiol* 1995;18:1540–1548.
73. Kühlkamp V, Khalighi K, Dörnberger V, et al. Single-incision and single-element array electrode to lower the defibrillation threshold. *Ann Thorac Surg* 1997;64:1177–1179.
74. Bardy G, Allen M, Mehra R, et al. An effective and adaptable transvenous defibrillation system using the coronary sinus in humans. *J Am Coll Cardiol* 1990;16:887–895.
75. Vlay S, Bilfinger T, Levy M, et al. Alternative locations for internal defibrillator electrodes. *Pacing Clin Electrophysiol* 1998;21:1309–1312.
76. Winkle A, Mead H, Ruder A, et al. Improved low energy defibrillation efficacy in man with the use of a biphasic truncated exponential waveform. *Am Heart J* 1989;117:122–127.
77. Fain E, Sweeney M, Franz M. Improved internal defibrillation efficacy with a biphasic waveform. *Am Heart J* 1989;117:358–364.
78. Block M, Hammel D, Böcker D, et al. A prospective randomized cross-over comparison of mono- and biphasic defibrillation using nonthoracotomy lead configurations in humans. *J Cardiovasc Electrophysiol* 1994;5:581–590.
79. Neuzner J, Pitschner HF, Huth C, et al. Effect of biphasic waveform pulse on endocardial defibrillation efficacy in humans. *Pacing Clin Electrophysiol* 1994;17:207–212.
80. Bardy G, Ivey T, Allen M, et al. A prospective randomized evaluation of biphasic versus monophasic waveform pulses on defibrillation efficacy in humans. *J Am Coll Cardiol* 1989;14:728–733.
81. Schuder J, Stoeckle H, West J, et al. Transthoracic ventricular defibrillation in the dog with truncated and untruncated exponential stimuli. *IEEE Trans Biomed Eng* 1971;18:410–415.
82. Tang A, Yabe S, Wharton M, et al. Ventricular defibrillation using biphasic waveforms: the importance of phasic duration. *J Am Coll Cardiol* 1989;13:207–214.
83. Natale A, Sra J, Krum D, et al. Relative efficacy of different tilts with biphasic defibrillation in humans. *Pacing Clin Electrophysiol* 1996;19:197–206.
84. Swartz J, Fletcher R, Karasik P. Optimization of biphasic waveforms for human nonthoracotomy defibrillation. *Circulation* 1993;88:2646–2654.
85. Walcott G, Walker R, Cates A, et al. Choosing the optimal monophasic and biphasic waveforms for ventricular defibrillation. *J Cardiovasc Electrophysiol* 1995;6:737–750.
86. Kroll M. A minimal model of the single capacitor biphasic defibrillation waveform. *Pacing Clin Electrophysiol* 1994;17:1782–1792.
87. Irnich W. Optimal truncation of defibrillation pulses. *Pacing Clin Electrophysiol* 1995;18:673–688.
88. Hahn S, Heil J, Lin Y, et al. Defibrillation strength-duration relationships for biphasic waveforms. *Pacing Clin Electrophysiol* 1996;19:654A.
89. Gold M, Shorofsky S. Strength-duration relationship for human transvenous defibrillation. *Circulation* 1997;96:3517–3520.
90. Block M, Hammel D, Bocker D, et al. Biphasic defibrillation using a single capacitor with large capacitance: reduction of peak voltages and ICD device size. *Pacing Clin Electrophysiol* 1996;19:207–214.
91. Natale A, Sra J, Krum D, et al. Comparison of biphasic and monophasic pulses: does the advantage of biphasic shocks depend on the waveshape? *Pacing Clin Electrophysiol* 1995;18:1354–1361.
92. Tomassoni G, Newby K, Deshpande S, et al. Defibrillation efficacy of commercially available biphasic impulses in humans: importance of negative-phase peak voltage. *Circulation* 1997;95:1822–1826.
93. Neuzner J, Pitschner HF, Schwarz T, et al. Effects of electrode polarity on defibrillation thresholds in biphasic endocardial defibrillation. *Am J Cardiol* 1996;78:96–97.
94. Shorofsky S, Gold M. Effects of waveform and polarity on defibrillation thresholds in humans using a transvenous lead system. *Am J Cardiol* 1996;78:313–316.
95. Usui M, Walcott GP, Strickberger SA, et al. Effects of polarity for monophasic and biphasic shocks on defibrillation efficacy with an endocardial system. *Pacing Clin Electrophysiol* 1996;19:65–71.
96. Strickberger SA, Man KC, Daoud E, et al. Effect of first-phase polarity of biphasic shocks on defibrillation threshold with a single transvenous lead system. *J Am Coll Cardiol* 1995;25:1605–1608.
97. Himmrich E, Liebrich A, Neuzner J, et al. Safety margin of low-energy shocks in patients with reduced left ventricular fraction and amiodarone therapy. *Pacing Clin Electrophysiol* 1998;21:931A.
98. Cates A, Wolf P, Hillsley R, et al. The probability of defibrillation success and the incidence of post shock arrhythmia as a function of shock strength. *Pacing Clin Electrophysiol* 1994;17:1208–1217.
99. Zivin A, Souza JPF, Flemming MKB, et al. Relationship between shock energy and post-defibrillation ventricular arrhythmias in patients with implantable defibrillators. *J Cardiovasc Electrophysiol* 1999;10:370–377.
100. Tokano T, Bach D, Chang J, et al. Effect of ventricular shock strength on cardiac hemodynamics. *J Cardiovasc Electrophysiol* 1998;9:791–797.
101. Winters S, Casale A, Inglesby T, et al. Setting of relatively low energy outputs may permit implantation of a nonthoracotomy automatic cardioverter defibrillator system when high energy outputs prove ineffective. *Pacing Clin Electrophysiol* 1996;19:1516–1518.
102. Marchlinski F, Flores B, Miller J, et al. Relation of the intraoperative defibrillation threshold to successful postoperative defibrillation with an automatic implantable cardioverter defibrillator. *Am J Cardiol* 1988;62:393—398.
103. Epstein A, Ellenbogen K, Kirk K, et al. Clinical characteristics and outcomes of patients with high defibrillation thresholds: a multicenter study. *Circulation* 1992;86:1206–1216.
104. Block M, Briethardt G. Relationship between acute defibrillation threshold and therapy outcome. In: Camm, AJ, Lindemans, FW, eds. *Transvenous defibrillation and radiofrequency ablation*. Armonk, NY: Futura Publishing, 1995:105.
105. Singer I, Lang D. Defibrillation threshold: clinical utility and therapeutic implications. *Pacing Clin Electrophysiol* 1992;15:932–949.
106. Lang D, KenKnight B. Implant support devices. In: Singer

I, ed. *Implantable cardioverter defibrillator.* Armonk, NY: Futura Publishing, 1994:223–252.
107. Hahn S, Winter J, Schumann C, et al. The relationship between the defibrillation threshold and the width of the defibrillation probability of success curve in humans. *Pacing Clin Electrophysiol* 1997;20:1215A.
108. Strickberger SA, Daoud EG, Davidson T, et al. Probability of successful defibrillation at multiples of the defibrillation energy requirement in patients with an implantable defibrillator. *Circulation* 1997;96:1217–1223.
109. Neuzner J, Liebrich A, Jung J, et al. Safety and efficacy of implantable defibrillator therapy with programmed shock energy at twice the augmented step-down defibrillation threshold: results of the prospective, randomized, multicenter Low-Energy Endotak Trial. *Am J Cardiol* 1999;83:34D–39D.
110. Neuzner J. Safety margins: lessons from the Low-Energy Endotak Trial (LEET). *Am J Cardiol* 1996;78:26–32.
111. Weiss R, Ostrow E, Malkin R, et al. Low Defibrillation Energy Dose (LoDED) trail: is a five Joule defibrillation safety margin enough? *Circulation* 1999;100:I-786A.
112. Olson W. Dual chamber sensing and detection for implantable cardioverter-defibrillators. In: Singer I, Barold SS, Camm AJ, eds. *Nonpharmocological therapy of arrhythmia for the 21st century: the state of the art.* Armonk, NY: Futura Publishing, 1998.
113. Britta S, Sperzel J, Schwarz T, et al. Temporal and exercise-related stability of a new "morphology-based" arrhythmia detection parameter in implantable defibrillators. *Pacing Clin Electrophysiol* 1999;22[Pt II]:823A.
114. Kuhlkamp V, Dornberger V, Suchalla R, et al. Specificity and sensitivity of a detection algorithm using patterns, AV-association and rate analysis for the differentiation of supraventricular tachyarrhythmias and ventricular tachyarrhythmias. *Pacing Clin Electrophysiol* 1999;22[Pt II]:823A.
115. Mirowski M, Reid PR, Mower MM, et al. Termination of malignant ventricular arrhythmias with an implanted automatic defibrillator in human beings. *N Engl J Med* 1980;303:322–324.
116. Gold MR, Hsu W, Marcovecchio AF, et al. A new defibrillator discrimination algorithm utilizing electrogram morphology analysis. *Pacing Clin Electrophysiol* 1999;22[Pt II]:179–182.
117. Connelly DT, de Belder MA, Cunningham D, et al. Long-term follow-up of patients with software based antitachycardia pacemaker. *Br Heart J* 1993;69:250–254.
118. Wellens HJ, Lau CP, Luderitz B, et al. Atrioverter: an implantable device for the treatment of atrial fibrillation. *Circulation* 1998;98:1651–1656.
119. Delfaut P, Saksena S, Prakash A, et al. Long-term outcome of patients with drug-refractory atrial flutter and fibrillation after single- and dual-site right atrial pacing for arrhythmia prevention. *J Am Coll Cardiol* 1998;32:1900–1908.
120. Gillis AM, Wyse DG, Connolly SJ, et al. Atrial pacing periablation for prevention of paroxysmal atrial fibrillation. *Circulation* 1999;99:2553–2558.
121. Lau CP, Tse HF, Yu CM, et al. Effect of dual site right atrial pacing on burden of atrial fibrillation in patients with drug-refractory atrial fibrillation. *J Am Coll Cardiol* 2000;35[Suppl A]:109A.
122. Tse HF, Lau CP, Yu CM, et al. Impact of dual site pacing on the natural history of symptomatic atrial fibrillation recurrence in patients without bradycardia. *J Am Coll Cardiol* 2000;35[Suppl A]:109A.
123. Bailin SJ, Adler SW, Guidici MC, et al. Prevention of chronic atrial fibrillation by pacing at Bachmann's bundle: results of a randomized prospective multicenter study. *Circulation* 1999;100[Suppl]:I-68A.
124. Touissaint JF, Ritter P, Lavergne T, et al. Biventricular resynchronization in end-stage heart failure: an eight-month follow-up by phase map radionuclide angioplasty. *Pacing Clin Electrophysiol* 1999;22[Pt II]:840A.
125. Nelson GS, Berger RD, Fetics BJ, et al. Left ventricular pre-excitation improves mechanoenergetics of patients with dilated cardiomyopathy and ventricular conduction delay. *J Am Coll Cardiol* 2000;35[Suppl A]:230A.
126. Stellbrink C, Auricchio A, Diem B, et al. Potential benefit of biventricular pacing in patients with congestive heart failure and ventricular tachyarrhythmia. *Am J Cardiol* 1999;83:143D–150D.
127. Gras D, Cazeau S, Ritter P, et al. Long term results of cardiac resynchronization for heart failure patients: the InSync clinical trial. *Circulation* 1999;100[Suppl I]:829.
128. Higgins S, Yong P, Scheck D, et al. Biventricular pacing may diminish ICD shocks. *Pacing Clin Electrophysiol* 1999;22[Pt II]:848A.
129. Dorian P, Newman D, et al. A randomized clinical trial of a standardized protocol for the prevention of inappropriate therapy using a dual chamber ICD. *Canadian Journal of Cardiology* 1999;15:136D.

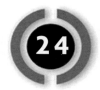

ATRIAL DEFIBRILLATORS

JOHAN E. P. WAKTARE, A. JOHN CAMM

Recurrent atrial fibrillation poses a challenge to the clinician. Patients may repeatedly revert to highly symptomatic atrial fibrillation despite optimal medical management. A newer therapeutic option, the implantable atrial defibrillator, has become available. Development began in the late 1980s, when the internal cardioversion of atrial fibrillation was described (1), with the transition of implantable cardioverter-defibrillators (ICDs) from investigational devices to routine clinical use. The marriage of the two technologies was a logical one, and in 1994, the first implantable atrial defibrillator, or atrioverter, was implanted at St. George's Hospital. The original atrioverter (Metrix, Guidant Corp., St. Paul, MN) (Fig. 24-1A) completed a phase III study (2), and atrial defibrillation has been incorporated into a conventional ICD with the addition of atrial pacing therapies to create a comprehensive arrhythmia management device (Jewel AF model 7250, Medtronic, Inc., Minneapolis, MN) (Fig. 24-1B).

Atrial defibrillators have provided a valuable additional therapeutic option for atrial fibrillation patients but their precise role has been brought into question by the simultaneous considerable advances in alternative therapies for atrial fibrillation. Following an original series of three cases (3) published in the same year as the first atrioverter was implanted, Haissaguerre and colleagues described the successful focal catheter ablation of atrial fibrillation in 50 patients (4). Their results are being reproduced by other investigators (5–8), and Lau and coworkers (9) described the successful catheter ablation of atrial foci in patients with recurrent, persistent atrial fibrillation, the very population best suited for atrioverter implantation. After many years of stagnation, a range of new antiarrhythmic agents have been launched or are approaching commercial release, including ibutilide, dofetilide, and azimilide.

The place of an implanted device in the management of a non–life-threatening arrhythmia has been called into question, but we believe that several definite roles do exist. In this chapter, we review the background of implantable atrial defibrillators, describe the available technologies, and assess the place of the device in atrial fibrillation management.

● THE ROLE OF RESTORATION OF SINUS RHYTHM

Atrial fibrillation increases in incidence with age and has previously been regarded as an almost normal manifestation of the ageing process. Although this is now accepted as being untrue with the recognition

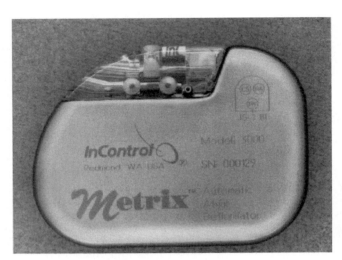 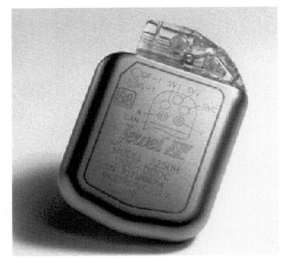

FIGURE 24-1. The Metrix 3020 (Guidant Corp.) and the Jewel AF 7250 (Medtronic, Inc.) devices.

of the numerous deleterious effects of atrial fibrillation (10), most of the harm from atrial fibrillation can be circumvented without restoring sinus rhythm. Thromboembolism may be prevented by appropriate anticoagulation (11,12) even though the restoration of sinus rhythm has never been shown to prevent thromboembolism, although it is commonly assumed to do so. Tachycardia-induced cardiomyopathy can be prevented by appropriate rate control using pharmacologic means or atrioventricular (AV) nodal ablation (13,14). The impairment in exercise capacity and quality of life can be at least partially reversed by the same rate control methods described previously (15). However, these broad findings from clinical studies belie the response of individual patients to the loss of sinus rhythm. Although symptom control may be an acceptable form of treatment for some patients, others demand maintenance of sinus rhythm.

In the management of patients with atrial fibrillation, the physician must decide about the optimal treatment strategy for individual patients. The hemodynamic and symptomatic benefits must be weighed against the inconvenience of repeated cardioversion. The atrial defibrillator allows the restoration of sinus rhythm to be performed with much greater convenience and earlier than if patients relied on clinical services.

Atrial fibrillation promotes its own persistence, a process often referred to as "atrial fibrillation begets atrial fibrillation" (16), and there is evidence that prompt restoration of sinus rhythm increases the period between atrial fibrillation recurrences (17,18). This observation implies an important potential long-term benefit from atrioverters, but direct evidence is lacking. A study of four patients with atrioverters *in situ* failed to show any reduction in the inducibility of atrial fibrillation, even after a prolonged atrial fibrillation-free period (19). Although there may be beneficial effects on atrial electrophysiology from implantable atrial defibrillators, such benefits have not been conclusively proven.

INTERNAL CARDIOVERSION OF ATRIAL FIBRILLATION

External cardioversion of atrial fibrillation achieves a reported cardioversion rate of 70% to 95% (20–23). Energy requirements are high, with acceptable cardioversion rates only achieved using energies of 200 to 360 J. Most of the energy is wasted. It is dissipated in skin or subcutaneous tissues, or is conducted to the anodal paddle through tissue other than the atrium. As a result, many patients with high transthoracic impedance due to obesity or emphysema fail to respond to external cardioversion (22).

Methodology

Internal cardioversion was originally developed for the treatment of ventricular arrhythmias (24,25), but it had also been used for terminating atrial arrhythmias (26). Lévy and colleagues (1), when performing low-energy AV nodal ablation for rate control in patients, observed that sinus rhythm was sometimes restored by the low-energy shock. They therefore prospectively assessed the efficacy of internal cardioversion in patients with prior failed external cardioversion. An ablation electrode was positioned at the AV node but then withdrawn to leave the electrode used for energy delivery free floating in the right atrial cavity. Shocks of 200 or 300 J were delivered between the catheter and a back plate, resulting in restoration of sinus rhythm in 9 of 10 patients. After this, development switched to defibrillation with lower energies between two intrathoracic electrodes, although results for a larger series of 112 patients were subsequently published and demonstrated the superiority of the original methodology for internal cardioversion over external cardioversion (23) (Fig. 24-2).

As with internal cardioversion of ventricular fibrillation, there are numerous variables that may be changed to optimize the efficacy of defibrillation shocks (Fig. 24-3). In a sheep model, Cooper and colleagues (27) demonstrated that internal cardioversion of atrial fibrillation can be achieved with mean energies as low as 1.3 J. This study evaluated the relative efficacies of different shock waveforms (monophasic versus biphasic) and shock durations. These data suggested the optimal configuration was a shock vector between the right atrial appendage and coronary sinus (Fig. 24-4).

Data (28,29) suggest that internal cardioversion is more effective at restoring sinus rhythm than conventional external cardioversion. However, biphasic defibrillation waveforms are now incorporated into external defibrillators (30–32), and the efficacy of these devices appears superior to conventional defibrillators (33). Ibutilide (34) and flecainide (35) have been shown to reduce the external defibrillation threshold. In particular, the use of ibutilide resulted in 100% efficacy of external cardioversion in the reported series (34). Because external defibrillation avoids the

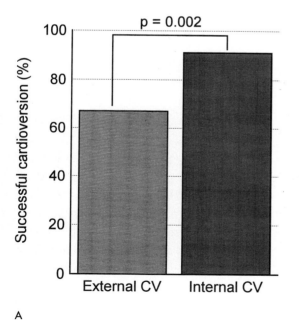
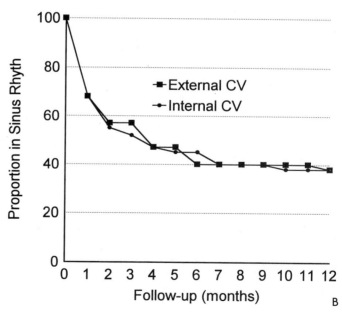

FIGURE 24-2. The outcome of external versus internal (i.e., right atrium to back plate) cardioversion in 112 patients who had failed previous external cardioversion. **A:** The success rate (91%) of internal cardioversion is higher than that (67%) for external cardioversion. **B:** The atrial fibrillation recurrence rate is significant despite amiodarone prophylaxis and irrespective of cardioversion modality.

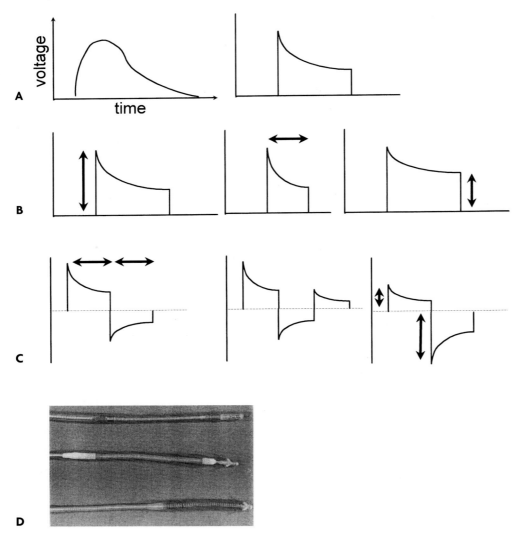

FIGURE 24-3. The possible variations for shock parameters are virtually infinite. **A:** Although external defibrillators have used a damped sine monophasic waveform until recently, implanted devices have used a truncated exponential waveform since their inception because of efficacy and design considerations. **B:** Although the energy delivered is a function of the leading-edge voltage, the shock duration and tilt (i.e., percentage of original voltage at which the waveform is truncated) also have an effect on energy and efficacy. **C:** Biphasic shocks are generally more efficient than monophasic shocks, and the tilt at which the polarity of the shock is changed can be optimized. Triphasic shocks and shocks using a larger leading-edge voltage for the second phase (by using two capacitors) have also been investigated. **D:** Numerous issues regarding the lead design and placement affect the efficacy of defibrillation. These include coil design and length, where the coil is positioned, and which coil is used as the active coil and which the indifferent.

cost of the internal cardioversion catheters and the small attendant risks of the invasive procedure, the pendulum may well swing back in favor of external cardioversion.

Pain Perception

External defibrillation shocks produce pain by direct nerve stimulation, cause profound muscle contraction and dissipation of energy at the defibrillator paddle–skin interface. The latter problem is avoided in internal cardioversion where much lower shock energies are used. Despite this, perceived pain is still significant (36). The threshold of shock that is perceived as painful exhibits significant interpatient variability and depends on perceived gain. In the series of Murgatroyd and coworkers (36), sedation was withheld initially but allowed at the patients' request as progressively greater energies were delivered. In all patients, discomfort increased with shock intensity, and there was great interindividual variation in the maximum energy tolerated, which was between 0.5 and 1.0 J in most cases. The actual shock energy that patients can tolerate in clinical practice is higher with most patients who have received the stand-alone atrioverter tolerating 6-J shocks. The discrepancy arises for several reasons. In the series of Murgatroyd and asso-

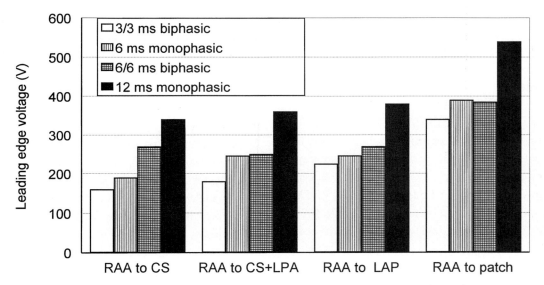

FIGURE 24-4. Comparison of the efficacies of different shock vectors and waveform configurations. In a sheep model, sustained atrial fibrillation (AF) was induced. The shock vectors tried were right atrial appendage to coronary sinus (RAA →CS), right atrial appendage to left pulmonary artery (RAA →LPA), right atrial appendage to a combined indifferent electrode (RAA →CS/LPA), and right atrial appendage to a subcutaneous patch (RAA →patch). This part of the study investigated 6- and 12-msec monophasic and 3/3- and 6/6-msec biphasic waveforms. All waveforms were truncated exponential waveforms generated using a 80-μF capacitor. (Adapted from Cooper RA, Alferness CA, Smith WM, Ideker RE. Internal cardioversion of atrial fibrillation in sheep. *Circulation* 1993;87:1673–1686, with permission.)

ciates, patients received multiple shocks in a step-up protocol, and there was anticipation of the higher-energy shocks. In practice, atrioverter patients usually receive a single shock that provides them with relief of the symptoms of atrial fibrillation. Clinical experience has demonstrated that patients prefer a single shock at an energy level above the previously demonstrated defibrillation threshold rather than requiring multiple shocks because of starting at an energy close to the defibrillation threshold.

Another tactic that has been explored to ameliorate internal cardioversion associated pain is the use of intranasal butorphanol. This synthetic opioid is rapidly absorbed from the vascular mucous membrane of the nasal cavity. Timmermans and colleagues (37) performed a step-up internal atrial defibrillation protocol in 47 patients to compare butorphanol with placebo if shocks had become uncomfortable. Symptom severity was assessed using a visual analogue scale and the McGill Pain Questionnaire. The investigators found that pain parameters, but not fear, were significantly reduced by butorphanol.

The pain associated with internal cardioversion does not prove a great issue in the clinical use of atrial defibrillators. The pain is, however, poorly tolerated by some individuals, and this issue must be explored before implantation. Although improvements in lead technology and defibrillation waveforms may bring the energy levels down further, the problem is unlikely to go away. Any shock capable of inducing depolarization of most atrial tissue can also depolarize some nerve fibers and skeletal muscle cells, thus causing pain and discomfort to the patient.

◉ IMPLANTED DEVICES

Two basic approaches have been taken to device design: 1) a stand-alone atrioverter with only backup ventricular pacing capabilities and 2) a dual-chamber defibrillator with pacing capabilities.

The Atrioverter

The atrioverter has three leads: a screw-in right atrial defibrillation lead, a self-retaining helical coronary sinus atrial defibrillation lead, and a conventional ventricular bipolar pacing lead for R-wave shock synchronization and backup VVI pacing (Fig. 24-5). The marketed model at the time of writing (Metrix 3020, Guidant Corp.) is a 53-cc device (weighs 82 g) containing a 160-μF capacitor. It delivers a 6/6-msec biphasic shock and has a maximum leading-edge voltage of 300 V, which equates to 6-J shock with typical impedances.

The device may be programmed into one of two modes for clinical use. In automated therapy mode, the device collects a few minutes of electrogram at preprogrammed intervals. If it detects atrial fibrillation, it charges and delivers an atrioversion shock. It is recommended that the wakeup interval be set to more than 12 hours to avoid battery depletion. There is an option for the device to deliver a low-energy "warning shock" in this mode. The alternative that is much more frequently employed in clinical practice is the patient-activated mode. With this, therapy is delivered only if atrial fibrillation is detected after the patient has activated the device using a magnet. This mode allows the patient control over the precise time of therapy delivery and prevents shocks occurring unexpectedly if atrial fibrillation onset is asymptomatic.

Arrhythmia detection is done in real time by the device, but because the algorithms are complex and therefore produce a significant current drain, electrograms are not collected continuously. During analysis, *quiet time* (i.e., proportion of time spent at near to 0 mV) and *baseline crossing* analysis on the right atrium–coronary sinus (RA–CS) channel are employed with automatic or programmable setting to determine the presence of atrial fibrillation (Fig. 24-6). Additional analysis is performed on the coronary sinus to right ventricular apex (CS–RVA) channel. If atrial fibrillation is detected, capacitor charging begins, and the defibrillation shock is delivered synchronous with an appropriate R wave.

Because the device has only backup ventricular pacing (VVI 40 bpm) and no ventricular defibrillation ability, avoidance of ventricular proarrhythmia is of paramount importance. Based on theoretical considerations and preliminary studies (38), the shock algorithm requires a RR interval of greater than 500 msec to deliver the shock. R-wave detection is done on the ventricular lead bipole and an electrogram generated between the right ventricle and the coronary sinus. Data for more than 11,000 shocks has failed to demonstrate a single ventricular proarrhythmic event (Table 24-1). To minimize the risk of proarrhythmia, the stand-alone atrioverter is only recommended in patients with no or minimal structural heart disease. This criterion excludes a significant number of patients who would otherwise be candidates for the atrioverter but for whom it may be unnecessary. A study of whether the atrioverter may be safely used in patients with structural heart disease is underway (39).

The published experience (2) with the atrioverter

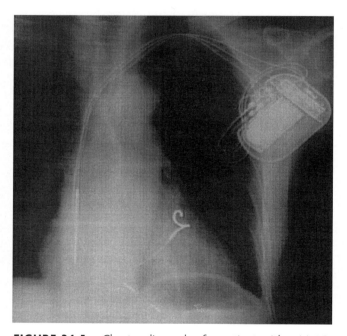

FIGURE 24-5. Chest radiograph of a patient with a Metrix atrioverter. The device is implanted at a left pectoral site. The right side may also be used because the device is not used as a defibrillation plate, unlike many implantable cardioverter-defibrillators. The coronary sinus coil has a corkscrew shape to reduce the probability of lead displacement. The other atrial coil is screwed into the low right atrium. A ventricular pacing lead is used for R-wave synchronization and backup VVI pacing.

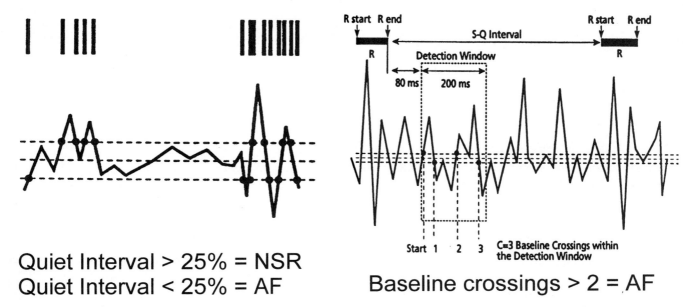

FIGURE 24-6. The quiet interval and baseline crossing atrial fibrillation detection algorithms from the Metrix.

in 51 patients with a mean follow-up of less than 9 months (261 ± 138 days). About 40% of patients who were screened were unsuitable for implantation because of high defibrillation threshold, but it is unclear how many of them were assessed at the stage when the model 3000 device was in use (it has a maximum output of 3 J, as opposed to the 6 J of the model 3020). Therapy for clinical episodes of atrial fibrillation was delivered in 41 of the patients, and successful defibrillation of atrial fibrillation occurred in 96% of atrial fibrillation episodes. However, early recurrence of atrial fibrillation (ERAF), successful defibrillation but atrial fibrillation recurrence within a minute resulting in a clinical failure (Fig. 24-7), was seen in 27% of episodes and occurred in 51% of patients. Various strategies have been suggested for the prevention of ERAF, including the use of atropine, flecainide, beta blockers, amiodarone, and atrial or dual-chamber pacing. It is likely that prompt defibrillation can prevent ERAF because no electrical remodeling has occurred and electrophysiologic changes due to neurohumoral activation remain limited for a while. However, ERAF may also result from firing from an atrial focus, which is amenable to radiofrequency ablation (9). This procedure renders the patient free from atrial fibrillation and obviates the need for an atrioverter.

A mixture of complications were seen, including lead repositioning, atrial dislodgement, rises in the de-

TABLE 24-1 • SAFETY DATA FOR THE GUIDANT METRIX ATRIOVERTER

Data to April 28, 1997 (52 patients)[a]
   3,488 shocks (2,502 therapeutic, 521 spontaneous AF)
   No proarrhythmia (VT/VF >150/min for 30 seconds or needing intervention) occasional aberrant conduction
      Upper level of 95% confidence limit: 0.08% chance of proarrhythmia
   Shock synchronization: 198,000 R waves—no failures
      Upper level of 95% confidence limit: 0.0002% chance of fail to synchronize
Data to September 1999 (latest available)
   More than 11,000 shocks given
   No proarrhythmia seen
      Upper level 95% confidence limit; 0.03% risk/shock

AF, atrial fibrillation; VF, ventricular fibrillation; VT, ventricular tachycardia.
[a] In each case, the 95% confidence interval for the probability of device failure to syndronize or to cause proarrhythmia has been calculated

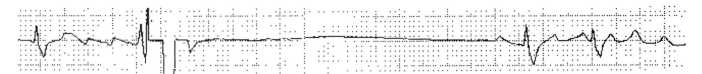

FIGURE 24-7. Early recurrence of atrial fibrillation (ERAF). The shock abolishes atrial activity, and a prolonged sinus pause is seen. There is a single sinus beat before atrial fibrillation restarts. ERAF has been a considerable problem in patients who receive an implantable atrial defibrillator but demonstrates much interpatient and interepisode variability.

fibrillation threshold, and a ventricular dislodgement that caused atrial fibrillation sensing difficulties, subclavian vein thrombosis (two patients), and implant-related infections (two patients). On the whole, the nature and level of complications were those that would be expected at the introduction of a new device, but of concern was an episode of cardiac tamponade that resulted from atrial perforation. With the benefit of hindsight, it was clear that the lead had dislodged and was free floating in the right atrium, but whether this was a chance occurrence or will prove to be a complication of multiple atrial defibrillations is unclear. Ten patients did not receive any shocks (five had no atrial fibrillation episodes, and five never attended hospital during episodes), but by the end of the study, all 47 patients who still had their devices implanted were in sinus rhythm.

The Dual-Chamber Defibrillators

An alternative approach to atrial defibrillators has been taken by another manufacturer. Jewel AF model 7250 (Medtronic, Inc., Minneapolis, MN) is a dual-chamber defibrillator that is also capable of delivering pacing therapies. It is marketed as an "arrhythmia management device."

Before discussing this device, it is worth considering whether atrial defibrillation coils are needed at all. A shock vector from the right ventricular apex to an active can or superior vena cava coil generates a defibrillation field encompassing both atria without greatly increasing the total volume of tissue to which energy is delivered. Although several modern ICDs have an atrial lead to allow sensing and pacing, the focus of this development has been on improving arrhythmia detection rather than clinical atrial defibrillation (40,41).

The Jewel AF can have a wide range of electrode arrangements, with defibrillation coils in the right ventricle, right atrium, and coronary sinus. The device can act as an active can, and subcutaneous patches can be incorporated. It is not envisaged that all be employed simultaneously. The 57-cc device provides a maximum shock energy of 27 J.

The arrhythmia detection is performed on a rather different basis than that employed in the stand-alone atrioverter. The Medtronic device can classify atrial fibrillation, atrial flutter or tachycardia, sinus and other 1:1 supraventricular tachycardias, ventricular tachycardia, ventricular fibrillation, and "dual" tachycardia and fibrillation (i.e., atrial and ventricular coexisting). Auto-adjusting atrial and ventricular sensing thresholds and short cross-chamber blanking periods are used to prevent undersensing. The RR interval is divided into four time zones. Atrial events during two successive RR intervals are used to generate interval codes representing the number and timing of P relative to R waves. The succession of interval codes defines the arrhythmia. The detection algorithms are employed in a hierarchic fashion to ensure that ventricular tachycardia and ventricular fibrillation detection always take precedence over other possible tachyarrhythmias (Figs. 24-8 and 24-9). Unlike the stand-alone atrioverter, the device has atrial pacing capabilities, including 50-Hz pacing (Fig. 24-10), that appear to have some value in the termination of early atrial fibrillation (42) (Table 24-2).

The device was initially used in patients with a conventional ICD indication coexistent with prior atrial fibrillation, but patients with atrial fibrillation alone are now being studied. Published data are not

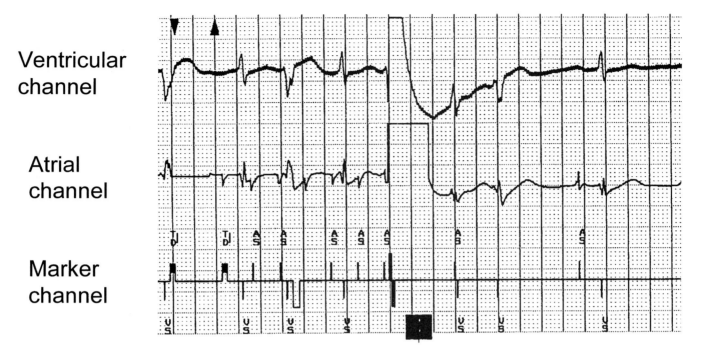

FIGURE 24-8. A stored electrogram from a Jewel AF shows a successful defibrillation of atrial fibrillation (AF) with an R-wave synchronous shock. The top line is the ventricular electrogram, and the middle one is the atrial electrogram. The marker channel shows all events detected outside blanking periods, along with the device interpretation of the event. AS, atrial sense; TD, tachycardia detect; VS, ventricle sense.

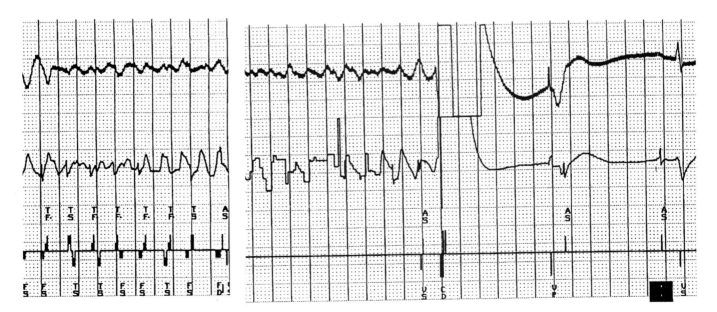

FIGURE 24-9. Simultaneous atrial (AF) and ventricular fibrillation (VF) in a patient with a Jewel AF. The VF is successfully treated by an 18-J shock, which also restores sinus rhythm to the atrium. AS, atrial sense; CD, capacitor discharge; FD, fibrillation detect; FS, fibrillation sense; TD, tachycardia detect; VP, ventricle pace; VS, ventricle sense.

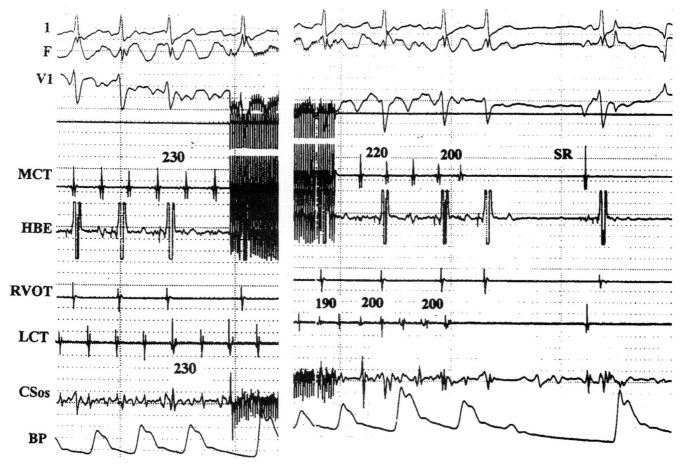

FIGURE 24-10. Termination of an atrial tachyarrhythmia by 50-Hz pacing during an invasive electrophysiologic study. Although the ventricular response is irregular, right atrial electrograms from the crista terminalis show a regular cycle length of 230 msec. The 50-Hz pacing results in acceleration of the atrial rhythm, which leads to arrhythmia termination just over 1 second later.

TABLE 24-2 • EFFICACY DATA FOR THE MEDTRONIC JEWEL AF 7250 FOR TREATING SPONTANEOUS EPISODES OF ATRIAL TACHYCARDIA AND TRIAL FIBRILLATION

Therapy	Atrial Tachycardia	Atrial Fibrillation
Antitachycardia pacing (ATP)	33/37 (89%)	Not applicable
50-Hz burst	22/95 (23%)	22/55 (40%)
Atrial shock	24/24 (100%)	139/151 (92%)

From Sulke N, Bailin SJ, Swerdlow CD, Investigators for WJA-O. Worldwide clinical experience with a dual-chamber implantable cardioverter defibrillator in patients with atrial fibrillation and flutter. *Eur Heart J* 1999;20:114, with permission.

yet available for this device at the time of writing, and impressions regarding the utility of the device are based on interim results and single-center experiences (42).

CONCLUSIONS

Atrial defibrillators have been extensively evaluated and are available for clinical use. The group of patients who benefit from the device is restricted (Table 24-3), but for many individuals, an atrioverter or dual-chamber defibrillator provides excellent therapy and improves quality of life. With the rapid advances in pacing, ablation, and drug therapy for atrial fibrillation, the precise role of implantable atrial defibrillators

TABLE 24-3 • PATIENTS CHARACTERISTICS RELEVANT TO SELECTION TO RECEIVE AN IMPLANTABLE ATRIAL DEFIBRILLATOR

Patient Characteristics	Atrioverter (Stand-alone Atrial Defibrillator)	Dual-Chamber Defibrillator
Normal heart or mild structural heart disease	+++	?
Significant structural heart disease	?	++
Documented ventricular arrhythmias	−	+++
Recurrent persistent atrial fibrilation	+++	
Long-duration paroxysmal atrial fibrillation	+	
Other patient characteristics	Intolerant of atrial fibrillation Capable of self-activating device Accepts defibrillation-associated discomfort (with or without buprenorphine or alternative analgesic strategy)	

is likely to evolve. In particular, the preventative atrial pacing strategies under evaluation will logically be incorporated into future devices.

REFERENCES

1. Lévy S, Lacombe P, Cointe R, Bru P. High energy transcatheter cardioversion of chronic atrial fibrillation. *J Am Coll Cardiol* 1988;12:514–518.
2. Wellens HJ, Lau CP, Luderitz B, et al. Atrioverter: an implantable device for the treatment of atrial fibrillation. *Circulation* 1998;98:1651–1546.
3. Haissaguerre M, Marcus FI, Fischer B, Clementy J. Radiofrequency catheter ablation in unusual mechanisms of atrial fibrillation: report of three cases. *J Cardiovasc Electrophysiol* 1994;5: 743–751.
4. Haissaguerre M, Jais P, Shah DC, et al. Spontaneous initiation of atrial fibrillation by ectopic beats originating in the pulmonary veins. *N Engl J Med* 1998;339:959–966.
5. Hwang C, Karagueuzian HS, Chen PS. Idiopathic paroxysmal atrial fibrillation induced by a focal discharge mechanism in the left superior pulmonary vein: possible roles of the ligament of Marshall. *J Cardiovasc Electrophysiol* 1999;10:636–648.
6. Chen SA, Hsieh MH, Tai CT, et al. Initiation of atrial fibrillation by ectopic beats originating from the pulmonary veins: electrophysiological characteristics, pharmacological responses, and effects of radiofrequency ablation. *Circulation* 1999;100: 1879–1886.
7. Chen SA, Tai CT, Yu WC, et al. Right atrial focal atrial fibrillation: electrophysiologic characteristics and radiofrequency catheter ablation. *J Cardiovasc Electrophysiol* 1999;10: 328–335.
8. Lau CP, Tse HF, Ayers GM. Defibrillation guided mapping and radiofrequency ablation of focal atrial fibrillation. *J Am Coll Cardiol* 1998;31[Suppl A]:61A.
9. Lau CP, Tse HF, Ayers GM. Defibrillation-guided radiofrequency ablation of atrial fibrillation secondary to an atrial focus. *J Am Coll Cardiol* 1999;33:1217–1226.
10. Waktare JE, Camm AJ. Atrial fibrillation begets trouble. *Heart* 1997;77:393–394.
11. Investigators S. Warfarin versus aspirin for prevention of thromboembolism in atrial fibrillation: Stroke Prevention in Atrial Fibrillation II study. *Lancet* 1994;343:687–691.
12. Petersen P, Boysen G, Godtfredsen J, et al. Placebo-controlled, randomised trial of warfarin and aspirin for prevention of thromboembolic complications in chronic atrial fibrillation: the Copenhagen AFASAK study. *Lancet* 1989;1:175–179.
13. Grogan M, Smith HC, Gersh BJ, Wood DL. Left ventricular dysfunction due to atrial fibrillation in patients initially believed to have idiopathic dilated cardiomyopathy. *Am J Cardiol* 1992; 69:1570–1573.
14. Van Den Berg MP, van Veldhuisen DJ, Crijns HJ, Lie KI. Reversion of tachycardiomyopathy after beta-blocker. *Lancet* 1993;341:1667.
15. Lundstrom T, Ryden L. Ventricular rate control and exercise performance in chronic atrial fibrillation: effects of diltiazem and verapamil. *J Am Coll Cardiol* 1990;16:86–90.
16. Wijffels MCEF, Kirchhof CJHJ, Dorland R, Allessie MA. Atrial fibrillation begets atrial fibrillation: a study in awake chronically instrumented goats. *Circulation* 1995;92: 1954–1968.
17. Sulke N, Kamalvand K, Tan K, et al. A prospective evaluation of recurrent atrial endocardial defibrillation in patients with refractory chronic atrial fibrillation and flutter. *Heart* 1996;75: 42A.
18. Timmermans C, Wellens HJJ. Effect of device-mediated therapy on symptomatic episodes of atrial fibrillation. *J Am Coll Cardiol* 1998;31:A331.
19. Rodriguez LM, Timmermans C, Wellens HJ. Are electrophysiological changes induced by longer lasting atrial fibrillation reversible? Observations using the atrial defibrillator. *Circulation* 1999;100:113–136.
20. Lown B, Perlroth MG, Kaidbey S, et al. "Cardioversion" of atrial fibrillation: a report on the treatment of 65 episodes in 50 patients. *N Engl J Med* 1963;269:325–331.
21. Morris JJJ, Peter RH, McIntosh HD. Electrical cardioversion of atrial fibrillation: immediate and long term results and selection of patients. *Ann Intern Med* 1966;65:216–231.
22. Dalzell GW, Anderson J, Adgey AA. Factors determining success and energy requirements for cardioversion of atrial fibrillation. *Q J Med* 1990;76:903–913.
23. Lévy S, Lauribe P, Dolla E, et al. A randomized comparison of external and internal cardioversion of chronic atrial fibrillation. *Circulation* 1992;86:1415–1420.
24. Mirowski M. Management of malignant ventricular tachyarrhythmias with automatic implanted cardioverter-defibrillators. *Mod Concepts Cardiovasc Dis* 1983;52:41–44.

25. Reid PR, Mirowski M, Mower MM, et al. Clinical evaluation of the internal automatic cardioverter-defibrillator in survivors of sudden cardiac death. *Am J Cardiol* 1983;51:1608–1613.
26. Nathan AW, Bexton RS, Spurrell RAJ, Camm AJ. Internal transvenous low energy cardioversion for the treatment of cardiac arrhythmias. *Br Heart J* 1984;52:377–384.
27. Cooper RA, Alferness CA, Smith WM, Ideker RE. Internal cardioversion of atrial fibrillation in sheep. *Circulation* 1993;87:1673–1686.
28. Sopher SM, Murgatroyd FD, Slade AK, et al. Low energy internal cardioversion of atrial fibrillation resistant to transthoracic shocks. *Heart* 1996;75:635–638.
29. Schmitt C, Alt E, Plewan A, et al. Low energy intracardiac cardioversion after failed conventional external cardioversion of atrial fibrillation. *J Am Coll Cardiol* 1996;28:994–999.
30. Morgan C. Advances in AED (automatic external defibrillator) technology. *JEMS J Emerg Med Serv* 1997;22:S12–S15.
31. Automated external defibrillators. *Health Devices* 1999;28:186–219.
32. Gliner BE, White RD. Electrocardiographic evaluation of defibrillation shocks delivered to out-of-hospital sudden cardiac arrest patients. *Resuscitation* 1999;41:133–144.
33. Gliner BE, Jorgenson DB, Poole JE, et al. Treatment of out-of-hospital cardiac arrest with a low-energy impedance-compensating biphasic waveform automatic external defibrillator: the LIFE Investigators. *Biomed Instrum Technol* 1998;32:631–644.
34. Oral H, Souza JJ, Michaud GF, et al. Facilitating transthoracic cardioversion of atrial fibrillation with ibutilide pretreatment. *N Engl J Med* 1999;340:1849–1854.
35. Boriani G, Biffi M, Capucci A, et al. Favorable effects of flecainide in transvenous internal cardioversion of atrial fibrillation. *J Am Coll Cardiol* 1999;33:333–341.
36. Murgatroyd FD, Slade AKB, Sopher SM, et al. Efficacy and tolerability of transvenous low energy cardioversion of paroxysmal atrial fibrillation in humans. *J Am Coll Cardiol* 1995;25:1347–1353.
37. Timmermans C, Rodriguez LM, Ayers GM, et al. Effect of butorphanol tartrate on shock-related discomfort during internal atrial defibrillation. *Circulation* 1999;99:1837–1842.
38. Ayers GM, Alferness CA, Ilina M, et al. Ventricular proarrhythmic effects of ventricular cycle length and shock strength in a sheep model of transvenous atrial defibrillation. *Circulation* 1994;89:413–422.
39. Timmermans C, Rodriguez LM, Ayers GM, et al. Design and preliminary data of the Metrix atrioverter expanded indication trial. *J Interv Card Electrophysiol* 2000;4[Suppl 1]:197–199.
40. Jung W, Wolpert C, Esmailzadeh B, et al. Long-term experience with the first dual-chamber implantable cardioverter-defibrillator. *Eur Heart J* 1997;18A.
41. Kouakam C, Klug D, Jarwé M, et al. Analysis of dual-chamber cardioverter-defibrillators electrograms for discrimination of ventricular from supraventricular tachycardia: implication for ICD specificity and programming. *Eur Heart J* 1999;20:115A.
42. From Sulke N, Bailin SJ, Swerdlow CD, Investigators for WJA-O. Worldwide clinical experience with a dual-chamber implantable cardioverter defibrillator in patients with atrial fibrillation and flutter. *Eur Heart J* 1999;20:114A.

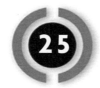

CLINICAL RESULTS WITH INVESTIGATIONAL IMPLANTABLE CARDIOVERTER-DEFIBRILLATORS
• • •

WERNER JUNG, BERNDT LÜDERITZ

Single-chamber ventricular defibrillator implantation has been shown to be an effective and safe treatment for patients with malignant ventricular tachyarrhythmias and to significantly reduce the incidence of sudden cardiac death. However, the high incidence of inappropriate implantable cardioverter-defibrillator (ICD) therapy due to supraventricular tachycardias (SVTs) is a major challenge that affects up to 25% of patients (1–2). Enhanced detection criteria such as rate stability, sudden onset, and morphology assessment improve the specificity of ICD therapy but may place the patient at risk of underdetection of ventricular tachycardia (3–8). It has been shown that algorithms using dual-chamber sensing can significantly improve differentiation between SVT and ventricular tachycardia (9–11). Another beneficial effect of dual-chamber ICD may be the opportunity to sense in the atrium and to pace in this chamber (12).

The overall prevalence of atrial fibrillation in the United States ranges from less than 1% in young, otherwise healthy individuals up to nearly 9% in elderly patients. Atrial fibrillation is a frequent and costly health care problem representing the most common arrhythmia resulting in hospital admission. Total mortality and cardiovascular mortality rates may be increased among patients with atrial fibrillation compared with controls. In addition to symptoms of palpitations, patients with atrial fibrillation have an increased risk of stroke and may develop decreased exercise tolerance and left ventricular dysfunction. All of these problems may be reversed with restoration and maintenance of sinus rhythm. Treatment of atrial fibrillation is warranted in hopes of eliminating symptoms, preventing complications, and possibly decreasing mortality associated with this commonly occurring arrhythmia. The high prevalence of atrial fibrillation and its clinical complications, the poor efficacy of medical therapy for preventing recurrences, and dissatisfaction with alternative modes of therapy stimulated interest in implantable atrial and combined atrioventricular (AV) defibrillators (13–19).

Congestive heart failure (CHF) is a syndrome that affects more than 3 million people in the United States, with 400,000 new cases diagnosed annually. Left ventricular dysfunction, reduced exercise tolerance, and ventricular arrhythmias accompany this condition. Prognosis is typically poor, with 1-year all-cause mortality rates of approximately 12% to 15%. The primary cause of death of these patients is typically pump failure from progressive heart failure or sudden death. The goals of therapy are to minimize symptoms, improve functional capacity, and increase survival. Multisite pacing has been explored as an alternative to conventional CHF drug therapy for improving hemodynamics by resynchronizing the ventricles in patients with intraventricular conduction delays. Preliminary findings suggest that acute hemodynamic improvement and increased functional capacity are possible with multisite pacing (20). It has been shown that the pacing location within the left ventricle is important for the best result and that midventricle to apex sites are preferred.

This chapter describes clinical experience with investigational ICDs providing dual-chamber detection algorithms for improved arrhythmia discrimination, prevention, tiered atrial detection and termination therapies, and biventricular pacing with ventricular defibrillation support.

⊙ DEFENDER DUAL-CHAMBER DEFIBRILLATOR

The Defender (ELA Medical, Montrouge, France) is a tiered-therapy dual-chamber ICD that provides dual-chamber sensing and pacing, antitachycardia pacing (ATP) modalities as well as low- and high-energy shock therapies (21). The Defender model 9001 and its successor model 9201 differ principally in size and weight, as well as in the function of their cans. The model 9001, with a weight of 230 g and a volume of 148 cc, has a passive housing and is used for implantation in an abdominal pocket, whereas the case of model 9201, with a weight of 140 g and a volume of 75 cc, serves as a defibrillation electrode and is intended for implantation in the pectoral region. To function properly, the model 9001 must be connected to at least two defibrillation leads and to one bipolar ventricular sensing and pacing lead. Adding a bipolar atrial lead to the system allows optimal functioning of the device because antibradycardia pacing and arrhythmia detection are performed in dual-chamber configuration. Because the active can of the model 9201 serves as a defibrillation electrode, this device must be connected to only one defibrillation lead and to a bipolar ventricular sensing and pacing lead as well as a bipolar atrial sensing and pacing lead. The following leads were proposed in the study: a ventricular lead for sensing, pacing, and defibrillation (model SL-ICD 60, Biotronik, Berlin, Germany) and an atrial lead for atrial sensing and pacing (model

Stela BS 45, ELA Medical, Montrouge, France). However, choice of the lead models and positioning of the leads were left to the discretion of the managing physician. Both ICD models offer an antibradycardia function that can be programmed in VVI, DDI, or DDD mode.

The Defender stores general quantitative information (i.e., statistics) concerning detected or paced events and number of delivered and successful tachycardia therapies since the last counter reset. More detailed information is also available in the Holter function that allows a complete review of the episode's mode of onset, evolution, and termination contained in 31-event log summaries of four selected tachyarrhythmia episodes. In general, the device stores the four most recent arrhythmia episodes. However, it can keep, in priority, the last episode of ventricular fibrillation, the last episode of ventricular tachycardia, and the last unsure or SVT episode. For each episode retained in the Holter memory, the device stores the time and date of the arrhythmia occurrence. It identifies the episode by storing the type of triggering rhythm. The device records a pre-AV and post-AV marker chain of 127 events each and an intracardiac pre-electrogram for a maximum duration of 3 to 4 seconds preceding the application of the first therapy and a post-electrogram for a maximum duration of six cycles after the device concluded that the applied therapy was successful.

PARAD Classification Algorithm

The Defender uses a sophisticated dual-chamber algorithm for tachyarrhythmia classification (9,22). A tiered arrhythmia detection analysis is performed in three consecutive steps: classification of ventricular cycles, majority rhythm identification, and persistence of rhythm. The device first classifies each ventricular cycle according to programmable cycle length criteria as ventricular fibrillation or ventricular tachycardia (Tachy) or slow rhythm (SR) cycle. Based on this cycle-to-cycle classification, the device applies the majority criterion (X% of Y cycles in a sliding window) to determine the predominant rhythm: ventricular fibrillation majority, Tachy majority, SR majority, or No majority. If the rhythm has been identified as Tachy majority, the device uses a new tachycardia sorting algorithm (PARAD) to differentiate among a sinus tachycardia; SVT including atrial fibrillation, atrial flutter, or atrial tachycardia; ventricular tachycardia; or unsure. Tachycardia sorting depends on the combination of three additional criteria: ventricular rate (RR) stability (stable or unstable), AV (PR) association (n : 1, 1 : 1, or none), and acceleration at the onset of the tachycardia (atrial origin, ventricular origin, or none). Therapy is applied only to sustained tachyarrhythmias, determined when the programmed number of cycles of the persistence counter is met.

The Defender uses the tachycardia sorting template to reclassify rhythms with Tachy majority into three categories: ventricular tachycardia (immediate therapy), SVT or sinus tachycardia (exempt from therapy), or unsure (deferred therapy). The Defender provides three predefined tachycardia sorting templates—rate only, standard V, and standard AV. The latter template takes into account all three criteria (i.e., RR stability, PR association, and acceleration) by using atrial and ventricular sensing together. In addition to the three standard templates, a "monitoring-only" device status can be selected without therapy delivery and a custom mode is available to the user that allows free programming of any combination of the recognition criteria. Table 25-1 summarizes the rhythm classification determined by the combination of these three criteria as a function of the three programmable standard tachycardia sorting templates.

The tachycardia recognition criteria are based on parameters programmed to X% of Y cycles in a sliding window. The Defender constructs a histogram of a programmable number of ventricular intervals and scans its RR interval histogram with a window set to the programmed RR stability window width (i.e., nominal setting of 63 msec). The stability criterion is fulfilled when the number of RR intervals contained in the window is equivalent to at least X% of Y cycles stored in the histogram. Only cycles faster than the ventricular tachycardia detection rate are considered for the calculation of the stability criterion. If the RR stability criterion is met, the device scans its PR interval histogram with a window set to the programmed PR association window width (i.e., nominal setting of 63 msec). It declares PR association when this number is at least X% of the number of stable RR intervals. If the number of PR intervals within this window represents at least X% of the cycles stored in the histogram, the device considers this as a 1 : 1 PR association. Otherwise, if X% of the number of stored PR intervals is not within the window, and it considers this as an N : 1 association. The device defines an accelerated cycle when its cycle length is shorter than the reference cycle (usually the preceding cycle) decreased by the programmed acceleration prematurity percentage (i.e., nominal setting of 25%) and when its cycle length is shorter than the programmed Tachy cycle length. Figure 25-1 depicts the tachycardia classification algorithm.

TABLE 25-1 • RHYTHM CLASSIFICATION ACCORDING TO PARAD PROGRAMMING

	Combination Of Criteria		PARAD Standard Programming		
RR Stability	PR Association	Acceleration	Std AV	Std V	Rate Only
Unstable	—	—	SVT/ST	SVT/ST	VT
Stable	N:1	Ventricular	SVT/ST	VT	VT
Stable	N:1	Atrial	SVT/ST	VT	VT
Stable	N:1	None	SVT/ST	SVT/ST	VT
Stable	1:1	Ventricular	VT	VT	VT
Stable	1:1	Atrial	SVT/ST	VT	VT
Stable	1:1	None	SVT/ST	SVT/ST	VT
Stable	None	Ventricular	VT	VT	VT
Stable	None	Atrial	VT	VT	VT
Stable	None	None	VT	SVT/ST	VT

AV, atrioventricular; SVT, supraventricular tachycardia; ST, sinus tachycardia; V, ventricle; VT, ventricular tachycardia.

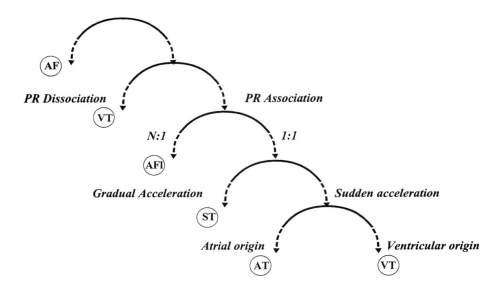

FIGURE 25-1. PARAD tachycardia classification algorithm programmed to the standard atrioventricular (AV) mode. The algorithm is based on ventricular stability (RR), AV association (PR), and atrial or ventricular acceleration. AF, atrial fibrillation; AFL, atrial flutter; AT, atrial tachycardia; ST, sinus tachycardia; VT, ventricular tachycardia.

Study Protocol

The criteria for inclusion in the study at the time of implantation were as follows: at least two consecutive successes at 23 J or less in the final lead configuration (providing a minimal defibrillation safety margin of 10 J), atrial and ventricular pacing thresholds of less than 2 V at a pulse duration of 0.37 msec, atrial sensing threshold of more than 0.5 mV obtained during sinus rhythm, and ventricular sensing threshold of more than 5 mV measured during sinus rhythm. If any of these implant criteria was not met, the lead system was repositioned. Determination of the defibrillation threshold was recommended, but not required. The ultimate decision to implant the ICD system was left to the investigator. This procedural flexibility allowed physicians to contend with the occasional patient who was not inducible into ventricular fibrillation or who deteriorated during the procedure before all testing could be completed. The ICD model 9001 was always implanted in an abdominal pocket because of its large size. The left subclavian or cephalic vein was preferentially used for lead insertion.

All parameters for pacing, detection, and therapies as well as the programming of the tachycardia classification algorithm were left to the discretion of the treating physician. However, in all cases when normal sinus activity was present and the P-wave sensing threshold was more than 2 mV, programming of the tachycardia classification algorithm in the standard AV mode was highly recommended. Patients were followed from the time of study entry to a common cutoff date of May 31, 1998 (for model 9001) or October 1, 1998 (for model 9201). Routine postimplantation evaluation and device interrogation was performed at predischarge, at 1 month, and every 3 months thereafter or whenever device therapy was experienced or in case of any adverse event. At prehospital discharge or at the 1-month follow-up visit, a noninvasive electrophysiologic study was highly recommended to assess the efficacy of pacing, sensing, and therapy of ventricular fibrillation and ventricular tachycardia, if applicable. However, postoperative electrophysiologic studies were not mandatory. Before hospital discharge, a 24-hour Holter recording was required to document the performance of the device, and a stress exercise test was suggested to evaluate the detection algorithm during a sinus tachycardia.

Results

Of the 128 patients eligible for therapy with a dual-chamber ICD, all patients received the device. In 95 patients, the Defender model 9001 was placed in an abdominal pocket. With the availability of the model 9201 by July 18, 1997, this smaller device was implanted in 33 patients, with most implanted in the pectoral region except for five replacements. Ninety-four patients (73%) received their first ICD system, and in 34 patients (27%), generator replacement was performed. Before the ICD insertion, 16 patients (13%) had a conventional antibradycardia pacemaker implanted that was removed at the time of ICD implantation. Overall, the final lead configuration consisted of a transvenous lead alone in 108 patients (87%), and 15 patients (12%) required a transvenous lead in conjunction with a subcutaneous patch electrode. Five patients (4%) had preexisting epicardial patch electrodes at the time of pulse generator replacement. Implantation duration ("skin-to-skin" time) was significantly shorter ($p < 0.001$) for pectoral implants (model 9201; average duration, 98 ± 34 minutes; range, 45 to 180 minutes) compared with abdominal implants (model 9001; average duration, 182 ± 64 minutes; range, 60 to 360 minutes). The mean hospital stay from the time of implantation to the predischarge evaluation was 6 ± 2 days (range, 2 to 12 days) for the model 9201 and 8 ± 3 days (range, 2 to 19 days) for the model 9001 ($p < 0.05$).

Of the 128 patients eligible for a dual-chamber ICD implantation, 4 patients (3%) with the model 9001 did not meet the required defibrillation implantation criterion, successful termination of ventricular fibrillation twice with consecutive 23-J or lower-energy shocks. Nevertheless, the treating physician decided to implant the Defender model 9001. In all patients, termination of induced ventricular fibrillation could be confirmed at least once at the maximum energy output of the implanted device. The clinical characteristics of these four patients did not differ significantly from the patients who received the dual-chamber ICD with respect to age, gender, type of structural heart disease, index arrhythmia, heart failure class, but they did have a lower mean left ventricular ejection fraction (0.27 ± 0.10, $p < 0.05$). At the last follow-up visit, 77% of the devices were programmed in DDD mode, 13% in DDI mode, and 10% in VVI mode. At the end of the study, device interrogation revealed that the predominant rhythm was dual-chamber pacing in 36% of the patients, atrial paced rhythm in 8%, and atrial tracking in 15%. In the remaining patients (41%), there was a predominant intrinsic rhythm.

Arrhythmia Detection and Therapy

The average follow-up period was 16 ± 9 months (range, 0 to 41 months), representing 1,990 device-months. During this follow-up, a total of 1,032 spontaneous tachycardia events among 84 patients (65%) were retrieved from the Holter memories of the devices: 555 confirmed ventricular tachycardia or ventricular fibrillation, 464 confirmed SVT or sinus tachycardia, 8 undetermined episodes, and 5 artifact episodes. Of these 1,032 tachycardia events, 555 were confirmed by the investigators to be ventricular fibrillation or ventricular flutter ($n = 59$ episodes; mean heart rate of 251 ± 49 bpm [range, 183 to 385 bpm]) in 22 patients (17%) or ventricular tachycardia ($n = 496$ episodes; mean heart rate of 167 ± 36 bpm [range, 101 to 319 bpm]) in 55 patients (43%). Thirty-three of the ventricular fibrillation episodes were not treated because they spontaneously ended within 4 seconds. Of the 496 ventricular tachycardia episodes, 129 were not treated mainly because they lasted less than 12 seconds.

ICD therapy was effective in 100% of documented episodes. Twenty-four episodes (92%) of ventricular fibrillation were terminated by a single high-energy shock, and two required additional device discharges. ATP restored sinus rhythm in 248 (84%) of 295 treated episodes of ventricular tachycardia, and cardioversion was successful in the remaining episodes. Pacing-induced acceleration of ventricular tachycardia was observed in eight instances (3%). Shocks were delivered as first therapy in 72 episodes of ventricular tachycardia, with a 95% termination rate by a single shock. Of the 367 treated episodes of confirmed ventricular tachycardia, 31 (8%) were dual tachycardias, consisting mainly of ventricular tachycardia and atrial fibrillation; all were correctly detected and successfully treated.

During follow-up, 464 episodes were classified by the investigators as confirmed SVTs. There were 300 episodes of sinus tachycardia at a mean rate of 126 ± 18 bpm (range, 101 to 183 bpm) among 41 patients (32%), who experienced an average of 7 ± 7 episodes (range, 1 to 34 episodes) and 164 episodes of SVT at a mean rate 163 ± 26 bpm (range, 101 to 226 bpm) among 37 patients (29%) who experienced an average of 3.2 ± 4 episodes (range, 1 to 18 episodes).

Sensitivity and Specificity

The mean cutoff rate for the ventricular tachycardia and ventricular fibrillation detection zones was programmed to 134 ± 25 bpm (range, 101 to 202 bpm) and 194 ± 17 bpm (range, 137 to 240 bpm), respectively. Of 1,032 spontaneous events, 199 among 47 patients (37%) were detected within the ventricular fibrillation zone, and 833 among 78 patients (61%) were detected within the tachycardia zone. Unnecessary therapy was delivered to 4 patients for five confirmed SVT episodes detected within the ventricular fibrillation zone. Five spurious episodes in 4 patients (3%) were detected and treated within the ventricular fibrillation zone for miscellaneous reasons, including sensing of ventricular noise because of lead fracture or dislodgement or electromagnetic interference due to electrocautery. In 8 (1%) of the 833 detected tachycardia events, the origin of the tachycardias could not be decisively classified by consensus of the tachycardia event committee and were excluded from further analysis. In 68 (8%) of the remaining 824 episodes, the atrial signal was absent, and these episodes were also excluded from analysis. Causes of permanent atrial undersensing included transition to permanent atrial fibrillation in one patient and loss of atrial signal without evidence of lead dislodgment in three patients. In nine other patients, proper atrial sensing could be restored by repositioning a dislodged atrial lead in three and reprogramming of the atrial sensitivity in six patients. Nine episodes of nonsustained unstable ventricular tachycardia that spontaneously ended in less than 12 seconds (average duration, 8.7 ± 3.2 seconds) were excluded from the analysis of sensitivity because the PARAD algorithm is not designed to treat unstable ventricular arrhythmias known to self-terminate or, if sustained, to evolve toward ventricular fibrillation.

Analysis of the sensitivity and specificity of the PARAD algorithm was based on the remaining 748 episodes detected within the tachycardia zone (23). An overall sensitivity of 99.1% was reached. Three episodes of ventricular tachycardia in three patients (2.3%) were inappropriately identified by the device. One ventricular tachycardia episode with 1 : 1 AV association started at a rate of 132 bpm, below the programmed rate cutoff of 154 bpm, and accelerated to 202 bpm. Sinus rhythm returned within 12 seconds. In this case, the acceleration criterion was not met because the acceleration occurred below the programmed tachycardia detection rate. A simulation test confirmed that a lower programmed tachycardia detection rate would have fulfilled the acceleration criterion. Another episode of ventricular tachycardia with a 1 : 1 AV association started at 120 bpm and accelerated to 142 bpm. The intrinsic sinus rate immediately before the onset of ventricular tachycardia was 100 bpm. In this case, the acceleration criterion programmed to a nominal setting of 25% was not met. This hemodynamically well-tolerated episode was treated by manual reprogramming of the ICD 15 minutes later. The third ventricular tachycardia episode was without AV association but with VA cross-talk, causing spurious 1 : 1 AV association detection. The rate of the ventricular tachycardia was hovering about the programmed tachycardia detection rate of 132 bpm. In this case, the acceleration criterion was lost because some of the cycles were below the programmed rate cutoff. In the absence of VA cross-talk, the rhythm would have been properly detected and treated. The ventricular tachycardia slowed below the rate cutoff within 2 minutes and later ended spontaneously.

The overall specificity was 92.9%. Limiting the analysis to episodes occurring during standard AV mode programming yielded a specificity of 90%. Inappropriate ICD therapy was delivered to 9 patients (7%) for 29 of 411 documented SVT or sinus tachycardia episodes detected within the tachycardia zone. One patient developed transient loss of atrial sensing while exercising, resulting in ATP without adverse consequences. In another patient, atrial tachycardia with 1 : 1 AV association was preceded by a premature ventricular beat. This episode was interpreted by the algorithm as stable, with 1 : 1 AV association and with ventricular acceleration, triggering the delivery of uncomplicated ATP. The remaining tachycardias consisted of one episode of atrial flutter and 25 episodes of atrial fibrillation among the nine patients. In each episode, the device interpreted the rhythm as stable and dissociated and therefore delivered therapy. In 23 episodes, ATP was delivered without complications. Four patients experienced inappropriate shocks for nine episodes as initial therapy or after ATP attempts. Sinus rhythm was restored in each instance.

VENTAK PRIZM DR DUAL-CHAMBER DEFIBRILLATOR

The VENTAK PRIZM DR (Guidant Corp., St. Paul, MN), with a volume of 39 cc and a weight of 98 g, is a downsized version of the VENTAK AV III (58 cc and 115 g) and is based on the same technical platform as the VENTAK AV III, which has been clinically evaluated in Europe and the United States. It contains a DR pacemaker for sensing and stimulation in the atrium and ventricle of the heart and a sensor for automatic adjustment of the heart rate under physical stress. The VENTAK PRIZM offers enhanced detection criteria for arrhythmia classification that allows for improved discrimination between ventricular tachycardia and SVT. The new detection enhancements may be programmed as therapy inhibitors, inhibitor overrides, and therapy accelerators (24). A therapy inhibitor causes a therapy to be delayed or inhibited if certain enhancement criteria are not satisfied at the end of the duration. *Onset* can be programmed to inhibit therapy if the patient's heart rate increases gradually. The *stability* parameter can be programmed to inhibit therapy if the ventricular rate is unstable. The *AFib Rate Threshold* and corresponding *AFib Stability* criterion can be programmed to inhibit ventricular therapy if the atrial rhythm is fast and the ventricular rate is unstable. An inhibitor override causes the therapy inhibitors to be bypassed if certain criteria are satisfied. The $V_{rate} > A_{rate}$ criterion can be used to override the therapy inhibitors, onset and stability, if the ventricular rate is faster than the atrial rate. The *sustained rate duration* parameter enables the pulse generator to override the therapy inhibitors, onset and stability, if the high rate continues over an extended period. A therapy "accelerator" accelerates the sequence of a therapy by skipping over or interrupting an antitachycardia scheme to initiate charging for the first programmed shock for the rate zone. The stability parameter can be programmed to accelerate delivery of shock therapy if the rhythm is declared to be unstable. The atrial rate may be used to inhibit therapy in the presence of atrial fibrillation and to bypass onset or stability as inhibitors if the ventricular rate is faster than the atrial rate. Table 25-2 shows detection enhancements that may be programmed in multizone configurations.

The multiple improvements implemented in the VENTAK PRIZM are expected to improve management of the device by the physician including noninvasive determination of the shocking lead impedance, the improvement of the detection algorithm for the differentiation between atrial and ventricular tachyarrhythmias, greatly enhanced user interface of the

TABLE 25-2 • DETECTION ENHANCEMENTS IN MULTIZONE CONFIGURATIONS OF VENTAK PRIZM DR

One-zone configuration		
Ventricular fibrillation		
No detection enhancements		
Two-zone configuration[a]		
Ventricular tachycardia	Ventricular fibrillation	
Onset		
Stability as an inhibitor	No detection enhancements	
Sustained rate duration		
Afib rate/AFib stability		
V rate > A rate or stability as an accelerator		
Three-zone configuration[a]		
Ventricular tachycardia-1	Ventricular tachycardia	Ventricular fibrillation
Onset		
Stability as an inhibitor	Stability as an accelerator	No detection enhancements
Sustained rate duration		
AFib rate/AFib stability		
V rate > A rate		

[a] Stability analysis cannot be programmed as an inhibitor and an accelerator in the same zone.

programmer and the addition of multiple special functions to facilitate the management of bradyarrhythmias. The atrial blanking period as well as the AFib Rate Threshold is programmable in the VENTAK PRIZM.

Study Protocol

The primary objective of the prospective, multicenter, randomized study was to document the appropriate performance of the system. The secondary objective was to compare the incidence of spontaneous episodes by randomizing patients to a programmed atrial blanking period of 45 or 85 msec. The goal of the randomization was to verify whether the atrial blanking period can be freely programmed in all patients implanted with the VENTAK PRIZM DR. The recruitment period was scheduled to start in the autumn of 2000. A minimum of 30 patients will be followed through to hospital discharge and then assessed at 1 and 3 months after discharge.

Results

Because the VENTAK PRIZM has the same detection, therapies, diagnostics, and electrophysiologic testing features as the VENTAK AV II DR system, the VENTAK AV II DR study was used to support the VENTAK PRIZM system. The VENTAK AV II DR was compared with a commercially available ICD (VENTAK AV) in an acute (nonimplant) paired study of 27 patients. An observational study of 52 patients implanted with the VENTAK AV II DR device was conducted. In the acute study, 27 patients (mean age, 69 years) with a mean left ventricular ejection fraction of 34% were enrolled in five centers of the United States. The acute study was performed in the operating room or in the electrophysiology laboratory without implanting the device. The mean ventricular fibrillation detection time for patients with inducible ventricular fibrillation was 2.86 ± 1.87 seconds using the VENTAK AV II DR and was not statistically different to the mean ventricular fibrillation detection time (2.35 ± 1.03 seconds) obtained in the patients using the VENTAK AV device.

In the observational study, 52 patients (mean age, 60 years) were enrolled in 18 European centers. Patients underwent standard ICD implantation procedure and were evaluated at predischarge and at 1 and 3 months after implantation. At the 1-month follow-up visit, an exercise test consisting of a 6-minute brisk walk or 6 minutes of stair climbing was required for all patients included in the study if the accelerometer sensor was programmed 'ON.' The purpose of the exercise test was to verify that there was an adequate rate response of the sensor under exercise conditions. After the test, the device was interrogated to verify if the rate response during activity functioned according to the patient need. If the rate response was insufficient, the trending function was used to optimize the sensor settings. In this study, all patients were implanted in a lead-alone configuration. The mean defibrillation threshold (DFT) for 26 patients tested with a step-down DFT protocol was 10.3 J. During a mean follow-up of 3.03 months, a total of 432 episodes of ventricular arrhythmias were treated, including 112 spontaneous and 320 induced episodes. Forty patients had the sensor programmed on and performed an exercise test. Nominal settings were appropriate for 80% of the patients tested. In all cases, the physician was able to program appropriate adaptive-rate settings to accommodate patient's needs.

● METRIX STAND-ALONE IMPLANTABLE ATRIAL DEFIBRILLATOR

A stand-alone implantable atrial defibrillator, the Metrix Atrioverter System (model 3000 and 3020, InControl Inc., Redmond, WA), has entered clinical investigation (13–15). The Metrix models 3000 and its successor 3020 differ principally in their maximum energy output: 3 J for the Metrix 3000 and 6 J for the Metrix 3020. Both deliver a biphasic, truncated exponential waveform of 3/3- and 6/6-msec duration, respectively, which accounts for the increased energy output of the model 3020. The device, with a weight of 79 g and a volume of 53 cc, is intended for implantation in the pectoral region like a conventional antibradycardia pacemaker. The model 3020 was introduced primarily because of the higher energy output. Graded shock therapy is available for up to 8 shocks (2 at each level) for each episode of atrial fibrillation. Biphasic shocks are programmable in 20-V increments up to 300 V. Atrial defibrillation is accomplished by a shock delivered between electrodes in the right atrium and the coronary sinus. The right atrial lead has an active fixation in the right atrium. The coronary sinus lead has a natural spiral configuration for retention in the coronary sinus and can be straightened with a stylet. Both leads are 7 Fr in diameter, and the defibrillation coils are each 6 cm long. The electrodes may be placed using separate leads or, in the near future, by using a single bipolar lead. A separate bipolar right ventricular lead is used for R-wave synchronization and postshock pacing. The Metrix defibrillator can be used to induce atrial fibrillation by using R-wave synchronous shocks and can store intracardiac electrograms for up to 2 minutes from the most recent six atrial fibrillation episodes (Fig. 25-2). The device can be programmed into one of the following operating modes: fully automatic, patient activated, monitor mode, bradycardia pacing only, and 'OFF.' Because atrial fibrillation is not life threatening, in the automatic mode, the device is only intermittently active in detecting and treating atrial fibrillation, and this "sleep-wake" cycle interval is programmable. At the end of the interval, it "awakens" and runs its detection algorithm. If atrial fibrillation is not detected it returns to the "sleep" mode for another cycle. The sleep mode significantly reduces energy consumption and prolongs device life. The patient activated mode differs from the automatic mode in that the device awakens only when a magnet is placed briefly over it. This allows the patient to control when the device is able to deliver therapy yet does not allow the patient to initiate a shock in the absence of atrial fibrillation.

The device employs extensive processing for detection and R-wave synchronization (13,14). The detection algorithms are run "off line" on digitally recorded, multichannel electrogram data. These data are first evaluated for integrity and quality, and the gains and sensitivities are set automatically. Two detection algorithms are run in series. The first algorithm, *Quiet Interval analysis*, is used to discriminate between a sinus and a nonsinus rhythm in the 8-second electrogram segment (Fig. 25-3). The second algorithm, the *Baseline Crossing* test, is invoked to detect atrial fibrillation (Fig. 25-4). This algorithm looks for electrical activity during parts of the cardiac cycle that are quiescent during sinus rhythm and most atrial arrhythmias, although not during atrial fibrillation when atrial activity is random and unrelated to the cardiac cycle. The *Quiet Interval* algorithm is very sensitive for detection of atrial fibrillation and highly specific for sinus rhythm. The *Baseline Crossing* algorithm is highly specific for atrial fibrillation. The result is a highly sensitive and extremely specific detector for

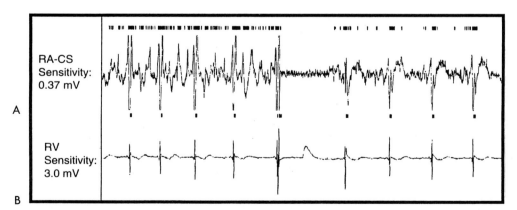

FIGURE 25-2. Stored electrogram of a successful conversion of atrial fibrillation with the automatic implantable atrial defibrillator. Sinus rhythm is restored by application of an internal automatic shock. **A:** Recordings of the intracardiac electrograms with their corresponding markers between a right atrial (RA) and a coronary sinus (CS) electrode using a sensitivity of 0.37 mV. **B:** Recordings of the right ventricular bipolar lead and marker signals with a sensitivity of 3.0 mV.

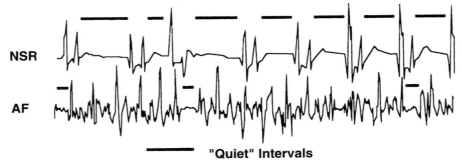

FIGURE 25-3. The first stage of the atrial fibrillation (AF) detection algorithm is the *Quiet Interval* test. It is highly specific for normal sinus rhythm (NSR). It scans the electrogram looking for periods when the atrial electrogram voltage is continuously at baseline for a minimum interval. Only NSR produces such periods. If the percentage of time spent at baseline exceeds a threshold, the algorithm classifies the rhythm as normal, and the detection process is terminated.

atrial fibrillation. The Metrix device uses a dual-channel synchronization algorithm (13,14). The objective of this algorithm is to be highly specific with little concern for sensitivity. It selects only R waves but may reject many as unsuitable even though they appear normal to casual inspection. The algorithm is designed to ensure that all shocks are delivered only to correctly synchronized R waves. Before synchronization is attempted, two electrograms are evaluated simultaneously in real time for integrity and data quality.

Study Protocol

In the phase I study, 51 patients from 19 centers in nine countries were enrolled. Patients had to meet the following inclusion criteria: prior episodes of atrial fibrillation that had spontaneously terminated or been converted to normal sinus rhythm with intervals of recurrence between 1 week and 3 months and treatment with at least one class I or III antiarrhythmic drug that proved ineffective or was not tolerated because of side effects. Preimplantation testing was per-

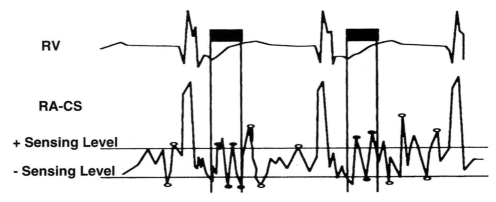

FIGURE 25-4. The second stage of the atrial fibrillation (AF) detection algorithm is the *Baseline Crossing* test. It is highly specific for AF. The algorithm looks for the number of times the electrogram crosses the voltage threshold *(Sensing Level)* in a window of time during the cardiac cycle. This window is synchronized to the R wave and positioned at a time in the cardiac cycle when atrial activity should be absent in rhythms other than AF. RA-CS, right atrium–coronary sinus electrogram; RV, right ventricular electrogram.

formed using designated temporary catheters. The purpose of this testing was to ensure that the atrial defibrillation level obtained was suitable for implantation of the device. Three endocardial catheters were positioned in the coronary sinus, the right atrium, and the apex of the right ventricle. Biphasic shocks were delivered between the catheters placed in the coronary sinus and the right atrium (Fig. 25-5). All leads were connected to the defibrillation system analyzer. Atrial fibrillation detection and synchronization tests were performed during sinus rhythm and during atrial fibrillation. Induction of atrial fibrillation was attempted by synchronized low-intensity shocks from the device or by rapid atrial pacing with the use of a separate catheter. To be eligible for implantation, two successes at 240 V had to be obtained during testing. Later, when the model 3020 became available, the implantation criterion was revised to allow one success in three attempts at 260 V for model 3000 and 240 V for model 3020.

At implantation, two of four successes at 240 V had to be attained at the final lead configuration. The atrial defibrillation threshold (ADFT) was determined starting with a 180-V shock. The shock intensity was increased in 20-V steps until successful defibrillation was achieved. After this initial success, atrial fibrillation was reinduced, and a shock 20 V less than the previously successful shock was delivered. Thereafter, the shock intensity was decreased in 20-V steps until a shock was delivered that failed to convert atrial fibrillation despite the delivery of two shocks at this intensity. Shocks were then delivered at 20-V steps of increasing intensity until atrial fibrillation was successfully converted with the delivery of two shocks at this intensity. To meet the implantation criterion, the ADFT had to be 240 V or less. Patients who did not meet the required implantation criterion did not undergo device implantation. Automatic mode operation, which consisted of atrial fibrillation detection, capacitor charge, atrial fibrillation redetection, syn-

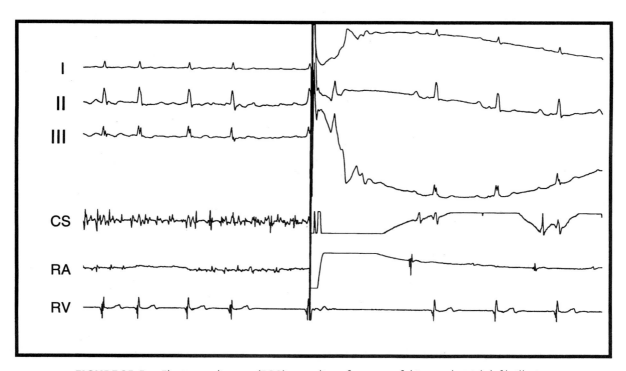

FIGURE 25-5. Electrocardiogram (ECG) recording of a successful internal atrial defibrillation. After delivery of a 2-J shock, atrial fibrillation (AF) is immediately converted to sinus rhythm. Shown is the surface ECG with leads I, II, and III and three intracardiac electrogram recordings from the coronary sinus (CS), right atrial appendage (RAA), and right ventricular apex (RVA).

chronization, shock delivery, and postshock pacing (if needed), was examined during the implantation procedure.

Postimplantation evaluation, including atrial fibrillation detection and R wave synchronization tests, was performed at predischarge, at 1, 3, and 6 months, and thereafter at 6-month intervals until completion of the study. Long-term ADFT testing was repeated at the 3-month follow-up visit. Device interrogation was performed at each follow-up visit. Specific electrophysiologic studies after device implantation were not mandatory. During the course of the study, no uniform programming of the shock intensities was required. It was highly recommended to program all shocks to the maximum output of the device or at least well above the ADFT obtained at the time of implantation. However, programming of the shock intensity for the first shock and for all remaining shock therapies was ultimately left to the discretion of the implanting physician. Some of the physicians preferred programming the first-shock intensity at the ADFT to allow for further investigation of the function of the device under controlled conditions.

Results

The first Metrix atrial defibrillator was implanted on October 30, 1995, and two other devices were implanted on November 7 and 10, 1995. Initial clinical experience with these three human implants has been reported elsewhere (25). In April 1996, the phase I Metrix multicenter clinical trial was started. The primary objective of this clinical study was to evaluate the device safety in terms of appropriate shock synchronization to avoid shock induced ventricular proarrhythmia. The secondary end point was to assess efficacy in detecting and terminating atrial fibrillation. As of May 1997, a total of 51 Metrix systems had been implanted as part of the phase I multicenter clinical trial (Fig. 25-6). Results of this phase I clinical trial have been published (26). These 51 patients were selected from 119 patients undergoing a screening test procedure. Of 50 patients screened, 17 received the model 3000, and 34 of 69 screened patients received the model 3020. Of the failed screenings, 43 were caused by high ADFTs. The remaining patients did

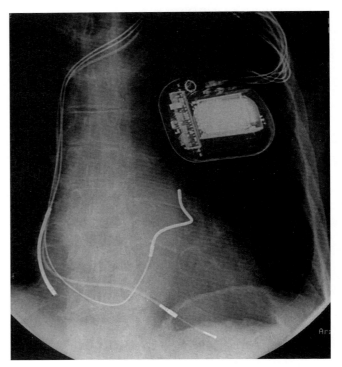

FIGURE 25-6. Posteroanterior chest radiograph of the implanted Metrix system. The pulse generator is implanted subpectorally in the left pectoral region and combined with an active fixation lead placed in the right atrium, a passive fixation lead advanced deep in the coronary sinus, and a conventional bipolar lead positioned in the right ventricle for proper R-wave synchronization and postshock VVI pacing.

not proceed to implantation because of a physician's or patient's decision or because of enrollment exclusions. In all patients eligible for device implantation, the coronary sinus lead could be properly placed. During phase I of this study, the device was programmed in the monitor mode, and shock therapy was delivered only by a physician in the hospital under controlled conditions.

Safety

A total of 3,719 shocks were delivered for atrial fibrillation induction, atrial defibrillation, testing, or termination of spontaneous atrial fibrillation episodes. Of these 3,719 shocks, 3,049 were delivered during testing, and 670 were delivered for treatment of spontaneous episodes of atrial fibrillation. Of the shocks delivered during testing, 1,065 were induction shocks, and 1,984 were therapeutic shocks. All shocks for spontaneous episodes were given during physician observation. There were no reported cases of induction of ventricular arrhythmias or inaccurately synchronized shocks during the study. A total of 242,435 R waves from 51 patients were analyzed for correct R-wave synchronization; 71,665 were obtained during sinus rhythm, and 170,770 were obtained during atrial fibrillation or atrial flutter; and 119,241 of the 242,435 R waves were marked as appropriate for shock delivery, 58,420 during sinus rhythm and 60,821 during atrial fibrillation. Correct synchronization was observed for all of the marked R waves. The accuracy of synchronization was 100% during sinus rhythm and atrial fibrillation or atrial flutter. A total of 2,240 tests of the detection algorithm were performed: 1,062 in sinus rhythm and 1,178 in atrial fibrillation; 1,069 of those obtained during atrial fibrillation or atrial flutter were true positives, and 109 were false negatives. Discrete atrial signals consistent with atrial flutter was the main reason for most false-negative detections. Of the 1,062 atrial fibrillation detections performed during sinus rhythm, there were no false-positive detections of atrial fibrillation. Analysis of the atrial fibrillation detection algorithm performance during observed operation revealed a 100% specificity for the recognition of sinus rhythm and 92.3% sensitivity for the detection of atrial fibrillation. From the same data, the positive predictive value of the atrial fibrillation detection algorithm was 100%, and the negative predictive value was 92.6%.

Frequency and Duration of Atrial Fibrillation Episodes

One or more valid monitoring periods were available from 46 of 51 patients, but one patient was excluded from further analysis because this patient had problems with detection since the time of implantation. The remaining five patients had no recorded detections of atrial fibrillation in the memory of their device during a mean follow-up of 164 ± 112 days. Five patients with a total of 29 episodes documented in the device memory did not seek therapy treatment for any of these episodes. The remaining 41 patients experienced 231 episodes of atrial fibrillation, with 190 of them falling within a valid monitoring period, defined as the time between interrogations of the device when a printout of the interrogation was made, and the device memory did not overflow because of too many individual atrial fibrillation detections during this interrogation period (>170 individual atrial fibrillation detections). A total of 1,161 valid episodes of atrial fibrillation were obtained from 45 patients during a mean follow-up period of 260 ± 144 days (average recurrence rate: 3.9 ± 5.0 episodes/patient-month). The median duration of the 190 treated episodes falling within a valid monitoring period was 17.6 hours and was 3 hours for the 971 nontreated episodes. Of the 190 treated episodes, 28% were about 8 hours long, compared with 78% of the nontreated episodes. These findings show that some patients have episodes of long duration requiring device treatment and short or asymptomatic episodes that are well tolerated or may even be ignored (27).

Efficacy

Forty-one of the 51 patients had a total of 231 spontaneous episodes of atrial fibrillation that were treated with device therapy (average, 5.6 episode per patient; range, 1 to 26 episodes). The mean follow-up duration for these 41 patients was 271 ± 144 days, or approximately 9 months. Because 4 of the 231 episodes were used for DFT testing, these episodes were excluded from further analysis. A total of 670 shocks were delivered for the treatment of the remaining 227 episodes, an average of three shocks per episode. For 1 of the 227 episodes of atrial fibrillation, a single 240-V shock was delivered and failed to convert atrial fibrillation. The episode converted spontaneously before the delivery of additional shock therapy, and therefore this episode was excluded from the calculation of efficacy. After shock delivery, 95.6% of the episodes were terminated. Of the 10 episodes that did not convert with device therapy, seven converted spontaneously, two were chemically cardioverted, and one was converted with external cardioversion after antiarrhythmic drug pretreatment. Atrial fibrillation recurred within 4 minutes after successful defibrillation during the treatment of 62 episodes (27%) observed in 51% of patients. Return of stable sinus rhythm with device therapy was prevented for 26 of the episodes. Six of these episodes were chemically converted before additional shock delivery (and were therefore excluded from the analysis), one was converted with external cardioversion, and 19 were allowed to convert spontaneously at a later time. Considering only those episodes for which sustained sinus rhythm was restored, the clinical efficacy of the defibrillation therapy for these spontaneous episodes was 86.3%.

Shock Tolerability

The use of sedation preceding shock delivery was left to the discretion of the treating physician in conference with the patient. No effort was undertaken to systematically collect data on patient tolerance of shock therapy and acceptability of the device during phase I of the study. Marked variability in shock tolerance between patients was reported by investigators. The interinstitutional variability in the level of sedation used made it impossible to address shock tolerance issue in detail. Specific quality of life questionnaires were not completed by the patients during phase I of the study but are one of the goals of a still ongoing study in the United States.

Complications

Two patients with the device implanted had subclavian vein thrombosis. One patient was treated successfully with urokinase. In five patients, the implantable atrial defibrillator was removed: two patients had infections, one patient developed cardiac tamponade because of a dislodged and penetrating atrial lead, one patient had frequent episodes of atrial fibrillation requiring His bundle ablation, and in one patient, early battery depletion caused telemetry loss. In six patients, lead repositioning procedures were necessary because of one atrial lead dislocation, three cases of an acute increase in defibrillation energy requirements, one case of a coronary sinus lead implanted in a small accessory coronary sinus vein and causing chest pain, and one right ventricular lead dislodgement, resulting in a change in signal quality, thus inhibiting appropriate shock delivery. No dislodgement of the coronary sinus lead was documented at completion of the study. The complications observed were mostly related to the use of intracardiac catheters and the implantation of a device, such as the necessity to reposition the lead (six patients), infection (two patients), and telemetry loss due to early battery depletion (one patient). A serious complication, atrial perforation with cardiac tamponade, occurred in one patient. In retrospect, inappropriate fixation of the atrial lead seems to be the explanation for this complication. The relatively high complication rate is probably related to the learning curve for using the device but may also be caused by its use in 19 centers with different techniques, practices, and levels of experience. This information resembles the early implantable ventricular defibrillator experience. Future improvements in technology may help to overcome most of the lead- and device-related problems observed with the first-generation systems.

Out of Hospital Treatment

As of October 1998, more than 200 Metrix systems had been implanted worldwide (28–30). Safety and efficacy data are available for the first 186 implants. Most Metrix patients have presented at implantation as highly symptomatic and refractory to or intolerant to conventional medical management. Many have experienced external cardioversion one or more times. Most patients implanted with the Metrix atrial defibrillator presented with a relatively healthy cardiovascular history. On average, this patient population has proven refractory to medical therapy for atrial fibrillation, which at presentation ranged from paroxysmal to long-standing and persistent. In general, the study has excluded patients whose atrial fibrillation episode frequency was greater than once per week or less than once per 3 months. Because atrial fibrillation is not acutely life threatening, it need not be treated immediately on detection. Unlike an implantable ventricular defibrillator, the Metrix system is designed to be highly specific and conservative in its detection and treatment decisions. In more than 3,300 atrial fibrillation detection tests, the "mirror" detection algorithm exhibited 100% specificity with a sensitivity of 90.8% using default values. No inappropriate shocks have been delivered. Of a total of 336,587 analyzed R waves, about one third (170,295) have been marked as suitable for potential shock delivery. Of 8,358 shocks delivered, no ventricular proarrhythmia or stroke has been observed. There has been no dislodgement of the coronary sinus lead. This lead plays a critical role in enhancing atrial fibrillation detection and lowering conversion energies. The number of shocks delivered per atrial fibrillation episode is 2.4 in the ongoing study versus 3.0 in the phase I clinical study. The conversion to sinus rhythm and the clinical success rates are similar in both studies, with electrical success rates of 93% and 96% and clinical efficacy rates of 84% and 86%, respectively.

Patient-Activated Mode

The Metrix system provides a programmable, patient-controlled mode. As of August 1998, 57 patients had their Metrix devices programmed to this mode. This treatment option enabled these patients to deliver therapy whenever and wherever it was appropriate and convenient for them. The 267 spontaneous episodes of atrial fibrillation have been treated in this way. Most patients have chosen to deliver cardioversion with no analgesia or sedation. Most atrial fibrillation episodes treated outside the hospital have been terminated with a single shock, with a mean number of shocks per episode of 1.7. No inappropriate shocks have been discharged. To allow patients to cardiovert themselves outside the hospital, implanting centers must complete an observed (in-hospital) therapy phase. Experience suggests that clinical success of the Metrix system does not depend on the setting in which therapy outside the hospital is administered. Patients administering therapy outside the hospital have successfully terminated 81% of spontaneous atrial fibrillation episodes, compared with 84% in the hospital. Overall, 202 patients received the Metrix system worldwide. Early in 1999, Guidant acquired InControl, and as a result, the stand-alone atrial defibrillator is only available for replacements but no longer for new implants. In the future, a more advanced atrial defibrillator with the capability of dual-chamber pacing and preventive pacing will be developed.

JEWEL AF ARRHYTHMIA MANAGEMENT DEVICE

Concern was raised about whether a stand-alone implantable atrial defibrillator is safe enough or should provide ventricular backup defibrillation in the rare case of shock induced ventricular proarrhythmia. In response, a dual-chamber defibrillator (Jewel AF model 7250, Medtronic, Inc., Minneapolis, MN) entered clinical investigation (14,17,31,32). The Jewel AF, with a weight of 93 g and a volume of 55 cc, is a multiprogrammable implantable medical device that detects and treats atrial tachycardia, atrial fibrillation, ventricular tachycardia, ventricular fibrillation, and bradycardia. The most important new features of the Jewel AF system include dual-chamber pacing, a dual-chamber detection algorithm (PR Logic) for rejection of SVTs, detection and painless treatment modalities of atrial arrhythmias, prevention strategies for atrial arrhythmias, automatic or patient-activated atrial defibrillation with complete ventricular backup (14,17,31,32). A patient-activated shock is delivered only if the Jewel AF confirms that atrial fibrillation or atrial tachycardia is present and only if it can synchronize to a ventricular event. The Jewel AF provides up to six defibrillation and up to six cardioversion shocks with a maximum energy of 27 J to treat a detected episode of ventricular fibrillation and ventricular tachycardia, respectively. Two detection zones can be programmed in the atrium. Treatment in these two zones includes ATP (burst and ramp), high-frequency (50-Hz) burst pacing (HFBP), and R-wave synchronous shock therapies ranging from 0.1 to 27 J. Time to delivery of pacing and shock therapies is independently programmable. Atrial shock therapy can be delivered within a specified time window, and the number of shocks can be limited. The Jewel AF has two prevention strategies for atrial arrhythmias: switchback delay and atrial rate stabilization. The first feature prolongs the time that the device is in DDI pacing mode after mode switching. The latter feature aims to eliminate the short-long PP intervals that often precede atrial arrhythmias. As soon as the device detects such intervals, it starts overdrive pacing the atrium. The device provides up to five or three automatic biphasic defibrillation shocks to treat detected episodes of atrial fibrillation or atrial tachycardia, respectively. Each defibrillation shock has a separately programmable energy, pathway, and synchronization. The Jewel AF requires an appropriate two- or three-lead system, consisting of the following: atrial pacing/sensing electrodes, ventricular pacing/sensing electrodes, supraventricular high-voltage electrodes, and a ventricular high-voltage electrode. An additional lead may be placed in the coronary sinus if needed to lower ADFT. Unlike the stand-alone implantable atrial defibrillator, the Metrix atrioverter, the housing of the Jewel AF system is an active electrode.

PR Logic Dual-Chamber Detection Algorithm

PR Logic, a patented dual-chamber detection algorithm, has been implemented in the Jewel AF system. The algorithm uses P : R pattern recognition and timing rules for rhythm classification and has been shown to provide improved dual-chamber detection (14,17,31,32). The dual-chamber tachyarrhythmia detection algorithm in the Jewel AF has been implemented such that detection of ventricular tachycardia or ventricular fibrillation always takes precedence to ensure timely therapies for these life-threatening arrhythmias. SVT detection has been designed to be highly specific to avoid overtreatment of nonsustained supraventricular arrhythmia episodes. Figure 25-7 presents the hierarchic structure of the dual-chamber detection algorithm. Based on the input A-V pattern and atrial and ventricular cycle lengths, the ventricular tachyarrhythmia detection rules are evaluated first. Specificity enhancing rules make use of A-V patterns to determine if a high ventricular rate results from atrial fibrillation or atrial tachycardia, sinus tachycardia, or some other 1 : 1 SVT. If the rules for ventricular tachycardia or ventricular fibrillation are satisfied and no specificity-enhancing rule is satisfied, ventricular tachycardia or ventricular fibrillation therapy is initiated. ventricular tachycardia or ventricular fibrillation therapy is also initiated if rules for dual-tachycardia detection are satisfied (e.g., ventricular tachycardia or ventricular fibrillation arising during SVT).

Supraventricular Tachyarrhythmia Detection

If ventricular tachycardia or ventricular fibrillation or dual tachycardia is not detected, the SVT detection rules are evaluated. The SVT detection rules are designed to detect and discriminate between atrial fibrillation and non-1 : 1 SVTs, including atrial tachycardia, using atrial cycle length thresholds and P : R pattern information. The median atrial cycle length is used to define three detection zones: the atrial fibrillation detection zone, the atrial tachycardia zone, and the Auto-discrimination zone formed by the overlap of the atrial fibrillation and atrial tachycardia zone. When the cycle length for a detected rhythm is in the Auto-discrimination zone, the rhythm is classified as atrial fibrillation if the atrial cycle lengths are "irregular" and atrial tachycardia if the cycle lengths are "regular." The criterion for atrial cycle length regularity is evaluated on each ventricular event. The P : R pattern information is incorporated into the algorithm by the atrial tachycardia or atrial fibrillation evidence counter, a pattern recognition algorithm that is specific for non-1 : 1 SVTs. This counter has

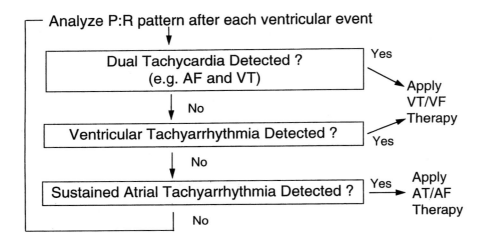

FIGURE 25-7. Hierarchy of dual-chamber detection in the Jewel AF. The device is constantly monitoring the rhythm in the atrium and the ventricle. When a dual tachycardia or a ventricular tachyarrhythmia is detected, the device delivers ventricular therapy. If not, the device looks for possible atrial arrhythmia, and it may deliver an atrial therapy. AF, atrial fibrillation; AT, atrial tachycardia; VF, ventricular fibrillation; VT, ventricular tachycardia.

up-down counting properties and is incremented on each ventricular event for which the P : R pattern shows evidence of a SVT. If there is no evidence, the counter is decremented. The counter has two stages of operation. The first stage is preliminary detection, which defines the start of an atrial tachycardia or atrial fibrillation episode when the evidence counter reaches a predefined threshold. After the start of an episode is defined, the episode duration timer begins incrementing, and the evidence counter switches to the sustained detection stage. During this stage, the evidence counter employs criteria that are less strict, allowing for some atrial undersensing.

Ventricular Tachyarrhythmia Detection

The dual-chamber ventricular tachycardia or ventricular fibrillation detection algorithm uses a hierarchic, rule-based approach to combine pattern and timing information and reach a rhythm decision. Atrial- and ventricular-sensed and -paced events are processed by the detection algorithm after ventricular events. Several timing statistics are computed and used in conjunction with P : R pattern information to determine whether a specific rhythm rule is satisfied. These time-based features include atrial and ventricular median intervals: PR dissociation; RR modesum, which is a measure of ventricular interval stability, and far-field R-wave count to assess whether far-field R waves are being sensed. Patterns of atrial and ventricular events are processed in the following manner: atrial events during a single RR interval are used to define interval codes that represent the number of atrial events and the relative timing of the P and R events. The RR interval is divided into four time intervals for the purpose of encoding atrial activity into interval codes (Fig. 25-8).

Atrial senses are expected to be observed in interval I and IV for junctional rhythms, premature atrial and ventricular contractions, and during atrial fibrillation or atrial tachycardia. Interval III is the normal conduction interval that extends from the midpoint of the RR interval to the beginning of interval IV. Atrial events are expected to be sensed primarily in interval III for normally conducted rhythms such as normal sinus rhythm and sinus tachycardia. Interval II is the retrograde conduction interval that extends from the end of interval I to the beginning of interval III. Atrial events resulting from retrograde conduction of a ventricular event are expected to be sensed in this inter-

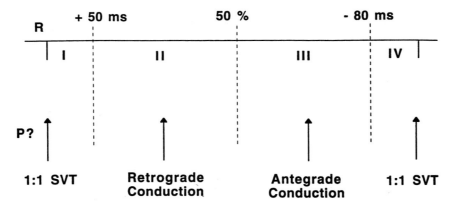

FIGURE 25-8. Definition of time intervals for interval codes. The detection algorithm looks for the position of the P wave relative to the R wave. The RR interval is divided into four time intervals, I through IV. Atrial senses are expected to occur in interval I and IV for junctional rhythms. Interval II (normal sinus rhythm, sinus tachycardia) is the normal antegrade conduction interval that extends from the midpoint of the RR interval to the beginning of interval IV. Atrial events resulting from retrograde conduction of a ventricular event are expected to be sensed in interval II. So-called couple codes, based on the interval codes of the current and previous RR intervals, are used to describe rhythm syntaxes. Sequences of those couple codes are used to classify the rhythm. SVT, supraventricular tachycardia.

val. Couple codes based on the interval codes of the current and previous RR intervals are the fundamental units used to describe rhythm syntaxes. These couple codes provide an abstract description of the activation pattern during adjacent RR intervals. Rhythm syntaxes are the sequences of couple codes that completely describe the patterns of P and R events that are characteristic of a particular tachyarrhythmia. After a couple code sequence matches one of the rhythm patterns for a syntax, the couple code sequence must continue to match that rhythm pattern for the sequence to be recognized as being generated by the particular rhythm. For further discussion of PR Logic, see Chapter 21.

Study Protocol

The Jewel AF 7250 investigation was a multicenter, prospective clinical study to evaluate safety and effectiveness of the model 7250 Jewel AF in preventing and treating atrial tachyarrhythmias and in treating ventricular tachyarrhythmias. There were two study groups: the ventricular tachycardia or atrial tachycardia subgroup and the ventricular tachycardia-only subgroup. The former group included patients with a history of ventricular tachycardia or ventricular fibrillation (or both) and at least two documented atrial fibrillation or atrial tachycardia episodes in the past year. The latter group included patients with a history of ventricular tachycardia and/or ventricular fibrillation only and no documented atrial fibrillation or atrial tachycardia episodes. The study design involved a two-period, two-arm, crossover design for the ventricular tachycardia or atrial tachycardia group. Patients were randomly assigned to have atrial prevention and termination therapies 'ON' or 'OFF' during the first 3 months of follow-up and then reversed during the second 3 months of follow-up to assess the ability of the atrial prevention and termination therapies to reduce the frequency and duration of atrial arrhythmias. The four primary objectives were as follows:

1. Overall safety as determined by complication-free survival at 6 months relative to the 7219C and 7219D systems
2. Efficacy of ATP and HFBP therapies in terminating spontaneous atrial tachycardia episodes
3. Efficacy of atrial defibrillation in terminating spontaneous atrial fibrillation episodes
4. Relative sensitivity of the dual-chamber detection algorithm

ADFT testing was performed on 42 patients according to the protocol requirements. A step-up protocol was used starting at 2 J, followed by 4, 6, 8, and 16 J. This protocol aimed at the E_{30} or E_{35} rather than for the E_{50} for the first-shock efficacy. It was therefore highly recommended to program the first shock at two times the ADFT, with a minimum of 10 J when no coronary sinus lead was used. In case the ADFT was measured at 16 J, all shocks should be programmed to maximal energy output of 27 J.

Results

The clinical study included 49 participating centers worldwide. The first implantation took place in Bonn, Germany, on January 10, 1997 (17). As of June 1998, 303 patients were enrolled in this study. The mean age was 64 years, and 80% of the patients were male. Of these patients, 293 (97%) were implanted with a Jewel AF device. Of the 10 patients who were not implanted with the Jewel AF device, 9 did not meet the ventricular DFT testing with the model 7250 and were implanted with an ICD having higher maximum output (34 J). The remaining patient died of heart failure during the implantation procedure. Of the 293 patients implanted with the model 7250, 221 (75%) were in the ventricular tachycardia or atrial tachycardia subgroup and 72 (25%) were in the ventricular tachycardia-only subgroup. Between July 1 and December 31, 1998, an additional 128 patients were enrolled. Overall, 89% of the patients enrolled in the study received a two-lead system, and less than 8% received a three-lead system. The mean ADFT obtained in the 42 patients who followed strictly the study protocol was 6.1 ± 4.3 J. During a mean follow-up of 7.9 ± 4.7 months, the therapy efficacy rate was 97.7% for 1,113 ($n = 84$ patients) appropriately detected and treated spontaneous ventricular tachycardia episodes and 100% for 309 ($n = 73$ patients) spontaneous ventricular fibrillation episodes. The positive predictive value for ventricular tachycardia or ventricular fibrillation detection approached 90.5%.

During the course of the study, 1,367 of 1,426 spontaneous atrial episodes detected by the device were classified as appropriate by the investigators. This resulted in a positive predictive value of 96% for the atrial fibrillation or atrial tachycardia detection algorithm (10,33). All 59 inappropriate detections resulted from far-field sensing. Fifty-seven patients had experienced a total of 789 spontaneous, appropriately treated atrial tachycardia episodes for which the last therapy to treat the episode was ATP (481 episodes [61%]) or HFBP (308 episodes [39%]). The adjusted efficacy rate of successfully terminated atrial tachycardia episodes was 70% and 20% with ATP and HFBP therapies, respectively. After adjusting for interpatient differences in success rates, 61% of spontaneous atrial tachycardia episodes were terminated by painless pacing therapies (i.e., ATP followed by HFBP). In 42 patients with 137 appropriately detected and treated spontaneous atrial fibrillation episodes, the efficacy rate for atrial defibrillation as a last therapy was 71.9% after adjusting for interpatient differences. Fifty-three ventricular tachycardia or atrial tachycardia patients were strictly randomized to all prevention and termination therapies programmed ON rather than OFF for the first two periods. Patients with prevention and termination therapies enabled experienced a significant reduction in the duration of spontaneous atrial tachycardia or atrial fibrillation episodes per week (average, 5.5-hour reduction per week), and the trend was toward a decrease in the frequency of spontaneous atrial tachycardia or atrial fibrillation episodes per day (mean, 44% reduction per day).

During the randomization period, quality of life status was assessed at 3 and 6 months after implantation. General health status and well-being were evaluated using the Medical Outcomes Study Short Form (SF)-36 questionnaire. The data suggest that patients' quality of life scores did not change during the two follow-up periods.

In an ongoing multicenter trial, the atrial fibrillation-only study, the safety and efficacy of the model 7250 was evaluated in patients with symptomatic and drug-refractory atrial tachycardia or atrial fibrillation episodes and no prior ventricular tachycardia or ventricular fibrillation episodes. The first patient was enrolled in this study on November 21, 1997. As of December 10, 1998, 51 patients were enrolled at 20 worldwide centers. The left ventricular ejection fraction was 55 ± 16%, and the left atrial dimension was 43 ± 9 mm. Thirty-five percent of the patients were categorized in New York Heart Association class II or III. During a mean follow-up of 3.2 ± 2.5 months, a total of 156 spontaneous atrial tachycardia and 206 atrial fibrillation episodes were detected in 13 and 28 patients, respectively. Overall efficacy of the Jewel AF system in terminating spontaneous atrial tachycardia and atrial fibrillation episodes using atrial shocks was 92% (163 of 175 episodes). An additional 41% (77 of 187 episodes) of spontaneous atrial tachycardia and atrial fibrillation episodes were terminated successfully by painless pacing therapies (ATP or HFBP) without the need for high-energy shocks (34).

● VENTAK AND CONTAK CD HEART FAILURE DEFIBRILLATOR

The VENTAK CHF AICD and the CONTAC CD CHFD pulse generator (Guidant Corp.) provide cardioversion and defibrillation therapy as well as biventricular ATP and dual-chamber, rate-adaptive bradycardia pacing. Both models provide biventricular pacing that allows simultaneous electrical stimulation of the right and left ventricles. The CONTAK CD CHFD is connected to a commercially available pace/sense and to a cardioversion/defibrillation lead. The EASYTRAK (Guidant Corp.) coronary venous pace/sense lead is to be used in conjunction with the CONTAK CD CHFD. The EASYTRAK is a steroid-eluting, unipolar, coronary-venous, pace/sense lead with an over-the-wire design that provides pacing and sensing of the left ventricle by inserting the lead through the coronary sinus and placing the lead in the cardiac vein branches. Ventricular sensing and detection occurs between the right ventricular defibrillation and the EASYTRAK electrode. The CONTAK CD CHFD system is indicated for use in patients who meet the general indication for ICD implantation, have symptomatic CHF despite optimal drug therapy, have left ventricular ejection fraction of 35% or less, and have a QRS duration of more than 120 msec. The clinical evaluation employs a randomized, two-period, crossover design with all patients receiving two consecutive treatments for CHF. At 1 month after implantation, patients are randomized to receive no pacing or biventricular pacing for 3-month intervals. Thereafter, patients are crossed over to the other treatment. On completion of these therapy phases, pacemaker programming is left to the discretion of the investigator.

The primary objectives of this clinical evaluation are improvement in peak oxygen uptake as measured by cardiopulmonary exercise testing and documentation of the safety of chronic biventricular pacing, sensing, and lead impedance. Cardiopulmonary exercise testing will be performed on a treadmill using a modified Naughton protocol. Comparisons for this end point will be made at the conclusion of two consecutive 3-month periods, one with biventricular pacing and the other with no pacing, administered in a randomized sequence. The secondary objectives of this trial are assessments of quality of life, efficacy rate of ATP, ventricular tachycardia detection time, severe device-related adverse events, operative mortality, and the evaluation of the EASYTRAK lead placement success rate. Patient recruitment started in early 1999 and ended on August 1999. A minimum of 168 patients will be followed through hospital discharge and at 30, 120, and 210 days after ICD implantation.

◉ INSYNC ICD HEART FAILURE DEFIBRILLATOR

The model 7272 InSync ICD (Medtronic, Inc.) is a device combining a state-of-the-art dual-chamber ICD with biventricular pacing capabilities to treat patients with CHF. The model 7272 device is a 64-cc, full-function ICD capable of delivering up to 34 J. The InSync ICD system incorporates an additional port in the header to accommodate the Attain lead for left ventricular pacing through the cardiac veins. In this system, all ventricular sensing and detection remains on the right side of the heart. This allows the coronary sinus lead to be disconnected by noninvasive reprogramming in case of any problems related to sensing or pacing through the coronary sinus electrode. The model 7272 also provides biventricular pacing to synchronize the myocardial contraction in patients with intraventricular or interventricular conduction delays. The device is designed to provide full biventricular DDD rate-responsive pacing. The 7272 ICD device is based on the model 7271 Gem DR and the model 7273 Gem II DR with additional biventricular pacing capabilities to provide cardiac resynchronization. The atrial pace/sense lead serves for atrial sensing and delivery of ATP. The right ventricular pace/sense lead serves for ventricular tachyarrhythmia detection, ventricular sensing, and delivery of bradycardia pacing and ATP. The left ventricular lead serves for delivery of bradycardia pacing and ATP. Right ventricular pacing takes place between the tip and the coil electrode. Left ventricular pacing takes place between the tip of the left electrode and the coil of the right electrode. The primary objective of this prospective, multicenter study is to evaluate the performance of this system. The InSync ICD system is indicated for use in patients who meet the general indication for ICD implantation and have symptomatic CHF despite optimal drug therapy with evidence of ventricular dyssynchrony demonstrated by a QRS duration of 130 msec or longer, a left ventricular ejection fraction of 35% or less, and a left ventricular end diastolic diameter of 55 mm or more. Clinical data are collected at baseline, implantation, before hospital discharge, at scheduled follow-up visits at 1, 3, and 6 months after implantation, and every 6 months thereafter until the study is terminated. The first implantation took place in Germany in June of 1999.

◉ CONCLUSIONS

Dual-chamber ICDs provide equivalent efficacy and safety compared with single-chamber ICDs. The new detection algorithms are highly efficacious in reducing the incidence of unnecessary ICD interventions without compromising the delivery of appropriate ICD therapy. Major issues that have to be addressed with an implantable atrial defibrillator are pain perception and the potential risk of inducing life-threatening ventricular arrhythmias during delivery of low-energy atrial shocks. Further efforts must be undertaken to reduce the patient discomfort associated with internal atrial defibrillation in an attempt to make this new therapy acceptable to a larger patient population with atrial fibrillation. Cost-effectiveness and quality of life analyses comparing an implantable atrial defibrillator with alternative therapeutic approaches will be needed. In particular, the early relapse of atrial fibrillation, which accounted for a decreased clinical success rate, has to be taken into consideration.

Shortcomings of the current implantable atrial defibrillator are the limited energy output of the device and the lack of ability to pace in the atrium and ventricle, especially if the subgroup of patients with sick sinus syndrome and atrial fibrillation is considered as potential candidates for future device implantation. A device that is equipped with a lead in the coronary sinus should ideally provide biatrial pacing for selected patients for the prevention of atrial fibrillation. Clinical experience with an implantable atrial defibrillator indicates stable ADFT, appropriate R-wave synchronization markers, no shock-induced ventricular proarrhythmia, and detection of atrial fibrillation with a specificity of 100%.

A new arrhythmia management system that combines detection and treatment in the atrium and the ventricle may represent an important milestone and a significant improvement in the management of patients with SVTs and ventricular tachyarrhythmias. Results of the Jewel AF worldwide multicenter, prospective clinical study demonstrate that the Jewel AF is highly effective in detecting and treating total atrial arrhythmias by painless pacing therapies. Jewel AF prevention and termination therapies resulted in a clinically significant reduction of spontaneous atrial tachyarrhythmia burden. Preliminary studies with multisite pacing demonstrated acute hemodynamic improvement and increased functional capacity. Long-term results with multisite devices providing biventricular pacing with additional ventricular defibrillation support are awaited.

REFERENCES

1. Hook BG, Marchlinski FE. Value of ventricular electrogram in the diagnosis of arrhythmias precipitating electrical device therapy. *J Am Coll Cardiol* 1991;19:490–499.
2. Grimm W, Flores BF, Marchlinski FE. Electrocardiographically documented unnecessary, spontaneous shocks in 241 patients with implantable cardioverter-defibrillators. *Pacing Clin Electrophysiol* 1992;15:1667–1673.
3. Swerdlow CD, Chen PS, Kass RM, et al. Discrimination of ventricular tachycardia from sinus tachycardia and atrial fibrillation in a tiered-therapy cardioverter-defibrillator. *J Am Coll Cardiol* 1994; 23:1342–1355.
4. Swerdlow CD, Ahern T, Chen PS, et al. Underdetection of ventricular tachycardia by algorithms to enhance specificity in a tiered-therapy cardioverter-defibrillator. *J Am Coll Cardiol* 1994;24:416–424.
5. Neuzner J, Pitschner HF, Schlepper M. Programmable VT detection enhancements in implantable cardioverter defibrillator therapy. *Pacing Clin Electrophysiol* 1995;18:539–547.
6. Schaumann A, von zur Mühlen F, Gonska BD, et al. Enhanced detection criteria in implantable cardioverter-defibrillators to avoid inappropriate therapy. *Am J Cardiol* 1996;78:42–50.
7. Higgins SL, Lee RS, Kramer RL. Stability: an ICD detection criterion for discriminating atrial fibrillation from ventricular tachycardia. *J Cardiovasc Electrophysiol* 1995;6:1081–1088.
8. Brugada J, Mont L, Figueiredo M, et al. Enhanced detection criteria in implantable defibrillators. *J Cardiovasc Electrophysiol* 1998;9:261–268.
9. Korte T, Jung W, Wolpert C, et al. A new classification algorithm for discrimination of ventricular from supraventricular tachycardia in a dual chamber implantable cardioverter defibrillator. *J Cardiovasc Electrophysiol* 1998;9:70–73.
10. Wolpert C, Jung W, Scholl C, et al. Electrical proarrhythmia: Induction of inappropriate atrial therapies due to far-field R wave oversensing in a new dual chamber defibrillator. *J Cardiovasc Electrophysiol* 1998;9:859–863.
11. Jung W, Lüderitz B. Clinical results with the fourth generation and investigational implantable cardioverter-defibrillators In: Singer I, Barold SS, Camm AJ, eds. *Nonpharmacological therapy of arrhythmias for the 21st century: the state of the art*. Armonk, NY: Futura Publishing, 1998:517–527.
12. Jung W, Lüderitz B. Should all candidates for ICD therapy receive a dual-chamber system? [Editorial]. *J Interv Card Electrophysiol* 1999;3:206–209.
13. Jung W, Wolpert C, Esmailzadeh B, et al. Specific considerations with the automatic implantable atrial defibrillator. *J Cardiovasc Electrophysiol* 1998;9:S193–S201.
14. Jung W, Lüderitz B. Implantable atrial defibrillator: quo vadis? [Editorial]. *Pacing Clin Electrophysiol* 1997;20:2141–2145.
15. Jung W, Wolpert C, Spehl S, et al. Clinical experience with implantable atrial and combined atrioventricular defibrillators. *J Interv Card Electrophysiol* 1999;3.
16. Jung W, Lüderitz B. Quality of life in atrial fibrillation. *J Cardiovasc Electrophysiol* 1998;9:S177–S186.
17. Jung W, Lüderitz B. Implantation of a new arrhythmia management system in patients with supraventricular and ventricular tachyarrhythmias. *Lancet* 1997;349:853–854.
18. Lüderitz B, Jung W, Deister A, et al. Patient acceptance of implantable cardioverter defibrillator devices: changing attitudes. *Am Heart J* 1994;127:1179–1184.
19. Lüderitz B, Jung W, Manz M. Antitachycardia pacing. In: Singer I, ed. *The implantable cardioverter-defibrillator*. Mount Kisco, NY: Futura Publishing, 1994:271–299.
20. Auricchio A, Stellbrink C, Block M, et al, for the Pacing Therapies for Congestive Heart Failure Group. Effect of pacing chamber and atrioventricular delay on acute systolic function of paced patients with congestive heart failure. *Circulation* 1999; 99:2993–3001.
21. Jung W, Wolpert C, Spehl S, et al. Does dual-chamber sensing improve ICD detection? *G Ital Cardiol* 1998;28[Suppl 1]: 589–592.
22. Nair M, Saoudi N, Kroiss D, et al, for the Participating Centers of the Automatic Recognition of Arrhythmia Study Group.

Automatic arrhythmia identification using analysis of the atrioventricular association. *Circulation* 1997;95:973–967.
23. Jung W, Wolpert C, Henry C, et al, for the Defender Investigators. Multicenter experience with a new dual-chamber defibrillator [Abstract]. *Eur Heart J* 1999;20:111.
24. Jung W, Spehl S, Wolpert C, et al. Improved arrhythmia classification with a new pectoral dual-chamber implantable cardioverter defibrillator [Abstract]. *Circulation* 1997;96:579.
25. Lau CP, Tse HF, Lok NS, et al: Initial clinical experience with an implantable human atrial defibrillator. *Pacing Clin Electrophysiol* 1977;20:220–225.
26. Wellens HJJ, Lau CP, Lüderitz B, et al, for the Metrix Investigators. The Atrioverter: an implantable device for treatment of atrial fibrillation. *Circulation* 1998;98:1651–1656.
27. Timmermans C, Lèvy S, Ayers G, et al, for the Metrix Investigators. Spontaneous episodes of atrial fibrillation after implantation of the Metrix Atrioverter: observations on treated and nontreated episodes. *J Am Coll Cardiol* 2000;35:1428–1433.
28. Jung W, Wolpert C, Herwig S, et al. Initial experience with the implantable atrial defibrillator. *G Ital Cardiol* 1998;28[Suppl 1]:592–594.
29. Jung W, Lüderitz B. Implantable atrial defibrillator: which results and indications In: Raviele A, ed. *Cardiac arrhythmias*. Heidelberg: Springer-Verlag, 1997:S100–109.
30. Jung W, Wolpert C, Spehl S, et al, for the Metrix Investigators. Worldwide experience with the Metrix implantable atrial defibrillator. In: Adornato E, ed. *Rhythm control from cardiac evaluation to treatment*. Rome: Ediziono Luigi Pozzi, 1998:139–143.
31. Jung W, Wolpert C, Spehl S, et al. Implantable atrial and dual-chamber defibrillators. In: Saoudi N, Schoels W, El-Sherif N, eds. *Atrial flutter and fibrillation*. Armonk, NY: Futura Publishing, 1998:327–348.
32. Jung W, Wolpert C, Spehl S, et al. Implantable atrial defibrillator with ventricular back-up. *G Ital Cardiol* 1998;28[Suppl 1]: 581–583.
33. Swerdlow CD, Schöls W, Dijkman B, et al, for the Worldwide Jewel AF Investigators. Atrial fibrillation and flutter detection by a dual-chamber implantable cardioverter defibrillator. *Circulation* 1999;100.
34. Sulke N, Bailin SJ, Swerdlow CD, for the Worldwide 7250 Jewel AF-Only Investigators. Worldwide clinical experience with a dual chamber implantable cardioverter defibrillator in patients with atrial fibrillation and flutter [Abstract]. *Pacing Clin Electrophysiol* 1999;22:871.

CLINICAL RESULTS WITH IMPLANTABLE CARDIOVERTER-DEFIBRILLATORS

• • •

SEAH NISAM

At the time this book comes out early in the 21st century, implantable cardioverter-defibrillator (ICD) therapy will be starting its 21st year. When Michel Mirowski and colleagues (1) implanted their first patient on February 4, 1980, few people believed that the therapy would ever be generally accepted. No one, except perhaps Dr. Mirowski, could have anticipated that, of all specific interventions, ICD therapy would have the single most significant impact on cardiovascular mortality over the next two decades. Deaths from cardiovascular disease are still the most dominant cause of mortality, with more than 600,000 victims annually in the United States and similar numbers in Europe (2,3). Because approximately one half of these deaths result from ventricular tachycardia or ventricular fibrillation (4), it is clear that the use of ICD therapy will continue to grow well beyond the 50,000 patients implanted within the past year (5,6). Part of this increased pool of ICD candidates will come from heart association initiatives aimed at significantly increasing the number of patients resuscitated from out-of-hospital sudden cardiac death (7,8). However, after the results of two major prospective, randomized studies (MADIT and MUSTT), the major increase will come from far greater prophylactic use of the ICD. These two studies showed that patients with previous myocardial infarction, depressed left ventricular function, and nonsustained ventricular tachycardia, but without previous arrhythmic events, achieve unequivocally better survival with ICDs compared with antiarrhythmic therapy or no (antiarrhythmic) therapy (9,10).

Because there are multiple substrates leading to sudden cardiac death, guidelines for the use of the ICD have been developed to address these multiple indications. In this chapter, we provide an overview of the ICD's impact on patient survival for specific classes of indications.

◉ EVOLUTION OF IMPLANTABLE CARDIOVERTER-DEFIBRILLATOR INDICATIONS

A task force, with representation from the American College of Cardiology, the American Heart Association, and the North American Society of Pacing and Electrophysiology, carefully reviewed data from clinical experience as well as prospective trials while preparing their guidelines, which were published in April 1998 (11). Before examining ICD results for each category, we present a brief chronologic review of the evolution of ICD guidelines (Table 26-1).

TABLE 26-1 • EVOLUTION IN GUIDELINES FOR CARDIOVERTER-DEFIBRILLATOR IMPLANTATION

Year	Indications For ICD Implantation
1980	Resuscitated from at least two episodes of cardiac arrest, neither associated with acute MI, and one of which had to occur despite AARx (1)
1982	One or more episodes of VF or hemodynamically unstable VT, not associated with acute MI (or other transient, reversible causes), but with evidence—from EP testing or Holter monitoring—of incomplete protection by AARx (12)
1986	Same, except relaxation of the requirement for initial EP inducibility and nonsuppressibility following AARx (13)

1991	A. Class I indications (14) (general concensus that ICD indicated):
	  1. ≥1 episodes of spontaneous sustained VT/VF in patients in whom EP testing and/or Holter monitoring could not be used to accurately predict efficacy of other therapies
	  2. Recurrent spontaneous sustained VT/VF, *despite* EP- or Holter monitoring-guided AARx
	  3. Spontaneous sustained VT/VF in case of a patient's noncompliance with or intolerance of AARx
	  4. Patients with spontaneous sustained VT/VF, who remain persistently inducible at EP study, while on "best" AARx or after VT surgery or catheter ablation
	B. Class II indication (ICD an acceptable option, but no concensus):
	  1. "Syncope of undetermined etiology in a patient with clinically relevant sustained VT or VF induced at EP study, in whom AARx is limited by inefficacy, intolerance, or noncompliance (14)"

1998	A. Class I indications (11) (general concensus that ICD indicated):
	  1. Cardiac arrest due to VT or VF, not due to a transient or reversible cause
	  2. Spontaneous sustained VT
	  3. Syncope of undetermined origin with clinically relevant, hemodynamically significant sustained VT or VF induced at EP study when drug therapy is ineffective, not tolerated, or not preferred
	  4. Nonsustained VT with coronary disease, prior MI, LV dysfunction, and inducible VF or sustained VT at EP study that is not suppressible by a class I AARx
	B. Class IIb indication (11) (ICD an acceptable option, but no concensus):
	  1. Cardiac arrest presumed due to VF when EP testing is precluded by other medical conditions
	  2. Severe symptoms attributable to sustained VT/VF while awaiting cardiac transplantation
	  3. Familial or inherited conditions carrying a high risk for life-threatening VT/VF, such as long QT syndrome or hypertrophic cardiomyopathy
	  4. Nonsustained VT with coronary artery disease, prior MI, and LV dysfunction, and inducible sustained VT/VF at EP study
	  5. Recurrent syncope of unknown origin in the presence of ventricular dysfunction and inducible VT/VF at EPS, when other causes of syncopy have been excluded

AARx, antiarrhythmic drug therapy; EP electrophysiologic; EPS, electrophysiologic study; ICD, implantable cardioverter-defibrillator; LV, left venticle; MI, myocardial infarction; VF, ventricular fibrillation; VT, ventricular tachycardia.

⊙ SURVIVAL RESULTS BY INDICATION

In the following sections, we present survival results for patients receiving ICDs according to current guidelines (11) (Table 26-1). Although the bibliography for each category is extensive, I usually selected the larger, better-known scientific studies as representative of the entire group.

Cardiac Arrest

The largest early ICD series ($n = 270$), reported by Winkle and colleagues, included 80% of patients with one or more cardiac arrests as the primary indication for ICD implantation (12). For patients in the entire series, the average age was 58 years, 80% were male, 78.2% had coronary artery disease, the mean left ventricular ejection fraction (LVEF) was 34%, and they had failed an average of 3.4 drug trials before ICD implantation. The Kaplan-Meier mortality results showed all-cause mortality of 7.7% at 1 year and 26.2% through 5 years. Powell and coworkers reported 331 survivors of cardiac arrest, of whom 150 received ICDs and 181 received antiarrhythmic drug therapy, surgical therapy, or both without ICD implantation (13). The patient characteristics were nearly identical to those in the Winkle series. At a mean follow-up of 31 months, 19.3% of the ICD-treated patients had died. The Kaplan-Meier results for the entire group were not given, but the 5-year mortality for ICD patients with LVEF >0.40 and ≤0.40 was 5.5% and 30.4%, respectively, significantly better than the 13.1% and 54.7%, respectively, for the nondefibrillator group. The Cardiac Arrest Study in Hamburg (CASH) included 99 survivors of cardiac arrest who received ICDs (14). The patients were similar in profile to those in the Winkle and Powell series, except that their LVEF was much better (0.46), with 9 patients (9%) showing no evidence of underlying heart disease. The 2-year sudden death and all-cause mortality rates for patients receiving ICDs were 4% and 14%, respectively.

Spontaneous Sustained Ventricular Tachycardia

The study with the largest number of patients with spontaneous sustained ventricular tachycardia was the Antiarrhythmics versus Implantable Defibrillator (AVID) trial, with 281 (55.4%) of the ICD-randomized group having sustained ventricular tachycardia as their presenting arrhythmia (15). The entire group had an average age of 65 years, 78% were male, 81% had coronary artery disease, and the mean LVEF was 0.32. At a mean follow-up of 18 months, the overall mortality rate was 15.8%, compared with 24.0% for the patients randomized to antiarrhythmic drugs (96% received amiodarone). A large, multicenter German study with 361 ICD patients included 158 (43.8%) whose presenting arrhythmias had been only ventricular tachycardia plus an additional 104 patients (28.8% who had had ventricular tachycardia and ventricular fibrillation) (16). The 262 patients, representing nearly three fourths of all patients in this study, had had sustained ventricular tachycardia before ICD implantation. The characteristics of the entire population resembled most of the series presented heretofore: the mean age was 59.5 years, 84.5% of patients were male, 69.5% had coronary artery disease, and the mean LVEF was 0.36. The Kaplan-Meier all-cause mortality rate was 6.8% at 1 year and an amazingly low 15.1% at 5 years. Analyzed on the basis of better or worse left ventricular function, the 5-year mortality for the patients with LVEF ≤0.30 was 26.1%, compared with 5.8% for patients with LVEF >0.30. Another large (n = 603), single-center series included 181 patients (30%) who had presented with ventricular tachycardia (without cardiac arrest) (17). For the entire group, the average age was 57.3 years, 77.4% were male, 85.5% had coronary artery disease, and the mean LVEF was 0.44. The Kaplan-Meier all-cause mortality rate for the entire study cohort reached 6.3% at 1 year and 25% by 5 years. Broken down by New York Heart Association (NYHA) class, the mortality rates at 5 years were 2.6% for NYHA 1, 13.0% for NYHA 2, and 44.1% for patients in NYHA class 3.

Syncope of Undetermined Origin

There are few studies on patients implanted with ICDs to treat syncope of undetermined origin. Link and associates reported 50 consecutive patients with syncope of undetermined origin, all of whom were inducible into ventricular tachycardia or ventricular fibrillation during electrophysiologic testing and implanted with ICDs (18). The mean age of these patients was 59 years, 80% were male, 92% had structural heart disease, 66% had coronary artery disease, and the mean LVEF was 0.36. During a mean follow-up of 23 months, there were four deaths (no data provided on actuarial rates). The primary outcome of this study was the demonstration that patients fitting this category have a "low incidence of sudden cardiac death and high incidence of appropriate defibrillator therapy." The actuarial probability of these patients receiving appropriate ICD shocks was 50% by 3 years. Another study of 213 patients with ICDs included 66 who had presented with syncope not associated with any identified causes who then underwent electrophysiologic testing (19). For these 66 patients were, the mean age was 61 years, 81% were male, 73% had coronary artery disease, and the mean LVEF was 0.30. The Kaplan-Meier curve showed an all-cause mortality rate of 10% at 24 months and 31% at 40 months of follow-up. The Canadian Implantable Defibrillator Study (CIDS) compared outcomes for patients randomized to ICDs (n = 328) or to amiodarone (n = 331) (20). The defibrillator cohort included 50 patients with "unmonitored syncope." The data available from the press release (20) (while awaiting publication of the study) provide the patient characteristics and survival data but are not broken down for each subgroup. For the entire population treated with ICDs, the Kaplan-Meier rate for all-cause mortality was 28% at 4 years.

Nonsustained Ventricular Tachycardia with Coronary Artery Disease, Left Ventricular Dysfunction, and Inducible Ventricular Tachycardia or Fibrillation

Thanks to the MADIT and MUSTT studies, there are substantial data on outcomes for patients with nonsustained ventricular tachycardia with coronary artery disease, left ventricular dysfunction, and inducible ventricular tachycardia or ventricular fibrillation and receiving ICDs prophylactically. Indication class I #4 requires evidence of nonsuppressibility by a class I antiarrhythmic drug (per MADIT), which differentiates it slightly from class II-B #4, for which nonsuppressibility is not required (per MUSTT). However, the patient characteristics and the outcomes of the two studies are otherwise so close that I have chosen to present both together. Table 26-2 summarizes the key patient characteristics for patients in both studies and shows how remarkably similar they are. The last column provides data from the AVID study, showing how closely the MUSTT and MADIT cohorts resemble patients with the classic indications for ICDs. For class II-B, with regard to the indications set out in Table 26-1, we focus here only on #2 and #3, because these are the only indications that differ significantly from those already presented.

Examining the Kaplan-Meier all-cause mortality rates at 2 years of follow-up for the ICD-randomized patients, MADIT reported 16% and MUSTT 12%. By 5 years, the mortality rates were 32% and 28%, respectively. The mortality rates for patients in the non-ICD limb for the two studies were 32% and 48% for MADIT at 2 years and 4 years, respectively, and 28% and 42% MUSTT at 2 and 4 years, respectively. The somewhat higher mortality in MADIT is logical, in light of the increased risk criteria compared with MUSTT (e.g., lower ejection fraction, repeat ventricular tachycardia inducibility after procainamide challenge).

Implantable Cardioverter-Defibrillators as a Bridge to Cardiac Transplantation

The various studies (21–24) that led the Guidelines Task Force to include patients using ICDs as a bridge

TABLE 26-2 • OVERVIEW OF MADIT, MUSTT, AND AVID STUDIES

Characteristic	MADIT (9)	MUSTT (10)	AVID (18)
Mean age (y)	63	67	65
Sex (% males)	92	90	80
Mean time p after MI[a] (months)	27	39	
Prior CABG/PTCA (%)	71	66	
LVEF (mean)	0.26	0.30	0.31
NSVT (mean number of beats)	9	5	N/A[b]
Pts. on BBI (ICD/controls) (%)	26/15[c]	37/51	42/17
CHF II–III (% patients)	65	64	58[d]
Randomization	ICD vs. Conv.	EP-guided vs. no Tx	ICD vs. (96%) amiodarone
Overall survival at 2 years			
ICD limb (%)	84	88	81.6
Control limb (%)	68	72	74.7

BBI, beta blockers; CABG, coronary artery bypass graft; CHF, congestive heart failure; EP, electrophysiology; LVEF, left ventricular ejection fraction; MI, myocardial infarction; NSVT, nonsustained ventricular tachycardia; PTCA, percutaneous transluminal coronary angioplasty; Tx, therapy.
[a] All MADIT and MUSTT study patients had previous MI (required by the protocol); in the AVID study, 65% of patients had previous MI.
[b] NSVT data are not available (not required for inclusion).
[c] Includes 7% on sotalol.
[d] For the AVID group, this figure includes the New York Heart Association classes I, II, and III.

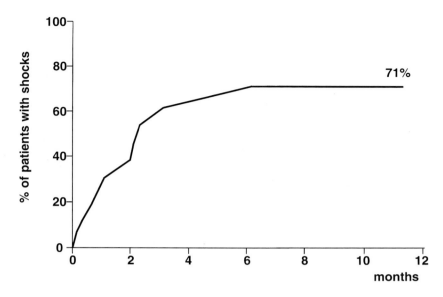

FIGURE 26-1. Incidence (Kaplan-Meier curve) of appropriate implantable cardioverter-defibrillator shocks in patients awaiting heart transplantation. (From Silka M, Kron J, Dunnigan A, Dick M. Sudden cardiac death and the use of implantable cardioverter-defibrillators in pediatric patients. *Circulation* 1993;87:800–807, with permission.)

to cardiac transplantation as potential ICD candidates focused on data showing high rates of mortality and sudden death for patients without ICDs, a demonstrated low rate of sudden deaths when such patients were treated with ICDs, and acceptably low morbidity and mortality related to ICD implantation in such patients. For example, in the retrospective study by Sweeney and colleagues, the 12-month sudden death rate for patients awaiting transplantation (mean NYHA class of 3.4) treated with ICDs was 9.2%, compared with 16% and 34.7% for patients treated without and with antiarrhythmic drugs, respectively (23). The investigators emphasized that, based on the far higher incidence of previous cardiac arrest in the ICD cohort, they would have been expected to have the highest incidence of sudden death. A later study of 19 patients awaiting heart transplantation demonstrated that such patients received appropriate ICD shocks for ventricular tachycardia or ventricular fibrillation early and often after ICD implantation (Fig. 26-1), with only one death and 18 of the 19 reaching transplantation (25,26).

Familial or Inherited Conditions

For the following indications, the series reported in the literature are relatively small, and the mortality when treated with ICDs so low that the investigators have focused their data on the appropriate shocks of the ICDs.

Hypertrophic Cardiomyopathy

Studies on the role of ICD therapy for patients with cardiac arrest or ventricular tachycardia and having hypertrophic cardiomyopathy (HCM) as the underlying disease have shown an incidence of appropriate ICD shocks ranging from a low of 21% at a mean follow-up of 40 months (27) up to 57% at a mean follow-up of 31 months (28). Borggrefe and Breithardt, in an editorial summarizing their and others' experience with ICD therapy for patients with HCM, concluded that "the patient with sustained ventricular tachyarrhythmias and HCM should undergo implantation of an ICD, unless there is a specific trigger that can be effectively targeted or a potential arrhythmogenic substrate that can be abolished effectively by myectomy . . . " (29).

Long QT syndrome

Two publications on patients with ventricular tachycardia or ventricular fibrillation suffering from long QT syndrome reported similar incidences of appropriate ICD shocks: 57% at a mean follow-up of 31 months in a series of 14 patients (28) and 60% at mean follow-up of 31 months in a series of 35 patients (30).

Most patients received ICDs because of cardiac arrest despite beta-blocker therapy. Dr. Arthur Moss reported that there are 88 long QT syndrome patients with ICDs in the worldwide registry, with no deaths in this group during an average 2-year follow-up (31).

Brugada Syndrome

The Brugada brothers described the clinical manifestations of a form of idiopathic ventricular fibrillation with a characteristic ST segment elevation as a marker for sudden death, and they examined the outcome of various therapies (32). For 63 patients (pooled from 33 centers worldwide), they reported an approximate 30% recurrence of ventricular tachycardia or ventricular fibrillation within 3 years, independent of whether the patients had previously presented with cardiac arrest ($n = 41$) or had been asymptomatic at the time of electrocardiographic identification ($n = 22$). Treatment consisted of ICDs for 35 patients, beta blockers and amiodarone for 15, and no specific treatment for the remaining 13. Although the incidence of arrhythmic events was similar for all three treatment groups, total mortality was zero for the ICD-treated patients, compared with 26% and 31% for the other two groups (log rank 0.0005). Nademanee and coworkers recognized this same syndrome as the cause of sudden death in young Thai men (33) and reported it as the most frequent cause of natural death in this population (34).

● EFFICACY OF IMPLANTABLE CARDIOVERTER-DEFIBRILLATORS

Studies evaluating ICD therapy versus other therapeutic options provide Kaplan-Meier survival curves, depicting the differences in outcome between patients treated by ICDs compared with medical treatment. We examined the survival curves from these various series and found a great similarity in outcomes for the patients treated without ICDs (Fig. 26-2A). The survival curves for the patients who received ICDs (Fig. 26-2B) are also fairly close together but superior to those who did not receive ICDs. Figure 26-2A demonstrates that overall survival for patients treated by amiodarone in the mid-1980s (35) or in later studies is remarkably similar: approximately 80%, 70%, and 60% at 1, 2, and 4 years, respectively. The importance of the MUSTT no-antiarrhythmic therapy limb is that it provides a "natural history" arm for such patients. In Figure 26-2A, this arm appears to adhere closely to (or is slightly better than) the results obtained with pharmacologic treatment. Figure 26-2B shows that patients treated with ICDs in the 1980s (12) seem to have essentially the same overall survival as those getting ICDs in more recent years: approximately 93%, 85%, and 80% at 1, 2, and 4 years, respectively. Over many years, the combined risk of dying from arrhythmias and all other causes has remained remarkably similar within each treatment group, with the ICD-treated patients showing approximately 50% lower mortality at each period of follow-up. A corollary, which we offer cautiously, is that neither the improvements in medical management nor those in ICD technology seem to have dramatically impacted the survival results, although we are not addressing quality of life and other aspects that have been affected.

An examination of the impact of ICDs on survival would be incomplete without summarizing the important lessons drawn from multicenter, prospective, randomized trials. Figure 26-3 illustrates the outcomes of these trials in terms of ICD impact on all-cause mortality. The left-hand histograms represent trials with patients who had already presented with life-threatening ventricular tachyarrhythmias; the right-hand side shows the "primary prevention" trials, aimed at examining the role of the ICD in populations deemed to be at risk but who had not presented with spontaneous, sustained ventricular tachycardia or ventricular fibrillation before the studies. These comparisons show that the ICD maintains a roughly 40% to 50% superiority over conventional medical management, and this advantage is maintained in the secondary and primary prevention trials. The Coronary Artery Bypass Graft (CABG)-Patch trial is the single deviant in these results (36), but there are understandable reasons, as previously reported by others and us (37–39). In contrast to all the other studies, the populations studied in CABG-Patch had never had sustained ventricular tachycardia, neither spontaneously nor induced, before the study. The

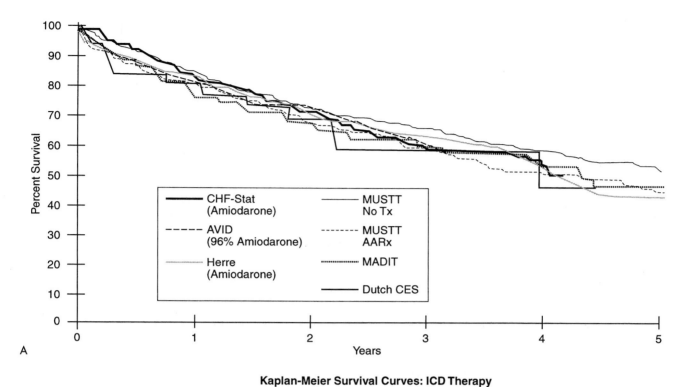
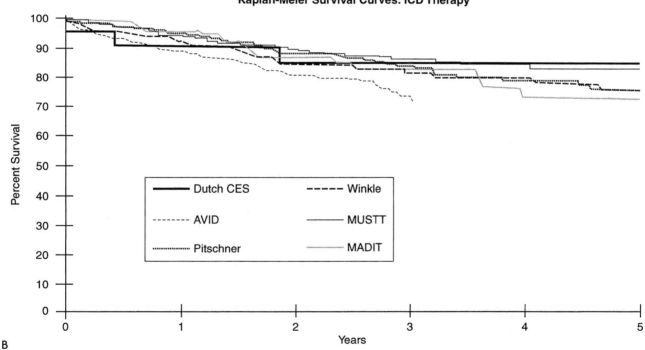

FIGURE 26-2. Overall survival (Kaplan-Meier curves) of patients treated with antiarrhythmic drugs or implantable cardioverter-defibrillators (ICDs). **A:** Antiarrhythmic drugs. Amiodarone was the only or primary antiarrhythmic drug in the CHF-Stat, MADIT, AVID, and Herre and colleagues studies. Two curves are given for MUSTT: No Tx for patients randomized to no antiarrhythmic therapy and AARx for patients provided antiarrhythmic drugs to which they responded (i.e., suppressed inducibility of ventricular tachycardia during electrophysiologic testing). **B:** ICDs. The MUSTT patients not responding to electrophysiologically guided antiarrhythmic drugs received ICDs. The remaining curves come from studies reported in this chapter.

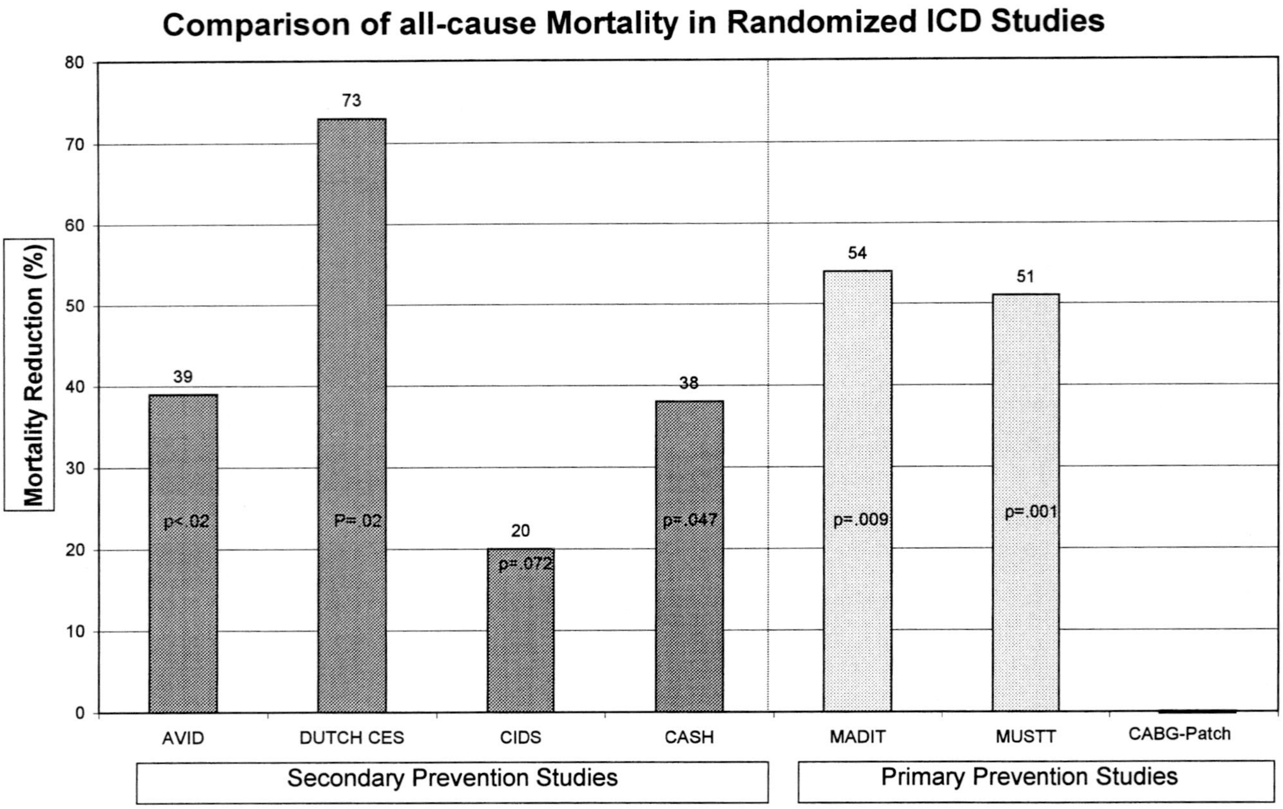

Comparison of all-cause Mortality in Randomized ICD Studies

[Bar chart showing Mortality Reduction (%) for Secondary Prevention Studies: AVID 39 (p<.02), DUTCH CES 73 (P=.02), CIDS 20 (p=.072), CASH 38 (p=.047); and Primary Prevention Studies: MADIT 54 (p=.009), MUSTT 51 (p=.001), CABG-Patch 0.]

FIGURE 26-3. Reductions in all-cause mortality in randomized, prospective implantable cardioverter-defibrillator (ICD) studies. Each histogram provides the percentage reduction in all-cause mortality in studies comparing survival outcomes for patients randomized to ICDs versus antiarrhythmic drugs (AVID, Dutch, CIDS, CASH, and MADIT studies) or no antiarrhythmic drugs (MUSTT and CABG-Patch studies).

great contribution of this study is to demonstrate that patients without significant (arrhythmic) risk do not benefit from defibrillator implantation. The mortality after the 30-day postoperative period was only 11% in the subsequent 24 months, a rate far below the 36.5% at 40 months hypothesized in the study (40) and far too low for ICD intervention to be able to affect.

We have presented the survival outcome for each of the categories formally accepted in the ICD guidelines. In general, the patient characteristics and their mortality risks are often widely divergent between these classes of indications. One study focused specifically on whether the presenting arrhythmia—cardiac arrest, stable ventricular tachycardia, or syncope of unknown origin—influenced the outcome for ICD recipients (19). They reported no differences in Kaplan-Meier survival curves for overall mortality among these three groups but found that patients presenting with cardiac arrest or syncope had later and fewer ICD therapies than the ventricular tachycardia group.

The bridge-to-transplant indication remains controversial. Despite the impressive reductions in sudden death rates observed in such patients when treated by ICDs, it is not clear that they benefit long term because of their high risk of death from pump failure (26,41). The study by Sweeney and colleagues (23) suggests that the ICD's impact on total mortality may be essentially nullified by the high incidence of non-sudden deaths. However, lack of randomization makes it impossible to draw any firm conclusions on what would have happened to the ICD-treated patients if they had not received ICDs and whether those remaining might not have fared better if they had received ICDs.

Although the superior efficacy of ICD therapy compared with other alternatives has been permanently and unambiguously demonstrated by the major prospective studies, we should give credit to some prominent researchers, who had already pronounced this same verdict years before, based on the accumulated clinical evidence in their own and others' experience (42,43).

⬤ CONCLUSIONS

The accepted indications for implanting ICDs have evolved significantly over the two decades since the ICD was clinically introduced. In addition to the expanded indications for patients who have already presented spontaneously with sustained life-threatening ventricular tachyarrhythmias, the latest guidelines also include indications for using the ICD as primary prevention in patients with previous myocardial infarction, compromised left ventricular function, and non-sustained but electrophysiologically inducible ventricular tachycardia. The landmark MADIT and MUSTT studies established the latter indications, demonstrating a more than 50% reduction in all-cause mortality for patients treated with ICDs compared with pharmacologic or no specific antiarrhythmic therapy. In general, the patients receiving ICDs in various series and prospective studies over the years have shown fairly similar survival results: approximately 95%, 85%, and 80% at 1, 2, and 4 years, respectively. This is roughly 50% lower mortality compared with those treated without ICDs, whose survival has been shown to be approximately 80%, 70%, and 60% at 1, 2, and 4 years, respectively. The prospective, randomized trials directly comparing ICDs to pharmacologic (or no antiarrhythmic) therapy have shown a similar 40% to 50% survival improvement for the patients randomized to ICD therapy.

⬤ ACKNOWLEDGEMENTS

The author wishes to recognize Ms. Yvonne Buysen for her excellent secretarial support, particularly her help with the computer-scanned artwork included with the manuscript.

REFERENCES

1. Mirowski M, Reid P, Mower M, et al. Termination of malignant ventricular arrhythmias with an implanted automatic defibrillator in human beings. *N Engl J Med* 1980;303:322–324.
2. Pisa Z. Sudden death: a worldwide problem. In: Kulbertus H, Wellens H, eds. *Sudden death, 3*. Boston: Martinus Nijhoff, 1980.
3. Myerburg R, Kessler K, Castellanos A. Sudden cardiac death: epidemiology, transient risk, and intervention assessment. *Ann Intern Med* 1993;119:1187–1197.
4. Myerburg R, Interian A, Mitrani R, et al. Frequency of sudden cardiac death and profiles of risk. *Am J Cardiol* 1997;80[Suppl 5B]:10F–19F.
5. Nisam S. Can implantable defibrillators reduce non-arrhythmic mortality? *J Interv Card Electrophysiol* 1998;2:371–375.
6. Cannom D. A review of the cardioverter defibrillator trials. *Curr Opinions Cardiol* 1998;13:3–8.
7. Weisfeldt M, Kerber R, McGoldrick R, et al. Public access defibrillation: a statement for healthcare professionals from the American Heart Association Task Force on Automatic External Defibrillation. *Circulation* 1995;92:2763.
8. Nichol G, Hallstrom A, Kerber R, et al. American Heart Association report on the second Public Access Defibrillation Conference, April 17–29, 1997. *Circulation* 1998;97:1309–1314.
9. Moss A, Hall J, Cannom D, et al, for the MADIT Investigators. Improved survival with an implanted defibrillator in patients with coronary disease at high risk of ventricular arrhythmias. *N Engl J Med* 1996;335:1933–19340.
10. Buxton A, Lee K, Fisher J, et al. A randomized study of the prevention of sudden death in patients with coronary artery disease. *New Engl J Med* 1999;341:1882–1890.
11. The ACC/AHA Task Force on Practice Guidelines. ACC/AHA guidelines for implantation of cardiac pacemakers and antiarrhythmia devices. *J Am Coll Cardiol* 1998;31:1175–1209.
12. Winkle R, Mead H, Ruder M, et al. Improved low-energy defibrillation efficacy in man with the use of biphasic truncated exponential waveform. *Am Heart J* 1989;117:122–127.
13. Powell A, Finkelstein D, Garan H, et al. Influence of implantable cardioverter-defibrillators on the long-term prognosis of survivors of out-of-hospital cardiac arrest. *Circulation* 1993;88:1083–1092.
14. Kuck K-H, Cappato R, Siebels J, et al. Randomized comparison of antiarrhythmic drug therapy with implantable defibrillators in patients resuscitated from cardiac arrest. *Circulation* 2000;102:748–754.
15. The Antiarrhythmic Versus Implantable Defibrillator (AVID) Investigators. A comparison of antiarrhythmic-drug therapy with implantable defibrillators in patients resuscitated from near-fatal ventricular arrhythmias. *N Engl J Med* 1997;337:1576–1583.
16. Pitschner H, Neuzner J, Himmrich E, et al. Implantable cardioverter-defibrillator therapy: influence of left ventricular function on long-term results. *J Interv Card Electrophysiol* 1997;1:211–220.
17. Böcker D, Bänsch D, Heinecke A, et al. Potential benefit from implantable cardioverter-defibrillator therapy in patients with and without heart failure. *Circulation* 1998;98:1636–1643.
18. Link M, Costeas X, Griffith J, et al. High incidence of appro-

priate implantable cardioverter-defibrillator therapy in patients with syncope of unknown etiology and inducible ventricular arrhythmias. *J Am Coll Cardiol* 1997;29:370–375.
19. Menz V, Schwartzman D, Hallamothu N, et al. Does the initial presentation of patients with implantable defibrillators influence the outcome? *Pacing Clin Electrophysiol* 1997;20:173–176.
20. Connolly S, Gent M, Roberts R, et al. A randomized trial of the implantable cardioverter defibrillator against amiodarone. *Circulation* 2000;101:927–1302.
21. Grimm M, Wieselthaler G, Avanessian R, et al. The impact of implantable cardioverter-defibrillators on mortality among patients on the waiting list for heart transplantation. *J Thorac Cardiovasc Surg* 1995;92:3273–3281.
22. Defibrilat Study Group. Actuarial risk of sudden death while awaiting cardiac transplantation in patients with atherosclerotic heart disease. *Am J Cardiol* 1991;68:545–546.
23. Sweeney M, Ruskin J, Garan H, et al. Influence of the implantable cardioverter/defibrillator on sudden death and total mortality in patients evaluated for cardiac transplantation. *Circulation* 1995;92:3273–3281.
24. Jeevanandam V, Bielefeld M, Auteri J, Sanchez J, et al. The implantable defibrillator: an electronic bridge to cardiac transplantation. *Circulation* 1992;6[Suppl II]:II-276–II-279.
25. Lorga-Filho A, Geelen P, Vanderheyden M, et al. Early benefit of implantable cardioverter defibrillator therapy in patients waiting for cardiac transplantation. *Pacing Clin Electrophysiol* 1998;21:1747–1750.
26. Brugada P. Personal communication, August 13, 1999.
27. Primo J, Geelen P, Brugada J, et al. Hypertrophic cardiomyopathy: role of the implantable cardioverter-defibrillator. *J Am Coll Cardiol* 1998;31:1081–1085.
28. Silka M, Kron J, Dunnigan A, Dick M. Sudden cardiac death and the use of implantable cardioverter-defibrillators in pediatric patients. *Circulation* 1993;87:800–807.
29. Borggrefe M, Breithardt G. Is the implantable defibrillator indicated in patients with hypertrophic cardiomyopathy and aborted sudden death? *J Am Coll Cardiol* 1998;31:1086–1088.
30. Groh W, Silka M, Oliver R, et al. Use of implantable cardioverter-defibrillators in the congenital long QT syndrome. *Am J Cardiol* 1996;78:703–706.
31. Moss A. Personal communication, August 28, 1999.
32. Brugada J, Brugada R, Brugada P. Right bundle-branch block and ST-segment elevation in leads V_1 through V_3: a marker for sudden death in patients without demonstrable structural heart disease. *Circulation* 1998;97:457–460.
33. Nademanee K, Veerakul G, Nimmannit S, et al. Arrhythmogenic marker for the sudden unexplained death syndrome in Thai men. *Circulation* 1997;96:2595–2600.
34. Brugada P, Brugada R, Brugada J, Geelen P. Use of the prophylactic implantable cardioverter defibrillator for patients with normal hearts. *Am J Cardiol* 1999:83:98–100.
35. Herre J, Sauve M, Scheinman M. Long-term results of amiodarone therapy with recurrent sustained ventricular tachycardia or ventricular fibrillation. *J Am Coll Cardiol* 1989;13:442–449.
36. Bigger JT, for the Coronary Artery Bypass Graft (CABG)-Patch Trial Investigators. Prophylactic use of implanted cardiac defibrillators in patients at high risk for ventricular arrhythmias after coronary artery bypass graft surgery. *N Engl J Med* 1997; 337:1569–1575.
37. Naccarelli G, Wolbrette D, Dell'orfano J, et al. A decade of clinical trial developments in postmyocardial infarction, congestive heart failure, and sustained ventricular tachyarrhythmia patients: from CAST to AVID and beyond. *J Cardiovasc Electrophysiol* 1998;9:864–891.
38. Domanski M, Exner D. Prevention of sudden cardiac death: a current perspective. *J Electrocardiol* 1999;31:47–53.
39. ICD trials: an *extraordinary* means of determining patient risk? *Pacing Clin Electrophysiol* 1998;21:1341–1346.
40. Bigger JT. Primary prevention of sudden cardiac death using implantable cardioverter-defibrillators. In: Singer I, ed. *Implantable cardioverter-defibrillators*. Armonk, NY: Futura Publishing, 1994:515–546.
41. Schmidinger H. The implantable cardioverter defibrillator as a "bridge to transplant": a viable clinical strategy? *Am J Cardiol* 1999;83:151–157.
42. Saksena S, Madan N, Lewis C. Implantable cardioverter-defibrillators are preferable to drugs as primary therapy in sustained ventricular tachyarrhythmias. *Prog Cardiovasc Dis* 1996;38: 445–454.
43. Böcker D, Block M, Borggrefe M, Breithardt G. Defibrillators are superior to antiarrhythmic drugs in the treatment of ventricular arrhythmias. *Eur Heart J* 1997;18:26–30.

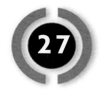

RANDOMIZED CLINICAL TRIALS OF IMPLANTABLE CARDIOVERTER-DEFIBRILLATORS FOR PROPHYLAXIS OF SUDDEN CARDIAC DEATH

DAVID S. CANNOM

In the past 25 years, American electrophysiology has gone through several eras. The era of the late 1970s and early 1980s documented the utility and reproducibility of intracardiac electrophysiology. Clinicians in Seattle identified the high rate of recurrence of sudden death in patients who had been resuscitated from a first episode. In the 1980s, electrophysiologic (EP) testing became increasingly popular for risk stratifying such high-risk patients, and electropharmacologic testing was employed in this patient group. The first implantable cardioverter-defibrillators (ICDs) were also implanted in the early 1980s. In the 1990s, a variety of prospective clinical trials—Antiarrhythmics Versus Implantable Defibrillator (AVID) (1), Canadian Implantable Defibrillator Study (CIDS) (2), and Cardiac Arrest Study Hamburg (CASH) (3)—conclusively demonstrated that the ICD is preferred therapy for most of these high-risk patients.

The next frontier in electrophysiology is the prophylactic use of ICDs in patients who have risk factors that predispose them to malignant cardiac arrhythmias (4,5). Trials such as the Sudden Cardiac Death–Heart Failure Trial (SCD-HeFT) (6), the Multicenter Automatic Defibrillator Implantation Trial II (MADIT II) (7), and the Defibrillators in Non-Ischemic Cardiomyopathy Treatment Evaluation (DEFINITE) trial (8) should define the role of the ICD in high-risk patients. Another frontier is the use of biventricular pacing in high-risk patients with congestive heart failure (9).

Each era in clinical medicine becomes shorter as the creation of superb technology drives new studies. A reasonable hope for the next decade is that ICD use will have a significant impact on the large number of Americans who still die suddenly from cardiac arrhythmias.

◉ SUDDEN CARDIAC DEATH

There has been no area in clinical electrophysiology that has undergone more intense study or whose clinical subtleties have been more clearly defined over the past decade than sudden cardiac death. To the clinician, it is arbitrary to separate the patient with sudden cardiac death from the patient with sustained monomorphic ventricular tachycardia. Some patients who die suddenly started with sustained monomorphic ventricular tachycardia and degenerate into ventricular fibrillation. However, there are clinical features unique to the patient with sudden cardiac death in terms of presentation, mechanism of arrhythmia, and therapy that make this area an important one to discuss and understand separately from the patient with sustained ventricular tachycardia.

Much of our understanding and approach to such patients is the result of seminal work in the 1990s by a variety of investigators, particularly the conceptual framework of Myerberg, Wellens, and Zipes (10,11). Sudden cardiac death has been defined as unexpected natural death from a cardiac cause occurring over a short period, generally less than 1 hour from the onset of symptoms. Sudden cardiac death is a natural death from cardiac causes that is heralded by the abrupt loss of consciousness, is unexpected, and whose key elements are that the death was "natural, rapid, and unexpected." The 1-hour definition refers to the duration of the terminal event and includes the pathophysiologic disturbances leading to cardiac arrest and the onset of the terminal event itself. Because 40% of sudden cardiac deaths are unwitnessed, the end point for any study of this subject must be mortality itself.

Sudden cardiac death accounts for 300,000 to 400,000 deaths in the United States annually, depending somewhat on the definition used. It is the most common and often the first manifestation of coronary disease and is responsible for 50% of the mortality from cardiovascular disease in the United States. A notable finding from the public health standpoint is that large population studies have demonstrated a 15% to 19% decline in the incidence of sudden cardiac death since early 1980s. At the same time, the absolute number of patients with congestive heart failure is increasing, with about 300,000 cases of congestive heart failure presenting each year. The pool of potential sudden cardiac death victims is increasing numerically.

As Myerberg eloquently pointed out, the public health challenge in population studies of sudden cardiac death is finding interventions that will influence the 1 of 1,000 patients who might experience sudden death while not intervening in the remaining 999 who will not experience sudden cardiac death. The screening of unselected large populations is impractical, and even current studies evaluating the impact of the prophylactic ICD on high-risk subsets will have little effect on the overall global problem of sudden cardiac death. The incidence of arrhythmic events is more frequent in populations who have powerful risk factors, but the total number of patients identified within these populations is relatively small.

The overall annual risk of death from ventricular arrhythmias in the general population is low. This is true even for survivors of myocardial infarction. Any intervention designed for a large-scale prophylaxis in the general population must be applied to the majority of the population who will never have the event, in order to have a possibility of influencing the minority of individuals who will suffer a cardiac event. Cost considerations and risk-benefit ratios make widespread application of even highly effective interventions prohibitive for all but the most simple and safe measures.

A tradeoff in targeting the progressively "higher-risk" subgroup exists. To increase the confidence with which a fatal event can be predicted in the target group, it is necessary to evaluate the increasing number of patients at lesser risk excluded from prior planned interventions. As the target group becomes smaller over time, it will contain a progressively smaller number of total fatal events experienced in the entire post-myocardial infarction population. Fatal events in the excluded population will occur at a much lower rate, but will constitute a progressively larger share of the total events in the population.

It is also important to consider timing of any particular study or intervention. Myerberg contends that high-risk patients, such as those surviving an episode of sudden cardiac death, such as those after myocardial infarction with high-risk markers or developing recent-onset congestive failure, have an attrition over time that is accelerated in absolute and relative terms for the initial 6 to 18 months. After this time, the slopes of the curves for the high-risk and the low-risk populations parallel each other, highlighting the early attrition and the attenuation of risk after 18 to 24 months. However, data from the MADIT and Multicenter Unsustained Tachycardia Trial (MUSTT) trials call this finding into question because patients, removed from their myocardial infarctions by many years, continued to be at high risk through the duration of those studies.

We know that 50% of patients who die of congestive heart failure die suddenly and that New York Heart Association class IV congestive heart failure patients have higher total death rates but a lower fraction of sudden death (12). We also know that most sudden cardiac deaths occur in the early morning, perhaps because of increased blood viscosity and platelet aggregation. Holter monitors recovered from patients who die suddenly show a tendency toward increases in sinus rate and ventricular premature beats before ventricular fibrillation which likely represents a change in autonomic activity or hemodynamic status. This data supports the concept of a role for active transient events in triggering the onset of a fatal arrhythmia. Other systemic abnormalities, such as hypoxemia, acidosis, or electrolyte imbalance, may also contribute to sudden death. Regional ischemia and acidosis may cause reentrant rhythms because of dispersion of refractoriness. Hypokalemia can cause torsades de pointes, and antiarrhythmic drugs can cause arrhythmias by prolonging the QT interval. Patients with left ventricular enlargement probably have sudden death caused by subendocardial ischemia. The underlying pathophysiology is a delicate balance between an abnormal substrate (usually scar), various triggers (e.g., premature ventricular contractions, nonsustained ventricular tachycardia), and modulating or transient risk factors (e.g., autonomic changes, ischemia, electrolytes, humeral factors).

The prevention of sudden cardiac death requires that we identify patients who have inherent characteristics that make the initiation of electrical instability likely. These clinical conditions can be determined genetically or on an acquired basis, such as a patient with the long QT syndrome whose sudden death is an interaction between a molecular abnormality, such as an ionopathy, and an inciting event, such as exercise in long QT-1 or sleep in long QT-3. Patients with acquired long QT may have their cardiac arrest only in response to certain drugs. Certain conditions such as hypertrophic cardiomyopathy and the Brugada syndrome may be a response to a genetic marker. I can think of no area in clinical electrophysiology where there has been a more exciting or important development than in our understanding of the pathophysiology of sudden cardiac death.

In the mid-1980s, considerable controversy existed about which end point to use to assess the benefit of therapy. Over time, total mortality emerged as the end point used in all major clinical trials for a variety of reasons. Potentially large inaccuracies exist in classifying other end points such as arrhythmic death or nonsudden cardiac death issues. Total mortality as an end point avoids ambiguity about the cause of death. Other end points used, such as quality of life and cost effectiveness, are clearly secondary end points.

Between 30% and 60% of post-myocardial infarction deaths are caused by primary arrhythmia. This figure represents the maximal proportion of device preventable deaths. From this total, other deaths must be subtracted, including those from device implantation, from nontreatable bradyarrhythmias, and from device failure and other competing causes of death such as recurrent myocardial infarction and congestive failure. The hope of any clinical trial is that the ICD may show a benefit of 20% to 50% reduction in total mortality, depending on patient selection. The next section explores screening techniques that can be employed to identify high-risk patients.

TESTS USED IN EVALUATION OF SUSTAINED VENTRICULAR ARRHYTHMIAS

Left Ventricular Function

Left ventricular function remains the single most important predictor of sudden death, regardless of the cause of left ventricular dysfunction. The 1-year cardiac mortality is less than 4% for post-myocardial infarction patients with a radionuclide-determined ejection fraction greater than 40%. The annual mortality rate for a patient with an ejection fraction of less than 20% is almost 50%, as shown by data gathered years ago by Moss (14).

Most studies suggest that Holter data and left ventricular ejection fraction (LVEF) are independent predictors of sudden cardiac death according to the Multicenter Post-Infarction Research Group and Multicenter Investigation of the Limitation of Infarct Size studies (15). All of the major studies evaluating the role of the ICD in primary prophylaxis of sudden death (i.e., SCD-HeFT, MADIT II, and DEFINITE) rely on the ejection fraction as the dominant and only risk factor in predicting future total mortality. Although use of thrombolytics in the treatment of acute myocardial infarction has reduced the number of patients postinfarction who have a very low ejection

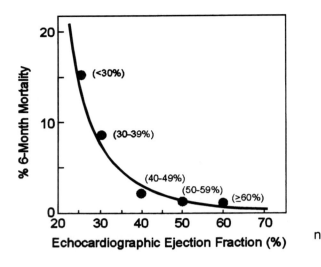 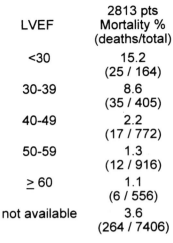

FIGURE 27-1. The GISSI-2 data show that there is a dramatic increase in 6-month mortality rates for patients receiving thrombolytic therapy after acute myocardial infarction as the ejection fraction falls below 30%. Correlation of high postinfarction mortality with low ejection fraction has not been altered during the era of thrombolytic therapy.

fraction (≤30%) (Fig. 27-1), thrombolysis has not changed the risk of future arrhythmic events posed by a low ejection fraction. The LVEF remains the most potent single predictor of survival. Subsequent mortality after myocardial infarction increases exponentially as LVEF decreases from 40% to 30%. Overall data suggest that the proportion of patients with severely impaired LVEF has decreased in the post-thrombolytic era, but the proportion of all deaths based on ejection fraction remains surprisingly similar over time. Using contemporary therapies, about 20% of the post-myocardial infarction population have an LVEF of less than 40%, and this subgroup accounts for 50% to 60% of all deaths over the subsequent few years.

The results from the AVID and CIDS studies, which were both major postevent randomized clinical trials, have focused on the importance of ejection fraction as a determinant of ICD benefit. In the AVID trial, the patients studied had survived an episode of ventricular fibrillation with an ejection fraction of less than 40%, an episode of sustained ventricular tachycardia with syncope, or an episode of symptomatic ventricular tachycardia with an ejection fraction of less than 40%. The mean ejection fraction of the AVID population was 31% to 32%. These postevent patients were randomized to the ICD or to drug therapy (i.e., amiodarone or sotalol) without the benefit of an EP study. For the overall AVID population the ICD statistically improved survival compared with drug therapy and led to the premature termination of the trial. Subsequent subset analysis of the AVID data has shown that there was benefit for the AVID patient only if the ejection fraction was less than 36% (16). This analysis showed that patients with the lowest ejection fraction (<20%) and intermediate ejection fractions (20% to 34%) have statistically significant benefit from the ICD. However, patients with the highest ejection fraction (≥35%) did not benefit from the ICD and did equally well with empirical drug therapy over the ICD (Fig. 27-2). In examining these survival curves, it is apparent that the high ejection fraction group did extremely well with a low 2-year mortality rate, making it difficult for the ICD to add additional survival benefit.

A subsequent analysis by the CIDS investigators showed comparable results. The CIDS investigators retrospectively stratified 659 study patients into four risk quartiles based on ejection fraction, advanced age, and poor New York Heart Association functional class. In the highest risk quartile, there was a 50% relative risk reduction in total mortality with ICD therapy compared with amiodarone. In the AVID and CIDS studies, there was benefit from the defibrillator only in the lowest ejection fraction group.

Further analysis by Moss (17) of the impact of ejection fraction on survival from the MADIT population confirmed the AVID data, albeit with small numbers. Although the eligibility criteria for MADIT was an ejection fraction of 35% or less, the median ejection

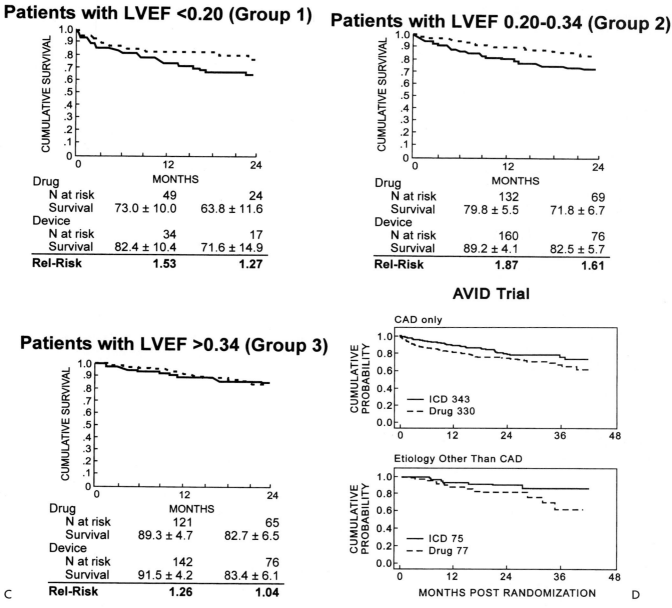

FIGURE 27-2. Shown are data from the AVID study, which was a study of postevent patients receiving an implantable cardioverter-defibrillator (ICD) or receiving amiodarone therapy. The Kaplan-Meier survival curves for the various ejection fractions (groups 1, 2, and 3) are shown. Patients with ejection fractions of less than 34% and having cardiac arrest or symptomatic, sustained ventricular tachycardia benefitted from the ICD *(dotted line)* compared with amiodarone or sotalol *(solid line)*. Patients with ejection fractions of more than 34% did not benefit from ICD implantation. This study of a postevent population confirms the importance of ejection fraction as a predictor of subsequent mortality. As is shown in D, the survival benefit of the ICD was documented whether cardiac arrhythmia occurred in a postinfarction population or a dilated cardiomyopathy population.

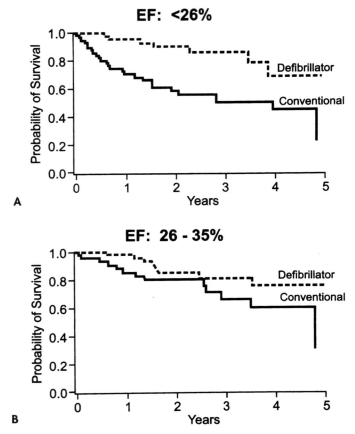

FIGURE 27-3. Probability of survival with implantable cardioverter-defibrillator (ICD) or conventional therapy in the MADIT population, which is divided by left ventricular ejection fraction. **A:** Patients with ejection fractions of less than 26% (defibrillator, $n = 46$; conventional, $n = 56$; $p = 0.001$). **B:** Patients with ejections fractions between 26% to 35% (defibrillator, $n = 49$; conventional, $n = 45$; p is not significant). The survival benefit from ICD therapy was significantly greater than from conventional therapy only in the subgroup with an ejection fraction of less than 26%.

fraction for the 196 enrolled patients was 26%. When the ejection fraction was dichotomized at the median value, the benefit from ICD therapy was most notable in those with an ejection fraction of less than 26% (Fig. 27-3). Four studies (i.e., AVID, CIDS, MADIT, and MUSTT) show that the chief determinant of poor outcome is a low ejection fraction ($\leq 35\%$) and that the ICD improves survival in all of these groups.

In designing a prophylactic ICD trial, if one is to show a benefit for the ICD in a low ejection fraction population, one needs to identify a patient group with a high 2-year mortality of which arrhythmic deaths constitute a large fraction of the total number of deaths (estimated at 50% in most studies). These data have overwhelming importance for anyone designing a prophylactic ICD trial at the millennium and suggest that future trials, such as MADIT II and SCD-HeFT, will show a benefit. Skeptics who thought that the ICD would not show a benefit in the lowest ejection fraction group ($\leq 30\%$) appear to be wrong, because the competing mortality risks in at least four studies have not overwhelmed the benefit of the ICD.

Electrophysiologic Testing

For more than two decades, EP testing has been used to judge drug efficacy in patients with sustained ventricular tachycardia and in survivors of cardiac arrest. The predictability of EP testing appears highest for patients with coronary disease. Ventricular tachycardia can be initiated in the EP laboratory in 90% of patients with sustained monomorphic ventricular tachycardia. In contrast, among sudden cardiac death survivors, sustained monomorphic ventricular tachycardia is induced in 50% to 60%, polymorphic ventricular tachycardia or ventricular fibrillation in another 10% to 20%, and nonsustained ventricular tachycardia or no arrhythmias in the remaining patients. The incidence of inducibility depends on the ejection fraction, the clinical arrhythmia at presentation, and which stimulation protocol is used. Patients who have neither structural heart disease nor dilated cardiomyopathy have a lower induction rate. Patients who have survived out-of-hospital cardiac arrest and have coronary disease have an approximately 60% arrhythmia induction rate in the EP laboratory.

Electrophysiologic-electropharmacologic testing was a very popular method of determining adequate antiarrhythmic therapy for patients with sustained tachyarrhythmias. However, it became clear in the early 1990s that even patients who were predicted to have a good result with successful arrhythmia suppression therapy in the laboratory had an unacceptably high mortality rate, particularly if the ejection fraction was less than 40% (17). This explains in large part the popularity of ICD therapy for patients with an ejection fraction of less than 40% and ventricular tachycardia, even if the arrhythmia was suppressed with drugs at EP testing. Although the data in early retrospective series suggested this, it was borne out in the prospective, randomized AVID trial in which device therapy was superior to drug therapy for patients with ejection fractions of less than 35%. Electrophysiologic testing was not part of the AVID protocol but was performed in more than 500 patients who were randomized in the AVID study. Inducibility in the EP laboratory did not select a group of patients who did poorly in either arm of the trial.

Among patients with coronary disease and a prior myocardial infarction who have clinical ventricular tachycardia, those who have inducible, sustained ventricular tachycardia have significantly poorer left ventricular function than those with polymorphic ventricular tachycardia or those who are noninducible. There is a strong correlation between persistent inducibility of sustained ventricular tachycardia on antiarrhythmic drugs and subsequent cardiac death and recurrent cardiac arrest. Those patients with an ejection fraction of less than 40% who remain inducible have a mortality rate approaching 50% at 4 years (17). Published in the late 1980s, these data were early observations leading to the increasing popularity of ICDs in this population.

In patients who have survived an uncomplicated myocardial infarction, EP testing has proven to be poorly predictive of future sudden cardiac death in unselected populations. For those patients who are considered at high risk, such as patients with congestive failure or conduction abnormalities observed on the electrocardiogram (ECG), EP testing is of benefit. In a meta-analysis of 12 series with a total of 926 patients with nonsustained ventricular tachycardia, most of whom had coronary artery disease, roughly one third had inducible, sustained arrhythmias (18). However, only 18% of the inducible patients had subsequent arrhythmic events in 19.4 months, whereas 7% of patients without inducible arrhythmias had events during the same follow-up. There is a relatively high negative predictive value in employing EP testing for such high-risk patients, but the positive predictive value is low.

There are a number of important considerations in terms of how the EP test is performed. These methodologic issues have largely been resolved in the large, prospective clinical trials such as MUSTT (19). In performing EP testing, a current strength of twice the diastolic threshold is employed using a pulse duration of 1 to 2 msec. The typical protocol involves introducing one to three extrastimuli at two sites and two drive cycles. If more than three extrastimuli are used, sensitivity increases but at the expense of specificity. In some patients atrial stimulation can induce ventricular tachycardia, especially those with left ventricular tachycardia and normal hearts. Sometimes, the use of burst pacing can initiate ventricular tachycardia, especially in those individuals with normal hearts and a tachycardia originating from the right ventricular outflow tract. Pharmacologic agents such as isoproterenol or epinephrine can be used to enhance the ability to induce ventricular tachycardia. These techniques are particularly useful in patients with normal hearts who have right ventricular outflow tract tachycardia. These techniques are routinely used in clinical practice, especially when a patient has a documented out-of-hospital clinical ventricular tachycardia that cannot be initiated with routine programmed stimulation.

Ambulatory Electrocardiography

Holter monitoring has also been applied to patients post-myocardial infarction in an effort to stratify them according to risk. One study placed Holter monitors on 160 post-myocardial infarction patients and found that a total of 14 patients who experienced sudden cardiac death during follow-up had frequent or complex ventricular ectopy (20). Other studies have reported similar findings. Although high-density or complex ventricular ectopy has prognostic significance in post-myocardial infarction patients, these findings are of little prognostic importance for patients with normal hearts. The use of the Holter monitor for post-myocardial infarction risk stratification has fallen into clinical disuse largely because of the results of the Cardiac Arrhythmia Suppression Trial (CAST), which demonstrated that Holter-guided suppression of ventricular premature contractions (VPCs) increased the patient's risk of dying suddenly rather than decreasing this risk (21).

However, as sobering statistics demonstrate, we have done little to reduce the number of patients dying suddenly other than by the routine use of thrombolytics (13). The Gruppo Italiano per lo Studio della Streptochinasi nell'Infarto miocardico 2

(GISSI-2) trial showed that, after thrombolytic therapy, the presence of ventricular arrhythmias decreased, although they still predicted a poor outcome and future sudden cardiac death. In this trial, the lower the ejection fraction, the worse was the prognosis (13). A Holter monitor predicted arrhythmias as it had in prethrombolytic studies. In the GISSI-2 study, 8,676 post-myocardial infarction patients were studied with Holter monitors. There were 256 deaths (3% of patients), of which 84 were sudden (33% of total deaths). Mortality rates were 2% for patients with no ventricular ectopic activity, 2.7% in patients with 1 to 10 VPCs, 5.5% in patients with more than 10 VPCs/hour, and 4.8% with complex ectopy. The presence of frequent VPCs remained a predictor of total mortality and sudden death mortality. However, the presence of nonsustained ventricular tachycardia was not associated with a worsening of the prognosis. Despite the decrease in mortality after myocardial infarction in patients treated with thrombolytic therapy, ventricular premature beats remain a marker of electrical instability.

Signal Averaged Electrocardiography

In addition to left ventricular function, other noninvasive parameters appear useful to identify patients at high risk for cardiac mortality. Signal-averaged electrocardiography (SAECG) is a technique that amplifies electrocardiographic signals and decreases the level of noise to identify abnormalities, for example, ventricular late potentials, that presumably identify areas of slowed conduction in abnormal ventricular tissue that is arrhythmogenic.

Several studies have supported the prognostic significance of SAECG for mortality after myocardial infarction. Sustained ventricular tachycardia in the first year after myocardial infarction occurred in 14% to 29% of patients with an abnormal SAECG compared with 0.8% to 4.5% with a normal SAECG (22). Unfortunately, the relatively low positive predictive accuracy of the SAECG limits it clinical applicability. In a variety of multivariate analysis the signal averaged ECG added significantly to the information provided by the ejection fraction alone. In one study, combining an abnormal signal averaged ECG and an ejection fraction of less than 40% was associated with a 34% incidence of arrhythmic events during a median follow-up of 14 months (23). These investigators also found the signal averaged ECG to be the most sensitive predictive of arrhythmic events in a prospective study of 155 post-myocardial infarction patients. The technique is less sensitive in an anterior wall than an inferior wall myocardial infarction.

Heart Rate Variability

Heart rate variability is another noninvasive test used for risk stratification. It is a noninvasive index of autonomic tone. The Multicenter Post-Infarction Group study demonstrated that decreased heart rate variability is an important indicator of prognosis after myocardial infarction (24). Farrell, in a study of 487 post-myocardial infarction patients, found that decreased heart rate variability was more predictive of arrhythmic events than the presence of late potentials, Holter-derived data, treadmills, or ejection fractions (25). The combination of late potentials and reduced heart rate variability is considered by many to be more predictive of future events than any other noninvasive tool.

A variety of approaches can be used. Respiratory sinus arrhythmia can provide a noninvasive measure of parasympathetic control of the sinus node and presumably reflects parasympathetic tone on other cardiac tissue. Determination of heart rate variability can be as simple as a 1- to 2-minute bedside breathing test or more complicated by evaluation of time-dependent or frequency-dependent values obtained during longer monitoring periods. Decreased vagal tone has been associated with increased mortality after myocardial infarction. However, the role of heart rate variability in risk stratification, as well as other noninvasive tests such as repolarization and QT dispersion, remains to be determined. At this juncture, heart rate variability must be considered an investigational tool and not a tool on which the clinician can make decisions on an individual basis regarding arrhythmic risk.

The era of the signal averaged ECG was clearly that of the 1980s. This was the time during which the CABG Patch trial was designed (26). As the CABG Patch investigators looked for a suitable electrical marker to indicate risk in low ejection fraction patients undergoing bypass surgery, a positive signal-averaged ECG was the criteria for entering into the study. This did not turn out to be a potent marker of risk. Overall mortality in the CABG Patch study was only 20%. This turned out to be as low a figure as any population that was studied in the era of prophylactic ICD trials.

Heart rate variability may prove to be a potent predictor of arrhythmic risk, but definitive studies have not confirmed this. Although heart rate variability is being measured in some of the prophylactic trials, it is not an entry criteria in any major trial at this juncture.

Electrical Alternans

Alteration in T-wave amplitude of the surface ECG has been reported in post-myocardial infarction patients to be a harbinger of sudden cardiac death. Rosenbaum employed signal analysis to quantify electrical alternans in a series of patients referred for EP study (27). Alternans of the ST segment and T wave is correlated with the induction of sustained arrhythmias at EP study. The absence of repolarization alternans correlated with an arrhythmia-free survival. This technique is being actively studied, and its utility will be defined on the basis of large-scale studies.

Electrical alternans has not been used as a dominant entry point into any of the major preevent trials. MADIT II investigators seriously considered using electrical alternans, and it is being studied by the DEFINITE investigators, although not as part of the clinical trial itself. If this technique proves to be of use clinically, it may well be incorporated into future trials.

⦿ ADJUNCTIVE THERAPY TO DECREASE MORTALITY

The concept of trial design assumes that the therapy under study can reduce cardiac mortality independent of other competing therapies. A lesson in the 1990s has been that the medical therapies available to high-risk patients have had potent and at times compelling effects on sudden death reduction independent of an intervention such as the defibrillator. Consequently, as we evaluate current ICD trials and plan future ICD trials, concurrent medical therapy crucially affects the overall improvement in patient outcome and the contribution that the ICD itself makes to this improvement (Fig. 27-4).

The therapies that have emerged during the past 20 years include a number that are accepted and others that are less widely understood and less widely applied. They are discussed in the following sections.

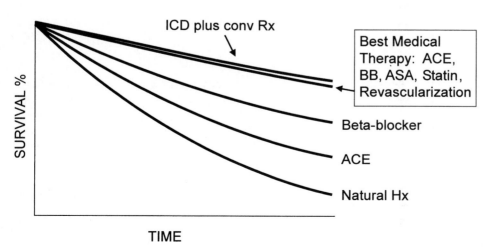

FIGURE 27-4. The theoretical construct attempts to show the importance of having any patient in an implantable cardioverter-defibrillator (ICD) trial on the best medical therapy. Background medical therapy, including angiotensin-converting enzyme (ACE) inhibitors, beta blockers, statins, and aspirin, improves survival. If the ICD is to provide additional survival benefit, patients must be aggressively treated with the best medical therapy so that the true survival advantage of the ICD can be measured. These therapies do not imply ICD benefit or can be overestimated, because the medical therapies themselves provide benefit.

Beta Blockade

There is no conjunctive therapy for the treatment of a post-myocardial infarction patient that is more important to patient's long-term survival than the judicious application of beta-blockade therapy. Numerous data sets confirm the utility of beta blockade in preventing future sudden cardiac death of the post-myocardial infarction survivor. A meta-analysis of clinical trials conducted in the prethrombolytic era that involved more than 27,000 patients indicate that beta blockade reduced mortality by 20% during the subsequent 2 to 3 years (28). The survival benefit appears mediated by a reduction in arrhythmia-related deaths (25% to 30% of all patients) and recurrent myocardial infarctions. Most trials showed that there is a beneficial effect from employing lipophilic drugs that have central nervous system activity. Drugs with simple sympathomimetic activity conferred no survival benefit. Patients with a history of congestive failure and depressed ejection fraction showed the greatest survival benefit.

The use of beta blockade in postinfarction patients has shown that there is a reduction in sudden cardiac death with this therapy. The benefit of beta blockade is greatest for those patients at highest risk for sudden death, namely patients with poor left ventricular function and complex ectopy. Holter data suggest that the suppression of ectopy is not a requisite for realizing the benefits of beta blockade.

Angiotensin-Converting Enzyme Inhibitors

Several trials have looked at the use of angiotensin-converting enzyme (ACE) inhibitors as prophylactic therapy to improve long-term survival in patients with left ventricular dysfunction. The SAVE and TRACE trials studied more than 7,500 patients with asymptomatic left ventricular dysfunction and demonstrated that survival was improved in patients with asymptomatic left ventricular dysfunction, significant wall motion abnormalities, or clinical heart failure after myocardial infarction (29). In these trials, ACE inhibitors were begun in the hospital and continued for several years. These studies showed a significant and progressive reduction in the late mortality rate of about 20% at 2 to 3 years. No particular ACE inhibitor seems preferred, and the benefit is probably mediated through a reduction in ventricular size with a subsequent reduction in reinfarction and new ischemic events.

The V-HeFT II trial showed a reduction in sudden death with enalapril that was significant compared with the use of hydralazine or nitrates in symptomatic patients with evidence of left ventricular dysfunction (30). A number of studies suggest that relatively asymptomatic patients appear to have a better prognosis from the standpoint of sudden death than patients with more severe symptoms and the same degree of left ventricular dysfunction. This finding was documented in the Studies of Left Ventricular Dysfunction (SOLVD) (31) and confirmed in the Cooperative North Scandinavian Enalapril Survival Study I (CONSENSUS I) (32), in which severely symptomatic patients with class IV congestive failure showed no benefit from ACE inhibitors in the prevention of sudden death. This is likely due to the fact that patients with more severe congestive failure tend to die of advanced failure, myocardial infarction, or bradyarrhythmias rather than suddenly. The patients

	Anti-platelet		Beta Blocker		Ace Inhibitor		Lipid Lowering	
	ICD	Conv	ICD	Conv	ICD	Conv	ICD	Conv
MADIT	??	??	27%	5%	57%	51%	??	??
CABG P	82%	85%	16%	20%	65%	55%	23%	23%
AVID	55%	55%	38%	11%	68%	66%	20%	18%

FIGURE 27-5. Use of adjunctive medical therapy in major trials that have been completed or are underway. The use of standard therapy such as beta blockers and angiotensin-converting enzyme (ACE) inhibitors is not as common as hoped but does parallel routine clinical practice. In future trials, every effort should be made to insist on this therapy before the implantable cardioverter-defibrillator is considered as a potential additional benefit.

with intermediate symptoms such as those studied in V-HeFT may be the most likely to benefit from therapy.

Although there is wide agreement that adjunctive therapy is very important clinically, in all clinical trials, the best medical therapy has been used sparingly. In the MADIT and CABG Patch trials, the rate of beta-blocker use was less than 30%, and ACE inhibitor use was less than 70%. Background medical therapy was better in CABG Patch (Fig. 27-5).

⦿ COMPLETED PREEVENT IMPLANTABLE CARDIOVERTER-DEFIBRILLATOR TRIALS

The goal of an ICD primary prevention trial is to help identify a patient population with a high enough annual mortality that the ICD can demonstrate improved survival for those patients in whom it is implanted. This study population must have a high enough sudden death rate that the defibrillator could be expected to decrease the sudden death mortality rate. During the past 15 years, a series of studies have emphatically and consistently identified the makeup of a high-risk population among the coronary artery disease population (33–38).

A series of trials designed in the late 1980s and early 1990s analyzed the role of the ICD in patients who have depressed ejection fractions and various electrical markers of risk but have not yet sustained a cardiac event. A number of these have recently been reported, and others are in progress (Tables 27-1 and 27-2).

The MADIT was a multicenter trial that studied a very carefully selected group of post-myocardial infarction patients who were at high risk for a future event (39). Published data from the 1980s suggested that the presence of nonsustained ventricular tachycardia on post-infarction Holter carried a mortality

TABLE 27-1 • IMPLANTABLE CARDIOVERTER-DEFIBRILLATOR STUDIES

Study	Investigators	Target Population	Therapies Employed	Sponsor
MUSTT (Multicenter Unsustained Tachycardia Trial)	Buxton	Post-MI (recent and late), LVEF ≤0.40, NSVT, SAECG (+)	EP-guided vs. no antiarrhythmic therapy	NIH
CAT (German Dilated Cardiomyopathy Trial)	Kuck	NICM, LVEF ≤0.30, NYHA class II/III	ICD vs. conventional	Guidant/CPI
MADIT-2	Moss	Late post-MI, LVEF ≤0.30	ICD vs. conventional	Guidant/CPI
SCD-HeFT (Sudden Cardiac Death Heart Failure Trial)	Bardy	NYHA class II/III, LVEF ≤0.35	ICD/admiodarone/ placebo	NIH and Medtronic
PRIDE (PRimary Implantation Cardioverter DEfibrillator)	Leon	Cardiomyopathy, VF or VT with syncope, NSVT	ICD vs. conventional	Guidant/CPI
BEST + ICD (Beta-blocker Strategy plus ICD trial)	Raviele	Recent post-MI, LVEF ≤0.35, HRV or NSVT or SAECG (+)	EP-guided (incl. ICDs in EP + pts. vs. conventional)	Guidant/CPI
DINAMIT (Defibrillator IN Acute Myocardial Infarction Trial)	Hohnloser, Kuck, Connolly, Dorian	Recent post-MI, LVEF ≤0.35, HRV or mean RR ≤750 msec	ICD vs. no ICD	St. Jude
DEFINITE (DEFibrillators in Non-ischemic Cardiomyopathy Treatment Evaluation)	Kadish	NICM, EF ≤0.35, NSVT or >10 PVCs/hour, symptomatic heart failure	Heart failure medications + beta blockers vs. ICD	St. Jude

CABG, coronary artery bypass grafting; EP, electrophysiologic study; ICD, implantable cardioverter-defibrillator; LVEF, left ventricular ejection fraction; MI, myocardial infarction; NICM, non-ischemic cardiomyopathy; NSVT, nonsustained ventricular tachycardia; NYHA, New York Heart Association classification; PVCs, premature ventricular contractions; SAECG, signal-averaged electrocardiography; VF, ventricular fibrillation; VT, ventricular tachycardia; (+), positive.

TABLE 27-2 • COMPLETED PRE-EVENT TRIALS

Trial	Design	Target Population	Therapies Employed	Outcome
MADIT	Randomized, total mortality	n = 196 coronary artery disease (MI >3 weeks) LVEF ≤35% NSVT EPS inducible PCA refractory CHF Cl I–III	ICD vs. conventional	ICD improved survival by 46%
CABG-Patch	Randomized, total mortality	n = 1000 CAD with ischemia LVEF <36% (+) SAECG CABG candidate	CABG in all ICD vs. no treatment	No survival benefit for ICD

CABG, coronary artery bypass grafting; CAD, coronary artery disease; CCM, congestive cardiomyopathy; CHF, congestive heart failure; EPS, electrophysiologic study; ICD, implantable cardioverter-defibrillator; LVEF, left ventricular ejection fraction; MI, myocardial infarction; PCA, procainamide; SAECG, signal-averaged electrocardiography.

risk of 14% at 12 months to 38% at 36 months (40). A widely heralded study by Wilber and colleagues (41) showed that the low-ejection-fraction coronary patient with nonsustained ventricular tachycardia who remained inducible in the EP laboratory after procainamide administration had a mortality of 40% at 2 years (Fig. 27-6). This is in contrast to the negligible mortality rate for patients who were noninducible or suppressed with procainamide. The MADIT trial took the Wilber data quite literally and designed a prospective study that recruited coronary artery disease patients who were 3 weeks removed from myocardial infarction, had nonsustained ventricular tachycardia evidenced on Holter (3 to 30 beats), had an ejection fraction of 35% or less, were inducible into sustained monomorphic ventricular tachycardia or

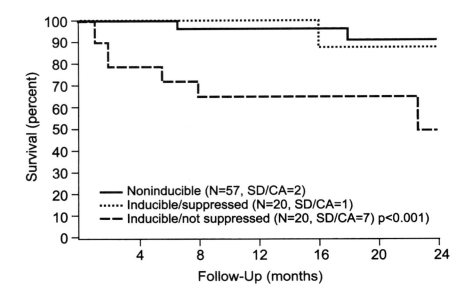

FIGURE 27-6. Shown is the Kaplan-Meier survival curve for patients with coronary disease, reduced ejection fraction, and nonsustained ventricular tachycardia who were studied in the electrophysiology laboratory. Patients whose conditions were noninducible or suppressed with procainamide did well, whereas the patients whose conditions were inducible and nonsuppressed had a markedly worse survival (dotted line) than either of the other groups. The construct was used in the design of the MADIT trial. (From Wilber DJ, Olshansky B, Moran JF, Scanlon PJ. Electrophysiological testing and nonsustained ventricular tachycardia. Circulation 1990;82:350–358, with permission.)

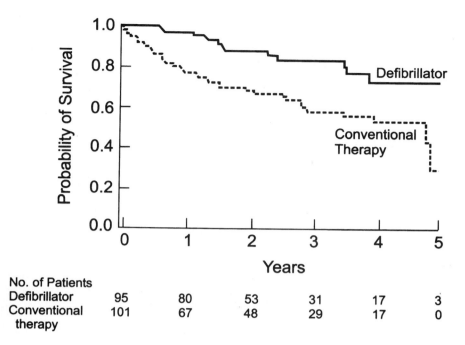

FIGURE 27-7. Kaplan-Meier survival curve from the MADIT trial. Implantable cardioverter-defibillator (ICD) therapy reduced mortality by 54% compared with best drug therapy. The two survival curves separated early and remained well separated throughout the 5-year study.

ventricular fibrillation, and were not suppressed with procainamide. This trial design assumed that the all cause mortality of the ICD group would be reduced from 20% to 8.8%, or a 46% reduction in the 2-year mortality rate based on the ICD. The ultimate outcome of the study was remarkably close to the initial projections.

The MADIT study enrolled 196 patients and randomized them to an ICD or to conventional therapy. At a mean follow-up of 27 months, the Data and Safety Monitoring Board (DSMB) terminated the trial prematurely at a time when the ICD showed marked survival benefit over conventional therapy. During the course of the trial, there were 39 deaths in the conventional therapy arm and 15 deaths in the ICD arm (Fig. 27-7). Thirteen of the deaths in the conventional arm were attributed to a primary arrhythmia, but only three deaths in the ICD arm were caused by a primary arrhythmia. There were 13 nonarrhythmic deaths in the conventional group, and 7 nonarrhythmic deaths in the ICD arm.

The MADIT population had the markers that suggested high risk. The mean ejection fraction of the conventional group was only 25% and that of the ICD group only 27%. The survival of all patients in the conventional group (all-cause mortality) was only 51% at 4 years. This survival is as poor as in any trial studying patients who have survived cardiac arrest or an episode of sustained ventricular tachycardia. The MADIT patients received frequent shocks from their ICDs, with 60% receiving device discharges at 2 years. The cause of these firings is not known because the devices were largely nondocumenting ICDs.

It is important to discuss the medications used in the conventional and ICD arms of the trials. This has been a source of great controversy since the trial was published (28). At 1 month after enrollment in the MADIT trial, 75% of the conventional-therapy group were receiving amiodarone, 8% were receiving beta blockers, and 10% were receiving class I antiarrhythmic drugs. In the ICD arm, only 2% were receiving amiodarone, 26% were receiving beta blockers, and 12% were receiving class I antiarrhythmic drugs. By the time of last contact before the trial was terminated, the amiodarone usage had fallen to only 45%, which was a 39% discontinuance rate. The incidence of the use of beta blockers and class I antiarrhythmics remained the same. The class I drugs used in the trial were not the agents that were shown in the CAST trial to cause harm (i.e., type IC antiarrhythmics), and the results of the trial cannot be explained on the basis of a proarrhythmic effect of the class I drugs used. However, there was a disproportionate use of beta blockers in the ICD arm that may have affected the outcome of the trial by enhancing the survival of the ICD group.

Results of the MADIT trial have been highly controversial, with several criticisms of the trial noted. Because no registry was kept, the total number of patients screened is unknown. Data were not kept on patients who were screened and were noninducible at EP study or were inducible and suppressed with procainamide. A small substudy from three centers in the trial suggested that the 2-year mortality rate in this subset was approximately 8% (42). A very high percentage of patients discontinued their amiodarone, and there was the aforementioned disproportionate use of beta blockers (3 : 1) in the ICD arm.

In the late 1990s, it was apparent that most clinicians were uncertain about what to do with the MADIT data (43). Although convincing in an investigational sense, it was not a trial that drew large numbers of patients into treatment after the data was published. The MADIT patients represented a small percentage of any post-myocardial infarction population (probably about 5%), and routine Holter monitoring had fallen out of favor in the mid-1990s. There were also issues of expense for the yield rate. The screening of potential MADIT patients was low.

All of the major prospective randomized trials have paid careful attention to the cost component of the ICD. In the MADIT trial, the cost analysis was done in an extremely careful fashion. Within the statistical confines of the trial, the average survival was 3.5 years for the ICD group and 2.7 years for the medication group, meaning that there was a 0.8-year extension of life with ICD use. The total per-patient cost for the ICD group was $90,000 over the duration of the trial, compared with $71,000 for the conventional group. The cost was $25,000/0.8 life-year saved, or $31,000/life-year saved. This cost of the ICD for extension of life is comparable to other lifesaving therapies.

Data from MUSTT showed, somewhat dramatically, that the findings from the MADIT trial were correct (44) (Table 27-3). The MUSTT trial was not a trial to evaluate therapeutic efficacy, but rather a trial to evaluate the efficacy of an EP testing approach to risk stratification and treatment of high-risk coronary artery disease patients. The hypothesis of this trial was that antiarrhythmic drug therapy that was guided by EP testing would reduce the risk of arrhythmic death and cardiac arrest in patients who had coronary artery disease, an ejection fraction of 40% or less, and nonsustained ventricular tachycardia as evidenced on Holter monitoring. Although not a trial to test therapeutic efficacy, the MUSTT trial in a surprising fashion turned out to verify the MADIT data. In the MUSTT trial, patients underwent EP testing. If the results were negative at testing, they were followed in the MUSTT registry. If results were positive at testing for inducible sustained monomorphic ventricular tachycardia, they were randomized to no antiarrhythmic therapy or EP-guided therapy (Fig. 27-8). Patients who were drug responders were followed; the nonresponders received a succession of antiarrhythmic drugs, and if no drug was successful, they received an ICD. The drug scheme was complicated and a product of the 1980s. It involved receiving a succession of antiarrhythmic drugs, including type IA, type IC, and type III drugs. Drug failure was predicted on the basis of EP testing, and those patients went on to receive ICD therapy.

The very ambitious MUSTT trial was sponsored by the National Heart, Lung, and Blood Institute. A total of 2,202 patients enrolled in 80 centers. The clinical characteristics of these patients were somewhat surprising in that the median ejection fraction was 30%, two thirds had New York Heart Association class II or III heart failure, one half had undergone bypass surgery, and fewer than 50% were not on beta blockers. As presented by Alfred Buxton at the 1999

TABLE 27-3 • COMPARISON OF MADIT AND MUST PATIENTS

Characteristic	MADIT	MUST
Heart disease	CAD	CAD
Qualifying EF	<36%	<40%
Mean number of VPCs in nonsust. VT	9	6
Mean EF	26	30
Percent inducible	100%	33%
Percent of inducible patients suppressed	100%	45%
Mortality in control group at 2 years	46%	30%
Reduction of death by ICD p value	0.09	0.001

EF, ejection fraction; ICD, implantable cardioverter-defibrillator; VPCs, ventricular premature contractions; VT, ventricular tachycardia.

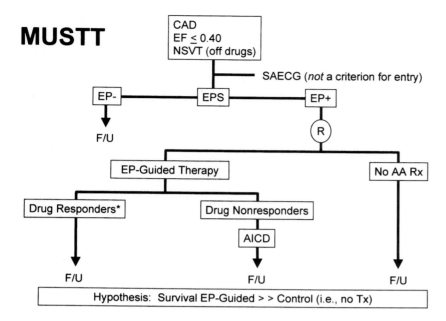

FIGURE 27-8. Study algorithm for the MUSTT trial. For the electrophysiologic responders (EP+), there was true randomization between EP-guided therapy and no antiarrhythmic drug therapy. Because a careful registry was kept, the outcome of patients in the EP-guided group (EP+) could be compared with the EP-negative (EP−) population.

American College of Cardiology meeting, 767 of the 2,202 patients were inducible. After the conclusion of antiarrhythmic drug testing in the EP-guided group, 45% of the patients received an antiarrhythmic drug, 46% received an ICD, and 7% refused an ICD. The statistical impact of the ICD was striking. The ICD reduced the risk of arrhythmic death or cardiac arrest with a p value of 0.001 and similarly improved overall mortality with a p value of 0.001. There was little doubt that EP-guided therapy reduced the risk of arrhythmic death, but it did so because of the use of ICDs and not antiarrhythmic drug use. What role, if any, drug proarrhythmia played in its differences is only speculative at this point.

When these data were presented to the North American Society of Pacing and Electrophysiology, the results showed that the EP-guided group and the control group (i.e., those inducible but not subjected to antiarrhythmic drug testing) had very similar arrhythmic death or cardiac arrest recurrences and total mortality rates. The total mortality rate was approximately 30% at 2 years (Fig. 27-9). However, the entire benefit of the survival of the EP-guided group was reflected in the significantly improved survival of the EP group who failed drugs and received an ICD. This group survival in terms of total mortality was roughly 90% at 2 years, a figure that is better than even the rate for the MADIT population. In an unintended fashion, a trial whose intent was to show that EP-guided therapy was preferable did so not on the basis of antiarrhythmic drug use but on the basis of ICD implantation.

Subsequent data from the MUSTT study were presented at the American Heart Association meeting in Atlanta in November 1999 (45). This evidence showed that the patients who were noninducible in the MUSTT algorithm as a whole had a survival that was better than those patients who were inducible. However, a number of clinical characteristics selected a particularly high-risk group. Patients with ejection fractions of less than 30%, runs of nonsustained ventricular tachycardia (six beats or more), and a positive signal-averaged ECG had the very highest risk and clearly should be treated with an ICD. However, survival in the inducible arm overall was comparable to the drug-treated group and raises the question of whether all MUSTT-eligible patients should receive an ICD. Further analysis of these data is necessary before a definitive conclusion can be reached.

A number of studies in the 1980s, including a coronary artery surgery study, showed improved survival for patients having double- and triple-vessel bypass surgery in terms of its impact on long-term sudden death. The hypothesis for the CABG Patch trial was

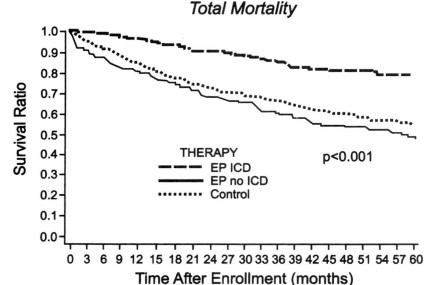

FIGURE 27-9. Kaplan-Meier survival curve derived from the MUSTT data. This fascinating curve shows that the control population and the electrophysiologic (EP)-guided therapy group with no implantable cardioverter-defibrillator (ICD) (among those patients who were inducible) did about the same in terms of survival but much less well ($p < 0.001$) than inducible patients who failed drugs and received an ICD. The EP-ICD group had a markedly improved survival over patients on antiarrhythmic drugs or on no drugs at all, and survival was remarkably similar to the survival data from the MADIT trial. The data suggest that the prime determinant of risk is a low ejection fraction and that the ICD can significantly modify that risk.

based on a seven-center retrospective survey in the late 1980s, which suggested that at least 40% of the patients who died after bypass surgery and had a low ejection fraction died because of an arrhythmia. The hypothesis was that prophylactic implantation of an ICD in this patient population might substantially decrease this mortality figure.

The randomization scheme developed was a simple one. The patient recruited into the trial had ischemic heart disease that warranted bypass surgery. Beyond this, the patient's age needed to be less than 80 years, and ejection fraction had to be less than 36%. A positive signal-averaged ECG was used as a marker of electrical instability. The patient underwent routine coronary artery revascularization, and at the conclusion of the case, the patient was randomized to receive or not receive an ICD (26).

The CABG Patch trial enrolled 1,055 patients over 4 years and was in its follow-up phase when the DSMB prematurely concluded the trial in April 1997, after a mean follow-up of 32 months. The DSMB concluded that there was no survival benefit because of ICD implantation and that the survival curves for the treated and untreated groups were identical (Fig. 27-10). The total number of deaths was 196, which was lower than projected. The DSMB encouraged the investigators to continue to follow the patients, but decided there was no indication to treat the control patients with ICD implantation.

The CABG Patch trial was the first trial that did not show positive result for the ICD, and the results have not been fully understood. The differences between this and other studies probably result from the design and the therapies chosen. Although the CABG Patch trial investigators thought that they had targeted a high-risk population, this was not the case. The mortality rate at 12 months was approximately 20% and held constant over the next 3 years (Fig. 27-10). It also appeared that the signal-averaged ECG was not as potent a predictor of arrhythmic risk as a positive EP study was in the MADIT population. It is not known what effect the revascularization procedure had on ejection fraction. Any improvement in ejection fraction might have overwhelmed the ability of the device to increase survival further. There was a 53% ICD firing rate at 2 years, but most discharges were probably for atrial arrhythmias, not for life-threatening arrhythmias.

Subsequent analysis of the deaths in the CABG Patch trial were of considerable interest. In the entire CABG Patch trial, there were 198 deaths (46). There were 79 (82%) deaths in the control group, and 76 (75%) of the 102 deaths in the ICD group were attributed to cardiac causes. In the control group, arrhyth-

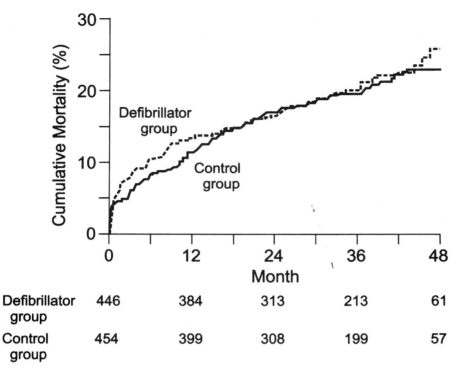

FIGURE 27-10. Survival data from the CABG Patch trial. The defibrillator group and the control group had comparable survival rates throughout the duration of the trial. The overall mortality in this trial is much less than encountered in other patient groups, pointing to the importance of the coronary revascularization procedure itself in predicting survival.

mic deaths constituted 17 of 59 witnessed cardiac deaths and only 9 of 56 witnessed deaths in the ICD group. There was a significant reduction by the ICD of arrhythmic death. Because there was little effect of the ICD on deaths from pump failure or cardiac procedures (as expected), the ICD reduction of arrhythmic death was not enough to affect overall total mortality in the ICD group. In the MADIT and CABG Patch trials, the proportion of all deaths that were arrhythmic were similar for the control groups of the two trials (29% for the CABG Patch trial versus 33% for the MADIT trial). The absolute arrhythmic death rate was lower in the CABG Patch trial and was 6.2% compared with 12.9% in the MADIT trial. Another difference in the MADIT trial was that the ICD effect on nonarrhythmic cardiac death and noncardiac deaths was substantially reduced in the ICD group, whereas in the CABG Patch trial mortality rates in these categories were slightly higher in the ICD group.

In a subsequent abstract presented at the American Heart Association meeting in November 1999, the CABG Patch investigators presented a substudy of 146 surviving CABG Patch patients who had postoperative EP studies (47). The qualifying clinical characteristics in the EP study group were similar to the 754 patients who did not have EP studies. Of these 146 patients, 40% were EP-study positive, demonstrating that the lack of benefit from the ICD in the CABG Patch trial was not because of recruitment of too few EP-positive patients but probably because of the benefit of the bypass operation itself. It is hypothesized that coronary revascularization might have unlinked the arrhythmic substrate from arrhythmic death, a finding that was not predicted by the positive signal averaged ECG but might have been predicted by a pre-CABG procedure EP study. These findings point to the importance of inducibility in such preevent populations and to the lack of impact of the signal-averaged ECG for stratification of risk.

⦿ ONGOING TRIALS OF IMPLANTABLE CARDIOVERTER-DEFIBRILLATORS FOR PRIMARY PREVENTION

The Sudden Cardiac Death Heart Failure Trial (SCD-HeFT) (6) is studying patients with a dilated cardiomyopathy or myopathy due to coronary disease who have an ejection fraction of less than 35% and

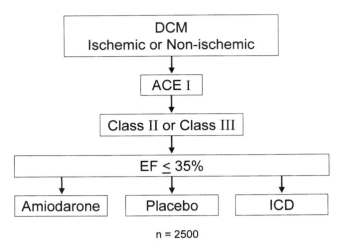

FIGURE 27-11. Randomization scheme for the SCD-HeFT trial. Patients with dilated cardiomyopathy (DCM) from ischemia or an idiopathic cause with class II or III heart failure are randomized to amiodarone or placebo or an implantable cardioverter-defibillator (ICD). The trial was expected to enroll 2,400 patients, with 800 in each arm. One controversial question about this randomization scheme is the inclusion of an amiodarone arm, given the negative results of the European Myocardial Infarct Amiodarone Trial (EMIAT) and Canadian Amiodarone Myocardial Infarction Arrhythmia Trial (CAMIAT) trials.

class II, or III heart failure. Patients are being randomized to receive conventional therapy, amiodarone, or an ICD (Fig. 27-11). The end point is total mortality, with strong cost and quality-of-life components. The trial assumes that the study population will have a mortality rate of 25% at 2.5 years, and that one half of these deaths will be sudden. The trial is designed to have a 95% power to detect a 25% reduction in mortality due to the ICD.

As of November 1999, the SCD-HeFT investigators enrolled 1,200 patients. The population is 78% male and 22% female, with a mean left ventricular ejection fraction of 24%. This is a study of patients with heart failure, and 70% have class II and 30% have class III heart failure. At this midpoint in enrollment, 62% have an ischemic myopathy, and 38% have a nonischemic cardiomyopathy. Regarding background medical therapy, 58% are taking beta blockers, 87% are taking ACE inhibitors, 30% are taking Warfarin, 60% are taking aspirin, and 40% are taking statins. This is the best usage of adjunctive therapy of any trial to date.

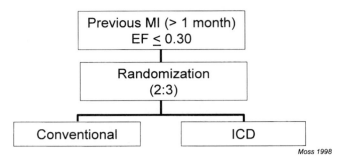

FIGURE 27-12. The MADIT II trial randomization scheme is similar to that for the MADIT I trial but lowers the ejection fraction to 30% and excludes noninvasive myocardial risk factors such as a ventricular ectopy, signal-averaged electrocardiogram, T-wave alternans, heart rate variability, or an electrophysiologic study. The projected total enrollment is 1,200 patients.

The MADIT II study (7) is testing a number of different hypotheses. This study is enrolling patients with coronary artery disease who have suffered a myocardial infarction and have an ejection fraction of less than 30%. They are being randomized to conventional therapy or to the ICD (Fig. 27-12).

The MADIT II trial is making assumptions similar to the SCD-HeFT (7). The assumption is that, for coronary patients with an ejection fraction of more than 30%, there will be a 19% 2-year mortality rate, and 50% of these deaths will be sudden. It is postulated that the ICD will improve survival and reduce mortality to 12% in the ICD population. Both groups will have similar therapy for heart failure and hopefully better therapy than in the MADIT I trial.

As of November 1999, 500 patients were enrolled in the MADIT II trial. Of this number, 84% of the patients are male. Seventy percent have had congestive failure in the previous 3 months, and 54% have been revascularized. Forty percent have undergone nonsurgical catheter revascularization. Of the patients enrolled, 52% have an ejection fraction of less than 25%, which makes this trial one with the lowest mean ejection fractions yet studied. A total of 60% of these patients are receiving beta blockers (Mary Brown: personal communication, 1999).

The patient selection criteria for MADIT II and SCD-HeFT studies are remarkably similar. MADIT II is studying only patients with coronary artery disease, and there is no amiodarone arm as there is in

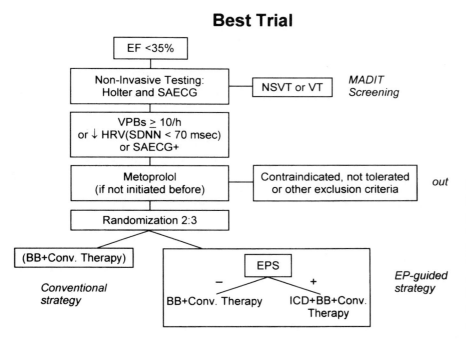

FIGURE 27-13. The BEST trial randomizes coronary patients with an ejection fraction in the 35% range after infarction with 10 ventricular premature contractions per hour or signs of decreased heart rate variability who are on beta blockers to conventional therapy or electrophysiologic-guided therapy. An appealing design feature of this trial is that all patients are on a beta blocker.

the SCD-HeFT trial. However, both these trials have the potential to prove that the ICD can benefit patient groups that are commonly seen clinically, enabling use of the ICD to reduce the total number of sudden deaths in this country.

Several smaller trials are also underway. The DEFINITE trial (8) is studying patients with dilated cardiomyopathy and randomizing them to ICD or best medical therapy. This multicenter, multinational trial has been slow to enroll. Its end point is total mortality, with strong cost-effectiveness and quality-of-life components.

The Beta-blocker Strategy Plus ICD (BEST + ICD) Trial is studying patients with a recent myocardial infarction who have an ejection fraction of 35% or less (48) (Fig. 27-13). They will be placed on a beta blocker and then randomized to a beta blocker plus conventional therapy or to EP-guided therapy that, depending on the patient's inducibility, could result in a beta blocker or an ICD plus a beta blocker plus conventional therapy. The appeal of this protocol is that it will ensure that both groups will be on a beta blocker, which has been a problem with other studies. A risk is that a strict adherence to beta blocker therapy may override some of the potential benefit of the ICD. The enrollment in the BEST + ICD trial has been slow in Italy, and other centers are being recruited for inclusion in the trial.

● TAKING CARE OF PATIENTS VERSUS READING CLINICAL TRIALS

A large number of patients have known high-risk factors or come from families with a strong history of sudden cardiac death. Regrettably, there are few data to guide individual clinical decisions when facing such a patient or a family member. This fact coupled with the ease of ICD implantation, makes it easier to recommend a prophylactic ICD in the absence of firm clinical data. Such high-risk patients include those with hypertrophic cardiomyopathy, the long QT syndrome, right ventricular dysplasia, and a dilated or ischemic cardiomyopathy who cannot be enrolled in a clinical trial. Family members at risk include brothers or sisters of such patients who have died suddenly.

One way to deal with such patients is to establish a national registry of patients with prophylactic ICDs looking at firing rates in high-risk populations. Such a study is being planned by one of the major device manufacturers. Eric Prystowsky has called caring for this group of patients "family-based medicine" rather than "trial-based medicine," because it emphasizes the personal relationship and the high stakes of such relationships. This is one of the undiscussed areas of modern electrophysiology that will become a prominent part of patient care in the next 10 years. My colleagues and I have a very low threshold for device implantation and have accrued about 60 prophylactic ICDs implanted between our trial patients and individual patients with a malignant clinical history.

⊙ TRENDS IN PRIMARY PREVENTION TRIALS

The next frontier in sudden death prophylaxis in the congestive heart failure population is to study the relationship between the effect of ventricular pacing on hemodynamics and any survival advantage that this may confer. Medtronic and Guidant have major congestive heart failure trials with biventricular pacing in the planning stages. The Guidant trial, which has been called the Companion trial, will randomize class II and III congestive heart failure patients into a medical therapy arm, a medical therapy with biventricular pacing arm, and an arm with medical therapy, biventricular pacing, and an ICD. The trial should be initiated in early 2001, and will have extraordinary implications for the field in terms of best therapies and patient survival. As medical therapy continues to improve at a dramatic level, the planning and time course of any such trial is critical because any device-based improvement could be equalled by drug therapy itself.

The short history of the ICD is an astounding one. We are now approaching the 21st anniversary of the first ICD, and about 40,000 new implantations are occurring per year, equalling a rate of 165 devices implanted per 1 million persons in the United States. There has never been any question that the ICD can successfully treat ventricular rhythms. However, prior studies, clinical practice, and the AVID, CASH, and CIDS studies have all shown the ICD confers an important survival benefit for the patients who has already suffered a cardiac arrest or an episode of ventricular tachycardia. One remaining challenge is that of finding appropriate pre-event populations that can benefit from ICD therapy. The challenge for the clinician will be to appropriately design trials that will show the ICD as a benefit. The challenge for the device manufacturer is to deliver devices that are effective and less costly, so large numbers of implantations can be done in pre-event patients without a catastrophic effect on the health care costs of the country.

Michel Mirowski and Morton Mower showed ingenious technical skills and incredible will power to bring the ICD to the bedside. I think, however, even these visionaries would be surprised by the extent of usage and the degree of acceptance of the ICD in the year 2001.

REFERENCES

1. The Antiarrhythmics Versus Implantable Defibrillators (AVID) Investigators. A comparison of antiarrhythmic drug therapy with implantable defibrillators in patients resuscitated from near-fatal sustained ventricular arrhythmias. *N Engl J Med* 1997;337: 1576–1583.
2. Connolly SJ, Gent M, Roberts RS, et al, for the CIDS Co-Investigators. Canadian Implantable Defibrillator Study (CIDS): study design and organization. *Am J Cardiol* 1993;72: 103F–108F.
3. Siebels J, Cappato R, Ruppel R, for the CASH Investigators. Preliminary results of the Cardiac Arrest Study Hamburg (CASH). *Am J Cardiol* 1993;72:109F–113F.
4. Domanski MJ, Zipes DP, Schron E. Treatment of sudden cardiac death: current understandings from randomized trials and future research direction. *Circulation* 1997;95:2694–2699.
5. Nisam S, Mower M. ICD trials: an extraordinary means of determining patient risk? *Pacing Clin Electrophysiol* 1998;21: 1341–1346.
6. Bardy GH, Lee KL, Mark DB, et al. SCD-HeFT: prevention of sudden cardiac death in patients with congestive heart failure trial. In: Singh S, Woosley R, eds. *Clinical trials (in press)*.
7. Moss AJ, Cannom DS, Daubert JP, et al, for the MADIT II investigators. Multicenter Automatic Defibrillator Implantation Trial II (MADIT II): design and clinical protocol. *Ann Noninvas Electrocardiogr* 1999;4:83–91.
8. Kadish A, Dyer A, Larson L, et al. The DEFINITE trial: pharmacoeconomic impact of prophylactic ICD implantation in nonischemic cardiomyopathy. *Cardiostim Conference*, Nice, France, June 17-20, 1998.
9. Aurrichio paper on biventricular pacing in CHF which may still be in abstract form. 1998 AHA, 1999 AHA.
10. Myerburg RJ, Castellanos A. Cardiac arrest and sudden cardiac death. In: Braunwald E, ed. *Heart disease: a textbook of cardiovascular medicine*. Philadelphia: WB Saunders, 1997:742–779.
11. Zipes DP, Wellens HJJ. Sudden cardiac death. *Circulation* 1998; 98:2334–2351.
12. Packer M, O'Connor CM, Ghali JK, et al, for the Prospective Randomized Amlodipine Survival Evaluation Study Group (PRAISE): effect of amlodipine on morbidity and mortality in severe chronic heart failure. *N Engl J Med* 1996;335:1107–1114.
13. Maggioni AP, Zuanetti G, Franzosi MG, et al. Prevalence and prognostic significance of ventricular arrhythmias after acute myocardial infarction in the fibrinolytic era: GISSI-2 results. *Circulation* 1993;87:312–322.
14. Moss AJ. Prognosis after myocardial infarction. *Am J Cardiol* 1983;52:667–669.

15. Kleiger RE, Miller JP, Bigger JT Jr, Moss AJ, for the Multicenter Post-Infarction Research Group. Decreased heart rate variability and its association with increased mortality after acute myocardial infarction. *Am J Cardiol* 1987;59:256–262.
16. Domanski MJ, Saksena S, Epstein A, et al, for the AVID Investigators. Relative effectiveness of the implantable cardioverter-defibrillator and antiarrhythmic drugs in patients with varying degrees of left ventricular dysfunction who have survived malignant ventricular arrhythmias. *J Am Coll Cardiol* 1999;34: 1090–1095.
17. Moss AJ. ICD therapy: the sickest patients benefit the most [Editorial]. *Circulation* 2000;101:1638–1640.
17. Powell AC, Fuchs T, Finkelstein DM, et al. Influence implantable cardioverter defibrillators on the long-term prognosis of survivors of out-of-hospital cardiac arrest. *Circulation* 1993;88: 1083–1092.
18. Kowey PR, Friehling TD. Uses and limitations of electrophysiology studies for selection of antiarrhythmic therapy. *Pacing Clin Electrophysiol* 1986;9:231–247.
19. Buxton AE, Fisher JD, Josephson ME, et al, for the MUSTT Investigators. Prevention of sudden death in patients with coronary artery disease: the Multicenter Unsustained Tachycardia Trial (MUSTT). *Prog Cardiovasc Dis* 1993;36:215–226.
20. Kotler M, Tabaznik B, Mower M, Tominaga S. Prognostic significance of ventricular beats with respect to sudden death in the late post-infarction period. *Circulation* 1973;47:959–966.
21. The Cardiac Arrhythmia Suppression Trial (CAST) Investigators. Preliminary report: effect of encainide and flecainide on mortality in a randomized trial of arrhythmia suppression after myocardial infarction. *N Engl J Med* 1989;321:406–412.
22. Gomes JA, Winters SL, Martinson M, et al. The prognostic significance of quantitative signal-averaged variables relative to clinical variables, site of myocardial infarction, ejection fraction and ventricular premature beats: a prospective study. *J Am Coll Cardiol* 1989;13:377–384.
23. Gomes JA, Winters SL, Stewart D, et al. A new noninvasive index to predict sustained ventricular tachycardia and sudden death in the first year after myocardial infarction: based on signal-averaged electrocardiogram, radionuclide ejection fraction and Holter monitoring. *J Am Coll Cardiol* 1987;10:349–357.
24. Kleiger RE, Miller JP, Bigger JT, Moss AJ, for the Multicenter Post-Infarction Research Group. Decreased heart rate variability and its association with increased mortality after acute myocardial infarction. *Am J Cardiol* 1987;59:256–267.
25. Farrell TG, Bashir Y, Cripps T, et al. Risk stratification of arrhythmic events in post-infarction patients based on heart rate variability, ambulatory electrocardiographic variables and the signal averaged electrocardiogram. *J Am Coll Cardiol* 1991;18: 687–697.
26. Bigger JT, for The CABG Patch Trial Investigators. Prophylactic use of implanted cardiac defibrillators in patients at high risk for ventricular arrhythmias after coronary artery bypass graft surgery. *N Engl J Med* 1997;337:1569–1575.
27. Rosenbaum DS, Jackson LE, Smith JM, et al. Electrical alternans and vulnerability to ventricular arrhythmias. *N Engl J Med* 1994; 330:235–241.
28. Yusef S, Peto R, Lewis J, et al. Beta blockade during and after myocardial infarction: an overview of the randomized trials. *Prog Cardiovasc Dis* 1985;27:335–371.
29. Lantini R, Maggioni AP, Flather M, et al. ACE inhibitor use in patients with myocardial infarction: summary of evidence from clinical trials. *Circulation* 1995;92:3132–3137.
30. Cohn JN, Archibald DG, Ziesche S, et al. Effect of vasodilator therapy on mortality in chronic congestive heart failure: results of a Veterans Administration cooperative study. *N Engl J Med* 1987;316:1429–1435.
31. The SOLVD Trial Investigators. Effect of enalapril on mortality and the development of heart failure in asymptomatic patients with reduced left ventricular ejection fractions. *N Engl J Med* 1992;327:6585–691.
32. The CONSENSUS Trial Group. Effects of enalapril on mortality in severe congestive heart failure: results of the Cooperative North Scandinavian Enalapril Survival Study. *N Engl J Med* 1987;316:1429–35.
33. Stevenson WG, Stevenson LW, Middlekauff HR, Saxon LA. Sudden death prevention in patients with advanced ventricular dysfunction. *Circulation* 1993;88:2953–2961.
34. Myerburg R, Kessler KM, Castellanos A. Sudden cardiac death: epidemiology, transient risk and intervention assessment. *Ann Intern Med* 1993;119:1187–1197.
35. Zipes DP. Implantable cardioverter defibrillator: lifesaver or a device looking for a disease. *Circulation* 1994;89:2934–2936.
36. Prystowsky EN, Heger JJ, Zipes DP. The recognition and treatment of patients at risk for sudden death. In: Eliot RS, Saenz A, Forker AD, eds. *Cardiac emergencies.* Mt Kisco, NY: Futura Publishing, 1982:353—384.
37. Saksena S. On MADIT and future clinical trials for prevention of sudden cardiac death. MADIT. *J Interv Card Electrophysiol* 1997;1:91–93.
38. Domanski MJ, Zipes DP, Schron E. Treatment of sudden cardiac death: current understandings from randomized trials and future research direction. *Circulation* 1997;95:2694–2699.
39. Moss AJ, Hall WJ, Cannom DS, et al, for the MADIT Trial Investigators. Improved survival with an implanted defibrillator in patients with coronary disease at high risk for ventricular arrhythmia. *N Engl J Med* 1996;335:1933–1940.
40. Bigger JT, Fleiss JL, Kleiger R, et al. The relationships among ventricular arrhythmias, left ventricular dysfunction, and mortality in the 2 years after myocardial infarction. *Circulation* 1984; 69:250–258.
41. Wilber DJ, Olshansky B, Moran JF, Scanlon PJ. Electrophysiological testing and nonsustained ventricular tachycardia. *Circulation* 1990;82:350–358.
42. Daubert JP, Higgins SL, Zareba W, Wilber DJ. Comparative survival of MADIT-eligible but non-inducible patients. *J Am Coll Cardiol* 1997;29[Suppl A]:78A.
43. Stevenson WG, Friedman PI. Unsustained ventricular tachycardia—to treat or not to treat [Editorial]. *N Engl J Med* 1985;335: 1984–1985.
44. Buxton AE, Fisher JD, Josephson ME, et al, for the MUSTT Investigators. Prevention of sudden death in patients with coronary artery disease: the Multicenter Unsustained Tachycardia Trial (MUSTT). *Prog Cardiovasc Dis* 1993;36:215–226.
45. Prystowsky EN, Hafley GE, Buxton AE. Are there subgroups of patients at high risk for sudden death and cardiac arrest without inducible sustained monomorphic ventricular tachycardia—results from the Multicenter Unsustained Tachycardia Trial (MUSTT). *Circulation* 1999;100[Suppl 1]:I-81.
46. Bigger JT, Whang W, Rottman JN, et al. Mechanisms of death in the CABG Patch trial: a randomized trial of implantable cardiac defibrillator prophylaxis in patients at high risk of death after coronary artery bypass graft surgery. *Circulation* 1999;99: 1416–1421.
47. Bigger JT, Rottman JN, Whang W, et al, for the CABG Patch Trial Investigators. CABG surgery unlinked the arrhythmic substrate from arrhythmic outcomes in the CABG Patch trial. *Circulation* 1999;100[Suppl 1]:I-366–I-367.
48. Raviele A, Bongiorni MG, Brignole M, et al. Which strategy is "best" after myocardial infarction? The beta blocker strategy plus implantable cardioverter defibrillator trial: rationale and study design. *Am J Cardiol* 1999;83:104–111.

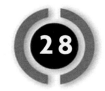

WHAT IS THE ROLE FOR PHARMACOLOGIC THERAPY FOR SUSTAINED VENTRICULAR TACHYARRHYTHMIAS?

L. BRENT MITCHELL

The patient who has experienced an episode of hemodynamically significant sustained ventricular tachycardia (VT) or ventricular fibrillation (VF) in the absence of a transient or reversible cause is at high risk for future VT/VF episodes. Recurrent VT/VF episodes also expose these patients to a high risk of sudden cardiac death. To date, seven therapeutic approaches have been proposed for the prevention of VT/VF and sudden cardiac death in this patient population. The primary goal of most of these proposed therapeutic alternatives, including the five pharmacologic approaches, is prevention of recurrences of VT/VF, with the expectation that success in this regard can also prevent sudden cardiac death. However, the primary goal of implantable cardioverter-defibrillator (ICD) therapy is to prevent sudden cardiac death, not by preventing VT/VF, but rather by reacting to VT/VF when it occurs to effect its termination and to reestablish normal rhythm. Clinical trial evidence has indicated that the ICD prevents death better than pharmacologic therapy. This observation raises the important question about the continuing roles, if any, of pharmacologic therapy for patients with a demonstrated propensity for VT/VF. This chapter examines this issue in detail.

● REVIEW OF THE PROBLEM

Sudden cardiac death is epidemic. Approximately 350,000 lives are claimed by sudden cardiac death each year in North America (1), making sudden cardiac death the most common nonaccidental cause of death of adults. Most result from VT/VF (2). The yearly incidence of sustained VT/VF or sudden death is approximately 0.1% for the general adult population, 1% to 2% for patients with multiple risk factors for atherosclerotic heart disease, 5% for patients with previous coronary events, and 20% for patients with congestive heart failure and left ventricular ejection fractions of less than 0.30 (3). Nevertheless, patients who have had a previous episode of sustained VT/VF in the absence of a transient or reversible cause are at the highest risk. Without treatment, these patients have a 1-year actuarial probability of VT/VF recurrence or sudden death of 30% and a 2-year actuarial probability of VT/VF recurrence or sudden death of 50% (3,4) (Fig. 28-1).

These estimates of the risk of VT/VF recurrence or sudden death were initially reported from early studies of the untreated natural history of patients who had been resuscitated from VT/VF (5–15). Since these early descriptions, ethical considerations have

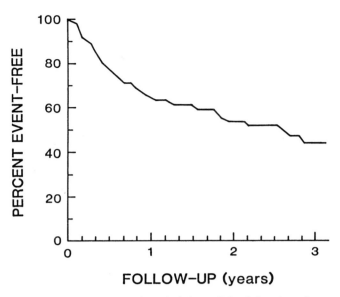

FIGURE 28-1. Actuarial probabilities (%) of freedom from death and ventricular fibrillation (VF) recurrence over 3 years of follow-up in patients who experienced an out-of-hospital VF cardiac arrest in the absence of a transient or reversible cause, most of whom received no specific antiarrhythmic therapy. (From Cobb LA, Baum RS, Alvarez H III, et al. Resuscitation from out-of-hospital ventricular fibrillation: 4 years of follow-up. *Circulation* 1975;52[Suppl III]:III-223–III-228, with permission.)

ensured that treatment is provided to patients with a history of VT/VF in the absence of a transient or reversible cause. Accordingly, contemporary estimates of the natural history of VT/VF patients are unavailable. Nevertheless, analyses of the follow-up probabilities of appropriate ICD therapy in patients treated with an ICD rather than with antiarrhythmic drug therapy have suggested that the estimates of the natural history studies are still relevant today (16,17). Most reports indicate that the follow-up probabilities of arrhythmia recurrence are higher for patients with ventricular tachycardia than patients with ventricular fibrillation. However, ventricular fibrillation recurrences are more likely to be fatal than ventricular tachycardia recurrences. The follow-up probabilities of sudden cardiac death for patients with hemodynamically significant ventricular tachycardia and patients with ventricular fibrillation are likely to be equivalent (4).

The high risk of VT/VF recurrence and sudden death of patients with sustained VT/VF in the absence of a reversible or transient cause indicates a need for specific long-term prophylactic treatment. The typical patient with VT/VF has significant structural heart disease, has depressed left ventricular function, and does not present an arrhythmia substrate that is readily curable with surgical or transcatheter ablative techniques. For these patients, the choice of therapy distills to chronic prophylactic pharmacologic therapy or ICD therapy.

CLARIFICATION OF THE GOALS OF THERAPY

The treatment of any patient with a significant arrhythmia requires consideration of the goals of therapy so that therapy capable of attaining the selected goals can be appropriately selected and administered. For patients who have experienced VT/VF, the dominant goals of therapy are to prevent VT/VF recurrences and to prevent the consequences of VT/VF recurrences, particularly sudden cardiac death. Pharmacologic therapies are designed to prevent VT/VF recurrences. To the extent that pharmacologic therapy is effective at preventing VT/VF recurrences, such therapy can also prevent sudden death. However, in its current form, ICD therapy does not prevent VT/VF recurrences. Instead, the goal of ICD therapy is to prevent sudden death by prompt termination of episodes of VT/VF when they occur.

The goals of prevention of VT/VF recurrence and the prevention of sudden death are not synonymous. Although it may seem obvious that both goals should be achieved in all patients, there are frequent instances when both goals are neither necessary nor advisable.

PHARMACOLOGIC TREATMENT APPROACHES

Empirical Standard Antiarrhythmic Drug Therapy

The first therapeutic approach recommended for patients with sustained VT/VF was the empirical use of the antiarrhythmic drug therapies that were in standard use at the time—predominantly agents from Vaughan Williams class I (18–20). However, applications of this approach were unable to demonstrate a beneficial effect even when using historical controls. Descriptions (21–24) of the outcomes of VT/VF patients treated empirically with these standard antiarrhythmic drug therapies indicate that the prognosis may actually be worsened by such therapy. Given these observations, the use of empirical antiarrhythmic drug therapy from Vaughan Williams class I or III (except for amiodarone) for the prevention of VT/VF in an otherwise unprotected high-risk patient has been abandoned.

Individualized Antiarrhythmic Drug Therapy

Failure of empirical standard antiarrhythmic drug therapy recommended the development of approaches to predict the ultimate efficacy of an antiarrhythmic drug regimen before trusting in its long-term use. Two potential approaches to such prediction been described: a noninvasive (electrocardiographic monitoring) approach (1,25–27) and an invasive (electrophysiologic study) approach (28–32).

The noninvasive approach and the invasive approach begin with the identification of an index of myocardial electrical instability in an antiarrhythmic drug-free state. Thereafter, a selected drug regimen is predicted to be effective in long-term use by virtue of its ability to suppress the index of myocardial electrical instability. The index of electrical instability used to guide the noninvasive approach is frequent, spontaneous ventricular premature beats. In general, an individual is considered to have sufficient ventricular ectopy to guide the noninvasive approach if 24-hour ambulatory electrocardiographic monitoring in an antiarrhythmic drug–free state demonstrates a mean of 30 or more ventricular premature beats per hour (33,34). Thereafter, an antiarrhythmic therapy is initiated, and after steady-state conditions have been reestablished, a drug-assessment 24-hour ambulatory electrocardiographic examination is performed. The most commonly used criterion for acceptance of a prediction of long-term antiarrhythmic drug efficacy is a decrease in the frequency of isolated ventricular

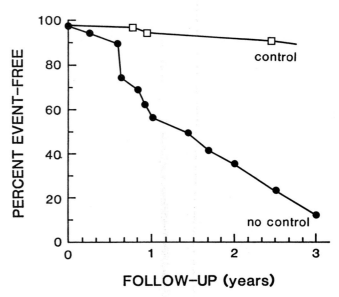

FIGURE 28-2. Actuarial probabilities (%) of freedom from sudden death over 3 years of follow-up for patients with hemodynamically compromising ventricular tachycardia or fibrillation (VT/VF) treated with antiarrhythmic drugs predicted to be effective by the noninvasive approach (*open box*, control) or predicted to be ineffective by the noninvasive approach (*solid circle*, no control). (From Graboys TB, Lown B, Podrid PJ, et al. Long-term survival of patients with malignant ventricular arrhythmia treated with antiarrhythmic drugs. *Am J Cardiol* 1982; 50:437–443, with permission.)

premature beats of 80% or more, a decrease in the frequency of ventricular couplets by 90% or more, and the elimination of ventricular triplets or longer repetitive forms on a drug-assessment 24-hour ambulatory electrocardiogram and a drug-assessment exercise tolerance test (1,26,35). A patient-drug combination receiving an efficacy prediction by the noninvasive approach has a lower probability of VT/VF recurrence or sudden death than a patient-drug combination not receiving an efficacy prediction by the noninvasive approach (27) (Fig. 28-2). The index of electrical instability used to guide the invasive approach is the induction of the patient's sustained VT/VF by programmed stimulation during an electrophysiologic study performed in an antiarrhythmic drug–free state. Of the various inducible ventricular tachyarrhythmias, the one that is most specific in its guidance of the invasive approach is the reproducible induction of sustained monomorphic ventricular tachycardia matching the previous spontaneous ventricular tachycardia in QRS morphology and rate (36). Antiarrhythmic therapy is initiated, and after steady-state conditions have been reestablished, a drug-assessment electrophysiologic study is performed. The most commonly used criteria for acceptance of a prediction of long-term antiarrhythmic drug efficacy is the inability to induce more than four repetitive ventricular responses using up to three extrastimuli applied to the stimulation site that permitted the induction of sustained VT/VF at the baseline study (32,37–42). A patient-drug combination receiving an efficacy prediction by the invasive approach has a lower probability of VT/VF recurrence or sudden death than does a patient-drug combination not receiving an efficacy prediction by the invasive approach (43) (Fig. 28-3).

Empirical Amiodarone Therapy

Empirical amiodarone therapy has been used for the treatment of ventricular arrhythmias for 30 years (44). Initially, amiodarone therapy was reserved for patients who had failed therapy with conventional antiarrhythmic drugs (45–47). Follow-up studies of VT/VF patients receiving amiodarone therapy demonstrated a low probability of VT/VF recurrence or sudden death rates compared with historical controls (45). The follow-up outcomes associated with empirical amiodarone therapy were apparently comparable to that of individualized standard antiarrhythmic therapy predicted to be effective by the noninvasive or invasive approach (Fig. 28-4). This observation was particularly impressive in that the patients who received empirical amiodarone therapy had already demonstrated a resistance to antiarrhythmic drug therapy. Early use of empirical amiodarone therapy was also characterized by the use of relatively high maintenance dosages (>400 mg daily). At these dos-

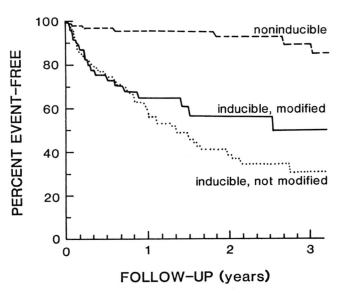

FIGURE 28-3. Actuarial probabilities (%) of freedom from sudden death and sustained ventricular tachycardia or fibrillation (VT/VF) over 3 years of follow-up for patients with inducible sustained VT/VF treated with antiarrhythmic drugs predicted to be effective by the invasive approach (*dashed line*, noninducible) or predicted to be ineffective by the invasive approach with modification of the inducible VT/VF (*solid line*, inducible, modified) or without modification of the inducible VT/VF (*dotted line*, inducible, not modified). (From Waller TJ, Kay HR, Spielman SR, et al. Reduction in sudden death and total mortality by antiarrhythmic therapy evaluated by electrophysiologic drug testing: criteria of efficacy in patients with sustained ventricular tachyarrhythmia. *J Am Coll Cardiol* 1987;10:83–89, with permission.)

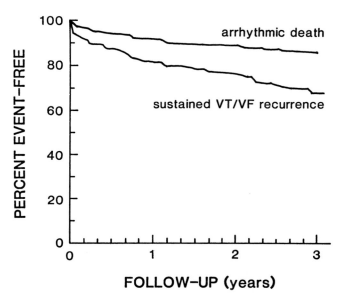

FIGURE 28-4. Actuarial probabilities (%) of freedom from arrhythmic death and freedom from recurrent sustained ventricular tachycardia or fibrillation (VT/VF) over 3 years of follow-up for patients with sustained VT/VF treated empirically with amiodarone therapy. (From Herre JM, Sauve MJ, Malone P, et al. Long-term results of amiodarone therapy in patients with recurrent sustained ventricular tachycardia or ventricular fibrillation. *J Am Coll Cardiol* 1989;13:442–449, with permission.)

ages, amiodarone therapy has a high probability of being associated with serious adverse effects (48,49). Subsequent experience (50–52) with lower dosages (200 to 400 mg/day) has suggested that the frequency of adverse effects from amiodarone therapy can be substantially reduced without loss of the antiarrhythmic efficacy of the therapy.

Accumulated evidence supports the contention that the ultimate efficacy of amiodarone therapy in patients with VT/VF can be predicted by the noninvasive approach (53–56) or invasive approach (53,55, 57–61) to individualized antiarrhythmic drug therapy. Nevertheless, most practitioners use amiodarone empirically, a convention that began when amiodarone therapy was prescribed to VT/VF patients with no other therapeutic alternative and for whom a prediction of therapeutic failure had no clinical value.

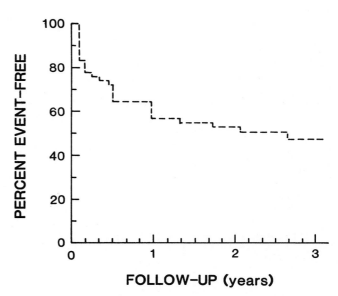

FIGURE 28-5. Actuarial probabilities (%) of freedom from sudden death and sustained ventricular tachycardia or fibrillation (VT/VF) over 3 years of follow-up for patients with sustained VT/VF or syncope with inducible VT/VF treated empirically with metoprolol therapy. (From Steinbeck G, Andresen D, Bach P, et al. A comparison of electrophysiologically guided antiarrhythmic drug therapy with beta-blocker therapy in patients with symptomatic, sustained ventricular tachyarrhythmias. *N Engl J Med* 1992;327:987–992, with permission.)

Empirical Beta-Blocking Drug Therapy

Isolated beta-blocking therapy for the goals of prevention of VT/VF and sudden death has been advocated for specific patient subgroups: those with VT/VF occurring in the setting of mitral valve prolapse (62), exercise (63–65), acute myocardial infarction (66–68), long QT interval syndromes (69), or the absence of identifiable structural heart disease (64,70, 71).

Steinbeck and colleagues (72) reported the outcomes associated with use of empirical beta-blocking drug therapy in 54 unselected patients with spontaneous VT/VF and inducible VT/VF who received metoprolol therapy as their only antiarrhythmic intervention. The metoprolol dosage was initially 25 mg twice each day and was then increased, as tolerated, to 100 mg twice each day. On follow-up, the 2-year probability of VT/VF recurrence or sudden death was approximately 45%, indistinguishable from that of historical, untreated patient populations (Fig. 28-5). Accordingly, isolated empirical beta-blocking drug therapy is not commonly used to prevent VT/VF recurrences in this patient population. Instead, isolated beta-blocking antiarrhythmic therapy for VT/VF patients requires an efficacy prediction from the noninvasive approach (73–75) or the invasive approach (76–78) to individualized antiarrhythmic drug therapy.

Substantial evidence supports using beta-blocking drug therapy in addition to specific antiarrhythmic therapy in VT/VF patients. First, many patients with VT/VF have sustained a remote myocardial infarction. There are numerous reports of a reduction in the follow-up probability of sudden death in postmyocardial infarction patients who are prescribed empirical beta-blocking drug therapy (79–83). Second, the electrophysiologic effects and antiarrhythmic benefits of predicted-effective standard antiarrhythmic drug therapy may be overcome by sufficient beta-adrenergic stimulation (84). Third, patients with sustained VT/VF may have a selective increase in arrhythmogenic cardiac sympathetic activity as suggested by measurements of total and cardiac norepinephrine spillover into plasma (85). For these reasons, the efficacy of individualized standard antiarrhythmic drug therapy may be enhanced by the concomitant administration of a beta-blocking drug (86–88). More evidence of this advantage comes from a retrospective multivariate analysis by Leclercq and coworkers (24). Patients with sustained ventricular tachycardia and left ventricular ejection fractions (LVEFs) of less than 30% treated with a variety of empirical antiarrhythmic therapies and whose therapy included a beta-blocking drug had a lower 2-year actuarial cardiac mortality probability (approximately 9%) than those whose therapy did not include a beta-blocking drug (approximately 34%) ($p < 0.01$).

● COMPARISONS OF PHARMACOLOGIC THERAPIES

Before the clinical trials comparing pharmacologic therapy and ICD therapy, a series of clinical trials of varying quality sought to determine the best of the pharmacologic approaches for the prevention of VT/VF and sudden death. First, the approach of empirical standard antiarrhythmic drug therapy was again dispatched by the Cardiac Arrest Study Hamburg (CASH) (89). This study randomized patients who had survived a ventricular fibrillation cardiac arrest to four separate therapeutic approaches: empirical propafenone therapy, empirical beta-blocking drug therapy, empirical amiodarone therapy, or an ICD. An interim report (89), after an average follow-up of 11 months, indicated that patients assigned to empirical propafenone therapy ($n = 56$) were experiencing recurrent cardiac arrest and all-cause mortality at rates that were higher that those of patients assigned to the other three study therapies. Accordingly, empirical use of propafenone in CASH was stopped. These results, taken in conjunction with less well controlled evaluations of empirical standard antiarrhythmic drug therapy, have convinced the electrophysiologic community that empirical standard antiarrhythmic drug therapy is not a viable approach to the goal of prevention of VT/VF recurrences or sudden death in otherwise unprotected VT/VF patients.

Two randomized clinical trials (41,42,90,91) compared the noninvasive and invasive approaches to selection of individualized antiarrhythmic drug therapy for the goal of prevention of VT/VF recurrence. Unfortunately, these two trials provide conflicting results. The small Calgary Trial (41,42) suggested that, in a drug-naïve ventricular tachycardia population, the invasive approach selects therapy that prevents VT/VF recurrence better than does that selected by the noninvasive approach (2-year actuarial probabilities of 7% versus 47%, respectively; $p = 0.02$). The larger Electrophysiologic Study Versus Electrocardiographic Monitoring (ESVEM) study (90,91) suggested that, in a drug-resistant VT/VF patient population, neither approach selects therapy that provides adequate protection from VT/VF recurrence; 2-year actuarial probabilities were approximately 50% in each group. Neither of these trials was designed to evaluate the efficacies of the two approaches relative to the goal of prevention of sudden death. Nevertheless, the ESVEM (91) study did report that the 4-year probability of sudden death was lower for patients randomized to the invasive approach to drug therapy selection than for patients randomized to the noninvasive approach to drug therapy selection (20% versus 25%, respectively) and that the 4-year probability of death from any cause was lower for patients randomized to the invasive approach to drug therapy selection than for patients randomized to the noninvasive approach to drug therapy selection (38% versus 47%, respectively). The statistical significance of these differences was not reported. However, application of a simple chi-square statistic to the data provided indicates that these differences are close to reaching standard statistical measures of significance.

The relative efficacies of empirical amiodarone therapy and of individualized class I antiarrhythmic drug therapy for the goal of prevention of VT/VF recurrences were compared in the Cardiac Arrest in Seattle: Conventional versus Amiodarone Drug Evaluation (CASCADE) study (92,93). Patients who survived an out-of-hospital ventricular fibrillation cardiac arrest were randomized to receive empirical amiodarone therapy or individualized standard antiarrhythmic drug therapy selected by the invasive approach if that approach was applicable and successful or, if not, by the noninvasive approach. During the CASCADE study, the protocol was changed to include the implantation of an ICD in each study subject. Thereafter, the primary outcome variable of the CASCADE study was the combined end point of sustained VT/VF recurrence, cardiac death, or syncope followed by an ICD discharge. An intention-to-treat analysis indicated that empirical amiodarone therapy prevents this outcome cluster better than individualized standard antiarrhythmic therapy (2-year actuarial probabilities of 18% versus 31%, respectively; $p = 0.007$). However, this conclusion is substantially weakened by the observation that, in the CASCADE study, at least 40% of the patients receiving individualized standard antiarrhythmic drug therapy were receiving therapy that was predicted to be ineffective. Nevertheless, many clinicians have accepted the notion that empirical amiodarone therapy, if not more effective than, is at least as effective as individualized standard antiarrhythmic drug therapy selected by the invasive approach.

The relative efficacies of empirical beta-blocking drug therapy and individualized standard antiarrhythmic drug therapy for the goal of prevention of VT/VF recurrences were examined by Steinbeck and associates (72). A total of 115 patients with VT/VF in the absence of a transient or reversible cause were randomized to receive empirical beta-blocking drug therapy or to receive individualized standard antiarrhythmic drug therapy selected by the invasive approach. An intention-to-treat analysis suggested that empirical metoprolol therapy and individualized antiarrhythmic drug therapy selected by the invasive approach were equivalent therapies for the prevention of VT/VF recurrence; each approach was associated with a 2-year actuarial probability of VT/VF recurrence or sudden death of approximately 50%. However, 52% of the patients randomized to receive individualized antiarrhythmic drug therapy selected by the invasive approach actually received therapy that that approach predicted would be ineffective. When each group is considered individually, the 2-year follow-up actuarial probability of VT/VF recurrence or sudden death was lowest (21%) for patients receiving antiarrhythmic drug therapy that was predicted to be effective by the invasive approach, intermediate (52%) for patients receiving empirical metoprolol therapy, and highest (66%) for patients receiving antiarrhythmic drug therapy that was predicted to be ineffective by the invasive approach. Accordingly, although beta-blocking drug therapy is still useful as adjunctive therapy, beta-blocking drug therapy is not often used as primary antiarrhythmic therapy for patients with VT/VF in the absence of a transient or reversible cause.

The combined results of these trials indicate that the most effective pharmacologic therapies for the goal of prevention of VT/VF are empirical amiodarone therapy and individualized antiarrhythmic drug therapy predicted to be effective by the invasive approach.

NONPHARMACOLOGIC THERAPIES

Nonpharmacologic therapies with reported efficacy in the treatment of patients with VT/VF include operative or transcatheter ablation or isolation of the arrhythmogenic substrate and use of an ICD. A tendency for recurrent ventricular tachycardia may be cured by ablation or electrical isolation of the arrhythmogenic ventricular substrate during open-heart surgery (94,95), by catheter approaches to the direct endocardial application of destructive energy sources (96,97), and by catheter approaches to the indirect transcoronary application of destructive materials (98, 99).

There have been no direct comparisons of electrosurgical or transcatheter ablative therapies to any other form of VT/VF therapy. Nevertheless, the concept of cure for the patient with ventricular tachycardia is attractive. Despite the absence of comparative trials, this form of therapy is already established as the preferred treatment modality for patients with idiopathic right ventricular outflow tract ventricular tachycardia (100), idiopathic left septal ventricular tachycardia (101), or bundle branch reentrant ventricular tachycardia (102). Developments in electrosurgical and transcatheter ablation techniques for ventricular tachycardia in patients with coronary heart disease are encouraging and suggest that these techniques may well mature into highly effective, curative therapies for patients with VT/VF, even in the presence of structural heart disease.

The final treatment approach for patients with a demonstrated propensity to VT/VF is use of the ICD (103–105). In its current form, the ICD does not prevent episodes of VT/VF from occurring. Instead, it reacts to their presence with pacing or direct current (DC) shock therapies that terminate the VT/VF and restore normal heart rhythm. In doing so the goal of ICD therapy is to prevent adverse consequences of

VT/VF, particularly that of sudden death. Many early reports (103–105) of the follow-up course of VT/VF patients treated with an ICD showed actuarial probabilities of sudden death that were much better than either those of historical, untreated control populations or those of pharmacologically treated patient populations—so much better as to suggest that ICD recipients were drawn from a different patient population than previous studies (106).

The initial comparative studies of pharmacologic therapy and ICD therapy for patients with VT/VF used nonrandomized controls (107–109) and reached conflicting conclusions. To study the relative efficacies of ICD therapy and pharmacologic therapy in a manner free from potential bias in the distribution of patients between therapeutic approaches, randomized studies were required. In 1987, CASH (89) began randomizing patients with out-of-hospital cardiac arrest to receive an ICD, empirical propafenone therapy, empirical metoprolol therapy, or empirical amiodarone therapy. The empirical propafenone arm of CASH was stopped in 1992, when it became apparent that the efficacy of propafenone therapy in this setting was significantly inferior to that of other therapies (89). The Canadian Implantable Defibrillator Study (CIDS) (110) began randomizing VT/VF patients to receive an ICD or to receive empirical amiodarone therapy in 1990. In 1993, the Antiarrhythmics Versus Implantable Defibrillator (AVID) trial (111) began randomizing VT/VF patients to receive an ICD or to receive drug therapy (i.e., individualized sotalol therapy predicted to be effective by the noninvasive or the invasive approach or empirical amiodarone therapy).

In 1997, the Data and Safety Monitoring Committee of the AVID trial recommended that the study be stopped early as the patients randomized to receive an ICD had a significantly lower probability of all-cause mortality during follow-up than did the patients randomized to receive pharmacologic therapy (98% of whom received empirical amiodarone therapy) (112). In the AVID trial, the 2-year actuarial probability of death in patients who received an ICD was 18%, and the 2-year actuarial probability of death in patients who received a pharmacologic therapy was 27% ($p < 0.02$) (Fig. 28-6). Overall, the relative risk reduction associated with use of an ICD rather than

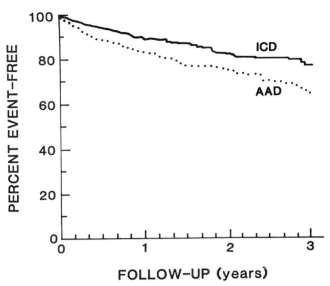

FIGURE 28-6. Actuarial probabilities of freedom from death (%) over 3 years of follow-up for patients resuscitated from ventricular fibrillation (VF) and patients with severely symptomatic ventricular tachycardia (VT) with a left ventricular ejection fraction of less than 0.40 who were randomly assigned to receive antiarrhythmic drug *(dotted line)* treatment (97% empirical amiodarone therapy, 3% sotalol therapy predicted to be effective by the invasive approach or the noninvasive approach) or to receive an implantable cardioverter-defibrillator *(solid line)*. (From The AVID Investigators. A comparison of antiarrhythmic drug therapy with implantable defibrillators in patients resuscitated from near-fatal sustained ventricular arrhythmias. *N Engl J Med* 1997;337:1576–1583, with permission.)

pharmacologic therapy in the AVID trial was 34% (95% CI, 16%–49%). However, use of an ICD was associated with an average extension of life of only 3.2 months after 3 years at an incremental cost of $27,500. These findings describe a cost per year of life saved of more than $100,000 (113). Recognizing that we cannot choose treatments based on cost issues alone, this cost per year of life saved is not attractive (114).

The results of CIDS and CASH were presented at a meeting of the American College of Cardiology (115). In CIDS, the 2-year actuarial probability of death in patients who received an ICD was approximately 15%, and the 2-year actuarial probability of death in patients who received a pharmacologic therapy was approximately 21% ($p = 0.14$). Overall, the relative risk reduction associated with use of an ICD rather than pharmacologic therapy in CIDS was 20% (95% CI,-8%–40%). In CASH, the 2-year actuarial probability of death in patients who received an ICD was 12%, and the 2-year actuarial probability of death in patients who received pharmacologic therapy (combining the empirical metoprolol and empirical amiodarone treatment groups) was 20% ($p < 0.05$). The data required to calculate the overall relative risk reduction associated with use of an ICD in CASH are not yet available. From the data that are available, the estimated relative risk reduction associated with use of an ICD in CASH is 39%. The 95% confidence intervals of these three point estimates of the mortality benefit of ICD therapy have substantial overlap. The results of these three trials are compatible and are consistent with a relative risk reduction of death associated with the use of an ICD rather than pharmacologic therapy in the range of 20% to 40%.

When the primary goal of therapy is the prevention of sudden death, ICD therapy is superior to the best that current pharmacologic therapy has to offer to VT/VF patients at high risk of sudden death.

ROLES OF PHARMACOLOGIC THERAPY FOR PATIENTS WITH VENTRICULAR TACHYCARDIA OR FIBRILLATION

The current roles of pharmacologic therapy in patients who have experienced sustained VT/VF in the absence of a transient or reversible cause are as primary antiarrhythmic drug therapy in a select group of VT/VF patients and as ancillary antiarrhythmic drug therapy in the other patients who have been treated with an ICD.

Primary Pharmacologic Therapy for Patients with Ventricular Tachycardia or Fibrillation

The randomized trials comparing pharmacologic therapy and ICD therapy selected for participation patients with VT/VF characteristics associated with a high risk of sudden death with subsequent VT/VF recurrences—patients with hemodynamically significant VT/VF. Patients at high risk of death for other reasons, including patients with functional New York Heart Association (NYHA) class IV congestive heart failure were excluded from participation. Accordingly, their results may not apply to patients who present with hemodynamically stable ventricular tachycardia or to patients with a concurrent illness that significantly affects longevity, including functional class IV congestive heart failure. In either patient population, it is probable that very few patients would benefit from ICD implantation because patients with hemodynamically stable ventricular tachycardia, especially those with preserved left ventricular function, are at low risk of sudden death and patients with functional class IV congestive heart failure are at high risk of death for other reasons. Given that the economics of ICD use in the general population of VT/VF patients are already problematic, cost-benefit considerations in VT/VF patient populations at low risk of sudden death or at high risk of death for other reasons suggest that pharmacologic approaches to therapy would be appropriate for these patients. In these settings, the primary goal of therapy is to prevent VT/VF recurrences rather than to prevent death. Pharmacologic therapies are capable of attaining this goal; ICD therapy is not.

When a patient's characteristics suggest a low risk of sudden death despite the probability of future VT/VF recurrences, therapies other than an ICD are appropriate. A few of these patients are amenable to cure by electrosurgery or catheter ablation of the arrhythmogenic substrate. Nevertheless, most necessitate a choice between empirical amiodarone therapy and individualized antiarrhythmic drug therapy predicted to be effective by the invasive approach. This choice is usually made by consideration of the relative advantages and disadvantages of the two therapeutic approaches. The major advantage of empirical amiodarone therapy is its initial simplicity. The major advantage of individualized standard antiarrhythmic drug therapy predicted to be effective by the invasive approach is the opportunity to avoid the adverse effect profile of long-term amiodarone therapy. Which of these two treatment alternatives is superior when both are applicable remains unknown.

When a patient's characteristics suggest a high risk of death for reasons other than VT/VF, therapies other than an ICD are appropriate. In this instance, the simplicity of empirical amiodarone therapy recommends its use.

When the goal of prevention of sudden death is required and advisable, ICD therapy has a therapeutic advantage. However, it is expensive. The cost of ICD therapy may be reduced by limiting the therapy to patients who are most likely to benefit from ICD therapy. Substudies of AVID (116) and CIDS (117) have reported that a depressed LVEF identifies a patient who will benefit from ICD therapy over pharmacologic therapy. For example, in AVID, the mortality benefit of the ICD over antiarrhythmic drug therapy appeared to be limited to patients who had substantially depressed left ventricular function (116). Patients with LVEF less than 0.20 had a lower 2-year actuarial probability of death if treated with an ICD than if treated with antiarrhythmic drug therapy (28.4% ± 14.6% versus 36.2% ± 11.6%). Similarly, patients with LVEFs in the range of 0.20 to 0.34 also had a lower 2-year actuarial probability of death if treated with an ICD than if treated with antiarrhythmic drug therapy (17.5% ± 5.7% versus 28.2% ± 6.7%). However, for patients with relatively preserved left ventricular function (LVEF ≥0.35), there was no difference in the actuarial probability of death between patients treated with an ICD and those treated with antiarrhythmic drug therapy (16.6% ± 6.1% versus 17.3% ± 6.5%). A more comprehensive analysis of the CIDS database suggested that essentially all of the benefit of ICD therapy over pharmacologic therapy was enjoyed by an subgroup of participants that was identifiable and small (118).

A multivariate analysis of predictors of the risk of death for the patients randomized to the amiodarone arm of CIDS identified three independent predictors of death: age of 70 years or older, LVEF of 0.35 or less, and NYHA class III heart failure. Follow-up of patients in CIDS (118) with none or only one of these characteristics showed no benefit of ICD therapy over empirical amiodarone therapy; the relative risk reduction in all-cause mortality with ICD therapy was −0.09 (95% CI, −0.62–0.27; p was not significant). The remaining 25% of sustained VT/VF patients had two or three of these risk factors and benefited greatly from ICD therapy over empirical amiodarone therapy with a relative risk reduction in all-cause mortality with ICD therapy of 0.50 (95% CI, 0.21–0.68) (118). Although these data clearly represent a post hoc subgroup analysis, they do support limiting ICD therapy to VT/VF patients with two or more risk factors for death despite amiodarone therapy (i.e., age ≥70 years, LVEF ≤0.35, and NYHA class III).

These considerations notwithstanding, the results of randomized trials of ICD therapy for patients with a demonstrated propensity to sustained VT/VF in the absence of a transient or reversible cause indicate that the dominant role of pharmacologic therapy in this setting should be as ancillary therapy provided in addition to ICD therapy.

Ancillary Antiarrhythmic Drug Therapy for Patients with Implantable Cardioverter-Defibrillators

The ancillary uses for antiarrhythmic drug therapy for VT/VF patients who have received an ICD include drug therapy designed to prevent VT/VF recurrences (119–121), drug therapy designed to render ventricular tachycardia more amenable to ICD pace-termination (122,123), drug therapy designed to prevent supraventricular tachyarrhythmias that are confusing the ICD (124,125), and drug therapy designed to lower the ventricular defibrillation threshold (126–144).

As predicted by the untreated natural history of patients with sustained VT/VF in the absence of a transient or reversible cause, approximately 50% of VT/VF patients who are treated with an ICD will have a recurrent VT/VF episode treated by their device within 2 years of its implantation (16,17,22, 103–105,119–121,144,145). Some of these patients have enough VT/VF recurrences that the frequency of ICD therapies becomes unacceptable, especially when DC shock therapies are required. For this reason, approximately 30% of ICD recipients are treated with antiarrhythmic drugs to reduce the frequency of VT/VF recurrences and enhance quality of life (16, 17,22,103–105,119–121,144,145). Because a VT/VF patient with an ICD does not necessarily require perfect antiarrhythmic drug therapy and because the ICD also provides relative protection from antiarrhythmic drug proarrhythmia, most antiarrhythmic drug therapies prescribed in this setting are given empirically.

The first prospective evaluation of the efficacy of class I or class III antiarrhythmic drug therapies for this purpose suggested no benefit from such therapy (119). Thirty-four patients with drug-resistant VT/VF who had received an ICD were randomized to also receive or not to receive open-label, prophylactic antiarrhythmic drug therapy that had favorably modified the patient's VT/VF as assessed by electrocardiographic monitoring or electrophysiologic study before ICD implantation. This study found that the 1-year probabilities of receiving an ICD shock were equivalent whether the patients were treated with a prophylactic antiarrhythmic drug or not (approximately 72% and 60%, respectively; $p = 0.66$). However, two larger randomized trials of sotalol therapy in this setting have reported that sotalol therapy effectively lowers the follow-up probability of VT/VF recurrences and ICD therapies (120,121). In the first of these studies, 93 patients with structural heart disease and drug-resistant VT/VF who received an ICD were randomized to receive or not to receive open-label, prophylactic sotalol therapy for the prevention of VT/VF recurrences (120). The 2-year actuarial probability of VT/VF recurrence was lower in the sotalol-treated patient group than in the untreated group (approximately 18% versus 50%, respectively; $p = 0.023$). Over the duration of the study, this benefit represented a relative risk reduction for sotalol prophylaxis of 0.39 (95% CI, 0.02–0.62).

This benefit was substantiated by a randomized, placebo-controlled trial of sotalol therapy (121). A total of 302 patients receiving an ICD for the treatment of life-threatening VT/VF were randomized to receive sotalol or its matching placebo in a double-blind fashion. The two treatment groups were well matched for baseline predictors of subsequent VT/VF recurrences. After 12 months of therapy, fewer sotalol-treated patients than placebo-treated patients had died or had experienced an appropriate ICD shock (27% versus 42%, $p < 0.001$) (Fig. 28-7). Sotalol prophylaxis was associated with a relative risk reduction of death or appropriate ICD shock of 0.38 (95% CI, 0.18–0.53). Similar benefits may result from prophylactic amiodarone therapy in this setting; however, this hypothesis has yet to be tested. Given these

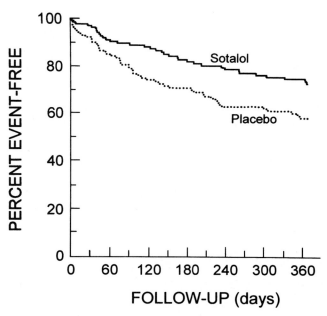

FIGURE 28-7. Actuarial probabilities (%) of freedom from death or the delivery of an appropriate implantable cardioverter-defibrillator (ICD) therapy for a ventricular tachyarrhythmia over 1 year of follow-up for patients with life-threatening ventricular tachyarrhythmias who had received an ICD randomly assigned to receive empirical sotalol therapy *(solid line)* or to receive its matching placebo *(dotted line)*. (Adapted from Pacifico A, Hohnloser SH, Williams JH, et al. Prevention of implantable-defibrillator shocks by treatment with sotalol. *N Engl J Med* 1999;340:1855–1862, with permission.)

data, it could be argued that all or most VT/VF patients who receive an ICD should receive ancillary prophylactic antiarrhythmic drug therapy to reduce the probability that an ICD would actually be required. However, restraint is advisable. Although 50% of VT/VF patients who are treated with an ICD will have a VT/VF recurrence within 2 years, 50% of VT/VF patients who are treated with an ICD will not have a VT/VF recurrence within 2 years. Because patients with an ICD are protected from sudden death as a consequence of VT/VF recurrence, the use of prophylactic antiarrhythmic drug therapy in this setting should await the demonstration of VT/VF recurrence. Even then, it could be argued that only patients with frequent VT/VF recurrences should receive antiarrhythmic drug therapy for the goal of decreasing VT/VF recurrences. However, given that ICD therapy does not prevent all VT/VF deaths (16,17,22,

103–105,119–121,144,145) and given the adverse psychologic and quality-of-life effects of multiple ICD shocks (146), patients with recurrent ICD therapies should receive prophylactic antiarrhythmic drug therapy earlier rather than later. The timing of such therapy is individualized based on consideration of the potential benefits of decreasing the frequency of VT/VF recurrences (i.e., improved quality-of-life and ICD longevity) and the potential disadvantages of prophylactic antiarrhythmic drug therapy (i.e., additional cost and the possibility of antiarrhythmic drug adverse effects).

Some VT/VF patients with an ICD also benefit in a quality-of-life sense from antiarrhythmic drug therapy designed to organize and slow VT/VF that requires an ICD shock for termination to a ventricular tachycardia that can be terminated painlessly by antitachycardia pacing (122,123). Although not yet studied prospectively, data from other settings suggest that this goal is most likely to be achieved safely with sotalol or amiodarone therapy.

Antiarrhythmic drug therapy may also benefit some VT/VF patients with an ICD who have been experiencing inappropriate ICD therapies as a result of sinus tachycardia or supraventricular tachyarrhythmias (124,125). Although newer ICDs are becoming quite accomplished in distinguishing ventricular tachyarrhythmias that need ICD therapy from supraventricular tachyarrhythmias that do not need ICD therapy, this distinction is still imperfect. For this reason, some patients require antiarrhythmic drug therapy that slows the supraventricular tachycardia below the rate cutoff for ICD therapy or to prevent supraventricular tachyarrhythmias altogether. In the placebo-controlled, randomized trial of sotalol therapy after ICD implantation discussed earlier (121), fewer sotalol-treated patients than placebo-treated patients had experienced an inappropriate ICD shock for supraventricular tachyarrhythmias during the first year of therapy (7% versus 19%, $p = 0.004$). Sotalol prophylaxis was associated with a relative risk reduction of inappropriate ICD shocks for supraventricular tachyarrhythmias of approximately 0.62 (95% CI, 0.32–0.79).

Ancillary antiarrhythmic drug therapy may be used for patients with VT/VF who have received an ICD with the goal of decreasing the defibrillation threshold. Antiarrhythmic drugs that work primarily by slowing ventricular conduction velocity are considered to be Vaughan Williams class I agents, and they increase defibrillation thresholds (126–131). Antiarrhythmic drugs that work primarily by prolonging ventricular action potential duration are considered to be class III agents, and they decrease defibrillation thresholds (132–137). Antiarrhythmic drugs with a balance of class I and class III actions (e.g., amiodarone) may increase or decrease defibrillation thresholds (138–142). These observations inform the selection of ancillary antiarrhythmic drug therapies in VT/VF patients with an ICD. Antiarrhythmic drugs with predominant class III action may be useful for the singular purpose of decreasing defibrillation energy requirements in patients with high ventricular fibrillation defibrillation energy requirements. One nonrandomized study reported that the lowest successful defibrillation energy during a step-down defibrillation testing protocol was significantly lower for 25 patients on sotalol at the time of an ICD implantation (5.9 ± 3.4 J) than for a concurrent control group of 23 patients not receiving sotalol at the time of an ICD implantation (16 ± 10 J) ($p < 0.01$) (143). Nevertheless, no prospective or randomized trials have yet quantified the advantages and disadvantages of using class III antiarrhythmic drug therapy for this purpose in ICD patients with high defibrillation energy requirements.

FUTURE OF ANTIARRHYTHMIC DRUG THERAPY

All other things being equal, an effective preventative therapy is superior to an effective reactive therapy. Nevertheless, the reactive therapy for life-threatening episodes of VT/VF prevents death better than the best that preventative pharmacologic therapies have to offer. The challenge for preventative pharmacologic therapies is to improve enough that their efficacy relative to the primary objective of VT/VF prevention is equal or superior to the standard that has been set by ICD therapy relative to the secondary goal of preventing death from VT/VF when it does occur.

In the interim, pharmacologic therapies will maintain an important role in the treatment of VT/VF patients. Pharmacologic therapies will continue to be used as primary therapy for VT/VF patients with a very low risk of sudden death and for VT/VF patients at very high risk of death from other causes unrelated to their VT/VF. Pharmacologic therapies will continue to be used as important ancillary therapy for VT/VF patients who have received an ICD to lessen the frequency of VT/VF recurrences, to render ventricular tachycardia more amenable to pace-termination attempts, to prevent supraventricular tachyarrhythmias that initiate inappropriate ICD therapies, and to lower the ventricular fibrillation defibrillation threshold.

REFERENCES

1. Lown B. Sudden cardiac death: the major challenge confronting contemporary cardiology. *Am J Cardiol* 1979;43:313–328.
2. Bayes de Luna AB, Coumel P, Leclercq J-F. Curriculum in Cardiology: ambulatory sudden cardiac death; mechanisms of production of fatal arrhythmia on the basis of data from 157 cases. *Am Heart J* 1989;117:151–159.
3. Myerburg RJ, Kessler KM, Castellanos A. Sudden cardiac death: epidemiology, transient risk, and intervention assessment. *Ann Intern Med* 1993;119:1187–1197.
4. Mitchell LB. Pharmacological therapy. In: Singer I, ed. *Implantable cardioverter defibrillator*. Armonk, NY: Futura Publishing, 1994:577–613.
5. Strauss MB. Paroxysmal ventricular tachycardia. *Am J Med Sci* 1930;179:337–345.
6. Lundy CJ, McLellan LL. Paroxysmal ventricular tachycardia: an etiological study with special reference to the type. *Ann Intern Med* 1934;7:812–836.
7. Williams C, Ellis LB. Ventricular tachycardia: an analysis of thirty-six cases. *Arch Intern Med* 1943;71:137–156.
8. Trevor Cooke W, White PD. Paroxysmal ventricular tachycardia. *Br Heart J* 1943;5:33–54.
9. Herrmann GR, Hejtmancik MR. A clinical and electrocardiographic study of paroxysmal ventricular tachycardia and its management. *Ann Intern Med* 1948;28:989–997.
10. Armbrust CA Jr, Levine SA. Paroxysmal ventricular tachycardia: a study of one hundred and seven cases. *Circulation* 1950;1:28–40.
11. Herrmann GR, Park HM, Hejtmancik MR. Paroxysmal ventricular tachycardia: a clinical and electrocardiographic study. *Am Heart J* 1959;57:166–176.
12. Liberthson RR, Nagel EL, Hirschman JC, et al. Prehospital ventricular fibrillation: prognosis and follow-up course. *N Engl J Med* 1974;291:317–321.
13. Baum RS, Alvarez H III, Cobb LA. Survival after resuscitation from out-of-hospital ventricular fibrillation. *Circulation* 1974;50:1231–1235.
14. Schaffer WA, Cobb LA. Recurrent ventricular fibrillation and modes of death in survivors of out-of-hospital ventricular fibrillation. *N Engl J Med* 1975;293:259–262.
15. Cobb LA, Baum RS, Alvarez H III, et al. Resuscitation from out-of-hospital ventricular fibrillation: 4 years of follow-up. *Circulation* 1975;52[Suppl III]:III-223–III-228.
16. Leitch JW, Gillis AM, Wyse DG, et al. Reduction in defibrillator shocks with an implantable device combining antitachycardia pacing and shock delivery. *J Am Coll Cardiol* 1991;18:145–151.
17. Bardy GH, Hofer B, Johnson G, et al. Implantable transvenous cardioverter-defibrillators. *Circulation* 1993;87:1152–1168.
18. Myerburg RJ, Conde C, Sheps DS, et al. Antiarrhythmic drug therapy in survivors of prehospital cardiac arrest: comparison of effects on chronic ventricular arrhythmias and recurrent cardiac arrest. *Circulation* 1979;59:855–863.
19. Myerburg RJ, Kessler KM, Estes D, et al. Long-term survival after prehospital cardiac arrest: analysis of outcomes during an 8-year study. *Circulation* 1984;70:538–546.
20. Vlay SC, Reid PR, Griffith LSC, et al. Relationship of specific coronary lesions and regional left ventricular dysfunction to prognosis in survivors of sudden cardiac death. *Am Heart J* 1984;108:1212–1220.
21. Goldstein S, Landis Jr, Leighton R, et al. Predictive survival models for resuscitated victims of out-of-hospital cardiac arrest with coronary heart disease. *Circulation* 1985;71:873–880.
22. Moosvi AR, Goldstein S, VanderBrug Medendorp S, et al. Effect of empiric antiarrhythmic therapy in resuscitated out-of-hospital cardiac arrest victims with coronary artery disease. *Am J Cardiol* 1990;65:1192–1197.
23. Willems AR, Tijssen JGP, van Capelle FJL, et al. Determinants of prognosis in symptomatic ventricular tachycardia or ventricular fibrillation late after myocardial infarction. *J Am Coll Cardiol* 1990;16:521–530.
24. Leclercq J-F, Coumel P, Denjoy I. Long-term follow-up after sustained monomorphic ventricular tachycardia: causes, pump failure, and empiric antiarrhythmic drug therapy that modify survival. *Am Heart J* 1991;121:1685–1692.
25. Winkle RA, Alderman EL, Fitzgerald JW, et al. Treatment of recurrent symptomatic ventricular tachycardia. *Ann Intern Med* 1976;85:1–7.
26. Lown B. Management of patients at high risk of sudden death. *Am Heart J* 1982;103:689–697.
27. Graboys TB, Lown B, Podrid PJ, et al. Long-term survival of patients with malignant ventricular arrhythmia treated with antiarrhythmic drugs. *Am J Cardiol* 1982;50:437–443.
28. Wu D, Wyndham CR, Denes P, et al. Chronic electrophysiological study in patients with recurrent paroxysmal tachycardia: a new method for developing successful oral antiarrhythmic therapy. In: Kulbertus HE, ed. *Reentrant arrhythmia: mechanisms and treatment*. Lancaster, PA: MTP Press, 1977:294–311.
29. Hartzler GO, Maloney JD. Programmed ventricular stimulation in management of recurrent ventricular tachycardia. *Mayo Clin Proc* 1977;52:731–741.
30. Fisher JD, Cohen HL, Mehra R, et al. Cardiac pacing and pacemakers. II. Serial electrophysiologic-pharmacologic testing for control of recurrent tachyarrhythmias. *Am Heart J* 1977;93:658–666.
31. Horowitz LN, Josephson ME, Farshidi A, et al. Recurrent sustained ventricular tachycardia. 3. Role of the electrophysiologic study in selection of antiarrhythmic regimens. *Circulation* 1978;58:986–997.
32. Mason JW, Winkle RA. Electrode-catheter arrhythmia induction in the selection and assessment of antiarrhythmic drug therapy for recurrent ventricular tachycardia. *Circulation* 1978;58:971–985.
33. Morganroth J, Michelson EL, Horowitz LN, et al. Limitations of routine long-term electrocardiographic monitoring to assess ventricular ectopic frequency. *Circulation* 1978;58:408–414.
34. Swerdlow CD, Peterson J. Prospective comparison of Holter monitoring and electrophysiologic study in patients with coro-

nary disease and sustained ventricular tachyarrhythmias. *Am J Cardiol* 1985;56:577–580.
35. Hohnloser SH, Raeder EA, Podrid PJ, et al. Predictors of antiarrhythmic drug efficacy in patients with malignant ventricular tachyarrhythmias. *Am Heart J* 1987;114:1–7.
36. Brugada P, Green M, Abdollah H, et al. Significance of ventricular arrhythmia initiated by programmed ventricular stimulation: the importance of the type of ventricular arrhythmia induced and the number of premature stimuli required. *Circulation* 1984;69:87–92.
37. Mason JW, Winkle RA. Accuracy of the ventricular tachycardia-induction study for predicting long-term efficacy and inefficacy of antiarrhythmic drugs. *N Engl J Med* 1980;303:1073–1077.
38. Swerdlow CD, Winkle RA, Mason JW. Determinants of survival in patients with ventricular tachyarrhythmias. *N Engl J Med* 1983;308:1436–1442.
39. Morady F, Scheinman MM, Hess DS, et al. Electrophysiologic testing in the management of out-of-hospital cardiac arrest. *Am J Cardiol* 1983;51:85–89.
40. Ruskin JN, Schoenfeld MH, Garan H. Role of electrophysiologic techniques in the selection of antiarrhythmic drug regimens for ventricular tachyarrhythmias. *Am J Cardiol* 1983;52:41C–46C.
41. Mitchell LB, Duff HJ, Manyari DE, et al. A randomized clinical trial of the noninvasive and invasive approaches to drug therapy of ventricular tachycardia. *N Engl J Med* 1987;317:1681–1687.
42. Mitchell LB, Duff HJ, Gillis AM, et al. A Randomized clinical trial of the noninvasive and invasive approaches to drug therapy for ventricular tachycardia: long-term follow-up of the Calgary trial. *Prog Cardiovasc Dis* 1996;38:377–384.
43. Waller TJ, Kay HR, Spielman SR, et al. Reduction in sudden death and total mortality by antiarrhythmic therapy evaluated by electrophysiologic drug testing: criteria of efficacy in patients with sustained ventricular tachyarrhythmia. *J Am Coll Cardiol* 1987;10:83–89.
44. Van Schepdael J, Solvay H. Étude clinique de l'amiodarone dans le troubles du rythme cardiaque. *Presse Med* 1970;78:1849–1850.
45. Herre JM, Sauve MJ, Malone P, et al. Long-term results of amiodarone therapy in patients with recurrent sustained ventricular tachycardia or ventricular fibrillation. *J Am Coll Cardiol* 1989;13:442–449.
46. Myers RJ, Peter T, Weiss D, et al. Benefits and risks of long-term amiodarone therapy for sustained ventricular tachycardia/fibrillation: a minimum of three-year follow-up. *Am Heart J* 1990;119:8–14.
47. Weinberg BA, Miles WM, Klein LS, et al. Five-year follow-up of 589 patients treated with amiodarone. *Am Heart J* 1993;125:109–120.
48. Fogoros RN, Anderson KP, Winkle RA, et al. Amiodarone: clinical efficacy and toxicity in 96 patients with recurrent, drug-refractory arrhythmias. *Circulation* 1983;68:88–94.
49. Mason JW. Drug therapy: amiodarone. *N Engl J Med* 1987;316:455–466.
50. Nicklas JM, McKenna WJ, Stewart RA, et al. Prospective, double-blind, placebo-controlled trial of low-dose amiodarone in patients with severe heart failure and asymptomatic frequent ventricular ectopy. *Am Heart J* 1991;122:1016–1021.
51. Singh BN, Fletcher RD, Fisher SG, et al. Amiodarone in patients with congestive heart failure and asymptomatic frequent ventricular ectopy. *N Engl J Med* 1995;333:77–82.
52. Vorperian VR, Havighurst TC, Miller S, et al. Adverse effects of low dose amiodarone: a meta-analysis. *J Am Coll Cardiol* 1997;30:791–798.
53. Horowitz LN, Greenspan AM, Spielman SR, et al. Usefulness of electrophysiologic testing in evaluation of amiodarone therapy for sustained ventricular arrhythmias associated with coronary heart disease. *Am J Cardiol* 1985;55:367–371.
54. Veltri EP, Griffith LSC, Platia EV, et al. The use of ambulatory monitoring in the prognostic evaluation of patients with sustained tachycardia treated with amiodarone. *Circulation* 1986;74:1054–1060.
55. Lavery D, Saksena S. Management of refractory sustained ventricular tachycardia with amiodarone: a reappraisal. *Am Heart J* 1987;113:49–56.
56. Kim S, Felder SD, Figure I, et al. Value of Holter monitoring in predicting long-term efficacy and inefficacy of amiodarone used alone and in combination with class Ia antiarrhythmic agents in patients with ventricular tachycardia. *J Am Coll Cardiol* 1987;9:169–174.
57. Kadish AH, Marchlinski FE, Josephson ME, et al. Amiodarone: correlation of early and late electrophysiologic studies with outcome. *Am Heart J* 1986;112:1134–1140.
58. Yazaki Y, Haffajee CI, Gold RL, et al. Electrophysiologic predictors of long-term clinical outcome with amiodarone for refractory ventricular tachycardia secondary to coronary artery disease. *Am J Cardiol* 1987;60:293–297.
59. Schmitt C, Brachmann J, Waldecker B, et al. Amiodarone in patients with recurrent sustained ventricular tachyarrhythmias: results of programmed electrical stimulation and long-term clinical outcome in chronic treatment. *Am Heart J* 1987;114:279–283.
60. Zhu J, Haines DE, Lerman BB, et al. Predictors of efficacy of amiodarone and characteristics of recurrence of arrhythmia in patients with sustained ventricular tachycardia and coronary artery disease. *Circulation* 1987;76:802–809.
61. Greenspon AJ, Volosin KJ, Breenber RM, et al. Amiodarone therapy: role of early and late electrophysiologic studies. *J Am Coll Cardiol* 1988;11:117–123.
62. Winkle RA, Lopes MG, Goodman DJ, et al. Propranolol for patients with mitral valve prolapse. *Am Heart J* 1977;93:422–427.
63. Wu D, Kou HC, Hung JS. Exercise-triggered paroxysmal ventricular tachycardia. *Ann Intern Med* 1981;95:410–414.
64. Palileo EV, Ashley WW, Swiryn S, et al. Exercise provocable right ventricular outflow tract tachycardia. *Am Heart J* 1982;104:185–193.
65. Sung RJ, Olukotun AY, Baird CL, et al. Efficacy and safety of oral nadolol for exercise-induced ventricular arrhythmias. *Am J Cardiol* 1987;60:15D–20D.
66. Stock JPP, Dale N. Beta-adrenergic receptor blockade in cardiac arrhythmias. *Br Med J* 1963;2:1230–1233.
67. Wasir HS, Mahapatra RK, Bhatia ML, et al. Metoprolol—a new cardioselective beta-adrenoceptor blocking agent for treatment of tachyarrhythmias. *Br Heart J* 1977;39:834–838.
68. Rydén L, Ariniego R, Arnman K, et al. A double-blind trial of metoprolol in acute myocardial infarction: effects on ventricular tachyarrhythmias. *N Engl J Med* 1983;308:614–618.
69. Moss AJ, Schwartz PJ, Crampton RS, et al. The long QT syndrome: a prospective international study. *Circulation* 1985;71:17–21.
70. Buxton AE, Waxman HL, Marchlinski FE, et al. Right ventricular tachycardia: clinical and electrophysiologic characteristics. *Circulation* 1983;68:917–927.
71. Brodsky MA, Sato DA, Allen BJ, et al. Solitary beta-blocker therapy for idiopathic life-threatening ventricular tachyarrhythmias. *Chest* 1986;89:790–794.
72. Steinbeck G, Andresen D, Bach P, et al. A comparison of electrophysiologically guided antiarrhythmic drug therapy

with beta-blocker therapy in patients with symptomatic, sustained ventricular tachyarrhythmias. *N Engl J Med* 1992;327: 987–992.
73. Woosley RL, Kornhauser D, Smith R, et al. Suppression of chronic ventricular arrhythmias with propranolol. *Circulation* 1979;60:819–827.
74. Podrid PJ, Lown B. Pindolol for ventricular arrhythmia. *Am Heart J* 1982;104:491–496.
75. Brodsky MA, Allen BJ, Bessen M, et al. Beta-blocker therapy in patients with ventricular tachyarrhythmias in the setting of left ventricular dysfunction. *Am Heart J* 1988;115:799–808.
76. Duff HJ, Mitchell LB, Wyse DG. Antiarrhythmic efficacy of propranolol: comparison of low and high serum concentrations. *J Am Coll Cardiol* 1986;8:959–965.
77. Brodsky MA, Allen BJ, Luckett CR, et al. Antiarrhythmic efficacy of solitary beta-adrenergic blockade for patients with sustained ventricular tachyarrhythmias. *Am Heart J* 1989;118: 272–280.
78. Leclercq J-F, Leenhardt A, Lemarec H, et al. Predictive value of electrophysiologic studies during treatment with the beta-blocking agent nadolol. *J Am Coll Cardiol* 1990;16:413–417.
79. Multicenter International Study. Reduction in mortality after myocardial infarction with long-term beta-adrenergic receptor blockade. *Br Med J* 1977;2:419–421.
80. The Norwegian Multicenter Study Group. Timolol-induced reduction in mortality and reinfarction in patients surviving acute myocardial infarction. *N Engl J Med* 1981;304:801–807.
81. Julian DG, Prescott RJ, Jackson FS, et al. Controlled trial of sotalol for one year after myocardial infarction. *Lancet* 1982;1: 1142–1147.
82. Beta-Blocker Heart Attack Study Group. A randomized trial of propranolol in patients with acute myocardial infarction. I. Mortality results. *JAMA* 1982;247:1707–1714.
83. Lichstein E, Morganroth J, Harrist R, et al. Effect of propranolol on ventricular arrhythmias: the Beta-Blocker Heart Attack Trial experience. *Circulation* 1983;67[Suppl I]:I-5–I-10.
84. Jazayeri MR, VanWyhe G, Avitall B, et al. Isoproterenol reversal of antiarrhythmic effects in patients with inducible sustained ventricular tachyarrhythmias. *J Am Coll Cardiol* 1989;14: 705–711.
85. Meredith IT, Broughton A, Jennings GL, et al. Evidence of a selective increase in cardiac sympathetic activity in patients with sustained ventricular arrhythmias. *N Engl J Med* 1991; 325:618–624.
86. Leahey EB Jr, Heissenbuttel RH, Giardina EGV, et al. Combined mexiletine and propranolol treatment of refractory ventricular tachycardia. *Br Med J* 1980;281:357–358.
87. Hirsowitz G, Podrid PJ, Lampert S, et al. The role of beta blocking agents as adjunct therapy to membrane stabilizing drugs in malignant ventricular arrhythmia. *Am Heart J* 1986; 111:852–860.
88. Deedwania PC, Olukotun AY, Kupersmith J, et al. Beta blockers in combination with class I antiarrhythmic agents. *Am J Cardiol* 1987;60:21D–26D.
89. Siebels J, Cappato R, Rüppel R, et al. ICD versus drugs in cardiac arrest survivors: preliminary results of the Cardiac Arrest Study Hamburg. *Pacing Clin Electrophysiol* 1993;16: 552–558.
90. The ESVEM Investigators. The ESVEM trial: electrophysiologic study versus electrocardiographic monitoring for selection of antiarrhythmic therapy of ventricular tachyarrhythmias. *Circulation* 1989;79:1354–1360.
91. Mason JW, for the ESVEM Investigators. A comparison of electrophysiologic testing with Holter monitoring to predict antiarrhythmic-drug efficacy for ventricular tachyarrhythmias. *N Engl J Med* 1993;329:445–451.
92. The Cascade Investigators. Cardiac arrest in Seattle: conventional versus amiodarone drug evaluation (the CASCADE study). *Am J Cardiol* 1991;67:578–584.
93. The Cascade Investigators. Randomized antiarrhythmic drug therapy in survivors of cardiac arrest (the CASCADE study). *Am J Cardiol* 1993;72:280–287.
94. Guiraudon G, Fontaine G, Frank R, et al. Encircling endocardial ventriculotomy: a new surgical treatment of life-threatening ventricular tachycardias resistant to medical treatment following myocardial infarction. *Ann Thorac Surg* 1978;26: 438–444.
95. Cox JL. Patient selection criteria and results of surgery for refractory ischemic ventricular tachycardia. *Circulation* 1989; 79[Suppl I]:I-163–I-177.
96. Klein LS, Miles WM. Ablative therapy for ventricular arrhythmias. *Prog Cardiovasc Dis* 1995;37:225–242.
97. Stevenson WG, Khan H, Sager P, et al. Identification of reentry circuit sites during catheter mapping and radiofrequency ablation of ventricular tachycardia late after myocardial infarction. *Circulation* 1993;88:1647–1670.
98. Brugada P, de Swart H, Smeets J, et al. Transcoronary chemical ablation of ventricular tachycardia. *Circulation* 1989;79: 475–482.
99. Nora MO, Miles WM, Klein LS, et al. Alcohol ablation of ventricular tachycardia. *J Cardiovasc Electrophysiol* 1991;2: 456–461.
100. Klein LS, Shih H-T, Hackett K, et al. Radiofrequency catheter ablation of ventricular tachycardia in patients without structural heart disease. *Circulation* 1992;85:1666–1674.
101. Wen M-S, Yeh S-J, Wang C-C, et al. Successful radiofrequency ablation of idiopathic left ventricular tachycardia at a site away from the tachycardia exit. *J Am Coll Cardiol* 1997; 30:1024–1031.
102. Miles WM. Bundle branch reentrant tachycardia: a chance to cure? *J Cardiovasc Electrophysiol* 1993;4:263–265.
103. Mirowski A. The automatic implantable cardioverter defibrillator: an overview. *J Am Coll Cardiol* 1985;6:461–466.
104. Manolis AS, Tan-Deguzman W, Lee MA, et al. Clinical experience in seventy-seven patients with the automatic implantable cardioverter defibrillator. *Am Heart J* 1989;118:445–450.
105. Winkle RA, Mead RH, Ruder MA, et al. Long-term outcome with the automatic cardioverter defibrillator. *J Am Coll Cardiol* 1989;13:1353–1361.
106. Connolly SJ, Yusuf S. Evaluation of the implantable cardioverter defibrillator in survivors of cardiac arrest: the need for randomized trials. *Am J Cardiol* 1992;69:959–962.
107. Fogoros RN, Fielder SB, Elson JJ. The automatic cardioverter defibrillator in drug-refractory ventricular arrhythmias. *Ann Intern Med* 1987;107:635–641.
108. Pinski SL, Sgarbossa EB, Maloney JD, et al. Survival in patients declining implantable cardioverter defibrillators. *Am J Cardiol* 1991;68:800–801.
109. Newman D, Sauve MJ, Herre J, et al. Survival after implantation of the cardioverter defibrillator. *Am J Cardiol* 1992;69: 899–903.
110. Connolly SJ, Gent M, Roberts RS, et al. Canadian Implantable Defibrillator Study (CIDS): study design and organization. *Am J Cardiol* 1993;72:103F–108F.
111. The AVID Investigators. Antiarrhythmics Versus Implantable Defibrillators (AVID)—rationale, design, and methods. *Am J Cardiol* 1995;75:470–475.
112. The AVID Investigators. A comparison of antiarrhythmic drug therapy with implantable defibrillators in patients resuscitated

from near-fatal sustained ventricular arrhythmias. *N Engl J Med* 1997;337:1576–1583.
113. Singh BN. Controlling cardiac arrhythmias: an overview with a historical perspective. *Am J Cardiol* 1997;80:4G–15G.
114. Goldman L, Gordon DJ, Rifkind BM, et al. Cost and health implications of cholesterol lowering. *Circulation* 1992;85:1960–1968.
115. Ferguson JJ. Meeting highlights: 47th Annual Scientific Sessions of the American College of Cardiology. *Circulation* 1998;97:2377–2381.
116. Domanski MJ, Sakseena S, Epstein AE, et al. Relative effectiveness of the implantable cardioverter-defibrillator and antiarrhythmic drugs in patients with varying degrees of left ventricular dysfunction who have survived malignant ventricular arrhythmias. *J Am Coll Cardiol* 1999;34:1090–1095.
117. Krahn AD, Klein GJ, Yee R, et al. The effect of ejection fraction on the relative benefit of the implantable defibrillator in the Canadian Implantable Defibrillator Study (CIDS) [Abstract]. *Circulation* 1998;98[Suppl 1]:I-93.
118. Sheldon RS, Connolly S, Krahn A, et al. Identification of patients most likely to benefit from ICD therapy: the Canadian Implantable Defibrillator Study. *Circulation* 2000;101:1660–1664.
119. Anderson JL, Karagounis LA, Roskelley M, et al. Effect of prophylactic antiarrhythmic drug therapy on time to implantable cardioverter defibrillator discharge in patients with ventricular tachyarrhythmias. *Am J Cardiol* 1994;73:683–687.
120. Kühlkamp V, Mewis C, Mermi J, et al. Suppression of sustained ventricular tachyarrhythmias: a comparison of D,L-sotalol with no antiarrhythmic drug treatment. *J Am Coll Cardiol* 1999;33:46–52.
121. Pacifico A, Hohnloser SH, Williams JH, et al. Prevention of implantable-defibrillator shocks by treatment with sotalol. *N Engl J Med* 1999;340:1855–1862.
122. Ip JH, Winters SL, Schweitzer P, et al. Determinants of pace-terminable ventricular tachycardia: implications for implantable antitachycardia devices. *Pacing Clin Electrophysiol* 1991;14:1777–1781.
123. Kantoch MJ, Green MS, Tang AS. Randomized cross-over evaluation of two adaptive pacing algorithms for the termination of ventricular tachycardia. *Pacing Clin Electrophysiol* 1993;16:1664–1672.
124. Manz M, Jung W, Lüderitz B. Interactions between drugs and devices: experimental and clinical studies. *Am Heart J* 1994;127:978–984.
125. Schmitt C, Montero M, Melichercik J. Significance of supraventricular tachyarrhythmias in patients with implanted pacing cardioverter defibrillators. *Pacing Clin Electrophysiol* 1994;17:295–302.
126. Dorian P, Fain ES, Davy J-M, et al. Lidocaine causes a reversible, concentration dependent in defibrillation energy requirements. *J Am Coll Cardiol* 1986;8:327–332.
127. Fain ES, Dorian P, Davy J-M, et al. Effects of encainide and its metabolites on energy requirements for defibrillation. *Circulation* 1986;73:1334–1341.
128. Peters W, Gang ES, Okazaki H, et al. Acute effects of intravenous propafenone on the internal ventricular defibrillation threshold in the anesthetized dog. *Am Heart J* 1991;122:1355–1360.
129. Echt DS, Gremillion ST, Lee JT, et al. Effects of procainamide and lidocaine on defibrillation energy requirements in patients receiving implantable cardioverter devices. *J Cardiovasc Electrophysiol* 1994;5:752–760.
130. Hernandez R, Mann DE, Breckinridge S, et al. Effects of flecainide on defibrillation thresholds in the anesthetized dog. *J Am Coll Cardiol* 1989;14:777–781.
131. Frame LH, Sheldon JH. Effect of recainam on the energy required for ventricular defibrillation in dogs as assessed with implanted electrodes. *J Am Coll Cardiol* 1988;12:746–752.
132. Wang M, Dorian P. DL and D sotalol decrease defibrillation energy requirements. *Pacing Clin Electrophysiol* 1989;12:1522–1529.
133. Dawson AK, Steinberg M, Shapland JE. Effects of class I and class III drugs on current and energy required for internal defibrillation [Abstract]. *Circulation* 1985;72[Suppl III]:III-384.
134. Dorian P, Wang M, David I, et al. Oral clofilium produces sustained lowering of defibrillation energy requirements in a canine model. *Circulation* 1991;83:614–621.
135. Echt DS, Black JN, Barbey JT, et al. Evaluation of antiarrhythmic drugs on defibrillation energy requirements in dogs: sodium channel blockade and action potential prolongation. *Circulation* 1989;79:1109–1117.
136. Tacker WA, Niebauer MJ, Babbs CF, et al. The effect of newer antiarrhythmic drugs on defibrillation threshold. *Crit Care Med* 1980;8:177–180.
137. Dorian P, Newman D, Sheahan R, et al. D-sotalol decreases defibrillation energy requirements in humans: a novel indication for drug therapy. *J Cardiovasc Electrophysiol* 1996;7:952–961.
138. Fogoros RN. Amiodarone-induced refractoriness to cardioversion. *Ann Intern Med* 1984;100:699–700.
139. Troup PJ, Chapman PD, Olinger GN, et al. The implanted defibrillator: relation of defibrillating lead configuration and clinical variables to defibrillation threshold. *J Am Coll Cardiol* 1985;6:1315–1321.
140. Frame LH. The effect of chronic oral and acute intravenous amiodarone administration on ventricular defibrillation thresholds using implanted electrodes in dogs. *Pacing Clin Electrophysiol* 1989;12:339–346.
141. Guarnieri T, Levine JH, Veltri EP, et al. Success of chronic defibrillation and the role of antiarrhythmic drugs with the automatic implantable cardioverter/defibrillator. *Am J Cardiol* 1987;60:1061–1064.
142. Fain ES, Lee JT, Winkle RA. Effects of acute intravenous and chronic oral amiodarone on defibrillation energy requirements. *Am Heart J* 1987;114:8–17.
143. Dorian P, Newman D. Effect of sotalol on ventricular fibrillation and defibrillation in humans. *Am J Cardiol* 1993;72:72A–79A.
144. Böcker D, Haverkamp W, Block M, et al. Comparison of D,L sotalol and implantable defibrillators for treatment of sustained ventricular tachycardia or fibrillation in patients with coronary artery disease. *Circulation* 1996;94:151–157.
145. Saksena S. Clinical outcome of patients with malignant ventricular tachyarrhythmias and a multiprogrammable implantable cardioverter-defibrillator implanted with and without thoracotomy: an international multicenter study. *J Am Coll Cardiol* 1994;23:1521–1530.
146. Morris PL, Badger J, Chmielewski C, et al. Psychiatric morbidity following implantation of the automatic implantable cardioverter defibrillator. *Psychosomatics* 1991;32:58–64.

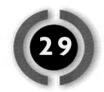

FUTURE IMPLANTABLE CARDIOVERTER-DEFIBRILLATOR TECHNOLOGIES

EDWIN G. DUFFIN

During the first decade of the new millennium, the primary areas of concentration for implantable cardioverter-defibrillator (ICD) advances will probably be size reduction, cost reduction, smaller, more flexible lead systems, greater detection specificity, tachycardia prevention, enhanced telemetry, ease of use through automaticity, improved follow-up tools, and comorbidity management capabilities. In this period, the implantable defibrillator will likely become a pacemaker-sized instrument used to help manage heart failure as well as atrial and ventricular bradyarrhythmias and tachyarrhythmias. Complementing this increased functionality, indwelling artificial intelligence will reduce the need for manual device programming and dramatically lessen the user's need to understand intricate device details. The implanted device will monitor and self-manage most of its functions, automatically signaling by standard communication channels if expert assistance is required. Prophylactic indications for use will expand dramatically, resulting in higher-volume production of devices with a resultant reduction in unit cost. A much higher percentage of patients who should receive these devices will do so. Eventually, biomedical and genetic engineering may eliminate the need for implantable defibrillators by creating artificial hearts, successful transplantation techniques using animal donors, or biologic repair of the original organ.

◉ ELECTRONICS

Capacitors

The greatest opportunity for continued ICD size reduction continues to be in the technology used for making the high-energy storage capacitors that represent a significant portion of the ICD's volume. Traditionally, defibrillators have used standard aluminum electrolytic capacitors that are built in large quantities for use in many commercial devices such as televisions, radios, and flash cameras. Because the medical device market for these capacitors constitutes an insignificant portion of their sales, their manufacturers have little incentive to optimize them for use in implantable defibrillators. These standard capacitors store up to 1.9 J/cc, come only in cylindrical form, and require reformation by periodic charging to ensure acceptable charge times.

Implantable device manufacturers of necessity have

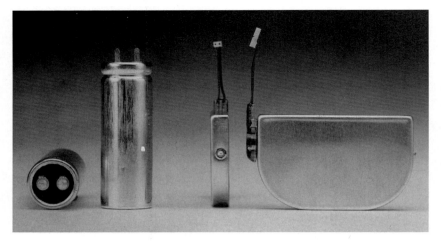

FIGURE 29-1. On the left are the general-purpose, cylindrical, aluminum electrolytic capacitors that are used in early defibrillators. To the right are custom-built, flat, aluminum electrolytic capacitors used in some of the most recent defibrillators. These proprietary designs provide higher stored energy density and flexibility in shaping to maximize efficiency when packaged in the housing of an implantable defibrillator.

resorted to designing and building capacitors specifically tailored for implantable defibrillator applications. Several of the latest commercially available ICDs use these new proprietary flat electrolytic capacitors. Figure 29-1 compares the flat capacitor with the cylindrical capacitor. With energy storage densities of approximately 2.5 to 3.0 J/cc, these capacitors allow construction of defibrillators having volumes of 34 to 39 cc with outputs of 30 J, and further refinement is likely.

An alternative electrolytic capacitor technology, the wet tantalum capacitor, has been developed by Wilson Greatbatch Limited. This proprietary design has been reported to offer an energy density of approximately 4.5 J/cc and to have the further benefit of not requiring regular reforming of the anode.

Eventually, electrolytic capacitors are likely to be replaced by advanced ceramic and metallized polymer film capacitors. The ceramic devices will probably become available first, eventually to be replaced by lighter and less-expensive polymer devices. It is conceivable that the energy storage density of the advanced capacitors will be a 10-fold improvement over that of the original cylindrical aluminum electrolytic capacitors.

Circuits

The various discrete components used to create an ICD continue to be scaled down in size. For example, the rather large, high-voltage MOSFET transistors used to protect ICDs from high-energy sources such as external defibrillators were reduced in size by 40%. Most importantly, the relentless drive to create integrated circuits with ever-smaller line size is a major boon to ICD developers, because current drain decreases in virtually direct proportion to line size and surface area decreases by approximately 75% for each halving of line size. For an ICD, these gains present the opportunity to reduce overall circuit size by providing higher degrees of integration with fewer discrete components and fewer external interconnection pathways; increase longevity or decrease battery size; increase device capability as a consequence of added functions; provide more efficient microprocessors that can be run faster and for longer periods to implement more powerful detection algorithms because the battery current drain is reduced; and increase reliability by virtue of reduced total part count. The designer is given the freedom to make many desirable tradeoffs as a result of these improved circuits.

Waveforms

Biphasic defibrillation waveforms are superior to monophasic waveforms, but the explanations about why this is so remain postulates, making rational design of improvements difficult and leading to slow, costly, trial-and-error testing of arbitrary new waveforms that offer a seemingly endless number of parameter

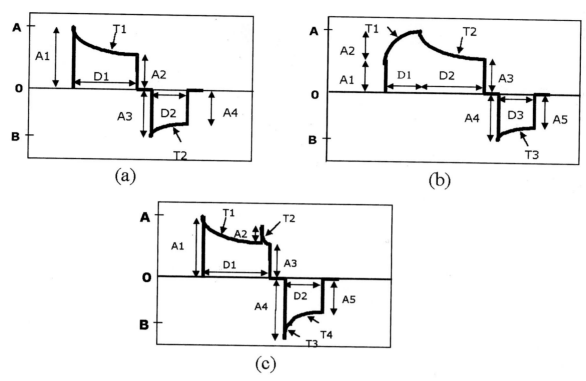

FIGURE 29-2. Variations on the biphasic waveform. The many possible combinations of parameters may alter waveform efficacy, but a well-grounded rationale for selecting the optimal form *a priori* has yet to be identified. The problem is compounded by opportunities to use multiple electrode configurations for delivery, options for varying timing of delivery relative to sensed activity, and the difficulty of measuring defibrillation thresholds in patients.

variations. Figure 29-2 illustrates three of the many possible biphasic waveforms. Each of these basic waveforms offers enormous adjustability by manipulation of the various component amplitudes, durations, and time constants. Waveform *a* is the generic basis for the biphasic waveforms used in current defibrillators. Waveform *b* is an example of a "softer" biphasic waveform that may be more efficient. Waveform *c* has extra voltage spikes added at the end of the first phase and the start of the second phase in an attempt to increase efficiency and efficacy. Compounding the difficulty of testing waveforms is the interaction between the impedances of the specific electrode configurations employed and the waveform. ICD waveform optimization efforts are somewhat reminiscent of past attempts to develop more effective waveforms for pacemakers (1), and the outcome could well be similar—moderate gains when weighed against the much larger opportunities afforded by advancing electronic circuit technology (e.g., integrated circuits, batteries, capacitors) and lead designs. Compared with waveforms in current clinical use, modified biphasic waveforms have demonstrated modest reductions in defibrillation threshold (DFT) energy ranging between 4% and 32% (2–6).

One aspect of device performance that is easily controlled in the design process, charge time, can significantly affect defibrillation success. On balance, it appears that charge time may outweigh waveform morphology improvements for determining the DFT, particularly when batteries have depleted and charge times increase. In patients, biphasic waveform DFTs have been shown to increase by 50% when ventricular fibrillation duration is prolonged from 5 to 20 seconds (7). ICDs should be designed with minimal charge times despite the very tempting option of minimizing device size at the expense of charge time. This often-underappreciated aspect of device performance has begun to receive more attention (8).

LEAD SYSTEMS

Leads

Lead development is accelerating to provide revolutionary functionality, which is urgently needed for the next generations of defibrillator systems. Although lead reliability will always be an essential focus, the lead development task is more challenging than ever given the coexisting goals to reduce lead size, increase pacing and defibrillation efficiency, provide easy and safe access to the left side of the heart, and add sensors for monitoring parameters relevant to multiple comorbidities afflicting many ventricular tachycardia or fibrillation patients.

The coming decade will see a major shift in lead design, away from stylet-based delivery systems and toward very small diameter, sheath-delivered leads. Sheath delivery allows significant reduction in lead diameter because the space-consuming hollow core needed to accommodate the stylet can be eliminated. Lead diameter reduction should help reduce the likelihood of crush failures and, in conjunction with the sheath delivery system, permits access to the left ventricle through the coronary venous system. Left-sided access may provide significant decreases in DFTs or may reduce the occurrence of high DFTs. Models have indicated as much as a 51% reduction in DFT when comparing a Middle Cardiac Vein–Can + superior vena cava (SVC) system with a conventional Right Ventricle (RV)–SVC + Can system (9,10), and animal studies have demonstrated a 30% lower DFT when comparing a lead system using the middle cardiac vein, right ventricle, and can to one using only the right ventricle and can electrodes (11). The addition of a supplemental low-energy shock on the left side may offer further reductions in DFT (12).

Significant improvements in lead technology are needed before left-sided systems can be accepted for routine clinical practice. Ease of placement, time for placement, flexibility of placement location, removability, and potential for damage as a consequence of the high energy shocks all need to be addressed. Current prototype systems are promising (13), but they add significant time to the procedure and cannot always be placed in the desired location that, it appears, may be critical (14). This will be especially likely for left-sided lead placement intended to provide improved pacing synchronization for supporting patients with heart failure.

Another major lead development effort is the incorporation of sensors (e.g., pressure, acceleration, oxygen saturation) (15–18) that may contribute to additional automaticity of pacing functions, enhanced arrhythmia detection, and patient monitoring to aid in the management of heart failure.

Connectors

The current IS-1/DF-1 connector standard has greatly simplified the use of ICDs, allowing minimal fuss when mixing and matching generators and lead systems or when replacing generators. However, standards can be a barrier to progress. Lead delivery techniques using introducer sheaths and the extension of ICD capabilities to include the treatment of atrial fibrillation, left-sided pacing for heart failure, and sensors for advanced monitoring render the current connector standard inadequate. It does not allow implementation of leads that offer isodiametric connectors that facilitate catheter delivery, but rather it requires the addition of more conventional ports leading to unwieldy lead bulk at the ICD implant pocket. The industry is working to develop the urgently needed new lead connection standard, and in a few years, we will undoubtedly view the IS-1/DF-1 system as absurdly oversized as we now do the four-prong plug that had long been the standard for U.S. telephone connections.

ARRHYTHMIA DETECTION ALGORITHMS

Despite the outstanding performance of current ICDs (19,20), considerable effort is being focused on improving arrhythmia detection algorithms. Dual-chamber devices offer detection algorithms that benefit from the additional information derived from electrograms reflecting atrial activity. This has been helpful with some devices (21), but it is still imperfect (22,23), and not all dual-chamber algorithms improve detection accuracy (24). Moreover, the atrial lead creates new possibilities for detection errors if far-field R waves are misinterpreted or the lead dislodges. There will always be a need for some single-chamber ICDs without an atrial electrogram, and their detection algorithms will be enhanced by ventricular waveform analysis. Several ventricular electrogram morphology analyses are now commercially available (25–27), but they have not been so successful as to halt the drive toward further improvements. Newer variants (28,29), although promising, have yet to be clinically proven. All morphology detection algorithms have been relatively crude, hampered by the limited computational power of microprocessors that are sufficiently energy efficient for use in implanted devices. As integrated circuit technology continues to migrate to finer line sizes, the gains in mathematical power and energy efficiency will support far more sophisticated morphology analyses and will then be used to analyze atrial and ventricular electrograms.

Perhaps the most important advance in detection algorithms will be the transition from user-programmed systems, which require considerable knowledge about device operation, to fully automatic algorithms that free the physician to simply prescribe therapies. Because today's automatic external defibrillators require no detection programming, it takes little imagination to extend this concept to the implanted defibrillators. Current and evolving ICD arrhythmia detection techniques are the building blocks that will make this possible.

AUTOMATICITY

The highly programmable nature and sophistication of current implantable defibrillators is a double-edged sword, allowing extensive tailoring to specific patient requirements at the expense of significant time and effort from the physician. Often, this is compounded when the physician faces a mix of devices from different eras and manufacturers. Managing the wide variety of detection algorithms, optimizing therapies for bradycardia and tachycardia, selecting optimal monitoring modes, tracking the various replacement indicators, and troubleshooting malfunctioning systems can be perplexing and time consuming. As device functions evolve to include management of atrial arrhythmias and heart failure, the challenges will be even greater. However, much of this complexity represents the initial wave of technologies that will ultimately coalesce to allow the device to manage many functions automatically.

In addition to automation of arrhythmia detection, future ICDs may also optimize shock waveform characteristics automatically, based on the specific configuration and impedances of the lead system that is connected to the generator (30,31). Antibradycardia pacing functions will become more automatic, advancing to include self-adjusting ventricular and atrial pacing output energies (32,33) for maximal longevity without compromising patient safety (34,35), automatically adapting or closed loop rate response algorithms (36,37), hemodynamic sensor driven adjustment of atrioventricular (AV) delays for optimal hemodynamics as the patient moves from sedentary to strenuous activities, and self-setting of amplifier sensitivities to ensure appropriate sensing while avoiding detection of interference. Current rudimentary problem alerts will continue to evolve into more comprehensive, automatic, self-diagnostic tools.

ARRHYTHMIA PREVENTION

Except for certain long QT syndrome patients (38), pacing has not been particularly successful in preventing ventricular arrhythmias. Rate-smoothing algorithms have been incorporated into some pacemakers and defibrillators, but definitive evidence of efficacy has yet to be presented.

Dual-chamber defibrillators make it possible to maintain AV synchrony and to minimize pacing the ventricles in patients with sinus abnormalities. In these patients, ventricular pacing is associated with a significantly higher incidence of atrial fibrillation than is seen with atrial pacing (39), but it is not clear whether atrial pacing prevents naturally occurring atrial fibrillation or merely avoids iatrogenic atrial fibrillation because of ventricular pacing.

Some success in preventing atrial fibrillation has been reported using bicameral or multisite right atrial pacing (40,41), although these techniques continue to be investigational and have not been widely endorsed (42). Two studies, both recently competed but as yet unpublished, Dual-Site Atrial Pacing to Prevent Atrial Fibrillation and Synchronous Biatrial Pacing (SYNBIAPACE) for atrial arrhythmia prevention, may help establish the proper role for pacing in the prevention of atrial fibrillation (43).

Arrhythmia prevention will probably require far more patient-specific techniques than termination. A high-energy shock deals effectively with virtually any ventricular fibrillation, but preventing arrhythmias may require multiple approaches even in a single patient. Options beyond direct cardiac stimulation may prove worthy of investigation. Drug delivery capability or neural stimulation coupled with suitable means to detect impending onset of arrhythmias may be added to future ICD systems.

◉ MONITORING

Implanted defibrillators have evolved from devices with no programmability and no stored data to systems that store 250,000 bytes of data and provide more than 40 programmable parameters, each with multiple options. There is no end in sight for the demands to increase data storage capacity and device flexibility. Just as lead connectors have become inadequate, so too have telemetry schemes. In the age of remote controls, cellular phones, and central monitoring of automobile functions by geopositioning satellite systems, it is no longer reasonable to ask that patients disrobe or be close by for connection to follow-up equipment, nor is it reasonable to expect busy clinicians to spend precious minutes with the patient standing by just to obtain data from implanted devices. Telemedicine is increasingly of interest and appears ready to blossom once outmoded medical licensing provisions are updated.

The technology to support these changes is at hand. Automobile manufacturers offer on-board monitoring and concierge service that uses the cell network and the geopositioning satellite system to direct assistance to motorists when the system detects problems such as a deployed air bag. Cellular phone technology has been incorporated in ambulatory electrocardiographic recorders and was used to provide up to 43 hours of continuous monitoring of patients as they traveled throughout Europe (44). It is already possible to buy a personal electronic tracker that provides a geopositioning satellite receiver and cellular phone

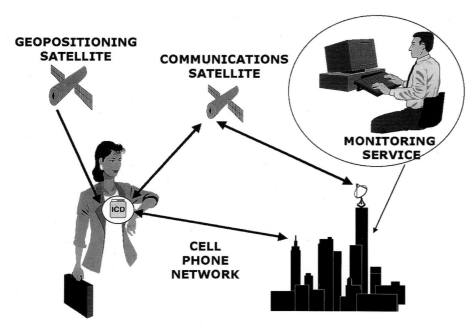

FIGURE 29-3. Advanced telemetry schemes will allow future implanted devices to communicate directly with follow-up personnel by means of the cell phone network and communications satellite linkages. Geopositioning satellites will be used to locate the patient.

circuits in a pager-sized package (45). This device is currently positioned as a personal tracking system for children, the elderly, house-arrest prisoners, or for travelers in dangerous environments, but it demonstrates how close we are to technology that could be embedded in implantable devices to link them directly to the world communication system. Figure 29-3 illustrates the use of advanced telemetry technology with current ICD patients, and it highlights the significant potential for extending the utility of diversified monitoring features in ICDs and other implanted devices designed to assist in the treatment of multiple pathologies, including atrial fibrillation, heart failure, and ischemia (46).

COMORBIDITY MANAGEMENT

Atrial Fibrillation Therapy

Implantable defibrillation therapy for atrial arrhythmias has been evaluated with two devices, one intended solely for atrial applications and no longer being produced (47) and the other designed to treat atrial and ventricular arrhythmias (48). These systems have demonstrated the ability to defibrillate the atria and, with atrial pacing techniques, to terminate atrial tachycardias, but their clinical role has yet to be determined. Of primary concern is patient acceptance of painful shocks for an arrhythmia that is not immediately life threatening. Without a means to provide pain-free defibrillation, this narrows the patient population to those having relatively infrequent episodes of atrial fibrillation.

Ablation techniques may eventually cure atrial fibrillation (49) or perhaps make it possible to alter the arrhythmic substrate sufficiently to produce pace-terminable rhythms instead of atrial fibrillation, thereby reducing or eliminating the need for painful high-energy therapies. Alternatively, pacing techniques for atrial fibrillation prevention may be developed and incorporated into these devices. Another possibility is development of an automatically triggered, implanted drug infusion system designed to terminate atrial fibrillation.

Heart Failure

Because many patients having ventricular arrhythmias also suffer some degree of heart failure, there is considerable interest in adding to the ICD features that would help manage and treat this coexisting condition. Efforts are focused on advanced pacing modalities and expanded monitoring features.

Considerable activity is being devoted to developing and evaluating multisite ventricular pacing as a means for improving cardiac function. Several investigational pacemakers and ICDs offer biventricular pacing capability designed to resynchronize ventricular activation in patients having significant conduction delays, and some investigators have creatively adapted standard ICDs to accomplish this function (50). Figure 29-4 is an example of an investigational ICD along with the small-diameter lead designed for catheter-assisted transvenous placement on the left ventricle through the coronary veins.

Preliminary results with investigational pacemakers suggest that biventricular pacing in patients with dilated cardiomyopathy, poor ejection fractions, and significantly prolonged QRS durations can reduce valvular regurgitation, decrease pulmonary capillary wedge pressures (51), improve 6-minute hall walk test times, enhance quality-of-life scores, decrease a patient's New York Heart Association (NYHA) class of heart disease (52,53), and reduce the need for compensatory support from sympathetic activation (54). Some have questioned whether these gains may be offset by impairment in renal function (55). Still others have suggested that pacing the left side alone may be sufficient (56,57). Studies of normal and pacing-induced heart failure in dogs have shown that pacing from the right ventricular apex is the least effective site for pacing and that stimulating the left and right ventricular apices and bases simultaneously significantly improves cardiac function compared with conventional right ventricular apical pacing (58). Although it is not clear what degree of complexity is required for effective pacing of the heart failure patient, it does appear that a lead will be required on the left side. Barring significant detrimental findings, pacing for heart failure will most likely become a standard feature of future ICDs.

Pacing therapy for heart failure will probably apply

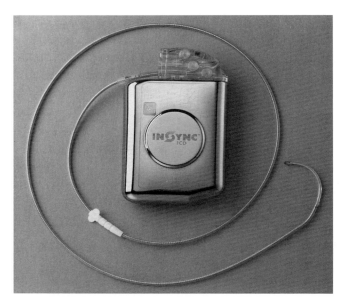

FIGURE 29-4. An investigational implantable cardioverter-defibrillator offering atrial-based multisite ventricular pacing for treatment of heart failure is shown along with an electrode designed for transvenous placement on the posterolateral wall of the left ventricle.

to a somewhat limited pool of heart failure patients—those with significant conduction disturbances—but virtually all heart failure patients would be candidates for intensive monitoring if such surveillance can be shown to improve patient outcomes. Investigational monitoring devices have been implanted in heart failure patients (15,16), and preliminary results suggest that stable sensor performance can be provided. It has also been shown that derivatives of right ventricular pressure measurements can provide a highly correlated analog of the pulmonary artery diastolic pressure (59). Studies are in progress to determine if these monitoring data can be used to reduce emergency admissions and improve patient management. Additional key elements to successful application of this technology will be advanced data management and communication techniques that can provide evidence of evolving problems in a sufficiently timely manner.

INDICATIONS

Many studies have demonstrated significant mortality reductions achieved by ICD implantation (60) in survivors of sudden cardiac death (Cardiac Arrest Study Hamburg) (61); patients after myocardial infarction (post-MI) with ejection fractions of less than 0.35 and nonsustained asymptomatic ventricular tachycardia (Multicenter Automatic Defibrillator Trial) (62); post-MI coronary artery disease patients with ejection fractions of less than 0.40 and nonsustained ventricular tachycardia inducible (Multicenter UnSustained Tachycardia Trial) (63); and patients with ventricular fibrillation or sustained ventricular tachycardia with syncope, or sustained ventricular tachycardia with presyncope or angina and depressed ejection fraction (Canadian Implantable Defibrillator Study [64], Antiarrhythmics Versus Implantable Defibrillators [65]).

Additional studies being planned or underway may significantly expand the indications for ICDs (66). The Sudden Cardiac Death in Heart Failure Trial (SCD-HeFT), a three-arm study with conventional heart failure therapy as a control and the addition of amiodarone or an ICD in the other two treatment limbs, is evaluating all-cause mortality in patients with coronary artery disease or cardiomyopathy and who are in NYHA class II or III failure with ejection fractions of less than 0.35. A positive finding for electrical therapy could dramatically expand the ICD patient population and give further impetus to the addition of ICD features specifically aimed at heart failure management. The Multicenter Automatic Defibrillator Trial II (MADIT II) is evaluating total mortality with and without an ICD in post-MI patients who have coronary artery disease and ejection fractions of less than 0.30 (67). The Defibrillators in Acute Myocardial Infarction Trial (DINAMIT) will examine prophylactic ICD usage in patients who have had an MI and who also have an ejection fraction below 35% along with abnormal heart rate variability indices (68).

The search for additional tools to select patients who are at risk of sudden cardiac death and should therefore be candidates for prophylactic ICD implantation continues. Current indicators, used alone or in combination, have at best a 30% positive predictive accuracy (69). Baroreceptor sensitivity, late potentials in the signal-averaged electrocardiogram, QT interval dispersion, heart rate variability, and T-wave alternans are among the potential screening measurements that are under scrutiny (70–72). Subanalyses of the MADIT II and SCD-HeFT trials should help determine the utility of a number of these risk indicators.

COSTS

Cost concerns are intensifying as the patient population indicated for defibrillators continues to expand. Rapid evolution of these devices has been a double-edged sword, decreasing costs by virtue of simplified implant procedures (73–75) and greater device longevities, yet causing costs to rise given the constant pressure to increase functional capabilities while reducing device size. Continued size reduction has driven device manufacturers more deeply into the electronic components business to create unique parts (e.g., capacitors, batteries, sensors) solely for ICD use, with consequent increased development costs and loss of economy of scale. Development costs are also under upward pressure given the short life cycle of these products in the market and the need to support increasingly costly outcome studies.

Studies comparing ICD with pharmacologic therapy have demonstrated that ICD economics range from incremental cost savings of $13,975 to additional incremental costs of $114,917 per life-year saved. Most of these studies have found ICD cost effectiveness to be consistent with other currently accepted therapies such as hemodialysis or diuretics for mild hypertension (76–82). The AVID study, which was terminated early after demonstrating significant mortality advantages with the ICD, reported an unusually large incremental cost ($114,917 per life-year saved). This finding must be considered in light of the truncated follow-up period associated with this study that precluded full amortization of up-front device and implant procedure costs. Nevertheless, as indications broaden, the total absolute costs to society are likely to be problematic (83), especially if the SCD-HeFT, MADIT II, and other study outcomes are positive for ICD therapy.

Some have proposed addressing costs by reusing explanted devices, an option not available in some countries because of device ownership and medical liability issues. Beyond these barriers, one analysis concluded that the impact of reuse on the cost of ICD therapy in general should be marginal (84).

Purchasers can exert significant control on the annualized costs of defibrillator therapy by selecting devices on the basis of longevity rather than size, especially now that devices are universally small enough for pectoral implantation in virtually any patient. The annualized cost of ICD therapy (excluding follow-up costs) can easily be reduced by one third by adding approximately 5-cc more battery to the volume of a typical device, thereby increasing longevity by 50%. Future device designs are strongly influenced by the customers' pocketbook votes on current devices.

CONCLUSIONS

The ICD is evolving to become a therapeutic instrument capable of addressing multiple cardiac pathologies. Consequently, its cost effectiveness should continue to increase. Advances in electronic technology are making this possible while continuing the dramatic size reductions that make the ICD an increasingly attractive option. Figure 29-5 shows a very early ICD, a current dual-chamber version, and the hypo-

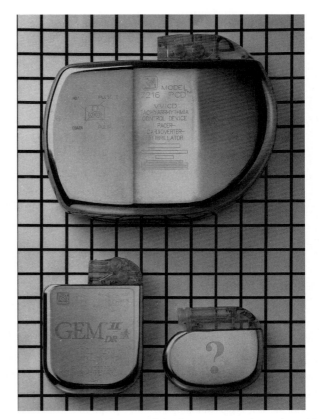

FIGURE 29-5. At the top of the figure is an early implantable defibrillator with a volume of 209 cc. At the bottom left is a 39.5-cc, dual-chamber implantable cardioverter-defibrillator (ICD) that was commercialized in 1999. The device at the bottom right represents a hypothetical ICD with a volume of less than 25 cc. Such a device may be developed before 2005.

thetical embodiment of a device that could be available in the first decade of the new millennium. In light of the incredible accomplishment of creating an implantable version of the defibrillator, it seems probable that eventually the defibrillator will be supplanted by even more impressive technology, perhaps an artificial heart (85), a genetically modified animal heart transplant (86,87), or genetically engineered repairs to the original organ (88–90).

REFERENCES

1. Roy OZ. The current status of cardiac pacing. *Crit Rev Bioeng* 1975;2:259–327.
2. Rist K, Tchou PJ, Mowrey K, et al. Smaller capacitors improve the biphasic waveform. *J Cardiovasc Electrophysiol* 1994;5:771–776.
3. Swerdlow CD, Kass RM, Davie S, et al. Short biphasic pulses from 90 microfarad capacitors lower defibrillation threshold. *Pacing Clin Electrophysiol* 1996;19:1053–1060.
4. Natale A, Sra J, Krum D, et al. Relative efficacy of different tilts with biphasic defibrillation in humans. *Pacing Clin Electrophysiol* 1996;19:197–206.
5. Alt E, Evans F, Wolf PD, et al. Does reducing capacitance have potential for further miniaturization of implantable defibrillators? *Heart* 1997;77:234–237.
6. Yamanouchi Y, Mowrey KA, Kroll MW, et al. Optimized first phase tilt in "parallel-series" biphasic waveform. *J Cardiovasc Electrophysiol* 1997;8:649–657.
7. Windecker S, Ideker R, Plumb V, et al. The influence of ventricular fibrillation duration on defibrillation efficacy using biphasic waveforms in humans. *J Am Coll Cardiol* 1999;33:33–38.
8. Mann DE, Kelly PA, Robertson AD, et al. Significant differences in charge times among currently available implantable cardioverter defibrillators. *Pacing Clin Electrophysiol* 1999;22:903–907.
9. Bonner M, Min X. Ventricular defibrillation from the cardiac veins: a modeling study [Abstract]. *Pacing Clin Electrophysiol* 1999;22:870.
10. de Jongh AL, Entcheva EG, Booker RS, et al. Optimizing electrode placement in a proposed ICD system incorporating LV electrodes: finite element analysis. *Comput Cardiol* 1998;25:281–284.
11. Roberts PR, Urban JF, Euler DE, et al. The middle cardiac vein—a novel pathway to reduce the defibrillation threshold. *J Interv Card Electrophysiol* 1999;3:55–60.
12. Walker RG, KenKnight BH, Ideker R. Reduction of defibrillation threshold by 50% with a low amplitude auxiliary shock [Abstract]. *Pacing Clin Electrophysiol* 1998;21:853.
13. Meisel E, Pfeiffer D, Butter C, et al. Left ventricle coronary vein accessibility for implantation of a defibrillating ICD and/or pacing lead system [Abstract]. *Eur Heart J* 1999;20:454.
14. Meisel E, Butter C, Philippon F, et al. Human defibrillation using a transvenous left coronary vein lead and dual shock waveform: effect of left ventricular lead position. *Pacing Clin Electrophysiol* 1999;22:699.
15. Steinhaus DM, Lemery R, Bresnahan DR, et al. Initial experience with an implantable hemodynamic monitor. *Circulation* 1996;93:745–752.
16. Ohlsson A, Nordlander R, Bennett T, et al. Continuous ambulatory haemodynamic monitoring with an implantable system: the feasibility of a new technique. *Eur Heart J* 1998;19:174–184.
17. Holmstrom N, Johnson P, Carlsten J, Bowald S. Long-term in vivo experience of an electrochemical sensor using the potential step technique for measurement of mixed venous oxygen pressure. *Biosens Bioelectron* 1998;13:1287–1295.
18. Yoon Y, Jenkins JM. Automated analysis of intracardiac blood pressure waveforms for implantable defibrillators. *Comput Cardiol* 1998;25:269–272.
19. Swerdlow CD, Chen PS, Kass RM, et al. Discrimination of ventricular tachycardia from sinus tachycardia and atrial fibrillation in a tiered-therapy cardioverter-defibrillator. *J Am Coll Cardiol* 1994;23:1342–1355.
20. Schaumann A, von zur Muhlen F, Gonska BD, Kreuzer H. Enhanced detection criteria in implantable cardioverter-defibrillators to avoid inappropriate therapy. *Am J Cardiol* 1996;78:42–50.
21. Swerdlow CD, Sheth NV, Olson WH. Clinical performance of a pattern-based, dual chamber algorithm for discrimination of ventricular from supraventricular arrhythmias [Abstract]. *Pacing Clin Electrophysiol* 1998;21:800.
22. Dijkman B, Wellens HJJ. The VT-SVT discrimination algorithms in dual chamber ICDs—improved but still not perfect automatic arrhythmia detection [Abstract]. *Pacing Clin Electrophysiol* 1999;22:853.
23. Wolpert C, Jung W, Spehl S, et al. Potential pitfalls of a new dual-chamber detection algorithm: implications for patient selection and device programming [Abstract]. *Eur Heart J* 1999;20:110.
24. Kuhlkamp V, Dornberger V, Mewis C, et al. Clinical experience with the new detection algorithms for atrial fibrillation of a defibrillator with dual chamber sensing and pacing. *J Cardiovasc Electrophysiol* 1999;10:905–915.
25. Brachmann J, Swerdlow CD, Mitchell B, et al, for the Worldwide 7218 ICD Investigators. Worldwide experience with the electrogram width feature for improved detection in an implantable pacemaker-cardioverter-defibrillator [Abstract]. *J Am Coll Cardiol* 1997;29:115A.
26. Duru F, Schonbeck M, Luscher T, Candinas R. The potential for inappropriate ventricular tachycardia confirmation using the intracardiac electrogram (EGM) width criterion. *Pacing Clin Electrophysiol* 1999;22:1039–1046.
27. Schulte B, Sperzel J, Schwarz T, et al. Temporal and exercise-related stability of a new morphology-based arrhythmia detection parameter in implantable defibrillators. *Pacing Clin Electrophysiol* 1999;22:823.
28. Gillberg JM, Koyrakh LA, Pearson AM, Olson WH. Wavelet transform based electrogram morphology discrimination for implantable cardioverter-defibrillators [Abstract]. *Pacing Clin Electrophysiol* 1999;22:825.
29. Gold MR, Hsu W, Marcovecchio AF, et al. A new defibrillator discrimination algorithm utilizing electrogram morphology analysis. *Pacing Clin Electrophysiol* 1999;22:179–182.
30. Walcott GP, Walker RG, Cates AW, et al. Choosing the optimal monophasic and biphasic waveforms for ventricular defibrillation. *J Cardiovasc Electrophysiol* 1995;6:737–750.
31. Swerdlow CD, Fan W, Brewer JE. Charge-burping theory correctly predicts optimal ratios of phase duration for biphasic defibrillation waveforms. *Circulation* 1996;94:2278–2284.
32. Splett V, Trusty JM, Hammill SC, Friedman PA. Discrimination of pacing capture in implantable defibrillators: evoked response detection using RV coil to can vector [Abstract]. *Pacing Clin Electrophysiol* 1999;22:803.
33. Bradley K, Sloman L, Bornzin GA. An atrial autothreshold algo-

rithm using the atrial evoked response [Abstract]. *Pacing Clin Electrophysiol* 1999;22:851.
34. Riddell F, Biosa R, Richardson V. How effective is autocapture? Clinical experience with Regency SR + 2400L pacemaker and 1450T lead [Abstract]. *Pacing Clin Electrophysiol* 1998; 21:955.
35. Schiller H, Kruse I, Svensson O, Mortensen P. Long-term benefit of autocapture—four years of follow-up [Abstract]. *Pacing Clin Electrophysiol* 1999;22:807.
36. Mianulli M, Crossley G, Wilkoff B, Benditt DG. The utility and stability of a new automatic rate response optimization algorithm to achieve desired rate behavior [Abstract]. *Pacing Clin Electrophysiol* 1998;21:874.
37. Alt E. What is the ideal rate-adaptive sensor for patients with implantable cardioverter defibrillators: lessons from cardiac pacing. *Am J Cardiol* 1999;83[Suppl 5B]:17D–23D.
38. Schwartz PJ. Long QT syndrome. *Cardiology* 1999;[Special Edition]:43–47.
39. Andersen H, Nielsen J, Thomsen P, et al. Long-term follow-up of patients from a randomised trial of atrial versus ventricular pacing for sick sinus syndrome. *Lancet* 1997;350:1210–1216.
40. Daubert C, Mabo P, Berder V, et al. Atrial tachyarrhythmias associated with high degree interatrial conduction block: prevention by permanent atrial resynchronization. *Eur J Card Pacing Electrophysiol* 1994;4:35–44.
41. Saksena S, Delfaut P, Prakash A, et al. Multisite electrode pacing for prevention of atrial fibrillation. *J Cardiovasc Electrophysiol* 1998;9[Suppl 8]:S155–S162.
42. Lévy S, Breithardt G, Campbell RWF, et al, for the Working Group on Arrhythmias of the European Society of Cardiology. Atrial fibrillation: current knowledge and recommendations for management. *Eur Heart J* 1998;19:1294–1320.
43. Sharif MN, Wyse DG. Atrial fibrillation: overview of therapeutic trials. *Can J Cardiol* 1998;14:1241–1254.
44. Schmidd JJ, Schiller A, Zuber M, et al. Long term monitoring of cardiac patients via digital cellular phone transmission [Abstract]. *Pacing Clin Electrophysiol* 1999;22:839.
45. Gendreau PR. This PET locates its master. *Portable Design* 1999; March(5):39–45.
46. Brunner M, Baron TW, Zehender M. Detection of myocardial ischemia is possible using implantable defibrillators [Abstract]. *Eur Heart J* 1999;20:112.
47. Tse H, Lau C, Sra J, et al, for the Metrix Investigators. Atrial fibrillation detection and R-wave synchronization by Metrix implantable atrial defibrillator: implications for long-term efficacy and safety. *Circulation* 1999;99:1446–1451.
48. Heisel A, Jung J. The atrial defibrillator: a stand-alone device or part of a combined dual-chamber system? *Am J Cardiol* 1999; 83[Suppl 5B]:218D–226D.
49. Guerra PG, Lesh MD. The role of nonpharmacologic therapies for the treatment of atrial fibrillation. *J Cardiovasc Electrophysiol* 1999;10:450–460.
50. Walker S, Levy T, Rex S, Paul VE. Biventricular implantable cardioverter defibrillator use in a patient with heart failure and ventricular tachycardia secondary to Emery-Dreifuss syndrome. *Europace* 1999;1:206–209.
51. Cazeau S, Ritter P, Lazarus A, et al. Multisite pacing for end-stage heart failure: early experience. *Pacing Clin Electrophysiol* 1996;19:1748–1757.
52. Gras D, Cazeau S, Ritter P, et al. Permanent cardiac resynchronization after sustained clinical improvement in heart failure patients: the In-Sync trial [Abstract]. *Pacing Clin Electrophysiol* 1999;22:901.
53. Gras D, Mabo P, Tang T, et al. Multisite pacing as a supplemental treatment of congestive heart failure: preliminary results of the Medtronic, Inc., In-Sync study. *Pacing Clin Electrophysiol* 1998;21:2240–2255.
54. Saxon LA, DeMarco T, Chatterjee K, et al. Chronic biventricular pacing decreases serum norepinephrine in dilated heart failure patients with the greatest sympathetic activation at baseline [Abstract]. *Pacing Clin Electrophysiol* 1999;22:830.
55. Chatoor R, Bucknall C, Holt P. Biventricular pacing may adversely affect renal hemodynamics and neurohormones in heart failure [Abstract]. *Pacing Clin Electrophysiol* 1999;22:854.
56. Auricchio A, Stellbrink C, Block M, et al. Effect of pacing chamber and atrioventricular delay on acute systolic function of paced patients with congestive heart failure. *Circulation* 1999; 99:2993–3001.
57. Bradley K, Florio J, Pianca A, Bornzin GA. Hemodynamic comparison of left ventricular and biventricular pacing [Abstract]. *Pacing Clin Electrophysiol* 1999;22:901.
58. Fei L, Wrobleski D, Groh W, et al. Effects of multisite ventricular pacing on cardiac function in normal dogs and dogs with heart failure. *J Cardiovasc Electrophysiol* 1999;10:935–946.
59. Chuang PP, Wilson RF, Homans DC, et al. Measurement of pulmonary artery diastolic pressure from a right ventricular pressure transducer in patients with heart failure. *J Card Fail* 1996; 2:41–46.
60. Cappato R. Secondary prevention of sudden cardiac death: the Dutch study, the Antiarrhythmics Versus Implantable Defibrillator trial, the Cardiac Arrest Study Hamburg, and the Canadian Implantable Defibrillator Study. *Am J Cardiol* 1999;83[Suppl 5B]:68D–73D.
61. Kuck KH, for the CASH investigators. The CASH study: final results. Oral presentation at the annual session of the American College of Cardiology. Atlanta, 1998.
62. Moss AJ, Hall WJ, Cannom DS, et al. Improved survival with an implanted defibrillator in patients with coronary disease at high risk for ventricular arrhythmia. Multicenter Automatic Defibrillator Implantation Trial Investigators. *N Engl J Med* 1996; 335:1933–1940.
63. Buxton A, Fisher JD, for the MUSTT Investigators. Update on recent clinical trials. Presented at the 20th Annual Scientific Sessions. NASPE. Washington, D.C., May 1999.
64. Connolly S, for the CIDS investigators. The CIDS study: final results. Oral presentation at the annual session of the American College of Cardiology. Atlanta, 1998.
65. Antiarrhythmics Versus Implantable Defibrillators (AVID) Investigators. A comparison of antiarrhythmic-drug therapy with implantable defibrillators in patients resuscitated from near-fatal ventricular arrhythmias. *N Engl J Med* 1997;337:1576–1583.
66. Klein H, Auricchio A, Reek S, Geller C. New primary prevention trials of sudden cardiac death in patients with left ventricular dysfunctions: SCD-HeFT and MADIT-II. *Am J Cardiol* 1999; 83[Suppl 5B]:91D–97D.
67. Moss AJ, Cannom DS, Daubert JP, et al, for the MADIT II Investigators. Multicenter automatic defibrillator implantation trial II (MADIT II): design and clinical protocol. *Ann Noninvas Cardiol* 1999;4:83–91.
68. Connolly S: Prophylactic antiarrhythmic therapy for the prevention of sudden cardiac death in high-risk patients: drugs and devices. *Eur Heart J* 1999;1:C31–C35.
69. Zipes DP, Wellens HJJ. Sudden cardiac death. *Circulation* 1998; 98:2334–2351.
70. Camm AJ, Kautzner J. Assessment of arrhythmias after myocardial infarction in the post-CAST era. *Can J Cardiol* 1996; 12[Suppl B]:9B–19B.
71. Armoundas AA, Rosenbaum DS, Ruskin JN, et al. Prognostic significance of electrical alternans versus signal averaged electro-

71. cardiography in predicting the outcome of electrophysiological testing and arrhythmia-free survival. *Heart* 1998;80:251–256.
72. Hohnloser SH, Klingenheben T, Li Y, et al. T wave alternans as a predictor of recurrent ventricular tachyarrhythmias in ICD recipients: prospective comparison with conventional risk markers. *J Cardiovasc Electrophysiol* 1998;9:1258–1268.
73. Anvari A, Stix G, Grabenwoger M, et al. Comparison of three cardioverter defibrillator implantation techniques: initial results with transvenous pectoral implantation. *Pacing Clin Electrophysiol* 1996;19:1061–1069.
74. Cardinal DS, Connelly DT, Steinhaus DM, et al. Cost savings with nonthoracotomy implantable cardioverter-defibrillators. *Am J Cardiol* 1996;78:1255–1259.
75. Bollmann A, Kanuru NK, DeLurgio D, et al. Comparison of three different automatic defibrillator implantation approaches: pectoral implantation using conscious sedation reduces procedure times and cost. *J Interv Card Electrophysiol* 1997;1:221–225.
76. Goldman L, Gordon DJ, Rifkind BM, et al. Cost and health implications of cholesterol lowering. *Circulation* 1992;85:1960–1968.
77. Kupersmith J, Hogan A, Guerrero P, et al. Evaluating and improving the cost-effectiveness of the implantable cardioverter-defibrillator. *Am Heart J* 1995;130:507–515.
78. Kupersmith J, Holmes-Rovner M, Hogan A, et al. Cost-effectiveness analysis in heart disease, part II: preventive therapies. *Prog Cardiovasc Dis* 1995;37:243–271.
79. Owens DK, Sanders GD, Harris RA, et al. Cost-effectiveness of implantable cardioverter defibrillators relative to amiodarone for prevention of sudden cardiac death. *Ann Intern Med* 1997;126:1–12.
80. Mushlin AI, Hall WJ, Zwanziger J, et al. The cost-effectiveness of automatic implantable cardiac defibrillators: results from MADIT. Multicenter Automatic Defibrillator Implant Trial. *Circulation* 1998;97:2129–2135.
81. Larsen GC, McAnulty JH, Hallstom A, et al. Hospitalization charges in the antiarrhythmics versus implantable defibrillators (AVID) trial: the AVID economic analysis study [Abstract]. *Circulation* 1997;96[Suppl 8]:I-77.
82. Stanton MS, Bell GK. Economic outcomes of implantable defibrillators. *Circulation* 2000;101:1067–1074.
83. Pathmanathan RK, Lau EW, Cooper J, et al. Potential impact of antiarrhythmic drugs versus implantable defibrillators on the management of ventricular arrhythmias: the Midlands trial of empirical amiodarone versus electrophysiologically guided intervention and cardioverter implant registry data. *Heart* 1998;80:68–70.
84. Block M, Breithardt G. Reuse of defibrillators—is it feasible? *Eur Heart J Suppl* 1999;1:G12–G14.
85. Weiss WJ, Rosenberg G, Snyder AJ, et al. Steady state hemodynamic and energetic characterization of the Penn State/3M Health Care total artificial heart. *ASAIO J* 1999;45:189–193.
86. Minanov OP, Itescu S, Michler RE. Recent advances and the potential for clinical use of xenotransplantation. *Curr Opin Cardiol* 1996;11:214–220.
87. DiSesa VJ. Cardiac xenotransplantation. *Ann Thorac Surg* 1997;64:1858–1865.
88. Dorfman J, Duong M, Zibaitis A, et al. Myocardial tissue engineering with autologous myoblast implantation. *J Thorac Cardiovasc Surg* 1998;116:744–751.
89. Atkins BZ, Lewis CW, Kraus WE, et al. Intracardiac transplantation of skeletal myoblasts yields two populations of striated cells in situ. *Ann Thorac Surg* 1999;67:124–129.
90. Atkins BZ, Hueman MT, Meuchel J, et al. Cellular cardiomyoplasty improves diastolic properties of injured heart. *J Surg Res* 1999;85:234–242.

IMPLANTATION TECHNIQUES FOR SINGLE- AND DUAL-CHAMBER PACEMAKERS
• • •

PETER H. BELOTT

The approach to cardiac pacemaker implantation has undergone considerable evolution over the past half century (1). The 1950s marked the beginning of the era of modern artificial pacing. In 1958, Seymour Furman and J. B. Schwedel performed the first transvenous endocardial electrode placement (2). At the same time, Rune Elmqvist and A. K. E. Senning developed a totally implantable pacemaker system. The device was placed in an epigastric pocket and the electrodes connected subcutaneously directly to the heart (3). Simultaneously, these two events introduced transvenous and epicardial approaches to cardiac pacing. To this day, these two distinctly different anatomic approaches have been demonstrated to be safe and reliable methods for pacemaker implantation (4–6).

Initially, the epicardium was the prime site for pacemaker implantation. Today, the cephalic vein by cutdown and the subclavian vein by a percutaneous puncture are the most popular sites for pacemaker implantation. The epicardium is now reserved for patients undergoing cardiac surgery. The epicardial approach was performed by a cardiothoracic surgeon with the patient under general anesthesia. This approach was frequently used because many pacemaker implantations were associated with open cardiac procedures such as valve replacements and repair of congenital defects. Earlier pacemakers were more easily placed in a subcutaneous abdominal pocket. The initial popularity of the epicardial approach was also reinforced by the lack of reliable endocardial lead systems. As the pacemaker size decreased and endocardial lead systems saw the development of fixation mechanisms to avoid dislodgement, the transvenous endocardial approach by cutdown soon replaced an open-chest procedure. This approach was also more desirable because it precluded the use of general anesthesia, but it required some form of imaging for electrode placement. The initial transvenous electrode systems were unreliable and associated with an extremely high dislodgement rate. The development of fixation mechanisms all but eradicated the complication of lead dislodgement. Integrated circuitry and modern battery technology allowed a radical reduction in the pacemaker size and the resultant surgical requirement. A pacemaker implantation that initially required a major open-chest procedure under general anesthesia could be carried out by a simple cutdown and minor surgery.

In the late 1970s, Littleford and Spector introduced the percutaneous sheath-set technique for venous access through the subclavian vein (7). This approach and variations on its theme have revolutionized modern pacemaker implantation. The percutaneous approach has not been without controversy regarding its safety. It has introduced concerns about vascular trauma and pneumothorax. With the percutaneous approach and implantation procedure, previously the exclusive role of the cardiovascular surgeon, had become the purview of the invasive cardiologist. The procedure that was traditionally performed in the operating room could be safely conducted in a cardiac catheterization laboratory or special procedures room. With the advent of conscious sedation techniques, the role of the anesthesiologist has disappeared from the pacemaker implantation theater. The procedure that once required a rather protracted hospital stay is now routinely performed on an ambulatory basis.

The percutaneous subclavian approach has been associated with the *subclavian crush phenomenon*. This has resulted in a shift to alternate and sometimes unusual venous access sites. It has also engendered new percutaneous techniques for access of the axillary vein. The transmyocardial or epicardial approach has seen little change over the years, although transthoracic endocardial lead placement techniques by atriotomy and limited thoracotomy have been developed for unusual pathophysiologic and congenital anomalies. Thoracoscopic techniques have also been used for the placement of epicardial leads. Since Mirowski and associates' initial implant of the implantable cardioverter-defibrillator (ICD) in 1980, its evolution with respect to implantation has been identical to that of the cardiac pacemaker (8).

During the past half century, modern cardiac pacing has seen radical changes in anatomic approach, preoperative planning, implanting personnel, and implant facility. The discipline that was once exclusively that of the cardiac surgeon has been passed on to the invasive cardiologist and electrophysiologist. A procedure that was initially reserved for the operating room, is now performed routinely in the special studies or cardiac catheterization laboratory. General anesthesia has been replaced by simple conscious sedation procedures. The procedure that once required a lengthy hospital stay is now routinely conducted on an ambulatory basis.

This chapter reviews old and new implantation techniques for pacemakers from a historical perspective and with respect to anatomic approach, concerns about safety, special applications, and potential complications. Solutions to problems and alternatives are also discussed. The management of complex implant situations and the ambulatory approach to permanent pacing are presented.

IMPLANTATION APPROACHES AND ACCESS FOR LEAD INSERTION

Anatomic Approach

There are two basic anatomic approaches to permanent cardiac pacing. The first is the epicardial approach, which requires general anesthesia and surgical access to the epicardial surface of the heart. The second is the transvenous approach, which involves passage of the lead through a vein into the endocardial surface of the heart. This latter approach is performed under local anesthesia with conscious sedation (5,6).

Initially, almost all pacemaker and ICD procedures were approached exclusively from the epicardial point of view; however, with the development of the transvenous approach, by cutdown or percutaneous techniques, almost all pacemaker procedures are approached on a transvenous or nonthoracotomy basis. Today, the epicardial approach is reserved for certain unique circumstances. This usually involves a subxiphoid incision and a limited thoracotomy or direct application of electrodes on the exposed heart. Mediastinoscopy and thoracoscopy have been used to apply permanent pacing and, in the case of the ICD, rate-sensing electrodes and patch electrodes.

The transvenous approach can be performed by venous cutdown, percutaneous venous access, or a combination of the two. A thorough understanding of venous anatomic structures of the head, neck, and upper extremity are imperative for safe venous access (9) Fig. 30-1). The precise location and orientation of the internal jugular, innominate, subclavian, and cephalic veins is important for safe venous access (10). Their anatomic relationship to other structures is crucial to avoiding complications.

The venous anatomy of interest from a cardiac pacing point of view starts peripherally with the axillary vein (11). The axillary vein is a large venous structure that represents the continuation of the basilic vein. It starts at the lower border of the teres major tendon and latissimus dorsi. The axillary vein terminates immediately beneath the clavicle at the outer border of the first rib, where it becomes a subclavian vein. The axillary vein is covered anteriorly by the pectoralis minor and pectoralis major muscles and costocoracoid membrane. It is anterior and medial to the axillary

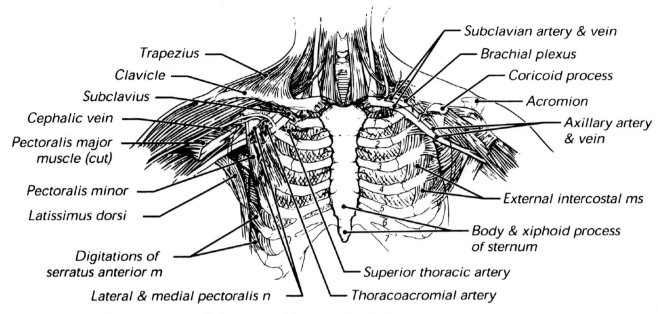

FIGURE 30-1. Detailed anatomy of the anterolateral chest, demonstrating the axillary vein with the pectoralis major and minor muscles removed. (From Belott PH, Reynolds WR. Permanent pacemaker and implantable cardioverter implantation. In: Ellenbogen K, Kay N, Wilkoff B, eds. *Clinical cardiac pacing and defibrillation.* Philadelphia: WB Saunders, 2000:586, with permission.)

artery, which it partially overlaps. At the level of the coracoid process, the axillary vein is covered by the clavicular head of the pectoralis major (Fig. 30-2). At this juncture, the axillary vein receives the more superficial cephalic vein.

The cephalic vein terminates in the deeper axillary vein at the level of the coracoid process, beneath the pectoralis major muscle. The cephalic vein commonly used for pacemaker venous access is classified as a superficial vein in the upper extremity. This vein, which commences near the antecubital fossa, travels along the outer border of the biceps muscle and enters the deltopectoral groove. The deltopectoral groove is an anatomic structure formed by the deltoid muscle and clavicular head of the pectoralis major. The cephalic vein traverses the deltopectoral groove and superiorly pierces the costocoracoid membrane, crossing the axillary artery, and terminates in the axillary vein just beneath the clavicle at the level of the coracoid process.

The subclavian vein is a continuation of the axillary vein. The subclavian vein extends from the outer border of the first rib to the inner end of the clavicle, where it joins the internal jugular vein to form the innominate vein. The subclavian vein is just inferior to the clavicle and subclavius muscle. The subclavian artery is located posterior and superior to the vein. The two structures are separated internally by the scalenus anticus muscle and phrenic nerve. Inferiorly, this vein leaves a depression in the first rib and on the pleura.

The juncture of the internal jugular and subclavian veins forms the brachiocephalic trunk or the innominate veins. These are two large venous trunks located on each side of the base of the neck. The right innominate vein is relatively short; it starts at the inner end of the clavicle and passes vertically down to join the left innominate vein just below the cartilage of the first rib. This junction forms the superior vena cava. The left innominate vein is larger and longer than the right, passing from left to right for approximately 2 inches, where it joins with the right innominate vein to form the superior vena cava. The left innominate vein is in the anterior and superior mediastinum.

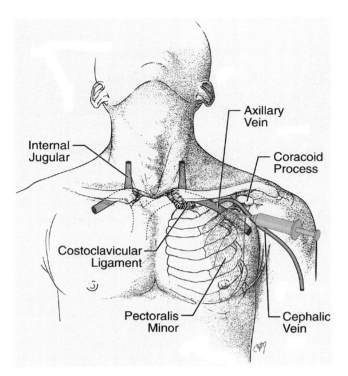

FIGURE 30-2. Anatomic relationship to the axillary vein to the pectoralis minor muscle; the pectoralis major has been removed. The cephalic vein drains directly into the axillary vein at approximately the first intercostal space. (From Belott PH. Unusual access sites for permanent cardiac pacing. In: Barold SS, Mugica J, eds. *Recent advances in cardiac pacing: goals for the 21st century*, vol 4. Armonk, NY: Futura Publishing, 1998:137–180, with permission.)

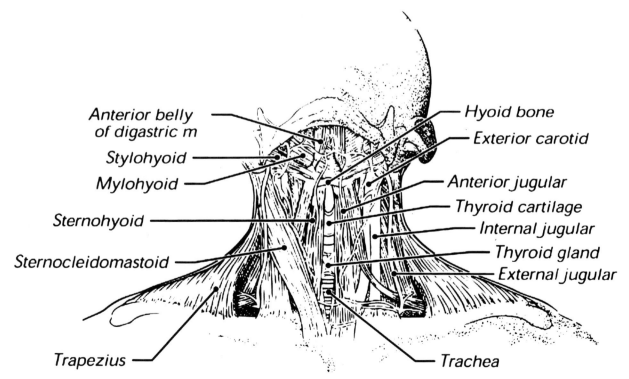

FIGURE 30-3. Detailed anatomy of the neck, demonstrating the relationship of venous anatomy to the superficial and deep structures. (From Belott PH, Reynolds WR. Permanent pacemaker and implantable cardioverter implantation. In: Ellenbogen K, Kay N, Wilkoff B, eds. *Clinical cardiac pacing and defibrillation*. Philadelphia: WB Saunders, 2000:586, with permission.)

The internal and external jugular veins have also been used for device venous access. The external jugular vein is a superficial vein of the neck receiving blood from the exterior cranium and face. This vein starts in the substance of the parotid gland at the angle of the jaw and runs perpendicular down the neck to the middle of the clavicle. In this course, it crosses the sternocleidomastoid muscle and runs parallel with its posterior border. At the sternocleidomastoid muscle's attachment to the clavicle, this vein perforates the deep fascia and terminates in the subclavian vein just anterior to the scalenus anticus muscle. The external jugular vein is separated from the sternocleidomastoid by a layer of deep cervical fascia. Superficially, it is covered by the platysma muscle, superficial fascia, and skin. The external jugular vein can be variable in size and even duplicated. Because of its superficial orientation, the external jugular vein is less frequently used for cardiac venous access.

The internal jugular vein, although an unusual site for pacemaker venous access, is used more frequently than the external jugular vein (Fig. 30-3) because of its large size and deeper and more protected orientation. The internal jugular vein starts just internal to the jugular foramen at the base of the skull. It drains blood from the interior of the cranium and from superficial parts of the head and neck. This vein is oriented vertically as it runs down the side of the neck. Superiorly, it is lateral to the internal carotid and inferolateral to the common carotid. At the base of the neck, the internal jugular vein joins the subclavian vein to form the innominate vein. The internal jugular vein is large and lies in the cervical triangle defined by the lateral border of the omohyoid muscle, the inferior border of the digastric muscle, and the medial border of the sternocleidomastoid. The superficial cervical fascia and platysma muscle cover the vein. It is usually identified just lateral to the easily palpable external carotid artery.

The concept of thoroughly understanding anatomy is underscored by Byrd's (12) description of the anteriorly and posteriorly displaced clavicles. The posteriorly displaced clavicle commonly seen in patients with chronic obstructive pulmonary disease can make percutaneous venous access extremely hazardous (Fig. 30-4). Similarly, in the anteriorly displaced clavicle, as found in elderly kyphoscoliotic patients with anteriorly bowed clavicles, renders percutaneous venous access next to impossible (Fig. 30-5). An appreciation of these anatomic variations is essential to

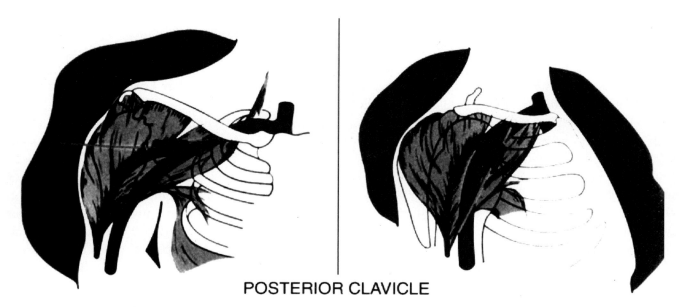

FIGURE 30-4. Posterior displacement of the clavicle, recognized by a horizontal rather than oblique position of the deltopectoral groove. (From Byrd CL. Current clinical applications of dual-chamber pacing. In: Zipes DP, ed. *Proceedings of a symposium*. Minneapolis: Medtronic, 1981:71, with permission.)

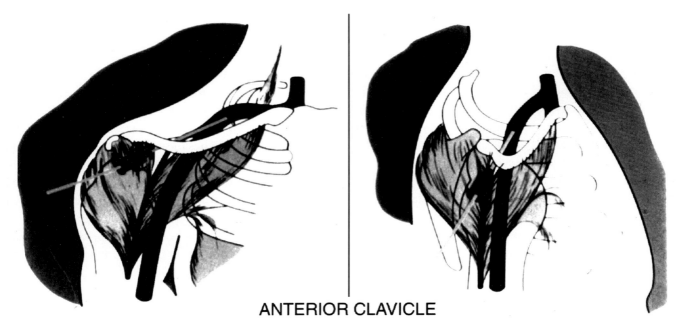

FIGURE 30-5. Anterior displacement of the clavicle. The deltopectoral groove is nearly vertical. (From Byrd CL. Current clinical applications of dual-chamber pacing. In: Zipes DP, ed. *Proceedings of a symposium.* Minneapolis: Medtronic, 1981:71, with permission.)

avoid the complications of pneumothorax, hemopneumothorax, and unsuccessful venipuncture. It should also be appreciated that the right ventricle is an anterior structure, the apex of which is usually located anteriorly and to the left (Fig. 30-6). Although the normal location is distinctly to the left of the midline, it occasionally can be rotated anteriorly and to the right. In extreme circumstances, this displacement rotates the right ventricular apex to the right of the midline. An example of this is seen in Figure 30-7. If this is not appreciated, lead placement can be extremely difficult or impossible. Appreciating this fact, ventricular lead placement can be expedited by using a right anterior oblique projection for fluoroscopy (Fig. 30-8). This maneuver helps define the apex of the right ventricle. The right ventricular apex is an anterior structure, but by using a right anterior oblique projection for fluoroscopy, the operator can create the illusion that the apex of the right ventricle is oriented toward the left lateral chest wall. An inexperienced operator can be frustrated for hours trying to position the ventricular electrode to the left of the spine when, in reality, the right ventricle is directly anterior. With simple rotation of the fluoroscopy unit into the right anterior oblique projection, the apex of the right ventricle becomes oriented in the left chest. This is the same maneuver that angiographers use when performing left ventriculography.

Transvenous Pacemaker Lead Placement

Historically, the venous cutdown technique has been the primary means of venous access for pacemaker electrode insertion (13). The cephalic vein has been commonly used in this approach from the right or left side. Occasionally, the more experienced surgeon has cannulated the internal jugular and the deeper axillary vein by this approach. Little departure from this pacemaker implantation technique had occurred until the late 1970s, when Littleford and Spector introduced the percutaneous sheath-set technique for venous access by means of the subclavian vein (14–17). This technique and variations on its theme have revolutionized pacemaker implantation. The percutaneous technique, however, has generated

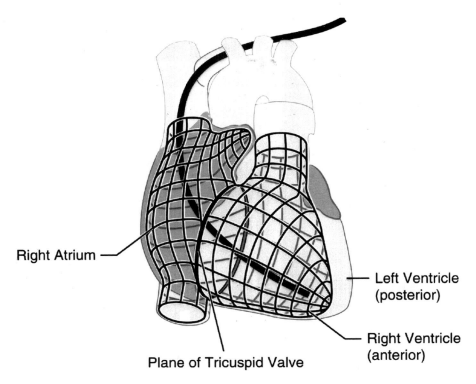

FIGURE 30-6. Spatial orientation of the right ventricle as an anterior structure in relation to the left or posterior ventricle or coronary sinus, which is also posterior. (From Belott PH, Reynolds WR: Permanent Pacemaker Implantation. In: Ellenbogen K, Kay N, Wilkoff B, eds. *Clinical cardiac pacing.* Philadelphia: WB Saunders, 1995:460–483, with permission.)

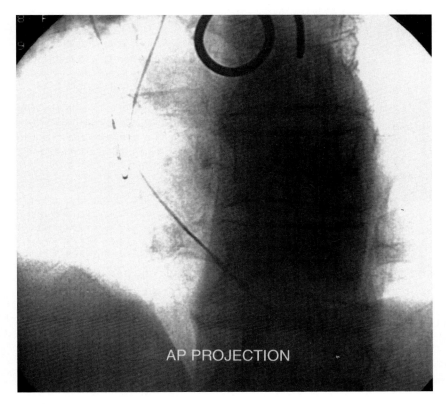

FIGURE 30-7. Digital cine-angiography, demonstrating extreme anterior orientation of the right ventricle. The pacemaker lead appears to be in the midline in the vicinity of the medial right atrium and tricuspid valve.

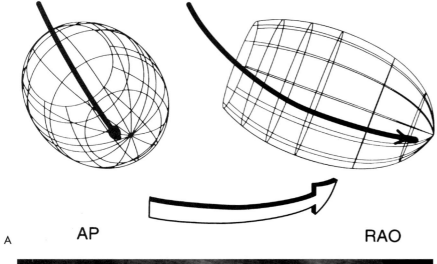

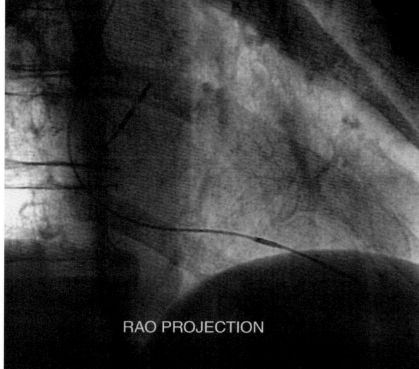

FIGURE 30-8. **A:** Wire frame, demonstrating the orientation of the lead in the right ventricular apex in the anteroposterior (AP) and right anterior oblique (RAO) projections. In the AP projection, the electrode appears to be vertical, whereas in the RAO projection, the lead is horizontal from right to left. **B:** Digital angiographic plate, using the RAO projection. The ventricular electrode is horizontal from left to right and is well to the left of the spine.

considerable controversy about its safety. The percutaneous sheath-set technique has proven to be especially efficacious for dual-chambered pacing. With the development of the peel-away sheath, the problem of sheath removal from the permanent electrode was resolved. All that remained was in puncturing the desired venous structure. A thorough knowledge of the normal and abnormal anatomy was essential.

A combination of cutdown and percutaneous technique has been used to successfully access the venous structure. This involves the cutdown on a vein for vascular control and subsequent direct percutaneous access to a vessel using the Seldinger technique. Common venous structures for pacemaker placement are listed in Table 30-1.

Dual-chamber pacing calls for the introduction of

TABLE 30-1 • VENOUS STRUCTURES FOR PACEMAKER LEAD INSERTION

Cephalic vein
Axillary vein
Subclavian vein
Internal jugular vein
External jugular vein
Femoral vein
Inferior vena cava

an atrial and a ventricular electrode. The cutdown technique is less suited for this approach because all too often the cephalic vein can hardly accommodate one electrode and even less frequently two. The percutaneous approach appears ideally suited for dual-chambered pacing because there is potential for unlimited access to the venous circulation. Various options for dual-chambered pacing venous access are listed in Table 30-2. There are five percutaneous approaches for dual-chambered pacing.

The first approach uses two separate percutaneous sticks and the application of two sheaths (18). This approach increases the risk of complications related to the venipuncture process in addition to possibly not finding the vessel a second time. There is also increased risk of pneumothorax, air embolism, bleeding, and vascular trauma.

The second technique uses one percutaneous stick and a large sheath set that can accommodate the passage of atrial and ventricular electrodes (19,20). The passage of two electrodes down one sheath is less desirable because the large sheath may increase the risk of air embolization and blood loss. There is also increased frustration from electrode dislodgement and entanglement.

The third approach, the retained guide wire technique, appears to be the most desirable approach. It also provides unlimited access to the central circulation (21–23). The operator is never committed or compromised. There is less risk of bleeding, pneumothorax, and air embolization. I prefer the retained guide wire technique. The ventricular electrode should be positioned first. This is safe and practical. It is safe because, once positioned, there is always electrical support of the ventricle in case asystole occurs. It is also preferred because the initially placed ventricular electrode is less susceptible to dislodgement during the positioning of the second (atrial) electrode. After the ventricular electrode is in position, it is stabilized by leaving the stylet in the vicinity of the lower right atrium. The electrode is also secured by use of a suture sleeve at the puncture site. After the ventricular electrode is stabilized, a second sheath set is applied to the retained guide wire (Fig. 30-9). The atrial electrode is introduced, positioned,

TABLE 30-2 • VENOUS ACCESS FOR DUAL-CHAMBERED PACING

Venous cutdown: isolate one or two veins
Percutaneous: two separate sticks and sheath applications
Percutaneous: two electrodes down one large sheath
Percutaneous: retained guide wire (Belott technique)
Cutdown with cephalic vein guide wire (Ong-Barold technique)

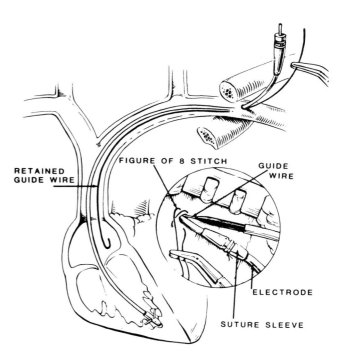

FIGURE 30-9. Retained guide wire technique. **Inset:** The secured ventricular electrode and suture sleeve, figure-of-eight stitch held by a clamp, and a second sheath set applied to the retained guide wire are shown. (From Belott PH, Byrd CL. Recent developments in pacemaker implantation and lead retrieval. In: Barold SS, Mugica J, eds. *New perspectives in cardiac pacing 2.* Armonk, NY: Futura Publishing, 1991:105–131, with permission.)

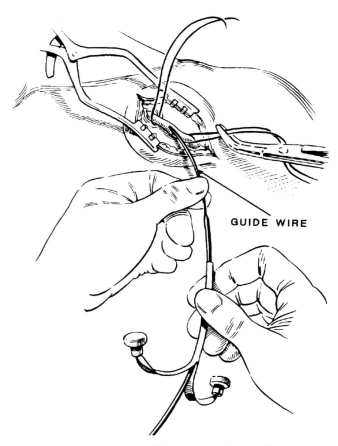

FIGURE 30-10. Ong-Barold technique. (From Belott PH, Byrd CL. Recent developments in pacemaker implantation and lead retrieval. In: Barold SS, Mugica J, eds. *New perspectives in cardiac pacing 2.* Armonk, NY: Futura Publishing, 1991:105–131, with permission.)

and secured. The retained guide wire is removed only after the operator is completely satisfied with both electrode positions and there is no need to exchange. Hemostasis is effected by a figure-of-eight suture stitch.

A fourth approach uses a combination of the sheath-set technique and a venous cutdown approach. Ong and colleagues described the cephalic–guide wire technique (24). This technique involves the cutdown and isolation of the cephalic vein (Fig. 30-10). Instead of performing a venotomy, the vein is punctured percutaneously, and a guide wire and sheath set are applied. Unlike the cutdown technique, the cephalic vein is completely sacrificed. If the guide wire is retained, multiple sheath set exchanges and lead placements can be carried out. Hemostasis is effected by compression, the application of a figure-of-eight suture stitch, or both techniques. Despite sacrificing the cephalic vein, there have been no reports of venous complications.

Venous Cutdown of the Cephalic Vein: Cephalic Venous Access

The cephalic vein is found in the deltopectoral groove. The deltopectoral groove is defined by the lateral border of the pectoralis major muscle and the medial border of the deltoid muscle at the level of the coracoid process. An incision is made along the deltopectoral groove extending approximately 1 to 2 inches. The incision is carried down directly through the dermis to the surface of the pectoralis muscle. The skin incision should be carried out in a single stroke. After the initial incision has been made, a Weitlaner self-retaining retractor can be applied for exposure. The deltopectoral groove is then clearly identified. The deltopectoral groove is opened using Metzenbaum scissors. Reapplication of the Weitlaner self-retaining retractor to the medial head of the deltoid and lateral head of the pectoralis major muscle affords excellent exposure. Careful dissection of the deltopectoral groove eventually exposes the cephalic vein. Sometimes, this vessel is extremely diminutive and atretic.

If the cephalic vein is too small, further dissection may be carried proximally. In rare instances, dissection may be carried to the deeper axillary vein. Once exposed, the cephalic vein is freed from its fibrous attachments and 0 silk ligatures are applied proximally and distally (Fig. 30-11). After adequate venous control has been obtained, a horizontal venotomy is made with iris scissors and a no. 11 scalpel blade (Fig. 30-12). The vein should be supported at all times with a smooth forceps. Using mosquito clamps, forceps, or a vein pick, the venotomy is opened and the electrodes introduced (Fig. 30-13). After venous access has been achieved, the electrodes are positioned in the appropriate chambers using standard techniques.

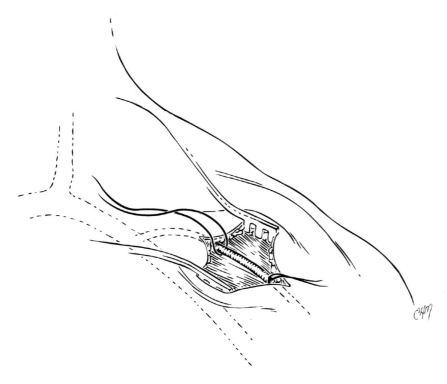

FIGURE 30-11. Cephalic vein cutdown technique. The cephalic vein is isolated and tied off distally. (From Belott PH, Reynolds WR. Permanent pacemaker implantation. In: Ellenbogen K, Kay N, Wilkoff B, eds. *Clinical cardiac pacing.* Philadelphia: WB Saunders, 1995:460–483, with permission.)

Percutaneous Access to the Subclavian Vein

The Seldinger technique has been used by cardiologists for percutaneous access for years. In this technique, a large-bore needle (18 gauge) is used to percutaneously puncture the vascular structure. A guide wire is introduced through the needle into the vessel, and the needle is removed over the wire and exchanged for a catheter or sheath. Prepackaged introducer sets commonly are used for this purpose (Fig. 30-14).

The operator must be completely familiar with normal anatomy and superficial anatomic landmarks. The traditional subclavian puncture is carried out in the middle third of the clavicle. This location is frequently associated with an increased risk of vascular trauma, pneumothorax, and lack of success. An alternate approach calls for the puncture at the apex of an angle formed by the clavicle and first rib (25) (Fig. 30-15). This location is remote from the apex of the lung, and the venous structure is generally much larger.

It is important to maintain the patient in the anatomic position. Maneuvers that artificially open the costoclavicular and infraclavicular spaces should be

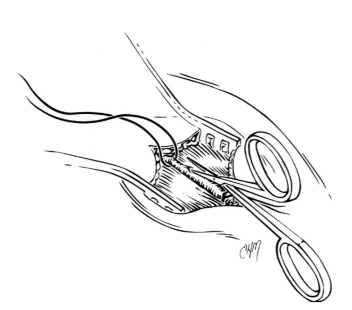

FIGURE 30-12. Venotomy is performed with an iris scissors. (From Belott PH, Reynolds WR. Permanent pacemaker implantation. In: Ellenbogen K, Kay N, Wilkoff B, eds. *Clinical cardiac pacing.* Philadelphia: WB Saunders, 1995:460–483, with permission.)

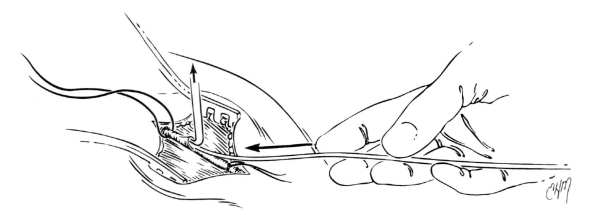

FIGURE 30-13. The lead is inserted while venotomy is held open with a vein pick. (From Belott PH, Reynolds WR. Permanent pacemaker implantation. In: Ellenbogen K, Kay N, Wilkoff B, eds. *Clinical cardiac pacing.* Philadelphia: WB Saunders, 1995:460–483, with permission.)

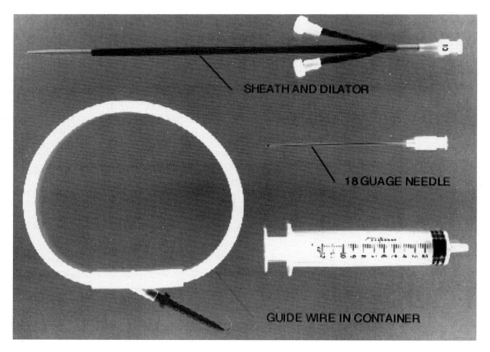

FIGURE 30-14. Percutaneous introducer set, prepackaged with a rubber dilator, sheath, guide wire, 18-gauge needle, and 10-mL syringe. (From Belott PH, Reynolds WR. Permanent pacemaker implantation. In: Ellenbogen K, Kay N, Wilkoff B, eds. *Clinical cardiac pacing.* Philadelphia: WB Saunders, 1995:460–483, with permission.)

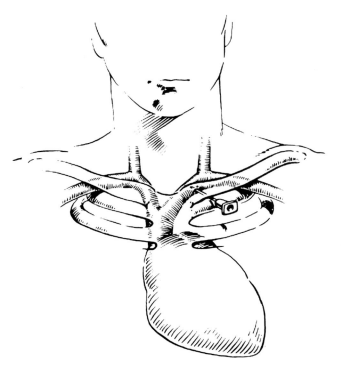

FIGURE 30-15. Extreme medial subclavian puncture. (From Belott PH, Byrd CL. Recent developments in pacemaker implantation and lead retrieval. In: Barold SS, Mugica J, eds. *New perspectives in cardiac pacing 2.* Armonk, NY: Futura Publishing, 1991:105–131, with permission.)

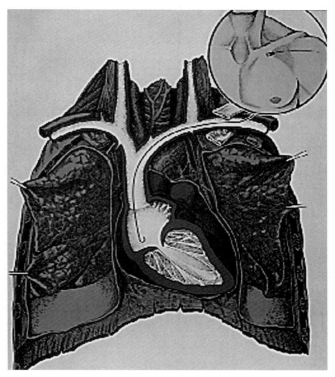

FIGURE 30-16. The guide wire is advanced to the middle right atrium.

avoided. Common practice of placing towels between the scapulae or extending the arm may result in undesirable puncture of the costoclavicular ligament or subclavius muscle. The medial venous puncture clearly increases the success rate as well as dramatically reducing the risk of pneumothorax and vascular injury.

An 18-gauge, thin-walled needle is used for venipuncture. After the vessel has been entered, the guide wire is inserted with its tip position in the middle right atrium (Fig. 30-16). Fluoroscopy should always be used to check position of the wire. The wire should never be forced; if resistance is encountered, re-advancement is advised. After venous access has been achieved, every effort should be made to retain it. If the guide wire tracks into the internal jugular vein, a subtle change in the needle angle should be effected and the guide wire retracted into the needle while the needle is still in the vascular structure. The wire is advanced again, usually resulting in passage through the innominate vein to the superior vena cava. If this maneuver fails, a small-gauge rubber dilator may be passed over the guide wire and used as a catheter to steer the guide wire into its proper trajectory. The dilator may also be used for injection of contrast material to define the venous anatomy.

After successful venous access has been achieved, the skin incision is created. The incision should be directed along anatomic lines. The skin incision is carried medially and inferiorly for approximately 2 inches. After the incision has been carried out, the Weitlaner self-retaining retractor is applied in a manner similar to that described for the venous cutdown. The Weitlaner retractor holds tissue under tension as broad-based scalpel strokes are carried around to the surface of the pectoralis muscle.

After the incision has been carried to the surface of the pectoralis muscle and there is good exposure of the puncture site, a figure-of-eight suture stitch is applied about the needle (Fig. 30-17). This stitch serves for hemostasis throughout the procedure. With the initial preparations of the wound completed, the

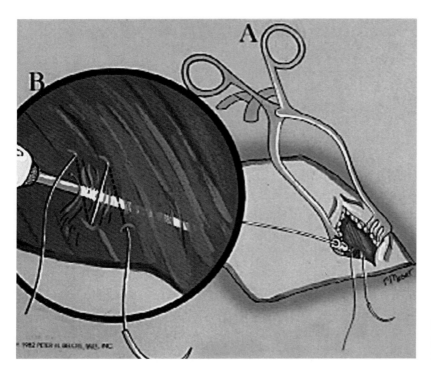

FIGURE 30-17. With the initial dissection complete, the figure-of-eight stitch is placed about the needle.

needle may be removed from the guide wire and a sheath set applied. The dilator and sheath are advanced over the guide wire with a continuous forward motion (Fig. 30-18). It is important to avoid twisting and rotating the dilator sheath, because this motion may result in tearing of the sheath's leading edge at the sheath dilator transition. The sheath should always be advanced under fluoroscopic observation. This avoids the inadvertent puncture or tearing of the right innominate vein and superior vena cava. After successful passage of the sheath set, the dilator is removed and the electrode passed down the sheath (Fig. 30-19). When the dilator is removed, the guide wire should be retained and the electrode passed alongside the guide wire. The sheath is then retracted and peeled away. Positioning of the electrode with the sheath *in situ* is unwise because it may result in air embolism or unnecessary blood loss. With the sheath removed, hemostasis is achieved by applying tension to the figure-of-eight stitch (26) (Fig. 30-20).

Retention of the guide wire is a variation of the standard introducer technique. The retained guide wire may provide unlimited venous access and the ability to exchange and introduce additional electrodes by simply applying another sheath to the guide wire. The retained guide wire should be held to the drape with a clamp to avoid inadvertent dislodgement. The retained guide wire can also serve as a ground for unipolar threshold analysis. It can also be used as an intracardiac lead for the recording of electrograms or for emergency pacing. The guide wire should be retained in single- and dual-chambered procedures until satisfactory lead position is attained.

Axillary Venous Access

Frequently, the solution to one problem creates another. A case in point is my proposal of the extreme medial subclavian percutaneous technique. Although this approach is safe, avoids the complication of pneumothorax, and expedites venous access, it has been implicated in causing of premature pacemaker lead failure by conductor fracture and insulation damage (27). Electrode failure as a result of an extreme medial approach has been called *the subclavian crush phenomenon*. Fyke was first to report insulation failure of two leads placed side by side in the percutaneous approach to the subclavian vein where there was a tight costoclavicular space (28,29). This phenomenon has since been extensively reported in the literature.

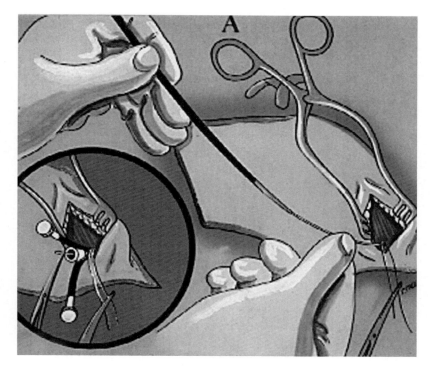

FIGURE 30-18. After the 18-gauge, thin-walled needle is removed, the sheath set is applied to the guide wire and advanced into the venous system.

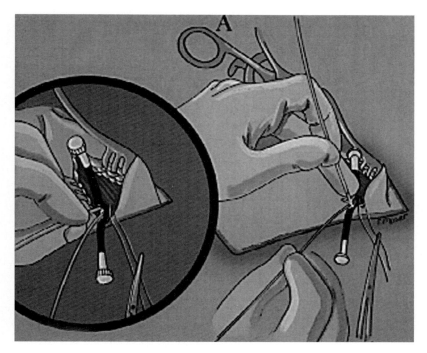

FIGURE 30-19. Pacemaker electrode entering the sheath.

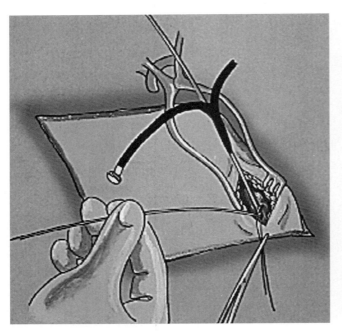

FIGURE 30-20. The sheath is retracted, and tension is applied to the figure-of-eight stitch. The guide wire is retained and clamped to the drape.

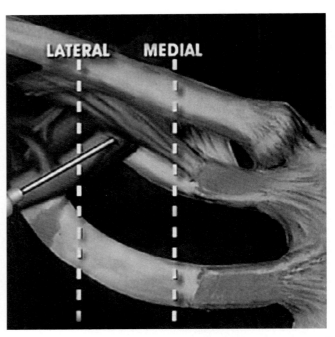

FIGURE 30-22. Safe access to the extrathoracic portion of the subclavian vein. (From Byrd CL. Recent developments in pacemaker implantation and lead retrieval. *Pacing Clin Electrophysiol* 1993:16;1781, with permission.)

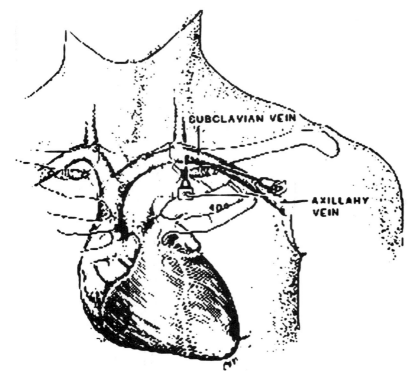

FIGURE 30-21. Anatomic orientation of the safety zone. (From Belott PH, Byrd CL. Recent developments in pacemaker implantation and lead retrieval. In: Barold SS, Mugica J, eds. *New perspectives in cardiac pacing 2.* Armonk, NY: Futura, 1991:105–131, with permission.)

There are several proposed mechanisms and potential solutions (1,30–32). Electrodes of a more complex design, such as bipolar coaxial construction, are most susceptible to this phenomenon. A more lateral percutaneous approach has been suggested to avoid the crush phenomenon. The axillary vein has been suggested as an alternate site of venous access to avoid the crush phenomenon. This was first suggested by Byrd in his proposed *safe introducer technique* (33).

Byrd defines a safety zone for percutaneous venous access similar to that for the subclavian window (Fig. 30-21). Several conditions must be fulfilled. An essential condition of puncture is adequate ease of needle insertion that avoids friction and puncture of bone, cartilage, or tendon (Fig. 30-22). If a puncture cannot be safely conducted within the safety zone, the axillary vein is then percutaneously cannulated. The axillary vein is actually a continuation of the subclavian vein after it exits the superior mediastinum and crosses the first rib. It is frequently called the extrathoracic portion of the subclavian vein. This vein is usually quite large. The axillary vein traverses the anterolateral chest wall into the axilla (Fig. 30-23). It crosses the deltopectoral groove at approximately the level of the coracoid process. At the level of the teres major and latissimus dorsi muscle, it becomes the basilic vein. The axillary vein is covered by pectoralis major and minor muscles. It runs medial and parallel to the deltopectoral groove for approximately 1 to 2 cm (Fig. 30-24).

The cephalic vein, a common venous access site for pacemaker implantation, drains directly into the axillary vein just superior to the pectoralis minor. The axillary vein is an excellent site for venous access but

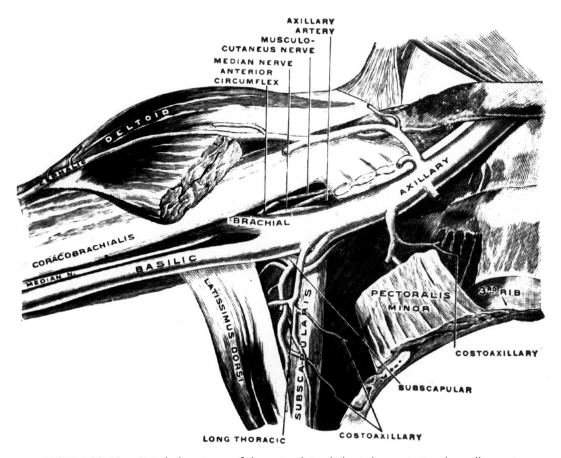

FIGURE 30-23. Detailed anatomy of the anterolateral chest demonstrates the axillary vein with the pectoralis major and minor muscles removed. (From Belott PH. Unusual access sites for permanent cardiac pacing. In: Barold SS, Mugica J, eds. *Recent advances in cardiac pacing: goals for the 21st century,* vol 4. Armonk, NY: Futura Publishing, 1998:137–180, with permission.)

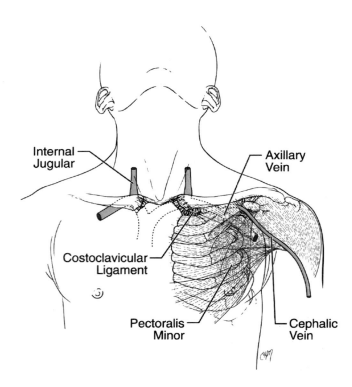

FIGURE 30-24. Relationship of the axillary vein to the pectoralis major and minor muscles, deltoid and cephalic vein. (From Belott PH. Unusual access sites for permanent cardiac pacing. In: Barold SS, Mugica J, eds. *Recent advances in cardiac pacing: goals for the 21st century*, vol 4. Armonk, NY: Futura Publishing, 1998:137–180, with permission.)

is usually not considered because it is a rather deep structure. Notable surface landmarks are the infraclavicular space, deltopectoral groove, and coracoid process.

The axillary venous approach was initially reported in 1987 by Nichalls as an alternate site of venous access for large central lines (34). Nichalls developed a technique from cadaver dissection by which he established reliable landmarks. He defined the axillary vein as an infraclavicular structure. In his technique, the needle is always anterior to the thoracic cavity, generally tangential to the chest wall to avoid pneumothorax and hemopneumothorax. Nichalls used the several landmarks subsequently described (Fig. 30-25). The vein starts medial at a point below the medial aspect of the clavicle, where the space between the clavicle and the first rib becomes palpable. The vein extends laterally to a point three fingerbreadths below the inferior aspect of the coracoid process. The skin is punctured along the medial border of the pectoralis minor muscle at a point above the vein as it is defined by surface landmarks. The axillary vein is punctured by passing the needle anterior to the first rib, maneuvering posteriorly and medially. It corresponds to the lateral to medial course of the axillary vein. The needle passes between the first rib and clavicle. In this technique, the arm is usually adducted 45 degrees.

The Nichalls' experience was further reinforced by Taylor and Yellowlees, who reported their experience with the technique in 102 consecutive patients (35). There were only four failures and one pneumothorax. In the technique described by Byrd, an 18-gauge, thin-walled needle is guided by fluoroscopy and directed to the medial portion of the first rib. The needle is held perpendicular to the first rib as it is walked laterally until the axillary vein is punctured, which is indicated by the aspiration of venous blood (Fig. 30-26). The guide wire is inserted, and the introducer is subsequently applied according to standard technique. The needle path is always directed anterior to the thoracic cavity to avoid the risk of pneumothorax. Byrd reported a series of 213 consecutive cases in which the extrathoracic portion of the subclavian vein (axillary vein) was successfully cannulated as a primary approach (36).

Magni and coworkers reported a new approach to percutaneous subclavian venipuncture to avoid lead fracture (37). This technique, very similar to Byrd's, uses only extensive surface landmarks for venipuncture (Fig. 30-27). The technique involves puncture

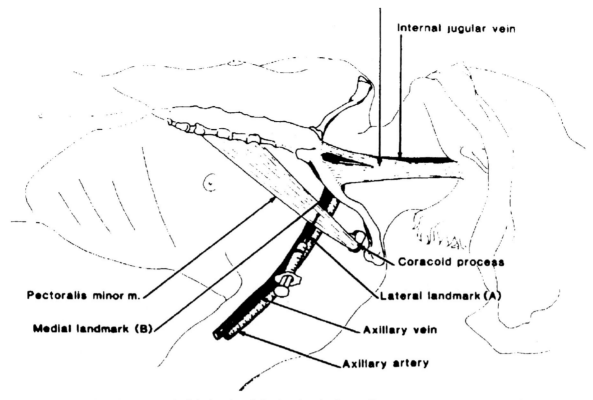

FIGURE 30-25. Nichalls' sketch of the landmarks for axillary vein puncture. (From Belott PH, Byrd CL. Recent developments in pacemaker implantation and lead retrieval. In: Barold SS, Mugica J, eds. *New perspectives in cardiac pacing 2*. Armonk, NY: Futura Publishing, 1991:105–131, with permission.)

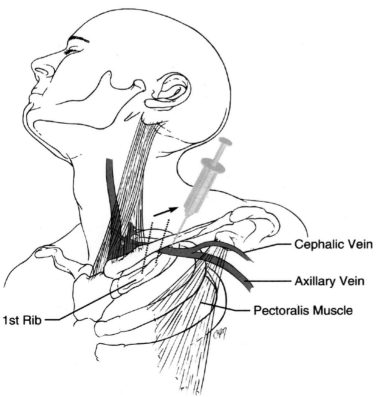

FIGURE 30-26. Byrd's technique for access of the extrathoracic portion of the subclavian vein. Sequential needle punctures are walked posterolaterally along the first rib until the vein is entered. (From Belott PH, Reynolds WR. Permanent pacemaker implantation. In: Ellenbogen K, Kay N, Wilkoff B, eds. *Clinical cardiac pacing*. Philadelphia: WB Saunders, 1995:460–483, with permission.)

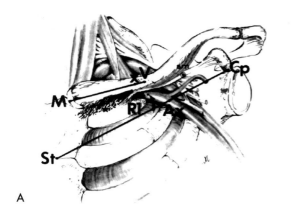

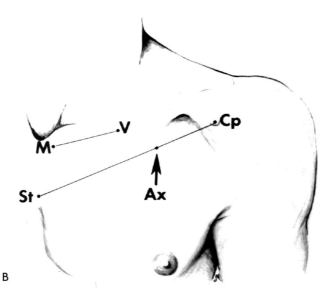

FIGURE 30-27. Deep (A) and superficial (B) anatomic relationships of the Magney approach to subclavian venipuncture. Point M indicates the medial end of the clavicle. X defines a point on the clavicle directly above the lateral edges of the clavicular/subclavius muscle (tendon complex). Point overlies the center of the subclavian vein as it crosses the first rib (R1). Ax, axillary vein; Cp, coracoid process; sm, subclavius muscle; St, center of the sternal angle; star, costoclavicular ligament; open circle with closed circle, costoclavicular ligament; open circle around closed circle, costoclavicular ligament. The arrow points to Magney's ideal point for venous entry. (Reproduced with permission from Magney JE, Staplin DH, Flynn DM, et al. A new approach for percutaneous subclavian venipuncture to avoid lead fracture or central venous catheter occlusion. *Pacing Clin Electrophysiol* 1993;16:2133, with permission.)

of the extrathoracic portion of the subclavian vein or axillary vein. The location of the axillary vein is defined as the intersection with a line drawn between the middle of the sternal angle and the tip of the coracoid process, which is generally near the lateral border of the first rib. I have described blind axillary venous access using a modification of the Byrd and Magni recommendations (38,39). In this technique, the deltopectoral groove and coracoid process are primary landmarks. The deltopectoral groove and coracoid process are palpated and the curvature of the chest wall noted (Fig. 30-28). An incision is made at the level of the coracoid process. It is carried medially for approximately 2 inches and is perpendicular to the deltopectoral groove (Fig. 30-29). The incision is carried to the surface of the pectoralis major muscle. The deltopectoral groove is directly visualized.

The needle is inserted at an angle of 45 degrees parallel to the deltopectoral groove and 1 to 2 cm medial (Fig. 30-30). If the vein is not entered, fluoroscopy is used to define the first rib. The needle is ad-

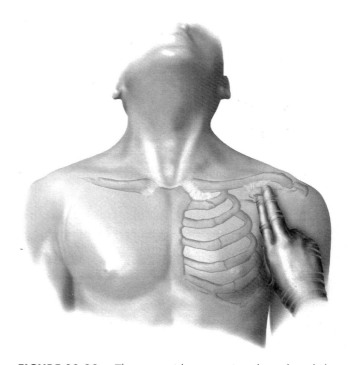

FIGURE 30-28. The coracoid process is palpated, and the angle of the deltopectoral groove is assessed. (From Belott PH, Reynolds WR. Permanent pacemaker and implantable cardioverter implantation. In: Ellenbogen K, Kay N, Wilkoff B, eds. *Clinical cardiac pacing and defibrillation.* Philadelphia: WB Saunders, 2000:586, with permission.)

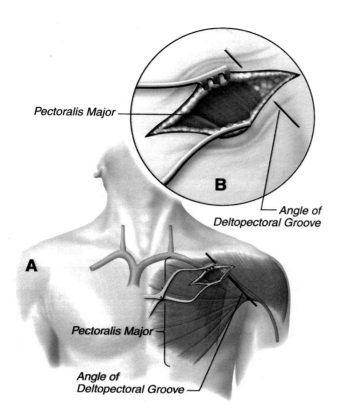

FIGURE 30-29. **A:** The incision is carried down to the surface of the pectoralis major muscle, and its orientation with respect to the deltopectoral groove is demonstrated. **B:** The inset shows the deltopectoral groove and orientation of the lateral border of the clavicular head of the pectoralis major. (From Belott PH, Reynolds WR. Permanent pacemaker and implantable cardioverter implantation. In: Ellenbogen K, Kay N, Wilkoff B, eds. *Clinical cardiac pacing and defibrillation.* Philadelphia: WB Saunders, 2000:595, with permission.)

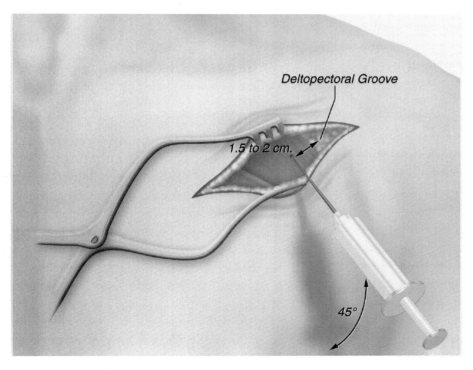

FIGURE 30-30. Needle trajectory and angle with respect to the deltopectoral groove, pectoralis major, lateral border of the cephalic head of the pectoralis major muscle, and the chest wall. (From Belott PH, Reynolds WR. Permanent pacemaker and implantable cardioverter implantation. In: Ellenbogen K, Kay N, Wilkoff B, eds. *Clinical cardiac pacing and defibrillation.* Philadelphia: WB Saunders, 2000:595, with permission.)

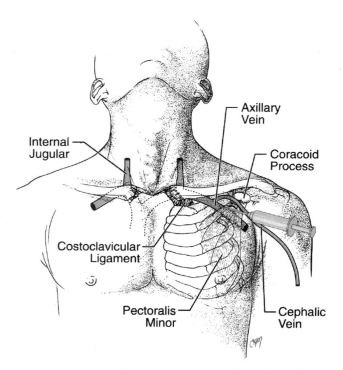

FIGURE 30-31. Axillary vein puncture and its relationship to surface landmarks and to the first rib. (From Belott PH. Unusual access sites for permanent cardiac pacing. In: Barold SS, Mugica J, eds. *Recent advances in cardiac pacing: goals for the 21st century,* vol 4. Armonk, NY: Futura Publishing, 1998:137–180, with permission.)

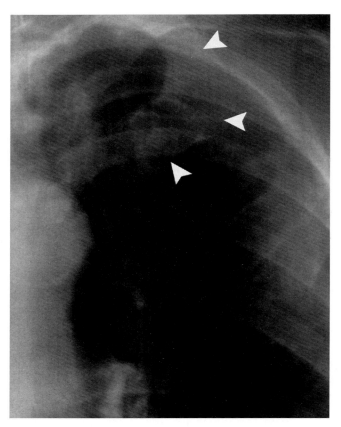

FIGURE 30-32. The radiograph shows the location of the first rib. (From Belott PH. Unusual access sites for permanent cardiac pacing. In: Barold SS, Mugica J, eds. *Recent advances in cardiac pacing: goals for the 21st century,* vol 4. Armonk, NY: Futura Publishing, 1998:137–180, with permission.)

vanced and touches the first rib. Sequential needle punctures are walked laterally and posteriorly until the vein is entered (Fig. 30-31). The physician usually cannot palpate the axillary artery pulse, and it is therefore not a reliable landmark. The axillary artery and brachial plexus are usually much deeper and more posterior structures. This simple technique using basic anatomic landmarks of the deltopectoral groove and a blind venous stick has been used successfully in 168 consecutive pacemaker and ICD procedures. There have only been three failures. These required an alternate approach. With a thorough knowledge of regional anatomy, the axillary vein can be safely used as a primary site for venous access. If the vein is not entered, fluoroscopy is used to define the first rib (Fig. 30-32). The needle is advanced and touches the first rib, and sequential needle punctures are walked laterally and posteriorly until the venous structure is entered. The axillary vein may also be isolated by direct cutdown (Fig. 30-33). Using Metzenbaum scissors, the fibers of the pectoralis major muscle are separated adjacent to the deltopectoral groove at the level of the coracoid process, which is a point just above the level of the superior border of the pectoralis minor. The pectoralis major is split in this area, and the fibers are gently teased apart. This is carried out in an access parallel to the muscle bundles. The axillary vein is found directly underneath the pectoralis major. A pursestring stitch is applied to the vein, and it can be cannulated by percutaneous or the cutdown approach. A pursestring stitch serves for hemostasis and ultimately assists in anchoring the electrodes after positioning.

A number of techniques have been developed to assist access of the axillary vein. Varnagy and associates described a technique for isolating the cephalic vein,

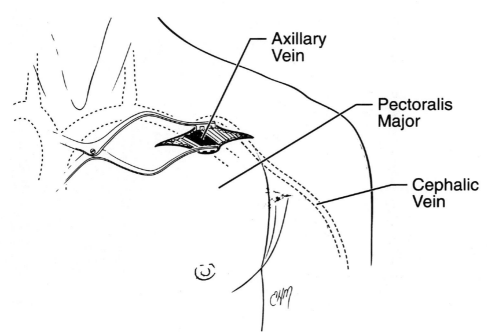

FIGURE 30-33. Cutdown on the axillary vein through the pectoralis major and minor muscles. (From Belott PH. Unusual access sites for permanent cardiac pacing. In: Barold SS, Mugica J, eds. *Recent advances in cardiac pacing: goals for the 21st century*, vol 4. Armonk, NY: Futura Publishing, 1998:137–180, with permission.)

axillary vein, or both (40). This technique consists of introducing a J-ended Teflon guide wire through the vein in the antecubital fossa under fluoroscopic control. The metal guide wire is then palpated in the deltopectoral groove or identified by fluoroscopy (Fig. 30-34). The palpated guide wire guides the subsequent cutdown for puncture of the vessel by fluoroscopy. The cutdown can be performed on the vein or the intravascular guide wire pulled out of the venotomy to allow application of an introducer. It is felt that this technique offers the benefits of rapid venous access while avoiding the hazard of pneumothorax associated with the percutaneous approach. If the percutaneous approach is used, the puncture can always be extrathoracic using fluoroscopy to guide the needle to the guide wire. Axillary venipuncture can also be facilitated by the use of contrast venography. The venous anatomy can be observed by fluoroscopy in the pectoral area and, if possible, recorded for repeat viewing. The needle trajectory and venipuncture are guided by contrast material in the axillary vein (41). Laboratories fortunate enough to have sophisticated imaging capabilities can create a mask. Spencer and colleagues reported the use of contrast venography for localizing the axillary vein in 22 consecutive patients (42,43). Similarly, Ramza and coworkers demonstrated the safety and efficacy of the axillary vein for placement of pacemaker and defibrillator leads when guided by contrast venography (44). Lead placement was successfully accomplished in 49 of 50 patients using this technique.

Contrast venography can facilitate percutaneous venous access to the subclavian and axillary veins. In

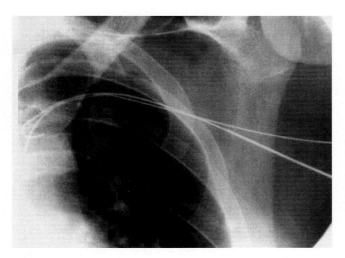

FIGURE 30-34. Percutaneous access to the axillary vein using a J wire introduced through the antecubital vein for reference. (From Belott PH. Unusual access sites for permanent cardiac pacing. In: Barold SS, Mugica J, eds. *Recent advances in cardiac pacing: goals for the 21st century*, vol 4. Armonk, NY: Futura Publishing, 1998:137–180, with permission.)

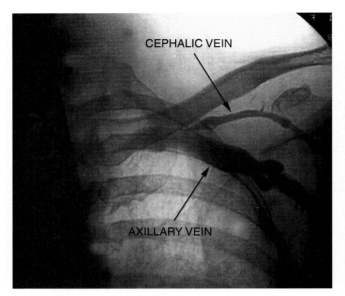

FIGURE 30-35. Contrast venography shows the larger axillary vein with a smaller cephalic vein draining into it at a right angle. (From Belott PH, Reynolds WR. Permanent pacemaker and implantable cardioverter implantation. In: Ellenbogen K, Kay N, Wilkoff B, eds. *Clinical cardiac pacing and defibrillation.* Philadelphia: WB Saunders, 2000:598, with permission.)

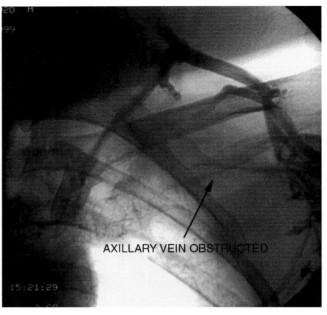

FIGURE 30-36. Complete absence of the axillary vein. Notice the plexus of veins draining over the clavicle into the external jugular and subsequently the innominate vein.

this technique, first described by Hayes and colleagues (41), a venous line is established on the side of planned venous access. It is advisable to use a large-gauge needle. Contrast material (10 to 20 mL) is injected rapidly into the intravenous line, followed by a saline flush. Occasionally, this is facilitated by a nonsterile assistant massaging the contrast material through the peripheral venous system underneath the sterile drape. Fluoroscopy is then used to direct the needle to the site of venous access as defined by the contrast material (Fig. 30-35). In the cardiac catheterization laboratory or special studies room, a mask or map may be obtained for guidance after the contrast material has dissipated. This technique has been extremely helpful in locating the subclavian and axillary veins and has been applied to other venous structures. When this technique is used regularly, the operator becomes aware of the extreme medial to lateral variability of the location of the axillary vein's course and location. Occasionally, this approach is used after multiple attempts at blind venipuncture where contrast venography demonstrates a proximal complete obstruction of the venous structure with collaterals to the internal jugular (Fig. 30-36).

Venous access of the axillary vein can also be guided by Doppler and ultrasound techniques. Fyke described a Doppler-guided extrathoracic introducer insertion technique in 59 consecutive patients (total of 100 leads) with a simple Doppler flow detector (45). A sterile Doppler flow detector is moved along the clavicle, and after the vein is defined, the location and angle of the probe are noted and the venipuncture carried out (Fig. 30-37). Care is taken to avoid directing the Doppler beam beneath the clavicle. Gayle and associates developed an ultrasound technique that directly visualizes the needle puncture of the axillary vein (46,47). A portable ultrasound device with sterile sleeve and needle holder are used. The ultrasound head is placed over the skin surface in the vicinity of the axillary vein. Once identified, the puncture and Seldinger technique are used. Because this technique directly visualizes the axillary vein, it has been used with considerable success for pacing and defibrillator electrodes. There have been no pneumothoraces. The technique can be carried out transcutaneously or through the incision on the surface of the pectoralis muscle (Fig. 30-38).

The axillary vein is becoming a common venous

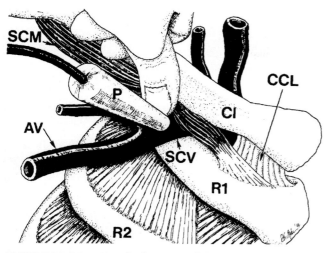

FIGURE 30-37. Doppler location of the axillary vein crossing the first rib. AV, axillary vein; CCL, costoclavicular ligament; CL, clavicle; P, Doppler probe; R1, first rib; R2, second rib; SMC, subclavius muscle; SCV, subclavian vein. (From Fyke FE III. Doppler-guided extrathoracic introducer insertion. *Pacing Clin Electrophysiol* 1995;18:1017, with permission.)

TABLE 30-3 • TECHNIQUES FOR AXILLARY VENOUS ACCESS

Blind percutaneous puncture using surface landmarks
Blind puncture through pectoralis major muscle using deep landmarks
Direct cutdown on the axillary vein
Fluoroscopy: needle the first rib for reference
Contrast venography
Doppler-guided
Ultrasound-guided

access site for pacemaker and defibrillator implantations, given the concerns of the subclavian crush and the requirement for insertion of multiple electrodes for dual-chambered pacing and a large complex electrode for transvenous nonthoracotomy defibrillation. There are now a number of reliable techniques for axillary venous access (Table 30-3).

Given the interest in the axillary vein, it is recom-

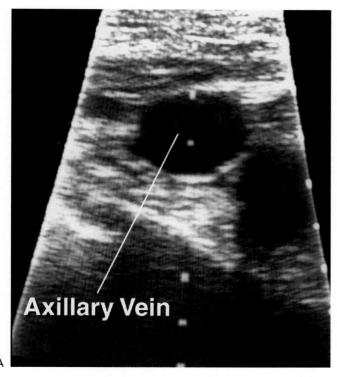
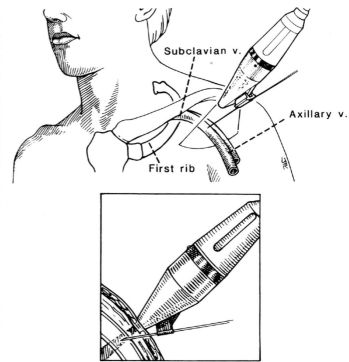

FIGURE 30-38. **A:** Ultrasonic image of the axillary vein. (From Gayle DD, Bailey JR, Haistey WK, et al. A novel ultrasound-guided approach to the puncture of extrathoracic subclavian vein for surgical lead placement. *Pacing Clin Electrophysiol* 1996;19:700, with permission.) **B:** Ultrasound-guided puncture of the axillary vein using the SiteRight device. (Courtesy of Dymax Corporation, Pittsburgh, PA.)

mended that the implanting physician become thoroughly familiar with the anatomy of the anterior thoracic wall, shoulder, and axilla. The physician should visit the anatomic laboratory to review the regional anatomy and surface landmarks.

Jugular Venous Access

The jugular vein has been used for permanent pacemaker implantation as an alternate cutdown site (48). As a rule, the jugular vein has not been used for nonthoracotomy lead systems. This is a large venous structure that lies in the cervical triangle defined by the lateral border of the omohyoid muscle, inferior border of the digastric muscle, and the medial border of the sternocleidomastoid (Fig. 30-39). It is covered by the superficial cervical fascia and platysma muscle. It can be identified by palpation as being located just lateral to the external carotid. Many investigators have described exotic and sophisticated landmarks to define its location when simple palpation of the carotid pulse can define the jugular vein. Punctures immediately lateral to the carotid pulse are frequently rewarded with success.

Historically, jugular venous access has been considered when traditional venous cutdown of the cephalic vein has been unsuccessful. This approach is somewhat less desirable than the subclavian, axillary, and cephalic vein placement because of increased risk of lead fracture and the potential for lead erosion. The acute angle that is created on the lead after it exits the venous structure as it is brought down over the clavicle to the pocket creates circumstances for this problem. This procedure is somewhat more involved, because tunneling is required to bring the lead to the pocket. If tunneling is performed under the clavicle, there is increased risk of pneumothorax and vascular injury. If the lead is tunneled over the clavicle, tissue is typically thin, and there is a greater risk of erosion. As a rule, the right internal jugular approach is preferred. In early reports, jugular venous access was performed by the cutdown technique. An alternate percutaneous approach has been proposed that requires little attention to anatomic landmarks and dissection. An initial supraclavicular incision is not required. This

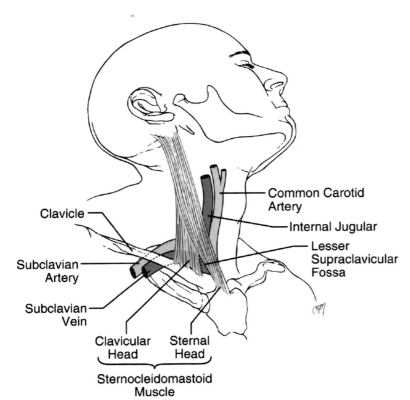

FIGURE 30-39. Anatomic relationships of the right internal jugular vein and common carotid artery. (From Belott PH, Reynolds WR. Permanent pacemaker implantation. In: Ellenbogen K, Kay N, Wilkoff B, eds. *Clinical cardiac pacing.* Philadelphia: WB Saunders, 1995:460–483, with permission.)

approach involves percutaneous access of the right internal jugular vein. Access to the internal jugular vein is best obtained with the patient in the normal anatomic position with the head facing anterior. Rotating the head to the left only distorts the anatomy. The carotid artery is palpated in the lower third of the neck. The internal jugular vein is lateral to the common carotid artery. The two structures are parallel. Addressing the patient on the right side for the right internal jugular approach, the implanting physician places the middle finger over the course of the common carotid artery. The course of the internal jugular is under the index finger. The index and middle fingers side by side are generally analogous to the size and orientation on the surface of the skin to the deeper internal jugular vein and common carotid artery as they run side by side underneath the skin. The venipuncture anywhere along the course should enter the internal jugular vein. If the puncture is made above the clavicle, pneumothoraces are avoided. The needle is generally held perpendicular to the plane of the neck rather than angled. This helps avoid infraclavicular puncture and potential pneumothorax. After the needle has entered the vein, it is gently angled inferiorly for the passage of the guide wire. If the internal carotid artery is inadvertently punctured, the needle is removed and pressure held. A repeat attempt at venipuncture is made slightly lateral to the initial stick.

After the internal jugular vein is entered, the technique is essentially identical to a standard procedure. A small incision is carried laterally down the shaft of the needle to the surface of the sternocleidomastoid muscle. If more tissue depth is required, the muscle can be split and the incision carried directly down over the vein. A small Weitlaner retractor is used for more adequate exposure. It is important to place a figure-of-eight suture for vascular control, hemostasis, and anchoring (Fig. 30-40). The retained guide wire technique may be used for placement of the atrial and ventricular electrodes. After adequate lead position, the figure-of-eight stitch is secured for hemostasis, and the lead is anchored to the muscle body using the suture sleeve. A second incision for the pocket formation is made infraclavicularly. The leads are then tunneled to the pocket by standard tunneling

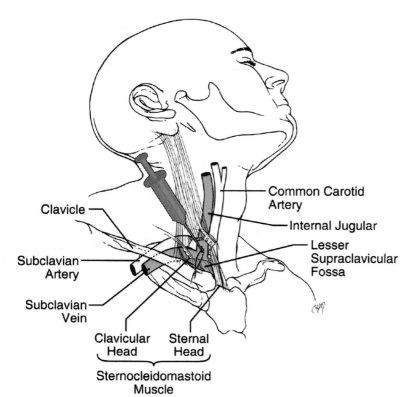

FIGURE 30-40. Percutaneous venous access to the right internal jugular vein. (From Belott PH. Unusual access sites for permanent cardiac pacing. In: Barold SS, Mugica J, eds. *Recent advances in cardiac pacing: goals for the 21st century*, vol 4. Armonk, NY: Futura Publishing, 1998:137–180, with permission.)

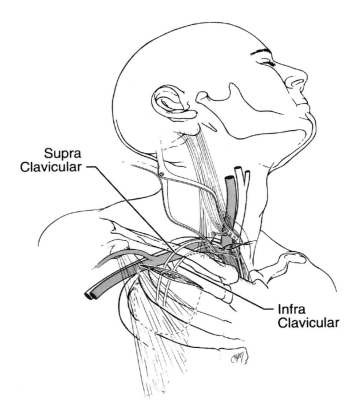

FIGURE 30-41. Pacemaker leads tunneled over and under the clavicle to the infraclavicular pocket. (From Belott PH. Unusual access sites for permanent cardiac pacing. In: Barold SS, Mugica J, eds. *Recent advances in cardiac pacing: goals for the 21st century*, vol 4. Armonk, NY: Futura Publishing, 1998:137–180, with permission.)

techniques (Fig. 30-41). When the electrodes are tunneled under the clavicle, care must be taken to avoid vascular trauma. Conversely, when tunneling over the clavicle, every effort should be made to ensure optimal tissue depth to avoid potential erosion.

The tunneling technique described by Roelke and colleagues for submammary pacemaker implantation may also be used for infraclavicular tunneling (49). A long, 18-gauge spinal needle can be passed from the infraclavicular incision to the supraclavicular incision. The guide wire is passed, and the sheath set is applied and tunneled to the supraclavicular incision. The rubber dilator is removed. The lead to be used is inserted in the distal end of the sheath and tied. Once secured, the lead and sheath are pulled through to the infraclavicular incision (Fig. 30-42).

The external jugular vein is less frequently used for venous access because it is more inferiorly located and there is higher risk of pneumothorax and vascular complications. It is less precise, and successful cannulation may be more frustrating.

Femoral Venous Access

The femoral vein has been reported as an alternate site for pacemaker implantation. If the venous structure is punctured from above Poupart's ligament, it is anatomically the iliac vein; below Poupart's ligament, it is designated as the femoral vein. Iliac venipuncture has been reported as an alternate source for single- and dual-chambered pacemaker implantation (50,51). It has not been used for defibrillator electrode placement. Ellestad and French reported their experience using the iliac vein in 90 patients. This vein can be used for transvenous lead placement when an abdominal pocket is desired. It is usually reserved for patients with little pectoral tissue, such as in the case of bilateral mastectomy, extensive pectoral radiation damage, or for a variety of other cosmetic reasons. A small incision is made above the inguinal ligament above the vein, just medial to the palpable femoral artery (Fig. 30-43). The incision is carried down to the surface above the vein. The vein is then punctured using the Seldinger sheath-set technique with the guide wire retained for dual-chambered implants. A figure-of-eight stitch or a pursestring suture is placed for hemostasis. The suture is placed through the fascia around the lead as it enters the vein. Special long (85-cm) leads are positioned in a conventional manner and secured to the fascia by use of a tie around the suture sleeve and lead. A horizontal incision is made at the second site, just lateral to the umbilicus. This is carried down to the surface of the rectus sheath. A pacemaker pocket is created in the conventional manner. Preparations are then made for tunneling the leads from the initial incision to the newly created pocket by use of one of the standard tunneling techniques. Active-fixation electrodes are recommended for atrial and ventricular lead placement. In the Ellestad experience, lead dislodgements have been reported as a major weakness in this approach. Venous

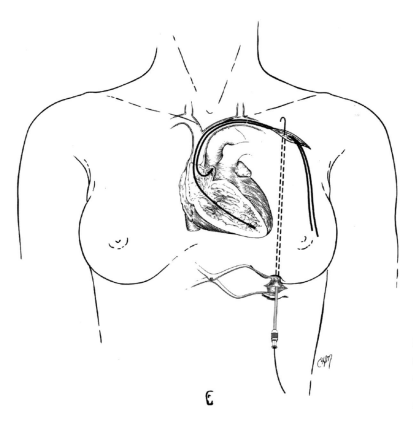

FIGURE 30-42. Subcutaneous tunneling with a guide wire and sheath. (Adapted from Roelke, Jackson G, Hawthorne JW. Submammary pacemaker implantation: a unique tunneling technique. *Pacing Clin Electrophysiol* 1994;17:1793, with permission.)

thrombosis and lead fracture do not appear to be a problem, although the published experience with this approach is relatively small and the latter is difficult to discern. The complication of pneumothorax associated with the percutaneous approach does not exist. Similarly, the complication of air embolism is not a problem.

Upgrading Techniques for Dual-Chambered Pacing and Defibrillator Systems

When approaching a patient for a permanent transvenous pacemaker or modern automatic ICD system, every effort should be made to preserve atrial and ventricular relationships. With physicians sensitive to this concept, most patients receive dual-chambered pacing and ICD systems. There is, however, a large group of patients who have previously received single-chamber, ventricular-demand pacing systems. There is also a smaller group of patients who have previously received single-chamber atrial pacing systems. Some individuals require an upgrade of their pacing system, which requires abandonment of a pacing system and the addition of an implantable defibrillator. Many of the patients with VVI pacing and single-chamber defibrillator systems have symptoms of the pacemaker syndrome. A small group of atrially paced patients who have previously received single-chamber atrial systems have symptoms of AV block. Many of the symptomatic patients with such systems require pacemaker system upgrade with the addition of an atrial electrode. Patients who are atrially paced and have symptoms of AV block require ventricular support with the addition of a ventricular electrode. A patient previously paced atrially or ventricularly who requires a defibrillator system will require the addition of a nonthoracotomy shocking lead. These groups of patients require system upgrades with the addition of one or more electrodes.

The conventional pacing system upgrade techniques and pacing and defibrillator upgrading tech-

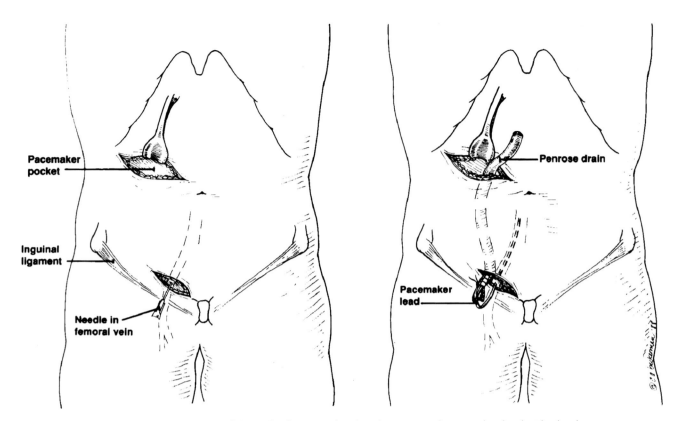

FIGURE 30-43. Use of the right iliac vein for the placement of pacemaker leads. The leads are ultimately tunneled using a Penrose drain to a pocket created in the right upper quadrant. (From Ellestad MH, French J. Iliac vein approach to permanent pacemaker implantation. *Pacing Clin Electrophysiol* 1986;12:1030, with permission.)

niques involve the placement of a second electrode. This procedure is combined with a pulse generator change. The dilemma with pacemaker and ICD system upgrade is the required supplemental venous access for placement of a second lead.

Venous access can be carried out by cutdown or the percutaneous approach. If the initial electrode has been placed by cutdown, the isolation of a second vein for venous access will prove extremely difficult. In this case, percutaneous approach should be attempted. Conversely, if the initial electrode has been placed percutaneously, a second percutaneous approach or a cutdown is always possible. The second percutaneous puncture is usually carried out just lateral to the initial venous entry site. The initial lead can be used as a marker of the venous anatomy. If any difficulty is encountered, fluoroscopy is used to guide the lead using the chronic ventricular lead for reference (52,53).

There is potential risk of damaging the initial electrode, and care should be taken to avoid its direct puncture. The use of radiographic materials can also help define the venous structure and its patency.

Occasionally, the vessel to be recanalized is thrombosed or obstructed, precluding venous access on the same side. In this case, contralateral venous access should be considered (54). The desired electrode is passed through the contralateral subclavian vein, positioned, and subsequently tunneled back to the original pocket (Fig. 30-44). The contralateral puncture site requires a limited skin incision of about 1 to 2 cm. It is carried down to the surface of the pectoralis muscle. The pectoralis muscle is used for anchoring the electrode with its suture sleeve. After the electrode has been positioned, it is anchored and secured. The proximal end of the electrode is then tunneled back to the original pocket.

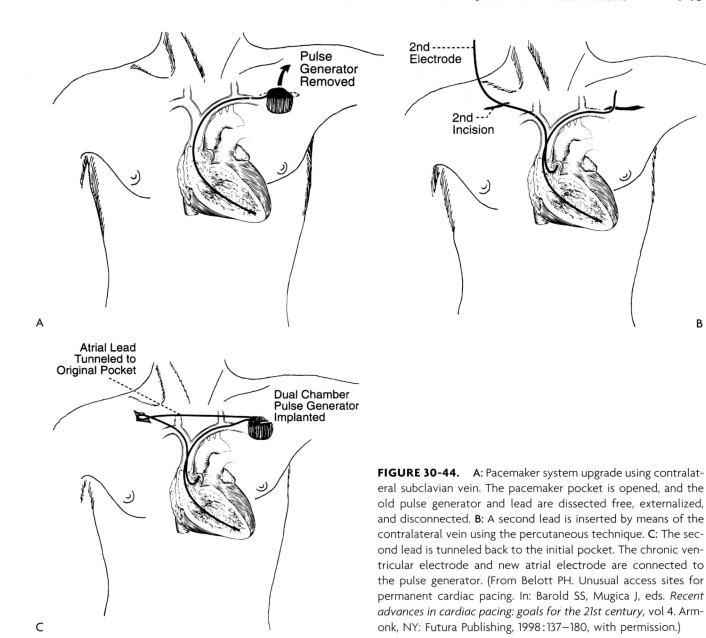

FIGURE 30-44. **A:** Pacemaker system upgrade using contralateral subclavian vein. The pacemaker pocket is opened, and the old pulse generator and lead are dissected free, externalized, and disconnected. **B:** A second lead is inserted by means of the contralateral vein using the percutaneous technique. **C:** The second lead is tunneled back to the initial pocket. The chronic ventricular electrode and new atrial electrode are connected to the pulse generator. (From Belott PH. Unusual access sites for permanent cardiac pacing. In: Barold SS, Mugica J, eds. *Recent advances in cardiac pacing: goals for the 21st century,* vol 4. Armonk, NY: Futura Publishing, 1998:137–180, with permission.)

Epicardial Lead Placement

Initially, epicardial pacemaker lead placement was the implant technique of choice because of the large size of the pacemaker pulse generator and unreliable leads for transvenous placement. Today, epicardial pacemaker lead placement is reserved for patients undergoing cardiac surgery. Even in this circumstance, the transvenous approach is frequently employed. This is largely because of the safety and efficacy of the transvenous approach. Today, only rare and unusual circumstances result in an epicardial pacemaker implant. These include patients undergoing cardiac surgery, patients with recurrent transvenous dislodgement, and patients with a prosthetic tricuspid valve or a congenital anomaly such as tricuspid atresia. The epicardial approach regained popularity with the development of the ICD. This system initially required placement of epicardial patch electrodes and rate-sensing leads. With development of the nonthoracotomy defibrillator lead, the epicardial approach again fell into disuse. There has been some

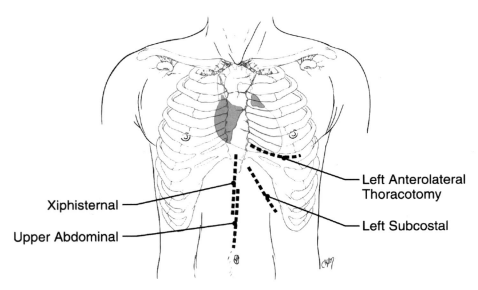

FIGURE 30-45. Location of surgical incisions for the placement of epicardial systems. The common median sternotomy is not shown. (From Belott PH, Reynolds WR. Permanent pacemaker implantation. In: Ellenbogen K, Kay N, Wilkoff B, eds. *Clinical cardiac pacing.* Philadelphia: WB Saunders, 1995:460–483, with permission.)

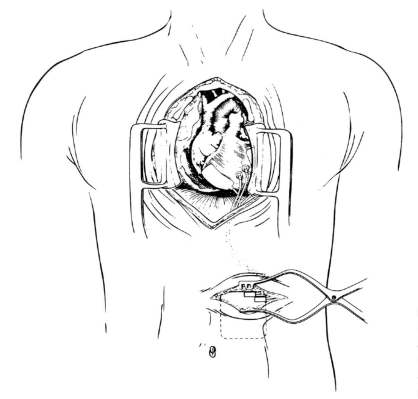

FIGURE 30-46. Median sternotomy. (From Belott PH, Reynolds WR. Permanent pacemaker and implantable cardioverter implantation. In: Ellenbogen K, Kay N, Wilkoff B, eds. *Clinical cardiac pacing and defibrillation.* Philadelphia: WB Saunders, 2000:630, with permission.)

resurgence of interest in this approach with the development of four-chamber pacing for dilated cardiomyopathy.

Epicardial approach does offer the advantage of mapping for ideal pacing thresholds and other electrophysiologic parameters. Leads or patch electrodes are directly attached to the epicardium and pulled through to a subcutaneous pocket. This pocket is usually in the upper abdomen. Historically, multiple epicardial approaches have been developed (Fig. 30-45). These include median sternotomy, left anterolateral thoracotomy, subxiphoid, left subcostal, and thoracoscopic approaches. The subxiphoid and the left subcostal approaches do not require a thoracotomy. General anesthesia is usually required for all epicardial pacemaker and ICD implantations. These procedures generally are performed in the operating room by the cardiothoracic surgeon.

Identical epicardial approaches have been used for pacing and ICD implantation. The more recent use of the epicardial approach for ICD implantation was necessitated to configure defibrillation patch electrodes around the heart for optimal defibrillation thresholds (DFTs) in the rare instances where satisfactory DFTs cannot be achieved with transvenous ICD leads. Similar to early pacemakers, ICD pulse generator were large and required an abdominal pocket for implantation. Because there is little call for epicardial pacemaker placement today, the following discussion reviews the epicardial approach as it applies to the rare instances when implantation of an ICD, requires an epicardial approach.

The median sternotomy is the most popular approach because it provides optimal exposure and access to the entire heart (55–57). It is used in patients undergoing an open-heart procedure who also require ICD implantation. The incision is well tolerated and associated with less patient discomfort. Two large patches may easily be placed extrapericardially (Fig. 30-46). Excellent exposure is achieved because the procedure is generally performed under cardiopulmonary bypass with the lungs deflated. The rate-sensing leads are directly screwed to the epicardial surface. The patch electrodes are sutured to the pericardium.

The left anterolateral thoracotomy also offers excellent exposure of the heart and left ventricle. An

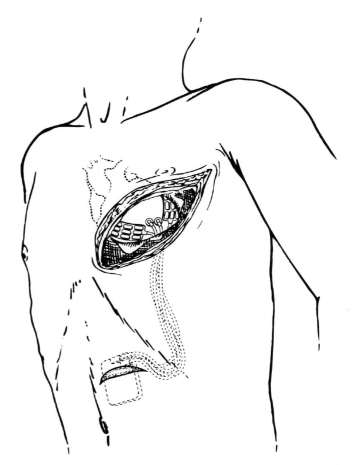

FIGURE 30-47. Left lateral thoracotomy with epicardial rate-sensing and patch electrodes tunneled to the subcutaneous pocket in the left upper quadrant. (From Belott PH, Reynolds WR. Permanent pacemaker and implantable cardioverter implantation. In: Ellenbogen K, Kay N, Wilkoff B, eds. *Clinical cardiac pacing and defibrillation.* Philadelphia: WB Saunders, 2000:630, with permission.)

incision is created in the fifth intercostal space (Fig. 30-47). This approach is ideal for extrapericardial placement of a large patch electrode over the posterior surface of the left ventricle and a smaller patch anteriorly between the sternum and pericardium. This approach is associated with considerable postoperative pain, which is its major drawback. This pain frequently results in atelectasis and transient pleural effusions. Today, a more lateral approach has been adopted that eliminates pain associated with division of the latissimus dorsi. The leads are tunneled to an abdominal pocket by use of a small chest tube or hemostat.

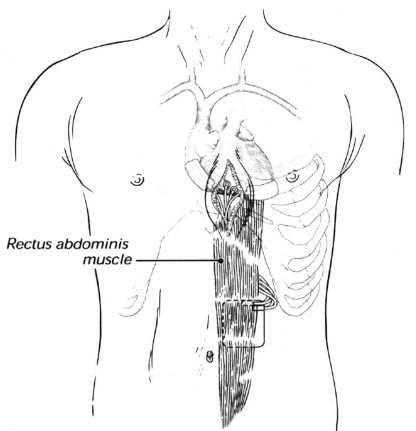

FIGURE 30-48. Subxiphoid epicardial approach with rate-sensing and patch electrodes tunneled to the subrectus pocket in the left upper quadrant. (From Belott PH, Reynolds WR. Permanent pacemaker and implantable cardioverter implantation. In: Ellenbogen K, Kay N, Wilkoff B, eds. *Clinical cardiac pacing and defibrillation.* Philadelphia: WB Saunders, 2000:631, with permission.)

The subxiphoid approach was developed for patients undergoing simple ICD implantation (Fig. 30-48). There is decreased morbidity and discomfort with this approach. There is, however, a slight increase in resultant DFTs compared to other epicardial approaches. Wound discomfort postoperatively is much less. The major disadvantage of this approach is limited surgical exposure and the absolute requirement for intrapericardial placement of patches. Frequently, because of unacceptable DFTs, an additional transvenous electrode is required. This approach is generally not used in patients who have undergone a prior cardiac surgical procedures.

The left subcostal approach was originally developed for placement of rate-pacing and -sensing leads. It is now also used for placement of ICD patches. This approach is associated with minimal morbidity (58,59). The left subcostal approach is carried out with an incision in the left subcostal area. This approach can also be used in patients who have had prior cardiac surgery (60,61). The left subcostal approach is extrathoracic and avoids the complications of a thoracotomy. There is, however, greater postoperative wound discomfort when compared with the subxiphoid approach. Occasionally, pacing leads and ICD patches have been placed using thoracoscopy. A small incision is made on the anterior chest, and the pacing leads or defibrillator patches are introduced into the left pleural space (Fig. 30-49). The thoracoscope is used to guide the leads and patches to the pericardial surface for attachment (62,63) (Fig. 30-50). Thoracoscopy, a relatively new approach, appears to be safe

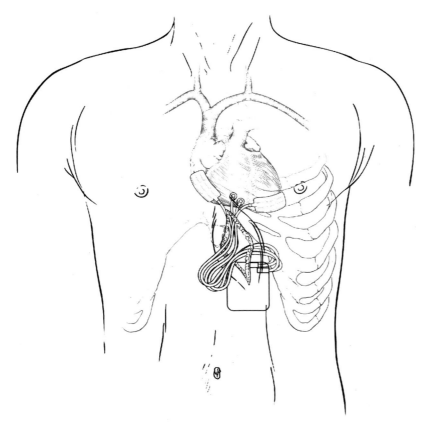

FIGURE 30-49. Left subcostal epicardial approach with rate-sensing and patch electrodes tunneled to the subcutaneous pocket in the left infracostal space. (From Belott PH, Reynolds WR. Permanent pacemaker and implantable cardioverter implantation. In: Ellenbogen K, Kay N, Wilkoff B, eds. *Clinical cardiac pacing and defibrillation.* Philadelphia: WB Saunders, 2000:631, with permission.)

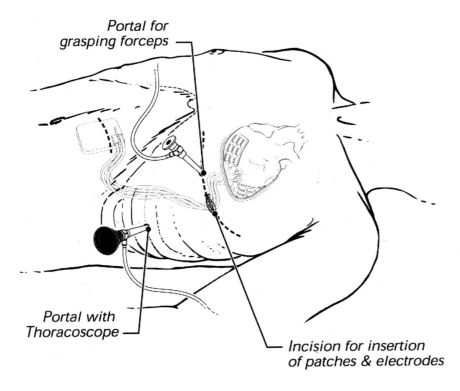

FIGURE 30-50. Thoracoscopic epicardial rate-sensing and patch electrode placement. Electrodes are tunneled subcutaneously to the cardioverter-defibrillator pocket in the left upper quadrant. (From Belott PH, Reynolds WR. Permanent pacemaker and implantable cardioverter implantation. In: Ellenbogen K, Kay N, Wilkoff B, eds. *Clinical cardiac pacing and defibrillation.* Philadelphia: WB Saunders, 2000:632, with permission.)

and efficacious. Because thoracotomy and sternotomy are avoided, it carries the lowest morbidity of all the epicardial approaches.

SPECIAL SITUATIONS

Use of the Coronary Sinus for Cardiac Pacing

The coronary sinus has been used for pacing by design and by misadventure (64,65) and more recently, for multisite pacing. In the past, this has proven to be an extremely unreliable site for ventricular pacing and has been avoided. When left atrial pacing is required, coronary sinus has proven to be an ideal location. The major problem with coronary sinus pacing has been a somewhat more challenging access, and lead stability. Before the development of reliable atrial electrodes, the coronary sinus was a popular site for lead placement for atrial pacing. The best position for atrial pacing is the proximal coronary sinus. Special coronary sinus leads have been developed to enhance position stability. When simultaneous right and left atrial pacing is desired, a distal coronary sinus location has been used. Primary coronary sinus catheterization requires experience, and there are a growing number of implanting electrophysiologists who routinely use the coronary sinus for diagnostic studies are also implanting pacemakers, the need for additional experience with this technique has become somewhat of a moot point. As a rule, placement of a coronary sinus lead is much easier from the left subclavian vein. A generous curve is required in the lead. Coronary sinus placement is confirmed by the posterior lead position on fluoroscopy in the lateral or left anterior oblique projections (66). Lead placement is not associated with ventricular ectopy as is the case when the lead is inadvertently placed in the pulmonary outflow tract where it may mimic the flouroscopic appearance of coronary sinus position in the AP view. Once a popular approach for atrial pacing, the coronary sinus is used infrequently today in this manner. However, as biatrial pacing becomes more important for control of atrial arrhythmias and four-chamber pacing is desired for management of cardiomyopathy, there has been a resurgence of interest in the use of the coronary sinus.

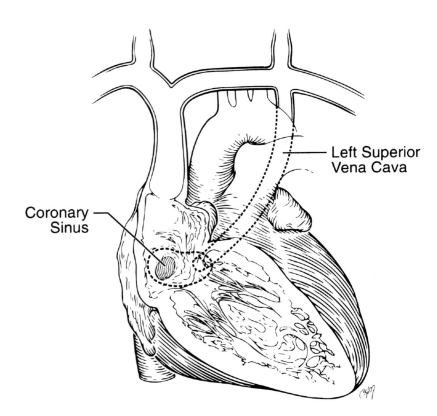

FIGURE 30-51. Persistent left superior vena cava. (From Belott PH. Unusual access sites for permanent cardiac pacing. In: Barold SS, Mugica J, eds. *Recent advances in cardiac pacing: goals for the 21st century,* vol 4. Armonk, NY: Futura Publishing, 1998:137–180, with permission.)

Electrode Placement through Anomalous Venous Structures

Occasionally, a patient has a persistent left superior vena cava. Embryologically, the left superior vena cava becomes atretic. In approximately 0.5% of the population, this structure persists. The persistent left superior vena cava connects directly to the coronary sinus. The persistent left superior vena cava represents failure in the development of the left innominate vein. This vein normally forms by communication of the right and left anterior cardinal veins. In this situation, the left anterior cardinal vein persists and continues to drain to the brachiocephalic veins and the sinus venosus. This ultimately develops into a left superior vena cava, which enters directly into the coronary sinus (Fig. 30-51). Normally, the left innominate vein develops as an anastomosis between the left and right

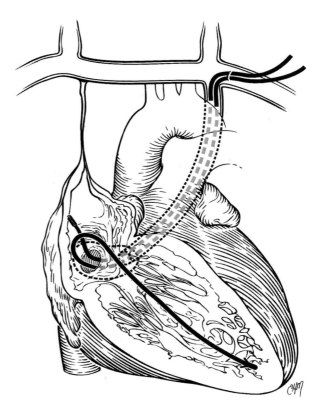

FIGURE 30-53. Placement of an atrial and ventricular electrode by means of a persistent left superior vena cava. (From Belott PH. Unusual access sites for permanent cardiac pacing. In: Barold SS, Mugica J, eds. *Recent advances in cardiac pacing: goals for the 21st century*, vol 4. Armonk, NY: Futura Publishing, 1998:137–180, with permission.)

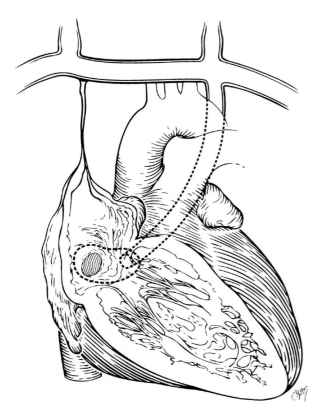

FIGURE 30-52. Persistent left superior vena cava with an absent right superior vena cava. (From Belott PH. Unusual access sites for permanent cardiac pacing. In: Barold SS, Mugica J, eds. *Recent advances in cardiac pacing: goals for the 21st century*, vol 4. Armonk, NY: Futura Publishing, 1998:137–180, with permission.)

anterior cardinal veins. With persistent left superior vena cava, there frequently is associated atresia and complete absence of the right superior vena caval system (Fig. 30-52). In this situation, venous access for pacing from the right atrial structures is virtually impossible.

Placement of electrodes through a persistent left superior vena cava can prove extremely challenging, if not impossible (67–72). It is important to appreciate that the lead or leads are advanced into the coronary sinus and out its ostium into the right atrium. If right ventricular apical positions are to be achieved, the lead must negotiate at an acute angle to cross the tricuspid valve. This is best accomplished by having a lead form a loop on itself using lateral right atrial wall for support (Fig. 30-53). This maneuver can prove extremely challenging. Depending on anatomy, occasionally such efforts prove unsuccessful, and an alternate site of venous access must be considered. At this point, it is prudent to assess the patency of the right venous system with contrast materials (73). If the surgeon encounters a persistent left superior vena cava, an assessment of the right superior vena cava by means of contrast injection may prove helpful. This can be carried out by advancing the standard end-hole catheter from the left superior vena cava to the vicinity of the right superior vena cava. Occasionally, such communication does not exist. If the right superior vena cava is absent, the iliac vein approach should be considered. Atrial electrode placement in the case of a persistent left superior vena cava is also challenging. It is recommended that positive-fixation, screw-in electrodes be used (74,75). The use of a preformed atrial J-ended wire will prove difficult or impossible. Dislodgement of the preformed J wire is also a concern.

Permanent pacemakers have also been implanted using the inferior vena cava with a retroperitoneal approach (76) (Fig. 30-54). This is usually done in the setting of complex congenital anomalies and subsequent corrective procedures. Venous access to the right atrium and ventricle is complicated by loss of continuity between the right atrium and the superior vena cava. Bipolar, active-fixation, screw-in electrodes are used for the atrium and ventricle. The pulse generator is usually implanted in a subcutaneous pocket formed on the anterior abdominal wall.

In a similar approach, pacemaker leads have been placed through transhepatic cannulation (77) (Fig. 30-55). Venous access is achieved percutaneously; with

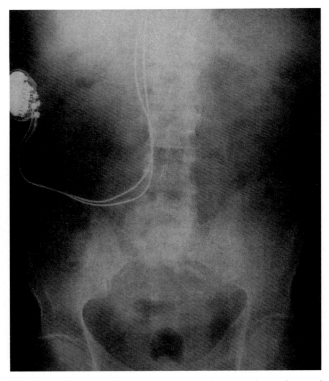

FIGURE 30-54. Posteroanterior abdominal radiograph shows the position of a pacemaker and generator lead inserted into the inferior vena cava using a retroperitoneal approach. (From West JNW, Shearmann CP, Gammange MD. Permanent pacemaker positioning via the inferior vena cava in a case of single ventricle with loss of right atrium–vena cava continuity. *Pacing Clin Electrophysiol* 1993;16:1753, with permission.)

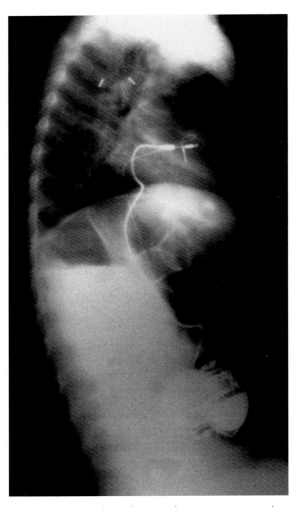

FIGURE 30-55. A lateral view demonstrates transhepatic lead placement. (From Belott PH, Reynolds WR. Permanent pacemaker and implantable cardioverter implantation. In: Ellenbogen K, Kay N, Wilkoff B, eds. *Clinical cardiac pacing and defibrillation*. Philadelphia: WB Saunders, 2000:625, with permission.)

the guide wire passed transhepatically, the sheath set is applied, allowing the subsequent introduction of a permanent pacing electrode. This procedure has been reserved for complex congenital anomalies that preclude venous access through a superior vein.

Inframammary Implantation

The principles of plastic surgery can be used for standard pacemaker implantation for an optimal cosmetic effect (78). This technique involves more surgery and is best performed under modified or complete general anesthesia. Because of more postoperative wound pain, an overnight stay is advised. Venous access is achieved percutaneously for single- and dual-chamber pacing. After the subclavian vein has been accessed, a limited 1- to 2-cm initial incision is made. The incision is carried to the surface of the pectoralis muscle. After the electrodes are placed, a second incision is made under the breast along the breast fold. A standard pocket is created under the breast (Fig. 30-56). The pacemaker leads are tunneled to the inframammary pocket. The pulse generator and electrodes are connected and the incision closed. It is recommended that active-fixation, screw-in electrodes be employed for the atrium and ventricle. It is also recommended that a Parsonnet pouch be used to avoid pulse generator migration and a twiddler syndrome.

An alternate approach calls for a second incision made in the axilla with the arm in abduction. The incision is carried to the depth that exposes the muscular fascia. In this case, the pulse generator is placed subpectorally.

Roelke and coworkers described a submammary pacemaker implantation technique using unique tunneling (49). Venous access is achieved percutaneously or by cephalic vein cutdown. The electrodes are positioned and anchored. A horizontal incision is made in the inframammary fold. A 20-cm-long, 18-gauge pericardiocentesis needle is directed from the inframammary pocket to the infraclavicular incision. A J wire is passed down the needle to the infraclavicular incision. The needle is removed, and using a retained guide wire technique, two 10-Fr introducer dilators are passed consecutively over the guide wire. The free ends of the atrial and ventricular electrodes from the infraclavicular incision are placed in the sheaths and secured with a tie. The sheaths are then withdrawn to the inframammary pocket.

A retropectoral transaxillary percutaneous tech-

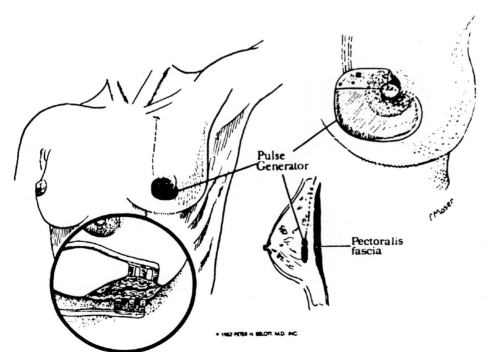

FIGURE 30-56. Inframammary incision and placement of a pulse generator with tunneled electrodes. (From Belott PH, Byrd CL. Recent developments in pacemaker implantation and lead retrieval. In: Barold SS, Mugica J, eds. *New perspectives in cardiac pacing 2.* Armonk, NY: Futura Publishing, 1991:105–131, with permission.)

nique has also been used for optimal cosmetic effect (79). This technique is performed under local anesthesia and conscious sedation. Venography is used to confirm the relationship of the axillary vein to the surface anatomy. A marker is placed in the axillary vein through the antecubital fossa (Fig. 30-57). This marker may be a temporary transvenous pacing wire or a standard 0.032-mm guide wire. Using the marker as a guide, the axillary vein is punctured. A longitudinal incision is made along the posterior border of the pectoralis major muscle in the axilla. A standard retropectoral pocket is created. One or two pacing elec-

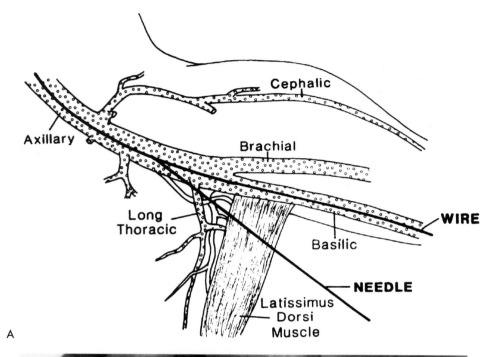

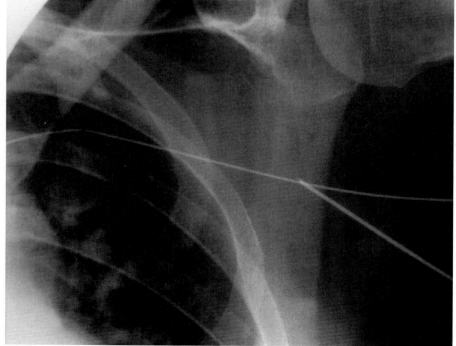

FIGURE 30-57. A: Stylized illustration of axillary venipuncture using the guide wire as a landmark. B: Radiograph of needle accessing the axillary vein using the guide wire as a landmark. (From Shefer A, Lewis SB. The retropectoral transaxillary permanent pacemaker: description of a technique for percutaneous implantation of an invisible device. *Pacing Clin Electrophysiol* 1996;16:1648, with permission.)

fied and the electrode is passed transatrially through an incision or by using a sheath set. Hemostasis is effected by a pursestring suture about the entry site. Fluoroscopy can be used for ventricular placement of a tined or screw-in electrode. All electrodes are then secured to the endocardial surface. Sutures placed under the tines secure the electrode. The electrodes are then driven through an atriotomy into the atrial cavity and out the atrial muscle at a point of desired endocardial fixation. The electrodes are pulled through the incision and snugged to the endocardium by pulling and tying the double-ended suture (Fig. 30-59). This approach is recommended over the epicardial approach because of the excellent thresholds that can be achieved.

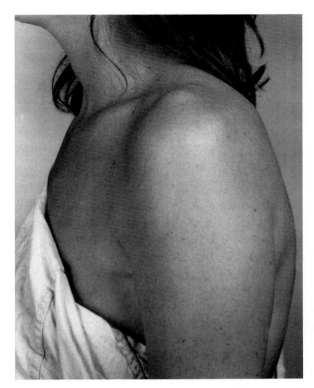

FIGURE 30-58. Lateral view of a patient after transaxillary retropectoral pacemaker implantation using the Shefer approach. (From Shefer A, Lewis SB. The retropectoral transaxillary permanent pacemaker: description of a technique for percutaneous implantation of an invisible device. *Pacing Clin Electrophysiol* 1996;16:1648, with permission.)

trodes can then be placed by conventional techniques. The electrodes are secured by their suture sleeve to the pectoralis fascia. The leads are then connected to the pacemaker and inserted into the retropectoral pocket. This technique offers optimal cosmetic results (Fig. 30-58), and there have been no restrictions in physical activity or movement of the shoulder joint.

Transthoracic Endocardial Lead Placement

Occasionally, transvenous endocardial lead placement is impractical, impossible, or contraindicated. Endocardial leads may be placed transthoracically under general anesthesia and through a limited thoracotomy (80). The pacemaker electrodes are passed and positioned transatrially through a limited thoracotomy in the sixth intercostal space. The right atrium is identi-

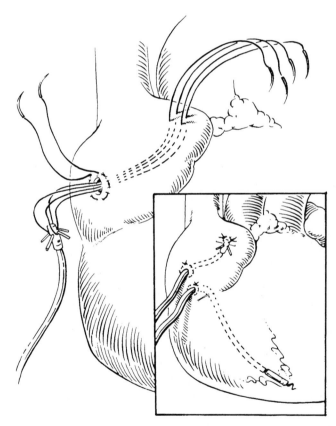

FIGURE 30-59. Atrial lead placement through atriotomy and pursestring suture. The atrial and ventricular electrodes are positioned, and the atriotomy is secured. (From Belott PH, Byrd CL. Recent developments in pacemaker implantation and lead retrieval. In: Barold SS, Mugica J, eds. *New perspectives in cardiac pacing 2.* Armonk, NY: Futura Publishing, 1991:105–131, with permission.)

Hayes and associates described a similar technique of endocardial electrode placement at the time of corrective cardiac surgery (81). In this procedure, epicardial pacing was avoided because of poor pacing and sensing thresholds. Traditionally, at the time of surgery, the patient requiring a dual-chamber pacing system would receive epicardial ventricular electrodes. The atrial electrode was placed transvenously later in the hospitalization. In the postoperative period, a dual-chamber system appeared crucial for optimal hemodynamics. Using the technique of Hayes and colleagues, a dual-chamber pacemaker patient with severe tricuspid regurgitation and chronic endocardial electrodes required removal of all endocardial electrodes and placement of a prosthetic tricuspid valve. New epicardial electrodes were placed in the ventricle. Stable atrial pacing and sensing was achieved by transatrial endocardial placement of the atrial appendage. The lead was secured by pursestring ligatures about the incision (Fig. 30-60).

A third transthoracic endocardial approach was described by Byrd (82). This technique allows conventional transvenous electrodes to be implanted in patients requiring an epicardial approach. It has been used in patients with superior vena cava syndrome, those with anomalous pulmonary venous drainage, and younger patients with innominate vein thrombosis. The technique involves a limited surgical approach under general anesthesia. A small incision is made in the third or fourth intercostal space. The third and fourth costal cartilages are excised and the atrial appendage exposed. An atriotomy is performed, and an introducer is placed inside an atrial pursestring suture and secured in a vertical position. The atrial and ventricular electrodes are passed down a standard sheath set into the atrium (Fig. 30-61). Using standard

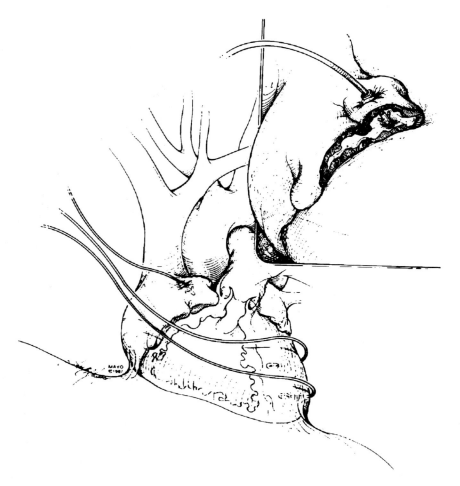

FIGURE 30-60. Atrial lead placement. *Inset:* The atrial endocardial lead is placed through the wall of the right atrial appendage, with the tip of the pacemaker lead abutting the endocardial surface. A pursestring suture is placed around the lead at the point of entry. The relationship of the atrial lead to the heart is also shown. (From Hayes DL, Vliestra RE, Puga FJ, et al. A novel approach to atrial endocardial pacing. *Pacing Clin Electrophysiol* 1989;12:125, with permission.)

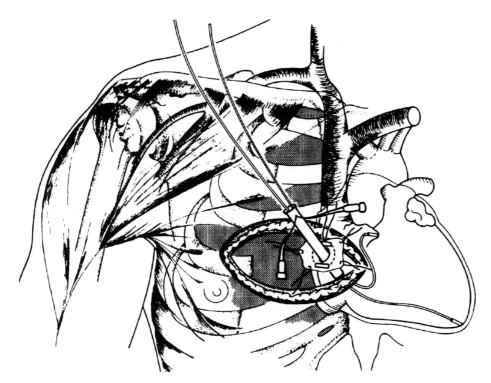

FIGURE 30-61. The Lemmon surgical approach consists of resection of the third costal cartilage through a small incision, reflection of the pleura, and opening of the pericardium. The introducer and transvenous sleeve are inserted through a right atrial pursestring suture. The leads are positioned in the right ventricle and right atrium using standard fluoroscopic techniques. Through the incision, the subcutaneous pocket is constructed over the pectoralis muscle on the anterior chest wall in its normal position. The leads are connected to the pacemaker without the need for an adapter or tunneling. (From Byrd CL. Transatrial implantation of transvenous pacing leads as an alternative to implantation of epicardial leads. *RBM* 1990;12:60, with permission.)

techniques, including fluoroscopy, the electrodes are positioned. After the electrodes are positioned, the introducer is removed, and the pursestring suture is used to close the atriotomy and secure the electrodes. The pacemaker is placed in a pocket adjacent to the incision on the right anterior chest wall. The advantage of this technique is minimal morbidity compared with the standard epicardial approach. The chest is never entered, and the time required for such procedure is similar to the transvenous approach. The technique, however, requires general anesthesia, violation of the epicardium, and an obligatory right-sided approach.

Ambulatory Approach

Historically, most pacemaker and ICD procedures have been performed on an inpatient basis. The patient has been formally admitted to the hospital. As a rule, the preoperative evaluation, procedure, and postoperative care are rendered in the hospital. In the case of permanent pacing and ICD implantation, individuals are generally admitted with major symptoms such as syncope. The patient is formally admitted, and the procedure is scheduled after a complete workup. After the procedure, the patient is observed briefly in the hospital and subsequently discharged and referred for outpatient device follow-up. In today's cost-containment environment, such an approach is inefficient. There has been an attempt to abbreviate the patient's hospital stay and render care on an ambulatory basis.

In the early days, when devices were large, surgery more involved, and catastrophic complications such as lead dislodgement, perforation, and wound infections frequent, hospitalizations were usually prolonged. The prospect of a brief hospital stay would have appeared heretical and unthinkable. Today, extensive experience and limited surgery have made complications rare. Most importantly, the major concern over lead dislodgement and potential for asystole is rare with the modern positive-fixation electrode systems. In the current pacemaker population, truly pacemaker-dependent patients are few. The patients are generally evaluated on an ambulatory basis, with symptoms of presyncope and syncope detected by outpatient ambulatory monitoring. They are subsequently admitted to the hospital for a permanent pacemaker implant. If this procedure were performed on an ambulatory basis and experienced total failure, the likely outcome would be a patient who is no better off than before the procedure. Today, when issues of cost containment are paramount the prospect of an ambulatory pacemaker procedure seems appealing.

The safety and efficacy of this approach has been demonstrated in Europe and in the United States (83, 84). However, concerns about potential complications continue to be expressed (85,86,87). Questions about lead selection, timing of discharge, and the intensity of follow-up are raised frequently. Economic benefit has yet to be fully appreciated. Although it is believed that more pacemaker procedures are being performed on an ambulatory basis, this has not been reflected in the literature. Since the original reports of Zegeleman and colleagues (83) and Belott (84), Haywood and associates reported a randomized control study of the feasibility and safety of ambulatory pacemaker procedures (88). Our experience includes more than 13 years with more than 1,474 pacemaker procedures, of which 1,043 have been performed on an ambulatory basis (89) (Table 30-4). Of these procedures, 967 were performed on a true ambulatory basis with the patient admitted and discharged on the same day. It appeared that over the 15-year period, 69% of all pacemaker procedures were ambulatory. From 1990 to 1995, 85% of the procedures were ambulatory. There were no pacemaker deaths or emergencies.

Two principles emerge from this experience. First, if there are any doubts or concerns, a patient's hospitalization can be extended. Second, it is thought that any operator is always aware of the problem patient, and for such a patient, who has potentially sustained a complication, hospitalization can always be extended.

Given the gratifying results of the 13-year experience, all elective permanent pacemaker procedures at our pacemaker center are performed on an ambulatory basis (90). This includes new implants, electrode repositioning, upgrade procedures, electrode extractions, and pulse generator changes. Because of the dramatically reduced ICD size and thus, the required surgery, as well as protocols for more expeditious device testing, even these procedures are now performed on an ambulatory basis.

Pacemaker Implantation in the Anticoagulated Patient

Management of surgery in the anticoagulated patient is a controversial topic. There is a paucity of information throughout the literature with respect to handling a patient requiring anticoagulation. The patient receiving anticoagulants, including heparin and platelet antagonists, is at risk for hematoma formation. It is commonly held that patients who require oral anticoagulants should have the prothrombin time brought to normal before the implantation. Anticoagulants can be resumed between 24 and 48 hours after the pacemaker procedure. Reducing the prothrombin time to normal in patients requiring anticoagulants, such as those with artificial heart valves, places the patient at grave risk for thromboembolic complications. Addressing this issue, many operators choose to admit the patient to the hospital and start intravenous heparin while the warfarin is withheld and the

TABLE 30-4 • AMBULATORY PACEMAKER PROCEDURE ANALYSIS, 1983 THROUGH 1995

Year	83	84	85	86	87	88	89	90	91	92	93	94	95	Total
TP	99	102	112	110	112	123	100	107	135	119	145	113	97	1474
TA	34	34	56	60	78	87	70	87	124	94	128	104	87	1043
TRUE	8	16	44	56	78	86	68	83	124	90	125	102	87	967
<24	26	18	12	4	0	1	2	4	0	4	3	2	0	76
%AMB	34	34	50	60	69	70	70	77	91	78	88	92	88	69

TP, total patients; TA, total ambulatory; TRUE, cases discharged the same day of procedure; <24, cases discharged within 24 hours (overnight hospitalization); %AMB, percent ambulatory procedure.

prothrombin time brought to normal values. This often takes days. After the prothrombin time has reached the control value, the patient is scheduled for surgery. On the day of surgery, the heparin is stopped and reversed, and the surgery is carried out. Several hours after surgery, heparin is resumed. After 24 to 48 hours with no evidence of significant hematoma, the warfarin is resumed. Once therapeutic, heparin is stopped, and the patient is discharged on oral warfarin therapy. In this age of cost control and managed care, this approach can prove to be quite expensive. Despite vigorous attempts at hemostasis, large hematomas have resulted from the use of heparin.

Although anecdotal, it is my impression that the greatest risk of bleeding complications—hemorrhage and hematoma—occur with the use of heparin and in patients on platelet antagonists such as aspirin. Having had the experience of a devastating thromboembolic complication from the withdrawal of warfarin and multiple large hematomas from the use of heparin in some patients under my care, I have chosen to perform pacemaker and ICD procedures with the patient fully anticoagulated on warfarin. This policy has been in effect for a minimum of 10 years. As a rule, the patient on oral anticoagulants has the international normalized ratio (INR) decreased to approximately 2. There have been no devastating hematomas or thromboembolic events with this policy. I think the pacemaker and ICD procedures can be performed quite safely with the anticoagulated patient. This approach has been supported by a 4-year experience reported by Goldstein and coworkers (91). There was no difference in the incidental bleeding complications between patients receiving warfarin and those not anticoagulated. There were no wound hematomas, blood transfusions, or clinically significant bleeding in any patient receiving warfarin. The interruption of anticoagulant therapy in pacemaker and ICD procedures to prevent hemorrhage is unfounded. The medicolegal risks from interrupted continuous anticoagulant therapy and the resultant thromboembolic event are real. Although there is a theoretical risk of hemorrhage after pacemaker procedures in patients with therapeutic levels of anticoagulation, the risk appears to be minimal. The bleeding can generally be treated by local measures or reoperation. The risk of bleeding is greatly outweighed by the risk of thromboembolism after withdrawal of anticoagulant therapy. If a major hemorrhage does occur, resulting in tamponade due to a perforation, such bleeding will not cease on the basis of thrombus formation, because it is mechanical and requires emergent surgical intervention. The issue of pacemaker and ICD surgery on anticoagulated patients will become more prevalent as more patients receive anticoagulation therapy for atrial fibrillation and for coronary artery interventions.

POTENTIAL COMPLICATIONS OF PACEMAKER IMPLANTATION

Venous Access

Complications of venous access are largely associated with the Seldinger percutaneous sheath-set technique (92–94). Such access has been associated with pneumothorax, hemopneumothorax, and air embolization and perforation of the innominate vein. The percutaneous needle can inadvertently damage or puncture the lung, subclavian artery, thoracic duct, and nerves. A pneumothorax may be asymptomatic and discovered on a routine postoperative chest radiograph. In almost every instance, the presence of a pneumothorax can be suspected by an alert operator when air is withdrawn into the probing percutaneous needle and syringe. The presence of pneumothorax may also be suspected by the patient's complaint of pleuritic pain, dyspnea, and cough. In rare circumstances, the patient may develop a tension pneumothorax. This can result in profound respiratory distress, hypoxemia, and cardiovascular collapse. Tension pneumothorax may be potentiated by the use of general anesthesia and positive-pressure ventilation. Management of pneumothorax depends on the severity. In the case of a tension pneumothorax, emergent chest tube insertion is mandatory. Whether a small asymptomatic pneumothorax should be managed with a chest tube or Heimlich valve is a matter of debate. As a rule, a pneumothorax greater than 10% should be managed surgically with a chest tube insertion.

Hemopneumothorax or hemothorax are rare and usually results from subclavian artery puncture and dissection. This may occur when the artery is punctured and a sheath applied to this vascular structure.

TABLE 30-5 • PERCUTANEOUS COMPLICATIONS

Pneumothorax
Hemothorax
Hemopneumothorax
Laceration, subclavian artery
Arteriovenous fistula
Nerve injury
Thoracic duct injury
Cheilothorax
Lymphatic fistula

TABLE 30-6 • PREVENTION OF AIR EMBOLISM DURING PERMANENT PACEMAKER PROCEDURES

Awareness of the potential problem
Well-hydrated patient, avoiding long periods of no oral intake
Awareness of when patient is at greatest risk—open sheath in vein
Assessment of hydration (take a peak)
For high-risk patient,
    Use increased hydration or wide-open intravenous lines
    Keep cooperative patients awake
    Elevate lower extremities or use a wedge
    Use Trendelenburg position (if available)
    Use expeditious lead placement and sheath removal
    Check for introduction of air
    Employ continuous monitoring (e.g., vital signs, oxygen saturation, blood pressure)
    For an extremely high-risk, uncooperative patient, intubation and temporary loss of consciousness may be required

Most hemopneumothoraces and hemothoraces require surgical drainage. In rare instances, a chronic hemothorax requires a decortication procedure.

There is an ongoing debate with respect to the safety and efficacy of blind subclavian puncture technique. Furman demonstrated remarkable efficiency of the cutdown approach for dual-chamber pacing, particularly with unipolar leads. The cutdown technique was less successful for bipolar leads through a single cephalic vein. Furman recorded no vascular or pleural complications in a series of 3,500 cases using the cutdown approach for single- and dual-chamber pacing implants. Furman emphasized that the complication rate of a blind subclavian puncture technique has probably been underestimated. A list of common complications associated with the percutaneous approach are shown in Table 30-5.

Air Embolism

Air embolism is a complication associated with the use of the Seldinger technique with a percutaneous sheath set. Air embolism is a well-known, well-documented complication of the percutaneous approach. To avoid this problem, it has been recommended that the patient be well hydrated and placed in the Trendelenburg position. Unfortunately, cases performed in the cardiac catheterization laboratory preclude this approach. The most important step in prevention is awareness on the part of the implanting physician for the risk of air embolization. There are many steps that may be taken to avoid this complication (95) (Table 30-6). The time of greatest risk is when the dilator is removed from the sheath set. In patients with a volume-overload state, there is little or no risk. However, an elderly dehydrated patient who has had no oral intake for many hours is at risk for serious air embolization. It is recommended that, before any percutaneous pacemaker or ICD procedure, the patient be maintained in a mild state of overhydration. The patient's state of hydration should be assessed just before removal of the dilator.

By careful withdrawal of the dilator from the sheath, one can assess the patient's state of hydration and venous pressure with the cycles of respiration. In a patient who is well hydrated or with a high venous pressure, there is a continuous flash of blood from the sheath despite the cycles of respiration. However, a dehydrated patient manifests no blood meniscus or flash of blood, and with each inspiration, retraction of the meniscus occurs. If the blood meniscus is observed to move inward, the dilator is rapidly advanced back into the sheath to avoid air embolism during this assessment. If the patient is deemed to be at high risk for air embolism, several precautions should be instituted. First, the lower extremities can be elevated by the insertion of a wedge to increase venous return. Second, if the patient is sleeping or oversedated, it is important to arouse the patient and achieve total patient cooperation with respect to the cycles of respira-

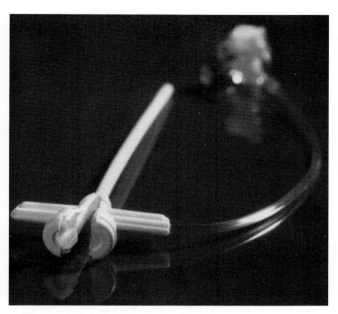

FIGURE 30-62. Pacemaker peel-away sheath with hemostatic valve. (Courtesy of Pressure Products, Inc., Rancho Palos Verdes, CA.)

TABLE 30-7 • COMPLICATIONS OF PACEMAKER INSERTION

Complication	Incidence (%)
Subclavian vein puncture leading to pneumothorax	1.0
Subclavian artery puncture	3.0
Wound or pocket hematoma	5.0
Hematoma requiring reoperation	0.1–0.5
Failure of wound healing	0.1
Infection	1.0

tion. Third, increased hydration can be initiated by increasing administration of intravenous fluids. Measures such as pinching the sheath with the lead have proven to be completely ineffective. Expeditious lead insertion is extremely important. The lead should be inserted rapidly and the sheath totally removed. The practice of slowly peeling the sheath away *in situ* should be avoided. The pacemaker electrode should never be positioned with the sheath set left in place.

A peel-away sheath with hemostatic valve has been developed. Use of this device completely avoids the problem of air embolization (Fig. 30-62).

A review of the complications associated with venous access suggests a 1% incidence of pneumothorax. Arterial puncture, somewhat more common, occurs at a rate of 3%. A list of pacemaker complications associated with insertion proposed by Sutton and Bourgeos (96) is found in Table 30-7.

Complications Associated with Manipulation of the Pacing Lead

The introduction and manipulation of pacing leads are frequently associated with tachyarrhythmias and bradyarrhythmias as a lead negotiates the chambers of the right heart. Ventricular tachycardia is extremely common as the pacing electrode or guide wire contacts the right ventricular myocardium. Withdrawal of these objects usually terminates the arrhythmia. In extreme cases, sustained monomorphic ventricular tachycardia or ventricular fibrillation may occur. Some institutions have instituted a policy of placing external defibrillation pads prophylactically in anticipation of required cardioversion.

The pacing lead, during the process of placement, may perforate the right ventricular free wall. The incidence of this complication is relatively low, occurring at a rate of approximately 0.1%. It is suspected that right ventricular perforation may be somewhat more common than reported because many patients remain clinically asymptomatic. This is because most perforations are self-sealing when the lead is withdrawn. If a life-threatening tamponade occurs, the implanting physician should be prepared to perform an emergency pericardiocentesis. It is advisable to have a pericardiocentesis tray readily available in case such a drainage procedure is required. Nonclinical perforations may be suspected by the presence of a friction rub and documented by two-dimensional echocardiography.

Sutton and Bourgois (96) compiled a list of complications associated with the pacing lead as well as their incidence (Table 30-8). Lead dislodgement, once the most common lead complication, has declined to a rate of 0.5% to 2% for the ventricular electrode and 1.5% to 5% for the atrial lead. This reduction largely reflects the genesis of fixation devices. Lead dislodgement is generally managed by reoperation and the lead

TABLE 30-8 • COMPLICATIONS OF PACING

Complications	Incidence (%)
Complications of the Pacing Lead	
Perforation of right ventricle	0.1
Ventricular lead displacement	0.5–2.0
Atrial lead displacement	1.5–5.0
Ventricular exit block (>5 years)	>1.0
Conductor fracture (>10 years)	0.1
Insulation fracture (>10 years)	0–0.15
Undersensing (ventricular)	Rare
Undersensing (atrial)	1–10
Oversensing (unipolar)	20–80
Oversensing (bipolar)	0
Diaphragmatic pacing	
Complications of the Vein Used for Pacing	
Axillary vein thrombosis	0.5–1.0
Partial great vein obstruction	≤100
Pulmonary embolism	Rare

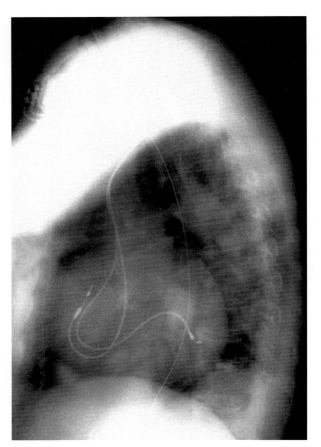

FIGURE 30-64. Lateral radiographic projection of the same patient as in Figure 30-63 clearly demonstrates the posterior placement of the ventricular lead in the left ventricle. (From Belott PH, Reynolds WR. Permanent pacemaker and implantable cardioverter implantation. In: Ellenbogen K, Kay N, Wilkoff B, eds. *Clinical cardiac pacing and defibrillation*. Philadelphia: WB Saunders, 2000:625, with permission.)

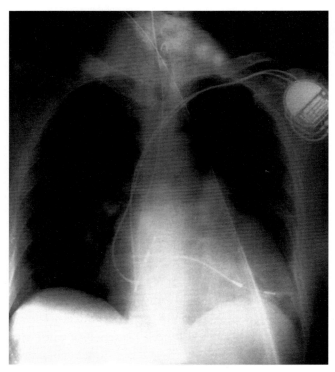

FIGURE 30-63. Anteroposterior chest radiograph with a ventricular electrode placed in the lateral wall of the left ventricle. This view can be deceiving. At first glance, the electrode appears to be appropriately placed in the apex of the right ventricle. The high takeoff across the tricuspid valve provides a clue that the lead is in reality crossing a patent foramen ovale. (From Belott PH, Reynolds WR. Permanent pacemaker and implantable cardioverter implantation. In: Ellenbogen K, Kay N, Wilkoff B, eds. *Clinical cardiac pacing and defibrillation*. Philadelphia: WB Saunders, 2000:626, with permission.)

repositioned. In rare instances, an electrode requires replacement, exchanging a passive-fixation for an active-fixation device.

Occasionally, the ventricular lead can be inadvertently placed in the left ventricle. This usually occurs if a lead is passed from the right atrium through a patent foramen ovale into the left atrium and then advanced into the left ventricle across the mitral valve. The radiographic appearance can be extremely deceptive in the anteroposterior projection (Fig. 30-63). A lateral radiographic projection is telling (Fig. 30-64). The electrocardiogram is also characteristic, with a right bundle branch QRS pattern during ventricular pacing. Acute left ventricular lead placement requires repositioning within the first 24 hours to avoid the potential complication of thromboembolic phenomenon. Chronic left ventricular lead placement usually requires long-term anticoagulant therapy because lead repositioning is inadvisable and extremely hazardous.

REFERENCES

1. Schecter DC. Modern era of artificial cardiac pacemakers. In: Schecter DC, ed. *Electrical cardiac stimulation*. Minneapolis: Medtronic, 1983:110–134.
2. Senning A. Discussion of a paper by Stephenson SE Jr, Edwards WH, Jolly PC, Scott HW: physiologic P-wave stimulator. *J Thorac Cardiovasc Surg* 1959;38:639.
3. Furman S, Schwedel JB. An intracardiac pacemaker for Stokes-Adams seizures. *N Engl J Med* 1959;261:948.
4. Mirowski M, Reid PR, Mower MM, et al. Termination of malignant ventricular arrhythmias with an implantable automatic defibrillator in human beings. *N Engl J Med* 1980;303:322–324.
5. Parsonnet V, Furman S, Smyth NP, Bilitch M. Optimal resources for implantable cardiac pacemakers: Pacemaker Study Group. *Circulation* 1983;68:226A.
6. Smyth NPD. Cardiac pacing. *Ann Thorac Surg* 1979;37:270.
7. Parsonnet V, Bernstein AD, Lindsay B. Pacemaker implantation complication rates: an analysis of some contributing factors. *J Am Coll Cardiol* 1989;13:917.
8. Littleford PO, Spector SD. Device for the rapid insertion of permanent endocardial pacing electrode through the subclavian vein: preliminary report. *Ann Thorac Surg* 1979;27:265.
9. Smyth NPD. Pacemaker implantation: surgical techniques. *Cardiovasc Clin* 1983;14:31.
10. Netter FH. *Atlas of human anatomy*. West Caldwell, NJ: Ciba Geigy Medical Education, 1992:174–176, 186, 200, 201.
11. Gray H, Pick TP, Howden RE. *1901 Edition: anatomy, descriptive and surgical*. Philadelphia: Running Press, 1974:609.
12. Byrd C. Current clinical applications of dual-chamber pacing. In: Zipes DP, ed. *Proceedings of a symposium*. Minneapolis: Medtronics, 1981:71.
13. Netter FH. *The Ciba collection of medical illustrations*, vol 5. Heart. Summit, NJ: Ciba Medical Education Division, 1981:22–26.
14. Furman S. Venous cutdown for pacemaker implantation. *Ann Thorac Surg* 1986;41:438.
15. Feiesen A, Kelin GJ, Kostuck WJ, et al. Percutaneous insertion of a permanent transvenous pacemaker electrode through the subclavian vein. *Can J Surg* 1977;10:131.
16. Littleford PO, Spector SD. Device for the rapid insertion of permanent endocardial pacing electrodes through the subclavian vein: preliminary report. *Ann Thorac Surg* 1979;27:265.
17. Littleford PO, Parsonnet V, Spector SD. Method for rapid and atraumatic insertion of permanent endocardial electrodes through the subclavian vein. *Am J Cardiol* 1979;43:980.
18. Miller FA Jr, Homes DR Jr, Gersh BJ, Maloney JD. Permanent transvenous pacemaker implantation via the subclavian vein. *Mayo Clin Proc* 1980;55:309.
19. Belott PH, Byrd CL. Recent developments in pacemaker implantation and lead retrieval. In: Barold SS, Mugica J, eds. *New perspectives in cardiac pacing 2*. Mt Kisco, NY: Futura Publishing, 1991:105–131.
20. Stokes K, Staffeson D, Lessar J, et al. A possible new complication of the subclavian stick: conductor fracture. *Pacing Clin Electrophysiol* 1987;10:748.
21. Fyke FE III. Simultaneous insulation deterioration associated with side by side subclavian placement of two polyurethane leads. *Pacing Clin Electrophysiol* 1988;11:1571.
22. Fyke FE III. Infraclavicular lead failure: tarnish on a golden route. *Pacing Clin Electrophysiol* 1993;16:445.
23. Jacobs DM, Fink AS, Miller RP, et al. Anatomical and morphological evaluation of pacemaker lead compression. *Pacing Clin Electrophysiol* 1993;16:373.
24. Magey JE, Flynn DM, Parsons JA, et al. Anatomical mechanisms explaining damage to pacemaker leads, defibrillator leads, and failure of central venous catheters adjacent to the sternoclavicular joint. *Pacing Clin Electrophysiol* 1993;16:445.
25. *Subclavian venipuncture reconsidered as a means of implanting endocardial pacing leads*. Angleton, TX: Issues Intermedics, December, 1987:1–2.
26. Subclavian puncture may result in lead conductor fracture. *Medtronic News* 1986–1987;16:27.
27. Byrd CL. Safe introducer technique for pacemaker lead implantation. *Pacing Clin Electrophysiol* 1992;15:262.
28. Nichalls RWD. A new percutaneous infraclavicular approach to the axillary vein. *Anesthesia* 1987;42:151.
29. Taylor BL, Yellowlees I. Central venous cannulation using the infraclavicular axillary vein. *Anesthesiology* 1990;72:55.
30. Magney JE, Staplin DH, Flynn DM, et al. A new approach to percutaneous subclavian needle puncture to avoid lead fracture or central venous catheter occlusion. *Pacing Clin Electrophysiol* 1993;16:2133.
31. Belott PH. Blind percutaneous axillary venous access. *Pacing Clin Electrophysiol* 1998;21:873.
32. Varnagy G, Velasquez R, Navarro D. New technique for cephalic vein approach in pacemaker implants. *Pacing Clin Electrophysiol* 1995;18:1807.
33. Spencer W III, Kirkpatrick C, Zhu DWX. The value of venogram-guided percutaneous extrathoracic subclavian venipuncture for lead implantation. *Pacing Clin Electrophysiol* 1996;19:700.
34. Spencer W III, Zhu DWX, Kirkpatrick C, et al. Subclavian venogram as a guide to lead implantation. *Pacing Clin Electrophysiol* 1998;21:499.
35. Ramza BM, Rosenthal L, Hui R, et al. Safety and effectiveness of placement of pacemaker and defibrillator leads in the axillar vein guided by contrast venography. *Am J Cardiol* 1997;80:892.
36. Fyke FE III. Doppler-guided extrathoracic introducer insertion. *Pacing Clin Electrophysiol* 1995;18:1017.
37. Gayle DD, Bailey JR, Haistey WK, et al. A novel ultrasound-guided approach to the puncture of the extrathoracic subclavian vein for surgical lead placement. *Pacing Clin Electrophysiol* 1996;19:700.
38. Nash A, Burrell CJ, Ring NJ, Marshall AJ. Evaluation of an ultrasonically guided venipuncture technique for the placement of permanent pacing electrodes. *Pacing Clin Electrophysiol* 1998;21:452.
39. Lamas GA, Fish DR, Braunwald NS. Fluoroscopic technique of subclavian venous puncture for permanent pacing: a safer and easier approach. *Pacing Clin Electrophysiol* 1987;11:1398.
40. Higano ST, Hayes DL, Spittell PC. Facilitation of the subclavian-introducer technique with contrast venography. *Pacing Clin Electrophysiol* 1992;15:731.
41. Belott PH. Implantation techniques—new developments. In: Barold SS, Mugica J, eds. *New perspectives in cardiac pacing*. Mt Kisco, NY: Futura Publishing, 1988:258–259.
42. Bognolo DA. Recent advances in permanent pacemaker implantation techniques. In: Barold SS, ed. *Modern cardiac pacing*. Mt Kisco, NY: Futura Publishing, 1985:206–207.

43. Parsonnet V, Werres R, Atherly T, et al. Transvenous insertion of double sets of permanent electrodes. *JAMA* 1980;243:62.
44. Bognolo PA, Vijayanagar RR, Eckstein PR, et al. Two leads in one introducer technique for A-V sequential implantation. *Pacing Clin Electrophysiol* 1982;5:217.
45. Vander Salm TJ, Haffajee CI, Okike ON. Transvenous insertion of double sets of permanent electrodes through a single introducer: clinical application. *Ann Thorac Surg* 1981;32:307.
46. Belott PH. A variation on the introducer technique for unlimited access to the subclavian vein. *Pacing Clin Electrophysiol* 1981;4:43.
47. Gessman LJ, Gallagher JD, MacMillan RM, et al. Emergency guide wire pacing: new methods for rapid conversion of a cardiac catheter into a pacemaker. *Pacing Clin Electrophysiol* 1984;7:917.
48. Ong LS, Barold S, Lederman M, et al. Cephalic vein guide wire technique for implantation of permanent pacemakers. *Am Heart J* 1987;114:753.
49. August DA, Elefteriades JA. Technique to facilitate open placement of permanent pacing leads through the cephalic vein. *Ann Thorac Surg* 1986;42:112.
50. Furman S. Venous cutdown for pacemaker implantation. *Ann Thoracic Surg* 1986;41:438.
51. Furman S. Subclavian puncture for pacemaker lead placement. *Pacing Clin Electrophysiol* 1986;9:467.
52. Belott PH. *A practical approach to permanent pacemaker implantation.* Mt Kisko, NY: Futura Publishing, 1995:59.
53. Sutton R, Bourgeois I. *The foundations of cardiac pacing, part I: an illustrated practical guide to basic pacing.* Mt Kisko, NY: Futura Publishing, 1991:235–243.
54. Barrold SS, Mugica J. *Recent advances in cardiac pacing: goals for the 21st century.* Mt Kisko, NY: Futura Publishing, 1998:213–231.
55. Bognolo DA, Vijaranagar RR, Eckstein PF, Janss B. Method for reintroduction of permanent endocardial pacing electrodes. *Pacing Clin Electrophysiol* 1982;5:546.
56. Bognolo DA, Vijay R, Eckstein P, Jeffrey D. Technical aspects of pacemaker system upgrading procedures. *Clin Prog Pacing Electrophysiol* 1983;1:269.
57. Belott PH. Use of the contralateral subclavian vein for placement of atrial electrodes in chronically VVI paced patients. *Pacing Clin Electrophysiol* 1983;6:781.
58. Parsonnet V. A stretch fabric pouch for implanted pacemakers. *Arch Surg* 1972;105:654.
59. Said SA, Bucx JJ, Stassen CM. Failure of subclavian venipuncture: the internal jugular vein as a useful alternative. *Int J Cardiol* 1992;35:275.
60. Roelke M, Jackson G, Hawthorne JW. Submammary pacemaker implantation: a unique tunneling technique. *Pacing Clin Electrophysiol* 1994;17:1793.
61. Ellestad MH, French J. Iliac vein approach to permanent pacemaker implantation. *Pacing Clin Electrophysiol* 1989;12:1030.
62. Antonelli D, Freedberg NA, Rosenfeld T. Transiliac vein approach to a rate-responsive permanent pacemaker implantation. *Pacing Clin Electrophysiol* 1993;16:1637.
63. Belott PH, Bucko D. Inframammary pulse generator placement for maximizing optimal cosmetic effect. *Pacing Clin Electrophysiol* 1983;6:1241.
64. Young D. Permanent pacemaker implantation in children: current status and future considerations. *Pacing Clin Electrophysiol* 1981;4:61.
65. Smith RT Jr. Pacemakers for children. In: Gillette PC, Garson A Jr, eds. *Pediatric arrhythmias: electrophysiology and pacing.* New York: Grune & Stratton, 1990:532–558.
66. Smith RT Jr, Armstrong K, Moak JP, et al. Actuarial analysis of pacing system survival in young patients. *Circulation* 1986;74[Suppl II]:120.
67. Gillette PC, Zeigler VL, Winslow AT, Kratz JM. Cardiac pacing in neonates, infants, and preschool children. *Pacing Clin Electrophysiol* 1992;15[Pt 2]:2046.
68. Guldal M, Kervancioglu C, Oral D, et al. Permanent pacemaker implantation in a pregnant woman with guidance of ECG and two-dimensional echocardiography. *Pacing Clin Electrophysiol* 1987;10:543.
69. Lau CP, Wong CK, Leung WH, et al. Ultrasonic assisted permanent pacing in a patient with severe pulmonary tuberculosis. *Pacing Clin Electrophysiol* 1989;12:1131.
70. Morris DC, Scott IR, Jamesson WR. Pacemaker electrode repositioning using the loop snare technique. *Pacing Clin Electrophysiol* 1989;12:996.
71. Westerman GR, Van Devanter SH. Transthoracic transatrial endocardial lead placement for permanent pacing. *Ann Thorac Surg* 1987;43:445.
72. Hayes DL, Vliestra RE, Puga FJ, et al. A novel approach to atrial endocardial pacing. *Pacing Clin Electrophysiol* 1989;12:125.
73. Byrd CL, Schwartz SJ. Transatrial implantation of transvenous pacing leads as an alternative to implantation of epicardial leads. *Pacing Clin Electrophysiol* 1990;13:1856.
74. Dosios T, Gorgogiannis D, Sakorafas G, et al. Persistent left superior vena cava: a problem in transvenous pacing of the heart. *Pacing Clin Electrophysiol* 1991;14:389.
75. Hussaine SA, Chalcravarty S, Chaikhouni A. Congenital absence of superior vena cava: unusual anomaly of superior systemic veins complicating pacemaker placement. *Pacing Clin Electrophysiol* 1981;4:328.
76. Ronnevik PK, Abrahamsen AM, Tollefsen J. Transvenous pacemaker implantation via a unilateral left superior vena cava. *Pacing Clin Electrophysiol* 1982;5:808.
77. Cha EM, Khoury GH. Persistent left superior vena cava. *Radiology* 1972;103:375.
78. Colman AL. Diagnosis of left superior vena cava by clinical inspection: a new physical sign. *Am Heart J* 1967;73:115.
79. Dirix LY, Kersscochot IE, Fiernen SH, et al. Implantation of a dual-chambered pacemaker in a patient with persistent left superior vena cava. *Pacing Clin Electrophysiol* 1988;11:343.
80. Giovanni QV, Piepoli N, Pietro Q, et al. Cardiac pacing in unilateral left superior vena cava: evaluation by digital angiography. *Pacing Clin Electrophysiol* 1993;14:1567.
81. Robbens EJ, Ruiter JH. Atrial pacing by unilateral persistent left superior vena cava. *Pacing Clin Electrophysiol* 1986;9:594.
82. Hellestrand KJ, Ward DE, Bexton RS, et al. The use of active fixation electrodes for permanent endocardial pacing via a persistent left superior vena cava. *Pacing Clin Electrophysiol* 1982;5:180.
83. Belott PH. Outpatient pacemaker procedures. *Int J Cardiol* 1987;17:169.
84. Dalvi B. Insertion of permanent pacemakers as a day case procedure. *Br Med J* 1990;300:119.
85. Hayes DL, Vliestra RE, Trusty JM, et al. Can pacemaker implantation be done as an outpatient? *J Am Coll Cardiol* 1986;7:199.
86. Hayes DL, Vliestra RE, Trusty JM, et al. A shorter hospital stay after cardiac pacemaker implantation. *Mayo Clin Proc* 1988;63:236.
87. Haywood GA, Jones SM, Camm AJ, et al. Day case permanent pacing. *Pacing Clin Electrophysiol* 1993;14:773.
88. Belott PH. Ambulatory pacemaker procedures: a 13-year experience. *Pacing Clin Electrophysiol* 1996;19:69.
89. Belott PH. Ambulatory pacemaker procedures. *Mayo Clin Proc* 1988;63:301.

90. Philip BK, Corvino BG. Local and regional anesthesia. In: Wetchler BV, ed. *Anesthesia for ambulatory surgery,* 2nd ed. Philadelphia: JB Lippincott, 1991:309–334.
91. Goldstin DJ, Losquadro W, Spotnitz HM. Outpatient pacemaker procedures in orally anticoagulated patients. *Pacing Clin Electrophysiol* 1998;21:1730.
92. Fishberger SB, Cammanas J, Rodriguez-Fernandez H, et al. Permanent pacemaker lead implantation via the transhepatic route. *Pacing Clin Electrophysiol* 1996;19:1124.
93. Moss AJ, Rivers RJ Jr. Atrial pacing from the coronary vein: ten-year experience in 50 patients with implanted pervenous pacemakers. *Circulation* 1978;57:103.
94. Greenberg P, Castellanet M, Messenger J, Ellestad MH. Coronary sinus pacing. *Circulation* 1978;57:98.
95. Hewitt MJ, Chen JTT, Ravin CE, Gallagher JJ. Coronary sinus atrial pacing: radiographic considerations. *Am J Radiol* 1981;136:323.
96. Levine PA, Balady GJ, Lazar HL, et al. Electrocautery and pacemakers: management of the paced patient subject to electrocautery. *Ann Thorac Surg* 1986;41:313.

CLINICAL TRIALS IN CARDIAC PACING

KENNETH A. ELLENBOGEN, MARK A. WOOD

Prospective clinical trials have become the cornerstone of clinical research in cardiology. The Thrombolysis in Myocardial Infarction (TIMI) and TAMI trials marked the beginning of the extension of clinical trial methodology on a large scale to the study of ischemic heart disease. Clinical trial methodology has been extended to cardiac pacing. The objectives of this chapter are to review the results of clinical trials enrolling patients with permanent cardiac pacemakers and to present the design and goals of ongoing clinical trials.

In the field of cardiac pacing, clinical research is largely focused in three different areas. The first is the effect of pacing mode on clinical outcomes such as survival, quality of life, congestive heart failure, and atrial fibrillation. A second focus of clinical research is the testing of different pacing algorithms and atrial pacing sites on the prevention of atrial fibrillation. A third area of research focuses on the use of alternate ventricular pacing sites to improve the exercise tolerance and quality of life in patients with congestive heart failure.

● CLINICAL TRIALS OF PACING MODE AND CLINICAL OUTCOMES

A large number of retrospective studies of pacing mode in patients have suggested that VVI pacing is associated with a higher incidence of atrial fibrillation, congestive heart failure, stroke, and death compared with physiologic pacing (e.g., AAI/AAIR or DDD/DDDR) (1–4). These retrospective studies have been criticized on the basis of their research methodology. Some of these studies, however, use fairly sophisticated statistical techniques for data analysis or clever study designs. For example, Sgarbossa and colleagues from the Cleveland Clinic performed a retrospective multivariate analysis of a large series of 507 patients with sick sinus syndrome with an average follow-up of 59 ± 38 months. They were able to show that VVI pacing was an independent predictor of stroke (relative risk [RR] = 2.61; $p = 0.008$) and chronic atrial fibrillation (RR = 1.98; $p = 0.003$) but not of congestive heart failure, cardiac mortality, or total mortality (5). Rosenqvist studied 168 patients from two separate centers; one center implanted all AAI pacemakers ($n = 89$), and the other center all VVI pacemakers ($n = 79$) (6). The baseline characteristics of the two patient groups were similar except for a lower age and less cardiomegaly in the patients who underwent AAI pacing. After 4 years, the group undergoing AAI pacing had a lower incidence of congestive heart failure, death, and chronic atrial fibrillation but not of stroke. Based on a retrospective chart review, Lamas demonstrated that Medicare beneficiaries receiving VVI pacemakers were older, sicker, poorer, and more likely to be women than patients receiving DDD pacemakers (7). In retrospective, nonrandomized studies there was likely bias in patient selection for different pacing modes, differences in therapy among patients with different pacing modes, and inconsistent follow-up. These limitations of retrospective trials stimulated the design of prospective clinical trials to assess the effect of pacing mode on mortality and morbidity (8,9). Despite more than 40 years of clinical pacing experience, fundamental questions such as the relative benefits of dual- or single-chamber pacing remain unresolved.

The first prospective, randomized trial of the effect of pacing mode on clinical outcomes was performed by Andersen and coworkers and initial results of this trial were published in 1994 (10). The trial design was a prospective, randomized trial enrolling 225 consecutive patients with sick sinus syndrome randomized to receive AAI ($n = 110$) or VVI ($n = 115$) single-chamber pacemakers. Patients were excluded from this trial (e.g., did not undergo AAI pacemaker implantation) if during pacemaker implantation 1:1 atrioventricular conduction was absent. The mean age of patients in this trial was 75.5 ± 8 years, and they were followed for a mean duration of 3.3 ± 1.5 years (range, up to 5 years). The primary end points of this study were atrial fibrillation, severity of congestive heart failure as judged by New York Heart Association (NYHA) classification and dose of diuretics, thromboembolism, and mortality. The initial report of the results of the Danish study showed an increased risk of thromboembolic events in patients with VVI pacemakers, but the frequency of other end points (e.g., mortality, congestive heart failure, atrial fibrillation) did not reach significance. Multivariate analysis showed that ventricular pacing was the only variable associated with an increased risk of thromboembolic events ($p = 0.039$), and tachycardia-bradycardia syndrome was the only variable associated with a significantly increased incidence of developing chronic atrial fibrillation during follow-up ($p = 0.016$).

Extended follow-up of the Danish trial was published in 1997 (11). The final duration of follow-up was 5.5 ± 2.4 years, with some patients assessed for up to 8 years. End points were the same as for the earlier reported follow-up, except the investigators also reported the incidence of atrioventricular block. At long-term follow-up, atrioventricular block occurred in only four patients in the AAI-paced group (0.6% annual risk) (12). The Wenckebach block point and atrioventricular conduction intervals as measured from the atrial pacing stimulus to the QRS complex remained stable. The cumulative risks of atrial fibrillation (documented on the 12-lead electrocardiogram during follow-up), chronic atrial fibrillation, thromboembolic events, cardiovascular death, and NYHA class of congestive heart failure and diuretic use were all decreased in patients with AAI pacing (Figs. 31-1 and 31-2). In multivariate analysis, atrial pacing was significantly associated with freedom from thromboembolic events (RR reduction = 47%; 95% CI, 0.24–0.92; $p = 0.028$) and survival from cardiovascular death (RR reduction = 52%; 95% CI, 0.30–0.91; $p = 0.022$) but not with freedom from chronic atrial fibrillation (RR reduction = 45%; 95% CI, 0.20–1.05; $p = 0.063$) or with better overall survival (RR reduction = 71%; 95% CI, 0.46–1.08; $p = 0.11$) (13,14).

This small trial underscores the importance of continued long-term follow-up of pacemaker patients enrolled in mode trials. Many of the important differences discovered were not observed until long-term follow-up, suggesting a potential detrimental effect for VVI pacing. This observation has prompted two large clinical trials (Mode Selection Trial [MOST] and Canadian Trial of Physiologic Pacing [CTOPP]) to propose extended follow-up of patients. The mechanism of this long-term increased risk of congestive heart failure and atrial fibrillation is presumed to be related to atrial remodeling caused by VVI pacing.

The Danish group has embarked on a follow-up study to answer the question of the importance of the physiologic pacing mode (15). The cause of the deleterious effect of ventricular pacing is unknown, but multiple mechanisms may play a role (16). Ventricular pacing leads to changes in cardiac blood flow, ventricular activation sequence, ventricular diastolic function, and alteration in neurohumoral agents (17, 18). It is unclear whether the deleterious effects of ventricular pacing may also occur with DDD pacing. Andersen and colleagues have initiated a prospective, multicenter randomized trial of AAI versus DDD

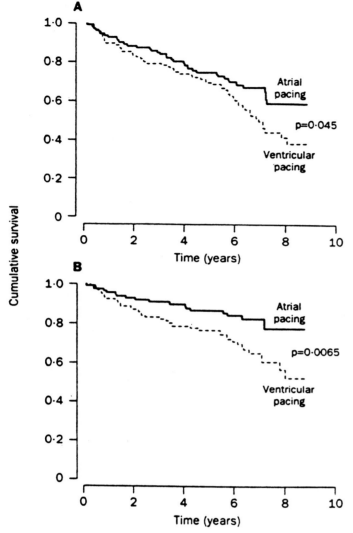

FIGURE 31-1. Kaplan-Meier survival plots of overall survival (A) and of survival from cardiovascular death (B). (From Andersen HR, Nielsen JC, Thomsen PEB, et al. Long-term follow-up of patients from a randomised trial of atrial versus ventricular pacing for sick sinus syndrome. *Lancet* 1997;350:1210–1216, with permission.)

pacing in sick sinus syndrome (the DANPACE trial). This trial is a national study involving all implanting centers in Denmark. A total of 1,900 patients will be randomized to AAIR or DDDR pacing. The major end point is total mortality. The study has been designed for a mean follow-up time of 5.5 years. The study result is expected to be available in 2008, and already more than 100 patients are enrolled (Henning Rud Andersen, Skejby University Hospital, Aarhus, Denmark: personal communication, 2000).

Mattioli and associates published the results of a study of 210 patients with no prior history of atrial fibrillation or stroke (19,20). Patients were randomized to receive physiologic pacing (AAI/DDD/DDDR/VDD) or single-chamber VVI/VVIR pacing for high-degree atrioventricular block ($n = 100$) or sick sinus syndrome ($n = 110$). Clinical characteristics were similar in the two patient groups. In this trial, all patients underwent computed tomography (CT) scan of the brain before study enrollment and

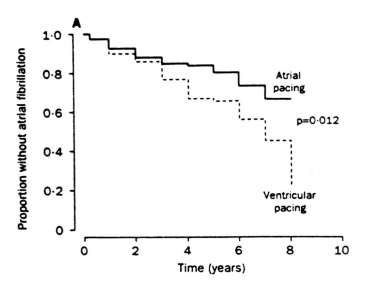

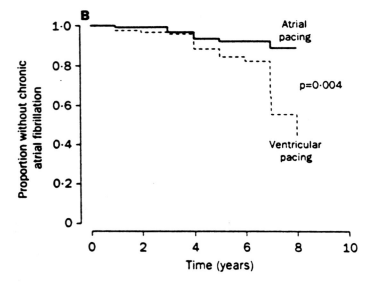

FIGURE 31-2. Kaplan-Meier plots of freedom from atrial fibrillation (A) and chronic atrial fibrillation (B) during follow-up. (From Andersen HR, Nielsen JC, Thomsen PEB, et al. Long-term follow-up of patients from a randomised trial of atrial versus ventricular pacing for sick sinus syndrome. *Lancet* 1997;350:1210–1216, with permission.)

then again after 12 and 24 months. The mean age of patients studied was 79 ± 9 years. The overall incidence of atrial fibrillation was 10% at 1 year, 11% at 2 years, 23% at 3 years, and 31% at 5 years. The incidence of chronic atrial fibrillation was higher in patients with VVI pacemakers ($p < 0.05$). The actuarial incidence of stroke was 15% at 1 year and 25% at 2 years. Nineteen of 105 patients with VVI pacing developed stroke, compared with 10 of 105 with physiologic pacing ($p < 0.05$). The risk of cerebral infarction was higher in patients with sick sinus syndrome; 9 of 100 atrioventricular block patients versus 20 of 110 sick sinus syndrome patients, $p < 0.05$. The investigators did not perform multivariate analysis, but univariate analysis showed that stroke was associated with ventricular pacing, mitral regurgitation, sick sinus syndrome, and left ventricular dysfunction. The CT scan showed cerebral ischemia in 12 patients without symptoms. A major limitation to this study is the inclusion of VDD pacemakers, which made up 21% of the pacemakers in patients who underwent physiologic pacing. Inclusion of these patients is problematic as it becomes difficult to evaluate these patients as "physiologically paced" when atrial pacing may be absent some of the time and VVI pacing at the lower rate may occur intermittently in some of these patients with sinus bradycardia.

Lamas and colleagues reported the results of the Pacemaker Selection in the Elderly (PASE) trial, a randomized, prospective, single-blind trial evaluating the effect of pacing mode on the quality of life in elderly patients (21). This study was a multicenter trial enrolling patients older than 65 who required pacemaker implantation for symptomatic bradycardia. All patients underwent implantation of a DDDR pacemaker and at the time of implant were randomized to VVIR ($n = 204$) or DDDR ($n = 203$). The PASE trial enrolled 407 patients, with a mean age of 76 years who were followed for a mean duration of 2.5 years. After initial quality-of-life measurements before pacemaker implantation, follow-up interviews took place at 3, 9, and 18 months of follow-up, as well as at the conclusion of the study. The primary end point was quality of life measured by the 36-item Medical Outcomes Study Short-Form General Health Survey (SF-36) and the Specific Activity Scale. The prespecified end points were death from all causes, first nonfatal stroke or death, first hospitalization for heart failure, development of atrial fibrillation, and development of pacemaker syndrome. Twenty-six percent of patients underwent crossover from VVIR to DDDR primarily for pacemaker syndrome. During follow-up at 3 and 9 months, quality of life was not different between the two pacing modes. At the 18-month follow-up visit, dual-chamber pacing was associated with a significant and sustained benefit in quality of life, which was even more marked for patients with sick sinus syndrome compared with patients with atrioventricular block. For patients with sick sinus syndrome, there was a trend toward a lower combined secondary end point ($p = 0.07$) of stroke, hospitalization for heart failure, or death from any cause. Sick sinus syndrome patients also demonstrated a trend toward a lower incidence of atrial fibrillation with dual-chamber pacing ($p = 0.06$). A major weakness of this trial is the small sample size to detect differences in clinical events (secondary end points) and the high rate of crossover from VVIR to DDDR.

The MOST trial (Mode Selection Trial) is a large multicenter prospective, randomized trial assessing DDDR versus VVVIR pacing for patients with sick sinus syndrome taking place at 100 centers in the United States. The patients will be followed for 1.5 to 2 years, although plans are being made to extend follow-up by at least 1 more year. The enrollment of 2,000 patients was completed in 1999, and follow-up continues. The primary end points are death and stroke, with secondary end points including quality of life, cost effectiveness, total mortality, cardiovascular mortality, total mortality for stroke or heart failure requiring hospitalization, heart failure score, health status in women and the elderly, and occurrence of pacemaker syndrome. The results of this trial are anticipated to be available in 2001 or 2002.

Another large, multicenter trial that has presented results is the CTOPP trial (Canadian Trial of Physiologic Pacing). This trial compares physiologic pacing (AAI/AAIR or DDD/DDDR to VVIR) with respect to its effect on cardiovascular death and stroke. To avoid increases in regional health care budgets, the proportion of VVI to physiologic pacemakers implanted was chosen from one of five ratios by the participating center: 67 : 33, 60 : 40, 50 : 50, 40 : 60, and 33 : 67. A total of 2,568 patients with sick sinus syndrome (37%), atrioventricular block (51%), or both (8%) or other indications for bradycardia pacing were enrolled in this study. Secondary end points were all-cause mortality, atrial fibrillation lasting for more than 15 minutes, and hospitalization for congestive heart failure. The mean age of patients in this trial was 73 years. The trial completed enrollment in 1998, and results were recently published (22). Overall, there was no significant difference between the group with physiologic pacing and the group with ventricular pacing with respect to primary end points, all-cause mortality, or hospitalization for congestive heart failure. There was a significant reduction in the annual risk of atrial fibrillation in the patients with physiologic pacing (RR reduction 19%; 95% CI, 1.4–32.9; $p = 0.034$). Comparison of the Kaplan-Meier curves for the risk of stroke or cardiovascular death showed a slight separation after 18 months, suggesting a possible delay in detrimental effects as seen in the Danish trial.

The United Kingdom Pacing and Cardiovascular Events (UKPACE) trial is an ongoing, large-scale, prospective, randomized trial designed to evaluate the all-cause mortality in a group of 2,000 patients older than age 70 who undergo implantation of a DDD (50%), VVI (25%), or VVIR (25%) pacemaker for high-grade atrioventricular block (23). Patients undergo evaluation with a quality-of-life assessment using the SF-36 and the EuroQoL EQ-5D questionnaires, 6-minute walk test, history, physical examination, and routine blood work. The patients are followed for a minimum of 3 years. The other outcome measures being assessed in this study are quality of life, exercise capacity, cardiovascular events, and cost utility. Substudies that are being undertaken include nuclear imaging to assess left ventricular function, Holter monitoring to record atrial arrhythmias, and more detailed analyses of quality of life and cognitive function.

The Rate Modulated Pacing and Quality of Life Study (RAMP) trial is a 38-center, prospective, randomized trial that compared DDD with DDDR pacemakers with respect to quality of life. In this study, 402 patients with sinus rhythm requiring a pacemaker for bradycardia underwent implantation with a Pacesetter (St. Jude Medical, Sylamar, CA) DDDR pacemaker with the sensor programmed to the passive mode. The primary end point is quality of life measured with the SF-36 and Specific Activity Scale questionnaires. Patients were randomized to DDD or DDDR after 1 month based on completion of an exercise test and reaching 60% of the maximum age predicted heart rate. Patient follow-up is for 2 years. The average age of patients was 72 years. The primary indication for pacemaker implantation was for sick sinus syndrome in about 40% and for atrioventricular block in about 50%.

The overall results from these trials are summarized in Tables 31-1 and 31-2.

TABLE 31-2 • PACING MODE TRIALS AND MORTALITY

Study	Total Mortality In VVI-Paced Patients	Total Mortality In Physiologically Paced Patients
Anderson	50%	35%
PACE (SSS)	20%	12%
CTOPP	20%	19%
PAC-A-TAC	6.8%	3.2%

SSS, sick sinus syndrome.

TABLE 31-1 • SUMMARY OF CLINICAL TRIALS OF PACING MODE

Study	Number Of Patients	Mean Age (years)	Diagnosis	Modes	Follow-up (months)	Status	Cross-overs (%)
Anderson (10,11)	225	76	SSS	VVI, AAI	66	Finished	1.7
PASE (21) (SSS)	175	76	Any brady	VVIR, DDDR	18	Finished	26
CTOPP	2,568	73	Any brady except CSH	VVI(R), DDD(R) or AAI(R)	36	Finished	<5
MOST	2,000	74	SSS	VVIR, DDDR	30	Finished	26
PAC-A-TACH (26)	198	72	SSS, tachy, brady	VVIR, DDDR	24	Finished	44
UK-PACE (23)	2,000	≥70	Second- or third-degree AV block	VVI, VVIR, DDD	50	Enrolling	<5

AV, atrioventricular; CSH, carotid sinus hypersensitivity; SSS, sick sinus syndrome.

STUDIES OF ATRIAL FIBRILLATION PREVENTION

A wide variety of studies are being undertaken to evaluate pacing for prevention of atrial fibrillation. We focus here on trials evaluating pacing from a single atrial site and the effect of different pacing algorithms and pacing modes. Available elsewhere (24) is a review of biatrial pacing for prevention of atrial fibrillation and more information on alternate atrial sites for pacing prevention of atrial fibrillation.

The Atrial Pacing Peri-Ablation of Atrial Fibrillation (PA3) trial is a multicenter Canadian trial comparing the effect of rate adaptive atrial pacing to prevent paroxysmal atrial fibrillation in the absence of symptomatic bradycardia (25). This trial has two phases. Phase I tests the effect of atrial pacing on patients without a symptomatic bradycardia or other indication for pacing. This phase tests the effect of atrial pacing on the frequency or duration of episodes of atrial fibrillation. Phase II was designed to compare the effects of DDDR versus VDD pacing on time to first recurrence of paroxysmal atrial fibrillation, intervals between consecutive episodes of atrial fibrillation, and frequency and duration of atrial fibrillation after atrioventricular junction ablation. Patients with paroxysmal atrial fibrillation who were intolerant of, or resistant to antiarrhythmic drug therapy, underwent implantation of a DDDR pacemaker 3 months before a planned atrioventricular junction ablation. Between 40% and 50% of patients had no structural heart disease. One third of patients were taking amiodarone, and 28% to 48% of patients were taking other antiarrhythmic agents. Ninety-seven patients were enrolled in this trial and underwent implantation of a Thera DR pacemaker (Medtronic, Minneapolis, Minnesota). They were then randomized to no pacing (DDI at 30 bpm) or atrial pacing (DDIR at 70 bpm). After a 2-week stabilization period, they were followed for an additional 10 weeks. Patients randomized to atrial pacing were paced about 63% of the time in the atria. Time to first episode of paroxysmal atrial fibrillation and the time between the first and second episodes of paroxysmal atrial fibrillation was similar in both groups, but the paroxysmal atrial fibrillation burden was lower in the no-pacing group. Ambulatory monitoring revealed that atrial pacing reduced the frequency of supraventricular premature beats from 3.8 to 0.5 per hour ($p < 0.01$), but this frequency remained unchanged in the no-pacing group. A small cohort of 11 patients who crossed over to a trial of atrial pacing after completing the 3-month phase in the no-pacing limb had an increase in their paroxysmal atrial fibrillation burden and shorter time to first episode of paroxysmal atrial fibrillation with atrial pacing. The results of this trial highlight the fact that atrial pacing in patients without bradycardia may suppress premature atrial beats but does not have a beneficial effect on paroxysmal atrial fibrillation burden, time to first episode of atrial fibrillation, and time to subsequent episodes of atrial fibrillation (Figs. 31-3 and 31-4).

The Pacemaker Modality on Atrial Tachyarrhythmia Recurrence in the Tachycardia-Bradycardia Syndrome (PAC-A-TACH) trial is a multicenter trial that prospectively evaluated the effect of DDDR ($n = 100$) and VVIR ($n = 98$) pacing modes on fre-

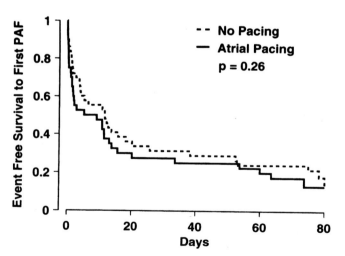

FIGURE 31-3. Event-free survival to first episode of sustained paroxysmal atrial fibrillation (PAF) in patients randomized to no-pacing therapy (*dashed line*, n = 48) or to atrial-pacing therapy (*solid line*, n = 49). Analysis was performed on the basis of intention to treat. (From Gillis AM, Wyse DG, Connolly SJ, et al. Atrial pacing periablation for prevention of paroxysmal atrial fibrillation. *Circulation* 1999;99:2553–2558, with permission.)

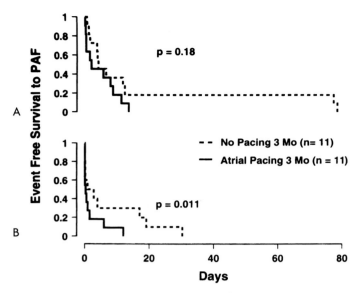

FIGURE 31-4. A: Event-free survival to first episode of sustained paroxysmal atrial fibrillation (PAF) in 11 patients who completed a trial of no-pacing therapy *(dashed line)* and then completed a trial of atrial-pacing therapy *(solid line)*. **B:** Event-free survival between the first and second episodes of PAF in 11 patients who completed at trial of no pacing *(dashed line)* and then a trial of atrial pacing *(solid line)*. (From Gillis AM, Wyse DG, Connolly SG, et al. Atrial pacing periablation for prevention of paroxysmal atrial fibrillation. *Circulation* 1999; 99:2553–2558, with permission.)

quency of atrial tachyarrhythmias in patients with tachycardia-bradycardia syndrome (26). The trial has concluded, and preliminary results were presented at the American Heart Association meeting in November 1998. The median age was 72 years; 55% were men, and 37% had coronary artery disease, and 55% had hypertension. The primary end point was the development of atrial tachyarrhythmias, and secondary end points were death, pacemaker syndrome, congestive heart failure, stroke, embolic events, and quality of life. After a median follow-up of almost 24 months, crossover from VVIR to DDDR occurred in 44% of patients, for most because of recurrent atrial tachyarrhythmias (13%) or pacemaker syndrome (28%). There was no statistically significant difference in recurrence of atrial tachyarrhythmias based on the intention to treat analysis (48% for DDDR versus 43% for VVIR). An unexpected and difficult to explain finding was the observation that mortality was signifi-

cantly decreased in the DDDR pacing group (6.8% versus 3.2%, $p = 0.007$).

Two other published trials deserve mention. Preliminary results from the Prevention of Atrial Arrhythmias by Overdriving and the Rest Rate (PROVE) trial were presented in August 1999 (27). The purpose of the PROVE study is to evaluate the effect of overdrive pacing and the lower programmed heart rate on the frequency of atrial arrhythmias in patients selected for pacemaker implantation. This trial included 39 patients, about two thirds with sick sinus syndrome or tachycardia-bradycardia syndrome and one third with atrioventricular block. All patients undergo pacemaker implantation (Chorum or Talent, Ela Medical, Montrouge, France) and undergo a 1-month phase of monitoring to identify the number of atrial arrhythmias at baseline. Mean age of patients was 72 years. About one half of the patients had a previous history of atrial arrhythmias, and about one half were taking antiarrhythmic drugs. Patients are then classified as class I patients if they have at least two atrial fibrillation episodes and class II patients are all other patients. There were 14 class I patients and 25 class II patients in this trial. Class I patients were programmed with a base rate of 60 bpm or to an atrial overdrive rate of 10 bpm above the mean atrial rate with the automatic rest rate being activated and the rate responsive mode enabled. Class II patients are programmed with a higher base rate of 70 bpm or a standard DDDR programming of 60 bpm. Within each group, the two pacemaker settings are applied in random order. The number of atrial arrhythmias was reduced by 58% and the total duration of episodes by 72% with atrial overdrive pacing in class I patients. In class II patients the number of atrial arrhythmias was too small to make a conclusion about the different algorithms. The statistical power of this study is too low to make definitive conclusions about atrial overdrive pacing. The second trial was also a small trial comparing biatrial pacing, right atrial pacing, and no pacing in patients with drug refractory atrial fibrillation (28). Nineteen patients with a mean age of 64 years and with at least three documented episodes of symptomatic atrial fibrillation in the previous year who were refractory to antiarrhythmic therapy underwent pacemaker implantation for arrhythmia prevention as the sole indication (84%) or for an additional clinically accepted indication. The number of atrial fibrillation episodes and their durations were obtained from the pacemaker memory. Comparison of the control period with right atrial pacing or no pacing showed a significant decrease in the duration of atrial fibrillation from 27 ± 35 days to 11 ± 27 days ($p = 0.04$), with no effect on the number of atrial fibrillation episodes (control at 79 ± 108 versus right atrial at 41 ± 80, $p = 0.11$). In this trial, pacing was at a base rate of 70 bpm (no pacing was a base rate of 40 bpm), and the right atrially paced group was paced $62 \pm 33\%$ of the time.

The Systematic Trial of Pacing to Prevent Atrial Fibrillation (STOP-AF) is a prospective, randomized trial of pacing mode in patients with sick sinus syndrome using the sequential trial design (29). The primary end point is reduction in the incidence of paroxysmal atrial fibrillation and chronic atrial fibrillation. Secondary end points include congestive heart failure, pacemaker syndrome, change of mode because of lead problems, and death. Enrollment is anticipated to be 350 patients. Sample size will be adjusted using sequential trial methodology. In this trial, all patients receive DDD pacemakers and then are randomized to receive VVI pacing (VDD with an atrioventricular delay of 300 msec to use atrial diagnostics) or DDD pacing. Prior atrial fibrillation is not a contraindication to enrollment, and 45% of patients have a history of prior atrial fibrillation. Those with chronotropic incompetence will be randomized separately to rate responsive features programmed ON. Patients will be followed for 2 years. Two substudies will analyze the effects of pacing mode on quality of life and cost benefit. Predictors of the development of atrial fibrillation will also be studied. A second trial studying this question is now being performed in patients with dual chamber ICDs.

Another study sponsored by Guidant (St. Paul, Minnesota) examines the effect of varying the lower rate limit of dual-chamber pacemakers in patients with bradycardias and a history of paroxysmal atrial fibrillation through the use of stored electrograms and an arrhythmia log book. The trial is designed to measure the effect of atrial pacing at two different rates on the frequency and duration of atrial fibrillation. The end points of this trial are the frequency, time to occurrence, and the burden of atrial fibrillation. Patients will be randomized to a lower rate of 60 or 80 bpm. Patients are seen at 1, 3, and 6 months. All patients will complete a 6-month follow-up visit. Enrollment is occurring at 30 centers and will include about 200 patients.

The Atrial Dynamic Overdrive Pacing Trial (ADOPT) (St. Jude Medical) is designed to investigate whether DDDR pacing at 60 ppm with the Dynamic Atrial Overdrive (DAO) pacing algorithm can prevent episodes of symptomatic atrial fibrillation more effectively than DDDR pacing at a base rate of 60 ppm in this group of patients. Patients will be enrolled who have symptomatic paroxysmal or persistent atrial fibrillation and sinus node dysfunction with one or more American College of Cardiology and American Heart Association Class I bradycardia pacing indications. All patients (a minimum of 226) receive a St. Jude Medical device incorporating the DAO algorithm. The patients are prospectively randomized to either DAO ON or DAO OFF for a six month period. The dynamic atrial overdrive algorithm prevents atrial fibrillation by providing an atrial pacing rate at or just above the intrinsic sinus rate, while at the same time allowing the sinus rate to demonstrate circadian patterns. In the presence of atrial extrasystoles, the algorithm would prevent the pause that commonly follows premature beats by pacing at a faster rate to help reduce the incidence of ectopy. In the presence of a stable atrial rhythm, the algorithm should pace the atrium only slightly faster than the intrinsic rhythm, and as that rate increases or decreases, the pacemaker will track this by modifying its rate. The primary end point of the study is to determine whether the algorithm decreases the number of episodes of symptomatic atrial fibrillation recorded with a patient-activated event recorder. Secondary end points include time to recurrence of atrial fibrillation, number of atrial fibrillation episodes documented by the mode switch algorithm in the pulse generator, total duration of mode switches, need for electrical or pharmacologic cardioversion, patient well-being as measured by the SF-36 quality-of-life questionnaire, and hospital admissions. A summary of atrial fibrillation trials is found in Tables 31-3 and 31-4.

TABLE 31-3 • CLINICAL TRIALS IN ATRIAL FIBRILLATION

Characteristic	PA3 (25)	PAC-A-TACH (26)	Lévy et al. (28)	PROVE (27)	STOP-AF (29)
Study design	Effect of atrial pacing on PAF episodes before and after AVJ ablation	Evaluate pacing mode for prevention of recurrent AF	Effect of pacing on recurrent, symptomatic, drug-refractory AF	Effect of atrial overdrive pacing and base rate on AF recurrence	Prospective, randomized, sequential trial of atrial-based pacing to prevent AF
Patient age	61	72	64	72	73
Number of patients	97	198	19	39	210 (350 expected)
Follow-up	10 weeks	24 months	6 months	6 months	2 years
Pacing modes	DDI (30 bpm) vs. DDIR (70 bpm)	DDDR vs. VVIR	DDD (40 bpm) vs. DDD (70 bpm)	DDDR with different base rates and overdrive algorithm	AAI(R), DDD(R) vs. VDD(R) with AV = 300 msec
Pacing indication	PAF	Tachy-brady syndrome	Refractory AF in 90%	SSS (SVT 50%) AV block in 50%, 50% with prev. AF and AAD	SSS
Comments	No difference in AF frequency or duration with atrial pacing	44% crossover rate; no difference in AF between DDDR and VVIR	Pacing at 70 bpm decreased duration but not frequency of AF	Overdrive pacing and automatic rest rate decreases AF frequency & duration	Trial in progress

AF, atrial fibrillation; AVJ, atrioventricular junction; PA3, Atrial Pacing Peri-Ablation of Atrial Fibrillation trial; PAC-A-TACH, Pacemaker Modality on Atrial Tachyarrhythmia Recurrence in the Tachycardia-Bradycardia Syndrome trial; PAF, paroxysmal atrial fibrillation; PROVE, Prevention of Atrial Arrhythmias by Overdriving and the Rest Rate trial; STOP-AF, Systematic Trial of Pacing to Prevent Atrial Fibrillation.

TABLE 31-4 • VARIABLES IN ATRIAL FIBRILLATION PACING TRIALS

Patient populations selected
   Paroxysmal atrial fibrillation with bradycardia
   Paroxysmal atrial fibrillation without bradycardia: sick sinus syndrome, atrioventricular block, tachycardia-bradycardia
Pacing modes
Pacing algorithms
   Overdrive pacing
   Other algorithms (e.g., prevent pauses)
Lower pacing rate
Site of atrial pacing
   Single site; atrial appendage vs. interatrial septum or Bachman's bundle
   Dual site
Episodes of sustained atrial fibrillation vs. episodes of nonsustained, self terminating atrial fibrillation
Frequency of episodes of atrial fibrillation; interepisode duration
Total duration or "burden" of atrial fibrillation
Premature atrial contractions or atria extrasystoles frequency

● CLINICAL TRIALS OF PACING AND CONGESTIVE HEART FAILURE PATIENTS

Much excitement has been generated by the observations of markedly improved hemodynamics in patients undergoing acute left ventricular and biventricular pacing in patients with dilated cardiomyopathy and bundle branch block. The history of pacing for congestive heart failure goes back to the 1980s, when a number of small, nonrandomized, noncontrolled studies suggested that DDD pacing (ventricular pacing site in the right ventricular apex) with short atrioventricular intervals may be of hemodynamic benefit in patients with dilated cardiomyopathy (30,31). These small, nonrandomized studies enrolled selected patients with cardiomyopathy, implanted pacemakers and followed the patients' clinical course. The potential placebo effect of pacemaker implantation and the simultaneous administration of other medical therapies to these patients made interpretation of patient outcome difficult (32). The variable natural history of cardiomyopathy patients could not be accounted for if all patients underwent pacemaker therapy. Two small, randomized trials of DDD pacing with short atrioventricular intervals failed to show any benefit to conventional pacing with short atrioventricular intervals (33,34).

Alternate sites of pacing to improve cardiac performance have become the focus of clinical interest in pacing trials in congestive heart failure. A variety of small trials in patients with right ventricular outflow tract (RVOT) pacing with single- or dual-chamber pulse generators have failed to demonstrate conclusively whether RVOT pacing is beneficial (35–40). Several acute studies showed an improvement in stroke volume and cardiac index with RVOT pacing compared with right ventricular apical (RVA) pacing (35–38). The completed long-term randomized trials of RVOT pacing are inconclusive at the present primarily as a result of small sample size (38,39).

The Right Ventricular Outflow versus Apical Pacing in Pacemaker Patients with Congestive Heart Failure and Atrial Fibrillation (ROVA) trial is a prospective, paired, case-crossover study to determine whether pacemaker recipients with chronic atrial fibrillation, congestive heart failure (NYHA class II or III), and left ventricular systolic dysfunction (LVEF <40%) will have better quality of life during VVIR pacing from the RVOT compared with the RVA. A secondary end point is left ventricular function measured by two-dimensional echocardiography and exercise performance. Patients must be more than 90% paced in the right ventricle as determined by telemetry. Patients are left in each pacing mode for 6 months and have a 3-month stabilization period. The study size is 150 patients, and 97 patients are already enrolled.

Acute hemodynamic trials of pacing from other sites in addition to the right ventricular apex and outflow tract have suggested "resynchronization" of the right and left ventricle by simultaneously pacing from the right ventricular apex and the left ventricle or only the left ventricle is associated with hemodynamic benefit (40–42). These trials have shown a wide variety of beneficial hemodynamic responses, including decreased mitral regurgitation, and improvement in physiologic parameters, including cardiac output, LV + dP/dT, pulse pressure, stroke volume, pulmonary capillary wedge pressure, and diastolic filling time. Preliminary results of several uncontrolled trials also suggest improved health status and NYHA improvement in functional class (41–44).

Follow-up from one initial European and Canadian multicenter trial of 96 patients with multisite pacing has been presented. The InSync study examined the safety and efficacy of a multisite pacemaker in 96 patients with NYHA class III or IV congestive heart failure, QRS duration of more than 150 msec, LVEF of less than 35%, left ventricular end-diastolic diameter of more than 60 mm, and absence of clinical improvement in heart failure despite stable, standard medical treatment for 1 month. Patients were followed with quality-of-life questionnaires, echocardiograms, and 6-minute walk tests. A transvenous left ventricular lead was placed through the coronary sinus. Over a 10-month period, the system was implanted successfully in 68 of 81 patients enrolled in the study. Initial clinical results showed improvement in NYHA functional class, quality of life, and 6-minute walk test (45). Additional follow-up was reported in August 1999. Mortality and follow-up was reported after a mean of 4 months, with some patients followed for up to 491 days after implantation. The survival was 82% at 6 months and improvements in NYHA functional class, quality of life, and 6-minute walk test in patients being paced was still evident. All patients were paced, and there was no placebo or no-pacing portion of this study (46).

Based on these exciting early results, several large, prospective, randomized, multicenter trials in pacing for congestive heart failure are in progress. One of the earliest trials of pacing in congestive heart failure was a trial performed from June 1995 through December 1998, the Pacing Therapies for Congestive Heart Failure (PATH-CHF) trial using univentricular and biventricular stimulation therapy (47). In this study, left ventricular pacing was performed through a thoracotomy to put the epicardial lead on the left ventricle. Forty-two patients from seven clinical sites were enrolled in the PATH-CHF trial. Patients were followed during each of four randomization periods. This multicenter prospective trial used a randomized crossover design evaluating two pacing modes over a 12-week period. The initial randomization scheme included two arms: one with univentricular pacing and the second with biventricular pacing. After 4 weeks of treatment, the devices were programmed OFF for 4 weeks. After this 4-week period, patients were then again programmed to pacing for another 4 weeks. The crossover arm is implemented during this phase. For patients previously programmed to univentricular pacing, they were programmed to biventricular pacing and *vice versa* for the other randomization arm. The primary end points are oxygen consumption, 6-minute walk test, quality-of-life score, LVEF, and NYHA classification. Patient enrollment criteria were dilated cardiomyopathy of idiopathic or ischemic origin, NYHA class III or IV, sinus rhythm, QRS duration of more than 120 msec, and PR interval longer than 150 msec.

VIGOR-CHF is a study of pacing therapy of patients with congestive heart failure being conducted at 25 centers with projected enrollment of up to 162 patients (48). The trial uses a sequential analysis consisting of two 6-week therapy phases (total, 12 weeks) and an additional therapy mode for 6 weeks until the 18-week visit. The purpose of the trial is to examine the effectiveness of biventricular pacing for improvement of congestive heart failure functional status. Patients are randomized to the VDD (atrial sensing, biventricular pacing) mode during phase I and II or to a no-pacing mode (ODO) in phase I and VDD pacing mode during phase II. Short-term (6-week) and long-term (18-week) data will be collected, and all patients will complete an identical follow-up schedule. The 18-week visit concludes the intensive evaluation phase of the study, after which investigators may program the pacemaker to the mode they feel will best help the patient. This study design allows for evaluation of a placebo effect, as has been observed in patients with hypertrophic cardiomyopathy after pacemaker implantation. End points are the clinical outcomes as measured by cardiopulmonary exercise testing using bicycle ergometry, 6-minute walk test, echocardiographic evaluation of chamber size, and quality of life. The primary end point is peak oxygen uptake during maximal exercise. Each patient will act as his or her own control. Patient enrollment criteria include symptomatic NYHA class II through IV congestive heart failure, sinus rhythm with a rate greater than 55 bpm, QRS complex duration $\geq$ 120 msec, PR interval or more than 160 msec, and a LVEF of less than 30%.

The VENTAK CHF/CONTAK CD is a multicenter trial with a prospective, randomized, two-phase crossover design to evaluate the efficacy of biventricular pacing to improve the functional status of congestive heart failure in patients indicated for an ICD. Initially, left ventricular pacing was performed with an epicardial lead and later from a transvenous approach through the coronary sinus. This study is being conducted at 35 centers and has enrolled 248 patients. All patients will receive optimal conventional therapy for congestive heart failure and ICD therapy. All patients are randomized after a 1-month stabilization period. During the initial phase, Treatment A consists of no pacing (VVI at 40 bpm), and Treatment B consists of biventricular therapy using the VDD mode. Patients will be randomized to either arm for 3 months. Crossover to the other arm will occur during the second period. After both periods are completed, programmed therapy is left to the discretion of the investigator. Enrollment criteria are similar to VIGOR CHF and include the presence of symptomatic NYHA class II through IV congestive heart failure, LVEF $\leq$ 35%, QRS complex duration $\geq$ 120 msec, and a clinically accepted indication for ICD implantation. Baseline and therapy follow-up consists of quality-of-life assessment, 6-minute walk test, cardiopulmonary exercise test, echocardiogram, measurement of neurohormonal levels, and 24-hour Holter monitoring. The primary end point of this trial is oxygen uptake with cardiopulmonary exercise testing. Secondary end points include quality of life, biventricular antitachycardia pacing efficacy and defibrillation therapy safety.

Another proposed study using the Guidant endocardial pacing system is the Comparison of Medical Therapy, Pacing, and Defibrillation in Congestive Heart Failure (COMPANION) study. This trial will enroll up to 2,200 patients at up to 80 United States centers and have a 1-year follow-up period. This trial is a multicenter, prospective, randomized, 1:2:2 design. Patients are randomized to one of three arms: optimal pharmacologic therapy of congestive heart failure, optimal pharmacologic therapy of congestive heart failure and biventricular pacing therapy with ICD support, or optimal pharmacologic therapy and biventricular pacing therapy without ICD support. The purpose of this study is to evaluate the long-term clinical benefits of biventricular stimulation in patients with symptomatic heart failure. The primary end point will be a composite of all cause mortality and all cause hospitalization, and secondary end points include cardiac morbidity and all cause mortality alone. Patient inclusion criteria are similar to those of the other trials described previously.

The Multicenter InSync Randomized Clinical Evaluation (MIRACLE) trial is a heart failure trial sponsored by Medtronic, and it is designed to evaluate biventricular pacing. Patient enrollment is expected to be between 225 and 300 patients from up to 41 investigative centers. Candidates for this study are patients with a QRS duration longer than 130 msec, LVEF greater than 35%, left ventricular end-diastolic dimension larger than 55 mm, NYHA class III or IV congestive heart failure, and no accepted indication for bradycardia pacing. Patients must be on a stable medical regimen for at least 1 month before enrollment. The medical regimen must include diuretics and angiotensin-converting enzyme (ACE) inhibitors or ACE inhibitor substitutes. The study design is a prospective, multicenter, randomized, double-blind, parallel-controlled clinical trial. After baseline evaluation that includes 6-minute hall walk test, quality-of-life assessment, cardiopulmonary exercise testing per modified Naughton protocol, and neurohormonal measurements, patients undergo implantation of a triple chamber pacemaker using the Medtronic transvenous Attain left ventricular lead system. Patients are randomized to the therapy arm (VDD at a lower rate of 30 bpm) or the control arm VDI at 30 bpm within 3 days after implantation. Patients are randomized to VDD or VDI for 6 months. After 6 months, all patients are programmed to VDD and will be followed in that mode for the remainder of the study. The primary end points of this trial are improved patient functional status as measured by quality of life, NYHA classification, and 6-minute hall walk test. Secondary objectives include measurement of synchrony of ventricular activation as determined by the QRS width on the surface electrocardiogram, functional capacity as assessed by cardiopulmonary testing, echocardiographic indices of cardiac function and dimensions, plasma neurohormones (i.e., BNP, aldosterone, renin, catecholamines, tumor necrosis factor, endothelin, cyclic GNP), patient survival, and health care use.

Two ongoing studies of left ventricular pacing are being supported by St. Jude Medical. The PAVE (Left Ventricular-based Cardiac Stimulation Post AV Node Ablation Evaluation) study is designed to compare cardiac function and clinical status associated with a variety of ventricular pacing sites including RV apex, left ventricle via a cardiac vein and biventricular. This will involve a total of 650 patients all of whom will have chronic atrial fibrillation and high grade atrioventricular block following AV nodal ablation with patients randomized to one of the ventricular pacing therapies. The primary endpoints will include functional ability as measured with the distance walked during the 6-minute walk test and a Quality of Life assessment using the Physical Component Study of the SF-36 instrument.

The other study is VecToR (VEntriCular Resynchronization Therapy Randomized Trial) is designed to evaluate the effect of resynchronization therapy utilizing biventricular pacing on cardiac function and clinical status in a series of 450 patients with congestive heart failure. All patients will be implanted with a biventricular dual-chamber pacing system (Frontier 3 x 2 pulse generator with left ventricle pacing accomplished using the Aescula left ventricle lead) and then be prospectively randomized to either resynchronization therapy ON or OFF. Study endpoints will include exercise capacity as measured by the distance walked in the 6-minute walk test, 6 month mortality and health related Quality of Life as assessed with the Minnesota Living with Heart Failure instrument. The design and goals of these trials are to provide clear objective evidence of pacing benefit in dilated cardiomyopathy and to help determine which patients are most likely to gain long-term benefit from pacing (49,50) (Tables 31-5 and 31-6).

TABLE 31-5 • RANDOMIZED CLINICAL TRIALS ENROLLING HEART FAILURE PATIENTS

Trial Characteristics	Miracle	Re-Le-Vent	Vigor CHF	Companion
Number of patients	225–300	>224	162	2,000
End point 1	Functional status (QOL, NYHA, 6-minute walk test)	Mortality	CPT testing (peak O_2 consumption)	Mortality
End point 2	CPT testing, echo, aldosterone, renin, BNP, catecholamines, health care utilization, survival	LV EDD, LV ESD, 6-minute walk test, QOL, hospitalization for CHF	6-minute walk test, echo, catecholamines, QOL	Hospitalization for CHF, morbidity
Therapy	VDD or VDI (no pacing)	No pacing, LV pacing, BiV pacing	VVDD vs. ODO for 6 weeks	Medical Rx; medical Rx + BiV pacing + ICD, Medical Rx + BiV pacing
Follow-up	6 months	>6 months	18 weeks	1 year

BiV, biventricular pacing; CHF, congestive heart failure; CPT, cardiopulmonary testing; echo, echocardiography; ICD, implantable cardioverter-defibrillator; LV, left ventricular pacing; NYHA, New York Heart Association; QOL, quality of life; Rx, therapy.

TABLE 31-6 • END POINTS IN CLINICAL TRIALS OF PACING FOR CARDIOMYOPATHY

New York Heart Association functional class
Change in number or dosage of heart failure medications
Cardiac mortality
Total mortality
Quality of life-measured by a variety of tests, surveys, questionnaires
Exercise duration, exercise capacity on treadmill with oxygen uptake analysis
Atrial fibrillation, stroke, thromboembolic events
Neurohumoral measurements—atrial natriuretic peptide, BNP, catecholamines, tumor necrosis factor, endothelin, aldosterone, plasma renin, cyclic GNP
Health care use; hospitalization, emergency room, and cardiology department visits
Six-minute walk test
Echocardiographic measurements—degree of mitral regurgitation, left ventricular chamber size, left ventricular end-diastolic diameter, left ventricular function, fractional shortening

ACKNOWLEDGMENTS

We acknowledge manuscript review by Charles Kerr, M.D., Gervasio A. Lamas, M.D., Paul A. Levine, M.D., Peggy Theisen Malikowski, R.N., M.S., Kenneth M. Riff, M.D., M.S.E.E., and Regina Rogers, R.N.

REFERENCES

1. Barlow M, Kerr CR, Connolly SJ. Survival, quality-of-life, and clinical trials in pacemaker patients. In: Ellenbogen KA, Kay GN, Wilkoff B, eds. *Clinical cardiac pacing and implantable cardiac defibrillators*, 2nd ed. Philadelphia: WB Saunders, 1999.
2. Tang CY, Kerr CR, Connolly SJ. Recent clinical trials of pacing mode selection. In: Ellenbogen KA, ed. *Update in cardiac pacing. Cardiology clinics*. Philadelphia: WB Saunders, 2000.
3. Barold SS, Santini M. Natural history of sick sinus syndrome after pacemaker implantation. In: Barold SS, Mugica J, eds. *New perspectives in cardiac pacing 3*. Mt Kisco, NY: Futura Press, 1993: 169–211.
4. Connolly SJ, Kerr C, Gent M, Yusuf S. Dual-Chamber versus ventricular pacing: critical appraisal of current data. *Circulation* 1996;94:578–583.
5. Sgarbossa EB, Pinski SL, Maloney JD, et al. Chronic atrial fibrillation and stroke in paced patients with sick sinus syndrome: relevance of clinical characteristics and pacing modalities. *Circulation* 1993;88:1045-—1053.
6. Rosenqvist M, Brandt J, Schuller H. Long-term pacing in sinus node disease: effects of stimulation mode on cardiovascular morbidity and mortality. *Am Heart J* 1988;116:16–22.

7. Lamas GA, Pashos CL, Normand S-LT, McNeil B. Permanent pacemaker selection and subsequent survival in elderly Medicare pacemaker recipients. *Circulation* 1995;91:1063–1069.
8. Lamas GA. Pacemaker mode selection and survival: a plea to apply the principles of evidence based medicine to cardiac pacing practice. *Heart* 1997;78:218–220.
9. Ovsycher IE, Hayes DL, Furman S. Dual-Chamber pacing is superior to ventricular pacing: fact or controversy? *Circulation* 1998;97:2368–2370.
10. Andersen HR, Thuesen L, Bagger JP, et al. Prospective randomised trial of atrial versus ventricular pacing for sick sinus syndrome. *Lancet* 1994;344:1523–1528.
11. Andersen HR, Nielsen JC, Thomsen PE, et al. Long-term follow-up of patients from a randomised trial of atrial versus ventricular pacing for sick sinus syndrome. *Lancet* 1997;350:1210–1216.
12. Andersen HR, Nielsen JC, Thomsen PEB, et al. Atrioventricular conduction during long-term follow-up of patients with sick sinus syndrome. *Circulation* 1998;98:1315–1321.
13. Nielsen JC, Andersen HR, Thomsen PEB, et al. Heart failure and echocardiographic changes during long-term follow-up of patients with sick sinus syndrome randomized to single-chamber atrial or ventricular pacing. *Circulation* 1998;97:987–995.
14. Andersen HR, Nielsen JC, Thomsen PEB, et al. Arterial thromboembolism in patients with sick sinus syndrome: prediction from pacing mode, atrial fibrillation, and echocardiographic findings. *Heart* 1999;81:412–418.
15. Andersen HR, Nielsen JC. Pacing in sick sinus syndrome—need for a prospective, randomized trial comparing atrial with dual chamber pacing. *Pacing Clin Electrophysiol* 1998;21:1175–1179.
16. Ellenbogen KA, Gilligan DM, Wood MA, Morillo CA. Should every patient with high-grade AV block have a DDD device? In: Rosenqvist M, ed. *Cardiac pacing: new advances*. London: WB Saunders, 1997:191–206.
17. Lee MA, Dae MW, Langberg JJ, et al. Effects of long-term right ventricular apical pacing on left ventricular perfusion, innervation, function and histology. *J Am Coll Cardiol* 1994;24:225–232.
18. Tse H, Lau C. Long-term effect of right ventricular pacing on myocardial perfusion and function. *J Am Coll Cardiol* 1997;29:744–749.
19. Mattioli AV, Vivoli D, Mattioli G. Influence of pacing modalities on the incidence of atrial fibrillation in patients without prior atrial fibrillation. *Eur Heart J* 1998;19:282–286.
20. Mattioli AV, Castellani ET, Vivoli D, et al. Prevalence of atrial fibrillation and stroke in paced patients without prior atrial fibrillation. *Clin Cardiol* 1988;21:117–122.
21. Lamas GA, Orav EJ, Stambler BS, et al. Quality of life and clinical outcomes in elderly patients treated with ventricular pacing as compared with dual-chamber pacing. *N Engl J Med* 1998;338:1097–1104.
22. Connolly SJ, Kerr CR, Gent M, et al. Effect of physiologic pacing versus ventricular pacing the risk of stroke and death due to cardiovascular cause. *N Engl J Med* 2000;342:1385–1391.
23. Toff WD, Skehan JD, de Bono DP, et al. The United Kingdom Pacing and Cardiovascular Events (UKPACE) trial. *Heart* 1997;78:221–223.
24. Saksena S, Mehra R, Ellenbogen KA. Pacing for the prevention of tachyarrhythmias. In: Ellenbogen KA, Kay GN, Wilkoff BL, eds. *Clinical cardiac pacing and implantable cardioverter defibrillators*. Philadelphia: WB Saunders, 2000.
25. Gillis AM, Wyse DG, Connolly SJ, et al. Atrial pacing periablation for prevention of paroxysmal atrial fibrillation. *Circulation* 1999;99:2553–2558.
26. Wharton JM, Sorrentino RA, Campbell P, et al. Effect of pacing modality on atrial tachyarrhythmia recurrence in the tachycardia-bradycardia syndrome: preliminary results of the pacemaker atrial tachycardia trial [Abstract]. *Circulation* 1998;98[Suppl I]:I-494.
27. Funck RC, Capucci A, Kappenberger L, et al. Prevention of atrial arrhythmias by overdriving and the rest rate; preliminary results from the PROVE study. *Eur Heart J* 1999;20:5A.
28. Lévy T, Walker S, Rochelle J, et al. Evaluation of biatrial pacing, right atrial pacing, and no pacing in patients with drug refractory atrial fibrillation. *Am J Cardiol* 1999;84:426–429.
29. Charles RG, McComb JM. Systematic Trial of Pacing to Prevent Atrial Fibrillation (STOP-AF). *Heart* 1997;78:224–225.
30. Hochleitner M, Hortnagl H, Ng C-K, et al. Usefulness of physiologic dual-chamber pacing in drug-resistant idiopathic cardiomyopathy. *Am J Cardiol* 1990;66:198–202.
31. Brecker SJ, Xiao HB, Sparrow J, et al. Effects of dual-chamber pacing with short atrioventricular delay in dilated cardiomyopathy. *Lancet* 1992;340:1308–1311.
32. Linde C, Gadler F, Kappenberger L, et al. Placebo effect of pacemaker implantation in obstructive hypertrophic cardiomyopathy. *Am J Cardiol* 1999;83:903–907.
33. Linde C, Gadler F, Edner M, et al. Results of atrioventricular synchronous pacing with optimized delay in patients with severe congestive heart failure. *Am J Cardiol* 1995.75:919–923.
34. Gold MR, Feliciano Z, Gottlieb SS, et al. Dual-chamber pacing with a short atrioventricular delay in congestive heart failure: a randomized study. *J Am Coll Cardiol* 1995;26:967–973.
35. Buckingham TA, Candinas R, Schlapfer J, et al. Acute hemodynamic effects of atrioventricular pacing at differing sites in the right ventricle individually and simultaneously. *Pacing Clin Electrophysiol* 1997;20:909–915.
36. Giudici M, Thornburg G, Buck D, et al. Comparison of right ventricular outflow tract and apical lead permanent pacing on cardiac output. *Am J Cardiol* 1997;79:209–212.
37. Barold S, Linhart J, Hildner F, et al. Hemodynamic comparison of endocardial pacing of outflow and inflow tracts of the right ventricle. *Am J Cardiol* 1969;23:697–701.
38. De Cock C, Meyer A, Kamp O, et al. Hemodynamic benefits of right ventricular outflow tract pacing: comparison with right ventricular apex pacing. *Pacing Clin Electrophysiol* 1998;21:536–541.
39. Schwab B, Frohlig F, Alexander C, et al. Influence of right ventricular stimulation site on left ventricular function in atrial synchronous ventricular pacing. *J Am Coll Cardiol* 1999;33:317–323.
40. Victor F, Leclercq C, Mabo P, et al. Optimal right ventricular pacing site in chronically implanted patients: a prospective randomized crossover comparison of apical and outflow tract pacing. *J Am Coll Cardiol* 1999;33:311–316.
41. Blanc JJ, Etienne Y, Gilard M, et al. Evaluation of different ventricular pacing sites in patients with severe heart failure: results of an acute hemodynamic study. *Circulation* 1997;96:3272–3277.
42. Etienne Y, Mansourati J, Gilard M, et al. Evaluation of left ventricular based pacing in patients with congestive heart failure and atrial fibrillation. *Am J Cardiol* 1999;83:1138–1140.
43. Auricchio A, Stellbrink C, Block M, et al. Effect of pacing chamber and atrioventricular delay on acute systolic function of paced patients with congestive heart failure. *Circulation* 1999;99:2993–3001.
44. Leclercq C, Cazeau S, le Breton H, et al. Acute hemodynamic effects of biventricular DDD pacing in patients with end-stage heart failure. *J Am Coll Cardiol* 1998;32:1825–1831.
45. Gras D, Mabo P, Tang T, et al. Multisite pacing as a supplemen-

tal treatment of congestive heart failure: preliminary results of the Medtronic, Inc., InSync study. *Pacing Clin Electrophysiol* 1998;21[Pt II]:2249–2255.

46. Tang A, Gras D, Mabo P, et al. Mortality evaluation in the InSync trial of cardiac resynchronization for heart failure [Abstract]. *Eur Heart J* 1999;20:3.

47. Aurichchio A, Stelbrink C, Sack S, et al. The Pacing Therapies for Congestive Heart Failure (PATH-CHF) study: rationale, design and endpoints of a prospective randomized multicenter study. *Am J Cardiol* 1999;83[Suppl 5B]:130D–135D.

48. Saxon LA, Boehmer JP, Hummel J, et al. Biventricular pacing in patients with congestive heart failure: two prospective randomized trials. *Am J Cardiol* 1999;83[Suppl 5B]:120D–123D.

49. Daubert C, Cazeau S, Leclercq C, et al. Outcome of patients chronically implanted with biventricular pacing systems for end stage congestive heart failure [Abstract]. *Pacing Clin Electrophysiol* 1997;20:1103.

50. Luttikhius HO, Gras D, Mabo P, et al. Long term performance of a transvenous system for atrio-biventricular pacing in patients with dilated cardiomyopathy and congestive heart failure [Abstract]. *Eur Heart J* 1999;20:579.

NEW AND EVOLVING INDICATIONS FOR CARDIAC PACING

S. SERGE BAROLD

Several new indications for pacing have emerged in the past decade (1–6). New indications for patients without conduction system disease include obstructive hypertrophic cardiomyopathy (OHCM), end-stage dilated cardiomyopathy with drug-refractory congestive heart failure (CHF), and orthostatic hypotension. With organic or functional conduction system disease, a very long PR interval (with unfavorable hemodynamic consequences), and neurally mediated (malignant vasovagal) syncope also constitute new indications for pacing. Pacing for malignant vasovagal syncope is discussed in Chapter 33.

◉ OBSTRUCTIVE HYPERTROPHIC CARDIOMYOPATHY

Many studies have shown that dual chamber pacing can be effective therapy for symptomatic relief in patients with OHCM (7–32) (Table 32-1). All these studies are observational except for three relatively small, controlled, crossover, randomized trials (18,23,27,30). Single-chamber right ventricular (RV) pacing is contraindicated because loss of atrioventricular synchrony in patients with left ventricular (LV) diastolic dysfunction results in hemodynamic compromise with decreased ventricular filling and increased left atrial and pulmonary capillary wedge pressures (33).

Acute Studies

Acute hemodynamic studies have shown that most patients develop a significant drop in the resting left ventricle outflow tract (LVOT) gradient during DDD pacing with an optimal (short) atrioventricular delay (8,9,17,19,34,35). The acute hemodynamic response during pacing studies does not reliably predict which patients will benefit from long-term DDD pacing, and such studies are generally no longer recommended (36). A few patients in most series demonstrated no hemodynamic improvement with temporary pacing (9,34,35,37,38). However, some of these patients improve on a long-term basis (35), suggesting that factors other than paradoxical septal motion, such as cellular and molecular modification of the myocardium, account for the hemodynamic changes. In some cases, lack of acute hemodynamic benefit may be caused by failure to achieve ventricular depolarization because of a short spontaneous PR interval.

TABLE 32-1 • WORLD-WIDE RESULTS OF DUAL-CHAMBER PACING IN 401 PATIENTS WITH OBSTRUCTIVE HYPERTROPHIC CARDIOMYOPATHY

Study	Center	No.	NYHA Before	NYHA After	LV Outflow Gradient Before	LV Outflow Gradient After	Exercise Duration (min) Before	Exercise Duration (min) After	Follow-up (mo)
McDonald et al (7)	Ireland	11	3	1.5	43	?	7.7	10.1	24
Jeanrenaud et al (9)	Switzerland	7	—	—	67 ± 42	17 ± 10	—	—	44 ± 11
Fananapazir et al (12)	NIH, Bethesda	84[a]	3.2 ± 0.5	1.6 ± 0.6	96 ± 41[b]	27 ± 31	5.3 ± 2.7	7.2 ± 2.8	26 ± 9
Gras et al (14)	France	30	3.2 ± 0.5	1.4 ± 0.5	112 ± 31	19 ± 12	—	—	34 ± 14
Yusvinkevich et al (15)	Russia	17	3.3 ± 0.9	1.6 ± 1.1	73 ± 39	38 ± 34	10.9 ± 4.4	12.9 ± 3.6	3
Umman et al (16)	Turkey	5	2.6 ± 0.5	1.6 ± 0.5	78 ± 20	42 ± 17	—	—	2.2 ± 3
Nishimura et al (18)	Mayo Clinic	19	2.9 ± 0.4	2.4 ± 0.7	76 ± 61	55 ± 38	5.7 ± 2.7	6.9 ± 2.2	3
Gambhir et al (17)	India	12	3	?	94 ± 29	39 ± 15	—	—	?
Slade et al (19)	England/France/Poland	56[c]	2.8 ± 0.5	1.7 ± 0.7	78 ± 31	36 ± 25	—	—	11 ± 11
Gadler et al (20)	Sweden	19	2.8 ± 0.4	1.8 ± 0.5	22 ± 6 (98 ± 31)[d]	(42 ± 26)[d]	—	—	12 ± 9
Gadler et al (20)	Sweden	22	3.0 ± 0.6	1.9 ± 0.5	86 ± 40	36 ± 24	—	—	12 ± 9
Sadoul et al (21)	France	16	—	—	79 ± 21	24 ± 17	—	—	18.7 ± 9.5
Kappenberger et al (23)[e]	Switzerland (PIC study)	83	Angina 1.4 Dyspnea 2.4	0.7 1.0	71 ± 62	28 ± 23	—	—	12
Sakai et al (25)	Japan	9	—	—	96	17	—	—	6
Iliou et al (26)	France	11	3.0 ± 0.4	2.3 ± 0.3	39 ± 19	14 ± 7	—	—	12

LV, left ventricular; No., number of patients in the study; NYHA, New York Heart Association.
[a] Seventy-four patients had resting obstruction, and 10 patients had provocable obstruction only.
[b] Gradients in patients with resting obstruction only.
[c] Two patients had provocable obstruction only.
[d] All patients had a provocable left ventricular outflow tract gradient, which is shown in parentheses.
[e] Double-blind study with the pacemaker turned OFF for 3 months.

Adapted from Fananapazir L, Atiga W, Tripodi D, et al. Therapy in obstructive hypertrophic cardiomyopathy: the role of dual chamber (DDD) pacing. In: Barold SS, Mugica J, eds. *Recent advances in cardiac pacing: goals for the 21st century.* Armonk, NY: Futura Publishing, 1998:35–50, with permission.

Permanent Pacing

Long-term pacing is beneficial in patients with drug-refractory OHMC with a resting gradient of ≥30 mm Hg or a provocable gradient of 30 to 50 mm Hg due to prominent basal septal hypertrophy (20,23,24). Reliable evaluation of pacemaker treatment is difficult because of the dynamic nature and variability of the LVOT gradient that occurs independently of the way it is measured. In 80% to 85% of patients with drug-refractory OHCM, permanent DDD pacing with a short atrioventricular interval (50 to 150 msec and often less than 100 msec) reduces symptoms (i.e., angina, dyspnea, presyncope, syncope and palpitations) and results in improvement of functional status (i.e., demonstrable by treadmill testing), long-term exercise capacity, and quality of life and reduction of pharmacotherapy (19,23). In most patients, the resting LVOT gradient eventually diminishes by about 50% during DDD pacing without significant alteration in blood pressure or cardiac output. There is no correlation between the magnitude of reduction of LVOT gradient and functional improvement (19, 23). In the absence of organic mitral valve abnormalities, DDD pacing reduces mitral regurgitation in parallel with reduction of LVOT gradient (39,40). Some studies have shown that acute pacing may cause deterioration of left ventricular diastolic function and increase in filling pressures (41–45). On a chronic basis, this does not seem to translate into a clinical problem despite the deterioration of certain indices of left ventricular diastolic function reported by some workers (43,46–50). Elderly patients seem to benefit from DDD pacing more than younger patients (51,52). However, about 10% of the patients with OHCM do not respond favorably to pacing, and about 10% may deteriorate. Significant mitral regurgitation caused by OHCM or left bundle branch block are not contraindications to DDD pacing.

Long-Term Pacing: Clinical Studies

Fananapazir and colleagues (8) (from NIH) first reported in 1992 the benefit of dual chamber pacing in 44 patients with OHCM refractory to verapamil and beta-adrenergic blocking drugs, and in 1994, they presented follow-up data on 84 patients; 74 patients had resting LVOT gradients greater than 30 mm Hg, and 10 patients had LVOT gradients greater than 55 mm Hg with provocation only (12). At a mean follow-up of 2.3 ± 0.8 years (maximum, 3.5 years), the New York Heart Association (NYHA) functional class improved ($p < 0.00001$) (Table 32-1). Symptoms were eliminated in 28 patients (33%), improved in 47 patients (56%), but remained unchanged in 7 patients (8%). Table 32-1 shows that pacing produced a significant drop in the mean LVOT gradient ($p < 0.00001$). In the patients with resting LVOT obstruction, the LVOT gradient was eliminated or insignificant in 65% and unchanged in 8%. Two patients died suddenly (97% cumulative 3-year survival rate). In both patients, symptoms and LVOT gradients had improved before sudden death. Symptoms and provocable LVOT gradients were also reduced in all 10 patients without significant resting, but provocable LVOT gradients. In the 84 patients, persistence of the LVOT gradient and symptoms were mostly related to an inability to preexcite the interventricular septum and onset of atrial fibrillation (12) (Table 32-2).

As documented in their 1992 report (8), Fananapazir and coworkers (12) demonstrated in follow-up cardiac catheterization studies a progressive reduction of the LVOT gradient during sinus rhythm compared with the baseline study during sinus rhythm when the pacemaker was turned off.

Jeanrenaud and associates (9) studied the chronic effects of pacing in OHCM in seven patients who received verapamil and beta blockers along with DDD pacemakers with an atrioventricular interval of 50 to 90 msec programmed to the optimal value (mean, 63 ± 18 msec) (Table 32-1). Observations were made at midterm (11 ± 10 months) and long-term (after 44 ± 11 months) follow-up. All seven patients had striking improvement, particularly with respect to angina. Dyspnea also improved, and two patients with previous syncope reported no further episodes. At the midterm assessment, the mean resting LVOT gradient during DDD pacing was 40 ± 31 mm Hg, rising to 65 ± 34 mm Hg when the pacemakers were switched off. The latter values during sinus rhythm were similar to those obtained during the acute baseline study. In contrast, Fananapazir and colleagues (8) observed a reduction of the resting

TABLE 32-2 • EXPLANATIONS FOR FAILURE OF DDD PACING TO IMPROVE SYMPTOMS OR TO RELIEVE LEFT VENTRICULAR OUTFLOW TRACT OBSTRUCTION

Inappropriate pacemaker programming
    Inadequate ventricular preexcitation: programmed AV delay too long
    Interference with left atrial emptying: programmed AV delay too short
Inadequate pacemaker trial period
Other Associated Abnormalities
    Proximal or high septal ventricular lead position
    Aberrant papillary muscle obstructing LV outflow
    Primary mitral valve regurgitation[a]
    Mid-cavity LV obstruction[b]
    Atrial and/or ventricular tachyarrhythmias
    LV diastolic dysfunction
    Inappropriate drug therapy

AV, atrioventricular; LV, left ventricular.
[a] The mitral valve regurgitation in obstructive hypertrophic cardiomyopathy may be primary and difficult to distinguish from severe mitral regurgitation due to systolic anterior motion of the mitral valve when the outflow obstruction is relieved.
[b] Pacing may relieve mid-cavitary obstruction.
From Fananapazir L, Atiga W, Tripodi D, et al. Therapy in obstructive hypertrophic cardiomyopathy: the role of dual chamber (DDD) pacing. In: Barold SS, Mugica J, eds. *Recent advances in cardiac pacing: goals for the 21st century.* Armonk, NY: Futura Publishing, 1998:35–50, with permission.

LVOT gradient as early as 6 weeks after pacemaker implantation during sinus rhythm when the pacemakers were switched off. However, in the study of Jeanrenaud and coworkers (9), at long-term follow-up, the mean resting LVOT gradient dropped to 17 ± 10 mm Hg during DDD pacing, significantly lower than at the midterm follow-up. When the pacemakers were switched off, the mean resting LVOT gradient rose to 31 ± 36 mm Hg, significantly lower than at the start of the study or the midterm follow-up evaluation (9).

A European double-blind, randomized study of DDD versus placebo AAI pacing (30 ppm) involving 83 patients with a resting LVOT gradient of more than 30 mm Hg clearly showed the benefit of DDD pacing (23). After 12 weeks, the pacing modes were inverted (i.e., crossover design) for another 12 weeks. Seventeen (20%) of 83 patients required early reprogramming from AAI to DDD because of persistent symptoms or deterioration. DDD significantly improved symptoms, quality of life, and exercise tolerance. The LVOT gradient fell from 59 ± 36 to 30 ± 25 mm Hg ($p < 0.001$) with DDD pacing. Seventy-nine (95%) of the 83 patients preferred DDD pacing. Subsequent follow-up of patients for 1 year showed that pacing was beneficial on pressure gradient and symptoms in 72 patients (87%) (29).

Therapeutic or Placebo Effect?

A placebo effect of pacing has been suggested by some workers (18,30). Baron and associates (30) conducted a prospective, randomized, double-blind, crossover study involving 48 patients with a LVOT gradient of 50 mm Hg or more. At 12 months, only 6 patients (12%) showed functional improvement, and most of these were in the 65- to 75-year-old group. The LVOT gradient decreased 40%. It was reduced in 57% of the patients and showed no change or an increase in 43%. There was no evidence of remodeling. Baron and colleagues (30) concluded that the perceived symptomatic improvement was consistent with a placebo effect. However, Linde and coworkers (28) showed that improvement was based on more than a placebo effect. They demonstrated that during inactive pacing there was a significant improvement in perceived chest pain, dyspnea, and palpitations associated with a statistically significant decrease of the LVOT gradient from 71 ± 32 to 52 ± 34 mm Hg. During active pacing, the perceived symptoms were similar, but there was improvement in alertness and "strenuous" exercise associated with a decrease of the LVOT gradient from 70 ± 24 to 33 ± 34 mm Hg.

Gadler and associates (27) analyzed the quality of life in patients from the Pacing in Cardiomyopathy (PIC) study to exclude a placebo effect during 1 year of follow-up. Patients were randomized to two study arms defining the sequence of pacemaker programming. In one arm, the pacemaker was inactive, and in the other, it was active. After 3 months, the pacemaker was reprogrammed to the alternate mode, and patients were followed for another 3 months. After this period, subsequent pacemaker programming corresponded to the mode preferred by the patient. A last assessment was made 1 year after baseline examinations. Eighty patients completed the first crossover period, and 75 completed the full 1 year of follow-up. Active pacing induced a significant improvement of 9% to 44% in the quality of life, regardless of programming sequence. Discontinuation of pacing after the first active period resulted in return of symptoms. Fourteen patients requested early reprogramming after having been programmed to inactive pacing after a first period of active pacing. Seventy-six patients preferred active pacing after the crossover period. Another 6 months of pacing induced progressive improvement in symptoms already favorably influenced.

Consequences of Prolonged Pacemaker Inactivation

Fananapazir and colleagues (46) evaluated the long-term (5.0 ± 0.7 years) results of DDD pacing therapy in 48 patients with OHCM and symptoms refractory to verapamil and beta blockers (mean age, 48 ± 15 years). The results are shown in Table 32-3. DDD pacing was switched off in six patients in whom the LVOT gradient had been reduced by more than 50% in sinus rhythm at the 5-year follow-up study. The bottom of Table 32-3 shows the results after another 6-month period without pacing during this period. It appears that left ventricular obstruction does not return in some patients after the pacemaker is switched off for a long time. This finding and the reduction in LVOT gradient recorded in sinus rhythm at the 5-year evaluation provide evidence of pacing-induced cardiac remodeling. In contrast, Gadler and coworkers (53) turned off the pacemakers of 10 patients successfully paced for 6 months or more and observed severe clinical deterioration in all of the patients. All required reactivation of pacing within 1 to 20 days. The LVOT gradient increased significantly, from 22 ± 21 to 47 ± 21 mm Hg, in all patients. The patients of Fananapazir and associates (46) exhibited a sustained reduction of the LVOT gradient possibly because they were studied after 5 years rather than about 6 months after pacemaker implantation.

Indications for Pacing

Implantation of dual-chamber pacing is relatively simple and seems to offer almost the same benefits as septal myectomy at lower cost and risk. It is not primary therapy and should not be considered as a replacement for drug therapy. Pacing allows augmentation of medical therapy with larger doses of drugs without concern for bradycardia. However, some patients may be able to discontinue drug therapy because pacing alone can produce striking clinical improvement (8). Pacing therapy should be weighed against the risk and efficacy of surgical left ventricular

TABLE 32-3 • FIVE-YEAR RESULTS OF DUAL-CHAMBER PACING IN OBSTRUCTIVE HYPERTROPHIC CARDIOMYOPATHY

		Sinus Rhythm			DDD Pacing		
Evaluation	NYHA	CO	PCW	LVG	CO	PCW	LVG
Pacing On[a]							
Baseline	3.1 ± 0.4	5.0 ± 1.1	15 ± 7	88 ± 51			
5 Years	1.7 ± 0.7	4.9 ± 1.0	13 ± 5	34 ± 39[b]	4.6 ± 1.1	13 ± 5	24 ± 30[b]
Pacing Off[c]							
Baseline	3.2 ± 0.4	5.0 ± 1.5	10 ± 4	71 ± 40			
5 Years	1.5 ± 0.6	4.9 ± 0.8	14 ± 4	14 ± 24[d]	5.0 ± 0.8	11 ± 3	12 ± 20[d]
6 Months	1.7 ± 0.8	4.7 ± 0.4	12 ± 3	18 ± 24[d]			

[a] The National Institutes of Health data included 48 patients with a mean age of 48 ± 15 years.
[b] $p < 0.0001$ compared with baseline.
[c] DDD pacing was switched off for 6 months at the 5-year follow-up for 6 patients.
[d] $p < 0.05$ compared with baseline.
From Fananapazir L, Tripodi D, McAreavey D. Five-year results of dual chamber pacing in obstructive hypertrophic cardiomyopathy patients with severe symptoms [Abstract]. *Pacing Clin Electrophysiol* 1998;21:791, with permission.

myectomy and percutaneous transcoronary septal myocardial ablation with ethanol injection into the first septal artery (i.e., chemical myectomy) (54–60). The latter procedure leads to pacing because of atrioventricular block in 15% to 20% of patients. There are no prospective, randomized studies comparing pacing with other therapeutic strategies.

The 1998 American College of Cardiology (ACC) and American Heart Association (AHA) guidelines for implantation of pacemakers (6) list medically refractory symptomatic hypertrophic cardiomyopathy with significant resting or provoked LVOT obstruction as a class IIb indication based on data from observational reports. Some workers believe that a class IIa designation would have been more appropriate, whereas others consider pacing controversial because favorable data were mostly derived from retrospective uncontrolled studies and the far less dramatic results obtained from three relatively small, randomized studies (54,55,58). The guidelines are vague on what constitutes a "significant resting or provoked gradient" in HOCM patients. As a rule, pacing should be considered only with a resting gradient ≥30 mm Hg and a provoked gradient ≥50 mm Hg (4).

Importance of Pacemaker Function and Programmability

The favorable response to pacing is closely tied to optimization of the atrioventricular interval (61).

Site of Ventricular Pacing

The ventricular lead must be positioned in the most distal part of the right ventricular apex. Pacing the proximal septum just beneath the tricuspid valve or high septal area produces no significant fall in the gradient (62,63). Lack of improvement sometimes necessitates repositioning of the RV pacing lead with the aid of echocardiographic imaging to ensure a distal apical position because fluoroscopy and electrocardiographic QRS configuration are imprecise markers of lead position.

Atrioventricular Interval

Dual-chamber pacemakers must be programmed with a short atrioventricular interval (occasionally as short as 50 msec) to avoid spontaneous ventricular depolarization and to ensure ventricular capture at all times to provide apical preexcitation.

The atrioventricular interval must therefore be carefully individualized. The optimal atrioventricular interval varies widely and has to be determined for each patient on the basis of Doppler-echocardiographic measurements, LVOT gradient, stroke volume, and parameters of the left ventricle filling such as transmitral flow and blood pressure (1,64). The atrial contribution to ventricular filling is crucial, and atrioventricular intervals that are too short may be deleterious (61,65,66). When the atrioventricular delay is too short, left ventricular diastolic filling becomes impaired despite a drop in the LVOT gradient, the left atrial pressure rises, and the cardiac output decreases.

The optimal paced atrioventricular delay may be significantly longer than the sensed atrioventricular delay (19). The optimal atrioventricular delay may occasionally vary with the passage of time and should be reevaluated at each follow-up visit.

The atrioventricular delay must be optimized at rest (and at several faster rates) and on effort. Patients must undergo a treadmill stress test to determine the optimal atrioventricular delay on exercise and whether they can maintain a paced ventricular rhythm at all times. The longest atrioventricular delay that achieves complete ventricular capture according to QRS configuration and duration may be inappropriate. An auto-adaptive atrioventricular interval that shortens automatically with exercise and acceleration of the atrial rate is important.

Negative atrioventricular interval hysteresis capability is designed to maintain full ventricular capture. The degree of shortening of AV nodal conduction during physiologic stress is not predictable. If the pacemaker senses spontaneous ventricular depolarization within the atrioventricular interval, it will automatically shorten the atrioventricular delay by a programmable value so that the atrioventricular delay becomes shorter than the Ap-Vs or As-Vs interval (67). A search function will ultimately restore the original atrioventricular delay if circumstances are appropriate.

When the PR interval is short, prolongation of

atrioventricular conduction by drugs or AV nodal radiofrequency catheter ablation may be useful to achieve the optimal atrioventricular interval to ensure pacemaker controlled ventricular depolarization in the absence of ventricular fusion (68–70). Ablation permits exclusive pacemaker activation of the left ventricle and longer, more flexible atrioventricular intervals to promote optimal left ventricular filling. Such an approach can produce significant improvement in patients who fail to benefit from pacing alone, even at short atrioventricular intervals.

Alternatively, the right and left atria can be paced simultaneously. Daubert and colleagues (71) used biatrial pacing (i.e., right atrial appendage and coronary sinus for left atrial stimulation) in conjunction with a DDD pacemaker in patients with OHCM with or without intraatrial or interatrial conduction delay. This arrangement of a triple-chamber pacemaker permits optimization of the mechanical atrioventricular delay on the left side of the heart. It allows shortening of the effective atrioventricular delay and avoids radiofrequency ablation to produce continual pacemaker controlled ventricular depolarization and pacemaker dependency.

Atrial Sensing

Atrial sensing is extremely important, and meticulous care must be taken at the time of implantation to ensure a good atrial signal. Atrial sensing should also be evaluated during exercise.

Polarity

Because patients can develop life-threatening ventricular tachyarrhythmias, a bipolar, dual-chamber pacemaker should be implanted on the right side in case a cardioverter-defibrillator (ICD) is required in the future. Such a pacemaker should be a dedicated bipolar device, and its reset to the VVI or VOO mode in response to electrical interference or battery depletion should always occur in the bipolar mode, because the unipolar mode may later interfere with detection of ventricular tachyarrhythmias if an ICD becomes necessary.

Rate-Adaptive Function

If cost is an issue, patients should be evaluated for atrial chronotropic incompetence, which is estimated to occur in about 30% of OHCM patients (72). Such patients would benefit from DDDR rather than less expensive DDD pacing (72). Ideally, all patients should receive a DDDR device because concurrent medications may blunt the atrial chronotropic response.

Automatic Mode Switching

Automatic mode switching is an important function. It prevents tracking of rapid atrial rates from atrial tachyarrhythmias, a common complication of OHCM.

Dual-Chamber Defibrillator Versus Pacemaker

Because the implantation procedure for a dual-chamber defibrillator is similar to that for a dual-chamber pacemaker, the question arises about whether it is preferable to implant a dual-chamber defibrillator (with DDDR pacing capability) because OHCM patients are at risk of malignant ventricular tachyarrhythmias and sudden death (73,74). At this juncture, a prophylactic ICD should at least be considered in high-risk patients (i.e., family history of sudden death, recurrent syncope, abnormal blood pressure response to exercise, septal or left ventricle thickness ≥ 30 mm and Holter-documented nonsustained ventricular tachycardia) (74). Atrial tachyarrhythmias often result in serious hemodynamic consequences, and an ICD with atrial defibrillation capability is also a consideration. Unfortunately, financial restrictions limit the application of an attractive universal mode of therapy.

Optimal Upper Rate

Myocardial Ischemia

Myocardial ischemia can occur in OHCM in the absence of coronary artery disease. Patients may develop angina and electrocardiographic abnormalities consistent with ischemia and infarction, and they frequently show replacement scarring at autopsy (75,76). Patients, especially those with previous cardiac arrest and syncope, may show exercise-induced reversible defects on thallium scintigraphy indistinguishable from those in patients with ischemia caused by coronary artery disease (77,78). Improvement of the scintigraphic abnormalities occur after surgical relief of LVOT obstruction (79). Preliminary studies suggest that dual-chamber pacing improves coronary blood flow and reduces myocardial ischemia (80–83). There are several mechanisms of myocardial ischemia in the absence of epicardial coronary artery disease:

1. Excessive myocardial oxygen demand can exceed the capacity of the coronary system to deliver oxygen. Atrial pacing can precipitate myocardial ischemia and abnormalities in lactate metabolism in susceptible patients with reduced coronary vasodilator response (84,85).
2. Abnormal (narrowed) intramural coronary arteries, which are components of the thickened myopathic ventricle, and inadequacy of capillary density with respect to the greatly increased left ventricular muscle mass may produce myocardial ischemia (75,76).
3. Systolic compression of large coronary arteries may be caused by myocardial bridges.
4. Diastolic occlusion of intramyocardial coronary arteries may result from marked elevations of left ventricular diastolic pressure.

Brinker (86) advocates establishing an upper rate limit that avoids ischemia during pacing. Myocardial scintigraphy on exercise should be considered in many and perhaps all OHCM patients evaluated for cardiac pacing. Such evaluation is particularly important in patients with atrial chronotropic incompetence, in whom excessive pacing rates during DDDR pacing should be avoided. Concomitant anti-ischemic therapy with beta blockers and verapamil may reduce or eliminate myocardial ischemia (78).

Wenckebach Upper Rate Response with Long Atrioventricular Intervals
The pacemaker should be programmed with a relatively high maximum rate and relatively short postventricular atrial refractory period (PVARP) to avoid a Wenckebach upper rate response. In some patients with retrograde ventriculoatrial conduction, a short PVARP requires an effective algorithm for the termination of endless-loop tachycardia almost as soon as it starts. A fast upper rate must be avoided in patients with demonstrable cardiac ischemia. Ideally, the maximum allowable sinus rate that avoids ischemia should be determined with a radionuclide stress test. When using beta blockers to prevent ischemia, the physician should program the upper rate accordingly.

Possible Mechanism of Beneficial Effect

The effect of DDD pacing is optimal only when RV apical stimulation is synchronized to atrial systole, producing optimal filling and activation of left ventricular apex before septal contraction, a mechanism called *inversion of ventricular contraction* (18) or *apical preexcitation* (24). The beneficial response may be related to altered or paradoxical motion of the ventricular septum, reduced systolic anterior movement of the mitral valve with widening of the LVOT, and reduction of the LVOT gradient associated with diminished mitral regurgitation (provided there is no primary abnormality of the mitral valve). There is also increased filling of the left ventricle and eventually reduced contractility as a result of discordant ventricular activation by pacing. Jeanrenaud and Kappenberger (87) observed a 12% reduction in septal motion (particularly the midportion) with atrioventricular pacing (without reduction in global ejection fraction) and paradoxical septal motion in only 1 of 9 patients, and Betocchi and coworkers (41) showed a decrease in septal ejection fraction.

There is a progressive reduction in the LVOT gradient with time (88). Some patients do not improve on a short-term basis and require several months to achieve significant improvement. When the pacemaker is switched off during follow-up of more than a few months, the original LVOT gradient in normal sinus rhythm remains reduced, at least on a short-term basis (8,9). All these observations suggest that factors other than paradoxical or altered septal motion account for the lower LVOT gradient and clinical improvement. There is perhaps pacing-induced remodeling of the myocardium resulting in left ventricular dilatation, depression of left ventricular systolic function producing permanent hemodynamic and possibly morphologic changes (89), or a mechanical memory effect (90,91).

In some studies, serial echocardiographic evaluation suggests localized thinning of the left ventricle wall and increase in the end-systolic volume (12,26, 50,88). Left ventricular remodeling and changes in hypertrophy and left ventricular systolic function may explain the progressive and sustained effect on the LVOT gradient (88).

Unresolved Questions About the Benefit of Pacing

The use of pacing in OHCM raises a number of questions. Long-term outcomes are not yet known. Is there some unrecognized harmful adaptation with dual-chamber pacing? Will left ventricular enlargement and depression of systolic and diastolic function (92) be detrimental long term and contribute to eventual heart failure? What are the cellular and biochemical changes in the myocardium? How does pacing influence ventricular remodeling and myocardial structure?

How can we identify noninvasively patients unsuitable for pacing? Obstruction other than subaortic or patients with anatomic abnormalities of the mitral valve may not respond to pacing. However, preliminary data suggest that patients with mid-cavity obstruction may also respond (24,93).

Is a combination of pacing with drugs better than pacing alone? Can conventional or two-site biatrial pacing prevent atrial fibrillation? Changes in the natural history and prevention of sudden death with pacing have not been determined.

Nonobstructive Hypertrophic Cardiomyopathy

Cannon and associates (94) reported the results of permanent dual-chamber pacing in 12 patients with symptomatic nonobstructive hypertrophic cardiomyopathy (i.e., no resting LVOT gradient and no LVOT gradient >30 mm Hg during a Valsalva maneuver, amyl nitrite inhalation, or isoproterenol infusion).

DDD pacing was associated with improvement in symptoms and effort tolerance, but there was a need for reinitiation of medical therapy, and no objective evidence of hemodynamic benefit was demonstrated. On this basis, Cannon and colleagues (94) concluded that chronic DDD pacing cannot be recommended for routine use in the management of patients with nonobstructive hypertrophic cardiomyopathy who are symptomatic despite medical therapy.

● CONGESTIVE HEART FAILURE

Hochleitner and coworkers (95) in 1990 reported the beneficial effects of DDD pacing (i.e., short atrioventricular interval of 100 msec) in the treatment of end-stage idiopathic dilated cardiomyopathy in 16 patients without atrioventricular block in whom conventional therapy had failed. They reported a striking improvement of dyspnea at rest and pulmonary edema, as well as a significant decrease in NYHA functional class, left atrial and RV dimensions, and reduced cardiothoracic ratio. The short atrioventricular interval appeared to reduce mitral regurgitation and improve left ventricular filling. Hochleitner and associates (96) subsequently reported the long-term efficacy of dual-chamber (DDD) pacing in the treatment of end-stage idiopathic dilated cardiomyopathy in a longitudinal study of 17 patients for up to 5 years. Critical analysis of these data suggests a less impressive benefit than the investigators' interpretation. Nevertheless, the work of Hochleitner and colleagues (95,96) fostered a number of short- and long-term studies in the past decade investigating the role of pacing in CHF caused by dilated cardiomyopathy. These reports yielded conflicting but mostly poor results with conventional dual-chamber pacing (with a short atrioventricular delay) for the treatment of CHF due to poor left ventricle function of various causes. Short-term improvement even in highly selected patients has been inconsistent (3,97–109). Long-term studies have also been disappointing (110–119), although the long-term study of Brecker and coworkers (102) suggests that limited improvement is possible in highly selected patients.

Mechanism of Beneficial Effect with Conventional Daul-Chamber Pacing

The role of mitral regurgitation was demonstrated by Rossi and associates (120) in a series of 20 patients with third-degree atrioventricular block and isolated mitral regurgitation. An optimally short atrioventricular delay (98 ± 7 msec) produced a significant reduction in the severity of mitral regurgitation and increase in stroke volume (120). Conventional pacing in patients with dilated cardiomyopathy and first-degree atrioventricular block abolishes presystolic mitral regurgitation and increases the time for forward flow. However, elimination of diastolic mitral regurgitation plays an undefined role in the hemodynamic improvement by pacing. Abolition of diastolic mitral regurgitation may cause more optimal hemodynamic performance because of a lower left atrial pressure and higher left ventricular preload at the onset of systole.

Identification of Patients Who May Benefit from Conventional Dual-Chamber Pacing with a Short Atrioventricular Interval

It does not make sense to consider conventional DDD pacing in unselected patients, but the 1998 ACC/AHA guidelines for pacemaker implantation (6) advocate conventional dual-chamber pacing as a class IIb indication in "symptomatic drug-refractory dilated cardiomyopathy with prolonged PR interval when acute hemodynamic studies have demonstrated hemodynamic benefit of pacing." Neither the degree of acceptable PR prolongation nor the QRS duration are stated. This recommendation is highly controversial, especially in the absence of a major left intraventricular conduction delay.

The following more acceptable recommendations are based on the work of Brecker and Gibson (117) and those of the Mayo Clinic workers (1). They should be considered in terms of limited clinical applicability because of the paucity of data and the promising results achieved with biventricular pacing currently undergoing intensive investigation:

1). A long PR interval in the resting electrocardiogram (ECG): As emphasized by Glickson and colleagues (1), some patients do not improve because atrial mechanical contraction may be poor or absent and the atrial contribution may be negligible in the presence of marked elevation of the pulmonary capillary wedge pressure. However, in some patients, a long interatrial conduction time and a long PR interval may already have appropriately timed mechanical left atrioventricular synchrony, and in such a situation, improvement would not be expected with pacing. In some patients, an attempt to optimize the atrioventricular interval may cause deterioration of left ventricular function because depression of left ventricular function resulting from paced (asynchronous) ventricular depolarization outweighs the benefit of optimized atrioventricular synchrony.

2). Substantial intraventricular conduction delay (QRS >140 msec) (117).

3). Prolonged functional mitral regurgitation of at least 450 msec, with a short ventricular filling time of less than 200 msec. According to The Mayo Clinic workers (1), patients who respond best exhibit early cessation of transmitral flow and diastolic mitral regurgitation. Abolition or diminution of mitral regurgitation may be an important factor in the beneficial effect of pacing.

4). Temporary pacing study: This should demonstrate hemodynamic benefit. According to The Mayo Clinic workers, during temporary pacing, "responders" have an increase in systolic blood pressure and an increase in peak mitral regurgitation velocity, reflecting a higher left ventricular systolic pressure and lower left atrial pressure (1). Patients should understand that initial hemodynamic benefit correlates poorly with long-term outcome.

⦿ BIVENTRICULAR PACING

In 1994, Cazeau and coworkers (121) reported the benefit of permanent four-chamber pacing in a single patient with refractory CHF, dilated cardiomyopathy, and left bundle branch block (QRS 200 msec). Simultaneous conventional RV and epicardial left ventricular pacing was used to achieve a more physiologic depolarization sequence, a process known as resynchronization. In this patient, biatrial (left atrial stimulation was from the coronary sinus) pacing was also undertaken to optimize atrioventricular synchrony because of a major interatrial conduction delay. This initial success with biventricular pacing generated a number of short-term studies showing that biventricular or left ventricular pacing improves indices of systolic function in patients with severe left ventricular systolic dysfunction, dilated cardiomyopathy, and a major left-sided intraventricular conduction disorder (122–130). In some patients, single-site pacing from the left ventricle provides better hemodynamics than simultaneous biventricular pacing. It appears that the atrioventricular delay has less influence on left ventricular function than the optimal left ventricular pacing site (125).

About 20% to 30% of class III and IV patients diagnosed with CHF have major left intraventricular conduction disorders (QRS >140 msec) that makes them potential candidates for long-term biventricular pacing. However, markers of left ventricular dyssynchrony more refined and sensitive than the simple electrocardiogram need to be investigated to extend the benefit of biventricular pacing to other CHF patients in the absence of an obvious left-sided intraventricular conduction disorder or even in the presence of right bundle branch block. Atrial fibrillation is not a contraindication (127). Intraventricular conduction delays may cause an inefficient pattern of contraction, with left ventricular segments contracting at different times. Delayed intraventricular depolarization or dyssynchrony impairs left ventricular function and causes a shorter diastole, overlapping systole and diastole, and aggravation of functional mitral regurgitation. Biventricular or left ventricular pacing can improve cardiac function by promoting a more coordinate and efficient left ventricular contraction, as well as reducing functional mitral regurgitation. One study demonstrated that left ventricular pacing reduces the MVO_2 in patients with dilated cardiomyopathy, depressed left ventricular systolic function, and a major left-sided intraventricular conduction disorder (129). The impact of chronic pacing on reverse left ventricular remodeling and the neurohumoral aspects of CHF are being investigated (131). Doppler imaging of tissue promises to be a useful technique to evaluate the effect of pacing on segmental contraction velocity in patients with left ventricular dyssynchrony (132,133).

Clinical Considerations in Biventricular Pacing

Preliminary long-term experience in a relatively small number of patients with CHF and major intraventricular conduction disturbances seems promising (134–155). Biventricular or left ventricular pacing (with or without biatrial pacing) is investigational in the United States, but not in Europe. Longer follow-up periods and controlled studies will be required to establish its place in the treatment of heart failure. Technology and patient selection remain problematic.

About 20% of patients fail to improve. The mortality rate is about 15% to 20% in the first year (156). This is not surprising, because pacing is used in a high-risk population. Sudden death accounts for about 40% of these deaths and is more common than progressive pump failure. Death is more common among class IV patients, those with coronary artery disease, and patients who fail to improve with pacing. The high incidence of sudden death suggests that some patients could benefit from a system that combines biventricular pacing and an ICD (157–163).

Patients with ischemic and idiopathic cardiomyopathy respond to pacing (139,154). Patients with chronic atrial fibrillation seem to benefit as much as patients in sinus rhythm (127,148,149). Mitral regurgitation decreases (141). Objective evaluation has not always shown change despite clinical improvement. Pacing may obviate the need for cardiac transplantation in selected patients or provide a bridge to transplantation. Studies are required to determine whether biventricular pacing can prevent ventricular arrhythmias in CHF patients (157–163).

A longer spontaneous QRS complex is correlated with a higher probability of hemodynamic improvement at least in acute studies (125). One study of biventricular pacing showed that, when patients are evaluated as a group, there is a correlation between the degree of QRS narrowing with the clinical response (136). In individual patients, the degree of QRS narrowing with biventricular pacing does not correlate with the maximal hemodynamic benefit (125).

Based on short-term data, it is possible that long-term, single-site left ventricular pacing may be hemodynamically equivalent or superior to biventricular pacing in some patients, probably because RV pacing may activate a substantial portion of the left ventricle, thereby interfering with the resynchronization process provided by left ventricular pacing alone (122, 123,125). This would have an enormous impact on the methodology of permanent pacing.

Many workers believe that a study of the acute hemodynamic response is unnecessary for most patients. The combination of spontaneous QRS duration and basal dP/dt (maximum) provides the best indicator of a maximal acute hemodynamic response during left ventricular pacing. A reliable way to screen potential nonresponders is required (125,164,165).

Clinical Results of Biventricular Pacing

Ventricular resynchronization has quickly generated much interest in the treatment of congestive heart failure (166–171). The Multisite Stimulation in Cardiomyopathy (MUSTIC) trial is a randomized, crossover, single-blind study of biventricular pacing in class III CHF patients with stable sinus rhythm, a major intraventricular conduction disorder (QRS >150 msec), left ventricular ejection fraction (LVEF) less than 35%, and left ventricular end-diastolic diameter of more than 60 mm (150). Biventricular pacing was activated for 3 months and turned OFF for 3 months. The study involving 58 randomized patients in sinus rhythm (LVEF $22 \pm 8\%$ and QRS 176 ± 19 msec), revealed statistically significant improvement in the following end points: 6-minute walking distance, NYHA class, quality-of-life score (Minnesota LWHF), peak VO_2, and reduction in hospitalizations. The mortality rate was low, but this was not a mortality trial. The left ventricular lead implantation success was 92%, and 88% of leads were functional at the end of the crossover. Biventricular pacing was preferred by 86% of patients, no pacing was preferred by 4%, and 10% voiced no preference in the mode of pacing. A second group of 46 patients with chronic atrial fibrillation showed the same benefit as those in sinus rhythm (148). No other randomized studies have yet been published.

Observational long-term results of biventricular pacing in patients with dilated cardiomyopathy and CHF (idiopathic or from coronary artery disease) are also encouraging (134–147,149,151–155). The InSync (Medtronic, Inc., Minneapolis, MN) trial (137,140) is an ongoing, prospective, nonrandomized multicenter study of ventricular resynchronization in patients with NYHA class III or IV heart failure and left ventricular dysfunction (i.e., LVEF ≤35%, left ventricular end-diastolic diameter ≥60 mm, and a ventricular conduction delay, with QRS ≥150 msec). From August 1997 to November 1998, 117 patients were enrolled, with a successful implantation rate of 88% using the coronary venous system for left ventricular pacing. Table 32-4 shows QRS duration, NYHA class, 6-minute hall walk distance, and quality-of-life score assessed at baseline and at 1, 6, and 12 months after implantation. The data suggest that the benefits of ventricular resynchronization are sustained through 12 months. The InSync Italian Registry (146,147) with 190 patients after a mean follow-up of 10 ± 5 months showed similar results. There were statistically improvements in the NYHA class (3.1 ± 0.6 to 2.1 ± 0.7), quality-of-life index, distance in the 6-minute hall walk test, and LVEF ($25 \pm 7\%$ to $31 \pm 8\%$).

The French Pilot study (134), conducted between August 1994 and January 1998, included 50 patients (68% in NYHA class IV) with severe drug-refractory heart failure (mean LVEF of $20\% \pm 6\%$, coronary artery disease in 48%, and idiopathic disease in 40%). Twenty patients had prior permanent pacemakers implanted for conventional indications. The mean QRS duration was 197 ± 32 msec (183 ± 29 msec in left bundle branch block and 221 ± 18 msec in patients with chronic pacing) and permanent atrial fibrillation was present in 28%. During a mean follow-up of 15.4 ± 10.2 months, 20 (40%) patients died, and all but 2 were categorized in class IV at the time of implantation. Death was sudden for 6 patients, and 11 died of progressive pump failure. In the 30 surviving patients, the mean NYHA class decreased from 3.5 ± 0.5 at the time of implantation to 2.2 ± 0.6 at 1 month ($p < 0.01$) and remained stable (2.2 ± 0.60) until the end of follow-up (20.2 ± 8.8 months). The

TABLE 32-4 • LONG-TERM OUTCOMES OF ADVANCED HEART FAILURE PATIENTS WITH CARDIAC RESYNCHRONIZATION THERAPY (InSync TRIAL)[a]

	QRS Duration			NYHA Class			6-Minute HWD			QoL Score		
	N	Base	FU	N	Base	FU	N	Base	FU	N	Base	FU
M1	82	180 ± 28	153 ± 26[b]	88	3.3 ± 0.5	2.4 ± 0.8[b]	62	304 ± 108	355 ± 105[b]	76	52 ± 18	32 ± 19[b]
M6	68	179 ± 27	154 ± 21[b]	73	3.3 ± 0.5	2.1 ± 0.8[b]	54	303 ± 109	367 ± 118[b]	68	53 ± 20	32 ± 23[b]
M12	42	180 ± 26	146 ± 23[b]	49	3.3 ± 0.5	2.2 ± 0.7[b]	24	309 ± 125	368 ± 93[b]	47	53 ± 21	29 ± 19[b]

FU, follow-up; HWD, hall walk distance; M, month (1, 6, and 12) of follow-up; N, number of patients; NYHA, New York Heart Association; QoL, quality of life.
[a] Entry criteria include NYHA class III or IV heart failure, left ventricular ejection fraction of 35% or less, left ventricular diameter of 60 mm or larger, and QRS of 150 msec or longer.
[b] $p < 0.001$.
From Gras D, Ritter P, Lazarus A, et al. Long-term outcome of advanced heart failure patients with resynchronization therapy [Abstract]. *Pacing Clin Electrophysiol* 2000;23:658.

echocardiographic data showed an increase in the LVEF from 20 ± 65% to 24 ± 10% ($p < 0.01$), but the left ventricular end-diastolic diameter was unchanged.

Methodologic and Technologic Considerations in Biventricular Pacing

Anatomic standardization of the various pacing sites is essential to permit meaningful comparison of data, because confusion already prevails. Biventricular pacing has been accomplished with slightly modified conventional hardware. Patients in sinus rhythm receive a triple-chamber pacemaker with two ventricular leads and one atrial lead. The left ventricle is often paced from one of the tributaries of the coronary veins over the epicardial surface of the left ventricle, usually at the site of latest activation according to the electrogram (151). A coronary venous angiogram is often performed to delineate the venous anatomy because the operator should aim to pass the lead into the lateral or posterolateral vein to pace the lateral left ventricle. In about one third of the patients, anatomic constraints require using less optimal coronary venous sites. The anatomic variability of the coronary venous system and operator skill account for this limitation (172). Some groups have experienced a relatively high incidence of displacement and threshold problems with coronary venous leads to the left ventricle, suggesting the presence of a definite learning curve and opportunity for advances in lead design. Initial success rates of about 50% for coronary venous lead implantation have improved to about 90% (173). Complications of coronary venous pacing include displacement in 5% to 10% of cases, a rise in pacing threshold, coronary sinus dissection, phrenic nerve stimulation, double counting of the spontaneous QRS complex (related to the temporal separation of RV and left ventricular electrograms and the relatively short ventricular blanking period of the device), and far-field oversensing of the P wave by the ventricular channel (146,147,174). Left ventricular pacing can also be established with a limited thoracotomy, an approach that provides the best exposure for mapping the most hemodynamically favorable site for left ventricular pacing.

A few patients have received two pacemakers: one conventional dual-chamber device and a second left ventricular device programmed to the VVT mode that discharges (triggers) its output immediately on detecting the RV stimulus. Such an arrangement provides simultaneous biventricular pacing. Some workers have implanted left ventricular leads by thoracoscopy. The placement of permanent endocardial left ventricular leads by transseptal puncture is feasible and requires long-term anticoagulation, but it is highly investigational because of the risk of catastrophic embolic complications (175–179). Some patients with severe CHF also have important atrial conduction abnormalities and require atrial resynchronization with dual-site atrial pacing, thereby creating a four-chamber pacing system as described in the original report of Cazeau and associates (121).

Technologic Considerations in Biventricular Pacing

Early Systems

Initial systems consisted of two separate unipolar leads with a wide distance between the two independent electrodes. One unipolar lead is the anode, and the other the cathode. With this arrangement, the leads are joined by a Y connector to the single bipolar ventricular port of the pacemaker so that the electrodes are connected in series. This arrangement has been called *split bipolar pacing* or *dual unipolar pacing*. Such systems were associated with high pacing thresholds (at the anodal site) and have been largely abandoned (169). Most workers favor a more effective divided pacemaker output or common dual-cathodal system (i.e., simultaneous dual-site cathodal stimulation with the leads connected in parallel) from a single pacemaker output by using a Y connector to produce a unipolar-unipolar or bipolar-bipolar system. There is a connection between the two cathodes and anodes, respectively. Unwieldy Y connector arrangements and composite electrode systems will disappear with the development of true multi-output or multiport pacemakers capable of independently stimulating two or more sites in the same electrical chamber, as in traditional unipolar or bipolar fashion. In the interim, the Y connector has been integrated into the pacemaker header.

Dual-cathodal unipolar stimulation generates a lot of current, especially if a high output has to be programmed. This may cause pectoral muscle stimulation requiring surgical correction and replacement with a bipolar system. One system allows unipolar left ventricular pacing with the anode on the ring electrode of the RV bipolar lead to eliminate muscle stimulation. A dual-cathodal system does not permit programming the output to a single ventricular chamber for testing purposes; the biventricular mode is committed. However, limited individual testing of one of the chambers or sites is often possible because the pacing thresholds of the two sites are different. Gradual reduction of output voltage and pulse duration causes loss of capture of the chamber with higher threshold before the chamber with the lower threshold. The pacemaker output must be programmed to accommodate the higher of the two stimulation thresholds because the leads are connected in parallel.

Conventional dual-chamber pacemakers can be used for biventricular pacing in patients with chronic atrial fibrillation with the "atrial" channel connected to the left ventricle and the ventricular channel to the right ventricle. The pacemaker should be connected to deliver stimulation to the left ventricle before the right ventricle. Few conventional pacemakers allow programming of an atrioventricular delay of zero or near zero. Consequently, conventional pacemakers used for biventricular pacing in patients with chronic atrial fibrillation and CHF may not provide an optimal delay between the two ventricles because the minimum atrioventricular delay (often between 25 and 30 msec) does not permit simultaneous activation. In such patients, radiofrequency ablation of the atrioventricular junction may be necessary before pacemaker implantation to ensure biventricular pacemaker-controlled activation. A conventional dual-chamber ICD modified with a Y connector for biventricular pacing may cause double sensing of the QRS complex, because marked delay in intraventricular conduction may deliver an adequate ventricular signal to the left ventricular electrode beyond the sensed refractory period initiated by the same QRS sensed in the right ventricle. This results in double counting and inappropriate firing of the ICD (180). Consequently, combined devices consisting of biventricular pacing and dual-chamber ICD capability, currently under investigation, sense only from the right ventricle to avoid double QRS sensing.

Future Systems

Multiport pacemakers

True multiport dedicated pacemakers will add a new dimension to biventricular pacing and do away with the inflexibility of the single output currently used for dual-site pacing. Complex circuitry will be needed to provide two timing cycles and different delays for optimal resynchronization between the two electrically connected ventricles according to pacing and sensing. This will require the development of new electronic clocks to provide a wide range of very small and precise delays between sequential stimuli. Current technology is unsuitable for the task because of too much tolerance and limitations by postblanking requirements. Preexcitation of one site may be more important than simultaneous activation for arrhythmia prevention rather than hemodynamic benefit (181).

Devices with three or more separate outputs will require larger battery capacity. A large pacemaker with two separate ventricular outputs and shorter longevity would be acceptable if it proves beneficial to CHF patients in view of their relatively short life expectancy. Resynchronization after sensing if it proves essential will require the use of a dedicated triggered mode (151). Extensive programmability will be essential to control new types of pacemaker arrhythmias engendered by a more complex electrophysiologic environment (146).

Leads

The leads used for biventricular pacing often impose the selection of pacing sites that represent a compromise among low thresholds, site accessibility, and lead stability. Improved and smaller leads are required (182–184). Characteristics of leads for biventricular pacing include easy and reliable cannulation of the coronary sinus os; visualization and maneuverability (i.e., small veins and angulation); and site selectability, which is important for a nonhomogeneous myocardium and for an optimal hemodynamic result (185–187). Experience suggests that a preimplantation retrovenogram is associated with improved site selection.

Lead hardware improvements will include novel steerable leads and guiding sheaths. Exploration of angioplasty guide wire–delivered devices is in process, and this technology may provide additional design alternatives to provide a full selection of lead technologies for implanters to choose from to accommodate the great variation in anatomy. The design of over-the-wire systems must address the acceptability of a center lumen filling with blood during and after implantation.

The leads should achieve immediate fixation but provide the capability for repositioning in the perioperative period if necessary. Stable, long-term fixation is necessary for sustained function and for the advantage of steroid-eluting leads for low stimulation thresholds. Acceptable threshold and sensing performance are needed for all implantation sites and device combinations. New designs must improve the ability to manage complications and enhance the ease of extraction.

Multi-output pacing requires a large header to accommodate additional ports. Leads of the future will require a downsized connector. Lack of connector standardization will be problematic if the patients live long enough.

FIRST-DEGREE ATRIOVENTRICULAR BLOCK

Schüller and Brandt defined the pacemaker syndrome in terms of "symptoms and signs present in the pacemaker patient which are caused by inadequate timing of atrial and ventricular contractions" (188). This characterization also applies to patients without an implanted pacemaker when "inadequate timing of atrial and ventricular contractions" causes a similar hemodynamic derangement (189,190). In this regard, Chirife and colleagues (191) called the hemodynamic disturbance produced by marked first-degree atrioventricular block the *pacemaker syndrome without a pacemaker,* and other workers have referred to this entity as the *pseudopacemaker syndrome* (192,193).

Several reports have documented the benefit of dual-chamber pacing in patients with symptomatic marked first-degree atrioventricular block and normal left ventricular function (191–196) (Table 32-5). A number of the reported patients developed their problem after ablation of the fast pathway for the treatment of AV nodal reentry tachycardia (192,193).

During markedly prolonged anterograde atrioventricular conduction, the close proximity of atrial systole to the preceding ventricular systole produces the same hemodynamic consequences as continual retrograde ventriculoatrial conduction. Patients with a markedly prolonged PR interval may or may not be symptomatic at rest. They are, of course, more likely to become symptomatic with mild to moderate levels of exercise when the PR interval does not shorten appropriately and atrial systole occurs progressively closer to the previous ventricular systole. Symptoms can be subtle. The hemodynamic disorder caused by

TABLE 32-5 • PACING FOR A LONG PR INTERVAL

Study	Year	Patients[a]	PR At Rest (msec)	Effect Of Exercise Or Faster Rate	Benefit Of Pacing
Chirife et al (191)	1990	1	400	NS	Improved
Zornosa et al (192)	1992	3	365, 380, 270	PR intervals lengthened progressively at rates >100 bpm	All improved
Mabo et al (196)	1993	8	410 ± 45	No shortening of PR interval	All improved; exercise duration ↑ 44%, cardiac output on exercise ↑ 29%, mean PCWP ↓ 33%
Kim et al (193)	1993	1	360[a]/160–180	NS	Improved

NS, not stated; PCWP, pulmonary capillary wedge pressure.
[a] Intermittent and sudden prolongation of PR interval associated with pacemaker syndrome.

a very long PR interval during exercise resembles the exercise-induced pacemaker syndrome produced by AAIR pacing when, for a variety of reasons, a paced atrioventricular interval lengthens disproportionately relatively early during exercise (197). PR prolongation often causes hemodynamically inconsequential diastolic mitral regurgitation in patients with preserved left ventricular function (198–203). Diastolic mitral regurgitation may play a more important role in patients with left ventricular systolic dysfunction and CHF.

Indication for Pacing

Wharton and Ellenbogen (204) have argued that "symptomatic first-degree atrioventricular block with symptoms suggestive of pacemaker syndrome" should be a class I indication for permanent pacing. They emphasized that "symptoms can be subtle in some patients or may be of sufficiently long duration that temporary pacing may be indicated to document improvement or reversal of longstanding problems." However, the 1998 ACC/AHA guidelines for pacemaker implantation state that "first-degree atrioventricular block with symptoms suggestive of pacemaker syndrome and documented alleviation of symptoms with temporary pacing" constitutes a class IIa indication (6). The PR interval should be ≥0.30 second. The class IIa recommendation does not apply to patients with CHF and dilated cardiomyopathy. The clinician must decide for the patient whether there will be a net benefit provided by two opposing factors: a positive effect from atrioventricular delay optimization and a negative effect of reduced left ventricular function from aberrant pacemaker-controlled depolarization. One study suggests that improvement with DDD pacing becomes evident with a PR interval of more than 0.28 second (205).

The necessity and appropriateness of a temporary atrioventricular pacing study are questionable, especially if the PR is very long and does not shorten on exercise. During a resting study, it may not be possible to demonstrate symptomatic improvement, and the execution of exercise studies with a temporary dual-chamber pacemaker in place is difficult. It is reasonable to implant a pacemaker in selected patients without a temporary pacing study that would add unnecessary risk and cost (4).

Pacemaker Technology

The pacemaker must prevent migration of the P wave into the postventricular atrial refractory period (PVARP), where it cannot be tracked.

Functional Atrial Undersensing

Bode and coworkers (206) reported the problems associated with first-degree atrioventricular block. They studied 255 patients with Holter recordings and found 9 patients with atrial undersensing despite an adequate atrial signal. The P waves fell continually in the PVARP of 276 ± 26 msec (without an active algorithm for automatic PVARP extension after a ventricular extrasystole). All 9 patients exhibited substantial delay of spontaneous conduction (284 ± 61 msec; range, 230 to 410 msec). The combination of a relatively fast sinus rate and prolonged atrioventricular conduction provides the appropriate setting for the development of functional atrial undersensing, during which the ECG shows sinus rhythm, a long PR interval, and conducted QRS complexes but no pacemaker stimuli. The conducted QRS complexes activate the ventricle while the P waves remain trapped in the PVARP. The pacemaker itself acts as a "bystander" in that it can initiate the pacemaker syndrome, but the ECG then shows no pacemaker activity (207).

Heart Rate

Bode and associates (206) recorded a mean sinus rate of 105 ± 3 bpm during functional atrial undersensing because a relatively fast atrial rate facilitates displacement of the P wave toward the PVARP. Some patients with a pacemaker for a long PR interval had marked sinus tachycardia during functional atrial undersensing. This appears to be a response to the hemodynamic derangement produced by the loss of atrioventricular synchrony, because the tachycardia subsides quickly on restoration of a physiologic atrioventricular delay by the pacemaker. As a rule, the PR interval does not shorten significantly in situations causing sinus tachycardia. During sinus tachycardia, the fixed PR interval can create a vicious cycle by pushing the P wave progressively closer to the preceding ventricular complex. This process may establish a more hemodynamically unfavorable ventricular-atrial (VA) relationship, and this can aggravate the sinus tachycardia.

Pacemaker Syndrome

Bode and colleagues (206) reported that five of their nine patients with functional atrial undersensing developed complaints suggesting the pacemaker syndrome. They prevented functional atrial undersensing in seven of their nine patients by shortening the PVARP and atrioventricular delay, and previously symptomatic patients became asymptomatic. The other two patients exhibited less atrial undersensing with a shorter PVARP.

Significance of Postventricular Atrial Refractory Period Extension

Functional atrial undersensing can occur with a short PVARP when a ventricular extrasystole activates an automatic PVARP extension. In this situation, an unsensed P wave within the extended PVARP gives rise to a conducted QRS complex that the pacemaker interprets as a ventricular extrasystole (208–211). Consequently, the pacemaker activates another PVARP extension. The extended PVARP is perpetuated from cycle to cycle as long as the pacemaker continues to interpret the conducted QRS complexes as extrasystoles.

Prevention of Functional Atrial Undersensing

A relatively short PVARP often can be programmed to prevent functional atrial undersensing because retrograde VA conduction is uncommon in patients with first-degree atrioventricular block. There are other measures (207):

1. Capability of programming off the automatic PVARP extension after a ventricular extrasystole.
2. Uncoupling of the PVARP extension when the pacemaker detects a P wave inside the PVARP preceding the next ventricular sensed beat.
3. Noncompetitive atrial pacing algorithm, which delivers a premature atrial stimulus 300 msec after the pacemaker detects atrial activity in the PVARP.
4. Prolongation of the atrial escape interval after a sensed ventricular extrasystole.
5. In difficult situations, ablation of the atrioventricular junction with resultant complete atrioventricular block (194,212).

ORTHOSTATIC HYPOTENSION

The use of atrial tachypacing (100/min) for the treatment of orthostatic hypotension was first proposed by Moss and coworkers (213) in 1980, but it never

TABLE 32-6 • PACING FOR ORTHOSTATIC HYPOTENSION

Study	Year	Patients	Pacemaker	Rate (ppm)	Drug Therapy	Follow-up	Benefit
Moss et al (213)	1980	1	AAI	100	?	10 mo	Yes
Goldberg et al (214)	1980	1	Temporary atrial	90–100	No	No	No
Kristinsson et al (215)	1983	2	AAI	95 (day) 55 (night)	Yes (all)[a]	2 yr	Yes
Cunha et al (216)	1990	1	AAI	96 (day) 60 (night)	?	9 mo	Yes
Weissman et al (217)	1992	5	3 AAI, DDD, DDDR	90–100 (95)	Yes (all)[a]	1 yr	4 Improved
Grubb et al (220)	1993	1	DDDR	RVPEP (sensor controlled)	?	4 mo	Yes
Clementy et al (218)	1995	5	DDDR	90–110	?	>3 mo	4 improved
Abe et al (219)	2000	2	DDD	100	?	5 & 6 mo	Yes

RVPEP, right ventricular preejection period.
[a] All on fludrocortisone.

became popular (Table 32-6). Soon afterward, Goldberg (214) described the unsuccessful use of temporary atrial pacing in a single patient. From 1980 to 1992, only three additional cases were reported. Kristinsson and associates (215) reported two cases of drug refractory orthostatic hypotension treated with permanent AAI pacing at a rate of 95 ppm during the day and 55 ppm at night (programming was done by the patient). The patients improved, with virtual disappearance of orthostatic hypotension for about 2 years, except when they forgot to program their pacemakers to 95 ppm/min in the morning (215). Both patients continued taking fludrocortisone acetate after pacemaker implantation. Cunha and colleagues (216) also reported in 1990 the marked improvement over a period of 9 months of a patient with drug-refractory orthostatic hypotension who received an atrial pacemaker designed to pace at 60 ppm at night and 96 ppm during the day, with rate programming performed by the patient.

Weissman and coworkers (217) renewed interest in the use of atrial tachypacing in a 1992 report of five cases of drug-refractory orthostatic hypotension treated with permanent pacemakers (three AAI, one DDD, and one DDDR) with a follow-up of 1 year (Table 32-6). After pacemaker implantation, all patients received fludrocortisone, and three also received propranolol. Three patients were able to lead a nearly normal life with virtually no orthostatic hypotension. One patient showed moderate improvement, but another one did not. The lower rate of the pacemakers varied from 90 to 100 ppm/min. In 1995, Clementy and associates (218) implanted DDDR pacemakers with an activity sensor in five patients, and four improved at least on a short-term basis. The devices were programmed to a daily minimal rate of 75 ppm and a sensor-mediated rate of more than 90 ppm during the movement from the seated or the supine position to the upright position. Two of the pacemakers allowed automatic decrease of the nocturnal pacing rate to 65 ppm. Patients and relatives were instructed to increase the pacing if necessary by tapping on the device. In 2000, Abe and colleagues (219) also reported two cases successfully treated with DDD pacemakers at a rate of 100 ppm.

It seems that most patients with idiopathic orthostatic hypotension have a markedly attenuated heart rate response to hypotension associated with the upright posture. The impaired chronotropic response may further accentuate the orthostatic hypotension by allowing a longer peripheral runoff during diastole (217). Tachypacing by reducing the duration of diastole augments the diastolic and mean blood pressure in patients with residual adrenergic activity. Weissman and coworkers (217) suggested that patients without adrenergic tone would probably not derive any benefit from tachypacing. A pacemaker for tachypacing should not be used as sole therapy for orthostatic hypotension. Adjunctive drug therapy with fludrocortisone seems essential and should be supplemented by beta blockers, added salt intake, and other measures (217).

Grubb and associates (220) reported the use of DDDR pacing with a sensor system controlled by the RV preejection period (i.e., systolic time interval from the onset of electrical ventricular depolarization to the onset of RV ejection) for the treatment of severe refractory orthostatic hypotension. The system adequately sensed the patient's fall in blood pressure when sitting or standing by a fall in RV filling, causing shortening of the preejection interval. The pacemaker augmented its rate (from 60 to 120 ppm) accordingly, thereby preventing syncope. No further orthostatic or syncopal episodes occurred over a 9-month follow-up period. (The report did not mention whether additional drug therapy was used.) This novel approach avoids continuous tachypacing and its potential harmful effects on the heart. This experience suggests that developments in sensor technology may allow earlier and more appropriate response to alterations in blood pressure and posture and greater applicability of this form of therapy.

All patients considered for atrial pacing should undergo repeated testing in the supine and upright positions, with or without pacing (90 to 100 ppm) by a temporary atrial or atrioventricular sequential pacing system. The procedure is best done on a tilt table so the patient is always supported. If rapid atrial pacing blunts the degree of hypotension, pacing therapy probably will be helpful, but the test has poor predictive value (218).

⊙ PREVENTION OF PAROXYSMAL ATRIAL FIBRILLATION

In patients with sick sinus syndrome, atrial pacing has proved more effective than VVI pacing in maintaining atrial electrical stability. New pacing techniques involving simultaneous stimulation at two atrial sites (i.e., right atrium–left atrium through the coronary sinus or two sites in the right atrium) have shown some degree of effectiveness in the long-term prevention of atrial fibrillation compared with single-site atrial pacing (221–242). Dual-site atrial pacing used for the prevention of atrial fibrillation was pioneered by Daubert and colleagues (241,242) for the treatment of sick sinus syndrome with advanced atrial conduction defects, a situation typically associated with atrial tachyarrhythmias, especially atypical atrial flutter. Atrial fibrillation develops in an electrically unstable atrial substrate characterized by regional conduction delays, increased dispersion of refractoriness, and anisotropic conduction. It is believed that arrhythmia prevention depends on resynchronization of the electrical activity of the two atria, with resultant near-normalization of the time difference of intraatrial and interatrial depolarization, reduction of dispersion of refractoriness, and to some extent, partial control of atrial ectopic activity, an important trigger of atrial fibrillation (243,244). With atrial conduction delay, resynchronization is expressed as normalization of P-wave configuration and duration. Single-site atrial septal pacing can also achieve atrial resynchronization, but its role in the prevention of atrial fibrillation remains to be determined (245–248).

Several studies have demonstrated the effectiveness of atrial pacing in the prevention of atrial fibrillation after coronary artery bypass surgery. Two of three studies have demonstrated the effectiveness of temporary or short-term dual-site atrial pacing in the prevention of atrial fibrillation immediately after coronary artery bypass surgery in the absence of technical problems related to epicardial left atrial pacing (249–251). The benefit of pacing when biatrial pacing is compared with no pacing in the postoperative period may be secondary to nonspecific overdrive suppression (252). Results of long-term studies are more problematic (221–242). Acute studies may not be predictive of long-term results. Delfaut and colleagues (221) used permanent bifocal atrial pacing (2 sites in the right atrium) in 30 patients with drug-refractory symptomatic atrial fibrillation (most with underlying bradycardia) and paced at rates of 80 to 90 ppm. The patients were not evaluated for interatrial conduction delay. The mean arrhythmia-free intervals increased from 9 ± 10 days in the control period preceding implantation to 143 ± 110 days ($p < 0.0001$) in single-site pacing and 195 ± 96 days in dual-site right atrial pacing ($p < 0.0001$ versus control). Single-site high right atrial pacing compared with coronary sinus os pacing did not differ in efficacy (221). Seventy-eight percent of patients at 1 year and 56% at 3 years remained free of symptomatic atrial fibrillation with permanent dual-site atrial pacing. A study of dual-site atrial pacing from Daubert's group (233), conducted between 1989 and 1997, enrolled 86 patients with drug-refractory atrial tachyarrhythmias and documented atrial conduction delay. The number of patients with atrial fibrillation or bradycardia was not specified, but previous reports from this group suggest that most patients had underlying bradycardia (1–3). After a mean follow-up time of 33 months, 55 patients (68%) remained in stable sinus rhythm, including 28 patients (32.6%) without any documented recurrence and 27 patients with one or more recurrences. Biatrial pacing allowed smaller doses of antiarrhythmic agents to be used. The only factor predictive of a positive response was a baseline P-wave duration of more than 160 msec.

The weight of the preliminary evidence suggests that dual-site atrial pacing may have a positive therapeutic effect in patients with paroxysmal atrial fibrillation and underlying bradycardia or interatrial block (253), and it may potentiate the effect of antiarrhythmic agents in these situations. In this respect, the 1998 ACC/AHA guidelines (6) for pacemaker implantation state that "dual-site right atrial pacing may offer additional benefits to single-site right atrial pacing in patients with symptomatic drug-refractory atrial fibrillation and concomitant bradyarrhythmias. In patients with sick sinus syndrome and intraatrial block (P wave >180 msec), biatrial pacing may lower recurrence rates of atrial fibrillation." These guidelines deserve two comments. First, the diagnosis of interatrial and intraatrial block can be made with a P wave greater than 120 msec rather than only greater than 180 msec. Second, the indication for pacing (class IIb) is stated in terms of "prevention of symptomatic drug-refractory recurrent atrial fibrillation," but this recommendation is vague because there is no mention of bradycardia, atrial conduction delay, or methodology of atrial pacing.

The efficacy and indications of permanent dual-site atrial pacing in patients without bradycardia for the prevention of atrial fibrillation in a variety of clinical circumstances need to be firmly established in multicenter, prospective, randomized trials. The role of atrial resynchronization is also being investigated in maintenance of sinus rhythm after cardioversion of chronic atrial fibrillation (254). Many multicenter trials are underway to evaluate a variety of new pacing techniques, including multisite atrial pacing for the prevention of atrial fibrillation in patients with or without the sick sinus syndrome. Pacemakers have been specifically designed with sophisticated overdrive algorithms for this purpose. The influence of several factors needs clarification: structural versus no heart disease, left atrial size, presence of intraatrial and interatrial conduction delay, bradycardia versus no bradycardia, symptomatic versus asymptomatic atrial fibrillation, and the efficacy of single-site atrial septal pacing in achieving the same degree of resynchronization as dual-site pacing. The stakes are huge because atrial fibrillation is a potentially disabling condition that can contribute to mortality and morbidity independently of associated heart disease.

REFERENCES

1. Glikson M, Hayes DL, Nishimura RA. Newer clinical applications of pacing. *J Cardiovasc Electrophysiol* 1997;8:1190–1203.
2. Hayes DL, Barold SS, Camm AJ, et al. Evolving indications for permanent cardiac pacing: an appraisal of the 1998 ACC/AHA guidelines. *Am J Cardiol* 1998;82:1082–1086.
3. Barold SS. New indications for cardiac pacing. In: Singer I, Barold SS, Camm AJ, eds. *Nonpharmacological therapy of arrhythmias for the 21st century: the state of the art.* Armonk, NY: Futura Publishing, 1998:775–795.
4. Hayes DL. Evolving indications for permanent pacing. *Am J Cardiol* 1999;83(5B):161D–165D.
5. Kappenberger L, Lyon X, Cox N, et al. Developing clinical indications for multisite pacing. *J Interv Card Electrophysiol* 2000; 4[Suppl I]:87–93.
6. Gregoratos G, Cheitlin MD, Freedman RA, et al. ACC/AHA guidelines for implantation of cardiac pacemakers and antiarrhythmia devices; a report of the American College of Cardiology/American Heart Association task force on practice guidelines (Committee on Pacemaker Implantation). *J Am Coll Cardiol* 1998;31:1175–1209.
7. McDonald K, McWilliams E, O'Keefe B, et al. Functional assessment of patients treated with permanent dual chamber pacing as primary treatment for hypertrophic cardiomyopathy. *Eur Heart J* 1988;9:893–898.
8. Fananapazir L, Cannon RO III, Tripodi D, et al. Impact of dual-chamber permanent pacing in patients with obstructive hypertrophic cardiomyopathy with symptoms refractory to verapamil and β-adrenergic blocker therapy. *Circulation* 1992; 85:2149–2161.
9. Jeanrenaud X, Goy JJ, Kappenberger L. Effects of dual-chamber pacing in hypertrophic obstructive cardiomyopathy. *Lancet* 1992;339:1318–1323.
10. McDonald KM, Maurer B. Permanent pacing as treatment for hypertrophic cardiomyopathy. *Am J Cardiol* 1991;68:108–110.
11. Richter T, Cserhalmi M, Lengyel M, et al. Changes in left ventricular hemodynamics of hypertrophic obstructive cardiomyopathy (HOCM) patients treated with VAT pacing. In:

Baroldi G, Camerini F, Goodwin JF, eds. *Advances in cardiomyopathies*. New York: Springer-Verlag, 1990:168–174.

12. Fananapazir L, Epstein ND, Curiel RV, et al. Long-term results of dual-chamber (DDD) pacing in obstructive hypertrophic cardiomyopathy: evidence for progressive symptomatic and hemodynamic improvement and reduction of left ventricular hypertrophy. *Circulation* 1994;90:2731–2742.
13. Gras D, Daubert C, Mabo P. Value of cardiac pacing in hypertrophic obstructive cardiomyopathy refractory to medical treatment. *Arch Mal Coeur* 1995;88:577–583.
14. Gras D, Pavin D, De Place C, et al. What is the status of patients with hypertrophic obstructive cardiomyopathy treated by DDD pacing for more than 1 year? [Abstract]. *Circulation* 1995;92[Suppl I]:I-780.
15. Yusvinkevich SA, Khirmanov VN, Domashenko AA, et al. Treatment of HOCM by short AV-delay DDD pacing [Abstract]. *Pacing Clin Electrophysiol* 1995;18:1807.
16. Umman S, Oncul A, Umman B, et al. Dual chamber pacemaker implantation in patients with hypertrophic obstructive cardiomyopathy [Abstract]. *Pacing Clin Electrophysiol* 1995;18:1813.
17. Gamhir DS, Arora R, Khalilullah M. Dual chamber pacing in hypertrophic obstructive cardiomyopathy [Abstract]. *Pacing Clin Electrophysiol* 1993;16:1525.
18. Nishimura RA, Trusty JM, Hayes DL, et al. Dual-chamber pacing for hypertrophic cardiomyopathy: a randomized, double-blind, crossover trial. *J Am Coll Cardiol* 1997;29:435–441.
19. Slade AKB, Sadoul N, Shapiro L, et al. DDD pacing in hypertrophic cardiomyopathy: a multicenter clinical experience. *Heart* 1996;75:44–49.
20. Gadler F, Linde C, Juhlin-Dannfelt A, et al. Long-term effects of dual chamber pacing in patients with hypertrophic cardiomyopathy without outflow tract obstruction at rest. *Eur Heart J* 1997;18:636–642.
21. Sadoul N, Simon JP, de Chillou C, et al. Intérêts de la stimulation cardiaque permanente dans les myocardiopathies hypertrophiques et obstructives rebelles au traitement medical. *Arch Mal Coeur* 1994;87:1315–1323.
22. Sadoul N, Slade AKB, Simon JP, et al. Dual chamber pacing in refractory hypertrophic obstructive cardiomyopathy: a two-centre European experience in 34 consecutive patients [Abstract]. *J Am Coll Cardiol* 1995;25:233A.
23. Kappenberger L, Linde C, Daubert C, et al. Pacing in hypertrophic obstructive cardiomyopathy: a randomized crossover trial. *Eur Heart J* 1997;18:1249–1256.
24. Fananapazir L, Atiga W, Tripodi D, et al. Therapy in obstructive hypertrophic cardiomyopathy: the role of dual chamber (DDD) pacing. In: Barold SS, Mugica J, eds. *Recent advances in cardiac pacing: goals for the 21st century*. Armonk, NY: Futura Publishing, 1998:35–50.
25. Sakai Y, Kawakami Y, Shimada S, et al. AV sequential pacing in hypertrophic obstructive cardiomyopathy, comparison between acute and chronic effects [Abstract]. *Circulation* 1996;94[Suppl I]:I-502.
26. Iliou MC, Lavergne TL, Hernigou A, et al. Left ventricular remodeling by long-term dual-chamber pacing in hypertrophic obstructive cardiomyopathy [Abstract]. *Circulation* 1996;94[Suppl I]:I-361.
27. Gadler F, Linde C, Daubert C, et al, for the Pacing in Cardiomyopathy (PIC) Group. Significant improvement of quality of life following atrioventricular synchronous pacing in patients with hypertrophic obstructive cardiomyopathy: data from 1 year of follow-up. *Eur Heart J* 1999;20:1044–1050.
28. Linde C, Gadler F, Kappenberger L, for the Pacing in Cardiomyopathy (PIC) Group. Placebo effect of pacemaker implantation in obstructive hypertrophic cardiomyopathy. *Am J Cardiol* 1999;83:903–907.
29. Jeanrenaud X. Rate of adverse cardiac events after one-year of dual chamber pacing in hypertrophic obstructive cardiomyopathy (HOCM): results of the PIC study group [Abstract]. *Circulation* 1997;96[Suppl I]:I-95.
30. Maron BJ, Nishimura RA, McKenna WJ, et al. Assessment of permanent dual-chamber pacing as a treatment for drug-refractory symptomatic patients with obstructive hypertrophic cardiomyopathy: a randomized, double-blind, crossover study (M-PATHY). *Circulation* 1999;99:2927–2933.
31. Park MH, Gilligan DM, Bernado NL, et al. Symptomatic hypertrophic obstructive cardiomyopathy: role of dual-chamber pacing. *Angiology* 1999;50:87–94.
32. Sakai Y, Kawakami Y, Hirota Y, et al. Dual-chamber pacing in hypertrophic obstructive cardiomyopathy: a comparison of acute and chronic effects. *Jpn Circ J* 1999;63:971–975.
33. Gross JN, Keltz TN, Cooper JA, et al. Profound "pacemaker syndrome" in hypertrophic cardiomyopathy. *Am J Cardiol* 1992;70:1507–1511.
34. Sadoul N, Simon JP, Chillon C, et al. Usefulness of temporary dual chamber pacing to determine indication for pacemaker implantation in patients with drug-resistant obstructive hypertrophic cardiomyopathy [Abstract]. *Pacing Clin Electrophysiol* 1993;16:1120.
35. McAreavey D, Fananapazir L. Acute pacing studies are not valuable in predicting long term benefits of DDD pacing for LV outflow obstruction in hypertrophic cardiomyopathy [Abstract]. *J Am Coll Cardiol* 1994;23:10A.
36. Daubert JC. Pacing and hypertrophic obstructive cardiomyopathy. *Pacing Clin Electrophysiol* 1996;19:1141–1142.
37. Jeanrenaud X, Kappenberger L. The optimal patient for pacemaker treatment of hypertrophic obstructive cardiomyopathy [Abstract]. *Pacing Clin Electrophysiol* 1993;16:1120.
38. Gross JN, Ben-Zur UM, Greenberg MA, et al. Acute hemodynamic assessment fails to identify hypertrophic cardiomyopathy patients responsive to DDD pacing [Abstract]. *J Am Coll Cardiol* 1994;23:324A.
39. Pavin D, de Place C, Le Breton H, et al. Effects of permanent dual-chamber pacing on mitral regurgitation in hypertrophic obstructive cardiomyopathy. *Eur Heart J* 1999;20:203–210.
40. Kappenberger L. Pacing in hypertrophic cardiomyopathy. *Eur Heart J* 1999;20:169–170.
41. Betocchi S, Losi MA, Piscione F, et al. Effects of dual chamber pacing in hypertrophic cardiomyopathy on left ventricular outflow tract obstruction and on diastolic function. *Am J Cardiol* 1996;77:498–502.
42. Nishimura RA, Hayes DL, Ilstrup DM, et al. Effect of dual-chamber pacing on systolic and diastolic function in patients with hypertrophic cardiomyopathy: acute Doppler echocardiographic and catheterization hemodynamic study. *J Am Coll Cardiol* 1996;27:421–430.
43. Betocchi S, Losi MA, Briguori C, et al. Long-term dual-chamber pacing reduces left ventricular outflow tract obstruction but impairs diastolic function in hypertrophic cardiomyopathy [Abstract]. *Circulation* 1997;96[Suppl I]:I-645.
44. Pak PH, Maughan L, Baughman KL, et al. Mechanism of acute mechanical benefit from VDD pacing in hypertrophied heart: similarity of responses in hypertrophic cardiomyopathy and hypertensive heart disease. *Circulation* 1998;98:242–248.
45. Elliott PM, Brecker SJ, McKenna WJ. Diastolic dysfunction in hypertrophic cardiomyopathy. *Eur Heart J* 1998;19:1261–1267.
46. Fananapazir L, Tripodi D, McAreavey D. Five-year results of dual chamber pacing in obstructive hypertrophic cardiomyop-

athy patients with severe symptoms [Abstract]. *Pacing Clin Electrophysiol* 1998;21:791.
47. Erwin J, McWilliams E, Gearty G, et al. Hemodynamic assessment of dual chamber pacing in hypertrophic cardiomyopathy using radionuclide angiography [Abstract]. *Br Heart J* 1986;55:507.
48. McDonald K, O'Sullivan JJ, King C, et al. Dual chamber pacing improves left ventricular filling in patients with hypertrophic cardiomyopathy [Abstract]. *Eur Heart J* 1989;10[Abstract Suppl]:401.
49. Pavin D, Llirbat ML, de Place C, et al. Optimized pacing therapy may prevent deterioration of left ventricular diastolic function in hypertrophic obstructive cardiomyopathy [Abstract]. *Pacing Clin Electrophysiol* 1998;21:792A.
50. Fananapazir L, McAreavey D. Therapeutic options in patients with obstructive cardiomyopathy and severe drug-refractory symptoms. *J Am Coll Cardiol* 1998;31:259–264.
51. McAreavey D, Fananapazir L. Ventricular pre-excitation is highly effective for elderly patients with obstructive hypertrophic cardiomyopathy and symptoms refractory to medication [Abstract]. *J Am Coll Cardiol* 1993;21:354A.
52. Meisel E, Rauwolf TP, Burkhard M, et al. Older patients with hypertrophic obstructive cardiomyopathy benefit most from pacemaker therapy: results from the PIC study [Abstract]. *Circulation* 1999;100[Suppl I]:I-78.
53. Gadler F, Linde C, Ryden L. Rapid return of left ventricular outflow tract obstruction and symptoms following cessation of long-term atrioventricular synchronous pacing for obstructive hypertrophic cardiomyopathy. *Am J Cardiol* 1999;83:553–557.
54. Gilligan DM, Maron BJ. Permanent pacing in patients with hypertrophic cardiomyopathy. *Card Electrophysiol Rev* 1999;2:384–388.
55. Spirito P, Maron BJ. Perspectives on the role of new treatment strategies in hypertrophic obstructive cardiomyopathy. *J Am Coll Cardiol* 1999;33:1071–1075.
56. Maron BJ. New interventions for obstructive hypertrophic cardiomyopathy: promise and prudence. *Eur Heart J* 1999;20:1292–1294.
57. O'Rourke RA. Cardiac pacing: an alternative treatment for selected patients with hypertrophic cardiomyopathy and adjunctive therapy for certain patients with dilated cardiomyopathy. *Circulation* 1999;100:786–768.
58. Erwin JP III, Nishimura RA, Lloyd MA, et al. Dual chamber pacing for patients with hypertrophic obstructive cardiomyopathy: a clinical perspective in 2000. *Mayo Clin Proc* 2000;75:173–180.
59. Gietzen FH, Leuner CJ, Hegselmann J, et al. hemodynamic effects of adjunct DDD pacing in patients with total AV block after transcoronary ablation of septum hypertrophy for hypertrophic obstructive cardiomyopathy [Abstract]. *Circulation* 1999;100[Suppl I]:I-464.
60. Ommen SR, Nishimura RA, Squires RW, et al. Comparison of dual-chamber pacing versus septal myectomy for the treatment of patients with hypertrophic obstructive cardiomyopathy: a comparison of objective hemodynamic and exercise end points. *J Am Coll Cardiol* 1999;34:191–196.
61. Gras D, Daubert C, Leclercq C, et al. Obstructive hypertrophic cardiomyopathy treated by DDD pacing: the major importance of AV synchrony [Abstract]. *J Am Coll Cardiol* 1994;23:11A.
62. Matsumato K, Saitou J, Mukosaka K, et al. Influences of changing the pacing site on the hemodynamic improvement by DDD pacing in patients with hypertrophic obstructive cardiomyopathy [Abstract]. *Circulation* 1993;88[Suppl 1]:I-210.
63. Gadler F, Linde C, Juhlin-Dannfeldt A, et al. Influence of right ventricular pacing site on left ventricular outflow tract obstruction in patients with hypertrophic obstructive cardiomyopathy. *J Am Coll Cardiol* 1996;27:1219–1224.
64. Glikson M, Espinosa RE, Hayes DL. Expanding indications for permanent pacemakers. *Ann Intern Med* 1995;123:443–451.
65. Gras D, de Place C, LeBreton H, et al. Importance of atrioventricular synchrony in hypertrophic obstructive cardiomyopathy treated by cardiac pacing. *Arch Mal Coeur* 1995;88:215–223.
66. Jeanrenaud X, Aebischer N, for the Pacing in Cardiomyopathy (PIC) Study Group. Importance of the AV interval during dual chamber pacing in hypertrophic obstructive cardiomyopathy: results from the PIC study group [Abstract]. *J Am Coll Cardiol* 1997;29[Suppl A]:111A.
67. Mayumi H, Kohno H, Yasui H, et al. Use of automatic mode change between DDD and AAI to facilitate native atrioventricular conduction in patients with sick sinus syndrome or transient atrioventricular block. *Pacing Clin Electrophysiol* 1996;19:1740–1747.
68. Chang AC, McAreavey D, Tripodi D, et al. Radiofrequency catheter atrioventricular node ablation in patients with permanent cardiac pacing systems. *Pacing Clin Electrophysiol* 1994;17:65–69.
69. Jeanrenaud X, Schlapfer J, Fromer M, et al. Dual chamber pacing in hypertrophic obstructive cardiomyopathy: beneficial effect of atrioventricular junction ablation for optimal left ventricular capture and filling. *Pacing Clin Electrophysiol* 1997;20:293–300.
70. Gadler F, Linde C, Darpo B. Modification of atrioventricular conduction as adjunct therapy for pacemaker treatment with hypertrophic obstructive cardiomyopathy. *Eur Heart J* 1998;19:132–138.
71. Daubert C, Gras D, Pavin D, et al. Biatrial synchronous pacing to optimize hemodynamic benefit of DDD pacing in hypertrophic obstructive cardiomyopathy [Abstract]. *Circulation* 1995;92[Suppl I]:I-780.
72. Slade AKB, Keeling PJ, Prasad K, et al. Acute evaluation of DDD versus DDDR mode predicts additional benefit of rate adaptive pacing in hypertrophic cardiomyopathy [Abstract]. *J Am Coll Cardiol* 1994;23:10A.
73. Maron BJ, Shen WK, Link MS, et al. Efficacy of Implantable cardioverter-defibrillators for the prevention of sudden death in patients with hypertrophic cardiomyopathy. *N Engl J Med* 2000;342:365–373.
74. Watkins H. Sudden death in hypertrophic cardiomyopathy. *N Engl J Med* 2000;342:42–43.
75. Louie EK, Edwards LC III. Hypertrophic cardiomyopathy. *Prog Cardiovasc Dis* 1994;36:275–308.
76. Maron BJ, Bonow, RO, Cannon RO III, et al. Hypertrophic cardiomyopathy: interrelations of clinical manifestations, pathophysiology and therapy. *N Engl J Med* 1987;316[Pt 1]:780–789.
77. O'Gara PT, Bonow RO, Maron BJ, et al. Myocardial perfusion abnormalities in patients with hypertrophic cardiomyopathy: assessment with thallium 201 emission computer tomography. *Circulation* 1987;76:1214–1223.
78. Dilsizian V, Bonow RO, Epstein SE, et al. Myocardial ischemia detected by thallium scintigraphy is frequently related to cardiac arrest and syncope in young patients with hypertrophic cardiomyopathy. *J Am Coll Cardiol* 1993;22:796–804.
79. Cannon RO III, Dilsizian V, O'Gara PT. Impact of surgical relief of outflow obstruction on thallium perfusion abnormalities in hypertrophic cardiomyopathy. *Circulation* 1992;85:1039–1045.
80. Thomson H, Fong W, Stafford W, et al. Reversible ischemia in hypertrophic cardiomyopathy. *Br Heart J* 1995;74:220–223.
81. Takeuchi M, Abe H, Kuroiwa A. Effect of dual chamber atrio-

ventricular sequential pacing on coronary flow velocity in a patient with hypertrophic obstructive cardiomyopathy. *Pacing Clin Electrophysiol* 1996;19:2153–2155.
82. Posma JL, Banksman PK, Van Der Wall EE, et al. Effects of permanent dual chamber pacing on myocardial perfusion in symptomatic hypertrophic cardiomyopathy. *Heart* 1996;76: 358–362.
83. Le Helloco A, Gras D, Devillers A, et al. Influence of DDD pacing on myocardial perfusion in patients with hypertrophic cardiomyopathy [Abstract]. *Pacing Clin Electrophysiol* 1997;20: 1592.
84. Cannon RO III, Rosing DR, Maron BJ, et al. Myocardial ischemia in patients with hypertrophic cardiomyopathy: contribution of inadequate vasodilator reserve and elevated left ventricular filling pressures. *Circulation* 1985;71:234–243.
85. Cannon RO III, Schenke WH, Maron BJ, et al. Differences in coronary flow and myocardial metabolism in rest and during pacing between patients with obstructive and patients with non-obstructive hypertrophic cardiomyopathy. *J Am Coll Cardiol* 1987;10:53–62.
86. Brinker JA. Permanent pacemakers: optimal choices for specific clinical scenarios. *Intelligence Rep Card Pacing Electrophysiol* 1992;2:1–4.
87. Jeanrenaud X, Kappenberger L. Regional wall motion during pacing for hypertrophic cardiomyopathy. *Pacing Clin Electrophysiol* 1997;20:1673–1681.
88. Pavin D, de Place C, le Breton H, et al. Long-term effects of DDD pacing on hypertrophic obstructive cardiomyopathy [Abstract]. *J Am Coll Cardiol* 1997;29[Suppl A]:388A.
89. Tavel ME, Fananapazir L, Goldshlager NF. Hypertrophic obstructive cardiomyopathy. Problems in management. *Chest* 1997;112:262–264.
90. Wigle ED, Rakowski H, Kimball BP, et al. Hypertrophic cardiomyopathy: clinical spectrum and treatment. *Circulation* 1995;92:1680–1692.
91. Nishimura RA, Symanski JD, Hurrell DG, et al. Dual-chamber pacing for cardiomyopathies: a 1996 clinical perspective. *Mayo Clin Proc* 1996;71:1077–1087.
92. Symanski JD, Nishimura RA. The use of pacemakers in the treatment of cardiomyopathies. *Curr Probl Cardiol* 1996;21: 385–444.
93. Hintringer F, Nesser HJ, Niel J, et al. Pacing in distal ventricular hypertrophic cardiomyopathy. *Pacing Clin Electrophysiol* 1998;21:1828–1830.
94. Cannon RO III, Tripodi D, Dilsizian V, et al. Results of permanent dual-chamber pacing in symptomatic nonobstructive hypertrophic cardiomyopathy. *Am J Cardiol* 1994;23:571–576.
95. Hochleitner M, Hortnagl H, Ng CK, et al. Usefulness of physiologic dual-chamber pacing in drug-resistant idiopathic dilated cardiomyopathy. *Am J Cardiol* 1990;66:198–202.
96. Hochleitner M, Hortnagl H, Hortnagel H, et al. Long term efficacy of physiologic dual-chamber pacing in the treatment of end-stage idiopathic dilated cardiomyopathy. *Am J Cardiol* 1992;70:1320–1325.
97. Kataoka H. Hemodynamic effect of physiologic dual-chamber pacing in a patient with end-stage dilated cardiomyopathy: a case report. *Pacing Clin Electrophysiol* 1991;14:1330–1335.
98. Auricchio A, Sommariva L, Salo RW, et al. Improvement of cardiac function in patients with severe congestive failure and coronary artery disease by dual-chamber pacing with shortened AV delay. *Pacing Clin Electrophysiol* 1993;16:2034–2043.
99. Hochleitner M, Hortnagl H, Gschnitzer F. Dual-chamber pacing in patients with end-stage ischemic cardiomyopathy [Letter]. *Lancet* 1993;341:1543.
100. Innes D, Leitch J, Fletcher P. VDD pacing at short atrioventricular intervals does not improve cardiac output in patients with dilated heart failure. *Pacing Clin Electrophysiol* 1994;17: 959–965.
101. Nishimura RA, Hayes DL, Holmes DR Jr, et al. Mechanism of hemodynamic improvement by dual-chamber pacing for severe left ventricular dysfunction: an acute Doppler and catheterization hemodynamic study. *J Am Coll Cardiol* 1995;25: 281–288.
102. Scanu P, Lecluse E, Michel L, et al. Effets de la stimulation cardiaque double chambre temporaire dans l'insuffisance cardiaque refractaire. *Arch Mal Coeur* 1994;89:1643–1649.
103. Shinbane J, Chu E, De Marco T, et al. Evaluation of acute dual-chamber pacing with a range of atrioventricular delays on cardiac performance in refractory heart failure. *J Am Coll Cardiol* 1997;30:1295–1300.
104. Brecker SJD, Xiao HB, Sparrow J, et al. Effects of dual-chamber pacing with short atrioventricular delay in dilated cardiomyopathy. *Lancet* 1992;340:1308–1312.
105. Mathew V, Chaliki H, Nishimura RA. Atrioventricular sequential pacing in cardiac amyloidosis: an acute Doppler echocardiographic and catheterization hemodynamic study. *Clin Cardiol* 1997;20:723–725.
106. Feliciano Z, Fisher ML, Corretti MC, et al. Acute hemodynamic effect of A-V delay in patients with congestive heart failure [Abstract]. *J Am Coll Cardiol* 1994;23:349A.
107. Paul V, Morris-Thurgood J, Cowell R, et al. Impaired ventricles: is short AV delay pacing beneficial and can we predict in whom? [Abstract]. *Pacing Clin Electrophysiol* 1994;17:776.
108. Shinbane JS, Chu E, DeMarco T, et al. Evaluation of dual-chamber pacing with a range of atrioventricular delays on cardiac performance in refractory heart failure. *J Am Coll Cardiol* 1997;30:1295–1300.
109. Sack S, Franz R, Dagres N, et al. Can right-sided atrioventricular sequential pacing provide benefit for selected patients with severe congestive heart failure? *Am J Cardiol* 1999;83(5B): 214D–129D.
110. Linde C, Gadler F, Edner M, et al. Results of atrioventricular synchronous pacing with optimized delay in patients with severe congestive heart failure. *Am J Cardiol* 1995;75:919–923.
111. Gold MR, Feliciano Z, Gottlieb SS, et al. Dual-chamber pacing with a short atrioventricular delay and congestive heart failure: a randomized study. *J Am Coll Cardiol* 1995;26: 967–973.
112. Brecker SJ, Kelly PA, Chua TP, et al. Effects of permanent dual chamber pacing in end-stage dilated cardiomyopathy [Abstract]. *Circulation* 1995;92[Suppl I]:I-7.
113. Greco O, Brofmann P, Khirmanov V, et al. Dilative cardiomyopathy and dual-chamber pacing with shortened AV delay: long-term results [Abstract]. *Pacing Clin Electrophysiol* 1997;20: 1574.
114. Occhetta E, Bortnik M, Francalacci G, et al. Dual-chamber DDD pacing in NYHA III-IV functional class dilated cardiomyopathy: short and middle-term evaluation. *Cardiologia* 1998; 43:1327–1335.
115. Ansalone G, Auriti A, Giannantoni P, et al. Physiological pacing with a short AV delay in patients with dilated cardiomyopathy, baseline first degree AV block and LBBB [Abstract]. *Pacing Clin Electrophysiol* 1997;20:1575.
116. Auricchio A, Salo RW, Klein H, et al. Problems and pitfalls in evaluating studies for pacing in heart failure. *G Ital Cardiol* 1997;27:593–599.
117. Brecker SJ, Gibson DG. What is the role of pacing in dilated cardiomyopathy? *Eur Heart J* 1996;17:819–824.
118. Paul V, Cowell R, Thurgood-Morris J, et al. Short atrioventricular delay pacing in heart failure: acute hemodynamic im-

provements do not predict long-term results [Abstract]. *Pacing Clin Electrophysiol* 1995;18:847.
119. Gold MR, Peters RW. Permanent pacemakers in patients with dilated cardiomyopathy. *Card Electrophysiol Rev* 1999;2:381–383.
120. Rossi R, Muia N Jr, Turco V, et al. Short atrioventricular delay reduces the degree of mitral regurgitation in patients with a sequential dual-chamber pacemaker. *Am J Cardiol* 1997;80:901–905.
121. Cazeau S, Ritter P, Bakdach S, et al. Four chamber pacing in dilated cardiomyopathy. *Pacing Clin Electrophysiol* 1994;17:1974–1979.
122. Blanc JJ, Etienne Y, Gilard M, et al. Evaluation of different ventricular pacing sites in patients with severe heart failure: results of an acute hemodynamic study. *Circulation* 1997;96:3273–3277.
123. Auricchio A, Stellbrink C, Block M, et al. Effect of pacing chamber and atrioventricular delay on acute systolic function of paced patients with congestive heart failure. The Pacing Therapies for Congestive Heart Failure Study Group. The Guidant Congestive Heart Failure Research Group. *Circulation* 1999;99:2993–3001.
124. Leclercq C, Cazeau S, Le Breton H, et al. Acute hemodynamic effects of biventricular pacing in patients with end-stage heart failure. *J Am Coll Cardiol* 1998;32:1825–1831.
125. Kass DA, Chen HC, Curry C, et al. Improved left ventricular mechanics from acute VDD pacing in patients with dilated cardiomyopathy and ventricular conduction delay. *Circulation* 1999;99:1567–1573.
126. Saxon LA, Kerwin WF, Cahalan MK, et al. Acute effects of intraoperative multisite ventricular pacing on left ventricular function and activation/contraction sequence in patients with depressed ventricular function. *J Cardiovasc Electrophysiol* 1998;9:13–27.
127. Etienne Y, Mansourati J, Gilard M, et al. Evaluation of left ventricular based pacing in patients with congestive heart failure and atrial fibrillation. *Am J Cardiol* 1999;83:1138–1140, A9.
128. Bakker PF, Meijburg H, De Jonge N, et al. Beneficial effects of biventricular pacing in congestive heart failure [Abstract]. *Pacing Clin Electrophysiol* 1994;17:820.
129. Nelson GS, Berger RD, Fetics BJ, et al. Left ventricular or biventricular pacing improves cardiac function at diminished energy cost in patients with dilated cardiomyopathy and left bundle branch block. *Circulation* 2000;102:3053–3059.
130. Kerwin WF, Botvinick EH, O'Connell JW, et al. Ventricular contraction abnormalities in dilated cardiomyopathy: effect of biventricular pacing to correct interventricular dyssynchrony. *J Am Coll Cardiol* 2000;35:1221–1227.
131. Hamdan MH, Zagrodzky JD, Joglar JA, et al. Biventricular pacing decreases sympathetic activity compared with right ventricular pacing in patients with depressed ejection fraction. *Circulation* 2000;102:1027–1032.
132. Mulukutla S, Stetten GD, Jacques DC, et al. Quantification of left ventricular regional phase asynchrony in patients with left bundle branch block using tissue Doppler echocardiography [Abstract]. *Circulation* 2000;102[Suppl II]:II-384.
133. Nelson GS, Fetics BJ, Murabayashi T, et al. Cardiac variability imaging enables detection of pacing-improved contractile coordination in patients with dilated cardiomyopathy and left bundle branch block [Abstract]. *Circulation* 2000;102[Suppl II]:II-539.
134. Leclercq C, Cazeau S, Ritter P, et al. A pilot experience with permanent biventricular pacing to treat advanced heart failure. *Am Heart J* 2000;140:862–870.
135. Leclercq C, Victor F, Alonso C, et al. Comparative effects of permanent biventricular pacing for refractory heart failure in patients with stable sinus rhythm or chronic atrial fibrillation. *Am J Cardiol* 2000;85:1154–1156.
136. Alonso C, Leclercq C, Victor F, et al. Electrocardiographic predictive factors of long-term clinical improvement with multisite biventricular pacing in advanced heart failure. *Am J Cardiol* 1999;84:1417–1421.
137. Gras D, Cazeau S, Ritter P, et al. Long-term results of cardiac resynchronization for heart failure patients: the InSync clinical trial [Abstract]. *Circulation* 1999;100[Suppl I]:I-515.
138. Tang ASL, Green M, Gras D, et al. Cardiac resynchronization: multicenter implant experience with atrio-biventricular pacing [Abstract]. *Pacing Clin Electrophysiol* 1999;22:701.
139. Leclercq C, Alonso C, Mabo P, et al. A comparison of the effects of cardiac resynchronization in patients with advanced heart failure of either ischemic or nonischemic origin [Abstract]. *Pacing Clin Electrophysiol* 2000;23:659.
140. Gras D, Ritter P, Lazarus A, et al. Long-term outcome of advanced heart failure Patients with resynchronization therapy [Abstract]. *Pacing Clin Electrophysiol* 2000;23:658.
141. Etienne Y, Valls-Bertault V, Mansourati J, et al. Permanent left ventricular-based pacing improves mitral regurgitation in patients with severe congestive heart failure [Abstract]. *Pacing Clin Electrophysiol* 2000;34:596.
142. Daubert JC, Ritter P, Cazeau S, et al. Pacing in congestive heart failure. In: Rosenqvist M, ed. *Cardiac pacing: new advances.* London: WB Saunders, 1997:3–25.
143. Daubert JC, Leclercq C, Pavin D, et al. Pacing therapy in congestive heart failure: present status and new perspectives. In: Barold SS, Mugica J, eds. *Recent advances in cardiac pacing: goals for the 21st century.* Armonk, NY: Futura Publishing, 1998:51–80.
144. Stellbrink C, Auricchio A, Butter C, et al. Pacing therapies in congestive heart failure II study. *Am J Cardiol* 2000:86[Suppl 1]:K138–K143.
145. Bakker PF, Meijburg HW, de Vries JW, et al. Biventricular pacing in end-stage heart failure improves functional capacity and left ventricular function. *J Interv Card Electrophysiol* 2000;4:395–404.
146. Ricci R, Ansalone G, Toscano S, et al. Cardiac resynchronization: materials, technique and results. The InSync Italian Registry. *Eur Heart J* 2000;2[Suppl J]:J6–J15.
147. Zardini M, Tritto M, Bargiggia G, et al. The InSync Italian Registry: analysis of clinical outcome and considerations on the selection of candidates to left ventricular resynchronization. *Eur Heart J* 2000;2[Suppl J]:J16–J22.
148. Daubert JC, Linde C, Cazeau S, et al. Clinical effects of biventricular pacing in patients with severe heart failure and chronic atrial fibrillation: results from the Multisite Stimulation in Cardiomyopathy (MUSTIC) Study Group II [Abstract]. *Circulation* 2000;102[Suppl II]:II-693.
149. Leclercq C, Alonso C, Victor F, et al. Long-term results of permanent biventricular pacing in patients with advanced heart failure: comparison of patients with stable sinus rhythm and chronic atrial fibrillation [Abstract]. *Pacing Clin Electrophysiol* 2000;23:635.
150. Daubert JC, Linde C, Cazeau S, et al. Clinical effects of biventricular pacing in patients with severe heart failure and normal sinus rhythm: results from Multisite Stimulation in Cardiomyopathy (MUSTIC) Group I [Abstract]. *Circulation* 2000;102[Suppl II]:II-694.
151. Daubert JC, Leclercq C, Alonso C, et al. Long-term experience with biventricular pacing in refractory heart failure. In: Ovsyshcher IE, ed. *Cardiac arrhythmias and device therapy: results*

and perspectives for the new century. Armonk, NY: Futura Publishing, 2000:385–392.
152. Auricchio A, Stellbrink C, Sack S, et al. Long-term benefit as a result of pacing resynchronization in congestive heart failure: results of the PATH-CHF Trial [Abstract]. *Circulation* 2000; 102[Suppl II]:II-693.
153. Walker S, Levy TM, Coats AJ, et al. Biventricular pacing in congestive cardiac failure: current experience and future directions. The Imperial College Cardiac Electrophysiology Group. *Eur Heart J* 2000;21:884–889.
154. Sack S, Auricchio A, Kadhiresan V, et al. Long-term improvement with ventricular resynchronization therapy in heart failure patients: does etiology of heart failure matter? [Abstract]. *Pacing Clin Electrophysiol* 2000;23:555.
155. Braunschweig F, Linde C, Gadler F, et al. Reduction of hospital days by biventricular pacing. *Eur J Heart Fail* 2000;2: 399–406.
156. Leclercq C, Alonso C, Pavin D, et al. Mortality in patients with permanent biventricular pacing for advanced heart failure: a 5-year single-center experience [Abstract]. *Pacing Clin Electrophysiol* 2000;23:596.
157. Kuehlkamp V, Doernberger V, Suchalla R, et al. Does biventricular pacing affect the incidence of ventricular tachyarrhythmias? [Abstract]. *Circulation* 2000;102[Suppl II]:II-761.
158. Ramaswamy K, Zagrodsky JD, Page RL, et al. Biventricular pacing decreases the inducibility of sustained monomorphic ventricular tachycardia [Abstract]. *Pacing Clin Electrophysiol* 2000;23:748.
159. Garrigue S, Barold SS, Hocini M, et al. Treatment of drug-refractory ventricular tachycardia by biventricular pacing. *Pacing Clin Electrophysiol* 2000:23:1700–1702.
160. Walker S, Levy T, Rex S, et al. Preliminary results with the simultaneous use of Implications for device interaction and development. *Pacing Clin Electrophysiol* 2000;23:365–372.
161. Higgins SL, Yong P, Sheck D, et al, for the Ventak CHF Investigators. Biventricular pacing diminishes the need for implantable cardioverter defibrillator therapy. *J Am Coll Cardiol* 2000;36:824–827.
162. Gaita F, Bocchiardo M, Porciani MC, et al. Should stimulation therapy for congestive heart failure be combined with defibrillation backup? *Am J Cardiol* 2000;86[Suppl 1]:K165–K168.
163. Walker S, Levy TM, Rex S, et al. Usefulness of suppression of ventricular arrhythmia by biventricular pacing in severe congestive cardiac failure. *Am J Cardiol* 2000;86:231–233.
164. Touiza A, Etienne Y, Gilard M, et al. Does acute hemodynamic evaluation predict long-term benefit of left ventricular-based pacing in patients with severe heart failure? *[Abstract].* Circulation 2000;102[Suppl II]:II-693.
165. Toussaint JF, Lavergne T, Darondel JM, et al. Early mechanical resynchronization predicts long-term right and left ejection fraction improvement in severe heart failure patients [Abstract]. *Circulation* 2000;102[Suppl II]:II-693.
166. Kay GN, Bourge RC. Biventricular pacing for congestive heart failure: questions of who, what, where, why, how, and how much. *Am Heart J* 2000;140:821–823.
167. Leclercq C, Daubert JC. Why biventricular pacing might be of value in refractory heart failure? *Heart* 2000;84:125–126.
168. Linde C. Biventricular pacing in patients with severe heart failure: has the time come? *Heart* 2000;84:123–124.
169. Barold SS, Cazeau S, Mugica J, et al. Permanent multisite cardiac pacing. *Pacing Clin Electrophysiol* 1997;20:2725–2729.
170. Cazeau S, Gras D, Lazarus A, et al. Multisite stimulation for correction of cardiac asynchrony. *Heart* 2000;84:579–581.
171. Barold SS. Biventricular cardiac pacing: promising new therapy for congestive heart failure. *Chest* 2000;118:1819–1821.
172. Daubert JC, Ritter P, Le Breton H, et al. Permanent left ventricular pacing with transvenous leads inserted into the coronary veins. *Pacing Clin Electrophysiol* 1998;21:239–245.
173. Ritter P, Gras D, Daubert C, for the MUSTIC Group. Implant success rate of the transvenous left ventricular lead in the MUSTIC trial [Abstract]. *Pacing Clin Electrophysiol* 2000;23:580.
174. Walker S, Levy T, Paul VE. Dissection of the coronary sinus secondary to pacemaker lead implantation. *Pacing Clin Electrophysiol* 2000;23:541–543.
175. Jaïs P, Douard H, Shah D, et al. Endocardial biventricular pacing. *Pacing Clin Electrophysiol* 1998;21:2128–2131.
176. Leclercq F, Hager FX, Marcia JC, et al. Left ventricular lead insertion using a transseptal catheterization technique: a totally endocardial approach for permanent biventricular pacing in end-stage heart failure. *Pacing Clin Electrophysiol* 1999;22:1570–1575.
177. Jaïs P, Takahashi A, Garrigue S, et al. Mid-term follow-up of endocardial biventricular pacing. *Pacing Clin Electrophysiol* 2000;23:1744–1747.
178. Gold MR, Rashba EJ. Left ventricular endocardial pacing: don't try this at home. *Pacing Clin Electrophysiol* 1999;22: 1567–1569.
179. Leclercq F, Kassnasrallah S, Macia JC, et al. Transcranial Doppler detection of microemboli during endocardial biventricular pacing in end-stage heart failure [Abstract]. *J Am Coll Cardiol* 2000;35[Suppl A]:141A.
180. Bocchiardo M, Padeletti L, Gasparini M, et al. Biventricular pacing in patients candidate to an ICD. *Eur Heart J* 2000; 2[Suppl J]:J36–J40.
181. Butter C, Auricchio A, Stellbrink C, et al. Non-simultaneous biventricular stimulation: a new paradigm of ventricular resynchronization therapy for heart failure patients [Abstract]. *Pacing Clin Electrophysiol* 2000;23:589.
182. Purefellner H, Nesser HJ, Winter S, et al. Transvenous left ventricular lead implantation with the EASYTRAK lead system: the European experience. *Am J Cardiol* 2000;86[Suppl 1]:K157–K164.
183. Curnis A, Neri R, Mascioli G, et al. Left ventricular pacing lead choice based on coronary sinus venous anatomy. *Eur Heart J* 2000;2[Suppl J]:J31–J35.
184. Walker S, Levy T, Rex S, et al. Initial results with left ventricular pacemaker lead implantation using a preformed "peel-away" guiding sheath and "side-wire" left ventricular pacing lead. *Pacing Clin Electrophysiol* 2000;23:985–990.
185. Butter C, Auricchio A, Stellbrink c, et al. Should stimulation site be tailored in the individual heart failure patient. *Am J Cardiol* 2000;86:K144–K151.
186. Auricchio A, Butter C, Stellbrink C, et al. Effect of left ventricular stimulation site on the systolic function of heart failure patients during ventricular resynchronization therapy [Abstract]. *Pacing Clin Electrophysiol* 2000;23:589.
187. Gras D, Mabo P, Bucknall C, et al. Does lead placement affect outcome of cardiac resynchronization in heart failure patients? Results from the InSync trial [Abstract]. *Pacing Clin Electrophysiol* 2000;23:580.
188. Schüller H, Brandt J. The pacemaker syndrome: old and new causes. *Clin Cardiol* 1991;14:336–340.
189. Brinker JA. Pursuing the perfect pacemaker. *Mayo Clin Proc* 1989;64:587–591.
190. Ellenbogen KA, Gilligan DM, Wood MA, et al. The pacemaker syndrome—a matter of definition. *Am J Cardiol* 1997; 79:1226–1229.
191. Chirife R, Ortega DF, Salazar AL. "Pacemaker syndrome" without a pacemaker: deleterious effects of first-degree AV block [Abstract]. *Rev Europ Technol Biomed* 1990;12:22.

192. Zornosa JP, Crossley GH, Haisty WK Jr, et al. Pseudopacemaker syndrome: a complication of radiofrequency ablation of the AV junction [Abstract]. *Pacing Clin Electrophysiol* 1992;15:590.
193. Kim YH, O'Nunain S, Trouton T, et al. Pseudo-pacemaker syndrome following inadvertent fast pathway ablation for atrioventricular nodal reentrant tachycardia. *J Cardiovasc Electrophysiol* 1993;4:178–182.
194. Kuniyashi R, Sosa E, Scanavacca M, et al. Pseudo-sindrome de marcapasso. *Arq Bras Cardiol* 1994;62:111–115.
195. Mabo P, Cazeau S, Forrer A, et al. Isolated long PR interval as only indication of permanent DDD pacing [Abstract]. *J Am Coll Cardiol* 1992;19:66A.
196. Mabo P, Varin C, Vauthier M, et al. Deleterious hemodynamic consequences of isolated long PR intervals: correction by DDD pacing [Abstract]. *Eur Heart J* 1992;13[Abstract Suppl]:225.
197. den Dulk K, Lindemans F, Brugada P, et al. Pacemaker syndrome with AAI rate-variable pacing: importance of atrioventricular conduction properties, medication and pacemaker programmability. *Pacing Clin Electrophysiol* 1988;11:1226–1230.
198. Rutishauser W, Wirz P, Gander M, et al. Atriogenic diastolic reflux in patients with atrioventricular block. *Circulation* 1966;34:807–817.
199. Schnittger I, Appleton CP, Hatle LK, et al. Diastolic mitral and tricuspid regurgitation by Doppler echocardiography in patients with atrioventricular block: new insight into the mechanism of atrioventricular valve closure. *J Am Coll Cardiol* 1988;11:83–88.
200. Appleton CP, Basnight MA, Gonzalez MS, et al. Diastolic mitral regurgitation with atrioventricular conduction abnormalities: relation of mitral flow velocity to transmitral pressure gradients in conscious dogs. *J Am Coll Cardiol* 1991;18:843–849.
201. Panidis IP, Ross J, Munley B, et al. Diastolic mitral regurgitation in patients with atrioventricular conduction abnormalities: a common finding by Doppler echocardiography. *J Am Coll Cardiol* 1986;7:768–774.
202. Ishikawa T, Kimura K, Miyazaki N, et al. Diastolic mitral regurgitation in patients with first-degree atrioventricular block. *Pacing Clin Electrophysiol* 1992;15:1927–1931.
203. Ishikawa T, Sumica S, Kimura K, et al. Critical PQ interval for the appearance of diastolic mitral regurgitation and optimal PQ interval in patients implanted with DDD pacemakers. *Pacing Clin Electrophysiol* 1994;17:1989–1994.
204. Wharton JM, Ellenbogen KA. Atrioventricular conduction system disease. In: Ellenbogen KA, Kay GN, Wilkoff BL, eds. *Clinical cardiac pacing*. Philadelphia: WB Saunders, 1995:304–320.
205. Iliev II, Yamachika S, Muta K, et al. Preserving normal ventricular activation versus atrioventricular delay optimization during pacing: the role of intrinsic atrioventricular conduction and pacing rate. *Pacing Clin Electrophysiol* 2000;23:74–80.
206. Bode F, Wiegand U, Katus HA, et al. Pacemaker inhibition due to prolonged native AV interval in dual-chamber devices. *Pacing Clin Electrophysiol* 1999;22:1425–1431.
207. Barold SS. Optimal pacing in first-degree AV block. *Pacing Clin Electrophysiol* 1999;22:1423–1424.
208. Greenspon AJ, Volasin KJ. "Pseudo" loss of atrial sensing by a DDD pacemaker. *Pacing Clin Electrophysiol* 1987;10:943–948.
209. Wilson JH, Lattner S. Undersensing of P waves in the presence of adequate P wave due to automatic postventricular atrial refractory period extension. *Pacing Clin Electrophysiol* 1989;12:1729–1732.
210. van Gelder BM, van Mechelen R, den Dulk K, et al. Apparent P wave undersensing in a DDD pacemaker post exercise. *Pacing Clin Electrophysiol* 1992;15:1651–1656.
211. Dodinot B, Beurrier D, Simon JP, et al. "Functional" loss of atrial sensing causing sustained first to high-degree AV block in patients with dual-chamber pacemakers [Abstract]. *Pacing Clin Electrophysiol* 1993;16:1189.
212. Pitney M, Davis M. Catheter ablation of ventriculoatrial conduction in the treatment of pacemaker mediated tachycardia. *Pacing Clin Electrophysiol* 1991;14:1013–1017.
213. Moss AJ, Glaser W, Topol E. Atrial tachypacing in the treatment of a patient with primary orthostatic hypotension. *N Engl J Med* 1980;302:1456–1457.
214. Goldberg MR, Robertson RM, Robertson D. Atrial tachypacing for primary orthostatic hypotension [Letter]. *N Engl J Med* 1980;303:885–886.
215. Kristinsson A. Programmed atrial pacing for orthostatic hypotension. *Acta Med Scand* 1983;214:79–83.
216. Cunha UG, Machado EL, Santana LA. Programmed atrial pacing in the treatment of neurogenic orthostatic hypotension in the elderly. *Arq Bras Cardiol* 1990;55:47–49.
217. Weissman P, Chin MT, Moss AJ. Cardiac tachypacing for severe refractory orthostatic hypotension. *Ann Intern Med* 1992;116:650–651.
218. Clémenty J, Gencel L, Garrigue S, et al. Permanent cardiac pacing in the treatment of orthostatic hypotension: literature data and five additional cases. In: Blanc JJ, Benditt D, Sutton R, eds. *Neurally mediated syncope*. Armonk, NY: Futura Publishing, 1996:127–136.
219. Abe H, Numata T, Hanada H, et al. Successful treatment of severe orthostatic hypotension with cardiac tachypacing in dual chamber pacemakers. *Pacing Clin Electrophysiol* 2000;23:137–139.
220. Grubb BP, Wolfe DA, Samoil D, et al. Adaptive rate pacing controlled by right ventricular preejection interval for severe refractory orthostatic hypotension. *Pacing Clin Electrophysiol* 1993;16:801–805.
221. Delfaut P, Saksena S, Prakash A, et al. Long-term outcome in patients with drug-refractory atrial flutter and fibrillation after single- and dual-site right atrial pacing for arrhythmia prevention. *J Am Coll Cardiol* 1998;32:1900–1908.
222. Mabo P, Daubert JC, Bohour A. Biatrial synchronous pacing for atrial arrhythmia prevention: the SYNBIAPACE study [Abstract]. *Pacing Clin Electrophysiol* 1999;22:755.
223. Neugebauer A, Mende M, Kolb HJ, et al. Long-term results of synchronous biatrial pacing for prevention of symptomatic atrial fibrillation [Abstract]. *Pacing Clin Electrophysiol* 1999;22:875.
224. D'Allones RG, Victor F, Pavin D, et al. Long-term effects of biatrial synchronous pacing to prevent drug refractory atrial tachyarrhythmias: a pilot study [Abstract]. *Pacing Clin Electrophysiol* 1999;22:755.
225. Lau CP, Tse HF, Yu CM, et al. Dual site right atrial pacing in paroxysmal atrial fibrillation without bradycardia (NIPP-AF Study) [Abstract]. *Pacing Clin Electrophysiol* 1999;22:804.
226. Friedman PA, Hill MR, Hammill SC, et al. Randomized prospective pilot study of long-term dual-site atrial pacing for prevention of atrial fibrillation. *Mayo Clin Proc* 1998;73:848–854.
227. Bondke H, Witte J, Reibis R, et al. Reduction of atrial fibrillation frequency by biatrial pacing [Abstract]. *Circulation* 1999;100[Suppl I]:I-151.
228. Witte J, Bondke HJ, Reibis R, et al. Biatrial pacing as an effective therapy for lone atrial fibrillation [Abstract]. *Pacing Clin Electrophysiol* 1999;22:A214.
229. Mirza I, Gill J, Bucknall C, et al. Prevention of refractory

paroxysmal atrial fibrillation with sequential biatrial pacing [Abstract]. *J Am Coll Cardiol* 1999;33:140A.
230. Daubert JC, Mabo P. Atrial pacing for the prevention of atrial fibrillation: how and where to pace? *J Am Coll Cardiol* 2000; 35:1423–1427.
231. Ramdat Misier AR, Beukema WP, Oude Luttikhuis HA, et al. Multisite atrial pacing: an option for atrial fibrillation prevention? Preliminary results of the Dutch dual-site right atrial pacing for the for the prevention of atrial fibrillation study. *Am J Cardiol* 2000;8[Suppl I]:K20–K24.
232. Leclercq JF, De Sisti A, Fiorello P, et al. Prevention of atrial fibrillation by dual-site vs. single-site atrial pacing [Abstract]. *Pacing Clin Electrophysiol* 2000;23:562.
233. D'Allones GR, Pavin D, Leclercq C, et al. Long-term effects of biatrial synchronous pacing to prevent drug-refractory atrial tachyarrhythmia: a nine-year experience. *J Cardiovasc Electrophysiol* 2000;11:1081–1091.
234. Levy T, Walker S, Rex S, et al. No incremental benefit of multisite atrial pacing compared with right atrial pacing in patients with drug-refractory paroxysmal atrial fibrillation. *Heart* 2001;85:48–52.
235. Tse HF, Lau CP, Yu CM, et al. Impact of dual site pacing on the natural history of symptomatic atrial fibrillation recurrence in patients without bradycardia [Abstract]. *J Am Coll Cardiol* 2000;35[Suppl A]:109A.
236. Lau CP, Tse HF, Yu CM, et al. Effect of dual site right atrial pacing on burden of atrial fibrillation in patients with drug-refractory atrial fibrillation [Abstract]. *J Am Coll Cardiol* 2000; 35[Suppl A]:109A.
237. Saksena S, Prakash A, Krol RB, et al. Dual site right atrial pacing is effective for long-term prevention of symptomatic chronic atrial fibrillation [Abstract]. *J Am Coll Cardiol* 2000; 35[Suppl A]:108A.
238. Saksena S, Prakash A, Boccadamo R, et al. Long-term safety and outcome of dual site right atrial pacing in patients with refractory paroxysmal and chronic atrial fibrillation [Abstract]. *Pacing Clin Electrophysiol* 2000;23:635.
239. Leclercq JF, De Sisti A, Fiorello P, et al. Prevention of atrial fibrillation by dual-site versus single-site Atrial pacing [Abstract]. *Pacing Clin Electrophysiol* 2000;23:582.
240. Beukema WP, Ramdat Misier AR, Luttikhuis HAO, et al. Dual versus single site right atrial pacing in patients with drug-refractory atrial fibrillation: a prospective r randomized trial [Abstract]. *Pacing Clin Electrophysiol* 2000;23:700.
241. Daubert C, Berder V, Gras D, et al. Atrial tachyarrhythmias associated with high degree interatrial conduction block: prevention by permanent atrial resynchronization. *Eur J Card Pacing Electrophysiol* 1994;1:35–44.
242. Daubert JC, D'Allonnes GR, Pavin D, et al. Prevention of atrial fibrillation by pacing. In: Ovsyshcher IE, ed. *Cardiac arrhythmias and device therapy: results and perspectives for the new century*. Armonk, NY: Futura Publishing, 2000:155–166.
243. Delfaut P, Saksena S. Electrophysiologic assessment in selecting patients for multisite atrial pacing. *J Interv Card Electrophysiol* 2000;4[Suppl 1]:81–85.
244. Nattel S, Li D, Yue L. Basic mechanisms of atrial fibrillation: new insights into very old ideas. *Annu Rev Physiol* 2000;62: 51–77.
245. Padeletti L, Porciani MC, Michelucci A, et al. Interatrial septum pacing: a new approach to prevent recurrent atrial fibrillation. *J Interv Card Electrophysiol* 1999;3:35–43.
246. Katsivas A, Manolis AG, Lazaris E, et al. Atrial septal pacing to synchronize atrial depolarization in patients with delayed interatrial conduction. *Pacing Clin Electrophysiol* 1998;21: 2220–2225.
247. Hermida JS, Carpentier C, Otmani A,, et al. Prevention of paroxysmal atrial fibrillation after resynchronization by atrial septal pacing: a prospective randomized study [Abstract]. *Circulation* 199;100[Suppl I]:I-152.
248. Padeletti L, Porciani C, Colella A, et al. Comparison of interatrial septum pacing with right atrial appendage pacing for the prevention of paroxysmal atrial fibrillation [Abstract]. *Pacing Clin Electrophysiol* 2000;23:582.
249. Fan K, Lee KL, Chiu CS, et al. Effects of biatrial pacing in prevention of postoperative atrial fibrillation after coronary artery bypass surgery. *Circulation* 2000;102:755–760.
250. Daoud EG, Dabir R, Archambeau M, et al. Randomized double-blind trial of simultaneous right and left atrial epicardial pacing for the prevention of post-open heart surgery atrial fibrillation. *Circulation* 2000;102:761–765.
251. Gerstenfeld EP, Hill MR, French SN, et al. Evaluation of right atrial and biatrial temporary pacing for the prevention of atrial fibrillation after bypass surgery. *J Am Coll Cardiol* 1999;33: 1981–1988.
252. Levy T, Fotopoulos G, Walker S, et al. Randomized controlled study of atrial fibrillation after coronary artery bypass surgery. *Circulation* 2000;102:1382–1387.
253. Sopher SM, Camm AJ. Atrial pacing to prevent atrial fibrillation. *J Interv Card Electrophysiol* 2000;4[Suppl]:149–153.
254. Fragakis N, Bostock J, Shakespeare C, et al. Reversion and maintenance of sinus rhythm in patients with permanent atrial fibrillation by internal cardioversion followed by biatrial pacing [Abstract]. *J Am Coll Cardiol* 2000;35[Suppl A]:108A.

IS THERE A ROLE FOR CARDIAC PACING IN VASODEPRESSOR SYNCOPE?

DAVID G. BENDITT, NEMER SAMNIAH, GERARD FAHY, KEITH G. LURIE, SCOTT SAKAGUCHI

Syncope most often occurs as a consequence of cerebral hypoperfusion caused by a transient but reversible period of arterial hypotension. Other potential mechanisms, such as global or regional cerebrovascular constriction, may also cause syncope, but it is believed that they are only infrequently the principal cause (1–3).

Vasodepressor syncope refers to those syncopal episodes in which the primary cause of systemic hypotension is an inappropriate fall in systemic vascular tone leading to a cerebrovascular perfusion pressure below the lower limit of the autoregulatory capacity of the cerebrovascular bed. In the so-called *pure neurally mediated vasodepressor faint,* the physiologic abnormality is a disturbance of neural control of peripheral vascular tone. In theory, other potentially contributing factors, such as bradycardia or cerebrovascular vasoconstriction is absent. Nevertheless, in most so-called vasodepressor faints, relative cardioinhibition is also evidenced by absence of an appropriate tachycardic response in the setting of severe hypotension. The magnitude of any concomitant cerebrovascular constrictive element is largely unknown.

In contrast to vasodepressor syncope, the cardioinhibitory form of the vasovagal faint is predominantly the result of cardiac slowing (often an asystolic pause exceeding 10 to 15 seconds) (Fig. 33-1). However, even in the presence of marked bradycardia, the practitioner cannot assume that the event is a pure cardioinhibitory faint. In such a circumstance, the absence of a driving force for blood flow (i.e., heart beat) makes it difficult to determine whether there is a concomitant contributing disturbance of vascular tone. Often, however, the latter may be suspected by observing a relatively slow recovery of systemic pressure after return of the heart beat (Fig. 33-2). Without inappropriate vasodilation, immediate restoration of blood pressure could be expected; "supernormal" pressure may be anticipated if appropriate reflex vasoconstriction has been evolving in the background.

Most supposedly vasodepressor or cardioinhibitory faints are not pure but exhibit mixed vasodilatation and bradycardic features (3). To the extent that it is possible, understanding the relative roles of these components in each patient may permit development of a more rational treatment strategy. Unfortunately, current diagnostic techniques do not permit such detailed assessment in most cases. It also remains uncertain whether spontaneous vasovagal events always exhibit the same balance of features in a given individual. Consequently, treatment plans must of necessity include consideration of both major pathophysiologic elements in essentially all cases.

This discussion focuses on the status of cardiac pac-

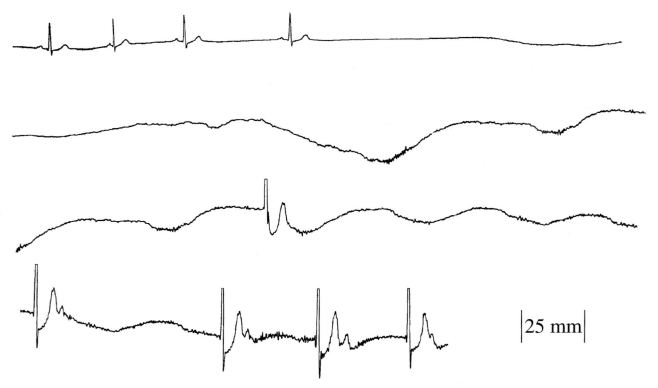

FIGURE 33-1. Electrocardiographic record obtained during a spontaneous vasovagal faint. Marked cardioinhibition is illustrated. Without a concomitant blood pressure trace, the magnitude of any coexisting vasodepressor element cannot be assessed.

ing in the treatment of the more common neurally mediated syncopal syndromes, especially the vasovagal faint. Particular attention is paid to strategies that have been incorporated into current-generation pacemakers to address the vasodepressor aspect of the faints. Consideration is also given to developments, which in the future may enhance the role of implantable devices in these settings.

TERMINOLOGY AND DEFINITIONS

Neurally mediated syncope (i.e., neurocardiogenic syncope) refers to any of a number of apparently related clinical conditions in which neural reflex–mediated disturbances of heart rate or vascular control contribute to systemic hypotension and inadequate cerebral perfusion and culminate in a faint or near-faint. Examples of some of the more common neurally mediated syncopal syndromes include the vasovagal faint, carotid sinus syndrome, postmicturition syncope, and cough syncope.

Vasovagal faint is a specific form of neurally mediated syncope, sometimes referred to as the *common* or *emotional faint*. As in the other forms of neurally mediated syncope, systemic hypotension may result from inappropriate neural reflex vasodilatation (i.e., vasodepressor form), marked bradycardia (i.e., cardioinhibitory form), or both (i.e., mixed form).

Vasodepressor syncope encompasses those neurally mediated syncopal events in which systemic hypotension predominantly results from inappropriate neural reflex vasodilatation. Unfortunately, this term occasionally is incorrectly employed as a synonym for vasovagal faint.

DIAGNOSTIC CRITERIA

Specific diagnostic criteria for separating vasodepressor, cardioinhibitory, and mixed forms of neurally

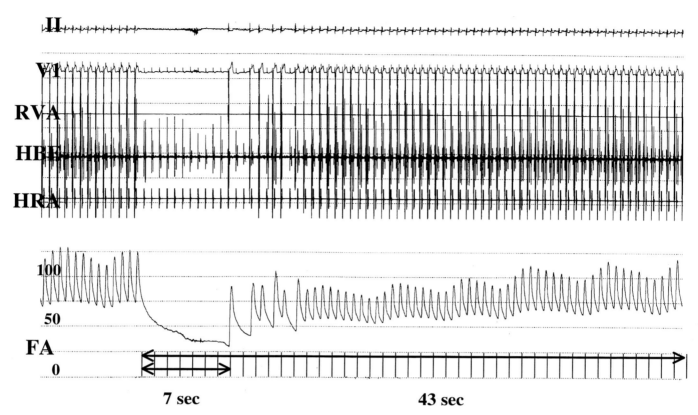

FIGURE 33-2. Recordings obtained during clinical laboratory tilt-table study of a patient with a clinical diagnosis of vasovagal syncope. Electrocardiographic, intracardiac, and blood pressure records are labeled. During the course of the study, the patient's blood pressure fell slightly with upright posture but stabilized at approximately 120/75 mm Hg just before the onset of a 7-second asystolic pause. Despite recovery of the heart rate after the pause, the blood pressure only slowly returned to normal values. Respiratory variation of blood pressure is also evident. These findings indicate the important vasodepressor physiology associated with this neurally mediated hypotensive event.

mediated syncope have not been developed. For the most part, current usage has evolved from the work of Franke (4) in which a drop of systemic arterial pressure of 50 mmHg with carotid sinus stimulation was deemed to indicate an abnormal vasodepressor response, and a pause of more than 3 seconds was taken to indicate abnormal cardioinhibition.

Although the Franke criteria suggest qualitatively the relative contributions of vasodepressor and cardioinhibitory components, they do not provide adequate diagnostic precision for identifying vasodepressor or cardioinhibitory faints. In this regard, it should be evident that a drop of 50 mm Hg of systemic pressure may or may not cause syncope, depending on the baseline arterial pressure from which the fall in pressure began, the autoregulatory status of the cerebrovascular bed, and the duration of the hypotensive period. Similarly, a pause of 3 seconds (or perhaps even 10 seconds) may not cause loss of consciousness, depending on factors such as the state of cerebral nutrient reserves and the posture of the patient.

The diagnostic criteria proposed for the Vasovagal International Study (VASIS) provide a workable basis for establishing the presence of a pure vasodepressor or pure cardioinhibitory response, although the investigators clearly recognize that the recommendations are arbitrary (3):

1. For the pure vasodepressor (VASIS type 3) diagnosis, the VASIS group focused almost exclusively

on heart rate issues and provided no quantitative assessment of the magnitude of abnormal blood pressure change required to establish the diagnosis. The criteria state that a pure vasodepressor response is present if during a tilt-induced (vasovagal-type) faint "heart rate rises progressively after adoption of a 60-degree head-up position and does not fall by more than 10% from its peak at the time of syncope. Blood pressure falls during tilt to cause syncope."

2. For cardioinhibitory syncope (VASIS type 2A and 2B), the VASIS definition states that the heart rate rises initially and then falls to a rate less than 40 bpm for more than 10 seconds or that asystole occurs for more than 3 seconds.

A physiologic basis for the VASIS standards was unfortunately not addressed by the VASIS investigators. It is perhaps as a result of that oversight that their seemingly sensible definitions have yet to become accepted worldwide. The investigators of the North American Vasovagal Pacemaker Study essentially ignored the VASIS definitions and adopted a more fanciful set of criteria (5,6). Specifically, for purposes of pacemaker eligibility, they required during tilt-table testing "a trough heart rate of less than 60 bpm if no isoproterenol was used, of more than 70 bpm if up to 2 μg/min of isoproterenol was used, or less than 80 bpm if more than 2 μg/min of isoproterenol was used." A physiologic rationale for these standards was not provided.

⊙ CAUSES OF VASODEPRESSOR SYNCOPE

The various neurally mediated syncopal syndromes are pathophysiologically closely related (2). Differences are largely related to the presumed trigger for the afferent neural signals, which initiate the reflex (e.g., cough in cough syncope, release of a distended bladder in postmicturition syncope). It is these afferent neural signals that set off a little-understood series of events within the medullary cardiovascular control areas, ultimately resulting in the efferent disturbances of heart rate and vascular control. The efferent neural reflex pathways comprise two elements: reduced sympathetic neural activity causing dilatation of skeletal muscle arterioles and splanchnic venules (vasodepressor component) and increased vagus nerve activity inducing bradycardia (cardioinhibitory component) and associated hypervagotonic symptoms such as nausea. The relative impact of the vasodepressor and cardioinhibitory elements may vary considerably among patients and perhaps even within patients at various times.

⊙ TREATMENT STRATEGIES FOR VASODEPRESSOR SYNCOPE

Excluding for the moment stress and anxiety management and education regarding avoidance of trigger events, the prevention of neurally mediated syncope recurrences (particularly in the case of the vasovagal faint but also to a somewhat lesser extent in carotid sinus syndrome) has focused on pharmacologic interventions (7–19). The two principal objectives have been to reduce susceptibility to the faint by use of agents such as beta-adrenergic blocking drugs or disopyramide and to prevent extreme manifestations of the episode by means of volume expanders (e.g., fludrocortisone, salt tablets), anticholinergics (e.g., scopolamine patches, disopyramide), or certain vasoconstrictor agents (e.g., midodrine). In essence, amelioration of the vasodepressor response has been a key target of pharmacologic strategies. Cardiac pacing has been used primarily for dealing with the cardioinhibitory element, especially in carotid sinus syndrome.

Not infrequently, combination therapy is needed. Education, volume expansion, drugs, and support hose may be necessary for patients who are very hard to treat. In some individuals, the addition of cardiac pacing to a pharmacologic regimen may also be of value. The latter is used primarily to ameliorate severe or relative bradycardia, but to a certain extent, it may also facilitate treatment of patients with predominant vasodepressor features. In the future, even more sophisticated implantable systems with pacing and drug-infusion capabilities may further enhance our ability to treat the most difficult cases.

CURRENT STATUS OF CARDIAC PACING

Carotid Sinus Syndrome

Cardiac pacing has proved highly successful in carotid sinus syndrome when bradycardia has been documented (20–26) and is the treatment of choice in all but the mildest forms of carotid sinus syndrome. The debate concerns the mode of pacing (i.e., single-chamber ventricular pacing versus dual-chamber pacing). In general, dual-chamber pacing with an abrupt rate-drop recognition feature and rapid pacing rate hysteresis response are desirable. The VVI or VVIR pacing mode should only be chosen if susceptibility to *ventricular pacing effect* (i.e., drop in systemic pressure as a result of ventricular pacing alone) and a substantial concomitant vasodepressor element can be clearly demonstrated to be absent. Single-chamber atrial pacing (AAI or AAIR) is contraindicated in carotid sinus syndrome and other forms of neurally mediated syncope because of the propensity for these conditions to be associated with paroxysmal high-grade atrioventricular (AV) block. In this regard, the presence of AV block may be masked by marked sinus bradycardia or asystole; it will, however, become immediately evident on pacing the atrium.

Despite the apparent clinical utility of cardiac pacing in carotid sinus syndrome, there is no convincing evidence that the vasodepressor component of the problem is adequately managed by conventional pacing. In this regard, Almquist and colleagues (28) studied eight patients with carotid sinus syndrome and did not find a significant difference in the drop in mean arterial pressure associated with carotid sinus stimulation in control (-60 ± 12 mmHg) or AV sequentially paced circumstances (-48 ± 19 mm Hg). In retrospect, the trend was perhaps encouraging, and the effects of higher rate pacing such as is employed in current *rate-drop response* devices might have been worth pursuing.

Vasovagal Syncope

Only within the past few years has the utility of cardiac pacing for treatment of recurrent vasovagal syncope become the subject of rigorous clinical study. Nevertheless, several professional societies, such as the American Heart Association and American College of Cardiology (29) and the British Pacing and Electrophysiology Working Group (30), have provided a class II indication for pacing in vasovagal syncope for some years.

In the longest follow-up study reported, Petersen and coworkers (31) examined the effectiveness of pacing in 37 patients in whom vasovagal syncope appeared to exhibit a predominantly cardioinhibitory character as assessed by tilt testing. Devices were programmed to the DDI mode to detect heart rates in the 40- to 50-bpm range and respond with pacing rates of 80 to 90 bpm. Patients were followed for 39 ± 19 months. Symptomatic improvement occurred in 84% of cases, with complete resolution of symptoms in 35%. The overall frequency of syncopal episodes (annual syncope burden) was reduced approximately 10-fold. In terms of prospective randomized studies, findings from the North American Vasovagal Pacemaker Study are available (5,6). The syncope recurrence rate was substantially less for the pacemaker group than control patients, resulting in an actuarial 1-year rate of recurrent syncope of approximately 18.5% for pacemaker patients and 59.7% for controls. However, the study was not without weaknesses (32), and a follow-up study addressing many of these limitations, particularly the potential placebo effect of a pacemaker implantation procedure, has been initiated. The results of the pacing arm of the VASIS trial (3,33) have also been reported, and are similar to those of the North American Study.

The studies described earlier focused on cardioinhibitory syncope primarily, but the entrance criteria did not absolutely exclude an important vasodepressor element. Consequently, a potential benefit of pacing in vasodepressor forms of the vasovagal faint remains possible. In reviewing the older literature, there is some suggestion, albeit indirect, that pacing benefit may exist in this setting. For example, in a prospective evaluation of the effects of temporary dual-chamber pacing in vasovagal syncope, Fitzpatrick and associates (34) examined hemodynamic and symptom status in seven patients with recurrent syncope and reproducible vasovagal reactions during tilt studies on 2 successive days. The pacing protocol in this study used a hysteresis feature in which the base rate was 50 bpm with an intervention rate of 90 bpm. With these settings, pacing was associated with greater cardiac index (baseline at 1.0 ± 0.2 L/min/m^2 versus paced at 1.6 ± 0.3 L/min/m^2), mean arterial blood pressure (baseline at 30 ± 11 mmHg versus paced at 48 ± 12 mmHg), and longer head-up tilt tolerance during induced vasovagal reactions. In five cases, syncope was prevented despite evident onset of a vasovagal reaction. In a somewhat larger study, Sra and colleagues (35) examined the impact of temporary cardiac pacing (at a rate approximately 20% higher than the supine resting heart rate) for prevention of tilt-induced hypotension in 22 patients for whom an initial tilt test was associated with at least modest bradycardia (heart rate nadir <60 bpm). Findings revealed that, despite pacing, mean arterial pressure fell significantly during upright tilt. However, the magnitude of tilt-induced hypotension was less during pacing than during tilt testing undertaken in the baseline untreated state (blood pressure decline paced at 41 ± 19 versus unpaced at 59 ± 16). Symptoms were much improved. Based on these studies, pacing at an elevated rate may ameliorate to some extent the hypotension associated with vasovagal episodes in patients who are not selected for having pure cardioinhibitory symptoms.

The optimal pacing algorithm for use during an impending vasovagal episode is unknown. Nevertheless, a form of rate hysteresis appears to offer benefit. Based on available clinical experience, the intervention rate probably needs to be in the range of 110 to 120 bpm. Periodically, the device needs to terminate pacing and to assess native heart rate and, if possible, systemic pressure. If these values have returned to normal, the pacing sequence terminates. If not, a further period of pacing support is initiated.

Vasovagal Syncope Detection and Pacing Interventions

Detection of any form of neurally mediated syncope by implantable pacing systems currently relies solely on recognition of relatively abrupt heart rate slowing (i.e., the cardioinhibitory element). For example, in the first vasovagal treatment algorithms introduced commercially, the Thera series of pacemakers (Medtronic, Inc., Minneapolis, MN) employed a rate-drop response feature, which may be characterized as a programmable *Window* used to identify heart rate changes compatible with an evolving vasovagal episode (36). The Window was defined by selectable upper (*Top Rate* in bpm) and lower (*Bottom Rate* in bpm) rate settings and by a similarly adjustable duration (*Width* in number of beats). During a period of evolving bradycardia, a vasovagal event was identified if the heart rate falls through the Window, beginning from a heart rate above the Top Rate and proceeding to a point below the Bottom Rate before expiration of the Width criterion (i.e., in a period less than a preprogrammed number of heart beats). A separate selectable confirmation criterion (*Confirmation* in programmable number of beats) must also be satisfied. This latter criterion required that the heart rate, after falling through the Window, remain less than the Bottom Rate for a programmable number of beats before pacing intervention can be initiated.

Subsequent evolution of the rate-drop response technique resulted in elimination of the programmable window. Instead, a *drop detect* feature was introduced (Fig. 33-3A). In this case, the concept was to increase diagnostic sensitivity by flagging any heart rate drop of a predetermined amount occurring within a given duration of time (i.e., *Detection Window*). In recent-model Kappa pacemakers (Medtronic, Inc.), the duration of the Detection Window is programmable for 2.5 to 10 minutes (Fig. 33-4). The device tracks peak rates, defined as the heart rate immediately below the fastest detected rate so as to avoid targeting premature cycles. If the drop in heart rate takes longer than this predetermined duration, a diagnosis is not made. Before treatment is initiated, however, a predetermined low rate (i.e., *Drop Rate*) must be achieved and confirmed. This same system also uses a second backup detection algorithm, referred to as the sustained low-rate pacing detection method (Fig. 33-3B). The physician is advised to program the *Low Rate* to a level lower than any expected conventional low heart rate in that patient. This may be difficult or impossible to do properly without also underestimating the heart rate nadir in vasovagal events.

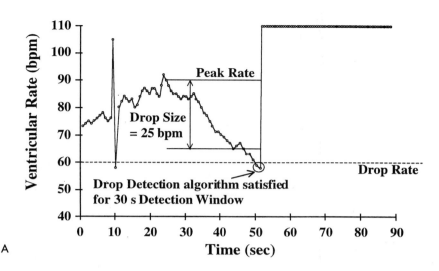

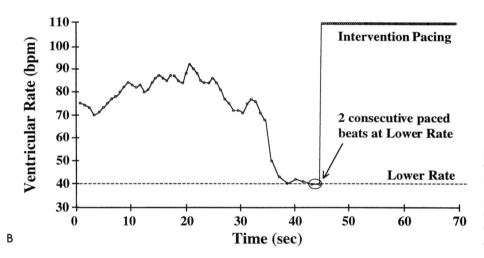

FIGURE 33-3. Recordings illustrate the detection methods for neurally mediated syncope employed in the Medtronic Kappa series of pacemakers. **A:** The drop detection aspect of the algorithm. **B:** The low rate detection method aspect of the algorithm.

The Thera and Kappa algorithms provide a programmable period of high-rate pacing after diagnostic criteria are fulfilled. The diagnostics are very cardioinhibitory dependent, but the treatment is aimed in part at overcoming the vasodepressor element of hypotension by forcing a relatively fast heart rate for a predetermined period. A similar effect can be obtained using recent Vitatron, Inc. (Dieren, The Netherlands), devices incorporating the so-called physiologic pacing band (37) (Fig. 33-4). In theory, this approach can take advantage of the frequently observed increase in atrial rate that precedes bradycardia in an evolving vasovagal faint. The increased rate forces the physiologic band to somewhat higher heart rates than would be customary in that patient. Consequently, subsequent development of abrupt bradycardia results in the device pacing at the lower end of the physiologic band. In this manner, the device averts the cardioinhibitory element and minimizes the additional hypotensive vasodepressor element by maintaining a relatively high pacing rate.

Rate-drop algorithms have been the most widely

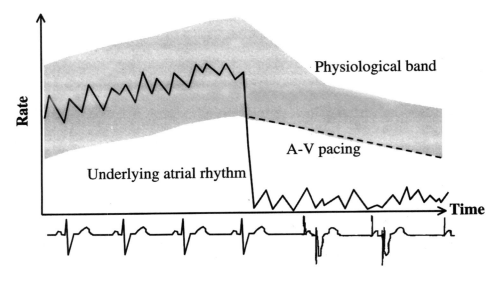

FIGURE 33-4. The schematic drawing shows the use of the Vitatron, Inc., physiologic band concept as a means of detecting neurally mediated bradycardia and of providing a pacing intervention.

adopted approach to detecting neurally mediated syncopal events by implantable pacing systems. Nevertheless, the methodology has limitations, and alternative methods are needed. This is especially the case when the event is primarily vasodepressor with little or no bradycardia. It would be desirable for implantable systems targeting the neurally mediated faints to recognize not only abrupt heart rate changes but other electrophysiologic, hemodynamic, and neurologic data. For example, several reports have examined the potential utility of assessing ventricular contractile state using an accelerometer in the distal end of the pacemaker electrode (BEST system, Sorin, Inc., Saluggia, Italy) (38–40) (Fig. 33-5). Petersen and coworkers examined the potential effect of dP/dt sensors for detecting pressure declines associated with vasodepressor faints (41). The results were too variable to be of immediate utility, but the concept is intriguing and may become of value in a combined sensor system.

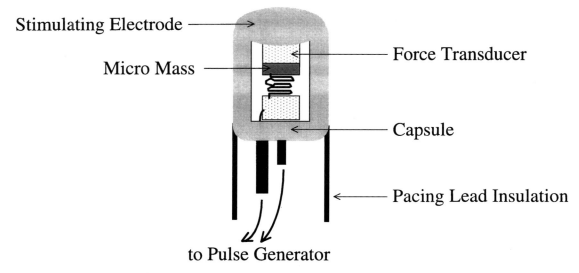

FIGURE 33-5. The schematic drawing shows the accelerometer sensor within the electrode of a pacing system (Sorin Inc, BEST system).

The concept of employing novel sensor strategies (perhaps in combinations) for triggering device therapy in severe recurrent neurally mediated syncope seems necessary to pursue. Along with heart rate assessment, the tracking of PR or QT interval variations or markers of change in systemic pressure, respiratory rate, or ventricular contractile state, may provide sensitive and specific recognition of vasovagal syndromes at an early stage. Treatment by pacing or drug delivery could then be initiated sooner and with greater confidence than is the case currently. Pacing interventions are initiated only after the onset of bradycardia. However, because vasodilatation tends to precede marked heart rate slowing (42), late-onset pacing may not be able to compensate sufficiently. Conceivably, pacing at an earlier stage could enhance treatment effectiveness. In this regard, the findings from Sra and associates (35), in which pacing was initiated in the supine posture before tilt, support this notion. Sutton and colleagues (43) had less success when pacing was manually triggered at what appeared to be an early stage of the vasovagal event. Further study of this concept is needed.

More effective sensor systems may permit extension of implantable device therapy, perhaps through a combined pacing and drug-delivery system, to patients who never develop severe bradycardia during their faints. Agents such as midodrine, ephedrine, phenylephrine or disopyramide could be candidates for parenteral delivery. However, before such an approach becomes feasible, considerable progress must be made in the development of diagnostic algorithms and in our understanding of drug dosing and routes of delivery.

CONCLUSIONS

Several lines of evidence suggest that cardiac pacing may be a useful adjunctive therapy in selected patients with recurrent vasovagal syncope. It appears that relative high pacing rates can be used to minimize the vasodepressor aspect of the vasovagal faint (i.e., prolong the warning phase and delay onset of the faint) and in other forms of neurally mediated syncope.

Despite the potential utility of cardiac pacing in vasodepressor faints, maximum benefit may not be attainable until several barriers are overcome. First, it is essential to develop implantable systems capable of recognizing vasovagal syncope at an early stage; in this regard, it is especially crucial to identify the occurrence of evolving hypotension in the absence of marked bradycardia. Second, better understanding of the most effective pacing algorithms is needed. Consideration needs to be given to combining pacing systems with evolving drug-infusion systems. Such a combined system may be better able to direct effective therapy to the cardioinhibitory and vasodepressor aspects of the neurally mediated faints.

ACKNOWLEDGMENT

The authors would like to thank Barry L. S. Detloff for technical assistance and Wendy Markuson for preparation of the manuscript.

REFERENCES

1. Kapoor W. Evaluation and outcome of patients with syncope. *Medicine (Baltimore)* 1990;69:160–175.
2. Benditt DG, Goldstein MA, Adler S, et al. Neurally mediated syncopal syndromes: pathophysiology and clinical evaluation. In: Mandel WJ, ed. *Cardiac arrhythmias,* 3rd ed. Philadelphia: JB Lippincott, 1995:879–906.
3. Sutton R, Petersen M, Brignole M, et al: Proposed classification for tilt induced vasovagal syncope. *Eur J Card Pacing Electrophysiol* 1992;2:180–183.
4. Franke H. *Uber das Karotissimus-Syndrome und den soy enannten hyperactiv en Karotissimus-Reflex.* Stuttgart: Friedrich-Kave Schattauer Verlag, 1963.
5. Sheldon RS, Gent M, Robert RS, Connolly SJ, for the NA-VAPC Investigators. North American Vasovagal Pacemaker study: study design and organization. *Pacing Clin Electrophysiol* 1997;20[Suppl II]:844–848.
6. Connolly SJ, Sheldon R, Roberts RS, Gent M, for the North American Vasovagal Pacemaker Study (VPS). A randomized trial of permanent cardiac pacing for the prevention of vasovagal syncope. *J Am Coll Cardiol* 1999;33:16–20.
7. Raviele A, Gasparini G, Di Pede F, et al. Usefulness of head-up tilt test in evaluating patients with syncope of unknown origin and negative electrophysiologic study. *Am J Cardiol* 1990; 65:1322–1327.
8. Benditt DG, Sakaguchi S, Schultz JJ, et al. Syncope: diagnostic considerations and the role of tilt table testing. *Cardiol Rev* 1993; 1:146–156.
9. Kosinski DJ, Grubb BP. Neurally mediated syncope with an update on indications and usefulness of head-up tilt table testing and pharmacologic therapy. *Curr Opin Cardiol* 1994;9:53–64.
10. Milstein S, Buetikofer J, Dunnigan A, et al. Usefulness of disopyramide for prevention of upright tilt-induced hypotension-bradycardia. *Am J Cardiol* 1990;65:1339–1344.
11. Fitzpatrick AP, Ahmed R, Williams S, Sutton R. A randomised

trial of medical therapy in "malignant vasovagal syndrome" or "neurally mediated bradycardia hypotension syndrome." *Eur J Card Pacing Electrophysiol* 1991;2:99–102.
12. Nelson S, Stanley M, Love C, et al. Autonomic and hemodynamic effects of oral theophylline in patients with vasodepressor syncope. *Arch Intern Med* 1991;90:2425–2429.
14. Sra JS, Murthy VS, Jazayeri MR, et al. Use of intravenous esmolol to predict efficacy of oral adrenergic blocker therapy in patients with neurocardiogenic syncope. *J Am Coll Cardiol* 1993;19:402–408.
15. Morillo C, Leitch JW, Yee R, Klein GJ. A placebo-controlled trial of intravenous and oral disopyramide for prevention of neurally mediated syncope induced by head-up tilt. *J Am Coll Cardiol* 1993;22:1843–1848.
16. Grubb BP, Wolfe D, Samoil D, et al. Usefulness of fluoxetine hydrochloride for prevention of resistant upright tilt induced syncope. *Pacing Clin Electrophysiol* 1993;16:458–464.
17. Kosinski DJ, Grubb BP, Temesy-Armos PN. The use of serotonin re-uptake inhibitors in the treatment of neurally mediated cardiovascular disorders. *J Serotonin Res* 1994;1:85–90.
18. Mahanonda N, Bhuripanyo K, Kangkagate C, et al. Randomized double-blind placebo-controlled trial of oral atenolol in patients with unexplained syncope and positive upright tilt table results. *Am Heart J* 1995;130:1250–1253.
19. Moya A, Permanyer-Miralda G, Sagrista-Sauleda J, et al. Limitations of head-up tilt test for evaluating the efficacy of therapeutic interventions in patients with vasovagal syncope: results of a controlled study of etilefrine versus placebo. *J Am Coll Cardiol* 1995;25:65–69.
20. Atiga WL, Rowe P, Calkins H. Management of vasovagal syncope. *J Cardiovasc Electrophysiol* 1999;10:874–886.
21. Fabian WH, Benditt DG, Lurie KG. Neurally-mediated syncope. *Curr Treat Options Cardiovasc Med* 1999;1:137–144.
22. Morley CA, Perrins EJ, Grant P, et al. Carotid sinus syncope treated by pacing: analysis of persistent symptoms and role of atrioventricular sequential pacing. *Br Heart J* 1982;47:411–418.
23. Madigan NP, Flaker GC, Curtis JJ, et al. Carotid sinus hypersensitivity: beneficial effects of dual-chamber pacing. *Am J Cardiol* 1984;53:1034–1040.
24. Brignole M, Sartore B, Barra M, et al. Is DDD superior to VVI pacing in mixed carotid sinus syndrome? An acute and medium-term study. *Pacing Clin Electrophysiol* 1988;11:1902–1910.
25. Brignole M, Sartore B, Barra M, et al. Ventricular and dual chamber pacing for treatment of carotid sinus syndrome. *Pacing Clin Electrophysiol* 1989;12:582–590.
26. Deschamps D, Richard A, Citron B, et al. Hypersensibilite sino-carotidienne: evolution a moyen et a long terme des patients traites par stimulation ventriculaire. *Arch Mal Coeur* 1990;83:63–67.
27. Brignole M, Menozzi C, Lolli G, et al. Validation of a method for choice of pacing mode in carotid sinus syndrome with or without sinus bradycardia. *Pacing Clin Electrophysiol* 1991;14:196–203.
28. Almquist A, Gornick CC, Benson DW Jr, Benditt DG. Carotid Sinus hypersensitivity: evaluation of the vasodepressor component. *Circulation* 1985;71:927–937.
29. Gregoratis G, Cheitlin MD, Conil A, et al. ACC/AHA guidelines for implantation of cardiac pacemakers and antiarrhythmia devices. *J Am Coll Cardiol* 1998;31:1175–1209.
30. British Pacing and Electrophysiology Group Working Party. Recommendations for pacemaker prescription for symptomatic bradycardia. *Br Heart J* 1991;66:185–191.
31. Petersen MEV, Chamberlain-Webber R, Fizpatrick AP, et al. Permanent pacing for cardio-inhibitory malignant vasovagal syndrome. *Br Heart J* 1994;71:274–281.
32. Benditt DG. Cardiac pacing for prevention of vasovagal syncope. *J Am Coll Cardiol* 1999;33:21–33.
33. Sutton R, Brignole M, Menozzi C, et al. Dual-chamber pacing is efficacious in treatment of neurally-mediated tilt positive cardioinhibitory syncope. Pacemaker versus no therapy: a multi-centre study. *Circulation* 2000;294–299.
34. Fitzpatrick A, Theodorakis G, Ahmed R, et al. Dual chamber pacing aborts vasovagal syncope induced by head-up 60 degree tilt. *Pacing Clin Electrophysiol* 1991;14:13–19.
35. Sra J, Jazayeri MR, Avitall B, et al. Comparison of cardiac pacing with drug therapy in the treatment of neurocardiogenic (vasovagal) syncope with bradycardia or asystole. *N Engl J Med* 1993:328;1085–1090.
36. Benditt DG, Sutton R, Gammage M, et al. "Rate-drop response" cardiac pacing for vasovagal syncope. *J Interv Card Electrophysiol* 1999;3:27–33.
37. Velimirovic D, Pavlovic S, Charles RG. A novel algorithm to detect sudden rate drop—initial experience [Abstract]. *Pacing Clin Electrophysiol* 1999;22:100.
38. Deharo J-C, Peyre J-P, Ritter PH, et al. A sensor-based evaluation of heart contractility in patients with head-up tilt induced neurally-mediated syncope [Abstract]. *Pacing Clin Electrophysiol* 1997;20:1096.
39. Deharo J-C, Peyre J-P, Ritter PH, et al. Adaptive rate pacing controlled by a myocardial contractility index for treatment of malignant neurally-mediated syncope [Abstract]. *Pacing Clin Electrophysiol* 1997;20:1192.
40. Gensini GF, Vaccari M, Plicchi G, et al. Temporary diagnostic utilization of endocardial acceleration sensor in critical setting. In: Santini M, ed. *Progress in clinical pacing 1996.* Armonk, NY: Futura Media Service, 1997:175–182.
41. Petersen ME, Williams TR, Erickson M, Sutton R. Right ventricular pressure, dP/dt, and preejection interval during tilt induced vasovagal syncope. *Pacing Clin Electrophysiol* 1997;20:806–809.
42. Chen M-Y, Goldenberg IF, Milstein S, et al. Cardiac electrophysiologic and hemodynamic correlates of neurally-mediated syncope. *Am J Cardiol* 1989;63:66–72.
43. Sutton R. Personal communication, 1999.

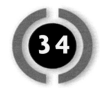

EXTRACTION OF TRANSVENOUS PACEMAKER AND DEFIBRILLATOR LEADS

• • •

AYMAN S. AL-KHADRA, BRUCE L. WILKOFF

The development of transvenous pacing and defibrillation systems represents an important milestone in arrhythmia management. With widening indications for such systems, the number of implants has risen dramatically. Transvenous leads are implanted in a hostile environment where they are exposed to tremendous physical stresses and host reactions. They are susceptible to bacterial colonization and infections as a consequence of transient bacteremias. A significant number of leads fail under such stresses and require removal. Explanting such leads would be an easy task if it were not for the considerable fibrous reaction that they elicit in the human body. Over the past few years, significant advances have been made in the area of transvenous lead extraction, allowing for controlled disruption of fibrosis and complete removal of the leads at an acceptable risk to the patient (1).

◉ PATHOLOGY OF THE HUMAN-LEAD INTERACTION: THE CHALLENGE OF EXTRACTION

The goal of the extraction procedure is the complete and safe removal of all transvenous leads. However, chronically implanted leads are fixed to the underlying myocardium by fibrous tissue. This process starts at the time of lead implantation and progresses over time. The initiating mechanism is endocardial and results from intimal damage triggered by mechanical trauma and possibly enhanced by host reaction to certain components of the lead itself. Certain patients appear to react more strongly than others. Other factors that determine the intensity of the fibrous reaction include the chamber in which the lead is implanted and the fixation mechanism. Leads implanted in the right ventricle are subjected to more mechanical stress, and significantly greater length of the lead is in contact with the endocardium. Passive fixation, compared with active fixation, appears to elicit more host reaction at the tip of the lead, possibly because of greater contact and movement between the tip and the endocardium. Nonthoracotomy implantable defibrillator leads (NTLs), which are characterized by their large size and rough shocking electrode surface, appear to incite intense endocardial fibrosis (2,3). The endothelial injury causes thrombus formation, which organizes into a fibrous capsule that surrounds the lead. This process is more exaggerated at sites of repeated contact between the lead and the endothelium. The resulting scar tissue thickens and its tensile strength increases with maturation of collagen. Over time, this fibrous tissue becomes calcified (Fig. 34-1).

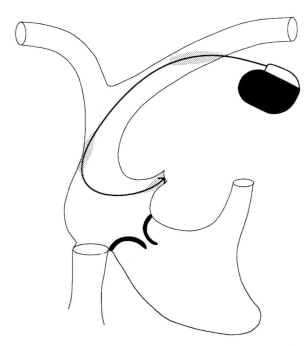

FIGURE 34-1. Fibrotic attachments of transvenous leads. Thrombotic and fibrotic tissue form along the length of the lead at sites of contact between the lead and the endovascular structures. Typical locations include the venous entry site, the superior vena cava wall, and at the electrode-endocardium interface. The strongest fibrosis is often found not at the lead tip but along the brachiocephalic vein or in contact with the other leads. This fibrotic tissue thickens and frequently becomes calcified with time.

Once held in place by the fibrosis, physical characteristics of the lead, particularly its basic construction and strength and its fixation mechanism, determine its handling characteristics when subjected to extraction forces. Leads with poor tensile properties are removed in pieces, whereas strong leads may refuse to breakup and can tear the myocardium. To avoid these situations, the operator must have control over every component of the lead, as well as the tools that are used to dissect the fibrosis. To control the lead, different tools are used to prepare the lead and apply equal pulling forces on the conductors, the tip, and the insulation. The challenge is that control of the tools dissecting the fibrous tissue is indirect. Such tools could be cutting through the lead or the vascular wall while giving little hint to the inexperienced operator of the gravity of the situation. Control of such tools can only be mastered with adequate training in a highly supervised environment.

⊙ INDICATIONS FOR EXTRACTION

The indications for transvenous lead extraction (Table 34-1) can be broadly divided into patient-related and lead-related indications. Patient-related indications can be further grouped as those related to an infection and those that are not related to an infection. The latter group includes cases of ineffective therapy (i.e., very high defibrillation thresholds) or the development of complications related to the lead placement, such as perforation, migration, embolization, and induction of arrhythmias, venous thrombosis, or the pain syndrome. Other patient indications include device interactions, device upgrades, change in the underlying disease (e.g., resolution of viral cardiomyopathy), or the presence of multiple abandoned leads.

TABLE 34-1 • INDICATION FOR PACEMAKER AND DEFIBRILLATOR LEAD EXTRACTION

I. Patient-related indications
  A. Infectious
    1. Localized pocket infections
    2. Sepsis
    3. Partially treated chronic infection
    4. Endocarditis
  B. Noninfectious
    1. Ineffective therapy (high pacing or defibrillation thresholds)
    2. Noninffectious complications
      a. Perforation
      b. Migration
      c. Embolization
      d. Induction of arrhythmia
      e. Venous thrombosis
      f. Pain syndrome
      g. Tricuspid valvular incompetence
    3. Device interactions
    4. System upgrades
    5. Change in the underlying indication or cardiac pathology (e.g., resolution of viral myocarditis)
    6. Prophylactic
      a. Presence of multiple leads
      b. Abandoned leads
      c. Telectronics J leads
II. Lead-related indications
  A. Lead recall
  B. Lead failure
    1. Insulation failure
    2. Conductor failure
    3. J-wire protrusion or fracture
  C. Lead interactions

Lead-related indications include lead recalls, lead failure, and the possibility of lead interactions (e.g., having two nonthoracotomy leads simultaneously) (4).

The indications for extraction can also be subgrouped into those mandating removal and those for which lead extraction is discretionary. For example, extraction of an infected system in a septic patient is mandatory, but extraction of a nonrecalled, abandoned, single-atrial lead that is being upgraded is discretionary. In most situations however, there is no clear dividing line between mandatory and discretionary indications, and the decision has to be made on a case-by-case basis. Age, sex, coexisting medical conditions, the number of leads traversing the superior veins, the age and type of the leads that need to be extracted, the potential for lead-lead interaction, the availability of venous access, the perceived risk of the operation, and the experience of the operator are all important factors. However, when the physical presence of pacing or defibrillation leads left in place pose a clear threat to the patient's health or life, extraction is indicated.

● OUTCOME OF LEAD EXTRACTION

The results of transvenous pacemaker lead extractions have been reported extensively in the literature (Table 34-2). However, there are limited reports describing procedural and overall success rates and risks associated with defibrillator lead extractions. Data from several published studies (5–10) using the superior vein approach without the laser tools revealed a success rate of 64% to 88% and risk of major complications of less than 1%. With the advent of laser extraction sheaths, success rates increased significantly (9). The Pacemaker Lead Extraction with the Laser Sheath (PLEXES) trial, a randomized trial of lead extraction with and without use of 12-Fr laser sheaths, enrolled 301 patients with 465 chronically implanted leads. Successful lead removal was achieved in 94% of attempts in the laser group and 64% in the nonlaser group ($p < 0.001$). Laser was successful in extracting 88% of leads that were not extracted using conventional tools. Extraction times were also significantly reduced in the laser group. Of the 244 patients who had laser extraction, three had complications, including one death (p was not significant). This complica-

TABLE 34-2 • LEAD EXTRACTION SUCCESS RATES

Clinical Characteristics	Complete (%)	Partial (%)	Failed (%)
Implant Duration			
1 year	98.9	0.8	0.3
2–4 years	97.8	1.9	0.3
5–7 years	94.1	5.1	0.9
8–24 years	83.6	12.6	3.8
Fixation			
Active	94.5	4.2	1.2
Passive	93.0	5.8	1.2
Placement			
Atrial	96.2	3.1	0.7
Ventricular	91.4	6.8	1.8
Total	93.8	4.9	1.2

Data from Cook Vascular Incorporated multicenter lead extraction registry. Presented at the annual scientific sessions of the North American Society for Pacing and Electrophysiology (NASPE). May 7, 1997. New Orleans. LA. Data were based on attempted extraction of 3,040 leads from 1,895 patients by 23 physicians who verified complete reporting of procedures from January 1994 through February 1997.

tion rate is consistent with the rate observed in the Cook Extraction Registry. Kennergren (11) and Levy (25) also reported similar results.

Attempts at extraction of NTLs have been met with similar rates of success (12–14). Our group from the Cleveland Clinic Foundation, accumulated the largest series of NTL extraction. Successful complete extraction of NTLs with and without use of laser tools, without major complications, was achieved in 92.7% of attempts to extract 110 leads. Clinical success was achieved in 97.8% of patients ($n = 94$). Failure, including development of major complications, occurred in two patients (15).

● TECHNIQUE OF TRANSVENOUS LEAD EXTRACTION

In the following sections, we describe techniques of transvenous pacemaker lead extraction, followed by a discussion of the variations necessary to extract certain pacemaker and defibrillator leads. At the Cleveland Clinic Foundation, the procedure is performed in the electrophysiology laboratory with immediate cardiothoracic surgical backup available. The procedure is performed under local anesthesia with deep intravenous sedation (16–18). This arrangement works for most patients presenting for transvenous lead extraction. However, when there are multiple leads to be extracted, when there is a large amount of debridement required, or if the patient is excessively anxious, it is appropriate to use general anesthesia. Most patients also undergo concomitant reimplantation of a new system unless there is evidence of infection or the indications for device implantation cease to exist.

The Patient

A detailed history and physical examination should be obtained for all patients, focusing on the original indication and the details of the pacemaker implantation procedure. Details about implanted hardware and the functional status of each of the components are essential to the construction of an extraction strategy. A chest radiograph, including overpenetrated posteroanterior and lateral x-ray films, should be obtained. Fluoroscopic views and venography of the leads and the superior veins may be necessary. The pacemaker system should be evaluated fully with pacing and sensing thresholds, including unipolar and bipolar thresholds. A detailed discussion of the strategy, possible outcomes, and possible risks should be conducted with the patient and his or her family. Informed consent can then be obtained.

The patient is brought to the electrophysiology laboratory in the postabsorptive state and is given a mild sedative. Supplemental oxygen is given as necessary.

The Operating Room

The operation can take place wherever the best environment exists for the extracting physician. Fluoroscopy is often far superior in the cardiac catheterization laboratory or the electrophysiology laboratory, whereas anesthesia and surgical support are better in the operating room. In either case, a comfortable environment with excellent fluoroscopy, including higher-magnification fluoroscopy, and anesthesia support must exist. Echocardiography, pericardiocentesis, peripheral cardiopulmonary bypass equipment, and thoracotomy instruments should be immediately available.

The Operator

Transvenous lead extraction is a technically complicated procedure that requires superior skills and judgment on part of the operator. Appropriate decision making and handling of potential complications demands that it is done only by well-trained physicians with adequate experience (Table 34-3). Even among those who were trained to perform lead extractions, it is appropriate to triage high-risk cases to more experienced operators. Every procedure is unique in some way, providing an opportunity to improvise and learn. A firm commitment to reporting each procedure to the national database enables the accumulated experience to contribute to the production of better leads, better understanding of failure mechanisms, avoidance of complications, and improved extraction techniques.

Preoperative Setup

The patient is prepped, and a large thoracic drape is placed from the neck to the groins, so that access to

TABLE 34-3 • COMPLICATIONS BY INTERVENTION

Complication[a]	Deaths	Total
Thoracotomy repair (tamponade or hemothorax)	2 (0.11%)	14 (0.74%)
Drainage—pericardiocentesis (hemopericardium or tamponade)	0	7 (0.37%)
Drainage—chest tube (hemothorax and pneumothorax)	0	4 (0.21%)
Transfusions	0	5 (0.26%)
Pulmonary embolism	0	1 (0.05%)
Subclavian AV fistula	1 (0.05%)	2 (0.11%)
Total	3 (0.16%)	28 (1.48%)

[a]Some patients have multiple events
Data from Cook Vascular Incorporated multicenter lead extraction registry. Presented at the annual scientific sessions of the North American Society for Pacing and Electrophysiology (NASPE). May 7, 1997. New Orleans, LA. Data were based on attempted extraction of 3,040 leads from 1,895 patients by 23 physicians who verified complete reporting of procedures from January 1994 through February 1997.

both deltopectoral areas and both groins is facilitated. Two large-bore intravenous lines, an arterial line, and a femoral venous line are placed to facilitate the administration of medications and fluids, monitoring of blood pressure, and insertion of temporary pacing lead if necessary, respectively. Placement of an additional central venous line is optional. The electrocardiogram (ECG) is continuously monitored. If the patient demonstrates pacemaker dependency, even if the ventricular lead is not to be removed, a temporary pacemaker is appropriate. The temporary pacing wire is placed at a stable position in the right ventricle away from the location of the soon-to-be-extracted ventricular lead. Sometimes, it is appropriate to place the pacing lead in the coronary sinus, which is conveniently located far from the ventricular leads.

Superior Venous Approach

Key Principles

Control of the tip and the body of the lead and controlled disruption of the fibrous tissue are the most important elements determining success of the extraction procedure while minimizing the risk to the patient. Control of the pacemaker lead body includes binding of its elements and applying uniform forces on the entire length of the lead so that it can be removed in one piece with minimal distortion or elongation. This control facilitates complete lead removal and helps with controlled disruption of the fibrous tissue along the lead.

Controlled disruption of the fibrous tissue is achieved through intravascular counterpressure, with the pulling force applied on the proximal end and the body of the lead assembly, against the tools dissecting through the fibrosis (Fig. 34-2). This force is applied tangentially to the vessel wall and adhering fibrous tissue. Counterpressure is therefore potentially associated with higher risk of vascular injury than other steps during lead extraction. By slowly advancing the sheaths over the electrode, only a modest degree of tensile integrity is required by the lead and by the vein leading to the heart. The risk of lead fragmentation and cardiovascular disruption is greatly reduced.

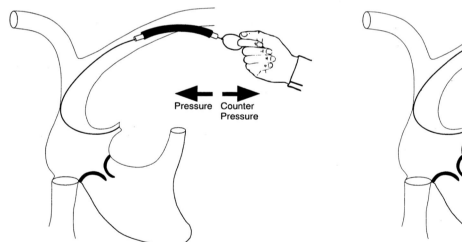 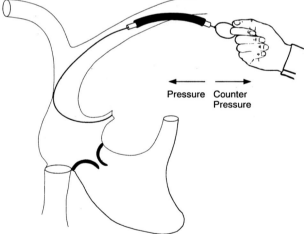

FIGURE 34-2. Appropriate counterpressure. The withdrawal force exerted on the looped end of the locking stylet should be minimal but equal to that necessary to prevent the force exerted on the sheaths from altering the course of the lead. Because the location and tenacity of the fibrotic tissue are unknown, moment to moment adjustment of the opposing forces and comparison with the high magnification fluoroscopic image are required. If the locking stylet slips, withdrawal force on the looped end of the stylet fails to counter the advancement force. It is safe only to advance the sheaths around a change in direction (e.g., from the left brachiocephalic vein to the superior vena cava) when the end is tethered by fibrosis and there is control of the lead body. In the drawings, notice that the pressure arrows are equal in size to the counterpressure arrows.

Telescoping sheaths have been used to effectuate the controlled disruption of the fibrous tissue. These cylindrical tools are made of two metal or polymer sheaths with beveled edges. Their use allows the operator to disrupt the fibrous attachments a few millimeters at a time. The inner sheath peels the lead away from the fibrous attachments. The outer sheath, which is just slightly larger than the inner sheath, shields the tool from the fibrous tissue and reduces friction. The outer sheath is protected from kinking because of the reinforcement of the inner sheath.

The principle of counterpressure is applied in a similar fashion with the Laser Extraction Sheath (Spectranetics Corp., Colorado Springs, CO). The difference is that the laser sheath replaces the inner sheath and is used with an outer polymer sheath. The outer sheath protects the laser sheath against buckling and kinking, which can sever the fiberoptics running along the sheath. The amount of force necessary to dissect the fibrosis is significantly less with the laser sheath. Application of excessive force or torque to the inner laser sheath can disrupt the fiberoptic conductors and reduce efficacy of the laser sheath.

One of the major sites for fibrosis is the lead-myocardium interface. After the lead has been peeled away from all of its endovascular contacts except the lead tip, most of the force applied to the end of the lead is transferred to the endocardial surface. This withdrawal force (i.e., traction) can invaginate the ventricular or atrial myocardium and cause hemodynamic compromise or cardiac laceration. However, by bracing the larger outer sheath against the endocardial surface (i.e., countertraction), the heart cannot invaginate when firm and nonsudden traction is applied. Instead, the lead is released from its endocardial entrapment. The force of countertraction is perpendicular to the endocardial surface and therefore is associated with lower risk of endovascular trauma than counterpressure.

The principles of control of the lead body, controlled counterpressure, and controlled countertraction are only good as long as certain assumptions are met. The basic assumption is that the lead travels through a normal venous route to the heart and remains intracavitary within the right heart. The incidence of patent foramen ovale, atrial septal defects, and ventricular septal defects should remind the physician that the lead may not always be on the venous side of the heart. Before the procedure, careful examination of the paced ECG should suggest this possibility to the clinician. Sometimes, a lead will migrate across the myocardium into the pericardial space. This can happen in the atrium, at the atrioventricular ring, or in the right ventricle. If one of these leads is extracted, tamponade can result. As long as the lead traverses the normal venous structures to the heart and as long as the chest radiograph, ECG, and other data support a diagnosis of normal lead positioning, it is appropriate to apply the tools as described in the next section.

Technique

We use a stepped approach to lead extraction, and at every step, an attempt is made to extract the lead using the minimum of tools. Recently implanted leads may require no more than simple traction, but older leads require some pull to be applied at the tip and can easily be extracted by applying a pulling force on a well-placed locking stylet. However, many leads, particularly those that are several years old, require multiple tools. The approach to extraction from the vein of implantation has been revolutionized by the advent of the excimer laser. However the technique depends on the skilled application of the traditional approach of counterpressure and countertraction. The traditional techniques are described first, followed by modifications for the laser technique.

The incision is made to optimize linear access to the vein of insertion, and the generator is explanted through that incision (Fig. 34-3). Particularly in infected cases, separate incisions may be necessary for debridement of the pocket, and removal of the electrodes from the vein. Dissection is carried down to the suture sleeves, which are identified and removed. The generator is then removed from the pocket, and the electrodes are removed. It is important to identify each lead, along with its model, course, and respective chamber, particularly in cases involving multiple leads. Serial numbers, printed on the proximal pin sleeve are helpful and should be documented before extraction. The terminal pin can be cut to facilitate withdrawal of the lead from the suture tie-down site, obviating the need for dissecting the lead free from the fibrous tissue. It is essential that all leads are dissected free of dense fibrous tissue to as close as possible to the leads' insertion into the vein. This firm extravascular fibrous tissue is frequently responsible for

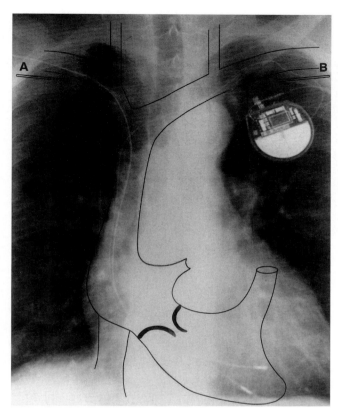

FIGURE 34-3. Chest radiograph shows the incision sites. Location and length of the incision should be optimized to permit linear access to the venous entry site. Particularly for the entry of the nonflexible steel sheaths, the incision should radiate from the venous entry site laterally to enable sheath orientation in all three axes to follow the course of the lead into the vein. The linear overlay drawings labeled A and B represent reasonable locations for incisions for this patient.

damage to the telescoping sheaths. However, the removal of too much of the softer or adventitial tissue could reduce hemostasis after the lead is removed.

One important point needs emphasis. Leads that are not to be removed should be tested before and after the extraction procedure. Although it is rare to damage the conductor or insulation of the other leads if attention is paid to their protection, these leads are at risk, particularly during the introduction of the steel sheaths at the level of the clavicle. Another source of possible trouble is created when the two leads are intertwined or wrapped around each other. When the sheaths are advanced under these circumstances, rotation of the outer sheath in both directions and withdrawal of the sheath after the lead is removed can dislodge the remaining lead. Fibrous attachments between the atrial and ventricular leads at the right atrium–superior vena cava junction can significantly bind the leads and prevent extraction or unintentionally dislodge the other lead.

After all leads have been dissected free, the proximal cut ends of the leads are prepared. Preparation of the leads consists of incising the insulation circumferentially about the lead (Fig. 34-4). For coaxial bipolar leads, the outer conductor is stretched and cut off, leaving the inner insulation and the inner conductor. The inner insulation is then incised circumferentially. The conical coil expander is used to expand the slightly crushed, most proximal tip of the inner conductor (Fig. 34-5). A standard pacemaker stylet is passed through the electrode to its distal tip to ascertain the distance that the locking stylet must travel and to clear the lumen of potential debris. The conductor coil is then sized with gauge pins, and the gauge of the largest gauge pin that snugly but freely enters the conductor coil lumen to its fullest extent corresponds to the gauge of the locking stylet to be

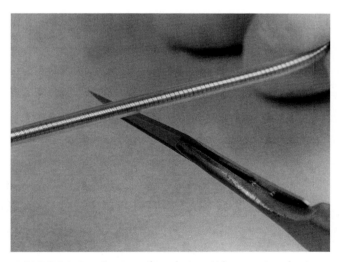

FIGURE 34-4. Cutting of insulation. When cutting the inner or outer insulation, the lead is grasped between the thumb and forefinger of both hands while the assistant positions the cutting edge of the no. 11 scalpel blade underneath the lead. The lead is rotated while dragging it over the sharp edge of the scalpel. The circumscribed fragment of insulation is removed from the lead, and the outer conductor is stretched over the cut end and trimmed off with the suture scissors. The inner insulation is then removed using a similar technique. It is important not to damage the remaining outer insulation and the inner coil, because they will be used to control the lead body with the locking stylet and suture.

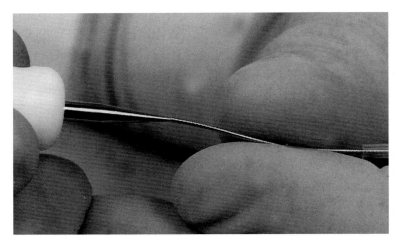

FIGURE 34-5. Coil expander. The conical coil expander is used to enlarge the cut tip of the conductor coil. The conductor coil is often distorted when it is cut. If not expanded, the gauge pins may undersize the coil, and the locking stylet may not grasp the lead strongly. Sometimes, the filament on the locking stylet becomes hung up on the partially crimped end or the damaged conductor coil.

employed (Fig. 34-6). It is necessary to size leads of the same make and model because there may be a difference of one to two sizes. The appropriate locking stylet is then passed all the way to the farthest reaches of the lead, optimally to the distal electrode. When the stylet locks farther down the lead, it produces shorter segments of the lead to elongate. Several designs of locking stylets are available.

The older locking stylet, manufactured by Cook Vascular, Inc. (Leechburg, PA), consists of a long stylet with a twisted thin flattened filamentous wire that runs back about 1.5 inches from its tip (Fig. 34-7). The filament braised to the tip of the locking stylet rubs against the conductor coil. When advancing the stylet down the lead, the stylet should be intermittently withdrawn slightly to roughen up the filament as it is advanced to the tip of the lead. If it is hard to advance the stylet after the slight withdrawal, this should be done less frequently, but if the stylet does not seem to be locking well, it should be done more frequently. Often, the locking stylet must be rotated clockwise to permit the passage to the lead tip. After the locking stylet is advanced to its farthest extent, the stylet must be rotated counterclockwise to activate the locking mechanism. The wire then becomes a strong fastener to the lead tip and compresses the conductor coil and prevents stretching of the lead during extraction efforts. Turning it counterclockwise four to ten times locks the stylet. A gentle tug is given, and then a repeat of the counterclockwise

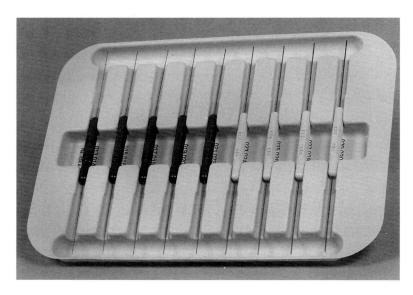

FIGURE 34-6. Gauge pin set. The gauge pins are manufactured in diameters of 0.013 to 0.030 inch to measure the internal diameter of the conductor coil. The corresponding locking stylet should fit snugly within the properly sized conductor coil.

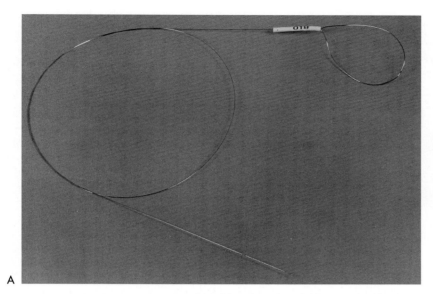

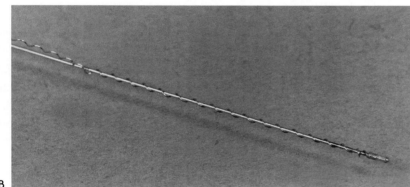

FIGURE 34-7. Locking stylet. **A:** The locking stylet is slightly thinner than the corresponding gauge pin. The filament braised to the tip of the locking stylet rubs against the conductor coil. When advancing the stylet down the lead, the stylet should be withdrawn slightly to roughen up the filament. If it is hard to advance the stylet after the slight withdrawal, this should be done less frequently, but if the stylet does not seem to be locking well, it should be done more frequently. **B:** The tip of the locking stylet has a thin, flattened filamentous wire braised to the tip. When properly sized, the filament uncoils when the locking stylet is rotated counterclockwise. Often, the locking stylet must be rotated clockwise to permit the passage to the lead tip. After the locking stylet is advanced to its farthest extent, the stylet must be rotated counterclockwise to activate the locking mechanism. The wire then becomes a strong fastener to the lead tip, compresses the conductor coil, and prevents stretching of the lead during extraction efforts.

rotation is performed. The most common reason that a locking stylet does not lock is undersizing, which is a consequence of damage to the proximal segment of electrode or failure to use the coil expander before sizing with gauge pins.

A newer and more easily used locking stylet is now available. This side-locking Wilkoff stylet (Cook Vascular, Inc.) is manufactured in five sizes to fit conductor coils of 0.017 to 0.019, 0.020 to 0.022, 0.023 to 0.025, 0.026 to 0.028, and 0.029 to 0.032 inch. The stylet has a barb at its distal tip that is angled to lock when the cylinder of the stylet is advanced (Fig. 34-8). The stylet is used in the same fashion as the traditional locking stylets but does not need to be sized as precisely, locks more strongly, and is more frequently reversible. Rotation of this stylet breaks the locking mechanism. If this occurs, another stylet can be introduced and securely locked. However, the original

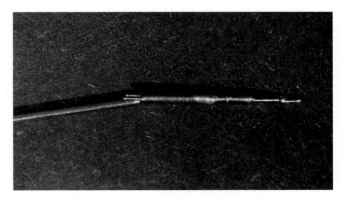

FIGURE 34-8. The Wilkoff stylet has a reversible side-locking mechanism, obviating the need for precise measurement of the inner diameter of the inner coil. It is manufactured in three sizes to fit conductor coils: 0.019 to 0.023, 0.024 to 0.027, and 0.028 to 0.030 inch. The stylet has a barb at its distal tip that is angled to lock when the cylinder of the stylet is advanced.

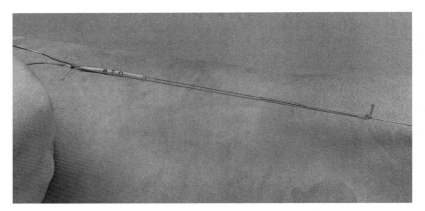

FIGURE 34-9. A strong suture is tied tightly to the insulation and to the looped end of the locking stylet to enhance the control of the lead body. If multiple conductor coils are available, a locking stylet should be introduced into each coil. Pulling on the insulation with the help of the suture facilitates advancement of the sheaths by minimizing the tendency of the insulation and attached fibrotic debris to bunch up and bind on the sheaths. This is particularly important for implantable cardioverter-defibrillator leads.

locking stylet is a better choice if rotation is desired, such as for a fixed, extended, screw-in lead.

A third locking stylet, the Lead Locking Device (Spectranetics Corp.) comes in three sizes fitting inner-coil diameters of 0.13 to 016, 0.017 to 0.026, and 0.027 to 0.032 inch. Although there is significantly less experience with this stylet, it appears that the locking mechanism firmly grabs the inner coil throughout its entire length. The locking mechanism is also frequently reversible, but it is not a good idea to rotate this locking stylet because the mechanism will break. This stylet is excessively long and interferes with the use of the suture as described subsequently.

After the locking stylet has been secured, a strong suture, usually 0-gauge, is securely tied around the outer insulation, compressing the insulation and the outer coil and inner coil as much as possible with a tight square knot (Fig. 34-9). The long end of the suture is tied taut between its attachment on the insulation to the looped end of the locking stylet, providing for parallel and simultaneous traction on the outer insulation and on the conductor coil. This latter step is performed on all leads except for Telectronics ACCUFIX J lead extractions. When determining which lead should be removed first, all of the available information regarding the number of leads in each vein, duration of implantation, intrinsic tensile strength of the leads, security of the locking stylet, and venous access is used. All factors that favor easy extraction point to the lead that should be removed first. The reasoning behind this is that, regardless of which lead is removed first, much of the interlead fibrosis is disrupted during that extraction. Consequently, more difficult lead removal becomes easier only after the first lead is removed.

Vessel entry is one of the key elements of lead extraction. The use of the straight, telescoping, stainless steel sheaths greatly facilitates this step, although this is no longer necessary when using laser sheaths, particularly in the absence of calcifications. The intent of these metal sheaths is to penetrate the fibrosis that is generally dense near the lead insertion into the vein (Fig. 34-10). These sheaths should not be advanced

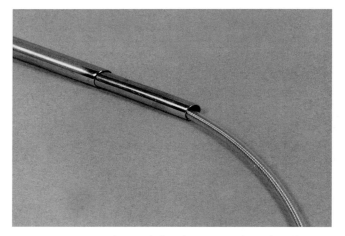

FIGURE 34-10. The steel sheaths are not sharp, but they are thinner and stronger than the Teflon or polypropylene sheaths. They prevent the use of excessive force during vein entry, especially if the lead enters through a narrow space under the clavicle or through fibrotic or calcified tissue. They can be safely passed as long as they can be maneuvered to follow the course of the lead. The steel sheaths can be used to separate leads from each other during their course through the left brachiocephalic vein.

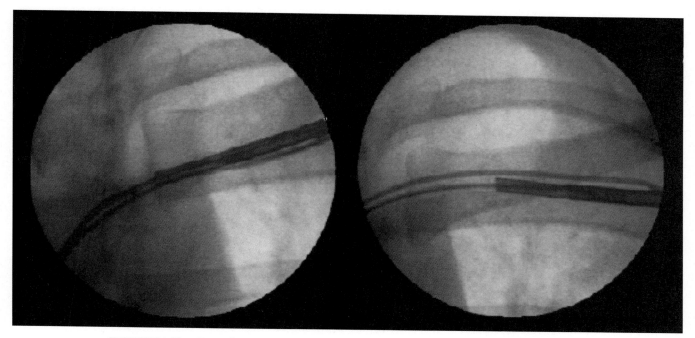

FIGURE 34-11. Triaxial positioning. The steel sheaths, in particular, are only safe and effective if they are oriented in the x, y, and z planes as they are advanced over the lead. Any lateral force is ineffective in producing sheath advancement and increases the likelihood of binding on the lead or produces an acute bend or crimp in the sheath. Comparison of the fluoroscopic image with the manipulation of the locking stylet and the sheaths is essential to effective lead extraction. The two fluoroscopic images demonstrate the reorientation of the steel telescoping sheaths as they are passed into the subclavian vein on the right and down the brachiocephalic vein on the left.

into the superior vena cava and should only be advanced during high-magnification fluoroscopy, looking for evidence of damage to the lead or the sheaths. It is not necessary to pull on the leads to any extent during this phase. All that is required is triaxial alignment of the sheaths with the course of the lead so that the sheaths slide over the monorail-like lead (Fig. 34-11). It is often necessary to rotate the inner and outer sheaths to disrupt the fibrosis surrounding the lead and to change the trajectory of the steel sheaths as the sheaths are advanced over the lead. These sheaths should be rotated and advanced slowly.

After the steel sheaths have been passed to the level where the lead starts to bend around a corner the steel sheaths need to be exchanged for Teflon or polypropylene sheaths (Table 34-4). This exchange should be performed quickly and while obstructing the outer sheath with the operator's fingertip to avoid air embolism. It is preferable to use relatively stiffer sheaths as long as there is strong control of the lead. These relatively stiffer high-barium-content or special polypropylene sheaths, labeled WIL, allow for greater strength along the lead as they are advanced. They tend to kink less and transfer the torque to the counterpressure site. Flexible and soft sheaths that are not strong enough to peel away the fibrosis are less safe than the more rigid sheaths. The retraction force on the looped end of the locking stylet should not be excessive. The force should be equal to that which allows advancement of the sheaths while holding the lead away from the outer arc of the insertion vein and into the heart. These sheaths should not be advanced directly against the vessel wall, but rather the leads should be peeled away from the wall of the vessel, bringing the lead into the center of the vascular lumen. Failure to advance the sheaths after initial progress probably is caused by damage to their leading edge and requires their replacement. The use of the

TABLE 34-4 • COUNTERTRACTION SHEATH CHARACTERISTICS

Material[a]	Color	Inner Sheath Length (inches)	Inner Sheath (Inner/Outer)	Outer Sheath Length (inches)	Outer Sheath (Inner/Outer)
Polypropylene	Yellow	15 and 18	8.4/10.7 Fr	13 and 16	11.6/13.9 Fr
Teflon B	Black	15 and 18	8.5/12.0 Fr	13 and 16	12.8/16.0 Fr
Teflon femoral	Black	36	8.5/12.0 Fr	27.4	12.8/16.0 Fr
Teflon C	Black	15 and 18	9.5/13.0 Fr	13 and 16	14.3/18.0 Fr
Polypropylene	White—special	15 and 18	9.7/12.3 Fr	13 and 16	13.3/15.6 Fr
Polypropylene	Green	15 and 18	10.0/12.1 Fr	13 and 16	13.1/15.2 Fr
Steel	Silver	10	10.4/11.9 Fr	7.75	12.7/13.7 Fr
Polypropylene	White—regular	15 and 18	11.4/13.6 Fr	13 and 16	14.1/16.1 Fr
Laser 12 Fr	Blue	15.7	8.3/12.4 Fr	12.6	13.4/17.0 Fr
Laser 14 Fr	Grey	15.7	10.2/14.5 Fr	12.6	15.5/19.3 Fr
Laser 16 Fr	Black	15.7	12.5/16.7 Fr	12.6	18.2/22.6 Fr

[a] Countertraction sheath pairs can be used singly, together, mixed, or exchanged to influence the strength, sharpness, flexibility, stiffness, and rotational torque of the system. An example of mixing two types of sheaths includes the use of an outer steel sheath to hold open the space between the clavicle and the first rib while an inner Teflon B sheath slides down to cover a protruding J wire of an Accufix lead. If the outer Teflon B sheath had been used, the clavicle and first rib would have pinched the sheaths, preventing advancement. If a polypropylene inner or both inner and outer sheaths were used, too much counterpressure would be required to redirect the sheaths from the brachiocephalic vein to the superior vena cava. This would have retracted the lead and potentially lacerated the venous structures.

pin vise is extremely advantageous in improving control of the sheaths and limiting fatigue while manipulating the relatively thin and frequently bloody and slippery telescoping sheaths (Fig. 34-12). The ability to rotate the sheaths often allows the sheaths to be advanced when simple pushing or direct advancement fails (Fig. 34-13).

It is not unusual for the lead to come free after the fibrosis in the subclavian vein is freed or as soon as the attachments between the leads all the way down to the atrial lead are released. Significant fibrous attachments exist at the endocardial surface, and at this level, patience and slow steady pressure are required. If the locking stylet is still locked and the control of

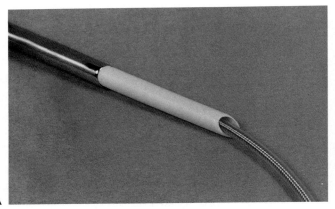
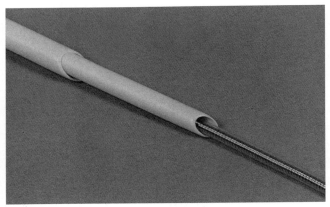

FIGURE 34-12. It is better to exchange one sheath at a time to maintain the progress produced with the previous sheaths. If the sheaths fail to progress, it may be caused by damage to the tip of the sheath. **A:** The steel inner sheath has been replaced by an inner polypropylene and high-barium-content sheath to maintain good strength and increase flexibility to advance the sheath into the superior vena cava. **B:** The steel outer sheath has been replaced by the matching outer polypropylene and high-barium-content sheath to continue counterpressure along the lead down to the endocardial surface for countertraction.

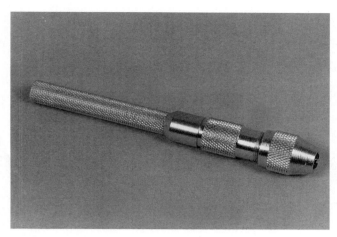

FIGURE 34-13. The pin vise can be mounted on any of the sheaths to improve the grip for rotational torque. This is particularly useful with the steel and high-barium-content polypropylene sheaths, because they are able to transmit the rotational torque to the sheath tip.

the lead is strong, the sheath can keep the cavity of the right heart from invaginating. No sudden or ripping actions should be applied. Sometimes, the lead releases from the myocardium, but the fibrosis is too large to enter the sheath. It is helpful to gently retract the lead and sheaths together periodically to see if the job is complete (Fig. 34-14). Because the relatively large-diameter fibrosis may inhibit its withdrawal from the subclavian vein, once withdrawn from the heart and into the superior vena cava, additional attempts at retraction of the inner sheath and lead into the outer sheath are usually successful. This limits the irritation and trauma to the subclavian, cephalic, or jugular veins as the lead is withdrawn.

After removal of the telescoping sheaths, bleeding can be controlled in most patients with simple pressure. Occasionally, a pursestring or figure-of-eight suture is required to control bleeding. Placement of the pursestring suture after lead preparation and before the use of the sheaths is advisable. If there is little or no bleeding, the suture can be removed.

Superior Venous Approach Using Laser Sheaths

Introduction of excimer laser sheaths by Spectranetics represented an important addition to the tools avail-

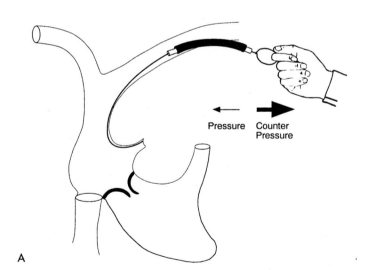
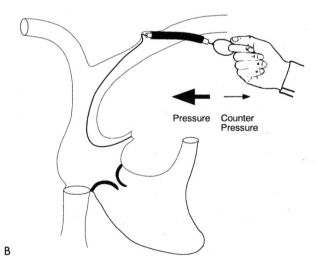

FIGURE 34-14. Two types of errors are made during counterpressure. When insufficient counter pressure is exerted on the locking stylet, the lead loses its properties that guide the sheaths safely down the center of the venous structures to the heart. Because the sheaths (even the softest) are relatively stiff and perfectly straight, the sheaths tend to scrape against the venous walls and increase the risk of laceration (**A**). If excessive counterpressure is applied, the lead will be withdrawn from the vein and from the heart without peeling of the fibrotic material from the lead. The opportunity for countertraction is lost, which increases the risk of myocardial avulsion and cardiac laceration and tamponade (**B**).

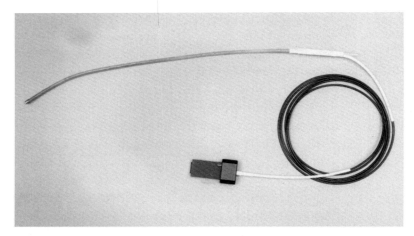

FIGURE 34-15. Laser extraction sheath. Excimer laser sheaths (Spectranetics Corp., Colorado Springs, CO) are used in conjunction with an outer Teflon sheath. The sheaths emit circumferential laser energy between the two stainless steel rings at the tip. These catheters come in 12-, 14-, and 16-Fr sizes and can therefore be used to extract implantable cardioverter-defibrillator leads. (From Wilkoff BL, Al-Khadra AS, et al. The technique of transvenous lead extraction. In: Singer I, Barold SS, Camm AJ, eds. *Nonpharmacological therapy of arrhythmias for the 21st century: the state of the art.* Armonk, NY: Futura Publishing, 1998:763, with permission.)

able for extraction of pacemaker leads (Fig. 34-15). These sheaths replace the inner telescoping sheaths and are used in conjunction with an outer Teflon sheath during the counterpressure phase of the extraction. By ablating fibrous tissue directly in contact and within 1 mm of the tip of the laser sheath, the amount of counterpressure necessary to cut through adhesions is greatly minimized. Because counterpressure is associated with the highest risk during lead extraction, it was reasonable to hope that the laser would reduce the morbidity and increase the likelihood of uncomplicated and complete lead extraction. However, the data do not support the conclusion that the laser can reduce complications. This is a difficult analysis because more difficult extraction situations with more, older, and larger leads have been approached with these techniques (19).

The laser sheath design is based on concepts similar to those used to devise laser coronary angioplasty systems. The catheters, which come in sizes of 12 to 16 Fr, are made of inner and outer polymer tubing. A single layer of optical fibers runs spirally between both layers of the tubing. At the distal end of the catheter, the tubing terminates in two stainless steel bands with beveled edges. In addition to protecting the catheter tip and the optical fibers, they serve as a radiopaque marker at the catheter tip. Between the two rings exits a single, circumferential ring of laser light. The CVX-300 Excimer XeCl system emits 135-ns pulses at a repetition rate of 25 to 40 Hz.

The steps involved in extraction of leads using laser sheaths are very similar to the standard techniques. The leads are dissected and prepared as described previously. The use of metal sheath is advisable when there is excessive calcification or dense fibrosis under the clavicles and at vein entry site. Before using the laser sheath, the system is calibrated. The ablation rate is determined by fluence (energy density per pulse) and repetition rate (pulses/sec). The fluence and repetition rate for this procedure are 60 mJ/mm^2 and 40 Hz, respectively. The maximum recommended laser firing time is 10,000 pulses (25 seconds at 40 Hz). Some preliminary data have been collected with higher fluence, repetition rates, and durations of exposure, which increase the power of the system. It is not clear what impact this makes on the safety of the procedure.

The laser catheter is used in conjunction with an outer sheath. Using a fish-tape device, the handle of the locking stylet is threaded through the inner lumen of the laser catheter, and the proximal end of the lead is pulled into the catheter. Using the same counterpressure technique described previously, the laser catheter and the outer sheath are advanced until an obstruction is met. The laser catheter is then activated, and gentle pressure is used to advance it by about 1- to 2-mm per second. As soon as the catheter passes through the obstruction, the laser is stopped. The outer sheath then is advanced over the laser catheter until the next obstruction is met. The tip of the laser catheter must always be within the fluoroscopy field. Both catheters should be manipulated only under fluoroscopic guidance. The laser is advanced from venous entry to within 0.5 to 1 cm of the myocardium. Laser energy should not be applied directly to the myocardium to free the lead tip, but countertraction may be used. As expected, laser sheaths may not be successful in areas where there is dense calcification. Unless this area can be freed using the outer sheath and then passed into the laser catheter, progress is unlikely and could cause vascular laceration. Resorting to larger laser or nonlaser sheaths may be necessary. Results using laser-assisted pacemaker lead extraction have been very promising. Data from the PLEXES trial (9) and others were discussed in the Outcome of Lead Extraction section.

The Transfemoral Approach

Transfemoral techniques are important adjuncts to the superior venous approach and are preferred by some operators. At the Cleveland Clinic, the use of polypropylene sheaths and laser sheaths permitted the removal of more than 95% of pacemaker leads by the superior vein approach. However, skill with the femoral technique is necessary to consistently and safely remove all leads.

The femoral approach is required when there is failure to progress with the telescoping sheaths or when the lead has been cut or retracted into the vein. Some operators may feel more comfortable with manipulating catheters from the femoral vein. The tools for femoral extraction have markedly improved as more femoral cases have been performed. The lead is prepared for extraction in a fashion similar to that described in the superior venous approach. The lead is freed, the suture sleeve is removed, and the lead is cut near the entry site into the subclavian vein. The femoral workstation is then introduced from the femoral vein, preferably on the right side.

The original Byrd Femoral Workstation is a 16-Fr Teflon sheath with a venous check-flow valve and a side port. Through this sheath, several tools can be passed to snare and retrieve the lead or lead fragment. Options include but are not restricted to the traditional Byrd Workstation countertraction sheath preloaded with a tip-deflecting guide wire, a Dotter basket in the straight or curved configuration, and the needle's-eye snare with a straight or curved sheath (Fig. 34-16). If the tip-deflecting wire and Dotter basket are used, the guide wire is looped around the lead so that the tip of the wire can be caught in the Dotter basket. The lead is then gently pulled down from the superior veins. The reversible nature of the loop formed by the tip-deflecting guide wire and Dotter basket around the lead allows the lead to be grasped at several levels and be progressively pulled down. Pulling the lead down and out of the subclavian vein is facilitated by the fact that the mediastinum resists downward movement. The lead is then pulled further into the countertraction sheath, and the sheath is advanced over the lead down to the endocardial surface for a countertraction procedure as described previously. Sometimes, the outer 16-Fr sheath of the Byrd Femoral Workstation can be advanced over the countertraction sheath and be used in conjunction with the inner sheath for countertraction.

As an alternative to the Dotter basket, the Amplatz gooseneck snare and tip-deflecting guide wire can be advanced through the Byrd Femoral Workstation without an inner sheath. The guide wire is looped over the lead and grasped by the snare. The lead can then be repetitively grasped and pulled down until it is pulled out of the superior venous structures. Countertraction is used to remove the lead. The Amplatz gooseneck snare is also good for removing leads that have retracted into the venous structures by loosening the free tip of the lead. Because there is no locking stylet, the lead often stretches and breaks before the lead is removed. It is then necessary to regrasp the lead and try again.

The needle's-eye snare is easier to use than the tip-deflecting guide wire and the Dotter basket if a significant loop is formed by the lead in the atrium. After the hook of the system is over the loop of the lead, the needle is advanced. Advancing the inner sheath traps the lead so that the outer sheath can be used for countertraction. Combining these newer tools with the new curved femoral sheaths allows better control over the lead all the way to the distal electrode and increases the rate of complete lead extraction from the femoral route.

The largest problem with the femoral techniques is that the tools are not easily steered in three dimensions. Except for the newer extraction devices, it is

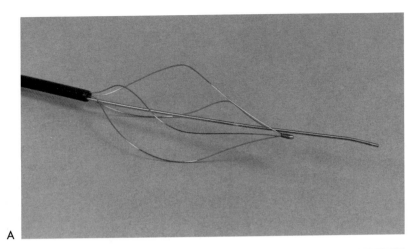
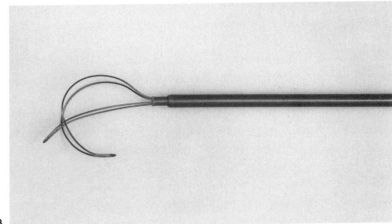
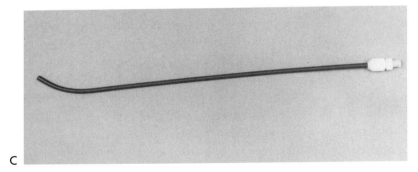

FIGURE 34-16. Femoral extraction tools. Extraction of leads using the femoral approach is more versatile but demands specially designed tools. An important first step is to be able to securely grasp the lead at particular points that will give mechanical advantage during counter traction. **A:** This can be accomplished using a Dotter basket snare and Cook deflection catheter. The deflection catheter encircles the lead, and the Dotter snare grasps the tip of the deflection catheter. The loop is then pulled into the workstation catheter. **B:** The needle's-eye snare also enables the operator to grasp and release the lead multiple times with ease and precision. Using this instrument, the lead is entrapped between the hook of the system and the needle. Advancing the inner sheath traps the lead so that the outer sheath can be used for countertraction. **C:** The use of curved femoral sheaths increases maneuverability and increases the ease of grasping the lead fragments. (From Wilkoff BL, Al-Khadra AS, et al. The technique of transvenous lead extraction. In: Singer I, Barold SS, Camm AJ, eds. *Nonpharmacological therapy of arrhythmias for the 21st century: the state of the art.* Armonk, NY: Futura Publishing, 1998:765, with permission.)

difficult to grasp the lead in a way that the lead can be released if the grasping does not produce an advantageous hold on the lead. Soft Teflon sheaths used with the femoral tools provide little power in breaking up fibrous tissue and have been particularly frustrating in the removal of defibrillator leads.

After lead removal using the femoral technique, it is advisable to allow slight back bleeding to remove whatever clot might have formed around the 16-Fr insertion site. Afterward, continuous pressure needs to be held for 10 minutes to prevent further bleeding. Care should be taken to watch the patient for deep venous thrombosis or pulmonary embolism. The inner and outer sheath system needs to be thoroughly flushed whenever the femoral countertraction sheath is removed and replaced to change or adjust the tools.

Reimplantation of New Leads and Generators

If the indication for lead removal is mechanical failure, there is no evidence of infection, and the patient continues to require arrhythmia therapy, pacemaker or defibrillator leads can be placed after completion of the extraction using the same vascular access (i.e., cephalic or subclavian). Vascular access is maintained by inserting a long J-shaped guide wire down into the inferior vena cava through the outer sheath, which is left in the superior veins after lead removal. Extreme care is exercised to avoid air embolism while this exchange is taking place. The outer sheath is then removed, and a long peel-away introducer is guided along the wire to the level of the right atrium. Long introducers permit access of the lead directly to the cardiac structures without catching on the stenotic, weakened, or torn fibrous tissue in the subclavian, brachiocephalic, and superior vena cava structures. Insertion of short introducers that end in the superior veins can increase the risk of extravascular lead insertion. If there is any resistance to reinsertion of the guide wire or the subsequent introduction of the pacing lead, this approach should be abandoned and a separate venous insertion planned. The new permanent lead, preferably an active-fixation lead, should be positioned in an area that is distant from the site that was occupied by the extracted leads to avoid areas of fibrosis.

POSTOPERATIVE CARE

Postoperative care involves control of pain and looking for signs of bleeding and infection. In the absence of infection, recovery is comparable to any other pacemaker procedure. The patient usually stays overnight and goes home the next day. Vigorous activities are limited for approximately 2 weeks. At 6 weeks, the patient returns for reprogramming of the new permanent pacemaker system for optimal efficiency of capture and sensing and to ensure that the situation has been resolved without complications. Late complications are rare, and in our experience, they have involved the subacute development of a modest hemothorax over 3 weeks, subclavian vein thrombosis, and poor function of the replacement pacemaker leads.

EXTRACTION OF IMPLANTABLE DEFIBRILLATOR LEADS

Defibrillator leads have design that differs significantly from that of pacemaker leads and directly influences the techniques used in their extraction. There are significant differences between different defibrillator leads, reflecting inherent differences in the approaches to defibrillation adopted by different companies (e.g., presence of two shocking electrodes, integrated and dedicated sensing circuits, requirement for additional superior vena cava lead). This results in each lead having its unique characteristics in terms of tensile strength, insulator, number of conductors, diameter, propensity toward marked fibrosis, and support during extraction.

Compared with pacemaker leads, implantable cardioverter-defibrillator (ICD) leads are larger in diameter, with multiple conductors increasing the rate of mechanical failure. One study from our institution showed a greater percentage of defibrillator leads extractions for lead failure compared with pacemaker lead extractions (20,21). Defibrillator leads have rough, large-surface-area electrodes that promote fibrosis (2). Each of these factors make removability more difficult and, at least in theory, increase the risk of lead extraction.

Steps for removal of defibrillator leads are very similar in principle to removal of pacemaker leads. The generator is removed, and the lead is dissected free of fibrous tissue. When extracting an abdominal system, it is important to isolate the yoke and any tiedowns before cutting the most proximal part of the lead. In the absence of infection, the lead is then pulled into the pectoral pocket, where the other tiedowns are removed and dissection into the infraclavicular region is performed. It is advisable to remove superior vena cava lead before removing the ventricular lead. The advantage is related to the relative ease of removal and that breaking up the fibrous tissue between the two leads facilitates the removal of the ventricular lead.

The ventricular Medtronic Transvene leads and the CPI Endotak leads have been implanted for longer time compared with other models. We discuss the approach to extraction of both of these leads and other defibrillator leads separately (22,23). The Endotak lead comes in several models with the same basic construction. These leads are Silastic-insulated, 10- to 12-Fr, tripolar leads. Two of the electrodes are shocking springs, and the third is a sensing- and pacing-tip electrode. There are two Teflon-coated wires that allow substantial pulling power to be placed on the lead. These Teflon-coated wires connect to the shocking electrodes. There is a standard pacing conductor coil. Advances in the construction have improved the tensile strength and reliability of these leads.

Extraction Technique

The pacing conductor coil is sized and instrumented with a locking stylet similar to the pacing electrodes. To take advantage of the two extra Teflon-coated wires to control the lead body, much of its length needs to be preserved. When the pulse generator is removed from the pocket, the lead is cut just distal to the Y branch in the lead. A second incision in the prepectoral area is necessary in patients with abdominal implants to facilitate release of the two suture sleeves and for passage of sheaths into the subclavian or cephalic vein. If there is no infection, the lead is pulled through the tissues to the pectoral incision. The insulation is circumscribed around the three conductors 6 to 8 cm from the venous insertion and removed from the lead. If there is an abdominal pocket infection, the lead is cut, leaving as much lead in the pectoral pocket. The lead remnant is removed from the abdominal incision. The locking stylet is secured by means of the standard approach. However, both Teflon wires are tied back to the looped end of the locking stylet and secured firmly and tautly to the locking stylet (Fig. 34-17). The suture is tied around the existing insulation and back to the looped end of the locking stylet as with pacemaker leads. Control of the lead body is maintained by traction on all four elements: the locking stylet, two Teflon-coated wires, and the suture.

The diameter of the Endotak lead is large enough

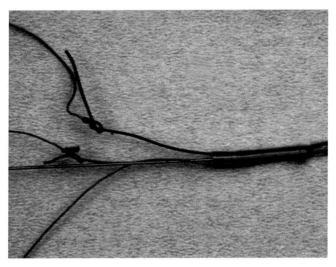

FIGURE 34-17. In preparation for the extraction of the Endotak defibrillator lead, sutures are tied to the exposed proximal ends of the Teflon-coated conductor cables and to the insulation. All three sutures are tied to the looped end of the locking stylet. This allows the force of traction exerted at the operator's end of the locking stylet to effect a coordinated withdrawal of the lead. The traction force is distributed among all four elements, which act as a unit during the counterpressure and countertraction maneuvers.

so that only the larger-diameter, steel, telescoping sheath and the larger-diameter, high-barium-content, telescoping polypropylene sheath can be advanced over the lead. When the steel sheath is advanced into the subclavian vein, the lead usually stretches so that the proximal coil pulls back into the brachiocephalic vein. Often, the steel sheath, with some encouragement, slides over the proximal spring, and because of the elastic nature of this lead, the spring exits the vein. The steel sheath must follow the course of the lead and change the trajectory of its insertion according to the path of the lead. It is necessary to rotate the sheath and align the lead to encourage the lead to pass through the steel sheath. Often, the coil is roughened and difficult to pass into the steel sheath. After this has been accomplished, the steel sheath is removed, and the larger-diameter or outer high-barium-content sheath is advanced over the lead. The high-barium-content sheath passes relatively easily to the middle brachiocephalic vein and down toward the superior vena cava. Use of the Pin Vise is helpful to advance the sheath over the distal spring. The lead usually disengages when the distal spring is peeled away from the inferior wall of the right ventricle. If there is failure to progress with the sheaths from above, laser sheath–assisted extraction is used if available. Otherwise, the lead is cut and snared using the transfemoral approach. Transfemoral countertraction is often a time-consuming approach because the femoral sheaths are softer and more malleable, requiring time and patience to pass through the fibrous attachments.

Extraction of the Transvene lead and other triaxial leads is different mainly because of the lack of Teflon-coated, high-voltage wires. The lead is prepared in a similar fashion to bipolar coaxial leads. Active-fixation leads are unscrewed. The lead is then cut with sufficient length in the prepectoral pocket to allow the insertion of the locking stylet and suture as with bipolar coaxial leads. Locking stylets are placed in the coaxial bipolar lead and in the superior vena cava lead (if applicable). It is advisable to remove the smaller-diameter superior vena cava lead before removing the right ventricular lead. Telescoping steel and polypropylene sheaths are required to remove the superior vena cava lead because of the considerable fibrosis that usually forms between the roughened surface of the superior vena cava lead, the ventricular lead, and the brachiocephalic vein. After the superior vena cava lead is removed, the ventricular lead is removed in a relatively standard fashion. The Transvene lead is an active-fixation electrode, and it is possible to unscrew the electrode by rotating the locking stylet and the inner conductor coil. This can be observed under fluoroscopy with separation of the radiopaque marker at the lead tip. Compared with the Endotak lead, there appears to be more fibrosis with the proximal shocking electrode of the Transvene lead. However, there is much less fibrosis around the ventricular shocking electrode. After the proximal electrode is removed, removal of the ventricular portion is generally less complicated.

Several adaptations to pacemaker lead extraction tools have been produced for the removal of ICD leads. Tangerine-colored, telescoping, polypropylene sheaths are sized so that they are long enough and large enough to be advanced over ICD leads as telescoping sheaths. These sheaths are relatively thin and kink easily. However, it is useful to be able to use the flexibility and strength of the telescoping mechanism in the removal of these leads.

A second useful tool is the 16-Fr excimer laser sheath used with the 22.6-Fr outer Teflon sheath. This sheath appears to be a major advantage in the removal of ICD leads. Its large diameter and relative inflexibility hamper it. Use of lubrication between the laser and the outer sheath and on the outer surface of the outer sheath helps to reduce the friction that sometimes impedes progress. In our experience, use of these tools permitted clinically successful removal of 108 ventricular ICD leads and failed extraction in only two patients (97.8%). Complications have occurred but not at an increased rate compared with those for pacemaker leads (15). These extractions are significantly more difficult than pacemaker leads implanted for the same duration.

Krishnan and Epstein (12) used 16-Fr laser sheaths to extract 14 defibrillator leads from 11 patients, 6 of whom had undergone failed previous extraction attempts using conventional tools. All 14 leads were successfully and completely removed using the superior venous approach. The mean time required for lead extraction once the locking stylet was in place was 7 ± 4 minutes. Major complications, including death, occurred in one patient (12).

Telectronics J Leads

There are three series of Telectronics J leads. Most of the publicity and problems have been directed toward the active-fixation models: Accufix 330-801, 329-701, and 033-802 and Accufix DEC 033-812. However, there are some passive-fixation J leads (Encor 330-854, 330-755, and 329-755A; Encor DEC 033-856 and 033-757) and atrial ICD leads (EnGuard/Atrial DF 040-112, 040-069, and 040-022). A number of older passive-fixation Cordis leads also used this construction and have not been identified with any reported injuries (Table 34-5). The original passive-fixation leads have a reinforcing J wire inserted within the inner conductor in the lumen usually reserved for the pacemaker stylets. The wire continues past the ring electrode and is connected to the distal electrode. The lead is protected from J-wire protrusion by the inner and outer conductors and by

TABLE 34-5 • TELECTRONICS LEAD MODELS WITH SHAPE RETAINING J WIRE

Model Name	Model Number	J Wire Location	J Wire Distal-Tip Location	Polarity	Fixation
Accufix	033-802[a]	Outside outer coil	Ring electrode	Bipolar	Retractable screw
Accufix DEC	033-812[a]	Outside outer coil	Ring electrode	Bipolar	Retractable screw
Accufix	329-701[b]	Outside outer coil	Ring electrode	Bipolar	Retractable screw
Accufix	330-801[b]	Outside outer coil	Ring electrode	Bipolar	Retractable screw
Encor DEC	033-856[a]	Inside inner coil	Tip electrode	Bipolar	Tines
Encor	327-747[b]	Inside inner coil	Tip electrode	Bipolar	Tines
Encor	327-754[b]	Inside inner coil	Tip electrode	Bipolar	Tines
Encor	329-749[b]	Inside inner coil	Tip electrode	Bipolar	Tines
Encor	329-754[b]	Inside inner coil	Tip electrode	Bipolar	Tines
Encor	330-848[a]	Inside inner coil	Tip electrode	Bipolar	Tines
Encor	330-854[b]	Inside inner coil	Tip electrode	Bipolar	Tines
Encor DEC	033-757[a]	Inside only coil	Tip electrode	Unipolar	Tines
Encor	327-745[b]	Inside only coil	Tip electrode	Unipolar	Tines
Encor	327-745P[b]	Inside only coil	Tip electrode	Unipolar	Tines
Encor	327-752[b]	Inside only coil	Tip electrode	Unipolar	Tines
Encor	327-752P[b]	Inside only coil	Tip electrode	Unipolar	Tines
Encor	328-752[b]	Inside only coil	Tip electrode	Unipolar	Tines
Encor	328-752P[b]	Inside only coil	Tip electrode	Unipolar	Tines
Encor	329-748[b]	Inside only coil	Tip electrode	Unipolar	Tines
Encor	329-748A[b]	Inside only coil	Tip electrode	Unipolar	Tines
Encor	329-748P[b]	Inside only coil	Tip electrode	Unipolar	Tines
Encor	329-755A[b]	Inside only coil	Tip electrode	Unipolar	Tines
Encor	330-748[b]	Inside only coil	Tip electrode	Unipolar	Tines
Encor	330-755[b]	Inside only coil	Tip electrode	Unipolar	Tines
EnGuard Atrial DF	040-022[a,c]	Inside inner coil	Tip electrode	ICD	Tines
EnGuard Atrial DF	040-069F[a]	Inside inner coil	Tip electrode	ICD	Tines
EnGuard Atrial DF	040-112[a,c]	Inside inner coil	Tip electrode	ICD	Tines

[a] Not distributed in the United States.
[b] U.S. and worldwide marketing.
[c] U.S. investigational device.

the outer insulation until it passes the ring electrode and by the inner conductor and outer insulation between the ring and tip electrodes. The active-fixation or Accufix leads were redesigned to have the J reinforcing wire moved from inside of the inner coil to outside of the outer conductor coil just internal to the outer insulation. The J wire is braised or crimped to the proximal edge of the ring electrode and travels under the outer insulation up to the straighter portion of the lead. There is less protection from protrusion and potential patient injury with the Accufix than with the passive-fixation Telectronics J leads. The estimated actual prevalence of J-wire fracture is 24.5% based on the results of the fluoroscopic examinations within the multicenter study and the known false-negative detection rate.

Special considerations for removal of active- and passive-fixation versions of the leads depend on the condition of the J wire. Sutures are tied to the exposed proximal ends of the Teflon-coated conductor cables and to the insulation. All three sutures are tied to the looped end of the locking stylet. This allows the force of traction exerted at the operators end of the locking stylet to effect coordinated withdrawal of the lead. The traction force is distributed among all four elements, which act as a unit during the counterpressure and countertraction maneuvers (Fig. 34-18).

There are two technical obstacles to extracting the Accufix lead. The first is the J wire, and the second is the very strong corkscrew, active-fixation mechanism. The most important principle in removing the Accufix lead is to keep the J wire shielded from the

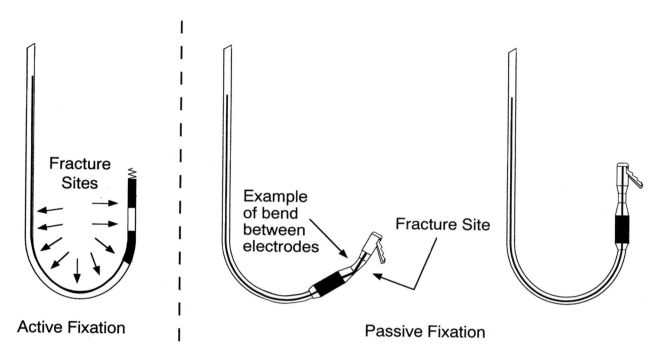

FIGURE 34-18. Telectronics J leads. The flattened J-shaped wire is located external to the outer conductor and connected to the proximal end of the ring electrode in the active-fixation J leads. The wire is located internal to the outer conductor and continues to the distal electrode in the bradycardia and implantable cardioverter-defibrillator passive-fixation J leads. Fractures and protrusion of the J wire usually occur at certain positions *(arrows)*.

vascular space by the lead's insulation or extraction sheaths. To accomplish this task, care is taken not to pull on the lead before advancing the sheaths over the ring electrode. Because even a small protrusion or a fracture without protrusion can be dangerous if the outer insulator is retracted or removed and because digital fluoroscopy is only about 50% sensitive and depends on the skill and experience of the observer, all leads when being removed should be treated as though there is a frank protrusion. Extreme care should be taken when dissecting the lead free in the pacemaker pocket and while removing the suture sleeve that a significant pulling force is not placed on the lead. During the extraction procedure, especially when the sheaths are not easily advanced, the condition of the lead, the J wire, and the sheaths must be evaluated. If protrusion is seen on the chest radiograph or on fluoroscopy, extra care should be taken not to withdraw the J portion out of the atrium into the smaller-diameter superior or inferior vena cava.

After dissection of the lead down to its insertion vein, the slotted stylet is advanced down to the lead tip. The atrial version of the slotted stylet promotes advancement around the J curvature of the lead. However, it is somewhat flimsy, and it is often easier to advance the ventricular version that is much stiffer. Considerable care is sometimes required to retract the screw mechanism. If the screw-in mechanism is not retracted, it is doubly important that retraction of the lead does not occur until after the sheaths are advanced. If a protrusion exists and the lead is rotated to unscrew the screw, the J wire may lacerate the circumference of the atrium. Because the screw is very strong, when unretracted, it is likely to tear a hole in the atrium. Often, use of an oblique fluoroscopic view is helpful in determining whether the screw has been retracted. After the screw is retracted, the locking stylet (0.026-inch or side-locking Wilkoff) is inserted and locked. A suture is tied around the outer insulation, binding the outer insulation and the outer coil with the J wire sandwiched between. The suture is cut and not extended up to the looped end of the locking stylet. If traction is exerted on the outer insulation by pulling on the suture, it is not uncommon to disassemble the lead at the level of the ring electrode.

The outer insulation, which was formerly acting as a sheath to the J wire, now exposes the J wire to the atrium. A formerly controlled protrusion then becomes an overt protrusion that could embolize. Taking care not to pull on the lead, the steel sheaths are advanced over the lead, peeling it away from the ventricular lead and the vascular space. It is often possible to pass the sheath several centimeters down the subclavian vein and into the brachiocephalic vein. These sheaths are then withdrawn, and Teflon B sheaths are used to pass over the lead. Teflon B sheaths are used because they are more flexible and permit little or no withdrawal force on the lead when rounding the corner at the superior vena cava. If the fibrosis succumbs to the Teflon sheaths and encases the lead to the level of the ring electrode, the J wire is within the sheaths and the lead can be removed. Often, there is significant fibrous attachment of the distal electrode porous tip to the atrium. Care should be taken in peeling the lead away from the atrial wall. There is often significant fibrosis to the ventricular lead.

If the Teflon sheaths cannot be passed without retracting the lead into the superior vena cava, a femoral approach is required. The lead must be grasped within the atrium and pulled into the femoral countertraction sheaths before withdrawing the lead into the inferior vena cava. The gooseneck Amplatz snare has proven to be particularly useful in this process (24). It is still necessary to retract the screw-in mechanism. The snare can then be used to grasp and withdraw just the protruded J wire or to grasp the protruded J wire and the lead proximal to the ring electrode and withdraw the entire lead into the Byrd Femoral Workstation sheath. The distal portion of the lead is not snared, because this action promotes disassembly of the lead. The fibrosis is likely to hold onto the outer insulation in the superior veins while the distal electrode and inner insulation and ring electrode slide out of the outer conductor and insulation. This could produce embolization of the J wire. There is much less room for error with extraction of these J leads, and constant observation of the relationship of the sheaths, J wire, lead, vascular space, and heart must be maintained. The 12-Fr laser sheath has been extremely effective in the removal of J wire leads and is the tool of choice for these leads.

The principles required for removing the passive-fixation version of this lead are similar except for the retraction of the active-fixation mechanism. However, it is less likely that the J-end wire will escape because it is within the confines of the outer conductor. Early reports suggest that distal-tip deformation (i.e., distortion of the segment of the lead between the ring and tip electrodes) has been observed in a few leads. Distal-tip deformation is more frequently seen with implantation techniques that employ right subclavian vein introducer implantation because of the acute angle and potential kinking of the introducer. If the lead is advanced against the kinked introducer, damage can be produced. Once bent, the J wire is more vulnerable. It is possible that a fractured J wire could protrude into the path of any stylet advanced through the inner conductor coil and force the J wire out of the lead and directly into the atrial wall. Although the experience is much more limited with this lead and the precise indications for removal not worked out, wisdom dictates that similar precautions are used as with the Accufix lead.

CONCLUSIONS

With the demonstrated safety and efficacy of current pacemaker and implantable defibrillator systems, criteria for implanting these devices became less stringent. The marked increase in the number and complexity of implanted systems uncovered the need for the development of technique and skills to remove these systems in many situations. Extraction of transvenous pacemaker and implantable defibrillator leads became a distinct clinical procedure, requiring specialized tools, techniques, and training. In experienced hands, this procedure improves outcome by preventing and treating potentially life-threatening situations and increases the number of options available to the treating physician. Removal is achieved with minimal risk to the patient during and after the procedure. The need for extracting defibrillator leads has added to the level of complexity of the procedure and required introduction of specialized instruments.

Introduction of laser extraction sheaths and other specially designed tools will lead to further improvement in success rates and reduction in the risk of complications. It needs to be emphasized, however, that judgment, adequate training, and careful patient selection are the more important factors in ensuring the success and safety of this procedure.

REFERENCES

1. Byrd CL. Management of implant complications. In: Ellenbogen KA, Kay GN, Wilkoff BL, eds. *Clinical cardiac pacing*. Philadelphia: WB Saunders, 1995:519–520.
2. Epstein AE, Kay GN, Plumb VJ, et al. Gross and microscopic pathological changes associated with nonthoracotomy implantable defibrillator leads. *Circulation* 1998;98:1517–1524.
3. Stokes KB, Anderson J, McVenes R, McClay C. The encapsulation of polyurethane-insulated transvenous cardiac pacemaker leads. *Cardiovasc Pathol* 1995;4:163–171.
4. Brodell GK, Wilkoff BL. A novel approach to determining the cause of pacemaker lead failure. *Cleve Clin J Med* 1992;59:91–92.
5. Brodell GK, Castle LW, Maloney JD, Wilkoff BL. Chronic transvenous pacemaker lead removal using a unique, sequential transvenous system. *Am J Cardiol* 1990;66:964–966.
6. Smith HJ, Fearnot NE, Byrd CL, et al. Five years' experience with intravascular lead extraction. *Pacing Clin Electrophysiol* 1994;17:2016–2020.
7. Myers MR, Parsonnet V, Bernstein AD. Extraction of implanted transvenous pacing leads: a review of a persistent medical problem. *Am Heart J* 1991;121:881–888.
8. Jarwe M, Klug D, LeFranc P, et al. Pacemaker lead extraction: mono-center comparison of lead removal via the implantation vein or via the femoral vein. *Pacing Clin Electrophysiol* 1997;20:1110A.
9. Wilkoff BL, Byrd CL, Love CJ, et al. Pacemaker lead extraction with the laser sheath: results of the PLEXES trial. *J Am Coll Cardiol* 1999;33:1671–1676.
10. Byrd CL, Wilkoff BL, Love CJ, et al. Intravascular extraction of problematic or infected permanent pacemaker leads: 1994–1996. *Pacing Clin Electrophysiol* 1999;22:1348–1357.
11. Kennergren C. First European experience using excimer laser for the extraction of permanent pacemaker leads. *Pacing Clin Electrophysiol* 1998;[Pt 2]:268–270.
12. Krishnan SC, Epstein LM. Initial experience with a laser sheath to extract chronic transvenous implantable cardioverter-defibrillator leads. *Am J Cardiol* 1998;82:1293–1295, A10.
13. Al-Khadra AS, Wilkoff BL, Byrd CL, et al. Extraction of nonthoracotomy defibrillator leads using the Spectranetics laser sheath: the US experience. *Pacing Clin Electrophysiol* 1998;21:889A.
14. Epstein LM, Byrd CL, Wilkoff BL, et al. Initial experience with larger laser sheaths for the removal of transvenous pacemaker and implantable defibrillator leads. *Circulation* 1999;100:516–525.
15. Al-Khadra AS, Niebauer MJ, Wilkoff BL. Non-thoracotomy implantable defibrillator lead extraction: results and comparison with extraction of pacemaker leads. *J Am Coll Cardiol (in press)*.
16. Geiger MJ, Wase A, Kearney MM, et al. Evaluation of the safety and efficacy of deep sedation for electrophysiology procedures administered in the absence of an anesthetist. *Pacing Clin Electrophysiol* 1997;20:1804–1808.
17. Natale A, Kearney MM, Brandon MJ, et al. Safety of nurse-administered deep sedation for defibrillator implantation in the electrophysiology laboratory. *J Cardiovasc Electrophysiol* 1996;7:301–306.
18. Bubien RS, Fisher JD, Gentzel JA, et al. NASPE expert consensus document: use of IV (conscious) sedation/analgesia by non-anesthesia personnel in patients undergoing arrhythmia specific diagnostic, therapeutic, and surgical procedures. *Pacing Clin Electrophysiol* 1998;21:375–385.
19. Wilkoff BL, Byrd CL, Love CJ, et al. Trends in intravascular lead extraction: analysis of data from 5339 procedures in 10 years. XIth World Symposium on Cardiac Pacing and Electrophysiology, Berlin. *Pacing Clin Electrophysiol* 1999;22[Pt II]:A207.
20. Niebauer MJ, Wilkoff BL, Van Zandt H, et al. Nonthoracotomy defibrillator lead extraction: comparison with ventricular pacing leads. *Pacing Clin Electrophysiol* 1997;20[Pt II]:1071.
21. Niebauer MJ, Al-Khadra A, Chung MK, et al. The Spectranetics laser sheath reduces extraction time for nonthoracotomy defibrillator leads. *J Am Coll Cardiol* 1998;31[Suppl 2]:1047–173, 120A.
22. Wilkoff BL, Smith HJ, Goode LB. Transvenous extraction of non-thoracotomy defibrillator leads: an emerging technical challenge. *Eur J Card Pacing Electrophysiol* 1994;4:132A.
23. Maloney JD, Wilkoff BL, Smith HJ, Zhu DWX. Feasibility of percutaneous extraction of defibrillator leads. *Circulation* 1995;92:I-151A.
24. Lloyd MA, Hayes DL, Holmes DR Jr, et al. Extraction of the Telectronics Accufix 330-801 atrial lead: the Mayo Clinic experience. *Mayo Clin Proc* 1996;71:230–234.
25. Levy T, Walker S, Paul V. Initial experience in the extraction of chronically implanted pacemaker leads using the Excimer Laser Sheath. *Heart* 1999;82:101–104.

INDEX

A

Ablation, 289–310. *See also* specific sites
  of accessory pathways, left-sided, 173–190
  of accessory pathways, right free wall, 193–206
  of anteroseptal and midseptal accessory pathways, 237–253
  of atrial fibrillation, 313–368
  of atrial tachycardia, 289–310
  of bundle branch reentrant tachycardia, 362–368
  of idiopathic ventricular tachycardia, 344–362
  of supraventricular tachycardia, 410–459
Accessory pathways. *See also* specific pathways, e.g., Posteroseptal accessory pathways
  anteroseptal and midseptal, 237–253 (*See also* Anteroseptal and midseptal pathways)
  congenital malformations in atrioventricular nodal region in, 22–23, 23f
    catheter placements for, 24f, 25
    classification conventions for, 23
    impulse direction of, 24–25
    slow and fast, 24
    surgical and ablation procedures for, 25–26, 25f, 26f
    Wolff-Parkinson-White syndrome and, 23, 26–27
  mapping of, 104
    orthogonal array catheters in, 105–106, 105f, 106f
  posteroseptal, 221–235 (*See also* Posteroseptal accessory pathways)
  right free wall, 193–206
Accessory pathways, left-sided, retrograde aortic *vs.* transseptal approach for, 173–190, 174f–178f
  ablation target mapping in, 185–187, 186f, 187f
  approach comparisons in, 187–189, 187t
  catheter ablation for, 179–185
    complications in, 189–190
    retrograde aortic approach in, 179–181, 180f, 181f
    suggestions for, 190
    transeptal approach in, 181–185, 182t, 183f–185f

diagnosis in, 173, 174f–178f
  anteroseptal pathway, 174f
  left lateral pathway, 174f
  left lateral pathway, with cycle length prolongation, 176f
  multiple pathways, 178f
  orthodromic atrioventricular reentrant tachycardia, 175f
  preexcited QRS, 177f
Accessory pathways, right free wall, ablation of, 193–206
  anatomic locations in, 193–196
    fluoroscopic view in, 194f
    muscular AV connections in, 194–196, 195f, 196f
    tricuspid valve *vs.* mitral valve annulus in, 194, 195f
  congenital anomalies in, 204–206
  electrocardiographic manifestations in, 196–197, 197f
  electrophysiologic testing in, 197–199, 199f
  historical perspectives in, 196
  intracardiac mapping in, 199–202
    target site criteria in, 200–202
    technique for, 199–200, 200f, 201f
  RF catheter ablation in, 202–204, 203t
ACE inhibitors
  with ICD, 671, 671t, 672–673, 672f
  in Sudden Cardiac Death Heart Failure Trial (SCD-HeFT), 680
Acetaminophen, 503
Acetylcholine, 39–40
Aconitine, 314
Activation map, endocardial right, 168f
Adaptive-duration shocks, 613
Adenosine
  on AVNRT, 256, 257f
  conduction block induction by, in accessory pathway, 211, 213f
  on idiopathic ventricular tachycardia, 344, 347, 347f
  on posteroseptal accessory pathways, 225
Adenosine-sensitive ventricular tachycardia, 344–362. *See also* Ventricular tachycardia, idiopathic
Aging
  on conduction system, 12–13
  DDD pacing and, 783

Air embolism, 758–759, 758t, 759f, 759t
Ambulatory electrocardiography, 669–670
Amiodarone
  in Canadian Implantable Defibrillator Study (CIDS), 666
  congenital heart disease surgery and, 34
  for early recurrence of atrial fibrillation (ERAF), 625
  vs. ICD, 655, 659f
  in MADIT trial, 675, 676
  for myocardial infarction, 18
  in Sudden Cardiac Death Heart Failure Trial (SCD-HeFT), 680, 680f
  for syncope of undetermined origin, 655–656
  for ventricular arrhythmia, 688–689, 688f, 692, 693–694, 696
  for ventricular tachycardia, with coronary heart disease, 373–374, 396, 400, 401
Amplatz catheters, 112, 113f, 833
Amyliodosis, 16
Anesthesia
  for ICD implantation, 495–497
    conscious sedation *vs.* general, 495–496
    fibrillation threshold testing and, 496–497
  for lead extraction, 821–822
  for vessel puncture, 78–79
Aneurysm, 97
Angiotensin-converting enzyme (ACE) inhibitors
  with ICD, 671, 671f, 672–673, 672f
  in Sudden Cardiac Death Heart Failure Trial (SCD-HeFT), 680, 680f
Anteroseptal accessory pathway, electrocardiogram of, 174f
Anteroseptal and midseptal accessory pathways, ablation of, 237–253
  ablation in, 244–248
    diagnostic studies for, 244–245, 245f, 246f
    electrode technique in, 247–248
    mapping in, 245–247, 247f, 248f
  anatomy in, 237–240
    atrioventricular junction in, 238–240, 240f
    classification system in, 237, 239f
    atrioventricular block risk in, 249–250, 249f

Anteroseptal and midseptal accessory pathways (*cont.*)
  efficacy and complications in, 250–253
    anteroseptal pathways, 250–253, 251t, 252f
    midseptal pathways, 253
  electrogram criteria in site selection for, 248–249
  electrophysiologic characteristics in, 240–244
    algorithms in, 241–244, 242f, 243f
    normal, 241, 241f, 242f
    para-Hisian, 244
  electrophysiologic classification of, 240, 241f
  power delivery in, 249–250, 249f
  research summary for, 238t
Antiarrhythmic drugs, 17–19. *See also* specific agents
Antiarrhythmics *versus* Implantable Defibrillator (AVID) trial, 655, 656t, 666, 666f, 667f, 669
  ejection fraction in, 666, 666f, 667f, 669
  termination of, 692
Antibiotics, for ICD implantation, 494–495
Anticholinergics, 812
Anticoagulated patient, 756–757
Antiemetics
  for electrophysiology laboratory ICD implantation, 496
  for outpatient ICD implantation, 503
Antitachycardia pacing, in tiered therapy, 611, 611f, 612f
Aortic annulus, 410, 412f
Arrhythmia. *See also* specific types, e.g., Supraventricular tachycardia
  after congenital heart disease surgery, 34
  aging process on, 13
  birth weights and, 6
  classification of, 4
  detection algorithms for, future of, 704–705
  familial, 19–21
  molecular substrates of, 17–21
    antiarrhythmic drugs in, 17–19
    connexins in, 20–21
    gap junctions in, 20–21
    genetic basis in, 19–20
  prevention of, future developments in, 705–706
Arrhythmogenic right ventricular dysplasia/cardiomyopathy (ARVD/C), 483
  genetic basis of, 14
  from infection, 14
Arterial dissection, from arterial puncture, 97
ARVD/C (arrhythmogenic right ventricular dysplasia/cardiomyopathy). *See* Arrhythmogenic right ventricular dysplasia/cardiomyopathy
Aspirin, 680
ASTRID trial, 614

Atherosclerosis, 15
Atresia, of sinoatrial node, 13
Atrial-axis discontinuity, 22
Atrial defibrillation, with implantable cardioverter-defibrillator (ICD), 571–591, 619–629. *See also* Atrial fibrillation
  clinical management strategies for, 573–574
  defibrillators for
    atrial fibrillation early recurrence in, 584–585
    atrial shock synchronization by, 581
    atrioverter in, 624–626, 624f–626f, 625t
    detection algorithms for, 579–580, 580f, 581f
    Guidant Metrix, 575–576, 576f
    Metrix defibrillation system in, 581–582, 582f
    Metrix phase I trial in, 582–583
    patient selection in, 629t
    threshold optimization in, 578–579
    thresholds of, 576–578, 577f
  defibrillators for, dual-chamber, 585–591, 626–628, 627f, 628f, 628t
    detection algorithms for, 586–588, 586f
    detection algorithms for, AV-ICDs, 586–589f, 588–590, 590f
    Jewel 7250 model, 590
    thresholds of, 585–586
  general considerations for, 619
  internal cardioversion in, 620–623
    vs. external, 620–621, 621f
    methodology for, 621–622, 621f–623f
    pain perception in, 622–623
  sinus rhythm restoration in, 619–620
Atrial defibrillation waveforms, 519
Atrial electrogram morphology, 528t, 529
Atrial extrastimulation pacing, on atrioventricular node reentry tachycardia (AVNRT), 206f, 259
Atrial extrastimuli
  of atriofascicular pathways, 208, 209f
  of right-sided accessory pathway, 199
Atrial fibrillation, 313–368. *See also* Atrial defibrillation
  atrial fibrillation in, 313–319
    initiation of, 313–314, 314f
    mechanisms of, 314–319
      automatic foci in, 314–316, 315f–318f
      persistent and chronic, 318–319
      pulmonary vein lesion creation in, 316–317, 318f
  catheter ablation in, 130–136, 319–336
    animal research in, 134–136, 134f
    catheter development in, 134–136, 134f
    clinical procedures in, early, 133–134, 134f
    direct, to prevent atrial fibrillation, 136

    direct, to terminate atrial fibrillation, 131–133, 131f, 132f
    experimental studies for, 320–336
      left atrium mechanical function in, 333–336, 334f–335f
      linear lesions in, 320–330
        animal model in, 320–322
        efficacy and outcomes of, 324, 328f–330f, 329–330
        loop catether design in, 322–324, 322f–327f
        for prevention, 331–333, 332t, 333f
      models in, 320
      rapid-pacing dog model in, 330–331, 331t
      general considerations in, 319–320, 321t
      left-sided, 136
      reduction of ventricular response in, 130–131, 130t, 131f
    catheter mapping of, 128–130, 129f
    dual-chamber sensing of, 524, 526–527, 526f
    future developments for, 707
    paroxysmal, 799–800
    prevalence of, 631
    radiofrequency ablation for, 37–40
    results and projections in, 336–340
      focal ablation in, 338
      future techniques in, 339
      gross and histologic findings in, 336–338, 336f, 337f
      linear lesion creation in, 338
      loop catheter design evaluation in, 339
      maze operation in, 338
      onging trials in, 338–339
    surgical ablation of, 420–428
      atrial functional anatomy in, 421
      atrial pathology in, 421
      clinical presentation in, 422
      mechanism in, 421–422, 421f
      results and applications in, 427–428
      surgical rationale in, 422, 423f
      surgical techniques in, 422–427
        corridor operation, 422–425, 524f
        fragmentation or compartment operation, 426
        left atrial isolation, 426
        maze operation, 425–426, 426f
        spiral operation, 426–427, 427f
        vertical transseptal approach, modified, 427
    surgical approach to, 433–469
      atrial fibrillation early explanations in, 433–434
      atrial mapping in, computerized, 434–437, 435f, 443–444
        methods of, 434
        results of, 434–437, 436f, 437f
        surgical intervention and, 443–444
      structural heart disease and, 451–459
        general considerations in, 451–452
        radial incision approach in, 454–459, 455f–459f, 458t

rheumatic mitral valve disease in, 452–454
surgical therapies in, 445–446, 445–451
ablative cure concept in, 446
electrophysiology and anatomy correlation in, 445–446
maze III procedure for, 449–451, 449f, 450t
maze procedure modifications for, 446–448, 447f, 448f, 448t
Atrial flutter, 124–128
in atrial tachycardia ablation
atypical, 297–298, 299f, 300f
typical, 290–297
ablation in, 296–297, 298f, 299f
animal models for, 290
flutter induction in, 296
mapping for, 291–296
activation, 292–293, 293f, 294f
entrainment, 294–296, 296f
split potentials, 293–294, 295f
substrate for, 291, 292f
catheter ablation of, 125–128
ectopic atrial tachycardia, 127–128, 128f
general considerations in, 125–127, 126t, 127f
catheter mapping of, 124–125, 124f, 125f
halo catheter for, 169, 169f
radiofrequency ablation for, 37–40
surgical approach to, 444–445
early explanations and, 433–434
mapping studies in, computerized, 437–443
activation maps in, dog, 442f, 443
clinical spectrum in, 443, 444f
electrodes and templates in, 439–441, 440f, 441f
reentrant circuits in, 437–438, 438f
right vs. left atrial anatomy in, 441f
slow conduction zone in, 438, 438f, 439f
surgical intervention and mapping data in, 443–444
Atrial free wall, folding over of onto ventricle, 195f
Atrial isomerism, 13
Atrial pacing
congenital heart disease surgery and, 34
decremental, 268–269
Atrial rate zones, 610
Atrial sensing, 787
Atrial tachycardia
atypical flutter in, 300f
and AVNRT, 270
dual chamber sensing and detection for, 543, 544f
ectopic, 127–128, 128f
Atrial tachycardia, ablation of, 289–310
atrial fibrillation, 305–306, 306f, 307f
focal, 301–304
mapping and ablation in, 301–304, 302f–304f
substrate in, 301

inappropriate sinus tachycardia in, 304, 305f
macro-reentrant, 290–301
atrial flutter in, atypical, 297–298, 299f, 300f
atrial flutter in, typical, 290–297
ablation in, 296–297, 298f, 299f
animal models for, 290
flutter induction in, 296
mapping for, 291–296
activation, 292–293, 293f, 294f
entrainment, 294–296, 296f
split potentials, 293–294, 295f
substrate for, 291, 292f
definitions in, 290, 291t
incisional reentry in, 298–301
mapping and ablation in, 301
mapping in, three-dimensional, 306–310, 308f, 309f
surgical, 418–420
atrial flutter, 418–419, 419f, 420f
ectopic, 418
intraoperative cardiac mapping for, 419–420
results and applications of, 420
sinus node, 418
surgical rationale for, 419
Atrial transport function, 454–455
Atrial undersensing, 796–797
Atriofascicular accessory pathways (Mahaim), ablation of, 206–217
clinical and electrophysiologic features in, 208
definition in, 206–208, 207f, 208f
electrophysiologic testing in, 208–211, 209f–213f
atrial extrastimuli in, 208, 209f
AVRT vs. AVNRT in, 209–211, 211f–213f
AVRT with LBBB pattern in, 209, 210f
historical perspective in, 206–208, 207f, 208f
mapping and RF catheter ablation in, 211–216
electrophysiologic criteria in, 214, 214f, 215f
results of, 214–216, 216f, 216t, 217f
summary of, 216–217
technique for, 211
Atriofascicular (His) connection, 23f
Atrioventricular attachment, 410–411, 411f
Atrioventricular block
in anteroseptal and midseptal accessory pathways ablation, 249–250, 249f
in congenital malformations, 21–22
Atrioventricular interval, 786–787
Atrioventricular junction, in anteroseptal and midseptal accessory pathways, 238–240, 240f
Atrioventricular nodal reentrant tachycardia, surgical ablation of, 416–418, 416f

Atrioventricular nodal region
accessory pathways in, 22–23, 23f
age-related changes of, 13
anatomy of, 9–11, 10f, 11f
conduction pathways of, 34–37, 36f
dissection of, 416f
Atrioventricular node reentry tachycardia (AVNRT)
atrioventricular nodal axis in, 10–11
conduction pathway morphology in, 34–37
node modification for, 255–283
catheter in, 270–283
fast pathway modification in, 280–281
historical background for, 270–271
slow pathway modification in, 271–280
electrogram-guided approach in, 272–273, 273f
electrogram-guided approach in, vs. stepwise anatomic, 274
electrophysiologic parameter changes in, 279–280, 279f
integrated approach in, 274f, 275–276, 275f, 276f
left-sided approach in, 276–277
mapping and imaging for, 277–278, 278f
other approaches in, 277
outcomes of, 280, 280t
stepwise anatomic approach in, 273–274
technique for, 271–272, 272f
therapeutic end points for, 278–279
unusual features and, 282–283
clinical presentation in, 255–256, 256f, 257f
concept evolution in, 256–266
AV node in, 256–259, 258f, 260f–261f
classification in, 263–266
fast/slow, 265–266, 267f
slow/fast, 263–265, 264f, 265f
slow/slow, 266, 267f
dual AV node physiology in
atrial extrastimulation pacing on, 206f, 259
fast vs. slow pathways of, 259–263, 262f
electrocardiographic findings in, 255–256, 256f, 257f
electrophysiologic study in, 267–270
catheter placement in, 267–268
decremental atrial pacing in, 268–269
decremental ventricular pacing in, 268
differential diagnosis in, 269–270
ventricular extrastimulation in, 268
vs. right-sided accessory pathway, 198–199
Atrioventricular septal defects (ASDs), 31–32

Atrium
    mapping studies of, computerized,
        434–444
        for atrial fibrillation, 437–443
            activation maps in, dog, 442f, 443
            clinical spectrum in, 443, 444f
            electrodes and templates in,
                439–441, 440f, 441f
            reentrant circuits in, 437–438, 438f
            right *vs.* left atrial anatomy in, 441f
            slow conduction zone in, 438,
                438f, 439f
        for atrial flutter, 437–443
            activation maps in, dog, 442f, 443
            clinical spectrum in, 443, 444f
            electrodes and templates in,
                439–441, 440f, 441f
            reentrant circuits in, 437–438, 438f
            right *vs.* left atrial anatomy in, 441f
            slow conduction zone in, 438,
                438f, 439f
        methods in, 437
        surgical intervention and, 443–444
    pulmonary vein insertion into,
        315–316, 318f
Atropine
    for early recurrence of atrial fibrillation
        (ERAF), 625
    for vasovagal reactions, 98
Automatic foci, in atrial fibrillation
    mechanisms, 314–316,
    315f–318f
AVNRT (atrioventricular node reentry
    tachycardia). *See* Atrioventricular
    node reentry tachycardia
Axillary vein
    anatomic considerations for, 714–715,
        716f
    percutaneous technique for, 751–752,
        752f
    venous access through, 726–738
        anatomical considerations in,
            729–730, 729f, 730f
        cephalic vein isolation in, 734–735,
            736f
        contrast venography in, 735–736,
            736f
        Doppler and ultrasound in, 736, 737f
        landmarks for, 730–734, 731f–735f
        safety zone for, 728f, 729, 729f
        techniques for, 737t

B

Bachmann's bundle, 4
    internodal tracts and, 9
Baseline crossing analysis, 624, 625f, 639,
    640f
Basket catheter arrays
    for atrial fibrillation, 128–129, 129f
        development of, 135–136
    for endocardial mapping, 169–170, 170f
    for ventricular tachycardia
        global, 137–140, 138f–141f
        regional, 140–142, 141f, 142f, 142t

Benzodiazepine, 351
BEST system, 816, 816f
Beta Blocker Strategy Plus ICD (BEST)
    Trial, 673t, 681, 681f
Beta blockers
    for early recurrence of atrial fibrillation
        (ERAF), 625
    for hypertrophic cardiomyopathy, 783,
        785
    with ICD, 671, 671t, 672, 672f
    in MADIT II trial, 680, 680f
    in MADIT trial, 675–676
    in Sudden Cardiac Death Heart Failure
        Trial (SCD-HeFT), 680
    for vasodepressor syncope, 812
    for ventricular arrhythmia, 689–690,
        689f, 691
    for ventricular tachycardia, idiopathic,
        349
    for ventricular tachycardia, with
        coronary heart disease, 401
Biphasic waveforms, 510–512, 511f, 512f,
    513–519, 520f
    action potential prolongation in,
        518–519, 519f, 520f
    for defibrillation, 612–613, 613f
    epicardial potential gradient distribution
        in, 513–515, 514f
    in external defibrillators, 621
    postshock activation in, 515, 515f
    resistor-capacitor model in, 516, 517f
    strength interval curves in, 518, 518f
    transmembrane potentials in, 515–516,
        516f
Bipolar electrograms, 95
    technical considerations in, 163–164,
        164f
    in ventricular arrhythmia, *vs.* unipolar,
        475f
Biventricular implantable cardioverter-
    defibrillator (ICD), 499–503,
    504f
Biventricular pacing, for congestive heart
    failure
        clinical considerations in, 790–791
        clinical results in, 792–793, 793t
        methodologic considerations in, 793
        technologic considerations in, 794–795
Blanking periods, in dual-chamber sensing,
    524–526, 525f
Brachial nerve, 99
Brevital (methohexital), 496
Brockenbrough needle, 85–86, 86f
Brugada syndrome, 350
    ICD and, 658
Bundle branch reentrant tachycardia,
    362–368
    ablation results in, 366–368
    ablation techniques for, 365–366, 367f
    tachycardia mechanism in, 362–365,
        364f, 365f
Bundle branches
    anatomy of, 11–12
    block of, right, and right accessory
        pathway, 198

Burst antitachycardia pacing, 611, 611f
Butorphanol, 623
Byrd Femoral Workstation, 833

C

Caffeine, 380
Calcium antagonists, mechanism of, 18–19
Calcium blockers, for ventricular
    tachycardia, idiopathic, 349
Calcium homeostasis, 18–19
Calgary Trial, 690
Canadian Amiodarone Myocardial
    Infarction Arrhythmia Trial
    (CAMIAT), 18
Canadian Implantable Defibrillator Study
    (CIDS), 655–656
    ejection fraction in, 666, 666f
    probability of death in, 692–693
Capacitors, 701–702, 702f
    defibrillation waveforms and, 510
Cardiac sarcoidosis, 14
Cardiac arrest, survival results for,
    654–655
Cardiac Arrest in Seattle: Conventional
    versus Amiodarone Drug
    Evaluation (CASCADE) study,
    690–691
Cardiac Arrest Study Hamburg (CASH)
    pharmacologic therapy in, 690
    probability of death in, 693
Cardiac Arrhythmia Suppression Trial
    (CAST)
    Holter monitoring in, 669–670
    sodium channel blockers in, 17
Cardiac catheterization, complications
    from, 96–98
Cardiac death
    ICD trials and, 663–682 (*See also under*
        Implantable cardioverter-
        defibrillator)
    prevalence of, 586f, 664, 685
Cardiac mapping. *See* Mapping, cardiac
Cardiac morphogenesis, 5–6
Cardiac myocytes, 6
Cardiac perforation, 97–98
Cardiac resynchronization, 499
Cardiac sarcoidosis, 14
Cardiac skeleton, 12, 12f
Cardiac transplantation, 656–657, 657f
Cardiomyopathy, 781–789. *See also*
    Hypertrophic cardiomyopathy,
    obstructive
Cardioplegic solutions, for ventricular
    arrhythmia, 471
Carotid sinus syndrome, in vasodepressor
    syncope, 813
CARTO system
    for atrial fibrillation, 320
    for right free wall accessory pathway
        mapping, 200, 201f, 204
Catecholamine-sensitive ventricular
    tachycardia, 344–362. *See also*
    Ventricular tachycardia,
    idiopathic

Catecholamines, 344
Catheter(s). *See also* Catheter designs; Catheterization
  adjustable-size loop, 110, 110f
  Amplatz, 112, 113f, 502
  basket array, 128–129, 129f
  coil-shaped regional array mapping, 131, 131f
  construction of, 106–107, 106f, 107f
  double-spline, 110, 111f
  halo, 169, 169f
  intracoronary, 108
  Judkins, 502
  large-tip, for atrial lesions, 126, 126t
  nonsteerable, 106–107, 107f
  open-lumen, 114, 114f
  orthogonal array, 105–106, 105f, 106f
  over-the-guide-wire, 110–111, 111f
  pigtail, 112, 112f
  reference, 104, 104f
  ring and coil, 322f, 331t
  ring and coil electrode, 322f
  small-size, 114–115, 115f
  steerability of, 107–108
  ultrasound location of, 155–156
Catheter designs, 103–156
  for atrial fibrillation, 128–136
    ablation of, 130–136
      animal research in, 134–136, 134f
      catheter development in, 134–136, 134f
      clinical procedures in, early, 133–134, 134f
      direct, to prevent atrial fibrillation, 136
      direct, to terminate atrial fibrillation, 131–133, 131f, 132f
      left-sided, 136
      reduction of ventricular response in, 130–131, 130t, 131f
    mapping of, 128–130, 129f
  for atrial flutter, 124–128
    ablation of, 125–128
      ectopic atrial tachycardia, 127–128, 128f
      general considerations in, 125–127, 126t, 127f
    mapping of, 124–125, 124f, 125f
  general considerations in, 103–104
  for intracardiac imaging, 153–156
    ultrasound alternatives in, 156
    ultrasound in, 154–156
  for supraventricular tachycardia, ablation of, 108–124
    anatomy-specific designs in, 110–114, 110f–114f
      adustable-size loop, 110, 110f
      Amplatz, 112, 113f
      double-spline, 110, 111f
      mitral valve annulus, 112, 112f, 113f
      open-lumen, 114, 114f
      over-the-guide-wire, 110–111, 111f
      pigtail, 112, 112f
      right coronary, 111–112
    electrodes in, 116–118, 116f–118f
    general considerations in, 108
    performance options in, 109
    sheaths in, 115–116, 116f
    size and shape in, 109
    small-size catheters in, 114–115, 115f
    temperature feedback alternatives in, 123–124
    temperature feedback in, 118–122, 118f–122f, 121t
    temperature sensors and placement in, 122–123, 123f, 123t
    in vivo adjustment in, 109–110, 109f, 110f
  for supraventricular tachycardia, mapping of, 104–108
    catheter construction in, 106–107, 106f, 107f
    electrodes in, 104–106, 105f, 106f
    enhanced graphics for, 108
    intracoronary catheters in, 108
    reference catheters in, 104, 104f
    steerability in, 107–108
    thermal, 108
  for ventricular tachycardia, ablation of, 143–152
    chemical, 152–153
    fluid-assisted, 146–152
      closed-loop system, 151–152, 151f, 152f, 152t
      general considerations in, 146–147, 146f–148f
      limitations and improvements in, 150–151, 150f
      open system, 147–150, 148f–150f
    large surface area electrodes in, 143–145, 144f, 145f
    multisite, 146
    special electrode design in, 145–146, 145f
  for ventricular tachycardia, mapping of, 137–143
    basket arrays in, global, 137–140, 138f–141f
    basket arrays in, regional, 140–142, 141f, 142f, 142t
    general considerations in, 137, 137f
    intravascular, 142
    thermal, 142–143
Catheterization, 77–93. *See also* Catheter(s)
  complications in, 96–100
    from cardiac catheterization, 96–98
    cerebrovascular, 99–100
    from radiofrequency catheter ablation, 100
    from subclavian stick technique, 98–99
  femoral artery puncture in, 78–79, 79f, 81–83, 82f
  femoral vein puncture in, 78–81, 79f–81f
  fluoroscopic views for, 87–89
    frontal, 87, 87f, 88f
    left anterior oblique, 88f, 89, 89f
    right anterior oblique, 87–89, 87f, 89f
  historical of, 77–78
  internal jugular vein puncture in, 84–85, 85f
  manipulation techniques for
    coronary sinus catheters, 91f
    intravascular sheaths in, 91f
    left ventricle in, 92–93, 93f
    sinus rhythm recordings in, 92, 92f
    steerable Livewire catheter, 89–90, 90f
  radiographic equipment for, 87
  subclavian vein puncture in, 83–84, 84f
  transeptal left atrial, 85–86, 86f
Cefazolin, 495
Cephalic vein
  anatomic considerations for, 715, 715f, 716f
  ICD leads and, 497–499, 497f, 498f
Cephalic vein cutdown technique, 722, 723f
Cephalic venous access, 722, 723f
Cephalosporin, 495
Cerebrovascular accidents, 99–100
Chest, anatomy of, 715f
Children, idiopathic ventricular tachycardia in, 348–349
Chloralose, 496–497
Chloroprocaine (Nesacaine), 79
Circuits, future of, 702
Clavicle, displaced, 717–718, 717f, 718f
Clindamycin, 495
Closed-loop temperature controlled RF ablation, 122, 122f
Clostridium difficile, 495
Coil expander, 825, 826f
Compartment operation, for atrial fibrillation, 426
Compazine (prochlorperazine), 496
Conduction system, morphology of, 3–45
  anatomy of, abnormal
    atresia, 13
    displacement, 13
    duplication, 13–14
    infarction, 14–16
    infection and inflammation, 14
    infiltration, 16–17
  anatomy of, normal, 6–13
    age-related changes on, 12–13
    atrioventricular nodal axis, 9–11, 10f, 11f
    bundle branches, 11–12
    cardiac skeleton, 12, 12f
    His bundle, 10f, 11–12
    internodal tracts, 9
    membranous septum, 12, 12f
    Purkinje fibers, 12
    sinus node, 6–9, 7f, 8f
  arrhythmia and
    after congenital heart disease surgery, 34
    classification of, 4
    molecular substrates of, 17–21
      antiarrhythmic drugs in, 17–19
      connexins in, 20–21
      gap junctions in, 20–21
      genetic basis in, 19–20

Conduction system (cont.)
  atrioventricular node in, pathways of, 34–37, 36f
  congenital malformations in, 21–34
    accessory pathways in
      atrioventricular nodal region in, 22–23, 23f
      catheter placements for, 24f, 25
      classification conventions for, 23
      impulse direction of, 24–25
      slow and fast, 24
      surgical and ablation procedures for, 25–26, 25f, 26f
      Wolff-Parkinson-White syndrome and, 23, 26–27
    arrhythmias, post-surgical, 34
    atrioventricular block, complete, 21–22
    Ebstein's anomaly, 30–31
    great arteries of, transposition of, 33–34
    Lown-Ganong-Levine syndrome, 27–30
    management of, 34
    septal defects, 31–32
    Tetralogy of Fallot, 32–33
    univentricular hearts, 33
  development of, 4–6
  historical synopsis of, 3–4
  radiofrequency ablation and
    for atrial fibrillation and atrial flutter, 37–41
      acetylcholine stimulation in, 39–40
      anatomical barriers in, 40–41, 40f
      AV node destruction and permanent pacing in, 39
      discontinuous lesions in, 38
      electrode tip length in, 38–39
      expandable loop catheters in, 39
      left atrium in, 37
      right atrium in, 37–38
    lesion pathology in, 41–44
      alternate energy sources in, 43–44
      animal models in, 41, 42f
      power regulation vs. temperature control in, 42–43
      tricuspid valve-inferior vena cava isthmus in, 42
Congenital complete atrioventricular block (CCAVB), 22
Congenital malformations, of conduction system, 21–34. *See also under* Conduction system, congenital malformations in
Congenitally corrected transposition of great arteries (CCTGA)
  Ebstein's anomaly in, 30
  morphological features of, 33–34
Congestive heart failure
  pacing for, 789–795
    beneficial effect mechanism in, 790
    biventricular pacing in, 790–791
    biventricular pacing in, clinical results of, 792–793, 793t
    biventricular pacing in, methodologic considerations in, 793
    biventricular pacing in, technologic considerations in, 794–795
    general considerations in, 789
    patient selection in, 789
  prevalence of, 631
Connectors, future developments in, 704
Connexins, 20–21
Conscious sedation, for ventricular tachycardia with CAD, 376
CONTAK CD CHFD pulse generator, 649–650
Continuous electrical activity electrograms, 95
Cooperative North Scandinavian Enalapril Survival Study I (CONSENSUS), 672
Coronary Artery Bypass Graft (CABG)-Patch trial, 658–660, 677–679, 679f
  adjunctive therapy in, 672f, 673
  heart rate variability and, 670–671
Coronary artery disease, ventricular tachycardia ablation in, 373–405
  case studies in, 388–404, 389f–404f
  electrophysiology laboratory for, 375–378
    intracardiac recordings in, 376
    patient preparation in, 376
    radiofrequency generators in, 377–378, 378f
    retrograde aortic approach in, 376
    tachycardia induction in, 376–377
  fluoroscopic technique in, 378–379, 379f
  indications for, 373–374
  limitations of, 404
  mapping and pacing response in, 381–387, 386t
    assessment of, 384–385, 384t
    bystander circuits in, 382, 382f
    common pathway in, 381, 381f
    entrainment in, concealed vs. classic, 383–385, 383f
    four-beat analysis in, 385, 386f
    loop diagram in, 381–382, 382f
    outcomes for, 385–387, 386t
    single-paced premature beats in, 387
  pacing technique in, 378–381, 379f, 380f
  preparation for, 374–375
  radiofrequency ablation in, 387–388
  recording technique in, 378–381, 379f, 380f
Coronary sinus
  cardiac pacing and, 748
  catheters for, 91f
  diverticulum of, 222, 222f
    mapping of, 229, 230f
  ostium of, as posteroseptal region landmark, 221–222, 222f
  in posteroseptal accessory pathway ablation, visualization of, 229, 230f
Coronary sinus diverticulum, 414, 414f
Coronary sinus ostium, 35, 36f
Corridor operation, 421
  for atrial fibrillation, 422–425, 524f
Coumel's tachycardia, 411, 414
Crista terminalis
  echocardiography of, 304f
  in inappropriate sinus tachycardia, 304
Cross-chamber blanking, 525–526, 525f
Cryoablation, 44
  for atrial fibrillation, 44
    maze procedure and, 459, 459f
  for atrioventricular nodal reentrant tachycardia, 417
  for ventricular arrhythmia, 470
  for ventricular tachycardia, 143

D

Danish Investigation of Arrhythmia and Mortality on Dofetilide (DIAMOND), 18
DCM
  fibrosis in, 16
  genetic basis of, 19
DDD pacing
  for congestive heart failure, 789–790
  for obstructive hypertrophic cardiomyopathy, 783–784, 784t
Decremental atrial pacing, for AVNRT, 268–269
Defender dual-chamber defibrillator, 632–636
  PARAD classification algorithm for, 632–633, 633t, 634f
  results of, 633–636
    arrhythmia detection and therapy in, 635
    sensitivity and specificity in, 636
  study protocol for, 633
Defibrillation patches, 494
Defibrillation threshold testing
  anesthesia and, 496–497
  for ICDs, 503
  shock polarity in, 512–513, 513f
  waveform tilt in, 510, 510f
Defibrillation waveforms, 507–520
  atrial and transthoracic, 519
  biphasic waveform efficacy in, 513–519, 520f
    action potential prolongation in, 518–519, 519f, 520f
    epicardial potential gradient distribution in, 513–515, 514f
    postshock activation in, 515, 515f
    resistor-capacitor model in, 516, 517f
    strength interval curves in, 518, 518f
    transmembrane potentials in, 515–516, 516f
  future developments in, 702–704, 703f
  morphology of, 507–513, 508f
    biphasic waveforms in, 510–512, 511f, 512f
    defibrillator capacitors and, 510
    shock polarity in, 512–513, 513f
    tilt and duration in, 507–510, 509f, 510f
  triphasic waveforms in, 519–520

Defibrillator, 58–59
DEFINITE trial, 673t, 681
Dehydration, 758–759, 758t
Detection parameters, for ICD tiered therapy programming, 609–611
Diprivan (propofol), 496
Direct current ablation, 67–68, 68f
Disopyramide, 812
Displacement, of sinoatrial node, 13
Dizziness, 344
Dofetilide, 18
Dotter basket, 833, 834f
Double-spline catheter, 110, 111f
Droperidol, 496
Dual-chamber implantable cardioverter-defibrillator (ICD), 499, 502f
  investigational, 631–651
    defender dual-chamber defibrillator in, 632–636
      PARAD classification algorithm for, 632–633, 633t, 634f
      results of, 633–636
      study protocol for, 633
    general consideration for, 631–632
    InSync ICD, 650
    Jewel AF 7250, 645–649
      PR logic algorithm for, 646–648, 646f, 647f
      results for, 648–649
      study protocol for, 648
      general considerations for, 638–640, 639f, 640f
      results for, 642–645, 642f
      study protocol for, 640–642, 641f
    VENTAK and CONTAK heart failure defibrillator, 649–650
    VENTAK PRIZM dual-chamber defibrillator, 637–638, 637t
  lead implantation for, 720–722, 721f, 722f
  sensing and detection for, 523–568 (See also under Implantable cardioverter-defibrillator)
Dual unipolar pacing, 794
Duplication, of sinoatrial node, 13–14
Duration, of waveform, 507–510, 509f, 510f

E

Early recurrence of atrial fibrillation (ERAF), 625–626, 626f
EASYTRAK, 649–650
Ebstein's anomaly, 30–31
  catheters for, 110–111, 111f
  of right free wall accessory pathways, 204–206, 204f, 205f, 206t
  in Wolff-Parkinson-White syndrome, 414
Echocardiography, of crista terminalis and right atrium, 304f
Economics, of ICD vs. pharmacologic therapy, 709
Ectopic atrial tachycardia, 127–128, 128f

Ectopic automaticity, 597–599
Ejection fraction
  in CABG Patch trial, 678–679
  in left ventricular evaluation, 665–668, 666f–668f
  in MADIT trial, 674, 674f
Electrical alternans, 671
Electrocardiograms
  of atrial fibrillation, ablation on, 325f–329f
  of atrial tachycardia, atypical flutter in, 300f
  of AVNRT, 256, 256f, 257f
    accelerated junctional rhythm in, 272f
    fast/slow, 266f
    His bundles in, 262f
    slow/slow, 267f
  bipolar, 95
    in supraventricular tachycardia mapping, 104–106, 105f, 106f
  bundle branch reentrant tachycardia, 364f, 365f
  of epicardial posteroseptal pathway, 228, 228f, 229f
    concealed, 231f
  of His bundle, 113, 113f
  of idiopathic ventricular tachycardia, verapamil-sensitive, 348f
  of posteroseptal accessory pathway, left, 223, 225f
  of posteroseptal accessory pathway, right, 223, 224f
  of sinus rhythm, in ventricular arrhythmia, 466–467, 467f
  unipolar, 94–95
    in supraventricular tachycardia mapping, 104–106, 105f, 106f
  of vasovagal syncope, 810f, 811f
  of ventricular arrhythmia, 472–476, 473f–477f
  of ventricular tachycardia
    after Tetralogy of Fallot repair, 375, 375f
    ST segment deviation in, 377, 378f
  of ventricular tachycardia, idiopathic
    isoproterenol-induced, 346f
    left fascicular, 358f–359f
    pre and post-ablation, 345f
    premature ventricular contractions in, 353f
    right overflow, 352f
    right ventricle, with pace map, 350, 350f
    right ventricular outflow, 361f
Electrocardiography
  ambulatory, 669–670
  signal averaged, 670
Electrodes
  split-tip, 105, 105f
  for supraventricular tachycardia ablation, 116–118, 116f–118f
Electronics, for ICD advancements
  capacitors, 701–702
  circuits, 702
  waveforms, 702–704, 703f

Electrophysiologic recordings, 93–100
  bipolar electrograms in, 95
  cardiac mapping with, 95
  complications in, 96–100
    from cardiac catheterization, 96–98
    cerebrovascular, 99–100
    from radiofrequency catheter ablation, 100
    from subclavian stick technique, 98–99
  physiologic recorders for, 93–94, 94f
  signal recording in, 95
  stimulator in, 95–96, 96f
  unipolar electrograms in, 94–95
Electrophysiologic Study Versus Electrocardiographic Monitoring (ESVEM), 690
Electrophysiologic testing, 668–669
Electrophysiology study database, 65–67, 66f, 67f
Embolism, air, 758–759, 758t, 759f, 759t
Emotional faint, 810
Encainide, 17
Endocardial balloon arrays, 137, 137f
  for cardiac mapping, 170, 170f
Endocardial lesions, morphometry of, 141, 142t
Endothelin, 6
Enterococcus, 495
Enteroviruses, 14
Epicardial pathway, 227–228, 228f, 229f
Epicardial sock arrays, 137, 137f
Epinephrine
  on idiopathic ventricular tachycardia, 351–352
  on ventricular tachycardia, 669
Etomidate, 496
European Myocardial Infarct Amiodarone Trial (EMIAT), 17–18
Exercise-induced ventricular tachycardia, 344–362. See also Ventricular tachycardia, idiopathic
Exit block, 474, 476f

F

Familial conditions, survival results for, 657–658
Fasciculoventricular fibers, 23f
Femoral arterial thrombosis, 97
Femoral artery puncture, 78–79, 79f, 81–83, 82f
  complications of, 97
Femoral vein puncture, 78–81, 79f–81f
  complications of, 97
Femoral venous access, 740–741, 742f
Femoral venous thrombosis, 97
Fentanyl
  for ICD implantation, 495–496
  in ventricular tachycardia with CAD, 376
Fibrosis
  in DCM, 16
  in myocardial ischemia, 20
  in transvenous leads, 819–820, 820f, 824–825

First-degree atrioventricular block, 795–797, 796t
Fistula, subclavian arteriovenous, 99
Fixed-duration shocks, 612–613
Flecainide
  in Cardiac Arrhythmia Suppression Trial (CAST), 17
  on defibrillation threshold, external, 621
  for early recurrence of atrial fibrillation (ERAF), 625
Fludrocortisone, 812
Fluid-assisted ablation, for ventricular tachycardia, 146–152
  closed-loop system, 151–152, 151f, 152f, 152t
  general considerations in, 146–147, 146f–148f
  limitations and improvements in, 150–151, 150f
  open system, 147–150, 148f–150f
Fluoroscopy
  for catheterization, 87–89
  in ventricular tachycardia ablation, with coronary artery disease, 378–379, 379f
Fontan operation, 33
Fossa ovale, 36f
Fractionated electrograms, 95
Fragmentation operation, 426

G

Gap junctions, 20–21
Gauge pin set, 825–826, 826f
Genetics, 19–20
Great arteries, transposition of, 33–34
Gruppo Italiano per lo Studio della Streptochinasi nell'Infarto Miocardico 2 (GISSI-2), 669–670
Guidant Metrix defibrillator, 575–576, 576f
Guidewire
  in femoral artery puncture, 83
  in femoral vein puncture, 81
  in internal jugular vein puncture, 85
  in subclavian vein puncture, 84, 84f
  in transeptal left atrial catheterization, 85

H

Halo catheter, 169, 169f
Halothane, 496
Heart rate variability, 670–671
Hemochromatosis, 16–17
Hemopneumothorax, 757–758, 758t
Hemorrhage, 97
Hemothorax, 757–758, 758t
  from catheterization, 98
Heparin
  implantation of ICDs and, 494
  pacemaker implantation and, 756–757
  in ventricular tachycardia with CAD, 376
Hepatanol, 15

His bundle
  anatomy of, 10f, 11–12
  in anteroseptal and midseptal pathway anatomy, 240
  electrograms of, 113, 113f
  in idiopathic ventricular tachycardia, 355–357
HNK-1 epitope, in internodal tracts, 9
Holter monitoring, 669–670
Hydration, 758–759, 758t
Hypertrophic cardiomyopathy
  genetic basis of, 19–20
  ICD and, 657
Hypertrophic cardiomyopathy, nonobstructive, 789
Hypertrophic cardiomyopathy, obstructive, pacing for, 781–789
  beneficial effect mechanism in, 788–789
  clinical studies in, acute, 781, 782t
  clinical studies in, long-term, 783–784, 784t
  indications for, 785–786
  pacemaker function and programmability in, 786–788
  pacemaker inactivation in, prolonged, 785, 785t
  permanent pacing in, 783
  placebo effect in, 784–785
  unresolved questions in, 789
Hypotension, 99

I

IART, 21
Ibutilide, 621
Idiopathic ventricular tachycardia, 344–362. See also Ventricular tachycardia, idiopathic
Impedance monitoring, 118–121, 118f, 119f, 121t, 123–124
Implantable cardioverter-defibrillator (ICD)
  atrial defibrillation with, 571–591, 619–629 (See also Implantable cardioverter-defibrillator (ICD), atrial defibrillation with)
  cardiac death prophylaxis trials of, 663–682 (See also Implantable cardioverter-defibrillator (ICD), cardiac death prophylaxis trials of)
  clinical results of, 653–661 (See also Implantable cardioverter-defibrillator (ICD), clinical results of)
  dual chamber sensing and detection for, 523–568 (See also Implantable cardioverter-defibrillator (ICD), dual chamber sensing and detection for)
  electrophysiology laboratory implantation of, 491–505
    anesthesia in, 495–497
      conscious sedation vs. general, 495–496

defibrillation threshold testing and, 496–497
  benefits of, 491–492
  device selection in, 492
  equipment for, 492–493, 492t, 493t
  outpatient implantation in, 503
  pectoral implantation technique in, 497–503
    for biventricular ICDs, 499–503, 504f
    for dual-chamber ICDs, 499, 502f
    general considerations in, 497–499, 497f, 498f, 500f, 501f
  personnel for, 493
  preoperative patient preparation in, 493–495
future technologies for, 701–710
  arrhythmia detection algorithms in, 704–705
  arrhythmia prevention in, 705–706
  automaticity in, 705
  comorbidity management in, 707–708, 708f
  costs in, 709
  electronics in, 701–704
    capacitors, 701–702
    circuits, 702
    waveforms, 702–704, 703f
  indications in, 708
  lead systems in, 704
  monitoring in, 706–707, 706f
implantation techniques for, 713–761 (See also Implantation techniques)
investigational, clinical results for, 631–651 (See also Implantable cardioverter-defibrillator (ICD), investigational, clinical results for)
leads for
  in cephalic vein, 497–499, 497f, 498f
  future developments in, 704
  unipolar, for pectoral ICDs, 498–499, 498f
tiered therapy for, 597–615
  clinical considerations in, 600–609
    antitachycardia pacing therapy delivery in, 602–605
    defibrillation in, 605–609, 607f, 608f
    detection in, 600–602
    low-energy cardioversion in, 605
  milestones in, 614–615
  programming in, 609–614
    detection parameters in, 609–611
    optimal outcomes in, 613–614
    therapy parameters in, 611–613, 611f–613f
  rationale for, 597–600
    ectopic automaticity in, 597–599
    tachyarrhythmia overview in, 599–600
  for ventricular tachycardia, 691–693, 692f, 694
    with coronary heart disease, 374

Implantable cardioverter-defibrillator
(ICD), atrial defibrillation with,
571–591, 619–629
  clinical management strategies for,
  573–574
  defibrillators for
    atrial fibrillation early recurrence in,
    584–585
    atrial shock synchronization by, 581
    atrioverter in, 624–626, 624f–626f,
    625t
    detection algorithms for, 579–580,
    580f, 581f
    Guidant Metrix, 575–576, 576f
    Metrix defibrillation system in,
    581–582, 582f
    Metrix phase I trial in, 582–583
    pain perception and discomfort in,
    583–584
    patient selection in, 629t
    threshold optimization in, 578–579
    thresholds of, 576–578, 577f
  defibrillators for, dual-chamber,
    585–591, 626–628, 627f, 628f,
    628t
    detection algorithms for, 586–588,
    586f
    detection algorithms for, AV-ICDs,
    586–589f, 588–590, 590f
    Jewel 7250 model, 590
    thresholds of, 585–586
  electrical cardioversion in, 574–575
  general considerations for, 571, 619
  health care burden and, 572–573, 573t
  internal cardioversion in, 620–623
    vs. external, 620–621, 621f
    methodology for, 621–622, 621f–623f
    pain perception in, 622–623
  rhythm disturbances in, 571–572
  sinus rhythm restoration in, 619–620
Implantable cardioverter-defibrillator
(ICD), cardiac death prophylaxis
trials of, 663–682
  adjunctive therapy in, 671–673, 671f,
  672f
  cardiac death in, sudden, 663–665
  patient care in, 681–682
  sustained ventricular arrhythmias,
  evaluation of, 665–671
    ambulatory electrocardiography in,
    669–670
    electrical alternans in, 671
    electrophysiologic testing in, 668–669
    heart rate variability in, 670–671
    left ventricular function, 665–668,
    666f–668f
    signal averaged electrocardiography
    in, 670
  trends in, 682
  trials in, completed, 673–679,
  673t–674t, 675f, 676t,
  677f–679f
  trials in, ongoing, 679–681, 680f, 681f
Implantable cardioverter-defibrillator
(ICD), clinical results of,
653–661

efficacy in, 658–661
guidelines for, evolution of, 653, 654t
survival results by indication in,
654–658
  as bridge to cardiac transplantation,
  656–657, 657f
  cardiac arrest, 654–655
  familial or inherited conditions,
  657–658
  nonsustained ventricular tachycardia,
  656, 656t
  spontaneous sustained ventricular
  tachycardia, 655
  syncope of undetermined origin,
  655–656
Implantable cardioverter-defibrillator
(ICD), dual chamber sensing and
detection for, 523–568
  clinical performance of, 561–568, 562f,
  564f, 565f
  dual chamber sensing considerations in,
  523–527
  PR logic blocks in, detailed, 534–550
    1:1 rhythms in, 535–543
      junctional tachycardia in
      ventricular tachycardia zone,
      539, 541f
      PR pattern analysis in, 538f–539f
      sinus tachycardia in ventricular
      tachycardia zone, 539, 540f
      spontaneous atrial tachycardia, 543,
      544f
      spontaneous ventricular
      tachycardia, 539, 542f, 543
    greater than 1:1 rhythms in, 543–550
      double tachycardia in, 546, 548f
      rapidly conducted atrial fibrillation/
      flutter in, 546, 548f
      sinus tachycardia with far-field R-
      wave, 549f, 550
    less than 1:1 rhythms in, 534–535,
    536f
  PR logic description in, advanced,
  550–561
    advanced examples in, 552–561
      double tachycardia in, 554, 557f,
      558
      nonsustained VT in, 554, 556f
      sinus tachycardia with FFRW
      oversensing, 560f, 561
      transition period on VT/FVT/VF
      detection, 552–554, 553f
      VT, not VT ;pl SVT, 558, 559f
      VT with 1:1 retrograde blocked
      conduction, 554, 555f
    comuputation flow in, 550–552,
    550f, 552t
  PR logic description in, basic, 529–534
    building blocks in, 530–531, 530t
    clinical inductive model in, 531–532,
    531f
    rhythm classification in, 532–534,
    533f
  tachycardia detection in, 527–529, 528t

Implantable cardioverter-defibrillator
(ICD), investigational, clinical
results for, 631–651
  defender dual-chamber defibrillator in,
  632–636
    PARAD classification algorithm for,
    632–633, 633t, 634f
    results of, 633–636
    study protocol for, 633
  general consideration for, 631–632
  InSync ICD, 650
  Jewel AF 7250, 645–649
    PR logic algorithm for, 646–648,
    646f, 647f
    results for, 648–649
    study protocol for, 648
  Metrix stand alone atrial defibrillator,
  638–645
    general considerations for, 638–640,
    639f, 640f
    results for, 642–645, 642f
    study protocol for, 640–642, 641f
  VENTAK and CONTAK heart failure
  defibrillator, 649–650
  VENTAK PRIZM dual-chamber
  defibrillator, 637–638, 637t
Implantation techniques, 713–761
  anatomic approach in, 714–718
    axillary vein in, 714–715, 716f
    cephalic vein in, 715, 715f, 716f
    clavicles in, 717–718, 717f, 718f
    epicardial vs. transvenous approach in,
    714, 715f
    jugular veins in, 715–717, 716f
    subclavian vein in, 715, 715f
  in atrial fibrillation, 447–448
  axillary venous access in, 726–738
    anatomical considerations in,
    729–730, 729f, 730f
    cephalic vein isolation in, 734–735,
    736f
    contrast venograhy in, 735–736, 736f
    Doppler and ultrasound in, 736, 737f
    landmarks for, 730–734, 731f–735f
    safety zone for, 728f, 729, 729f
    techniques for, 737t
  cephalic venous access in, 722, 723f
  complications of, 757–761
    air embolism, 758–759, 758t, 759f,
    759t
    pacing lead manipulation in,
    759–761, 760f, 760t
    venous access in, 757–758, 758t
  epicardial lead placement in, 743–748
    general considerations for, 743–745
    incisions for, 744f, 745
    sternotomy in, median, 744f, 745
    subcostal approach for, 746–747, 747f
    subxiphoid approach for, 746, 746f
    thoracotomy in, left lateral, 745, 745f
  femoral venous access in, 740–741, 742f
  general considerations for, 713–714
  jugular venous access in, 738–740,
  738f–741f
  for obstructive hypertrophic
  cardiomyopathy, 786

Implantation techniques (*cont.*)
  percutaneous access to subclavian vein in, 723–726
    extreme medial puncture in, 725t
    guide wire insertion in, 725, 725f
    patient positioning in, 724–725
    placement technique in, 725–726, 726f–728f
  special situations in, 748–757
    ambulatory approach in, 755–756, 756t
    anomalous venous structures in, 748f, 749–751, 749f, 750f
    anticoagulated patient in, 756–757
    coronary sinus for cardiac pacing in, 748
    inframammary implantation in, 751–753, 751f–753f
    transthoracic endocardial lead placement in, 753–755, 753f–755f
  transvenous lead placement in, 718–722
    approaches for, 721–722, 721f, 722f
    venous access in, for dual chamber pacing, 721t
    venous structures in, 721t
  upgrading techniques for dual chambered ICD, 741–742, 743f
Impulse direction, of accessory pathways, 24–25
Inappropriate sinus tachycardia, 304, 305f
Inapsine (droperidol), 496
Inderal, 400
Infarction, 14–16
Infection, 14
Inferior vena cava-tricuspid annulus isthmus, 40–41
Infiltration, 16–17
Inflammation, 14
Inframammary implantation, 751–753, 751f–753f
Inherited conditions, survival results for, 657–658
InSync ICD, 650
Internal jugular vein puncture, 84–85, 85f
Internodal tracts, 9
Interventional laboratory, 57–75
  equipment for, 58–72, 59t
    ablation equipment, 67–72
      direct current, 67–68, 68f
      radiofrequency, 68–70, 68t, 69f, 70f
      radiofrequency modes, 70–72, 71f
    computer requirements, 65–67, 66f, 67f
    defibrillator, 58–59
    imaging system, 64–65
    interconnection of, 74–75, 74f
    physiologic recorders, 59–64, 60t, 61f
      input channels of, 59–60
      signal sampling in, 62–64, 62f, 63t
    physiologic stimulator, 64, 64t, 65f
    radiographic, 87

  sedation monitoring, 59
  general requirements for, 57–58, 57t, 58t
  layout of, 72–74, 72f
  staffing requirements for, 57–58, 57t, 58t
Intracardiac echo ultrasound (ICE), 154–155
Intracardiac imaging, 153–156
  ultrasound alternatives in, 156
  ultrasound in, 154–156
Intranodal bypass tract, 23f
Intravascular sheaths, in catheterization, 91f
Investigational implantable cardioverter-defibrillator (ICD). *See under* Implantable cardioverter-defibrillator (ICD)
Iodophor, 494
Iron, 16–17
Isochronal mapping, 465, 465f
Isoflurane, 496
Isoproterenol
  for vasodepressor syncope, 812
  on ventricular tachycardia, 669
  on ventricular tachycardia, idiopathic, 346–347, 346f
    induction of, 351–352
  for ventricular tachycardia with CAD, 377, 380, 394
Isuprel, 377
Isuprel (isoproterenol), for ventricular tachycardia with CAD, 377

J
Jewel AF 7250 defibrillator, 590, 619, 620f, 645–649
  efficacy data for, 628t
  electrogram of, 627f
  PR logic algorithm for, 646–648, 646f, 647f
  results for, 648–649
  study protocol for, 648
Jugular veins, 715–717, 716f
Jugular venous access, 738–740, 738f–741f

K
Kappa pacemaker, 814–815, 815f
Kent bundles/potentials, 24
  in accessory pathways, 214, 214f, 215f
Koch's triangle
  in anteroseptal and midseptal pathway ablation, 239–240, 240f
  in atrioventricular nodal axis, 9–10, 10f, 11f
  in AVNRT, 258–259, 258f
  in RF ablation site location, 36, 36f, 37

L
Laser catheter, 832–833
Laser extraction sheath, 832, 832f
Leads. *See also* Implantation techniques; Leads, extraction of
  in cephalic vein, 497–499, 497f, 498f

  for congestive heart failure, 795
  future developments in, 704
  for obstructive hypertrophic cardiomyopathy, 786
  unipolar, for pectoral ICDs, 498–499, 498f
Leads, extraction of, 819–841
  implantable defibrillator leads in, 835–840
    general considerations in, 835–836
    technique for, 836–837, 836f
    Telectronics J leads in, 837–840, 838t, 839f
  indications for, 820–821, 821t
  outcome of, 821, 821t
  pathology of, 819–820, 820f
  postoperative care after, 835
  transvenous lead extraction in, 821–835
    operating room in, 822
    operator in, 822, 822t
    patient in, 822
    preoperative setup in, 822–823
    reimplantation in, 835
    superior venous approach in
      key principles for, 823–824, 823f
      technique for, 824–831, 825f–831f, 830t
    superior venous approach in, with laser sheaths, 831–833
    transfemoral approach in, 833–834, 834f
Left lateral accessory pathway, 174f
Left ventricular outflow tract, in hypertrophic cardiomyopathy, 781–789. *See also* Hypertrophic cardiomyopathy
Left ventricular function, evaluation of, 665–668, 666f–668f
Lemmon surgical approach, 755f
Lidocaine
  in defibrillation threshold testing, 496–497
  for ICD implantation, 495–496
  for vessel puncture, 79
Local conduction failure, 474, 476f
Locking stylet, 826–828, 827f, 828f
Long QT syndrome, 657–658
Low-energy cardioversion, 613
Lown-Ganong-Levine syndrome, 27–30
Lyapunov exponent, 329–330

M
MADIT II study, 680, 680f
MADIT study, 656, 656t, 673–676, 673t, 674t
  adjunctive therapy in, 672f, 673
  ejection fractions in, 666–668, 668f
  high risk populations in, 664
Mahaim pathway, 23–25, 23f. *See also* Atriofascicular accessory pathways
  ablation of, 113–114
  mapping of, 113, 113f

Mapping, cardiac, 95
  for accessory pathways, left-sided, 185–187, 186f, 187f
  for accessory pathways, right free wall, for ablation of, 199–202
    target site criteria in, 200–202
    technique for, 199–200, 200f, 201f
  for anteroseptal and midseptal accessory pathway ablation, 245–247, 247f, 248f
  for atrial fibrillation, 128–130, 129f, 437–443
    activation maps in, dog, 442f, 443
    clinical spectrum in, 443, 444f
    cryoablative technology in, 317
    electrodes and templates in, 439–441, 440f, 441f
    methods in, 437
    reentrant circuits in, 437–438, 438f
    right vs. left atrial anatomy in, 441f
    slow conduction zone in, 438, 438f, 439f
    surgical intervention and, 443–444
  for atrial flutter, 124–125, 124f, 125f, 437–443
    activation maps in, dog, 442f, 443
    clinical spectrum in, 443, 444f
    electrodes and templates in, 439–441, 440f, 441f
    methods in, 437
    reentrant circuits in, 437–438, 438f
    right vs. left atrial anatomy in, 441f
    slow conduction zone in, 438, 438f, 439f
    surgical intervention and, 443–444
  atrial tachycardia ablation, atrial flutter, typical, 291–296
    activation, 292–293, 293f, 294f
    entrainment, 294–296, 296f
    split potentials, 293–294, 295f
  for atrial tachycardia ablation, three-dimensional, 306–310, 308f, 309f
  for atrium, computerized
    for atrial fibrillation
      activation maps in, dog, 443
      clinical spectrum in, 444f
      electrodes and templates in, 440f, 441f
      reentrant circuits in, 438f
      slow conduction zone in, 438f, 439f
    for atrial flutter
      activation maps in, dog, 443
      clinical spectrum in, 444f
      electrodes and templates in, 440f, 441f
      reentrant circuits in, 438f
      slow conduction zone in, 438f, 439f
      methods in, 437
      surgical intervention and, 443–444
  for coronary sinus diverticulum, 229, 230f
  for His bundle, 113, 113f
  for idiopathic ventricular tachycardia ablation
    activation, 352–353, 352f
    pace mapping in, 353–354, 353f
  for inappropriate sinus tachycardia, 304
  retrograde, of orthodromic atrioventricular reentrant tachycardia, 175f, 179f
  right, disadvantages of, 111–112
  for supraventricular tachycardia, 104–108
    catheter construction in, 106–107, 106f, 107f
    electrodes in, 104–106, 105f, 106f
    enhanced graphics for, 108
    intracoronary catheters in, 108
    reference catheters in, 104, 104f
    steerability in, 107–108
    thermal, 108
  for tachyarrhythmias, 163–171
    technical considerations in, 163–164, 164f, 165f
    techniques for, 165–171
      computer assisted, 167–171
      plunge needles in, 165–167, 166f
      in surgical suite, 167
  for tricuspid valve annulus region, 110–112, 110f, 111f, 124–125, 125f
  for ventricular arrhythmia
    sinus rhythm in, 466–467, 467f
    ventricular pace mapping in, 467–469, 468f, 469f
  for ventricular tachycardia, 137–143
    basket arrays in, global, 137–140, 138f–141f
    basket arrays in, regional, 140–142, 141f, 142f, 142t
    general considerations in, 137, 137f
    intravascular, 142
    thermal, 142–143
Maze procedures
  anatomic representation of, 131–132, 132f
  for atrial fibrillation, 425–426, 426f, 446–448, 447f, 448f, 448t
    Maze III, 449–451, 449f, 450t
    vs. radial approach, 455, 455f, 456f
  in atrial fibrillation ablation, 338
  for atrial fibrillation and atrial flutter, 37, 131–132, 131f
  pacemaker cells and, 9
  schematic representation of, 131–132, 131f
Membranous septum, 11f, 12, 12f
Mesotheliomas, 17
Methohexital
  in defibrillation threshold testing, 496
  for ICD implantation, 496
Metoclopramide, 496
Metoprolol, 689–690, 689f, 691, 692

Metrix 3020, 619, 620f
  chest radiograph of, 624f, 642f
Metrix stand alone atrial defibrillator, 638–645
  general considerations for, 638–640, 639f, 640f
  results for, 642–645
    complications, 644
    efficacy, 643–644
    fibrillation episodes in, 643
    out of hospital treatment, 644–645
    patient-activated mode, 645
    safety, 642–643
    shock tolerability, 644
  study protocol for, 640–642, 641f
Microwave ablation, 43–44
Midazolam
  hypotension from, 99
  for ICD implantation, 495–496
  in ventricular tachycardia with CAD, 376
Midodrine, 812
Midseptal accessory pathways, ablation of, 237–253
  ablation in, 244–248
    diagnostic studies for, 244–245, 245f, 246f
    electrode technique in, 247–248
    mapping in, 245–247, 247f, 248f
  anatomy in, 237–240
    atrioventricular junction in, 238–240, 240f
    classification system in, 237, 239f
  atrioventricular block risk in, 249–250, 249f
  efficacy and complications in, 253
    anteroseptal pathways, 251t, 252f
  electrogram criteria in site selection for, 248–249
  electrophysiologic characteristics in, 240–244
    algorithms in, 241–244, 242f, 243f
    normal, 241, 241f, 242f
    para-Hisian, 244
  electrophysiologic classification of, 240, 241f
  power delivery in, 249–250, 249f
  research summary for, 238t
Mitral valve annulus
  catheter-tip stability in, 112, 112f, 113f
  left anterior oblique projection of, 239f
Mitral valve disease, atrial fibrillation and, 428, 452
  maze procedure for, modified, 452–454, 453t
Moricizine, 17
Morillo technique, 320
Morphology algorithms, 610–611
Mortality, in ICD trials, 660f
Mullins sheath, 376
Multicenter Post-Infarction Group study, 670

Multicenter Unsustained Tachycardia Trial (MUSTT), 656, 656t, 673t
electrophysiologic testing and, 669
EP testing in, 676–678, 676t, 677f, 678f
high risk populations in, 664
Multielectrode basket array, 128–129, 129f
development of, 135–136
Multiple wavelet reentry, 318–319
Multiport pacemakers, 794–795
Multisite ablation, for ventricular tachycardia, 146
Multisite Stimulation in Cardiomyopathy (MUSTIC) trial, 792
Mustard operation, 33–34
Myocardial infarction
antiarrhythmic drugs for, 17–18
conduction system disturbance from, 14–16
during electrophysiologic intervention, 99–100
on QT dispersion, 15
with ventricular tachycardia, surgical techniques for, 483–486
current approach in, 485–486
patient selection in, 484–485
surgical status in, 484
Myocardial ischemia, in obstructive hypertrophic cardiomyopathy, 787–788

N

Narcotic antagonists, in idiopathic ventricular tachycardia, 351
Narcotics, 503
Neck, 716f
Nesacaine (chloroprocaine), 79
Neural crest cells, 5
Neurally mediated syncope, 810
Nodoventricular fibers, 23f
Nonobstructive hypertrophic cardiomyopathy, 789
Nonsteerable catheters, 106–107, 107f
Nonsustained ventricular tachycardia, 656, 656t
North American Vasovagal Pacemaker Study, 812, 813
Nyquist sampling theory, 62–64, 62f, 63t

O

Obstructive hypertrophic cardiomyopathy, 781–789. See also Hypertrophic cardiomyopathy, obstructive
Ong-Barold technique, 722, 722f
Onset threshold, 610
Open-lumen catheters, 114, 114f
Oral D-Sotalol (SWORD), 18
Orthodromic atrioventricular reentrant tachycardia
electrophysiologic study of, 270
with left bundle branch block, 176f
retrograde mapping of, 175f
with ventricular extra stimulus, 179f

Orthodromic reciprocating tachycardia, 198, 199f
in posteroseptal accessory pathways, 223–224, 226f–227f, 227
Orthogonal array catheters, 105–106, 105f, 106f
Orthostatic hypotension, 797–799, 798t
Over-the-guide-wire catheters, 110–111, 111f

P

P-wave, 324, 324f, 325f
Pacemaker cells, in atrial fibrillation, 447
Pacemaker implantation, 713–761. See also Implantation techniques
Pacemaker Lead Extraction with the Laser Sheath (PLEXES) trial, 821
Pacemaker syndrome, 797
Pacing. See also Implantable cardioverter-defibrillator (ICD)
atrial decremental, for AVNRT, 268–269
atrial extrastimulation, in AVNRT, 206f, 259
for atrial fibrillation
rapid atrial pacing model in, 320
rapid-pacing dog model in, 330–331, 331t
future developments for, 707–708, 708f
implantation techniques for, 713–761 (See also Implantation techniques)
lead extraction in, 819–841 (See also Leads, extraction of)
new indications for, 781–800
congestive heart failure, 789–795
beneficial effect mechanism in, 790
biventricular pacing in, 790–791
biventricular pacing in, clinical results of, 792–793, 793t
biventricular pacing in, methodologic considerations in, 793
biventricular pacing in, technologic considerations in, 794–795
general considerations in, 789
patient selection in, 789
first-degree atrioventricular block, 795–797, 796t
hypertrophic cardiomyopathy, nonobstructive, 789
hypertrophic cardiomyopathy, obstructive, 781–789
beneficial effect mechanism in, 788–789
clinical studies in, acute, 781, 782t
clinical studies in, long-term, 783–784, 784t
indications for, 785–786
nonobstructive, 789
pacemaker function and programmability in, 786–788
pacemaker inactivation in, prolonged, 785, 785t

permanent pacing in, 783
placebo effect in, 784–785
unresolved questions in, 789
orthostatic hypotension, 797–799, 798t
paroxysmal atrial fibrillation, 799–800
para-Hisian, for posteroseptal accessory pathways, 224–225, 226f–227f
rapid atrial pacing model in, 320
for vasodepressor syncope, 809–817 (See also Vasodepressor syncope)
ventricular decremental, for AVNRT, 268
for ventricular tachycardia ablation, with coronary artery disease, 378–381, 379f, 380f
Pacing in Cardiomyopathy (PIC) study, 784–785
Pacing modes, 64, 64t, 65f
Pain perception, 583–584, 622–623
Palpitations
in bundle branch reentrant ventricular tachycardia, 368
in idiopathic ventricular tachycardia, 344
Papillary muscle of conus, 10f
Para-Hisian pathway
anteroseptal, 240, 241f
ECG characteristics of, 244
pacing for, 224–225, 226f–227f
PARAD classification algorithm, 632–633, 633t, 634f
Paroxysmal atrial fibrillation, 799–800
Patient sedation, 59
Pectoralis major, 499, 500f
Pediatrics, 114–115, 115f
Peel-away sheath, 759, 759f
Pentobarbital, 496
Percutaneous introducer set, 723, 724f
Percutaneous sheath-set technique, 718–720, 721t
complications in, 757–758, 758t
Pericarditis, sterile, 320
Permanent junctional reciprocating reentrant tachycardia (PJRT), 24–25
Permanent junctional reciprocation tachycardia, 231–232, 232f
Physiologic recorders, 59–64, 60t, 61f, 93–94, 94f
input channels of, 59–60
signal sampling in, 62–64, 62f, 63t
Pigtail catheter, 112, 112f
Pin vise, 830, 831f
Placebo effect, 784–785
Plunge needles, 165–167, 166f
Pneumothorax, 84, 98, 757, 758t
Polarity
for obstructive hypertrophic cardiomyopathy pacing, 787
programming of, 613
Population-based programming, 614
Posteroseptal accessory pathways, ablation of, 221–235
anatomic considerations in, 221–222, 222f
complications in, 234
electrocardiographic findings in, 223, 224f, 225f

electrophyiologic diagnosis in, 223–231
    adenosine block in, 225
    coronary sinus visualization in, 229, 230f
    epicardial pathway identification in, 227–228, 228f, 229f
    orthodromic reciprocating tachycardia in, 223–224, 226f–227f, 227
    right vs. left pathway in, 225–227, 228f
    site selection criteria in, 229–231, 231f
overview of, 234–235
permanent junctional reciprocation tachycardia in, 231–232, 232f
radiofrequency delivery techniques for, 232–234
    ablation site distribution in, 233–234
    catheter ablation efficacy in, 233
surgical delineation in, 222–223, 223f
Postventricular atrial refractory period, 796–797
PR logic algorithm, 646–648, 646f, 647f
Preexcitation
    and anteroseptal and midseptal pathways, 244
    in Ebstein's anomaly, 30–31
    in obstructive hypertrophic cardiomyopathy, 788
    in Wolff-Parkinson-White syndrome, 413–414
Primordium, 5
Proarrhythmia, 624–625, 625t
Procainamide
    in MADIT trial, 674, 674f
    in MUSTT study, 656
    on ventricular arrhythmia, 473
    for ventricular tachycardia, with coronary heart disease, 404
Prochlorperazine, 496
Propafenone, 692
Propofol
    for ICD implanatation, 496
    in ventricular tachycardia with CAD, 376
Psuedopacemaker syndrome, 795
Pulmonary veins, and atrial fibrillation
    angiogram of, 317f
    experimental lesion creation in, 316–317, 318f
    foci points in, 314–316, 315f–318f
Pulse timing, 64, 64t
Purkinje fibers
    anatomy of, 12
    hepatanol on, 15
    in idiopathic ventricular tachycardia, 355–357
    myogenic vs. neurogenic origin of, 5–6

Q
QT dispersion, 15
QT syndrome, genetic basis of, 19
Quiet interval analysis, 639, 639f, 640f
Quiet time, 624, 625f

R
Radiofrequency ablation. *See also* Catheters; Catheter designs; Catheterization; specific sites
    of accessory pathways, 24–26, 24f–26f
        for Ebstein's anomaly, 31
        postoperative issues in, 27–30
            autonomic nervous system, 29–30
            AVNRT, 30
            catheter positioning, 28
            electrode temperature, 28–29
            mechanical trauma, 29
            right free wall, 202–204, 203t
    for atrial fibrillation and atrial flutter, 37–40
        acetylcholine stimulation in, 39–40
        anatomical barriers in, 40–41, 40f
        AV node destruction and permanent pacing in, 39
        discontinuous lesions in, 38
        electrode tip length in, 38–39
        expandable loop catheters in, 39
        left atrium in, 37
        right atrium in, 37–38
    complications from, 100
    equipment for, 68–70, 68t, 69f, 70f
    intravascular, for ventricular tachycardia, 153
    lesion pathology in, 41–44
        alternate energy sources in, 43–44
        animal models in, 41, 42f
        power regulation vs. temperature control in, 42–43
        tricuspid valve-inferior vena cava isthmus in, 42
    for supraventricular tachycardia, in children, 37
Radiofrequency modes, 70–72, 71f
Ramp antitachycardia pacing, 611, 612f
Rapid atrial pacing model, 320
Rate zones
    in ICD tiered therapy programming, 609
    programming of, 613–614
Reentry circuits, 599
    atrioventricular node in, 34–37, 36f
Reglan (metoclopramide), 496
Repetitive monomorphic ventricular tachycardia, 344–362. *See also* Ventricular tachycardia, idiopathic
Respiratory sinus arrhythmia, 670
Respiratory syncytial virus, 14
Retained guide wire technique, 721–722, 721f
Rhabdomyomas, 17
Right ventricular tachycardia, 344–362. *See also* Ventricular tachycardia, idiopathic
RR interval analysis, 527, 528t
RR regularity, 527, 528t

S
Safe introducer technique, 728f, 729
Salt tablets, 812
Sarcoidosis, cardiac, 14
SAVE trial, 672
Scan antitachycardia pacing, 611, 612f
Scopolamine, 812
Sedation, 59
    conscious, 376
Sedatives, 99
Senning operation, 33–34
Septal defects, congenital, 31–32
Septal myectomy, vs. ICD, 785–786
Sheaths, in supraventricular tachycardia, 115–116, 116f
Shock polarity, 512–513, 513f
Sick sinus syndrome, 452
Signal averaged electrocardiography, 670
Signal recording, of electrograms, 95
Signal sampling, 62–64, 62f, 63t
Signal-to-noise ratio, 104–105
Sinoatrial node
    age-related changes of, 12–13
    atresia of, 13
    displacement of, 13
    duplication of, 13–14
Sinoauricular node, 4
Sinus node
    ablation of, 418
    anatomy of, 6–9, 7f, 8f
        photomicrograph of, 8f
        posterior-septal view of, 7f
        sinus impulse origin in, 9
        sinus node artery, 8f, 9
Sinus rhythm, 92, 92f
    anteroseptal accessory pathway
        normal, 241f
        vs. para-Hisian, 244
    in atrial fibrillation, maintenance of, 573, 574–575
    atrial fibrillation to normal conversion of, 333f
    in AVRNT, 256, 256f, 257f
    mapping of
        for, 467f
        for ventricular arrhythmia, 466–467, 467f
    normal vs. antidromic AVRT, 207f
Sinus tachycardia, inappropriate, 304, 305f
Situs ambiguous, 13
Situs inversus, 13
Situs solitus, 13
Small-size catheters, 114–115, 115f
Sodium channel blockers, 17
Sotalol, for ventricular arrhythmia, 692, 695–696
D-Sotalol, vs. oral D-Sotalol, 18
Spiral operation, 426–427, 427f
Split bipolar pacing, 794
Spreadsheets, 65–67, 66f, 67f
Staphylococcus aureus, 495
Staphylococcus epidermidis, 495
Statins
    with ICD, 671, 671t
    in Sudden Cardiac Death Heart Failure Trial (SCD-HeFT), 680
Steerable Livewire catheter, 89–90, 90f
Step-down defibrillation threshold testing (DFT), 496

Sterile pericarditis, 320
Stimulators, 95–96, 96f
Stroke, 313, 572, 574
Studies of Left Ventricular Dysfunction (SOLVD) trial, 672
Subclavian arteriovenous fistula, 99
Subclavian artery puncture, 83–84, 84f
Subclavian crush phenomenon, 714
  axillary venous access and, 726, 729
Subclavian vein, 724f–726f
  anatomic considerations for, 715, 715f
  percutaneous access to, 723–726, 724f–726f
    extreme medial puncture in, 725t
    guide wire insertion in, 725, 725f
    patient positioning in, 724–725
    placement technique in, 725–726, 726f–728f
  puncture of, 99
  stick technique for, complications, 98–99, 758
Sudden cardiac death
  ICD trials and, 663–682 (See also under Implantable cardioverter-defibrillator)
  prevalence of, 586f, 664, 685
Sudden Cardiac Death Heart Failure Trial (SCD-HeFT), 679–681, 680f
Sudden infant death syndrome (SIDS), 6
Superior vena cava, maze I incisions in, 448f
Supraventricular tachycardia. See also specific types, e.g., Atrioventricular nodal reentrant tachycardia (AVNRT)
  catheter ablation of, 108–124
    anatomy-specific designs in, 110–114, 110f–114f
      adustable-size loop, 110, 110f
      Amplatz, 112, 113f
      double-spline, 110, 111f
      mitral valve annulus, 112, 112f, 113f
      open-lumen, 114, 114f
      over-the-guide-wire, 110–111, 111f
      pigtail, 112, 112f
      right coronary, 111–112
    electrodes in, 116–118, 116f–118f
    general considerations in, 108
    performance options in, 109
    sheaths in, 115–116, 116f
    size and shape in, 109
    small-size catheters in, 114–115, 115f
    temperature feedback alternatives in, 123–124
    temperature feedback in, 118–122, 118f–122f, 121t
    temperature sensors and placement in, 122–123, 123f, 123t
    in vivo adjustment in, 109–110, 109f, 110f
  catheter mapping of, 104–108
    catheter construction in, 106–107, 106f, 107f
    electrodes in, 104–106, 105f, 106f
    enhanced graphics for, 108
    intracoronary catheters in, 108
    reference catheters in, 104, 104f
    steerability in, 107–108
    thermal, 108
  in children, 37
  classification of, 4
  mapping of, 104–108
    catheter construction in, 106–107, 106f, 107f
    electrodes in, 104–106, 105f, 106f
    enhanced graphics for, 108
    intracoronary catheters in, 108
    reference catheters in, 104, 104f
    steerability in, 107–108
    thermal, 108
  surgical ablation of, 409–428
    atrioventricular nodal reentrant tachycardia, 416–418, 416f
    general considerations in, 409–410
  surgical ablation of, atrial fibrillation, 420–428
    atrial functional anatomy in, 421
    atrial pathology in, 421
    clinical presentation in, 422
    mechanism in, 421–422, 421f
    results and applications in, 427–428
    surgical rationale in, 422, 423f
    surgical techniques in, 422–427
      corridor operation, 422–425, 524f
      fragmentation or compartment operation, 426
      left atrial isolation, 426
      maze operation, 425–426, 426f
      spiral operation, 426–427, 427f
      vertical transseptal approach, modified, 427
  surgical ablation of, atrial tachycardias, 418–420
    atrial flutter, 418–419, 419f, 420f
    ectopic, 418
    intraoperative cardiac mapping for, 419–420
    results and applications of, 420
    sinus node, 418
    surgical rationale for, 419
  surgical ablation of, Wolff-Parkinson-White syndrome, 410–416
    accessory atrioventricular connection in, 410–411, 411f
    results and applications of, 415–416, 416f
    surgical technique in, 411–415
      atypical intramembranous pathways in, 413
      cardiac lesions in, 414–415
      coronary sinus diverticulum in, 414, 414f
      endocardial approach, 412–413
      epicardial approach, 413, 413f
      junctional reciprocating tachycardia in, permanent form, 414
      multiple accessory pathways in, 414
      variant preexcitation in, 413–414
Sustained ventricular arrhythmias. See also Ventricular arrhythmia, sustained
  evaluation of, 665–671
  pharmacologic therapy for, 685–697

Syncope
  in bundle branch reentrant ventricular tachycardia, 368
  in idiopathic ventricular tachycardia, 344
  of undetermined origin, survival results for, 655–656
  vasodepressor, 809–817 (See also Vasodepressor syncope)

T
Tachycardia(s). See also specific types, e.g., Supraventricular tachycardia
  antitachycardia pacing for, 611, 611f, 612f
  dual chamber sensing of, 527–529
  implantable cardioverter-defibrillator (ICD) and, 599–600
Telectronics J leads, 837–840, 838t, 839f
Telemetry systems, 706–707, 706f
Temperature feedback, in supraventricular tachycardia ablation, 118–122, 118f–122f, 121t
  alternatives to, 123–124
  temperature sensors and placement in, 122–123, 123f, 123t
Tetralogy of Fallot
  morphologic features of, 32–33
  ventricular tachycardia in, 375, 375f
Thermistors, 123, 123t
Thermocouples, 123, 123t
Thoracoacromial neurovascular bundle, 499, 500f, 501f
Thromboembolism
  from atrial lesions, left, 37
  in ICD implantation, 494
  pacemaker implantation and, 757
  sinus rhythm restoration and, 620
Thrombosis, 97
Tilt, 507–510, 509f, 510f, 612
  in biphasic shock, 622f
Tilt table
  for vasovagal syncope, 811f
  in vasovagal syncope, 813–814
Tocainide, 400
Todaro's tendon, 10, 10f, 11f
  in AVNRT, 258–259, 258f
Torsades des pointes
  afterdepolarization and, 598
  detection parameters for, 610
TRACE trial, 672
Transeptal puncture, 183f
Transesophageal echo ultrasound (TEE), 154
Transfemoral approach, 833–834, 834f
Transhepatic cannulation, 750, 750f
Transitional cells, 11
Transthoracic defibrillation waveforms, 519
Transthoracic endocardial lead placement, 753–755, 753f–755f
Transvenous lead extraction, 821–835. See also under Leads, extraction of

Tricuspid valve annulus, 10, 10f
  catheter for
    adjustable-size loop, 110, 110f
    double-ablation electrode, 124–125, 125f
    double-spline, 110, 111f
  in Ebstein's anomaly, 204–205, 204f
  left anterior oblique projection of, 239f
Triphasic defibrillation waveforms, 519–520
Tumors, 17

U

Ultrasound ablation, 43
  for atrial fibrillation, 317
Ultrasound imaging, 154–156
Unipolar electrograms, 94–95
  technical considerations in, 163–164, 164f
  in ventricular arrhythmia, vs. bipolar, 475f
Unipolar leads, 498–499, 498f
Univentricular hearts, 33
Urokinase, 644

V

V-HeFT II trial, 672, 673
Vagal stimulation, 528t
  atrial fibrillation and, 320
Vagal tone, 670
Valsalva maneuver, 247
Vancomycin, 495
Vasodepressor syncope, pacing for, 809–817
  carotid sinus syndrome in, 813
  causes of, 812
  diagnostic criteria in, 810–812
  general considerations for, 809–810, 810f, 811f
  terminology in, 810
  treatment for, 812
  vasovagal syncope in, 813–814
  vasovagal syncope in, detection and pacing interventions for, 814–817, 815f, 816f
Vasovagal faint, 810
Vasovagal International Study (VAIS), 811–812
Vasovagal reactions, 98
Vasovagal syncope, 813–814
  detection and pacing interventions for, 814–817, 815f, 816f
Vena cava, implantation through inferior, 750, 750f
  persistent left superior, 748f, 749–750, 749f
Venous structures, anomalous, electrode placement through, 748f, 749–751, 749f, 750f
VENTAK CHF AICD pulse generator, 649–650
VENTAK PRIZM dual-chamber defibrillator, 637–638, 637t

Ventricle, left
  catheterization manipulation techniques for, 92–93, 93f
  evaluation of, 665–668, 666f–668f
  outflow tract, in hypertrophic cardiomyopathy, 781–789
Ventricle, right
  ablation techniques for, 350–355
    activation mapping for, 352–353, 352f
    catheter positioning for, 354–355, 355f, 356f
    general considerations in, 350, 350f
    induction of, 350–352, 351f
    pace mapping for, 353–354, 353f
  lead placement for, 718, 719f, 720f
Ventricular arrhythmia
  sodium channel blockers for, 17
  surgery and intraoperative mapping for, 463–478
    mapping equipment in, 465, 465f
    mapping necessity in, 471–472
    mapping techniques in, 465–471
      ablation and, 470–471
      activation mapping, 466, 466f
      sinus rhythm mapping, 466–467, 467f
      ventricular pace mapping, 467–469, 468f
      ventriculotomy and, 471
    preoperative mapping studies in, 471
    problems with, 472–476, 473f–477f
    substrates in, 463–465, 464t
  sustained
    evaluation of, 665–671
      ambulatory electrocardiography in, 669–670
      electrical alternans in, 671
      electrophysiologic testing in, 668–669
      heart rate variability in, 670–671
      left ventricular function, 665–668, 666f–668f
      signal averaged electrocardiography in, 670
    nonpharmacologic therapy for, 691–693
    pharmacologic therapy for, 685–697
      approaches to, 686–690
        comparisons of, 690–691
        empirical amiodarone therapy in, 688–689, 688f
        empirical beta-blocking therapy in, 689–690, 689f
        empirical standard therapy in, 686–687
        individualized, 687–688, 687f, 688f
      future of, 696–697
      vs. nonpharmacologic therapies, 691–693
      problem review in, 685–686, 686f
      role of, 693–696
      therapy goals in, 686
Ventricular contraction, inversion of, 788

Ventricular electrogram morphology, 527, 528t
Ventricular extrastimulation, 528, 528t
  for atrioventricular node reentry tachycardia (AVNRT), 268
Ventricular fibrillation, 612–613, 613f
Ventricular pace mapping, 467–469, 468f
Ventricular pacing, decremental, 268
Ventricular pacing effect, in carotid sinus syndrome, 813
Ventricular RR interval regularity, 609–610
Ventricular tachycardia, ablation of, 143–152
  catheter mapping in, 137–143
    basket arrays in, global, 137–140, 138f–141f
    basket arrays in, regional, 140–142, 141f, 142f, 142t
    general considerations in, 137, 137f
    intravascular, 142
    thermal, 142–143
  chemical, 152–153
  with coronary artery disease, 373–405
    case studies in, 388–404, 389f–404f
    electrophysiology laboratory for, 375–378
      intracardiac recordings in, 376
      patient preparation in, 376
      radiofrequency generators in, 377–378, 378f
      retrograde aortic approach in, 376
      tachycardia induction in, 376–377
    fluoroscopic technique in, 378–379, 379f
    indications for, 373–374
    limitations of, 404
    mapping and pacing response in, 381–387, 386t
      assessment of, 384–385, 384t
      bystander circuits in, 382, 382f
      common pathway in, 381, 381f
      entrainment in, concealed vs. classic, 383–385, 383f
      four-beat analysis in, 385, 386f
      loop diagram in, 381–382, 382f
      outcomes for, 385–387, 386t
      single-paced premature beats in, 387
    pacing technique in, 378–381, 379f, 380f
    preparation for, 374–375
    radiofrequency ablation in, 387–388
    recording technique in, 378–381, 379f, 380f
  fluid-assisted, 146–152
    closed-loop system, 151–152, 151f, 152f, 152t
    general considerations in, 146–147, 146f–148f
    limitations and improvements in, 150–151, 150f
    open system, 147–150, 148f–150f
  idiopathic ventricular tachycardia in, 344–362

Ventricular tachycardia (cont.)
  ablation techniques for, 350–357
    left septal, 355–357, 358f, 359f
    results of, 357–360
    right ventricle, 350–355
      activation mapping for, 352–353, 352f
      catheter positioning for, 354–355, 355f, 356f
      general considerations in, 350, 350f
      induction of, 350–352, 351f
      pace mapping for, 353–354, 353f
      right ventricular outflow tract mimics in, 360–362, 361f, 362f
  characteristics of, 344–347, 344t, 345f–347f
  in children, 348–349
  left, 347–348, 348f
  management and differential diagnosis of, 349–350, 349t
  large surface area electrodes in, 143–145, 144f, 145f
  multisite, 146
  special electrode design in, 145–146, 145f
Ventricular tachycardia, nonsustained, 656, 656t
Ventricular tachycardia, surgical techniques for, 481–486
  arrhythmogenic right ventricular dysplasia in, 483
  arrhythmogenic substrate in, 481–482
  post myocardial infarction, 483–486
    current approach in, 485–486
    patient selection in, 484–485
    surgical status in, 484
  therapeutic triad in ("target, bullet, and gun"), 482–483
Ventricular tachycardia onset, 610
Ventriculoatrial block, from adenosine, 225
Ventriculoatrial dissociation, 363
Verapamil
  for hypertrophic cardiomyopathy, 783, 785
  on idiopathic ventricular tachycardia, 344, 347
Verapamil-sensitive ventricular tachycardia, 344–362. See also Ventricular tachycardia, idiopathic
Versed (midazolam), 495–496
Vertical transseptal approach, 427
Vitatron, 815–816, 816f
Volume expanders, 812

W

Warfarin
  implantation of ICDs and, 494
  pacemaker implantation and, 756–757
  in Sudden Cardiac Death Heart Failure Trial (SCD-HeFT), 680
Waveforms, defibrillation, 507–520. See also Defibrillation waveforms
Waveforms, future of, 702–704, 703f
Wilkoff stylet, 827, 827f
Wolff-Parkinson-White syndrome
  accessory pathways in, 23, 26–27
    anteroseptal and midseptal pathway, 240
  activation maps of, 437f
  antidromic reciprocating tachycardia in, 198
  coronary sinus diverticulum in, 223f
  surgical ablation of, 410–416
    accessory atrioventricular connection in, 410–411, 411f
    results and applications of, 415–416, 416f
    surgical technique in, 411–415
      atypical intramembranous pathways in, 413
      cardiac lesions in, 414–415
      coronary sinus diverticulum in, 414, 414f
      endocardial approach, 412–413
      epicardial approach, 413, 413f
      junctional reciprocating tachycardia in, permanent form, 414
      multiple accessory pathways in, 414
      variant preexcitation in, 413–414